Textbook of Surgery

Textbook of Surgery

EDITED BY

Julian A. Smith

MBBS, MS, MSurgEd, FRACS, FACS, FFSTRCSEd, FCSANZ, FAICD
Head, Department of Surgery (School of Clinical Sciences at Monash Health), Monash University
Head, Department of Cardiothoracic Surgery, Monash Health
Editor-in-Chief, *ANZ Journal of Surgery*

Andrew H. Kaye AM

MBBS, MD, FRACS
Head, Department of Surgery, The University of Melbourne

Christopher Christophi AM

MBBS (Hons), MD, FRACS, FRCS, FACS
Head of Surgery (Austin Health), The University of Melbourne

Wendy A. Brown

MBBS (Hons), PhD, FRACS, FACS
Head, Department of Surgery (Central Clinical School, Alfred Health), Monash University
Director, Centre for Obesity Research and Education (CORE), Monash University

FOURTH EDITION

WILEY Blackwell

Registered Offices
John Wiley & Sons, Inc., 111 River Street, Hoboken, NJ 07030, USA
John Wiley & Sons Ltd, The Atrium, Southern Gate, Chichester, West Sussex, PO19 8SQ, UK

Editorial Office
9600 Garsington Road, Oxford, OX4 2DQ, UK

For details of our global editorial offices, customer services, and more information about Wiley products visit us at www.wiley.com.

Wiley also publishes its books in a variety of electronic formats and by print-on-demand. Some content that appears in standard print versions of this book may not be available in other formats.

Library of Congress Cataloging-in-Publication Data

Names: Smith, Julian A., editor. | Kaye, Andrew H., 1950– editor.
Title: Textbook of surgery / edited by Julian A. Smith, MBBS, MS, MSurgEd, FRACS, FACS, FFSTRCSEd, FCSANZ, FAICD Head, Department of Surgery (School of Clinical Sciences at Monash Health), Monash University, Head, Department of Cardiothoracic Surgery, Monash Health, Editor-in-Chief, ANZ Journal of Surgery, Andrew H. Kaye, AM, MBBS, MD, FRACS, Head, Department of Surgery, The University of Melbourne, Christopher Christophi, AM, MBBS (Hons), MD, FRACS, FRCS, FACS, Head of Surgery (Austin Health), The University of Melbourne, Wendy A. Brown, MBBS (Hons), PhD, FRACS, FACS, Head, Department of Surgery (Central Clinical School, Alfred Health), Monash University Director, Centre for Obesity Research and Education (CORE), Monash University.
Other titles: Surgery
Description: Fourth edition. | Hoboken, NJ : Wiley-Blackwell, 2020. | Includes bibliographical references and index.
Identifiers: LCCN 2019030070 (print) | LCCN 2019030071 (ebook) | ISBN 9781119468080 (paperback) | ISBN 9781119468172 (adobe pdf) | ISBN 9781119468165 (epub)
Subjects: LCSH: Surgery.
Classification: LCC RD31 .T472 2020 (print) | LCC RD31 (ebook) | DDC 617–dc23
LC record available at https://lccn.loc.gov/2019030070
LC ebook record available at https://lccn.loc.gov/2019030071

Cover image: © gchutka/Getty Images
Cover design by Wiley

Set in 9/11.5pt Sabon by SPi Global, Pondicherry, India
Printed and bound in Singapore by Markono Print Media Pte Ltd

10 9 8 7 6 5 4 3 2 1

Contents

Contributors

Alexios A. Adamides
BMedSci, BMBS, MRCS (Edin), MD, FRACS
Clinical Senior Lecturer, University of Melbourne
Neurosurgeon, Royal Melbourne Hospital
Melbourne, Victoria, Australia

Ahmad Aly
MBBS, MS, FRACS
Clinical Associate Professor of Surgery, University of
Melbourne
Head, Upper Gastrointestinal Surgery, Austin Health
Melbourne, Victoria, Australia

Mark W. Ashton
MBBS, MD, FRACS
Clinical Professor of Surgery, University of Melbourne
Plastic Surgeon, Royal Melbourne Hospital
Melbourne, Victoria, Australia

Roger Berry
MBBS, FRACS
Senior Lecturer in Surgery, Monash University
Upper Gastrointestinal and Hepatobiliary Surgeon,
Monash Health
Melbourne, Victoria, Australia

Robert J.S. Briggs
MBBS, FRACS, FACS
Clinical Professor of Surgery, University of Melbourne
Clinical Executive Director of Otolaryngology; Head,
Otology and Medical Director, Cochlear Implant Clinic,
Royal Victorian Eye and Ear Hospital
Melbourne, Victoria, Australia

Wendy A. Brown
MBBS (Hons), PhD, FRACS, FACS
Head, Department of Surgery (Central Clinical School,
Alfred Health), Monash University
Director, Centre for Obesity Research and Education
(CORE), Monash University
Melbourne, Victoria, Australia

Timothy Buckenham
MBChB, FRANZCR, FRCR, FCIRSE, EBIR
Professor of Vascular Imaging and Intervention, Monash
University
Head, Vascular Services, Department of Imaging,
Monash Health
Melbourne, Victoria, Australia

Andrew Bui
MBBS, MSc, FRACS
Lecturer in Surgery, University of Melbourne
Colorectal Surgeon, Austin Health
Melbourne, Victoria, Australia

Adele Burgess
BMedSci (Hons), MBBS, FRACS
Senior Lecturer in Surgery, University of Melbourne
Head, Colorectal Surgery, Austin Health
Melbourne, Victoria, Australia

David Burnett
BSc, MBBS, FRACS
Hepatopancreaticobiliary Surgeon
John Hunter Hospital
Newcastle, New South Wales, Australia

Paul Burton
MBBS(Hons), PhD, FRACS
Senior Lecturer in Surgery, Monash University
Upper Gastrointestinal Surgeon, Alfred Health
Melbourne, Victoria, Australia

John F. Cade AM
MD, PhD, FRACP, FANZCA, FCICM
Professorial Fellow, Department of Medicine, University
of Melbourne
Emeritus Consultant in Intensive Care, Royal Melbourne
Hospital
Melbourne, Victoria, Australia

Paul A. Cashin
MBBS, FRACS
Clinical Associate Professor of Surgery, Monash
University
Director of General Surgery, Monash Health
Melbourne, Victoria, Australia

Steven T.F. Chan
MBBS, PhD, FRACS
Professor of Surgery, University of Melbourne
Upper Gastrointestinal Surgeon, Western Health
Melbourne, Victoria, Australia

Raaj Chandra
MBBS, BMed Sci, MEd, FRACS
Adjunct Senior Lecturer in Surgery, Monash University
Colorectal Surgeon, Royal Melbourne Hospital
Melbourne, Victoria, Australia

Christine Chen
MBBS, PhD, FRANZCO
Clinical Associate Professor of Surgery, Monash University
Head, Department of Ophthalmology, Monash Health
Melbourne, Victoria, Australia

Peter F. Choong
MBBS, MD, FRACS, FAOrthA, FAAHMS
Professor of Surgery, University of Melbourne
Director of Orthopaedics, St. Vincent's Hospital
Chair, Bone and Soft Tissue Sarcoma Service
Peter MacCallum Cancer Centre
Melbourne, Victoria, Australia

Britt Christensen
BSc, MBBS(Hons), MPH, FRACP
Head, Inflammatory Bowel Disease Unit, Department of
Gastroenterology, Royal Melbourne Hospital
Melbourne, Victoria, Australia

Christopher Christophi AM
MBBS (Hons), MD, FRACS, FRCS, FACS
Head of Surgery (Austin Health), University of
Melbourne
Melbourne, Victoria, Australia

S.C. Sydney Chung
MD, FRCS (Edin), FRCP (Edin)
Formerly Dean, Faculty of Medicine, Chinese University
of Hong Kong
Senior Consultant in Surgery, Union Hospital
Hong Kong

Heather Cleland
MBBS, FRACS
Director, Victorian Adult Burns Service and Plastic
Surgeon, Alfred Health
Melbourne, Victoria, Australia

Anthony J. Costello AM
MBBS, MD, FRACS, FRCSI (Hon)
Professorial Fellow, University of Melbourne
Head, Department of Urology, Royal Melbourne Hospital
Melbourne, Victoria, Australia

Daniel M. Costello
MBBS, DipSurgAnat
Surgical Resident, St. Vincent's Hospital
Melbourne, Victoria, Australia

Scott K. D'Amours
BSc, MDCM, FRCSC, FRACS, FRCS(Glasg), FACS
Conjoint Senior Lecturer in Surgery, University of New
South Wales
Director, Department of Trauma Services, Liverpool
Hospital
Sydney, New South Wales, Australia

Helen V. Danesh-Meyer
MBChB, MD, PhD, FRANZCO
Professor of Ophthalmology, School of Medicine,
University of Auckland
Auckland, New Zealand

Andrew Danks
MBBS, MD, FRACS
Associate Professor of Surgery, Monash University
Head, Department of Neurosurgery, Monash Health
Melbourne, Victoria, Australia

Anthony Dat
MBBS, MS
Urology Registrar, Eastern Health
Melbourne, Victoria, Australia

Rajiv V. Dave
MBChB, FRCSEd, MD, BSc(Hons)
Fellow in Oncoplastic Breast and Endocrine Surgery,
Royal Melbourne Hospital
Melbourne, Victoria, Australia
The Nightingale Centre, Manchester University NHS
Foundation Trust
Manchester, UK

Stephen A. Deane AM
MBBS, FRACS, FACS, FRCSC, FRCSEd (ad hom),
FRCSThailand (Hon)
Associate Dean, Clinical Partnerships, Macquarie
University, Sydney
Conjoint Professor of Surgery, University of Newcastle
Honorary Consultant Surgeon, Hunter and New
England Local Health District
New South Wales, Australia

Peter De Cruz
MBBS, PhD, FRACP
Senior Lecturer in Medicine, University of Melbourne
Gastroenterologist and Director, Inflammatory Bowel
Disease Service, Austin Health
Melbourne, Victoria, Australia

Peter Devitt
MBBS, MS, FRCS, FRACS
Associate Professor of Surgery, University of Adelaide
General and Upper Gastrointestinal Surgeon, Royal
Adelaide Hospital
Adelaide, South Australia, Australia

Michael A. Fink
MBBS, MD, FRACS
Senior Lecturer in Surgery, University of Melbourne
Hepatopancreatobiliary and Liver Transplant Surgeon,
Austin Health
Melbourne, Victoria, Australia

Jonathan Foo
MBChB, DipGrad(Arts), PhD, FRACS
Upper Gastrointestinal Surgery Fellow, Austin Health
Melbourne, Victoria, Australia

David M.A. Francis
BSc (Med Sci), MS, MD, PhD (Arts), FRCS (Eng), FRCS
(Edin), FRACS
Renal Transplant Surgeon, Department of Urology, Royal
Children's Hospital, Melbourne, Victoria, Australia
Visiting Professor of Surgery and Renal Transplant
Surgeon, Department of Surgery, Tribhuvan University
Teaching Hospital, Kathmandu, Nepal

Michael J. Grigg
AM, MBBS, FRACS
Professor of Surgery, Monash University
Director of Surgery, Eastern Health
Melbourne, Victoria, Australia

Ian Hastie
MBBS, FRACS
Senior Lecturer in Surgery, University of Melbourne
Colorectal Surgeon, Royal Melbourne Hospital
Melbourne, Victoria, Australia

Ian Hayes
MBBS, MS, MEpi, FRCS(Gen Surg), FRACS
Clinical Associate Professor of Surgery, University of
Melbourne
Head, Colorectal Surgery Unit, Royal Melbourne
Hospital
Melbourne, Victoria, Australia

Andrew G. Hill
MBChB, MD, EdD, FRACS, FACS
Professor of Surgery, University of Auckland
Colorectal Surgeon, Middlemore Hospital
Auckland, New Zealand

Thomas J. Hugh
MD, FRACS
Professor of Surgery, University of Sydney
Head, Upper Gastrointestinal Surgery Unit, Royal North
Shore Hospital
Sydney, New South Wales, Australia

Frederick Huynh
BSc(Hons), MBBS(Hons), FRACS
ANZHPBA Fellow, Alfred Health
Melbourne, Victoria, Australia

Nigel B. Jamieson
MBChB, BSc(Hons), FRCS, PhD
Lecturer in Surgery and Cancer Research UK Clinician
Scientist, University of Glasgow
Honorary Consultant in HPB Surgery, Glasgow Royal
Infirmary
Glasgow, UK

Yazmin Johari
MBBS(Hons)
General Surgery Registrar, Alfred Health
Melbourne, Victoria, Australia

Ian T. Jones
MBBS, FRCS, FRACS, FASCRS
Clinical Professor of Surgery, University of Melbourne
Colorectal Surgeon, Royal Melbourne Hospital
Melbourne, Victoria, Australia

Rodney T. Judson
MBBS, FRACS, FRCS
Associate Professor of Surgery, University of Melbourne
Head of Trauma Service, Royal Melbourne Hospital
Melbourne, Victoria, Australia

Andrew H. Kaye AM
MBBS, MD, FRACS
Head, Department of Surgery, University of Melbourne
Neurosurgeon, Royal Melbourne Hospital
Melbourne, Victoria, Australia

John Laidlaw
MBBS, FRACS
Clinical Associate Professor of Surgery, University of
Melbourne
Neurosurgeon, Royal Melbourne Hospital
Melbourne, Victoria, Australia

Michael Levitt
MBBS, FRACS
Colorectal Surgeon, St. John of God Healthcare, Subiaco
Perth, Western Australia, Australia

Jacob McCormick
BMedSci, MBBS, FRACS
Colorectal Surgeon, Royal Melbourne Hospital and Peter
MacCallum Cancer Centre
Melbourne, Victoria, Australia

Christopher MacIsaac
MBBS (Hons), PhD, FRACP, FCICM
Associate Professor in Medicine
Director, Intensive Care Unit, Royal Melbourne Hospital
Melbourne, Victoria, Australia

Valerie B. Malka
MBBS, FRACS, MIPH, MA
Senior Lecturer in Surgery, University of New South Wales
General and Trauma Surgeon, Deputy Director of
Trauma, Liverpool Hospital
Sydney, New South Wales, Australia

G. Bruce Mann
MBBS, PhD, FRACS
Professor of Surgery, University of Melbourne
Director of Breast Tumour Stream, Victorian
Comprehensive Cancer Centre
Melbourne, Victoria, Australia

Vijayaragavan Muralidharan
BMedSci, MBBS (Hons), MSurgEd, PhD, FRACS
Associate Professor of Surgery, University of Melbourne
Hepatopancreatobiliary Surgeon, Austin Health
Melbourne, Victoria, Australia

Sonal Nagra
MBBS, MMed(Surg), FRACS
Senior Lecturer in Rural General Surgery
Deakin University
Consultant Surgeon, University Hospital Geelong
Geelong, Victoria, Australia

Mehrdad Nikfarjam
MD, PhD, FRACS
Associate Professor of Surgery, University of Melbourne
Hepatopancreatobiliary Surgeon, Austin Health
Melbourne, Victoria, Australia

Stephen O'Leary
MBBS, BMedSci, PhD, FRACS
Professor of Otolaryngology, University of Melbourne
Ear, Nose and Throat Surgeon, Royal Victorian Eye and
Ear Hospital
Melbourne, Victoria, Australia

Geraldine J. Ooi
MBBS, BMedSci (Hons)
Senior Registrar, Centre for Obesity Research and
Education (CORE), Monash University
Senior Registrar in General Surgery, Alfred Health
Melbourne, Victoria, Australia

Kurvi Patwala
MBBS(Hons)
General Medical Registrar, Austin Health
Melbourne, Victoria, Australia

Marcos V. Perini
MD, PhD, FRACS
Senior Lecturer in Surgery, University of Melbourne
Hepatopancreaticobiliary and Liver Transplant Surgeon,
Austin Health
Melbourne, Victoria, Australia

William R.G. Perry
BSc, MBChB, MPH, FRACS
Senior Clinical Fellow, Department of Colorectal Surgery,
Oxford University Hospitals NHS Foundation Trust
Oxford, UK

Jeffrey J. Presneill
MBBS(Hons), PhD, MBiostat, PGDipEcho, FRACP, FCICM
Associate Professor in Medicine
University of Melbourne
Deputy Director, Intensive Care Unit
Royal Melbourne Hospital
Melbourne, Victoria, Australia

Raffi Qasabian
BSc(Hons), MBBS(Hons), FRACS
Vascular and Endovascular Surgeon, Royal Prince Alfred
Hospital
Sydney, New South Wales, Australia

Kenny Rao
MBBS, MS
Urology Registrar, Eastern Health
Melbourne, Victoria, Australia

Fairleigh Reeves
MBBS (Hons), DipSurgAnat
Urology Registrar, Royal Melbourne Hospital
Melbourne, Victoria, Australia

Arthur J. Richardson
MBBS, DClinSurg, FRACS, FACS
Associate Professor of Surgery, University of Sydney
Head, Hepatopancreatobiliary Surgery, Westmead
Hospital
Sydney, New South Wales, Australia

Jeffrey V. Rosenfeld AC, OBE
MBBS, MS, MD, FRACS, FRCS(Ed), FACS, IFAANS,
FRCS (Glasg, Hon), FCNST(Hon), FRCST(Hon),
FACTM, MRACMA
Director, Monash Institute of Medical Engineering
Senior Neurosurgeon, Alfred Health
Melbourne, Victoria, Australia

Peter S. Russell
BSc, PGDipSci, MBChB
Research Fellow, Department of Surgery, University of
Auckland
Auckland, New Zealand

Hani Saeed
MD, BPharm
Vascular Surgery Registrar, Eastern Health
Melbourne, Victoria, Australia

Gurfateh Singh Sandhu
BSc (Advanced), MBBS
Vascular Surgery Registrar, Royal Prince Alfred Hospital
Sydney, New South Wales, Australia

Alan C. Saunder
MBBS, FRACS
Senior Lecturer in Surgery, Monash University
Vascular and Transplant Surgeon and Medical
Director, Surgery and Interventional Services Program,
Monash Health
Melbourne, Victoria, Australia

Shomik Sengupta
MBBS, MS, MD, FRACS
Professor of Surgery, Monash University
Urologist, Eastern Health
Melbourne, Victoria, Australia

Jonathan Serpell
MBBS, MD, MEd, FRACS, FACS, FRCSEd (ad hom)
Professor of Surgery, Monash University
Director of General Surgery and Head, Breast, Endocrine
and General Surgery Unit, Alfred Health
Melbourne, Victoria, Australia

Rose Shakerian
MBBS, DMedSci, FRACS
General Surgeon, Royal Melbourne Hospital
Melbourne, Victoria, Australia

Susan Shedda
MBBS, MPH, FRACS
Colorectal Surgeon, Royal Melbourne Hospital and
Royal Women's Hospital
Melbourne, Victoria, Australia

Julian A. Smith
MBBS, MS, MSurgEd, FRACS, FACS, FFSTRCSEd,
FCSANZ, FAICD
Head, Department of Surgery (School of Clinical
Sciences at Monash Health), Monash University

Head, Department of Cardiothoracic Surgery,
Monash Health
Melbourne, Victoria, Australia

John Spillane
MBBS, FRACS
Lecturer in Surgery, University of Melbourne
Surgical Oncologist, Division of Cancer Surgery, Peter
MacCallum Cancer Centre
Melbourne, Victoria, Australia

David Story
MBBS (Hons), MD, BMedSci (Hons), FANZCA
Chair of Anaesthesia, Centre for Integrated Critical Care,
University of Melbourne
Melbourne, Victoria, Australia

James Tatoulis AM
MBBS, MS, MD, FRACS, FCSANZ
Professor of Cardiothoracic Surgery, University of
Melbourne
Director of Cardiothoracic Surgery, Royal Melbourne
Hospital
Melbourne, Victoria, Australia

Jin W. Tee
BMSc, MBBS, MD, FRACS
Associate Professor of Surgery, Monash University
Complex Spine and Neurosurgeon, Spine Oncology
Surgery, Alfred Health
Head, Spine and Neurotrauma, National Trauma
Research Institute
Melbourne, Victoria, Australia

Robert J.S. Thomas OAM
MBBS, MS, FRACS, FRCS(Eng)
Professorial Fellow and Special Advisor on Health,
University of Melbourne
Melbourne, Victoria, Australia

Benjamin N.J. Thomson
MBBS, DMedSci, FRACS, FACS
Clinical Associate Professor in Surgery, University of
Melbourne
Head, Department of General Surgical Specialties
Royal Melbourne Hospital
Melbourne, Victoria, Australia

Ioana Tichil
MD
Burns Fellow, Victorian Adult Burns Service, Alfred Health
Melbourne, Victoria, Australia

Joe J. Tjandra (deceased)
MBBS, MD, FRACS, FRCS(Eng), FRCPS, FASCRS
Formerly Associate Professor of Surgery, University of
Melbourne
Colorectal Surgeon and Surgical Oncologist, Royal
Melbourne Hospital
Melbourne, Victoria, Australia

Val Usatoff
MBBS(Hons), MHSM, FRACS, FCHSM
Associate Professor of Surgery, University of Melbourne
Head, Upper Gastrointestinal and
Hepatopancreatobiliary Surgery, Western Health
Melbourne, Victoria, Australia

Neil Vallance
MBBS, FRACS
Senior Lecturer in Surgery, Monash University
Emeritus Head, Department of Otolaryngology, Head
and Neck Surgery, Monash Health
Melbourne, Victoria, Australia

David A.K. Watters AM, OBE
BSc (Hons), ChM, FRCSEd, FRACS
Professor of Surgery, Deakin University
Alfred Deakin Professor of Surgery
Deakin University and Barwon Health
General and Endocrine Surgeon
University Hospital Geelong
Geelong, Victoria, Australia

John A. Windsor
BSc, MBChB, MD, FRACS, FACS
Professor of Surgery, University of Auckland
General, Pancreatobiliary, Gastro-oesophageal and
Laparoscopic Surgeon, Auckland City Hospital
Auckland, New Zealand

Homayoun Zargar
MBChB, FRACS
Senior Lecturer in Surgery, University of Melbourne
Urologist, Royal Melbourne Hospital
Melbourne, Victoria, Australia

Preface

Medical students and trainees must possess an understanding of basic surgical principles, a knowledge of specific surgical conditions, be able to perform a few basic procedures and be part of a multidisciplinary team that manages the patient in totality. All students of surgery must also be aware of the rapid developments in basic sciences and technology and understand where these developments impinge on surgical practice.

The *Textbook of Surgery* is intended to supply this information, which is especially relevant given the current content of the surgical curriculum for undergraduates. Each topic is written by an expert in the field from his or her own wisdom and experience. All contributors have been carefully chosen from the Australasian region for their authoritative expertise and personal involvement in undergraduate teaching and postgraduate training.

In this textbook we have approached surgery from a practical viewpoint while emphasising the relevance of basic surgical principles. We have attempted to cover most aspects of general surgery including its subspecialties and selected topics of other surgical specialties, including cardiothoracic surgery, neurosurgery, plastic surgery, ophthalmology, orthopaedic surgery, otolaryngology/head and neck surgery, urology and vascular surgery.

Principles that underlie the assessment, care and treatment of surgical patients are outlined, followed by sections on various surgical disorders. The final section presents a practical problem-solving approach to the diagnosis and management of common surgical conditions. In clinical practice, patients present with symptoms and signs to the surgeon who then has to formulate care plans, using such a problem-solving approach. This textbook provides a good grounding for students in surgical diseases, problems and management. Apart from forming the core curriculum for medical students, surgical trainees will also find the *Textbook of Surgery* beneficial in their studies and their practice.

The fourth edition of the *Textbook of Surgery* includes new or extensively revised chapters on the assessment of surgical risk, the management of surgical wounds, introduction to the operating theatre, emergency general surgery, obesity and bariatric surgery, lower gastrointestinal surgery, endovascular therapies, benign urological conditions, genitourinary oncology, sudden-onset severe headache and the red eye.

With ever-expanding medical knowledge, a considerable amount of instructive and up-to-date information is presented in a concise fashion. Important leading references of classic publications or up-to-date literature have been provided for further reading. It is our aim that this textbook will stimulate students to refer to appropriate reviews and publications for additional details on specific subjects.

We have presented the textbook in an attractive and easily readable format by extensive use of tables, boxes and illustrations. We hope that this fourth edition will continue to be valuable to undergraduate, graduate and postgraduate students of surgery, and for general practitioners and physicians as a useful summary of contemporary surgery.

Julian A. Smith
Andrew H. Kaye
Christopher Christophi
Wendy A. Brown
Melbourne, Australia

Acknowledgements

This book owes its existence to the contributions of our talented surgeons and physicians from throughout Australia, New Zealand and Asia. We are indebted to the staff of Wiley in Australia (Simon Goudie) and in Oxford (Claire Bonnett, Jennifer Seward, Deirdre Barry and Nick Morgan) for their support and diligence. We thank Associate Professor David Francis, Mr Alan Cuthbertson and Professor Robert Thomas for their assistance with previous editions, which laid the foundation for this fourth edition.

Our patients, students, trainees and surgical mentors have all been an inspiration to us, but above all we owe a debt of gratitude to our loving families, specifically our spouses and partners – Sally Smith, Judy Kaye, Helena Fisher and Andrew Cook – as it was precious time spent away from them which allowed completion of this textbook.

The editors wish to dedicate this edition to two highly esteemed previous editors, the late Joe J. Tjandra and the late Gordon J.A. Clunie. Both were inspirational surgical educators who left an enduring legacy amongst the many students, trainees and colleagues with whom they interacted over many years.

Section 1
Principles of Surgery

1 Preoperative management

Department of Surgery (School of Clinical Sciences at Monash Health), Monash University and Department of Cardiothoracic Surgery, Monash Health, Clayton, Victoria, Australia

Introduction

This chapter covers care of the patient from the time the patient is considered for surgery through to immediately prior to operation and deals with important generic issues relating to the care of all surgical patients. Whilst individual procedures each have unique aspects to them, a sound working understanding of the common issues involved in preoperative care is critical to good patient outcomes. The important elements of preoperative management are as follows.

- History taking: the present surgical condition and a general medical review.
- Physical examination: the present surgical condition and a general examination.
- Reviewing available diagnostic investigations.
- Ordering further diagnostic and screening investigations.
- Investigating and managing known or discovered medical conditions.
- Obtaining informed consent.
- Scheduling the operation and any special preparations (e.g. equipment required).
- Requesting an anaesthetic review.
- Marking the operative site/side.
- Prescribing any ongoing medications and prophylaxis against surgical site infection and deep venous thrombosis.
- Planning postoperative recovery and possibly rehabilitation.

Informed consent

Although often thought of in a purely medico-legal way, the process of ensuring that a patient is informed about the procedure they are about to undergo is a fundamental part of good-quality patient care. Informed consent is far more than the act of placing a signature on a form. That signature in itself is only meaningful if the patient has been through a reasonable process that has left them in a position to make an informed decision.

There has been much written around issues of informed consent, and the medico-legal climate has changed substantially in the past decade. It is important for any doctor to have an understanding of what is currently understood by informed consent. Although the legal systems in individual jurisdictions may differ with respect to medical negligence, the standards around what constitutes informed consent are very similar.

Until relatively recently, the standard applied to deciding whether the patient was given adequate and appropriate information with which to make a decision was the so called Bolam test – practitioners are not negligent if they act in accordance with practice accepted by a reasonable body of medical opinion. Recent case law from both Australia and overseas has seen a move away from that position. Although this area is complex, the general opinion is that a doctor has a duty to disclose to a patient any material risks. A risk is said to be material if 'in the circumstances of that particular case, a reasonable person in the patient's position, if warned of the risk would be likely to attach significance to it or the medical practitioner is, or should reasonably be aware that the particular patient, if warned of the risk would attach significance to it'. It is important that this standard relates to what a person in the patient's position would do and not just any reasonable person.

Important factors when considering the kinds of information to disclose to patients include the following.

- The nature of the potential risks: more common and more serious risks require disclosure.
- The nature of the proposed procedure: complex interventions require more information as do procedures when the patient has no symptoms or illness.

Textbook of Surgery, Fourth Edition. Edited by Julian A. Smith, Andrew H. Kaye, Christopher Christophi and Wendy A. Brown.
© 2020 John Wiley & Sons Ltd. Published 2020 by John Wiley & Sons Ltd.

- The patient's desire for information: patients who ask questions make known their desire for information and they should be told.
- The temperament and health of the patient: anxious patients and patients with health problems or other relevant circumstances that make a risk more important for them may need more information.
- The general surrounding circumstances: the information required for elective procedures might be different from that required in those conducted emergently.

Verbal discussions concerning the therapeutic options, potential benefits and risks along with common complications are often supplemented with procedure-specific patient explanatory brochures. These provide a straightforward illustrated account for the patient and their relatives to consider and may be a source of clarification and/or further questions about the proposed operation.

What does this mean for a medical practitioner? Firstly, you must have an understanding of the legal framework and standards. Secondly, you must document how appropriate information was given to patients – always write it down. If discussion points are not documented, it may be argued that they never occurred. On this point, whilst explanatory brochures can be a very useful addition to the process of informed consent they do not remove the need to undertake open conversations with the patient.

Doctors often see the process of obtaining informed consent as difficult and complex, and this view is leant support by changing standards. However, the principles are relatively clear and not only benefit patients but their doctors as well. A fully informed patient is much more likely to adapt to the demands of a surgical intervention, and should a complication occur, they and their relatives almost invariably accept such misfortune far more readily.

Preoperative assessment

The appropriate assessment of patients prior to surgery to identify coexisting medical problems and to plan perioperative care is of increasing importance. Modern trends towards the increasing use of day-of-surgery admission even for major procedures have increased the need for careful and systematic preoperative assessment, much of which occurs in a pre-admission clinic (PAC).

The goals of preoperative assessment are:
- To identify important medical issues in order to
  - optimise their treatment
  - inform the patient of additional risks associated with surgery

  - ensure care is provided in an appropriate environment.
- To identify important social issues which may have a bearing on the planned procedure and the recovery period.
- To familiarise the patient with the planned procedure and the hospital processes.

Clearly the preoperative evaluation should include a careful history and physical examination, together with structured questions related to the planned procedure. Simple questions related to exercise tolerance (such as 'Can you climb a flight of stairs without being short of breath?') will often yield as much useful information as complex tests of cardiorespiratory reserve. The clinical evaluation will be coupled with a number of blood and radiological tests. There is considerable debate as to the value of many of the routine tests performed, and each hospital will have its own protocol for such evaluations.

Common patient observations, investigations and screening tests prior to surgery include:
- vital signs (blood pressure, pulse rate, respiratory rate, temperature) and pulse oximetry
- body weight
- urinalysis
- full blood examination and platelet count
- urea and electrolytes, blood sugar, tests of liver function
- blood grouping and screen for irregular antibodies ('group and hold')
- tests of coagulation, i.e. international normalised ratio (INR) and activated partial thromboplastin time (APTT)
- chest X-ray
- electrocardiogram (ECG).

On the basis of the outcomes of this preoperative evaluation a number of risk stratification systems have been proposed. One in widespread daily use is the relatively simple ASA (American Society of Anesthesiologists) system (see Chapter 3, Table 3.3).

The preoperative assessment and work-up will be guided by a combination of the nature of the operation proposed and the overall 'fitness' of the patient. Whilst there are a number of ways of looking at the type of surgery proposed, a simple three-way classification has much to commend it.
- **Low risk:** poses minimal physiological stress and risk to the patient, and rarely requires blood transfusion, invasive monitoring or intensive care. Examples of such procedures would be groin hernia repair, cataract surgery and arthroscopy.
- **Medium risk:** moderate physiological stress (fluid shifts, cardiorespiratory effects) and risk.

Usually associated with minimal blood loss. Potential for significant problems must be appreciated. Examples would be laparoscopic cholecystectomy, hysterectomy and hip replacement.
- **High risk:** significant perioperative physiological stress. Often requires blood transfusion or infusion of large fluid volumes. Requires invasive monitoring and will often need intensive care. Examples would be aortic surgery, major gastrointestinal resections and thoracic surgery.

A low-risk patient (ASA I or II) will clearly require a far less intensive work-up than a high-risk patient (ASA III or IV) undergoing a high-risk operation.

Areas of specific relevance to perioperative care are cardiac disease and respiratory disease. It is important that pre-existing cardiorespiratory disease is optimised prior to surgery to minimise the risk of complications. Patients with cardiac disease can be stratified using a number of systems (New York Heart Association Functional Class for angina or heart failure; Goldman or Detsky indices) and this stratification can be used to guide work-up and interventions and provide a guide to prognosis. One of the most important respiratory factors is whether the patient is a smoker. There is now clear evidence that stopping smoking for at least 4 weeks prior to surgery significantly reduces the risk of respiratory specific or generic complications.

Evaluation of the healthy patient

Patients with no clinically detectable systemic illnesses except their surgical problem are classified into ASA class I. Mortality for low-risk surgical procedures in this group is very low and complications are likely to be due to technical errors. The mortality for major high-risk surgical procedures in such patients is also low, of the order of a few per cent.

All such patients require detailed systems review by history and physical examination prior to the operation. Preoperative special tests may be added in order to detect any subclinical disease that may adversely affect surgery and to provide baseline values for comparison in the event of postoperative complications. These tests should be sufficiently sensitive to detect an abnormality, yet specific enough to avoid the chances of over-diagnosis. The prevalence of the disease or condition being looked for is likely to be low in a healthy asymptomatic patient population. Thus, most tests are likely to be within the normal range. Inappropriate and excessive tests increase the likelihood of a false-positive result due to chance. With extensive multiphasic screening profiles of healthy individuals, about 5% of healthy normal people will show one abnormal result.

Evaluation of the elderly asymptomatic patient

Ageing increases the likelihood of asymptomatic conditions and screening investigations are therefore more stringently applied to older, apparently healthy patients. Elderly patients (aged over 70 years) have increased mortality and complication rates for surgical procedures compared with young patients. Problems are related to reduced functional reserve, coexisting cardiac and pulmonary disease, renal impairment, poor tolerance of blood loss and greater sensitivity to analgesics, sedatives and anaesthetic agents.

Complications of atelectasis, myocardial infarction, arrhythmias and heart failure, pulmonary emboli, infection and nutritional and metabolic disorders are all more frequent. Separation of the effects of ageing, frailty and of associated diseases is difficult. Most of the increased mortality and morbidity is due to associated disease.

Special attention needs to be paid to the assessment of cardiac, respiratory, renal and hepatic function along with patient frailty before operation in elderly patients.

Patient safety (see also Chapter 12)

Once in hospital, and particularly once under anaesthetic, patients rely upon the systems and policies of individuals and healthcare institutions to minimise the risk of inadvertent harm. Whilst every hospital will have slightly different policies the fundamental goals of these include the following.
- The correct patient gets the correct operation on the correct side or part of their body. An appropriate method of patient identification and patient marking must be in place. It must be clear to all involved in the procedure, particularly for operations on paired limbs or organs when the incorrect side could be operated upon.
- The patient is protected from harm whilst under anaesthetic. When under a general anaesthetic the patient is vulnerable to a number of risks. Important amongst these are pressure effects on nerves, for example those on the common peroneal nerve as it winds around the head of the fibula.
- Previous medical problems and allergies are identified and acted upon.
- Protocols for the prevention of perioperative infection and venous thromboembolism are followed.

Prophylaxis

Infection

Infections remain a major issue for all surgical procedures and the team caring for the patient needs to be aware of relevant risks and act to minimise such risks.

Before discussing the use of prophylactic antibiotics for the prevention of perioperative infection, it is very important that issues of basic hygiene are discussed (see also Chapters 9 and 12). Simple measures adopted by all those involved in patient care can make a real difference to reducing the risk of hospital-acquired infection. The very widespread and significant problems with antibiotic-resistant organisms such as meticillin-resistant *Staphylococcus aureus* (MRSA) and vancomycin-resistant *Enterococcus faecalis* (VRE) have reinforced the need for such basic measures.

- Wash your hands in between seeing each and every patient.
- Wear gloves for removing/changing dressings.
- Ensure that the hospital environment is as clean as possible.

These measures, especially hand hygiene, should be embedded into the psyche of all those involved in patient care.

In addition to the very important matters of hygiene and appropriate sterile practice, antibiotics should be used in certain circumstances to reduce the risk of perioperative surgical site infection. Each hospital will have individual policies on which particular antibiotics to use in the prophylactic setting (see also Chapters 9 and 12). The antibiotics are usually administered at or shortly before the induction of anaesthesia and continued for no more than 24 hours postoperatively. It is also important to state that whilst the use of prophylactic antibiotics can, when used appropriately, significantly reduce infectious complications, inappropriate or prolonged use can leave the patient susceptible to infection with antibiotic-resistant organisms such as MRSA or VRE.

Factors related to both the patient and the planned procedure govern the appropriate use of antibiotics in the prophylactic setting.

Patient-related factors

Patients with immunosuppression and pre-existing implants and patients at risk for developing infective endocarditis must receive appropriate prophylaxis even when the procedure itself would not indicate their use.

Procedure-related factors

Table 1.1 indicates the risk of postoperative surgical site infections with and without the use of prophylactic antibiotics. In addition to considering the absolute risk of infection, the potential consequences of infection must also be considered; for example, a patient undergoing a vascular graft (a clean procedure) must receive appropriate antibiotic cover because of the catastrophic consequences of graft infection.

Venous thromboembolism

Deep vein thrombosis (DVT) is a not uncommon and potentially catastrophic complication of surgery. The risk for developing DVT ranges from a fraction of 1% to 30% or greater depending on both patient- and procedure-related factors. Both patient- and procedure-related factors can be classified as low, medium or high risk (Table 1.2). High-risk patients undergoing high-risk operations will have a risk for DVT of up to 80% and a

Table 1.1 Risks of postoperative surgical site infection.

Type of procedure	Definition	Wound infection rate (%)	
		Without prophylactic antibiotics	With prophylactic antibiotics
Clean	No contamination; gastrointestinal, genitourinary or respiratory tracts not breached	1–5	0–1
Clean-contaminated	Gastrointestinal or respiratory tract opened but without spillage	10	1–2
Contaminated	Acute inflammation, infected urine, bile, gross spillage from gastrointestinal tract	20–30	10
Dirty	Established infection	40–50	10

Table 1.2 Prevention of deep vein thrombosis.

		Operative risk factors		
		Low (e.g. hernia repair)	Medium (e.g. general abdominal surgery)	High (e.g. pelvic cancer, orthopaedic surgery)
Patient risk factors	Low (age <40, no risk factors)	No prophylaxis	Heparin	Heparin and mechanical devices
	Medium (age >40, one risk factor)	Heparin	Heparin	Heparin and mechanical devices
	High (age >40, multiple risk factors)	Heparin and mechanical devices	Heparin and mechanical devices	Higher-dose heparin, mechanical devices

pulmonary embolism risk of 1–5% when prophylaxis is not used. These risks can be reduced by at least one order of magnitude with appropriate interventions.

Whilst a wide variety of agents have been trialled for the prevention of DVT, there are currently only three widely used methods.

- Graduated compression stockings: these stockings, which must be properly fitted, reduce venous pooling in the lower limbs and prevent venous stagnation.
- Mechanical calf compression devices: these work by intermittent pneumatic calf compression and thereby encourage venous return and reduce venous pooling.
- Heparin: this drug can be used in its conventional unfractionated form or as one of the fractionated low-molecular-weight derivatives. The fractionated low-molecular-weight heparins offer the convenience of once- or twice-daily dosing for the majority of patients. It must however be remembered that the anticoagulant effect of the low-molecular-weight heparins may not easily be reversed, and where such reversal may be important, standard unfractionated heparin should be used.

The three methods are complementary and are often used in combination, depending on the patient and operative risk factors (Table 1.2).

The systematic use of such measures is very important if optimal benefit is to be gained by the potential reduction in DVT.

Preoperative care of the acute surgical patient

A significant number of patients will present with acute conditions requiring urgent or emergency surgical operations. There may be little time for an in-depth preoperative preparation. Whilst the principles already outlined are still valid, a number of additional issues are raised.

Informed consent

Whilst there is still a clear need to ensure that patients are appropriately informed, there are fewer opportunities to discuss the options and potential complications with the patient and their family. In addition, the disease process may have resulted in the patient being confused. The team caring for the patient needs to judge carefully the level of information required in this situation. Although it is very important that family members are kept informed, it has to be remembered that the team's primary duty is towards the patient. This sometimes puts the team in a difficult position when the views of the patient's family differ from those which the team caring for the patient hold. If such an occasion arises then careful discussion and documentation of the decision-making process is vital. Increasingly, patients of very advanced years are admitted acutely with a surgical problem in the setting of significant additional medical problems. It is with this group of patients that specific ethical issues around consent and appropriateness of surgery occur. It is important that as full as possible a picture of the patient's overall health and quality of life is obtained and that a full and frank discussion of the options, risks and benefits takes place.

Preoperative resuscitation

It is important that wherever possible significant fluid deficits and electrolyte abnormalities are corrected prior to surgery. There is often a balance to be made between timely operative intervention and the degree of fluid resuscitation required. An early discussion between surgeon, anaesthetist and, when required, intensivist can help plan the timing of surgical intervention.

Pre-existing medical comorbidities

There is clearly less time to address these issues and it may not be possible to address significant ongoing medical problems. Clearly such comorbidities should be identified, and all involved with planning the operation should be informed. The issues are most acute for significant cardiac, respiratory, hepatic or renal disease.

Preoperative nutrition

An awareness of the nutritional status of patients is important and such awareness should guide the decisions about nutritional support (see Chapter 7). The well-nourished adult patient should be fasted for at least 6 hours prior to anaesthesia to minimise the risk of aspiration. Where possible regular medications, especially those for cardiovascular and respiratory conditions, should be continued.

Before an operation the malnourished patient should, whenever possible, be given appropriate nutritional support. There is no doubt that significant preoperative malnutrition increases the risk of postoperative complications (>10–15% weight loss). If possible, such nutrition should be given enterally, reserving parenteral nutrition for the minority of patients in whom the gastrointestinal tract is not an option. Parenteral nutrition is associated with increased costs and complications and is of proven benefit only in the seriously malnourished patient, when it should be given for at least 10 days prior to surgery for any benefits to be seen. There is increasing evidence that enteral feeds specifically formulated to boost certain immune parameters offer clinical benefits for patients about to undergo major surgery.

After operation any patient who is unable to take in normal diet for 7 days or more should receive nutritional support, which as before operation should use the enteral route whenever possible.

Specific preoperative issues

Allergies

A history of adverse or allergic reactions to medications or other substances must be documented and repeat administration and/or exposure avoided as a life-threatening anaphylaxis may result. Examples of allergens within surgical practice include antibiotics, skin preparations (e.g. iodine), wound dressing adhesives and latex. A complete latex-free environment is required for those patients with a known latex allergy.

Diabetes mellitus

Diabetes mellitus is one of the most frequently seen medical comorbidities that complicate perioperative care. It is clearly important that patients with diabetes mellitus are appropriately worked up for surgery.

In the weeks leading up to elective surgery the management of the diabetes should be reviewed and blood glucose control optimised. Particular attention should be paid to HbA1c levels as an index of diabetic control as well as cardiovascular and renal comorbidities during the preoperative assessment.

Generally, patients with diabetes should be scheduled for surgery first case in the morning. Diet-controlled patients require no special preoperative preparation. For patients taking oral hypoglycaemic drugs, the drugs should be stopped the night before surgery and the blood glucose monitored. Patients with insulin-dependent diabetes should receive a reduced dose of insulin and/or a shorter-acting insulin or be commenced on an intravenous insulin infusion. There are two approaches to this.

- Variable-rate insulin infusion: the patient's blood glucose levels are monitored regularly and the rate of insulin infusion adjusted. An infusion of dextrose is continued throughout the period of insulin infusion.
- Single infusion of glucose, insulin and potassium (GIK): whilst this method has the advantage of simplicity, it is not possible to adjust the rates of glucose and insulin infusion separately and the technique can lead to the administration of excessive amounts of free water.

The variable-rate infusion is the most widespread approach and although more involved in terms of monitoring offers better glycaemic control. This in itself is associated with better patient outcomes.

Cardiac disease

Surgical risk is increased in the presence of cardiac disease. Consideration must be given to balancing the risk to the patient if the procedure is abandoned or delayed with the additional risk caused by the presence of cardiac disease. Emergency operations for life-threatening conditions should proceed regardless but elective surgery should be deferred in the presence of recent-onset angina, unstable angina, recent myocardial infarction, severe aortic valve stenosis, high-degree atrioventricular block, severe hypertension and untreated congestive cardiac failure. Time should be spent investigating the condition and optimising therapy, frequently with cardiological assistance. The introduction of beta-blocker therapy to slow heart rate and occasionally myocardial revascularisation (by percutaneous coronary intervention or coronary artery bypass grafting) may be required in advance of surgery on another system.

Anticoagulant or antiplatelet therapy

Patients on warfarin should be transferred to heparin or enoxaparin well in advance of surgery to ensure that the warfarin effect has worn off. Heparin can be ceased for a short time in the perioperative period: withhold an infusion 4 hours before surgery and recommence once the risk of postoperative bleeding is low. Subcutaneously administered heparin or enoxaparin is withheld the day or evening before surgery and recommenced later that day or the day after. Warfarin recommences once the patient can take oral medication. Rapid reversal of warfarin prior to an emergency operation may be achieved with vitamin K, pooled fresh frozen plasma or clotting factors.

The new oral anticoagulants (dabigatran, apixaban or rivaroxaban) are difficult to reverse acutely and need to be ceased 2–5 days preoperatively. A specific dabigatran reversal agent has recently become available. A bridging regimen such as that described above is also required.

The antiplatelet agents (aspirin, clopidogrel or ticagrelor) taken alone or in combination should be ceased at least 5 days prior to an operation. Bleeding will be highly problematic at the time of surgery especially if multiple antiplatelet agents are continued. Combined usage often follows coronary artery stenting and so their withdrawal in the context of surgery should be discussed with the treating interventional cardiologist. Elective surgery may need to be postponed if dual antiplatelet therapy cannot be safely ceased.

Active smoking and respiratory disease

All active smokers should be encouraged to cease for at least 4 weeks in advance of elective surgery in order to lessen the risk of respiratory problems (atelectasis, acute pneumonia and respiratory failure) in the postoperative period. Patients unwilling or incapable of stopping smoking should be referred to a dedicated support service to assist with such.

Patients with chronic obstructive pulmonary disease (COPD), asthma and obstructive sleep apnoea require a detailed respiratory assessment (including peak flow, spirometry and arterial blood gas estimation) especially if the patient reports significant exercise limitation. Elective surgery should be deferred in the presence of an active respiratory infection or an acute exacerbation of asthma or COPD.

Additional respiratory preparation may include chest physiotherapy, postural drainage, antibiotics for an acute infection with a positive sputum culture and inhaled bronchodilators or corticosteroid therapy. A formal preoperative pulmonary rehabilitation program may be indicated. Regional anaesthesia is frequently preferred in patients with severe respiratory dysfunction.

Long-term corticosteroid therapy

Long-term corticosteroid therapy results in adrenal suppression and an impaired response to surgical stress. High-dose intravenous hydrocortisone administration (100 or 250 mg every 6 hours) will be required during the perioperative period and when the patient is unable to take their regular medication or in the presence of postoperative complications especially infection.

Cerebrovascular disease

Stroke may complicate major surgery especially in elderly patients with severe intracranial or extracranial atherosclerotic disease faced with fluctuations in blood pressure or cerebral blood flow. An asymptomatic carotid bruit related to an internal carotid artery stenosis confirmed with Doppler ultrasonography may be the first indicator of such disease. Patients with symptomatic carotid disease (e.g. transient ischaemic attacks) should undergo carotid endarterectomy prior to the planned surgery. However, there is no evidence that a prophylactic carotid endarterectomy is of benefit in the asymptomatic patient.

Chronic liver disease and obstructive jaundice

Chronic liver disease of any cause may predispose the patient to surgical complications such as poor wound healing, sepsis, excessive bleeding, renal impairment and acute delirium. Each of the previously discussed screening investigations will be required in addition to specific liver and biliary tree imaging and possibly liver biopsy. The decision to operate on a patient with severe liver insufficiency must be carefully considered. Elective surgery should be deferred whilst liver function is optimised. Emergency surgery can often result in acute liver decompensation especially in the presence of sepsis, haemorrhage, electrolyte disturbances, hypoxia and hypoglycaemia.

Patients with obstructive jaundice (see Chapter 67) frequently have an abnormal coagulation profile and require vitamin K, coagulation factors or pooled fresh frozen plasma to correct the defect. Close attention needs to be paid to the patient's fluid and electrolyte status in order to prevent acute renal failure. The hepatic clearance of some commonly administered medications may be impaired.

Chronic kidney disease

All patients aged over 40 years should have their kidney function evaluated (urinalysis, serum creatinine, estimated glomerular filtration rate and serum albumin) when major surgery is planned. Documented chronic kidney disease does not mandate deferral of elective surgery. Patients with chronic kidney disease may experience an acute deterioration in kidney function if they become water or saline depleted. Acute kidney failure is the most significant complication of chronic kidney disease: prevention demands strict attention to fluid and electrolyte balance (especially avoiding dehydration and maintaining a stable level of serum potassium), maintaining kidney perfusion and accurate replacement of blood loss during surgery. Apart from acute kidney failure, the main complications of surgery in patients with chronic kidney disease are sepsis (including urinary tract infection), poor wound healing and cardiovascular complications (myocardial infarction and stroke).

Anaemia

As a general rule mild anaemia does not increase the risk of surgery. However, if time permits the cause of the anaemia should be identified before elective surgery. Iron deficiency anaemia is best detected early and treated by oral or intravenous iron. Patients with the anaemia of renal injury are an exception to the general rule and can cope with quite low haemoglobin levels, due to an increase in red cell 2,3-diphosphoglycerate (2,3-DPG) that promotes better transfer of oxygen at the tissue level. However, in all patients the combination of any degree of anaemia with decompensated cardiovascular disease (e.g. angina or obstructive airways disease) warns that intensive perioperative care will be necessary.

Preoperative haemoglobin measurement should be performed as a routine examination in all patients. Patients may have significant anaemia but no symptoms if the anaemia has developed slowly over a period of months and the body has compensated for the decreased oxygen-carrying capacity through such physiological mechanisms as increased cardiac output. The signs and symptoms of anaemia vary with its severity and are more marked if the anaemia has developed over a short period. Symptoms of weakness and tiredness, breathlessness, palpitations and angina can occur with moderate or severe anaemia. Pallor is the outstanding physical sign. Pallor of the conjunctiva and the palmar creases becomes apparent when the haemoglobin level falls below 10 g/dL. Tachycardia and cardiac failure may accompany severe anaemia. Patients with significant or symptomatic anaemia should be evaluated by a specialist physician or haematologist, frequently in a dedicated anaemia clinic.

In the surgical patient, it is often possible to institute iron therapy prior to admission to hospital. Anaemia is thus always best diagnosed and its cause determined during the first office consultation in patients needing elective surgery. For iron deficiency anaemia caused by blood loss, oral iron therapy begins immediately so that anaemia can be safely corrected prior to surgery. Patients with moderate iron deficiency or haemolytic anaemias do not pose an excessive risk provided the haemoglobin level and the blood volume are adequate (>10 g/dL) and cardiorespiratory function is normal.

In patients with megaloblastic anaemia surgery should be deferred, if possible, until specific therapy such as vitamin B_{12} or folic acid has repaired the generalised tissue defect. In these cases, transfusion alone may not render surgery safe, as protein metabolism of all cells is affected by the vitamin deficiency that causes the macrocytic anaemia. Adequate tissue levels can be achieved with 1–2 weeks of oral treatment with vitamin B_{12} or folic acid or both.

If it is not possible to correct the anaemia in a timely manner, the patient may be given concentrated red cells prior to surgery. A period of 3 days should be allowed to elapse before operation as the transfused blood will not reach its maximum oxygen-carrying capacity until at least 2 days following transfusion. This period allows the transfused red cells to accumulate normal levels of 2,3-DPG, necessary for efficient delivery of oxygen to the tissues, and allows plasma dispersal restoring normovolaemia. Elective surgery should seldom be undertaken when the haemoglobin concentration is less than 9–10 g/dL. Patients with long-standing anaemia are able to tolerate a reduced level of haemoglobin better than those who have become acutely anaemic. This tolerance in chronic anaemia is a result of altered 2,3-DPG concentration in the red cells, with a favourable shift in the oxyhaemoglobin dissociation curve to the right.

Psychological preparation and mental illness

All surgical patients must be in a relaxed state of mind irrespective of the nature of the procedure they are about to undergo. Anxiety and a fear of the unknown or of the potential complications of surgery are common, especially in the context of life-threatening illnesses or procedures. Reassurance can be achieved by empathetic surgeon communication with the patient and their relatives and, in certain instances, by the provision of specialised input from other healthcare professionals such as support nurses or psychologists.

Patients with pre-existing mental illness such as anxiety, depression, psychoses, substance abuse or dementia who are preparing for an operation require guidance from their treating healthcare professionals such that their condition is optimally managed in the perioperative period. The stress of surgery may worsen or unmask any pre-existing mental condition. Care must be taken in the prescription of analgesics, anxiolytics, sedatives, antidepressant and antipsychotic medications in these patients.

Further reading

Smith JA, Yii MK. Pre-operative medical problems in surgical patients. In: Smith JA, Fox JG, Saunder AC, Yii MK (eds) *Hunt and Marshall's Clinical Problems in Surgery*, 3rd edn. Chatswood, NSW: Elsevier, 2016:348–70.

Wilson H. Pre-operative management. In: Falaschi P, Marsh DR (eds) Orthogeriatrics. *Springer International Publishing*, 2017:63–79.

Woodhead K, Fudge L (eds) *Manual of Perioperative Care: an Eessential Guide*. Oxford: Wiley Blackwell, 2012.

MCQs

Select the single correct answer to each question. The correct answers can be found in the Answers section at the end of the book.

1 Without the use of prophylaxis the risk of deep calf vein thrombosis in a patient undergoing an anterior resection for rectal cancer is likely to be at least:
   a 10%
   b 20%
   c 30%
   d 50%

2 Which of the following measures is most likely to reduce the risk of postoperative wound infection with MRSA?
   a 5 days of broad-spectrum prophylactic antibiotics
   b ensuring the patient showers with chlorhexidine wash prior to surgery
   c a policy of staff hand washing between patients
   d screening patients for MRSA carriage prior to surgery

3 Which of the following constitutes the legal standard for the information that should be passed to a patient to meet the requirements of 'informed consent'?
   a what a patient in that position would regard as reasonable
   b what a reasoned body of medical opinion holds as reasonable
   c a list of all possible complications contained within a patient explanatory brochure
   d all serious complications that occur in more than 1% of patients

2 Assessment of surgical risk

Benjamin N.J. Thomson

University of Melbourne, Royal Melbourne Hospital Department of Surgery and Department of General Surgery Specialties, Royal Melbourne Hospital, Melbourne, Victoria, Australia

Introduction

This chapter reviews the assessment of risk for patients being considered for surgery or other invasive interventions.

Surgical risk

The definition of surgical risk is complex and differs depending on the point of view of the assessor. The risks of a particular surgical procedure may have a different value when considered by the surgeon, anaesthetist, intensivist, patient or family member.

What a surgeon may consider to be a small complication may be devastating to a patient depending on their personal circumstances. For example, a very rare risk of a unilateral recurrent laryngeal nerve injury leading to vocal cord palsy is well tolerated by the majority of patients but is a disaster for a professional singer. From a patient's perspective surgical risk encompasses the mortality and morbidity relevant to their circumstances as well as the chance of successfully achieving the desired outcome.

The General Medical Council (GMC) of the UK defines the risk of a proposed investigation or treatment using three criteria as well as the potential outcome of taking no action (Box 2.1). This is an integral component of the consent process required for each intervention or surgical procedure and allows the patient and clinician to make a consensual decision after considering the benefits of a procedure balanced against the associated risks. However, there may be a number of treatment options for each surgical pathology so the assessment of surgical risk also facilitates surgical decision-making.

For most surgical procedures the benefits of performing surgery far outweigh the risks and the decision is easier, but for complex surgical procedures the risks may outweigh any benefit. As outlined by the General Medical Council document the risks of not performing surgery also need to be considered. Another important aspect is the likely outcome from surgery. For example, most patients with adenocarcinoma of the head of the pancreas are not suitable for surgical management due to the presence of metastatic disease or involvement of the major adjacent blood vessels. After appropriate preoperative staging only 5–10% of patients are suitable for surgery. Resection of the pancreatic head (pancreaticoduodenectomy or Whipple's procedure) had a mortality of 50% in the 1950s, whereas in 2018 the reported mortality in specialist centres was 0.0–6.0%. Furthermore, operative morbidity is close to 50%. Despite the high morbidity and mortality, the median survival for those patients undergoing successful resection is only 14–24 months even in high-volume centres. Clearly any patient being considered for surgery needs also to understand the likelihood of successful treatment and to be able to balance this against their own personal circumstances as well as the likelihood of morbidity and mortality.

Another reason to assess surgical risk is identification of high-risk patients who may benefit from risk reduction measures such as preoperative and intraoperative optimisation as well as postoperative management in intensive care or high-dependency units.

Assessment of surgical risk

There are three components to assessment of surgical risk. The first is the associated mortality and morbidity of all surgical procedures. This can be

Textbook of Surgery, Fourth Edition. Edited by Julian A. Smith, Andrew H. Kaye, Christopher Christophi and Wendy A. Brown.
© 2020 John Wiley & Sons Ltd. Published 2020 by John Wiley & Sons Ltd.

obtained from multiple data sources that include personal audit, hospital audit, regional health data or specialty group audits. Furthermore, there is extensive published data available detailing the mortality and morbidity of surgical procedures or interventions, although this is often reflective of leading high-volume centres. Therefore, publications that report pooled data from all possible sources may offer a clearer representation of surgical risks. A brief overview of surgical risk is outlined in Table 2.1.

The next two components of surgical risk assessment involve both subjective and objective parameters. Subjective assessment includes information taken from the history and examination of a patient as well as recognition of patterns, clinical experience and intuition of the assessor. Often the experience of the assessor in surgical practice may be pivotal in identifying those patients at greater risk. Objective risk assessment includes biochemical and haematological testing as well as assessment of physiological function, particularly cardiac and respiratory function. Assessment of comorbidities also plays a role. There are also many risk prediction models and scoring systems available that can be general or surgery specific.

Discussing the risks of surgery

The General Medical Council of the UK has published guidance on the consent process and in particular on the discussion of the side effects,

complications and other risks of surgery or interventions. It details the need for clear, accurate information about the risks of a proposed procedure being presented in a way that the patient understands to enable them to make an informed decision. It is important to understand the patient's views and preferences as well as the adverse outcomes that they are most concerned about. It is impossible to cover every possible side effect or adverse outcome for each procedure but discussion of the common adverse outcomes whether severe or less serious is required as well as any possible serious adverse outcomes.

There are a number of resources available to aid in the discussion, such as procedure-specific information pamphlets produced at a hospital level, surgical regulatory authorities or government agencies.

Risk scoring systems

Many tools have been developed to estimate both mortality and morbidity rates for individual patients prior to a surgical procedure or intervention. Most are scoring systems that estimate risk for all patients whilst others are specific for high-risk patients or particular surgical procedures or disciplines. Like all tools they only provide an estimated risk and none are perfect. Most incorporate both physiological and comorbid data selected from large databases of patients. These have then been analysed with regression techniques to identify the key variables. Often a weighting is added to each of the variables. Ideally these scoring systems should be validated in multiple other centres to analyse their usefulness for particular patient groups.

ASA

One of the first scoring systems developed was by the American Society of Anesthesiologists (ASA) in 1963. It was a five-point classification system for assessment of a patient prior to surgery. It was

Table 2.1 Overview of the morbidity and mortality of common surgical procedures.

Surgical procedure	Morbidity (%)	Mortality (%)
Inguinal hernia repair	8–32	0–0.5
Appendicectomy	3.0–28.7	0.9–2.8
Laparoscopic cholecystectomy	14.7–21.4	0.3
Pancreaticoduodenectomy	20–54	0–6.0
Oesophagectomy	25–45	0.7–10.0
Coronary artery bypass grafting	30	1.5–2.5

Table 2.2 American Society of Anesthesiologists classification of mortality rates.

ASA rating	Number	Deaths (%)
1	92 227	0.001
2	367 161	0.002
3	195 829	0.028
4	45 118	0.304
5	353	6.232
1E	3 018	0.000
2E	12 188	0.033
3E	7 109	0.155
4E	5 000	3.280
5E	899	19.911

Source: Hopkins TJ, Raghunathan K, Barbeito A *et al.* Associations between ASA physical status and postoperative mortality at 48 h: a contemporary dataset analysis compared to a historical cohort. *Perioper Med* 2016;5:29.

subsequently revised with a sixth category coding for emergency patients. It is a combination of subjective anaesthetic opinion with an objective assessment of the patient's fitness for surgery. The majority of hospitals and anaesthetists in Australia use it routinely.

The ASA classification is as follows.

- ASA I: a normal healthy patient.
- ASA II: a patient with mild systemic disease.
- ASA III: a patient with severe systemic disease.
- ASA IV: a patient with severe systemic disease that is a constant threat to life.
- ASA V: a moribund patient who is not expected to survive without the operation.
- ASA VI: a declared brain-dead patient whose organs are being removed for donor purposes.

The coding for emergency patients is marked with the addition of an E.

The ASA system correlates with mortality, as outlined in Table 2.2 that details the outcome of 732,704 patients.

APACHE

First introduced in 1979, the Acute Physiology And Chronic Health Evaluation (APACHE) system was developed to measure the severity of illness in intensive care patients. It consisted of both acute physiological abnormalities as well as a chronic health evaluation measure. This was updated in 1985 with APACHE II with a reduction in the physiological values from 34 to 12 as well as adding a points score for diminished physiological reserve due to immune deficiency and ageing as well as chronic cardiac, pulmonary, renal or liver disease. Further

expansion and improvement in the prognostic estimates led to the development of APACHE III.

APACHE was never designed to predict mortality in individual patients. Furthermore, the ability to predict an individual's probability of survival depends upon response to therapy over time. The APACHE system is predominantly a guide for intensive care patients and therefore assessment of critically ill patients rather than a guide for elective surgery.

POSSUM

The Physiological and Operative Severity Score for the enumeration of Mortality and morbidity (POSSUM) was first described in 1991. Rather than a system for intensive care patients it was designed as a scoring system to estimate morbidity and mortality following surgery. It provides a risk-adjusted prediction of outcome. It is the most widely used surgical risk scoring system in the UK. Various modifications have been described and validated for colorectal, oesophagogastric and vascular patient groups. The Portsmouth P-POSSUM was developed in 1998 and is now the most commonly used in the UK.

Pre-admission clinics

Pre-admission clinics have been established for more than 20 years. They have many different roles that include administration, surgical clerking, consent, preoperative education as well as anaesthetic review. They provide an excellent environment for assessing surgical risk as well as for optimising patients' medical conditions prior to surgery. There are very few studies assessing the efficacy of pre-admission clinics in determining a patient's fitness but there are studies demonstrating increased patient satisfaction as well as a decrease in hospital length of stay.

Risk scoring systems lack sensitivity and specificity when applied to individuals. Assessment by an anaesthetist in a pre-admission clinic allows any scoring system to be used as an adjunct to information obtained through clinical assessment of each individual patient. The three objectives of an anaesthetic preoperative assessment are firstly to identify the risk of the patient developing an adverse outcome. The second is to assess any comorbidities that may be optimised prior to surgery. The third objective is to individualise perioperative management to attempt to minimise any remaining adverse outcomes.

There are a number of common comorbidities that should be assessed to minimise surgical risk.

Cardiac disease

Ischaemic heart disease is the commonest cause of serious cardiac adverse outcomes at the time of surgery. There is a greater risk amongst patients with a past history of myocardial infarction, particularly within 3–6 months. The presence of angina is less clear as a marker of increased risk but congestive cardiac failure has consistently been found to be an indicator of worse outcomes.

There are a number of investigations that can be used to assess cardiac risk, the commonest being an electrocardiogram. Non-invasive assessments of reversible cardiac ischaemia that may allow optimisation prior to surgery include exercise electrocardiogram, radionuclide stress cardiac imaging and stress echocardiography.

Respiratory disease

Patients with pulmonary disease are at risk of perioperative complications such as hyperreactive airways, prolonged ventilation, atelectasis, pneumonia and respiratory failure. The site of the surgical incision is important in determining risk due to impairment of pulmonary function. Median sternotomy, upper abdominal incisions and thoracotomy are associated with the greatest risk.

Pulmonary function tests are the main investigation for assessment of pulmonary disease and treatment of reversible airway disease may be required prior to surgery.

Renal risk assessment

Acute renal failure after surgical procedures is associated with a higher mortality rate. Many tertiary referral hospitals also have large nephrology services and surgical procedures on patients with end-stage renal failure are common. Again optimisation of the biochemical consequences of renal failure with preoperative renal dialysis is often required for those patients with end-stage renal failure.

Hepatic risk assessment

There are a number of risk assessments for chronic liver disease, including the Child–Pugh classification and the Model for End-stage Liver Disease (MELD). Patients with liver failure are at a high risk of death even following basic surgical procedures so management in a specialist centre is required to reduce the risk of an adverse outcome.

Neurological risk assessment

There are a number of risk factors for cerebrovascular complications in the postoperative period that include age, cerebrovascular disease, hypertension, atrial fibrillation and the type of surgery.

Haematological risk assessment

A past history of deep venous thrombosis, pulmonary embolism or haematological disorders (i.e. protein C and S deficiency) increases the risk of thromboembolism in the postoperative period.

Operative risk in the elderly

Operative risk is greater in the elderly, with a two to five times greater risk of death in comparison with younger patients. In general, elderly patients have a lower reserve when challenged by a surgical procedure or complication. In the original National Confidential Enquiry into Patient Outcome and Death (NCEPOD) released in 1987, 79% of perioperative deaths occurred in the over-65 age group, although that only represented 22% of the surgical population.

Summary

Assessment of surgical risk is a key component to both preoperative surgical and anaesthetic care. The assessment of surgical risk is critical in providing consent as well as for identifying those at risk who can be optimised prior to surgery or managed in an appropriate environment to allow for the best possible outcome.

Further reading

Burnand KG, Young AE, Lucas J, Rowlands BJ, Scholefield J (eds) *The New Aird's Companion in Surgical Studies*, 3rd edn. Edinburgh: Elsevier Churchill Livingstone, 2005.

Paterson-Brown S (ed.) *A Companion to Specialist Surgical Practice: Core Topics in General and Emergency Surgery*, 6th edn. Edinburgh: Elsevier, 2018.

MCQs

Select the single most appropriate answer to each question. The correct answers can be found in the Answers section at the end of the book.

1 Discussion of the risks of a surgical procedure should include:
   a the side effects
   b likely complications

c failure of the proposed surgery to achieve the desired outcome

d the potential outcome if no action is taken

e all of the above

2 The American Society of Anesthesiologists (ASA) risk scoring system:

a consists of 12 acute physiological abnormalities as well as a chronic health evaluation measure

b was designed for assessment of critically ill intensive care patients

c can be adjusted according to various different surgical procedures

d is a 6-point classification system for assessment of patients prior to surgery

e is assessed by the surgical team prior to surgery

3 Optimisation of cardiac ischaemia prior to surgery:

a is not necessary as ischaemic heart disease does not increase operative risk

b can be adequately assessed by electrocardiography alone

c is not required if the patient continues to smoke

d is only required for high-risk cardiac surgical patients

e may involve assessment of reversible cardiac ischaemia with radionuclide stress cardiac imaging or stress echocardiography

4 Operative risk in patients over 65 years of age is:

a no greater than for younger patients

b dependent on regular aspirin intake

c greater than younger patients

d only a greater risk if surgery is required for trauma

e greater for procedures performed under local anaesthesia rather than general anaesthesia

3 Anaesthesia and pain medicine

David Story

Centre for Integrated Critical Care, University of Melbourne, Melbourne, Victoria, Australia

Introduction

Anaesthetists aim to minimise the risks of surgery and anaesthesia for individual patients and provide optimal operating conditions leading to the best possible surgical outcomes. This requires direct patient care before, during and after surgery. The foundations of anaesthesia practice are general anaesthesia, regional anaesthesia, airway management, perioperative medicine, pain medicine, resuscitation crisis management, and safety and quality. In contemporary anaesthesia these all centre on evidence-based cost-effective practice.

Before surgery

The aim of preoperative assessment is to identify and reduce risks and develop an individualised plan for the patient for the perioperative period (before, during and after surgery) to achieve the goals of care, including being (ideally) cured of the surgical condition (particularly cancer) and returning to the best possible quality of life. About 20% of adult patients undergoing surgery and anaesthesia are at high risk of postoperative complications, disability or death after surgery. Preoperative factors increasing the risk of poor outcome range from severe heart disease to severe anxiety to long-term complex pain syndromes. However, for patients with robust health, failure to achieve an expected return to competitive sport or full employment would be a poor outcome.

Preoperative assessment

All patients should receive timely appropriate preoperative assessment. Increasingly, this includes a team approach including not only surgeons and anaesthetists but also general practitioners, general physicians, specialty physicians, pain medicine specialists, and nursing and allied health practitioners such as physiotherapists and cancer support nurses. The anaesthetist's assessment will include reviewing assessments from others including the surgical team and physicians. Anaesthetists want to know about coexisting conditions (comorbidity), including (i) the nature and extent of the patient's condition, (ii) the preferred treatment for this condition, and (iii) whether the patient is maximally optimised. Anaesthetists are experts in translating this information into a perioperative plan. As with all good clinical assessment, anaesthetists consider history, examination and tests.

The history often starts with a health questionnaire and then follow-up questions during a face-to-face meeting. Current medications and any adverse reactions to medications, particularly allergic reactions, are important. Another important area is prior experience of surgery and anaesthesia. The initial focus of anaesthesia assessment is ABC (airway, breathing and circulation) or, more specifically, potential airway problems and respiratory or cardiovascular dysfunction. Examination will focus on these areas. Tests will depend on the patient's comorbidity, age and planned surgery.

Airway

The aim is to detect potential airway problems that may adversely affect the intraoperative and/or postoperative period. An increasing number of patients have anatomy and disease states that may make intraoperative airway management both difficult and risky. Several factors (Box 3.1) are associated with difficult endotracheal intubation, and which are also associated with difficult mask ventilation and airway obstruction during sedation.

Textbook of Surgery, Fourth Edition. Edited by Julian A. Smith, Andrew H. Kaye, Christopher Christophi and Wendy A. Brown.
© 2020 John Wiley & Sons Ltd. Published 2020 by John Wiley & Sons Ltd.

Box 3.1 Factors associated with difficulty of airway management including during sedation

- Previous difficult endotracheal intubation
- Poor mouth opening
- Poor jaw advancement
- Prominent teeth
- Large tongue
- Limited neck movement
- Short, large neck (bull neck)
- Extreme obesity
- Obstructive sleep apnoea
- Large breasts

Box 3.2 Preoperative fasting recommendations

- For adults having an elective procedure, limited solid food may be taken up to 6 hours prior to anaesthesia and clear fluids may be taken up to 2 hours prior to anaesthesia. Clear fluids are regarded as water, pulp-free fruit juice, clear cordial, black tea and coffee. This excludes particulate or milk-based drinks.
- Prescribed medications may be taken with a sip of water less than 2 hours prior to anaesthesia unless otherwise directed (e.g. oral hypoglycaemics and anticoagulants).

Breathing (lung disease)

The most common lung conditions are asthma, chronic obstructive pulmonary disease (COPD) and recent cigarette smoking. Patients with severe asthma can deteriorate progressively or suddenly during the perioperative period; however, endotracheal intubation that directly stimulates the trachea can be a strong trigger for asthma. Patients with COPD may have a reactive asthma-like component as well as underlying structural lung disease. Oxygen saturation on finger pulse oximetry of less than 92% on room air is associated with severe lung disease and is a strong predictor of postoperative pulmonary complications including pneumonia. The anaesthesia plan will depend on the severity of the asthma or COPD and the nature of the surgery, with a preference for regional anaesthesia where possible for patients with severe lung disease. Care of patients with severe disease will often require coordination with optimisation plans, including preoperative oral steroids. While cigarette smoking is associated with perioperative respiratory complications, smoking is also associated with surgical site infection and patients should be supported with smoking cessation plans. Patients with very severe lung disease who may require prolonged mechanical ventilation in the intensive care unit (ICU) need very careful consideration of whether to proceed with surgery.

Another factor in respiratory assessment is aspiration risk. Aspiration occurs when stomach contents are vomited or passively regurgitated and contaminate the trachea and lower airways. Aspiration can be acidic gastric fluid and/or bile and/or food. Aspiration may be associated with chemical pneumonitis, bacterial pneumonia or airway obstruction and is a medical emergency. Aspiration continues to be an important cause of complications and death before and after surgery.

The greatest aspiration risk is for patients undergoing emergency surgery particularly abdominal surgery and in patients with known gastrointestinal obstruction, pain requiring opioids, and active vomiting. A relatively new aspiration risk is previous gastric banding for obesity (see Chapter 18). When possible, patients are fasted before surgery, including all elective surgery, to reduce the risk of aspiration, particularly from large amounts of solid material. Over the last 10 years fasting guidelines have been relaxed and fasting is not a barrier for patients receiving their regular medications (Box 3.2). However, patients with vomiting or gut obstruction often need parenteral drug substitution for important medications and pharmacist advice should be sought.

Cardiovascular

Symptomatic heart disease caries significant perioperative risk of complications and death, usually in the first few days after surgery. Cardiac complications are more common in patients with symptomatic ischaemic heart disease, heart failure or severe heart valve disease. The aim of cardiac assessment is to identify and minimise the risks of cardiac complications, such as myocardial injury after non-cardiac surgery including myocardial infarction, worsening cardiac failure and significant arrhythmia notably atrial fibrillation. Previous stroke is a risk factor for both further stroke and cardiac complications. Several drugs for cardiovascular disease may be withheld prior to surgery depending on individual circumstances, including opinion from the patient's cardiologist, to reduce perioperative risks, for example anticoagulants (including aspirin) to reduce bleeding risk and some antihypertensives (ACE inhibitors and angiotensin receptor blockers) to reduce the risk of persisting hypotension. Patients with significant cardiovascular disease often require more intensive monitoring and intervention during surgery, such as continuous monitoring of intra-arterial pressure and use of vasopressors and then ongoing care in high dependency or ICU after surgery.

Other frequent and important comorbidities include diabetes, anaemia and kidney disease.

Diabetes

Type 2 diabetes now affects up to 30% of surgical patients, with many previously undiagnosed. Poorly controlled diabetes in surgical patients is associated with increased complications including infection. Patients with type 2 diabetes frequently have, or need to be screened for, chronic kidney disease and cardiovascular disease. Preoperative assessment includes measurement of haemoglobin (Hb)A1c to screen for diabetes in patients aged over 50 years and for diabetes control in those with known diabetes. The key to managing diabetes in the perioperative period is to frequently measure the blood sugar and respond to both hyperglycaemia and hypoglycaemia. To avoid hypoglycaemia, most oral diabetes drugs will be withheld before surgery and insulin dosing will be modified. Many patients undergoing major surgery will need temporary change to insulin while in hospital in collaboration with the diabetes team.

Chronic kidney disease

Even mild chronic kidney disease, defined as an estimated glomerular filtration rate (eGFR) of less than 60 mL/min per m^2, carries a significant increase in the risk of death after surgery. Patients should be on optimal treatment for the severity of their kidney disease. Maintaining adequate hydration is the most important strategy in reducing the risks of chronic kidney disease.

Anaemia

Identifying preoperative anaemia, and the underlying cause, by measuring the haemoglobin and often undertaking iron studies is important for risk minimisation. Some surgical conditions, particularly colorectal cancer, have a high incidence of anaemia (see Chapter 1). Preoperative anaemia carries an increased risk of complications and mortality after surgery, in addition to an increased risk of red cell transfusion which also carries risks of complications. The risks of anaemia and transfusion may be reduced by identifying and managing preoperative iron deficiency and minimising intraoperative blood loss: patient blood management. The most effective way to treat iron deficiency is with iron infusion. However, some patients will have functional anaemia, also known as anaemia of chronic disease, which is harder to treat.

Postoperative nausea and vomiting

Postoperative nausea and vomiting (PONV) is called the 'big little problem'. PONV is common but usually preventable and treatable. However, patients find PONV distressing and may have delayed mobilisation and prolonged admission and occasionally serious complications such as pneumonia. The Apfel risk score for PONV includes four factors: (i) female sex; (ii) history of motion sickness or PONV; (iii) non-smoker; and (iv) planned postoperative opioid treatment. The incidence of PONV ranges from 10% with no Apfel factors to 80% with four factors. Patients at high risk will often receive multimodal intraoperative anti-emetic prophylaxis. Further, the anaesthesia and analgesia plan will have greater emphasis on non-opioid modalities, particularly regional analgesia. Patients at high risk of PONV will also have regular rather than just rescue postoperative anti-emetics.

Pain

Preoperative pain syndromes, particularly those treated with opioids and often requiring orthopaedic or spinal surgery, require close attention and specific planning. Multimodal pain management plans with regional analgesia blocks should be discussed with patients before surgery to outline risks and benefits. Chronic post-surgical pain is an under-recognised complication of surgery. Approximately 10% of patients have chronic pain (months to years) after major surgery, with about one-third of these patients having severe pain. This incidence is higher in specific types of surgery, notably thoracic and breast surgery. Pain management plans individualised to the patient and the surgery are important for reducing these risks. Some drugs, such as gabapentin, will need to be started preoperatively. The pain plan must include rescue for both poor postoperative pain control and complications of pain control such as excessive sedation.

Quantifying risk of complications and mortality

While we often focus on the risks of complication, death and disability, patient-focused outcomes also include pain, nausea and safe return to activities of daily living, as well as anaesthesia-specific risks including regional anaesthesia and adverse drug reaction. Following comprehensive anaesthesia

Table 3.1 American Society of Anesthesiologists Physical Score (ASA-PS).

ASA-PS class	Definition	Examples
ASA I	Healthy	Healthy, non-smoking, minimal alcohol use
ASA II	Mild systemic disease	Current smoker, well-controlled hypertension, or mild asthma
ASA III	Severe systemic disease	Poorly controlled diabetes, active hepatitis, or moderate reduction of left ventricular ejection fraction
ASA IV	Severe systemic disease that is a constant threat to life	Ongoing cardiac ischaemia, sepsis, end-stage cirrhosis
ASA V	A moribund patient who is not expected to survive without the operation	Examples include ruptured abdominal aneurysm, or gut ischaemia with septic shock

Source: https://www.asahq.org/
http://www.google.co.uk/url?sa=t&rct=j&q=&esrc=s&source=web&cd=1&cad=rja&uact=8&ved=2ahUKEwjX__
LSmLPeAhWlTt8KHRBzDX0QFjAAegQICBAC&url=http%3A%2F%2Fwww.asahq.org%2F~%2Fmedia%2Fsites
%2Fasahq%2Ffiles%2Fpublic%2Fresources%2Fstandards-guidelines%2Fasa-physical-status-classification-system.
pdf&usg=AOvVaw2VpwTL1ioJ7-XXfFM7Smwq Reproduced with permission of American Society of
Anesthesiologists.

assessment, patients should be allocated a score using the American Society of Anesthesiologists Physical Score (ASA-PS) (Table 3.1). This single-variable score is a remarkably strong predictor of postoperative complications and mortality. However, increased accuracy can be achieved by including other risk factors for complications and mortality such as increasing age, frailty and emergency surgery. Risk calculators, such as the American College of Surgeons online risk calculator (Box 3.3), allow quantitative risk assessment of complications and mortality, usually the risk of dying within 30 days of surgery (30-day mortality). Patients with a 5% or greater risk of 30-day mortality require higher levels of specialised care including admission to ICU after surgery. Patients with a 5% risk of mortality are likely to have a risk of major complications exceeding 20% and risk of poor functional recovery. Increasingly, in assessing the goals of care these high-risk patients undergo more limited surgery or non-surgical treatment.

Intraoperative care

The intraoperative care plan will depend on the nature and extent of the surgery and the patient. The broad aspects of anaesthesia are one or more of pain relief, sleep or sedation, no memory (amnesia), muscle relaxation and stable physiology, particularly haemodynamic stability. The fundamental keys to safe anaesthesia are appropriate intravenous access and control of the airway.

The broad options for anaesthesia involve one or more of the following: local anaesthesia, sedation, regional anaesthesia (spinal, epidural or nerve

---

Box 3.3 Example of calculating risks for patients and related decisions

Risk calculation for a 74-year-old woman for elective partial colectomy with colostomy using the American College of Surgeons Risk Calculator

- If assessed as ASA 2 (e.g. has hypertension), risk of death within 30 days of surgery is at least 0.5% and risk of complications is 20%. This patient is suitable for ward care.
- If assessed as ASA 4 (e.g. has diabetes, cardiac failure and chronic renal impairment), risk of death is at least 5% and risk of complication 35%. Clinicians should strongly consider critical care admission after surgery.
- If assessed as ASA 4, frail and having emergency surgery (a growing number of patients), risk of death is 13% and risk of complications 42%. The goals of care should be discussed with the patient (and family) and some may decide for supportive care only or limitations on medical treatment if she deteriorates after surgery.

---

block) and general anaesthesia, all of which have many additional options.

Intravenous access

For many procedures intravenous access is predominantly used to administer drugs to provide appropriate and safe anaesthesia, with fluid therapy being a minor component. The small cannulas (blue, 22G, 0.41 mm diameter) have a maximum flow rate of about 30 mL/min but because flow is related to the fourth power of the radius, a large cannula (orange,

14G, 1.6 mm diameter) has 10 times the flow (300 mL/min). Flow is enhanced in cannulas sited in larger veins. For adult trauma patients, the standard of care is two 16-gauge cannulas in large cubital fossa veins with a total flow of up to 400 mL/min (2 × 200 mL/min). This would be similar to intravenous access for major surgery. Long catheters placed in central veins (central lines), particularly the internal jugular vein, are used for reliable and robust intravenous access for drugs that could cause harm if they passed into interstitial tissue through damaged peripheral veins or if the drugs were suddenly stopped. Such drugs include potent vasoconstrictors whose sudden cessation can lead to severe shock and where extravasation can lead to tissue necrosis. Central lines also allow easy venous blood sampling for analysis and for measurement of central venous pressure.

Intraoperative monitoring

The most important intraoperative monitor is the pulse oximeter, which allows continuous non-invasive measurement of blood oxygen saturation and heart rate. Falling oxygen saturation is most frequently due to inadequate ventilation or inadequate inspired oxygen in patients who are anaesthetised but spontaneously breathing. Other fundamental monitoring includes ECG to detect changes or abnormalities in heart rate and rhythm, and blood pressure monitoring with either intermittent non-invasive cuff measurements (usually the brachial artery) or continuous invasive arterial monitoring (usually the radial artery).

Contemporary anaesthesia machines can perform extensive electronic monitoring of multiple patient and machine variables. In addition to the fundamental monitoring previously outlined, anaesthesia machines monitor inspired and expired gases (oxygen, carbon dioxide and anaesthetic gases). Further, anaesthesia machines have complex alarm systems that enhance safety monitoring individualised to the patient and procedure. Modern machine ventilators allow both full mechanical ventilation and assisted spontaneous ventilation. Depth of anaesthesia can be routinely monitored with specialised EEG, and depth of muscle relaxation with neuromuscular monitoring

Oxygen therapy and airway interventions

Intraoperative airway interventions range from supplemental oxygen via nasal prongs through to endotracheal intubation. Even patients undergoing procedures under local anaesthesia and sedation, such as minor plastic surgery, or those undergoing major surgery under spinal anaesthesia may require some supplemental oxygen due to respiratory depression or in order to wash out carbon dioxide and to reduce claustrophobia under drapes. Contemporary supplemental oxygen is often accompanied by continuous monitoring of expired carbon dioxide. This safety measure detects hypoventilation and airway obstruction due to apnoea.

Postoperative pain medicine

All anaesthetists, and many surgeons, are trained in acute pain medicine. Advanced pain medicine is now a medical speciality with many practitioners also being anaesthetists. Good pain control after surgery is a central part of postoperative care. The most important cause of chronic post-surgical pain is severe acute postoperative pain.

Pharmacological therapy will be combined with strategies such as physiotherapy and proactive nursing care to effectively and efficiently return the patient to the best possible function and recovery from their surgical condition. Other aims include minimising the risks of pain therapies for the individual and the spread of drugs of addiction (particularly opioids) into the broader community. Collaboration with an anaesthetist-led acute pain service greatly facilitates these aims. Further, acute pain medicine is more complex at extremes of age and in those with complex comorbidity, those suffering from opioid tolerance or dependence, obese patients and those with complex pain syndromes.

While anaesthetists will usually plan and establish a postoperative pain management plan, ward clinicians need to measure a patient's pain, often with a 0–10 visual analogue scale and alter the plan if patients have poor pain control or side effects, particularly excess sedation. Postoperative care also involves weaning from analgesia as appropriate and moving the patient to oral pain relief appropriate for community discharge and subsequent cessation. Chronic post-surgical pain is an important complication after surgery. While some operations, particularly surgery via thoracotomy, carry a major risk of chronic post-surgical pain, one in ten patients will have chronic pain after abdominal surgery.

Multimodal analgesia aims to combine the benefits of different mechanisms to treat pain to provide high-quality pain relief and minimise side effects. The following list gives an indication of the postoperative analgesic options that can be individualised to patients and operations.

- Paracetamol: regular paracetamol is an effective foundation for multimodal analgesia. With appropriate dosing paracetamol has minimal side effects.

- Non-steroidal anti-inflammatory drugs (NSAIDs): these drugs form the next tier of analgesics. While being very effective analgesics, NSAIDs can increase the risk of bleeding and acute kidney injury. For most patients the benefits greatly outweigh these relatively rare risks.
- Opioids: morphine has been a mainstay of pain relief for centuries. In contemporary practice morphine is administered in many ways: oral, subcutaneous, intramuscular, intravenous, epidural and spinal. Many patients receive morphine via patient-controlled analgesia (PCA) that aims to empower the patient and reduce risks. All routes of morphine administration carry the risk of life-threatening respiratory depression and death. Hospital protocols aim to minimise these risks. However, far more frequent complications include nausea, constipation and itch. Other frequently used alternative opioids are fentanyl and oxycodone. Tramadol is an atypical opioid with less respiratory depression, constipation and potential for abuse. However, tramadol can have important drug interactions that can limit its use, including a serotonin syndrome with some antidepressants. There is a strong trend towards minimising use of opioids around the time of surgery to reduce the frequency of in-hospital opioid complications (nausea and vomiting, constipation and itch), reduce long-term opioid use and reduce community opioid abuse.
- Ketamine: this drug acts on different receptors from the opioids and provides complementary but different analgesia and is opioid sparing. Ketamine infusion is often introduced for inadequately treated pain after major surgery and for patients at significant risk with opioid analgesia. The major complication with ketamine is hallucinations.
- Anticonvulsants: gabapentin and pregabalin are two anticonvulsants used to treat chronic as well as acute pain from nerve injury, which can occur in many types of surgery. These drugs are also opioid sparing and reduce opioid side effects.
- Local anaesthetics: increasingly, patients on wards have infusions of local anaesthetic through specialised catheters placed by anaesthetists that provide direct analgesia to major nerves and nerve plexuses, or wound catheters placed by surgeons. Epidural infusions are still used in some major thoracic and abdominal surgery, usually on an individualised basis. These infusions may provide better postoperative analgesia, less opioid use and less PONV, itch and sedation than only using systemic analgesia. The most important side effects of local anaesthetics are fitting, cardiac arrhythmias and cardiac arrest but are dose related and rare with contemporary practice.

Further reading

American College of Surgeons. Surgical Risk Calculator. Available at https://riskcalculator.facs.org/RiskCalculator/

National Institute for Health and Care Excellence. *Routine Preoperative Tests for Elective Surgery*. Nice Guideline NG45. London: NICE, 2016. Available at https://www.nice.org.uk/guidance/ng45

Schlug SA, Palmer GM, Scott DA, Halliwell R, Trinca J. Acute pain management: scientific evidence, fourth edition, 2015. *Med J Aust* 2016;204:315–17.

Thilen SR, Wijeysundera DN, Treggiari MM. Preoperative consultations. *Anesthesiol Clin* 2016;34:17–33.

MCQs

Select the single most appropriate answer to each question. The correct answers can be found in the Answers section at the end of the book.

1 A fit and healthy patient having their anterior cruciate ligament repaired:
  a has no cardiopulmonary perioperative risks
  b is American Society of Anesthesiologists Society Physical Status 1
  c will require minimal analgesia
  d will require a postoperative critical care bed and prolonged hospital stay
  e is likely to have obstructive sleep apnoea

2 Anaesthesia assessment:
  a is usually just before induction of anaesthesia
  b requires blood tests
  c excludes patients with complex pain syndromes
  d requires history, examination and further tests
  e is independent of surgical assessment

3 Which of the following risk factors for postoperative nausea and vomiting (PONV) is *incorrect*?
  a old age
  b gender
  c previous nausea and vomiting
  d non-smoking
  e use of opioids

4 Opioids:
  a are the foundation of all pain management plans
  b have excitation as a major side effect
  c cause diarrhoea
  d can be administered by several routes
  e are contraindicated for patients taking paracetamol

4 Postoperative management

Peter Devitt

Department of Surgery, University of Adelaide and Royal Adelaide Hospital, Adelaide, South Australia, Australia

Introduction

Good postoperative management will have started before the procedure with appropriate counselling and preparation (see Chapter 1). This preparation will have included an assessment of fitness for the procedure and identification and management of any risk factors. The patient will have been provided with a clear explanation of the procedure (emergency or elective), the risks and benefits, and the likely outcome. This will have included a description of what the patient should expect in terms of short- and long-term recovery from the procedure, possible complications and the necessity for any drains, stomas, catheters or other bits of tubing, the details of which would be alien to most of the population. The anticipated length of time in hospital will have been discussed, as well as details of how long it will take to make a full recovery from the procedure and how long the patient will be away from or unable to participate in their usual activities. The patient will have been reassured about pain control measures and, perhaps most difficult of all, the doctor will have tried to ensure that the patient's expectations match those of the health professional.

This chapter will focus on the care of the patient in the immediate postoperative period, up until the time of discharge from hospital. The immediate and short-term needs of the patient and care to be provided will depend on the magnitude and type of surgery.

Immediate management of the patient

Pain management

Pain relief is of paramount importance (see Chapter 3) and an appropriate drug regimen will have been prescribed by the surgeon and/or anaesthetist by the end of the procedure. In checking the charts of the patient after the procedure, care will be taken that these and any other medications required are prescribed and administered. These may include antibiotics (prophylactic or therapeutic), sedatives, anti-emetics and anticoagulants.

Monitoring

Depending on the nature of the procedure and the underlying state of health of the patient, the vital signs (blood pressure, pulse and oxygen saturation) will be measured and recorded regularly. If an arterial catheter has been inserted, blood pressure and pulse readings can be observed on a monitor constantly. The intensity and frequency of monitoring will be maximal in the recovery room and this level of scrutiny maintained if the patient is in an intensive care or high-dependency area.

Measurement of the central venous pressure may be required for patients with poor cardiorespiratory reserve or where there have been large volumes of fluid administered or major fluid shifts are expected.

The patient chart will also record all fluid that has been given during and since the operation, together with fluid lost. Ideally, these figures will have been balanced by the end of the procedure, so that the duty of the attending doctor will be to monitor ongoing losses (digestive and urinary tracts, drains, stomas) and replace these. The normal daily fluid and electrolyte requirements will also be provided. If there has been major fluid shifts or if renal function is precarious, a urinary catheter will be inserted and regular (hourly) checks made of fluid losses. Serum electrolytes and haematological values will be checked frequently, again the frequency depending on any abnormalities present and the magnitude of any fluid and electrolyte replacement.

Textbook of Surgery, Fourth Edition. Edited by Julian A. Smith, Andrew H. Kaye, Christopher Christophi and Wendy A. Brown.
© 2020 John Wiley & Sons Ltd. Published 2020 by John Wiley & Sons Ltd.

Mobilisation

Early mobilisation is encouraged. Unless there are specified orders to the contrary, all patients are encouraged to get up and move around as much as their underlying condition will allow. Obvious exceptions to this policy include patients with epidural catheters and those with severe multiple injuries. The aim of early mobilisation is to encourage good pulmonary ventilation and to reduce venous stasis. For those who cannot mobilise, physiotherapy should be provided to help with breathing and measures taken to either increase venous flow (pneumatic calf compression devices) or reduce risks of deep vein thrombosis (heparin). The timing of any planned heparin administration will depend on the nature of the procedure and the risks of haemorrhage from that procedure.

Communication

When problems arise, they are frequently compounded by a failure of communication. Whilst the doctor's duty of care is to the patients themselves, the needs of the relatives must be taken into account. Simple things – which are often forgotten – include a reassuring telephone call to the nearest relative after a procedure, informing them (usually in general terms) of how the procedure went. Whilst this is most obvious in the paediatric setting, the same principles should be followed with adult healthcare. The patients themselves will seek some form of reassurance in the immediate postoperative period. They will want to know how the procedure went and how they are progressing. They will also want reassurance that all the tubes, lines and equipment to which they are attached are quite normal and not an indication of impending disaster. Ideally, this will have been discussed with them prior to the procedure. Any unexpected findings or complications encountered during the procedure should be discussed with the patient. The timing and detail of this discussion is a matter of fine judgement and may be best done in the presence of the patient's relatives and by the individual who performed the procedure.

Further care in the postoperative period

This covers the time from recovery from anaesthesia and initial monitoring to discharge from hospital. Wound care is discussed in Chapter 6.

Prophylaxis against venous thromboembolism

This is a key part of the management of any hospitalised individual, particularly the surgical patient. A risk analysis will have been performed preoperatively (see Chapter 1) and depending on the nature of the procedure and the individual's risk, some form of chemoprophylaxis may be started in the postoperative period. This will require day-to-day monitoring and for major procedures, such as hip joint replacement or many cancer operations, the prophylaxis may be continued after discharge from hospital. For patients being managed in intensive care settings and who, for various reasons, will have limited or no mobility, intermittent mechanical calf compression will be used in addition to chemoprophylaxis.

Enhanced recovery after surgery (ERAS) programs

These structured programs are starting to replace traditional surgical practices, with implementation of protocols for early postoperative feeding, early mobilisation and more effective pain control measures. Evidence now exists showing that these ERAS systems can significantly reduce length of hospital stay and complications rates, with overall reduction in healthcare costs.

Respiratory care

In the otherwise fit and healthy patient, maintenance of respiratory function is usually not a problem, particularly if there is optimal management of pain. Even with upper abdominal or thoracic procedures, most patients will require little respiratory support provided they are able to mobilise themselves and breathe unimpeded by pain. When assistance is required simple breathing exercises, with or without the help of a physiotherapist, is usually sufficient. Mechanical ventilation may be required in the early phase of recovery from a particular procedure. This can vary from prolonged endotracheal intubation, to intermittent positive pressure ventilation, to supplemental oxygenation by face mask or nasal prongs. In these instances the patient may require prolonged monitoring in an intensive care or high-dependency unit with regular assessment of oxygen saturation (pulse oximetry and arterial blood gas analysis).

For less fit patients, and particularly those with chronic obstructive pulmonary disease (COPD), the risks of respiratory failure will be considerable and measures such as epidural local anaesthesia will be employed. Control of pain, attention to regular hyperinflation (inhalation spirometry and physio-therapy) and early mobilisation are the keys to preventing respiratory complications.

Fluid balance

The three principles of management of fluid balance are:
- correct any abnormalities
- provide the daily requirements
- replace any abnormal and ongoing losses.

Ideally, any abnormalities will have been identified and corrected before or during the surgical procedure. In the calculation of a patient's fluid requirements, there is a distinction to be made between the volume required to *maintain* the body's normal functions and that required to *replace* any abnormal losses. The normal maintenance fluid requirements will vary depending on the patient's age, gender, weight and body surface area.

Basic requirements

The total body water of a 70-kg adult comprises 45–60% of body weight. Lean patients have a greater percentage of their body weight as body water and older patients a lesser proportion. Of the total body water, two-thirds is in the intracellular compartment and one-third is divided between plasma water (25% of extracellular fluid) and interstitial fluid (75% of extracellular fluid). Therefore, a lean individual weighing 70 kg would have a plasma water of 3 L, an interstitial volume of 11 L and an intracellular volume of 28 L, making a total volume of 42 L.

The normal daily fluid requirement to *maintain* a healthy 70-kg adult is between 2 and 3 L. The individual will lose about 1500 mL in the urine and about 500 mL from the skin, lungs and stool. Loss from the skin will vary with the ambient temperature.

The electrolyte composition of intracellular fluid (ICF) and extracellular fluid (ECF) varies (Table 4.1). Sodium is the predominant cation in ECF while potassium predominates in the ICF. The normal daily requirements of sodium and potassium are 100–150 mmol and 60–90 mmol, respectively. This will balance the daily loss of these two cations in the urine.

Replacement

If an otherwise healthy adult is deprived of the normal daily intake of fluid and electrolytes, suitable intravenous maintenance must be provided. One

Table 4.1 Electrolyte concentrations.

Electrolyte	Extracellular fluid (mmol/L)	Intracellular fluid (mmol/L)
Sodium	135	10
Potassium	4	150
Calcium	2.5	2.5
Magnesium	1.5	10
Chloride	100	10
Bicarbonate	27	10
Phosphate	1.5	45

relatively simple regimen is 1 L of 0.9% saline and 1–2 L of 5% dextrose solution.

Both these solutions are isotonic with respect to plasma. The electrolyte solution contains the basic electrolyte requirements (154 mmol/L of sodium and 154 mmol/L of chloride) and the total volume can be adjusted with various amounts of dextrose solution. Potassium can be added as required. Other solutions (e.g. Ringer's lactate) may contain a more balanced make-up of electrolytes, but are rarely needed for a patient who is otherwise well and only requires intravenous fluids for a few days.

In the immediate postoperative period there is an increased secretion of antidiuretic hormone (ADH), with subsequent retention of water. In an adult of average build, maintenance fluids can be restricted to 2 L per day with no potassium supplements until a diuresis has occurred. This is not an absolute rule, and potassium supplements can be given early, provided the patient has normal renal function.

Fluid and electrolyte *replacement* is that required to correct abnormalities. Volume depletion and electrolyte abnormalities are relatively common in surgical patients, particularly those admitted with acute illnesses. Volume depletion usually occurs in association with an electrolyte deficit, but can occur in isolation. Reduced fluid intake, tachypnoea, fever or an increase in the ambient temperature may all lead to a unilateral volume loss. This will cause thirst and dehydration, which may progress to a tachycardia, hypotension and prostration. In severe cases there may be hypernatraemia and coma. Intravenous administration of 5% dextrose is used to correct the problem.

More often volume depletion is accompanied by an electrolyte deficit. Excessive fluid and electrolyte may be lost from the skin (e.g. sweating, burns), the renal tract (e.g. diabetic ketoacidosis) and the gastrointestinal tract (e.g. vomiting, ileus, fistula, diarrhoea). There is considerable scope for abnormal fluid losses in a surgical patient, particularly after a major abdominal procedure.

Table 4.2 Approximate electrolyte concentrations.

Secretions	Sodium (mmol/L)	Potassium (mmol/L)	Chloride (mmol/L)	Bicarbonate (mmol/L)	Hydrogen (mmol/L)
Salivary	50	20	40	50	—
Gastric	50	15	120	20	70
Duodenal	140	5	80	—	—
Biliary	140	10	100	40	—
Pancreatic	140	10	80	80	—
Jejuno-ileal	130	20	105	30	—
Faeces	80	10	100	25	—
Diarrhoea	100	30	50	60	—

There may be pooling of fluid at the operation site itself, an ileus might develop, fluid could be lost through a nasogastric tube or drains, and there might be increased cutaneous loss if there is a high fever.

The source of fluid loss will determine the type of electrolyte lost. There is considerable variation in the electrolyte content of different gastrointestinal secretions (Table 4.2). Loss from the upper digestive tract tends to be rich in acid, while loss from the lower tract is high in sodium and bicarbonate. Thus, patients with severe and prolonged vomiting from gastric outlet obstruction may develop a metabolic alkalosis.

While the management of maintenance fluid requirements can often be done on a daily basis, the fluid and electrolyte replacement needs of an acutely ill surgical patient is likely to be more involved and necessitate close monitoring and adjustment. Clinical assessment and appreciation of the types of fluid loss will give an approximate guide to the scale of the problem, but regular biochemical electrolyte estimations will be required to determine the precise composition of what needs to be replaced. In most instances, measurement of plasma electrolyte concentrations will provide sufficient information, but occasionally it may be necessary to estimate the electrolyte contents of the various fluids being lost.

Drains and catheters

Drains serve a number of purposes. They may be inserted into an operative site or into a wound as it is being closed to drain collections or potential collections. Drains may also be put into the chest cavity to help the lungs re-expand. They may be put into ducts and hollow organs to divert secretions or to decompress that structure. Examples of decompression include insertion of a tube into the common bile duct after duct exploration or nasogastric intubation to decompress the stomach after surgery for intestinal obstruction. Sump drains are used to irrigate sites of contamination or infection.

Drains can act as a point of access for infection, and whilst this may be of little consequence if the tube has been placed to drain an abscess cavity, all efforts are made to reduce contamination of any wound. There is increased use of closed drainage systems and dressings around drains are changed regularly. Any changes to tubes or bags on drains must be carried out using aseptic techniques. Once a drain has served its purpose, it should be removed. The longer a drain stays *in situ*, the greater the risk of infection.

The contents and volumes discharged through a drain must be recorded. Large volumes, such as those from the gastrointestinal tract, may need the equivalent amount replaced intravenously.

Gut function

Some degree of gut atony is common after abdominal surgery, particularly emergency surgery. The condition is usually self-limiting and of little clinical consequence. There are three conditions that can produce massive gut dilatation and pose serious problems for the patient:
- gastric dilatation
- paralytic (small intestine) ileus
- pseudo-obstruction (large intestine).

Gastric dilatation

Gastric dilatation is rare and when it occurs tends to be associated with surgery of the upper digestive tract. It may occur suddenly 2–3 days after the operation and is associated with massive fluid secretion into the stomach, with the consequent risk of regurgitation and inhalation. Treatment is by insertion of a nasogastric tube and decompression of the stomach. Unfortunately, when gastric dilatation does occur, often the first indication of the problem is a massive vomit and inhalation after the dilatation has occurred. By then the damage is done and the value of a nasogastric tube at this stage is questionable. Traditionally, nasogastric tubes were used routinely for patients following laparotomy, particularly in the emergency setting. However, the nasogastric tube is often the patient's major source of irritation and discomfort in the postoperative period and its routine use is gradually being abandoned.

Paralytic ileus

Paralytic ileus is less sinister and more common. In the acutely ill patient who has undergone surgical intervention for peritonitis, paralytic ileus may be present from the first postoperative day. Otherwise, it tends to make its presence felt about 5 days after operation, and the patient may have been making an apparently uneventful recovery. Abdominal distension occurs and the patient may vomit. Oral fluid restriction should be instituted and intravenous replacement may be required. Most cases resolve spontaneously. Occasionally a prokinetic agent may be considered.

Pseudo-obstruction

Classically, pseudo-obstruction occurs in the elderly patient who has recently undergone surgery for a fractured neck of femur. The condition is also often seen where there has been extensive pelvic or retroperitoneal injury and sometimes the condition appears to be more related to the use of opiate analgesia rather than the type of surgery itself. The atony, with abdominal distension and absence of bowel function, tends to occur 2–3 days after surgery (or from the time the injury was sustained). Pseudo-obstruction is often mistaken for mechanical obstruction and the dilatation of the colon and caecum can be massive. If the condition does not resolve spontaneously, colonoscopic decompression is usually successful. Occasionally, surgical intervention is required to prevent caecal perforation.

Important postoperative complications

Respiratory complications

Deterioration or impairment of respiratory function is the commonest and more important postoperative complication, occurring with greatest frequency in the patient undergoing an emergency procedure. The preoperative assessment will have judged the individual's risk and measures that might need to be taken to minimise respiratory problems (see Chapter 1). Apart from any comorbidities, such as COPD, the likely cause of a patient's hypoxaemia will vary with the time of onset (Box 4.1).

Measures must be taken to minimise the risks of postoperative pulmonary complications, including judicious use of pain medications, where local wound infiltration or nerve blocks may be more appropriate than systemic measures. Early mobilisation and encouragement to cough and breathe deeply must be actively promoted.

Depending on the initial state of respiratory function and the degree of deterioration, the patient may require anything from supplemental oxygen supplied by face mask to endotracheal intubation. A P_{CO_2} above 45 mmHg, a P_{O_2} below 60 mmHg and a low tidal volume all indicate that mechanical ventilation will be required. Once appropriate ventilatory support has been achieved, the cause of the respiratory failure can be addressed.

Wound failure

Provided the surgical procedure has a minimal risk of infection (see Chapter 9) and has been performed in an uneventful manner in a low-risk patient, then the chances of problems with the wound are minimal and most such wounds can be left undisturbed

---

Box 4.1 Factors contributing to postoperative hypoxaemia

Immediate
Respiratory depression (anaesthetic agents, opioids)

Within first 24 hours
Established respiratory disease (e.g. COPD)
Obesity
Excessive sedation
Opiates
Aspiration
Pneumothorax

Between days 2 and 5
Infection
Diaphragmatic splinting (secondary to abdominal distension)
Pleural effusion
Acute respiratory distress syndrome

After day 5
Pulmonary embolus

until the patient leaves hospital. If there are identifiable risks the wounds may need to be attended to regularly. The problems that are likely to occur with wounds relate to:

- discharge of fluid
- collection of fluid
- disruption of the wound.

Risk factors that may contribute to these problems include those that:

- increase the risk of infection (see Chapter 9)
- increase the risk of wound breakdown.

There are general and local factors that increase the risk of breakdown of a wound. General factors include those that interfere with wound healing, such as diabetes mellitus, immunosuppression, malignancy and malnutrition. Local factors include the adequacy of wound closure, infection and anything that might put mechanical stress on the wound. For example, abdominal wound failure is a potential problem in the obese, and in those with chest infections, ascites or ileus.

In the early stages of wound healing any abnormal fluid at the wound site is likely to discharge rather than collect. The fluid may be blood, serous fluid, serosanguinous fluid or infected fluid of varying degrees up to frank pus. As discussed elsewhere in this chapter, the discharge of blood from a wound may have all sorts of consequences for the patient, which will vary from prompt opening of the neck wound of a patient with a primary haemorrhage after a thyroidectomy to evacuation of a haematoma after a mastectomy.

Serous fluid may be of little significance and be the result of a liquefying haematoma from within the depths of the wound. However, a serosanguinous discharge from an abdominal or chest wound may herald a more sinister event, particularly if it occurs between 5 and 8 days after the operation. The discharge may have been preceded by coughing or retching. Such a wound is in imminent danger of deep dehiscence with evisceration. Should such an event occur, the wound must be covered in sterile moist packs and arrangements made to take the patient to the operating room for formal repair of the wound.

Collections in and under a wound may be blood, pus or seroma. As mentioned, the rapidity with which a haematoma appears and any pressure effects such a haematoma may cause will determine its treatment. Collections of pus must be drained. Depending on its proximity or distance from the skin surface, an abscess may be drained by opening the wound or inserting (under radiological control) a drain into a deeper-lying cavity. Seromas tend to occur where there has been a large area of dissection in subcutaneous tissues (e.g. mastectomy) or where lymphatics may be damaged (e.g. groin dissections). The seroma may not appear a week after the procedure. Seromas will lift the skin off the underlying tissues and impede wound healing. They also make fertile ground for infection. Seromas should be aspirated under sterile conditions and the patient warned that several aspirations may be required as the seroma may re-collect.

Confusion

Confusion in surgical patients is common and has many causes. Often the confusion is minor and transient and does not need treatment. The patient is typically elderly, has become acutely ill and in pain, is removed from the security and familiarity of their home surroundings, is subject to emergency surgery and more pain, is put in a noisy environment with strangers bustling around and is sleep-deprived. These factors alone would make many otherwise healthy individuals confused. Add to that recipe the deprivation of the patient's regular medications (particularly alcohol), the upset to their body biochemistry, the presence of hypoxia and a variety of postoperative medications such as opioids, and it becomes understandable that some degree of confusion is very common in the postoperative period. Confusion combined with restlessness, agitation and disorientation is referred to as delirium.

Important causes of confusion include:

- Sepsis (operative site, chest, urinary tract)
- Hypoxia (chest infection, pulmonary embolus, pre-existing pulmonary disease)
- Metabolic abnormalities (hyponatraemia, hyperglycaemia/hypoglycaemia, acidosis, alkalosis)
- Cardiac
- Hypotension (haemorrhage, dehydration)
- Cerebrovascular event
- Drug withdrawal (alcohol, opiates, benzodiazepines)
- Drug interaction (opiate sedation)
- Exacerbation of pre-existing medical conditions (dementia, hypothyroidism).

When a patient does become confused in the postoperative period, it is important to ensure that no easily correctable cause has been overlooked. Confusion is often secondary to hypoxia, where chest infection, over-sedation, cardiac problems and pulmonary embolism need to be considered. Other important causes to consider include sepsis, drug withdrawal, metabolic and electrolyte disturbances and medications.

The management of the confused patient will include a close study of the charts, seeking information on any coexisting disease (particularly cardiorespiratory), drug record, alcohol consumption and the progress of the patient since the operation. Current medications should be noted, together with the nursing record of the vital signs.

If possible, try to take a history and examine the patient. Ensure that the patient is in a well-lit room and give oxygen by face mask. Attention should be focused on the cardiorespiratory system, as this may well be the site of the underlying problem. Some investigations may be required to help determine the cause of the confusion. These might include arterial blood gas analysis, haematological and biochemical screens, blood and urine cultures, a chest X-ray and an electrocardiogram (ECG).

Most patients with postoperative confusion do not require treatment other than that for the underlying cause. However, the noisy violent patient may need individual nursing care, physical restraint or sedation. Sedation should be reserved for patients with alcohol withdrawal problems, and either haloperidol or diazepam should be considered in such circumstances. Most hospitals have clearly defined protocols for the management of patients going through alcohol withdrawal. These correlate the anxiety, visual disturbances and agitation of the patient with the degree of monitoring and sedation required.

Pyrexia

The normal body temperature ranges between 36.5 and 37.5°C. The core temperature tends to be 0.5°C warmer than the peripheral temperature. Thus an isolated reading of 37.5°C has little meaning by itself and needs to be viewed in context with the other vital signs. Changes in temperature and the pattern of change are more important. A temperature that rises and falls several degrees between readings suggests a collection of pus and intermittent pyaemia, while a persistent high-grade fever is more in keeping with a generalised infection.

Fever can be due to infection or inflammation. In determining the cause of the fever the following should be considered:
- the type of fever
- the type of procedure which the patient has undergone
- the temporal relationship between the procedure and the fever.

Perhaps the most useful factor in trying to establish the cause of a patient's fever is the relationship between the time of onset of the fever and the procedure. Fever within the first 24 hours of an operation is common and may reflect little more than the body's metabolic response to injury.

A fever that is evident between 5 and 7 days after an operation is usually due to infection. While pulmonary infections tend to occur in the first few days after surgery, fever at this later stage is more likely to reflect infection of the wound, operative site or urinary tract. Cannula problems and deep vein thrombosis (DVT) should also be considered.

A fever occurring more than 7 days after a surgical procedure may be due to abscess formation. Apart from infection as a cause of fever, it is important to remember that drugs, transfusion and brainstem problems can also produce an increase in body temperature.

A careful history, review of the charts and physical examination will usually determine the cause of the fever. The next stage in management will depend on the state of health of the patient. The fever of a septic process, which has led to circulatory collapse, will require resuscitation of the patient before any investigation. Otherwise, appropriate investigations may include blood and urine cultures, swabs from wounds and drains, and imaging to define the site of infection.

Treatment will depend on the severity and type of infection. The moribund patient will require resuscitation and empirical use of antibiotics, the choice varying with the likely source of infection. Surgical or radiological intervention (e.g. to drain an abscess) may be required before the patient improves. However, the well patient may have antimicrobial therapy deferred until an organism has been identified (e.g. Gram stain or culture).

Deep vein thrombosis and pulmonary embolism

These complications can still occur despite prophylaxis (see Chapter 1). Presentation of DVT may be silent (60%) or as a clinical syndrome (40%). If suspected on clinical grounds (painful, tender and swollen calf), duplex ultrasonography is the investigation of choice, with a sensitivity and specificity greater than 90%. In cases of suspected pulmonary embolism, a CT pulmonary angiogram is the appropriate investigation.

The treatment of DVT has now moved from unfractionated heparin infusion to subcutaneous low-molecular-weight heparin. This is maintained until the patient is fully anticoagulated on warfarin and the latter is continued for 3–6 months to minimise the risk of further thrombosis and the development of complications (see Chapters 73 and 75). A caval filter might have to be considered, particularly for clot extending into the iliofemoral segments.

The treatment of a pulmonary embolus will depend on the severity of the event. A relatively minor episode, with no cardiovascular compromise, can be managed with heparinisation, whereas a more serious embolus may need surgical intervention (embolectomy) or use of a fibrinolytic agent.

Oliguria

Oliguria is a common problem in the postoperative period and is usually due to a failure by the attending medical staff to appreciate the volume of fluid lost by the patient during the surgical procedure and in the immediate postoperative period. For example, the development of an ileus will lead to a large volume of fluid being sequestered in the gut and this 'loss' not being immediately evident. Before the apparent oliguria is put down to diminished output of urine, it is important to ensure that the patient is not in urinary retention. Such an assessment can be difficult in a patient who has just undergone an abdominal procedure. If there is any doubt, a urinary catheter must be inserted. Alternately, most wards are now equipped with ultrasonographic devices capable of providing an accurate estimation of the bladder content.

Diminished output of urine may be due to:
- poor renal perfusion (pre-renal failure due to hypovolaemia and/or pump failure)
- renal failure (acute tubular necrosis)
- renal tract obstruction (post-renal failure).

In the assessment of a patient with poor urine output (<30 mL/h), these three possible causes must be considered. Major surgery with large intraoperative fluid loss and periods of hypotension during the procedure might suggest renal tissue damage (acute tubular necrosis), while severe peritonitis with large fluid shifts and no hypotension would be more in keeping with inadequate fluid replacement.

The treatment of oliguria depends on the cause. Pre-renal hypovolaemia is treated by fluid replacement, while poor output secondary to pump failure requires diuretic therapy and perhaps medications (e.g. inotropes, antiarrhythmics) to improve cardiac function. To give a hypovolaemic patient a diuretic in an attempt to improve urine output may be counterproductive and detrimental.

In acute renal failure the oliguria will not respond to a fluid challenge. Management demands accurate matching of input to output, monitoring of electrolytes and even dialysis.

In summary, most cases of postoperative oliguria are secondary to hypovolaemia, and should be considered due to hypovolaemia until proven otherwise.

Hyponatraemia

Any reduction in the sodium concentration in the ECF may be absolute or secondary to water retention. Loss of the major cation from the ECF leads to a shift of water into the ICF. Any clinical manifestation will reflect the expansion of the ICF (e.g. confusion, cramps, and coma secondary to cerebral oedema) or the contraction of the ECF in absolute hyponatraemia (e.g. postural hypotension, loss of skin turgor).

Hyponatraemia due to a total body deficiency of sodium ions is an unusual scenario in the postoperative surgical patient. Any hyponatraemia that occurs tends to be due to dilution and is caused by the administration of an excessive amount of water. While this is a fairly frequent biochemical finding, it rarely leads to any clinically significant problem.

Any hyponatraemia secondary to dilution may also occur with inappropriate ADH secretion. The trauma of major surgery will produce an increase in ADH secretion and intravenous fluid must be administered judiciously in the immediate postoperative period. A safe rule of thumb is to restrict the patient to 2 L per day of maintenance fluid until a diuresis has been established. Hyponatraemia can usually be corrected by the administration of the appropriate requirements of isotonic saline. If the patient has a severe hyponatraemia and associated mental changes, an infusion of hypertonic sodium solution may be required.

Hypernatraemia

Hypernatraemia in the postoperative patient is a less common problem than hyponatraemia. Any hypernatraemia is usually relative rather than absolute and occurs secondary to diminished water intake. Patients with severe burns or high fever may also develop hypernatraemia. An increase in the plasma sodium concentration will lead to a loss of ECF volume and relative intracellular desiccation. The first clinical manifestation is thirst and if the hypernatraemia is allowed to persist, neurological problems (e.g. confusion, convulsions, coma) may ensue. Treatment is by administration of water by mouth or intravenous 5% dextrose.

Hyperkalaemia

With normal renal function, severe and life-threatening hyperkalaemia is rare. High concentrations of potassium in the ECF can be associated with cardiac rhythm disturbances and asystole. Hyperkalaemia may occur in severe trauma, sepsis and acidosis. Emergency treatment of arrhythmia-inducing hyperkalaemia consists of rapid infusion of a 1 L solution of 10% glucose with 25 units of soluble insulin. The insulin will help drive potassium into the cells and the glucose will help counteract the hypoglycaemic effect of the insulin. At the same time 20 mmol of calcium gluconate can be given to help stabilise cardiac membranes. If an arrhythmia has already developed, the calcium gluconate should be given before the dextrose and insulin. Sodium bicarbonate (20–50 mmol) can be given if the patient is acidotic. If the level of potassium is not too high, an ion-exchange resin (resonium) can be given. These resins can be administered by enema and they exchange potassium for calcium or sodium. Alternatively, the patient may be dialysed (peritoneal or haemodialysis). In the management of hyperkalaemia it is obviously as important to treat the cause as it is to treat the effect.

Hypokalaemia

Low levels of potassium in postoperative patients are common but hypokalaemia is rarely so severe as to produce muscle weakness, ileus or arrhythmias. Patients with large and continuous fluid loss from the gastrointestinal tract are prone to develop hypokalaemia. If potassium supplements are required they may be given either orally or intravenously. If by the latter route, the rate of infusion should not exceed 10 mmol/h. Faster rates may precipitate arrhythmias and should only be undertaken on a unit where the patient can be monitored for any ECG changes.

Haemorrhage

The management of haemorrhage in the postoperative period may be approached in several ways. In broad terms, bleeding may be classified as either localised or generalised. If the former, it may be classified as follows:
- primary (bleeding which occurs during the operation)
- reactionary (bleeding within the first 24 hours of the operation)
- secondary (bleeding occurring at 7–10 days after the operation).

If localised, the bleeding is usually related to the operative site and/or the wound. Occasionally, the bleeding may be at a point removed from both these areas, for example gastrointestinal haemorrhage from a stress-related gastric erosion. Bleeding from the wound site is usually indicative of a mechanical problem or local sepsis. Generalised bleeding may reflect a coagulation disorder and may be manifest by the oozing of fresh and unclotted blood from wound edges and with bleeding from sites of cannula insertion.

Most cases of reactionary (and primary) haemorrhage are from a poorly ligated vessel or one that has been missed, and are not secondary to any coagulation disorder. The bleeding point may go unnoticed during the operation if there is any hypotension, and makes itself known only when the patient's circulating volume and blood pressure have been restored to normal. The bleeding in secondary haemorrhage is due to erosion of a vessel from spreading infection. Secondary haemorrhage is most often seen when a heavily contaminated wound is closed primarily, and can usually be prevented by adopting the principle of delayed wound closure.

Postoperative haemorrhage can also be classified according to its clinical presentation. The most common forms are wound bleeding, concealed intraperitoneal bleeding, gastrointestinal haemorrhage and the diffused ooze of disordered haemostasis.

The approach to management will depend on the overall condition of the patient and the assessment of the type of bleed. A stable patient with a localised blood-soaked dressing will be managed differently from a hypotensive patient with 2 L of fresh blood in a chest drain, who in turn will be managed differently from a patient with a platelet count of 15×10^9/L and fresh blood oozing from all raw areas.

In the first case the tendency might be to apply another dressing in an attempt to achieve control by pressure. A more positive approach is to remove the dressing and inspect the wound. In most instances, a single bleeding point can be identified and controlled. In the next case, the patient has a major bleed and this is probably from a bleeding vessel within the operative site. Return to the operating room and formal re-exploration must be seriously considered. In the third case, the prime problem is an anticoagulation defect requiring urgent correction.

The diagnosis of postoperative haemorrhage is a clinical one, based on knowledge of the surgical procedure, the postoperative progress and an assessment of the patient's vital signs. The blood loss may not always be visible and could be concealed at the operative site or within the digestive tract. The treatment of postoperative haemorrhage depends on the severity of the bleed and the underlying cause. Hypovolaemia and circulatory failure will demand urgent fluid replacement and consideration of the likely cause and site of bleeding. Careful consideration must be given to control of localised haemorrhage and whether re-operation is warranted.

Vomiting

The causes of vomiting after surgery are many, and can be best determined by establishing the relationship between onset of vomiting and the time of the operation. The two most common causes of postoperative vomiting are drug-induced and gut atony.

Vomiting that occurs in the immediate postoperative period is usually drug related. If it is due to the effects of anaesthesia, vomiting will usually settle within 24 hours. Current anaesthetic techniques and modern anti-emetics have rendered nausea and vomiting a relatively minor postoperative problem for most patients.

Vomiting that occurs several days after operation may still be drug related, but in this instance is usually due to an opiate rather than an anaesthetic agent. Vomiting may be secondary to gut stasis, and this atony is usually self-limiting. If prolonged, a prokinetic agent can be effective.

If vomiting starts 7 days or so after abdominal surgery, a mechanical cause for the problem should be considered.

Further reading

Abeles A, Kwasnicki RM, Darzi A. Enhanced recovery after surgery: current research insights and future directions. *World J Gastrointest Surg* 2017;9:37–45.

Marcantonio ER. Delirium in hospitalized older adults. *N Engl J Med* 2017;377:1456–66.

MCQs

Select the single correct answer to each question. The correct answers can be found in the Answers section at the end of the book.

1 A previously well 56-year-old businessman is admitted with a perforated peptic ulcer and undergoes surgery and repair of the perforation. He is making a satisfactory recovery but 3 days after the operation becomes aggressive, shouting and demands to be let home. He is still requiring intravenous fluids for slow return of gut function. Which one of the following is the most likely explanation for his behaviour?
   a anxiety over work commitments
   b opiate toxicity
   c pneumonia
   d alcohol withdrawal
   e intravenous fluid overload

2 A 21-year-old man undergoes a laparoscopic appendicectomy for appendicitis. At operation, the dissection is difficult and the appendix is found to be perforated and 100 mL of purulent fluid aspirated from the abdominal cavity, after which a saline lavage is performed. The patient cannot void postoperatively and requires a urinary catheter for 24 hours. He is kept on intravenous antibiotics for 3 days and then discharged home on a 5-day course of oral antibiotics. Three days after discharge he goes to see his family doctor complaining of persistent diarrhoea. Which one of the following is the most likely diagnosis?
   a resolving paralytic ileus
   b prostatitis
   c *Clostridium difficile* enteritis
   d leakage from the appendix stump
   e urinary tract infection

3 A 56-year-old man undergoes a laparoscopic cholecystectomy 2 days after being admitted with acute cholecystitis. At operation some acute inflammatory changes are found around the gallbladder, which makes the procedure more difficult than expected. A drain is placed in the gallbladder bed at the end of the operation. The following day the patient does not look well and is complaining of right upper quadrant pain. He has required regular morphine overnight to control his pain. His blood pressure is 120/70 mmHg, heart rate 110 beats/min and temperature is 38.2°C. He has passed 100 mL of urine since the operation. On pulmonary auscultation there are bibasal crackles and there is guarding in the right upper quadrant. Nothing has come out of the drain. Which one of the following would be the most likely explanation for his current problem?
   a aspiration pneumonia
   b acute retention of urine
   c bile leak
   d duodenal perforation
   e pulmonary embolism

4 A 68-year-old man undergoes a semi-elective laparoscopic cholecystectomy for acute cholecystitis. The procedure is uncomplicated. Twelve hours later his blood pressure is 114/72 mmHg and his urine output since operation has been 90 mL. He has intravenous isotonic saline running at 80 mL/h. Which one of the following is the most appropriate next step in management?
   a continue current management
   b intravenous frusemide
   c infusion of dopamine
   d infusion of noradrenaline
   e 1 L isotonic saline over 4 hours

5 Surgical techniques

Benjamin N.J. Thomson[1] and David M.A. Francis[2]

[1] University of Melbourne, Royal Melbourne Hospital Department of Surgery and Department of General Surgery Specialties, Royal Melbourne Hospital, Melbourne, Victoria, Australia
[2] Department of Urology, Royal Children's Hospital, Melbourne, Australia and Department of Surgery, Tribhuvan University Teaching Hospital, Kathmandu, Nepal

Introduction

This chapter reviews techniques used in surgical practice and invasive procedures.

The operating room (see also Chapter 12)

The operating room is a dedicated area for surgical procedures and must be conducive to performing surgery to the highest standards of safety for patients and staff. The principal purpose of such a dedicated area is to reduce the risk of infection of patients. The operating room must be large enough for complex procedures to be undertaken, for storage of appropriate equipment, movement of staff, as well as the maintenance of a sterile area around the operative field. By changing the operating room air 20–25 times each hour at positive pressure relative to outside the room, low concentrations of airborne bacteria and particulate matter can be maintained. The number of people in the room and their movement should be minimised. Ambience within the operating theatre should be calm and professional, and procedures should be performed in a manner that is respectful to the patient and to all the staff involved. The air temperature should be such that inadvertent patient hypothermia does not occur. The operative field must be well illuminated; surgeons sometimes wear a head light for procedures in body cavities that cannot be illuminated easily by standard operating room lights.

The surgeon's assistant has the important role of assisting and supporting the surgeon in the smooth conduct of operations. It is important to concentrate on the task at hand, to carry out the surgeon's instructions with speed and accuracy, to have a sense of anticipation, and to notify the surgeon of any potential problem during the operation.

A face mask, which covers the nose and mouth, prevents droplet spread of secretions and bacteria, is worn for any invasive procedure and is changed after each case. Eye protection in the form of plain plastic glasses or a visor attached to the face mask must be worn to protect against droplet spray of infected body fluids. Gloves are worn if there is a possibility of coming into contact with patients' body fluids. Clean theatre attire, dedicated theatre shoes and a disposable hair cover are worn while in the operating suite.

Aseptic techniques

Joseph Lister, in 1865, first demonstrated the reduction in surgical site infections with disinfection techniques. Aseptic techniques are clinical practices that aim to prevent infection occurring in the patient as a result of the surgical procedure by:
- preparation and cleaning the patient's skin with antiseptic fluid before it is incised or punctured
- use of sterilised instruments, equipment or surgical materials which might come into contact with the operative field and surgical wound.

Personnel involved directly in the operative procedure (surgeon, surgical assistant and 'scrub' nurse) wash their hands and forearms with antiseptic soap for 5 minutes before the first operation of the day and for 3 minutes before each subsequent case to reduce skin flora. More recently, alcohol-based hand rubs have been developed that require application for 1 minute. Hands are dried with sterile towels, and a moisture-impermeable sterile gown is worn. One or two pairs of sterile gloves prevent transfer of bacteria from the surgeon's hands to the patient and also protect the surgeon from infected blood and body fluids from the patient.

After induction of anaesthesia, hair is removed from the operative site by shaving with a razor

Textbook of Surgery, Fourth Edition. Edited by Julian A. Smith, Andrew H. Kaye, Christopher Christophi and Wendy A. Brown.
© 2020 John Wiley & Sons Ltd. Published 2020 by John Wiley & Sons Ltd.

or electric clippers. The skin is cleansed with an antiseptic solution starting at the site where the incision will be made and working away from the area, so that approximately 10–20 cm of skin around the incision site is prepared. The patient is covered with sterile linen or impermeable drapes, leaving exposed only the cleansed area around the incision site, which may be covered by a sterile adhesive plastic drape.

Surgical antiseptics

The commonest source of bacterial contamination in the operating room is from the patient. Therefore, topical antiseptic agents are used to reduce the number of skin organisms prior to any skin incision or puncture, and include the following.

- Aqueous chlorhexidine (0.5%) is used to disinfect mucous membranes and parts of the body adjacent to structures which would be adversely affected by more stringent antiseptics (e.g. the skin around the eyes). Aqueous chlorhexidine is bactericidal and has low tissue toxicity.
- Cetrimide (2%) is bactericidal.
- Iodine-based antiseptics, such as povidone iodine 10% (Betadine) and alcoholic iodine solution, destroy a wide range of bacteria, especially staphylococci, by iodisation of microbial proteins.
- Alcohol-based (70%) antiseptics kill bacteria by evaporation.
- Chlorhexidine 2% can also be used in combination with 70% alcohol.

Sterility

Anything that comes into contact with the surgical wound must be sterile. The method of sterilisation depends on the item being sterilised (Box 5.1).

Universal precautions

The risk of transmission of infectious agents from patients to staff (and vice versa) is reduced by practising universal precautions. Thus, it is assumed that all patients harbour potentially dangerous pathogens (e.g. hepatitis C, HIV) no matter how innocuous they appear, because carrier status cannot definitely be excluded without repeated, expensive and time-consuming investigations. The principle of universal precautions is to establish a physical barrier between the patient and the carer to prevent direct contact with any potentially infected body fluid or tissue in either direction (Box 5.2).

Hazards

In addition to infection, there are many potential sources of hazard in the operating environment.

Box 5.1 Methods of sterilisation

Autoclave
Uses superheated steam at high pressure to reach a temperature of 121°C. Sterilisation is achieved when droplets of superheated water evaporate immediately upon reduction of pressure, thereby destroying microorganisms and leaving instruments dry. Most surgical instruments and linen drapes are sterilised by autoclaving.

Dry heat
Items which tolerate heat but not moisture can be sterilised by dry heat, but it is less efficient and takes longer than autoclaving.

Ethylene oxide gas
Takes several hours and is used for heat-sensitive items such as endoscopes, electrical and optical equipment and some plastics.

Glutaraldehyde
A 2% solution is used to sterilise equipment that can tolerate moisture but not heat, such as urological catheters, plastics and rubber.

Ionising radiation
Uses gamma rays and is particularly useful for sterilising single use disposables such as plastics, dressings, scalpel blades and synthetic conduits.

Hazards, other than those intrinsic to the anaesthetic and surgical operation, are organisational or related to operating room equipment or the transfer and positioning of the patient on the operating table.

Organisational hazards

Organisational hazards should be entirely preventable. A full history and examination of the patient must be made before surgery, including the past medical history, drug history and allergies, so that elementary errors are not made (e.g. unwittingly operating on a patient with a pacemaker or who is anticoagulated, or prescribing a drug to which the patient is allergic). Before surgery commences, the reason for and nature of the operation, together with its potential common and serious complications, and the reasonable expectations from the procedure, are discussed with the patient and family who are free to ask any questions. A consent or request for treatment form, which states the nature of the operation and the side on which the operation is to be performed if the operation is a unilateral procedure, is signed by the patient and the surgeon or deputy.

Once in the operating suite, a check is made to confirm that all the necessary safeguards have been

Box 5.2 Universal precautions

Barrier protection
Appropriate protective barriers are used during invasive procedures and handling contaminated materials: gloves, face mask, eye shield, impermeable gown, shoe covers, hair cover.

Minimising potential exposure
Decrease the risk of spreading potentially infected body fluids by avoiding spillages, careful disposal of materials and equipment contaminated by body fluids, having only essential personnel present during invasive procedures, excluding personnel with open wounds or abrasions, using impermeable dressings to cover wounds, and using closed rather than open drains.

Elimination of needlestick injuries
Do not handle uncapped needles, never re-sheath used needles, and never remove a used needle from a syringe. Use needles as little as possible. Immediately dispose of used needles in a designated 'sharps' disposal container which has a one-way opening.

Elimination of other penetrating injuries
Sharp objects (e.g. scalpels, needles) are transferred between operating personnel in a 'sharps dish', not from hand to hand. Hand-held needles are not used. Blunt suture needles are used where possible. Sharp instruments are not placed on the operative field or anywhere on the patient. Alert personnel to the presence of any sharp object in the operative field.

performed for the patient. The World Health Organization surgical safety checklist or variations are now mandatory in most Australian hospitals. The checklist can be used at three stages: before the induction of anaesthesia ('sign in'), before the incision of the skin ('time out') and before the patient leaves the theatre ('sign out'). The varied processes in each hospital include checklists that ensure the correct patient is having the correct procedure, the correct site or side of the operation has been marked, that relevant equipment is available and that the relevant imaging and clinical notes are available. At the start of each theatre list the 'time out' for the first patients also includes an introduction of all present in the theatre. Discussion of all anticipated surgical and anaesthetic concerns are also discussed along with plans for prevention of deep venous thrombosis during and after theatre.

Equipment

Diathermy is used universally in surgical practice. High-frequency alternating current passes from a small point of contact (active electrode) through the patient to a large contact site (indifferent electrode or 'diathermy plate') to produce localised heat which coagulates protein. Diathermy produces (i) coagulation (haemostasis with a small amount of adjacent tissue damage), (ii) cutting (tissue cutting with minimal tissue damage), or (iii) fulguration (haemostasis with considerable tissue necrosis). Potential dangers include electrocution, inadvertent burn to the patient at a remote site and to the surgeon, fire associated with pooled alcohol-based antiseptics, explosion of flammable anaesthetic gases, and interference with the function of cardiac pacemakers.

A variety of lasers with different wavelengths and effects on cells and tissues are used in surgical practice for highly accurate tissue destruction (e.g. mucosal surgery, CNS tumours, dermatological lesions, aerodigestive tumours), coagulating blood vessels (e.g. gastrointestinal tract, retinal photocoagulation), and for photoactivation of intra-tumour haematoporphyrin for malignant tumour destruction (photodynamic therapy). Hazards include eye damage, explosion of anaesthetic gases, and shattering and destruction of other equipment.

Limb tourniquets are used to provide a bloodless field in which to operate. The limb is elevated and exsanguinated by a rubber bandage or compressive sleeve, and the proximal tourniquet inflated to 50 mmHg (upper limb) or 100 mmHg (lower limb) above systolic blood pressure. A tourniquet should not be kept inflated for more than 60–90 minutes. A record should be kept during the operation of how long the tourniquet has been inflated. Tourniquet complications include arterial thrombosis, distal ischaemia, nerve compression and skin traction.

Positioning of the patient

The patient is positioned on the operating table in such a way that the procedure is facilitated and the airway can be protected. Pressure points are padded, and limbs are positioned so that peripheral nerves, major blood vessels, joints and ligaments are not stretched or compressed. The anaesthetised patient must be in a stable position on the operating table and may need to be strapped in position with broad adhesive tape. There must be no contact between the skin and any metallic surface because of the risk of diathermy burn and pressure necrosis. Sections of the operating table can be angled so that the patient is optimally positioned for the particular procedure (e.g. flexed while lying supine or on one side, head-down, head-up).

Endoscopy

Endoscopy is performed by inserting a fibre-optic telescope containing a light source and instrument channels into the gastrointestinal, respiratory and urinary tracts. The operator undertakes the procedure by manipulating the endoscope while viewing a video screen but occasionally the eyepiece of the instrument may be used.

Gastrointestinal endoscopy

Endoscopy of the gastrointestinal tract allows the endoscopist to view the lumen of the oesophagus, stomach and proximal half of the duodenum (oesophagogastroduodenoscopy or upper gastrointestinal endoscopy or gastroscopy), colon (colonoscopy), rectum and distal sigmoid colon (sigmoidoscopy), and distal rectum and anal canal (proctoscopy). It is usually performed under sedation. Intestinal endoscopy can also be performed at laparotomy (enteroscopy) by making a small incision in the intestine and passing the endoscope along the intestinal lumen. Procedures such as dilatation of strictures, biopsy and diathermy ablation of polyps, injection of adrenaline around bleeding gastric and duodenal ulcers, cholangiopancreatography, removal of common bile duct calculi, biliary dilatation or stenting, injection of haemorrhoids and tumour phototherapy can be performed using fibre-optic endoscopes.

Bronchoscopy

The upper airway, trachea and proximal bronchi can be inspected by bronchoscopy, which may be performed under local or general anaesthesia. Bronchoscopy is used for diagnosis (e.g. inspection and biopsy of lung tumours) or therapy (e.g. removal of foreign bodies, aspiration of secretions). Anaesthetists occasionally use the fibre-optic bronchoscope to facilitate difficult endotracheal intubation.

Urological endoscopy

The urethra (urethroscopy), bladder (cystoscopy) and ureters (ureteroscopy) can be inspected for diagnostic purposes. Extensive therapeutic procedures (e.g. resection of the prostate, diathermy and excision of bladder tumours, extraction of calculi) can be performed safely with far less morbidity than the equivalent open procedures.

Endoscopic surgery

There are two forms of endoscopic surgery that both involve the insertion of a microchip video camera with a light source into the lumen or through the wall of the aerodigestive tract into a body cavity. The latter is performed through an incision in the wall of the gastrointestinal tract with placement of specially crafted surgical instruments into a body cavity. For both techniques the surgeon undertakes the procedure by manipulating the instruments while viewing a video screen. Some forms of endoscopic surgery utilise endoscopic ultrasound for guidance of incisions or placement of internal drains. Examples of endoscopic surgical procedures include resections of larger gastrointestinal tumours (endoscopic mucosal resection), drainage of infected pancreatic collections into the stomach (endoscopic cystgastrostomy), oesophageal myotomy (per oral endoscopic myotomy or POEM), endoscopic sinus surgery and natural orifice transluminal endoscopic surgery (NOTES).

The advantages of endoscopic or 'closed' surgery are reduced postoperative pain and analgesic requirements, earlier discharge from hospital and earlier return to normal function. However, many surgical procedures either cannot be undertaken endoscopically because of their very nature, or cannot be completed endoscopically because of difficulty or patient safety, in which case the operation is converted to an 'open' procedure. Some procedures use endoscopic techniques to assist with the procedure and an incision is made to either complete the operation or deliver the resected specimen. The range of endoscopically performed operations in many surgical specialties has increased enormously over the last 20 years.

Open surgery

Open surgery is the traditional or conventional method of operating. In general terms, open surgery involves making a surgical wound, dissecting tissues to gain access to and mobilise the structure or organ of interest, completing the therapeutic procedure, ensuring haemostasis is complete, and then closing the wound with sutures. Open surgery is performed more with the hands and direct touch than endoscopic procedures, and fingers may be used for 'blunt' dissection. The surgical wound accounts for much of the morbidity of open surgery, particularly the cutting of muscle. The range of open operations is extremely wide, as evidenced by the procedures described throughout this book.

Minimally invasive surgery

Minimally invasive surgery avoids the larger incisions of open surgery to minimise morbidity. Different types of microchip video cameras can be used to visualise the required cavity or space within the body. The cameras vary in size and their complement of different angled lenses, which are either fixed or manoeuvrable. Magnification of the image often provides a superior view to that obtained at open surgery.

Abdominal surgery

Laparoscopy refers to the technique of insufflating the peritoneal cavity with gas, inserting a camera through most commonly a 10–15 mm subumbilical incision and inspecting the abdominal contents. Usually additional ports are inserted through 5–10 mm incisions in the abdominal wall and instruments (e.g. scissors, grasping devices, retractors, staplers, needle holders, energy devices) are introduced and manipulated by the surgeon to perform the operation. Procedures such as cholecystectomy, gastric fundoplication, hiatus hernia repair, division of adhesions, appendicectomy, splenectomy, adrenalectomy, nephrectomy, oophorectomy, tubal ligation, bariatric surgery and hernia repair can be undertaken laparoscopically with less morbidity than if undertaken as an open or conventional operation. Endoscopic surgery has allowed some procedures to be undertaken as day cases, whereas the same procedure performed as an open operation would require an inpatient stay of several days (e.g. cholecystectomy, hernia repair).

Thoracic surgery

Thorascopy involves inserting a camera with a light source and instruments into the thoracic cavity. The technique is used diagnostically and therapeutically for procedures such as drainage of the thoracic cavity (haemothorax, pleural effusion and empyema), lung biopsy, pleurodesis and excision of lung bullae. The mediastinum can be inspected and mediastinal lymph nodes can be biopsied by mediastinoscopy, which may prevent the need for an exploratory thoracotomy.

Orthopaedic surgery

Large joints (e.g. knee, hip, ankle, shoulder, wrist) can be inspected by arthroscopy. Therapeutic procedures include removal of bone chips, cartilage excision and removal, and ligament repair. Arthroscopic surgery has been enormously beneficial for orthopaedic patients and has allowed far more rapid return to function.

Robotic surgery

Robotic surgery is a form of minimally invasive surgery where the surgeon is positioned remote to the patient but usually within the operating theatre. A robotic system operated by the surgeon is used to control the camera as well as the instruments that are placed through multiple ports. A surgical assistant still makes the port site incisions and a theatre nurse is scrubbed to change to robotic instruments when required. The robot is particularly useful for work in cramped narrow spaces where robotic suturing is far superior to laparoscopic suturing techniques in such instances. The commonest example of robotic surgery is radical prostatectomy with the robotic reconstruction of the bladder and urethra in a narrow male pelvis. Other common examples include partial nephrectomy and thoracic surgery. However, nearly all abdominal, thoracic and some upper aerodigestive and cardiac operations have been described using robotic techniques. Recently, transaxillary breast, thyroid and parathyroid surgery have also been described.

Surgical methods

Surgical operations are performed by well worked out, standardised steps which progress in logical sequence. An operative plan is determined by the surgeon for every operation.

Surgical instruments

There are literally thousands of surgical instruments, some simple and others extremely complex, but each designed for a specific function. The surgical incision is made with a scalpel, which consists of a reusable handle and a disposable blade. Scissors are used to cut other tissues and sutures, and for blunt dissection with the blades closed. Diathermy is used for haemostasis and to cut through tissue layers beneath the skin. Tissues are held with dissecting or tissue-grasping forceps rather than the fingers. Hand-held forceps either have teeth for better grasping ability or are non-toothed for handling delicate tissues. Needle holders are used to hold needles for suturing and eliminate the need for hand-held needles, and are therefore safer. They have a ratchet so that the needle can be contained securely in the holder while not in the surgeon's hand. Retractors allow the surgeon to operate in an adequately exposed field. Self-retaining retractors keep the wound edges apart without the aid of an assistant. Retractors held by the assistant provide tissue retraction in awkward parts of the wound and in situations where retraction of specific tissues is required so that intricate parts of the operation can be performed. A sucker is used to aspirate blood and body fluids from the operative field and to remove smoke created by the diathermy. There are many instruments designed specifically for surgical specialties and procedures.

Incisions

Surgical incisions are made so that:
- the operation can be undertaken with adequate exposure of the area or structure of interest
- the procedure can be performed and completed safely and expeditiously
- the wound heals satisfactorily with a cosmetically acceptable scar.

Thus, incisions are to be of adequate but not excessive length and, if possible, placed in skin creases, particularly when operating on exposed areas of the body such as the face, neck and breast. Parallel skin incisions ('tram tracking') and V- or T-shaped incisions are avoided because of ischaemia of intervening tissue and pointed flaps.

Tissue dissection

Ideally, surgical dissection should be performed along tissue planes, which tend to be relatively avascular. The aim is to isolate (mobilise) the structure(s) of interest from surrounding connective tissue and other structures with the least amount of trauma and bleeding. Tissues should be handled with great care and respect and as little as possible. Dissection is undertaken by using a scalpel or scissor (sharp dissection), a finger, closed scissor, gauze pledget or scalpel handle (blunt dissection), or the diathermy. Gentle counter-traction on tissues by the assistant facilitates the dissection.

Haemostasis

Surgical haemostasis refers to stopping bleeding which occurs with transection of blood vessels. The majority of cases of operative and postoperative bleeding are due to inadequate surgical haemostasis rather than disorders of clotting and coagulation. Haemostasis is essential in order to prevent blood loss during surgery and haematoma formation postoperatively. Methods of surgical haemostasis include the following.
- Application of a haemostatic clamp to a blood vessel and then ligation with a surgical ligature.
- Suture ligation of a vessel: under-running a bleeding vessel with a figure-of-eight suture which is tied firmly.
- Application around a blood vessel of small metal U-shaped clips that are then squeezed closed.
- Diathermy coagulation.
- Localised pressure for several minutes to allow coagulation to occur naturally.
- Application of surgical materials (e.g. oxidised cellulose, Surgicel) which promote coagulation.
- Application of topical agents to promote vasoconstriction (e.g. adrenaline) or coagulation (e.g. thrombin).
- Packing of a bleeding cavity with gauze packs as a temporary measure until definitive haemostasis can be achieved.

Sutures and wound closure

Sutures have been used to close surgical wounds for thousands of years, and initially were made from human or animal hair, animal sinews and plant material. Today, a wide variety of material is available for suturing and ligating tissues (Box 5.3).

Sutures are selected for use according to the required function. For example, arteries are sutured together with non-absorbable polypropylene or polytetrafluoroethylene (PTFE) sutures, which are non-thrombogenic, cause virtually no tissue reaction and maintain their intrinsic strength indefinitely so that the anastomotic scar (which is under constant arterial pressure) does not stretch and become aneurysmal. Skin wounds, for example, are sutured with either non-absorbable sutures, which are removed after several days, or absorbable sutures hidden within the skin (subcuticular sutures) and which are not removed surgically but are absorbed after several weeks.

Sutures are available in diameters ranging from 0.02 to 0.50 mm. The minimum calibre of suture should be used, compatible with its function. Non-absorbable sutures are avoided for suturing the luminal aspects of the gastrointestinal and urinary tracts because substances within the contained fluids (e.g. bile, urine) may precipitate on persisting sutures and produce calculi.

Box 5.3 Sutures

Substance	Description*	Duration†	Trade name	Uses
Plain catgut	Nat, Multi, Ab	1–2 weeks	—	Subcutaneous fat
Chromic catgut	Nat, Multi, Ab	2–3 weeks	—	Subcutaneous fat, gastrointestinal and urinary tract anastomoses
Silk and linen	Nat, Multi, Non	Prolonged	—	Skin and cardiac sutures, ligatures
Stainless steel	Nat, Mono, Non	Prolonged	—	Sternum, skin and gastrointestinal staples, orthopaedic wire
Polyglycolic acid	Syn, Multi, Ab	3–4 weeks	Dexon	Gastrointestinal and urinary tracts, muscle, fascia, subcutaneous fat
Polyglactin	Syn, Multi, Ab	4–6 weeks	Vicryl	Gastrointestinal and urinary tracts, muscle, fascia, subcutaneous fat
Polypropylene	Syn, Mono, Non	Indefinite	Prolene	Ophthalmology, vascular sutures, abdominal closure, neurosurgery, fascia, skin
Polyamide	Syn, Mono, Non	Years	Nylon	Abdominal and skin closure, hernia repair
Polytetrafluoroethylene (PTFE)	Syn, Mono, Non	Indefinite	Gore-Tex	Vascular anastomoses, hernia repair

* Ab, absorbable; Mono, monofilament; Multi, multifilament; Nat, natural; Non, non-absorbable; Syn, synthetic.

† Time during which tensile strength is maintained.

The requirements of suture material are as follows.

- Tensile strength: the suture must be strong enough to hold tissues in apposition for as long as required.
- Durability: the suture must remain until either healing is advanced or indefinitely if the healed tissue is under constant pressure.
- Reactivity: tissue reaction (i.e. an inflammatory response) allows absorbable sutures to be removed by phagocytosis but results in chronic inflammation if non-absorbable sutures remain *in situ*.
- Handling characteristics: sutures must be easy to grasp, handle and tie.
- Knot security: sutures must be able to be tied effectively so that knots do not come undone or slip. Sutures are classified as follows.
- Absorbable or non-absorbable: the rate of absorption of absorbable sutures depends on their composition and their thickness. Disappearance of the suture occurs through inflammatory reaction, hydrolysis or enzymatic degradation.
- Synthetic or natural material: sutures of natural (animal) origin are being phased out of surgical practice because of the very minimal risk of disease transmission. A wide variety of synthetic suture materials are available.

- Monofilament or multifilament: monofilament sutures pass through tissues easily, are generally less reactive, and are more difficult to handle and knot securely. Multifilament sutures are braided or twisted thread, and are easier to handle and knot, but are more likely to harbour microorganisms within the suture.

Recently, cyanoacrylate adhesives ('superglue') have been used to seal small leaks in blood vessels and vascular suture lines, and for closure of small superficial skin wounds. The adhesive polymerises and hardens rapidly on contact with tissues.

Surgical knots

Knots are tied to ensure that ligatures and sutures remain in place and do not slip or unravel. The ability to tie a secure knot is a fundamental technique in surgery, and patients' lives literally depend on knot security (e.g. the knot in a ligature used to tie off an artery). Knot security depends on friction between the throws of the ligature material, the number of throws used to tie the knot, the strength of the ligature material and the tightness of the knot. Usually, multiple throws are used to secure the knot (e.g. two reef knots, one on the other).

Suturing

The technique of suturing depends on the tissue and wound being sutured. Sutures may be either continuous (e.g. subcuticular skin sutures, abdominal closure, vascular anastomosis) or interrupted (e.g. skin sutures, sternal wires). The function of sutures is to hold the adjacent edges of sutured tissues in apposition and to immobilise them in that position so that wound healing (i.e. neovascularisation, connective tissue ingrowth and collagen formation) is facilitated. It is essential that sutures are not tied so tightly that the tissues encompassed by them become ischaemic. Skin sutures may be supported by adhesive paper tapes.

Retention sutures (incorrectly referred to as *tension sutures*) are used to close abdominal incisions that are thought to be at increased risk of dehiscence, and are inserted to encompass a large amount of fascial tissue and are placed 3–5 cm apart. Retention sutures have now been replaced by techniques using lateral incisions of the abdominal wall, mesh reconstruction and negative pressure wound devices.

Within the last two decades, stainless steel staples have been used to close skin wounds and to perform gastrointestinal anastomoses. Staples are quicker to use than sutures, but are relatively expensive and produce a worse cosmetic result for skin closure than subcuticular absorbable sutures.

Suture removal

Sutures are removed as early as possible to minimise the risk of infection and scarring, so long as tissue healing is sufficiently advanced that the wound will not open when the sutures are removed. Sutures are therefore removed at different times, depending on tissue and general patient factors (Box 5.4). For example, sutures are left *in situ* for a longer time in patients who are immunosuppressed, malnourished, jaundiced or undergoing chemotherapy; in those who have renal failure; and in tissues judged to be relatively ischaemic, subject to increased stress and tension, and which have been irradiated.

Box 5.4 Timing of suture removal at various sites

Face	3–5 days
Neck (skin crease)	5–7 days
Scalp	7–10 days
Abdomen	10 days
Extremity	10–14 days
Amputation stump	21 days

Surgical drains

Drains are used widely in surgical practice to:
- Remove blood or serous fluid, which would otherwise accumulate in the operative area (e.g. wound drain)
- Provide a track or line of minimal resistance so that potentially harmful fluids can drain away from a particular site (e.g. drain placed into an intra-abdominal abscess cavity).

Several different methods of drainage may be used depending on the required function.
- Open drainage: a drain tube or strip of soft flexible latex rubber is placed so secretions or pus can drain along the track of the drain into gauze or other dressing covering the external end of the drain tube (e.g. drain placed in an abscess cavity, drain placed prophylactically near a bowel anastomosis in case of subsequent anastomotic leak).
- Closed drainage: a tube is placed into an area or viscus to drain fluid contents into a collecting bag so that there is no contamination of the drained area from outside the system (e.g. chest drain, urinary catheter, cholecystostomy drain).
- Closed suction drain: the drain tube is connected to a bottle at negative atmospheric pressure so that fluid is sucked out of the area (e.g. wound drain, drain under skin flaps).

It is important to note both the amount and the type of fluid that drains. Large volumes of fluid drainage may need to be replaced as intravenous fluids (e.g. duodenal fistula fluid). Depending on the particular situation, it may be necessary to culture drain fluid or send it for estimation of haemoglobin, creatinine, electrolytes, amylase or protein. A radiological contrast study may be performed along the drain tube, for example to estimate the size of a cavity being drained.

Drain tubes are removed when they are no longer required, for example when there is minimal fluid being drained, or when a cavity being drained has contracted and is small. Drains are removed simply by cutting the suture which anchors them to the skin and withdrawing the tube from the patient.

Venepuncture

Venepuncture involves removing blood from a superficial vein, usually in the antecubital fossa or dorsum of the hand, by inserting a needle attached to a syringe or collection tube at negative pressure (Vacutainer system). A venous tourniquet is applied around the arm, which is hung in a dependent position; the patient vigorously opens and closes the hand, and the vein is gently patted to encourage venous dilatation. The skin is cleansed with antiseptic and the needle is inserted through the skin into the dilated vein at an angle of 30–45°. Once the required volume is aspirated, the tourniquet is released, the needle withdrawn, the puncture site immediately covered with a cotton wool swab, and light pressure applied for 1–2 minutes. The site is covered with an adhesive dressing. Complications include bruising, haematoma and, rarely, infection and damage to deeper structures. Inadvertent needlestick injury to the venepuncturist is avoided by careful technique.

Intravenous cannulation

Intravenous (i.v.) cannulation is used commonly for administration of fluids and drugs. Superficial veins on the forearms and dorsum of the hands are used for i.v. cannulation. Antecubital fossa veins are best avoided for cannulation because the elbow has to be kept extended to avoid kinking of the cannula. Leg veins may have to be used in the absence of useable upper limb veins. Cannulas have a soft outer Teflon sheath attached to a hub, and a central hollow needle attached to a small chamber.

A suitable vein is identified as for venepuncture. Local anaesthetic cream is applied to the skin overlying the vein or local anaesthetic (1% lidocaine without adrenaline) is injected intradermally next to the vein after cleansing the skin with antiseptic. The cannula (needle and sheath) is inserted through the skin into the vein at an angle of 10–30°. The small chamber fills with blood when the needle is in the lumen of the vein. The cannula is then advanced into the vein. The needle is removed from the sheath and a closed three-way tap or i.v. giving set is joined to the hub of the sheath. The cannula is secured to the skin with adhesive tape.

Intravenous infusion is painful when the infusate is cold or contains irritants (e.g. potassium, calcium, drugs of low or high pH), or if the cannula pierces the vein wall and fluid extravasates subcutaneously. Thrombophlebitis develops at the insertion site after about 3 days, and i.v. cannulas should be re-sited if infusions are required for longer periods.

Central venous catheterisation

Percutaneous catheterisation of a central vein is used for:
- Short- or long-term venous access when peripheral veins are unsuitable or cannot be used (e.g. prolonged fluid infusion, total parenteral nutrition, ultrafiltration, haemodialysis, plasma exchange, chemotherapy)
- Short-term monitoring of central venous pressure. A central venous catheter (CVC) may be inserted into the internal or external jugular vein or the subclavian vein. Temporary CVCs are made of semi-rigid Teflon, are approximately 25 cm in length and, depending on their function, are between 1 and 4 mm in diameter and have one, two or three lumens. Long-term CVCs are made of barium-impregnated silastic and are quite flexible. They have a Dacron cuff bonded to the part of the catheter which lies subcutaneously and becomes incorporated by fibrous tissue after several weeks so that organisms cannot track along the catheter from the skin into the circulation.

Some long-term single-lumen CVCs are available with a small-volume chamber attached to the extravenous end of the catheter (Portacath, Infusaport). The catheter and chamber are implanted subcutaneously after the vein is catheterised and can be accessed for chemotherapy or blood sampling by inserting a needle into it through the skin.

CVC insertion is best performed in an operating theatre, under local or general anaesthesia, and with ultrasound localisation of the central vein. The patient is placed in a supine, slightly head-down position, and the surface anatomy of the vein is marked. Aseptic technique is essential. A hollow wide-bore needle is inserted into the vein, a guidewire is passed down the needle and the needle is removed. The guidewire position is checked radiologically. A plastic dilator is passed over the guidewire to dilate a track for the catheter and is then removed, and the CVC is passed over the guidewire which is removed after the CVC is in place. A chest X-ray is performed to check the final position of the CVC and also to ensure that a pneumothorax or haemothorax has not occurred due to inadvertent puncture of the pleura or lung. The catheter is sutured to the skin to prevent dislodgement and the exit site is dressed with an adhesive dressing.

Peripherally inserted central catheters are now placed under radiological guidance for the majority of patients who require long-term venous access for parenteral nutrition or antibiotics, or for those patients with difficult peripheral venous access.

Further reading

Cochran A, Braga R (eds) *Introduction to the Operating Room*. New York: McGraw-Hill, 2017.
Keen G, Farndon JR (eds) *Operative Surgery and Management*, 3rd edn. Oxford: Butterworth-Heinemann, 1994.

MCQs

Select the single correct answer to each question. The correct answers can be found in the Answers section at the end of the book.

1 Universal precautions:
   a protect operating theatre staff from electric shocks
   b prevent polluted air from entering the operating theatre
   c impose a physical barrier between patients and carers
   d are only to be used when operating on patients
   e protect only against bacterial pathogens

2 Laparoscopic surgery:
   a has a very limited role in general surgical practice
   b is inherently unsafe because the surgeon cannot touch the structures being operated on
   c is associated with greater postoperative pain and immobility
   d enables cholecystectomy to be performed as day-case surgery in some patients
   e can only be used for part of an operation

3 Sutures:
   a should be left in the skin for a minimum of 1 week
   b often need to be removed with local anaesthetic
   c must be tied tightly so that arterial inflow into tissues is not possible
   d made of Prolene will dissolve
   e of all types must eventually be removed

4 Surgical drains:
   a are removed when they are no longer necessary
   b should always be removed the day after surgery
   c are removed under general anaesthesia
   d are not necessary with modern surgical techniques
   e are required after the majority of general surgery procedures

6 Management of surgical wounds

Rodney T. Judson

University of Melbourne and Royal Melbourne Hospital, Melbourne, Victoria, Australia

Introduction

Surgery entails gaining access to deeper body structures usually necessitating a surgical incision, which may be performed by a scalpel or the use of diathermy. The final step in the surgical procedure is closure of the surgical incision (wound). Rapid complication-free healing is anticipated. Unfortunately, infection of the wound, described as surgical site infection (SSI), remains the most common healthcare-associated infection among surgical patients. While advances have been achieved in infection control practices, operating room design, sterilisation techniques and appropriate use of antibiotics preoperatively and perioperatively, SSI remains a common cause of morbidity and even mortality. The development of an SSI increases hospital length of stay by approximately 7–8 days. SSIs account for up to 16% of healthcare infections, of which most are related to bowel surgery (10%) with fewer than 1% from orthopaedic procedures. Other wound complications that affect patient recovery include haematoma formation and development of seromas, both of which increase the likelihood of wound infection. An SSI is also a common precursor to wound dehiscence or separation, which if involving the full thickness of the wound may lead to evisceration of the abdominal contents requiring urgent surgical intervention. Minimisation of these complications is achieved by (i) preoperative minimisation of any patient factors that might impede wound healing; (ii) choosing the most appropriate wound closure technique, be that primary wound closure or a method of delayed closure; (iii) selection of a wound dressing that will protect and support the wound while removing excessive fluid exudate and potentially reducing seroma formation; and (iv) providing wound surveillance to detect and intervene if any signs of complications develop. To achieve this aim a careful preoperative assessment is made based on clinical history and examination supported by special tests as indicated. Intraoperative assessment as to the health and perfusion of the wound edges and the extent of bacterial contamination informs decisions regarding the best wound closure technique. Decisions regarding the wound dressing are usually made based on whether the wound is closed and appears dry or whether the wound is to be left open. Postoperative care is centred on continuing to address those risks identified in the preoperative assessment that are likely to affect wound healing.

Preoperative assessment

A number of important factors affect wound healing and these should be assessed and corrected preoperatively if possible.
- Poor glycaemic control in diabetics is associated with a twofold increase in SSI.
- Smoking, with its effect on the cutaneous circulation, increases the likelihood of SSI.
- Obesity, with increased dead space in the wound, favours seroma formation and SSI.
- Malnutrition delays wound healing.
- Medications such as corticosteroids and immunosuppressive drugs increase infection risk.
- Systemic anticoagulants increase haematoma formation and subsequent SSI.
- Serious comorbidities, especially cardiorespiratory disease and decrease in oxygen saturation.

Steps should be taken to address any reversible adverse factors if possible. In emergency situations time may preclude any meaningful intervention, which is reflected in an increased risk of SSI following urgent surgery. Persistent risk factors need to be considered when deciding on the best method of wound management. Primary closure of wounds in the presence of adverse patient factors and bacterial contamination is associated with a high incidence of SSI, which delays healing and possibly results in severe systemic sepsis.

Classification of surgical wounds

Simple or complex

The commonest surgical wounds are linear incisions involving the skin, subcutaneous tissue and deeper fascial layers. These incisions are performed using a sharp scalpel to gain access to deeper structures which are the focus of the surgical procedure. Operations, especially for malignant disease, occasionally require excision of the skin and subcutaneous tissues overlying the tumour. These complex wounds may require complicated surgical techniques to achieve wound closure.

Clean

If the procedure is performed under sterile conditions and no contamination of the wound occurs, the wound is described as a clean incised wound. Such wounds have minimal bacterial contamination and under ideal circumstances would be expected to have a low SSI rate of 1–2%.

Clean contaminated

If the respiratory, alimentary, genital or urinary tracts are entered under surgically controlled conditions and without unusual contamination, the wound is classified as a clean contaminated wound. Such wounds would result from procedures including appendicectomy and cholecystectomy where no major break in technique was encountered. These wounds have a higher rate of SSI.

Contaminated

Operations involving gross spillage of intestinal contents or where major breaks in sterile technique have occurred are described as contaminated.

Dirty or infected

Wounds with signs of clinical infection such as neglected traumatic wounds or wounds in association with perforated viscera are described as dirty wounds.

Preoperative wound preparation

Skin care

Bathing or showering using soap the day before surgery is recommended. Preoperative bathing or showering using antiseptics has not shown any conclusive reduction in postoperative SSI. Preoperative hair removal such as shaving the day before surgery may increase infection risk due to colonisation of the resulting minor abrasions. If hair removal is deemed necessary, this should occur immediately prior to surgery.

Antibiotic prophylaxis

An important preoperative decision is the need for perioperative antibiotic coverage to reduce the likelihood of development of an SSI. This decision is based on an assessment of the potential wound, whether any prosthetic material is to be implanted at the time of surgery and the burden of patient risks factors.

The consensus of opinion is that a clean incised wound in a healthy patient performed in a well-vascularised area does not require antibiotic prophylaxis. For all other wounds, when prosthetic material is implanted and in patients with risk factors for SSI, preoperative antibiotics should be used.

For greatest effectiveness antibiotics should be administered parenterally approximately 1 hour prior to surgery to allow appropriate wound concentration of the antibiotic at the time of the incision.

The choice of antibiotic depends on the suspected or anticipated nature of bacterial contamination. Most hospitals have agreed antibiotic guidelines based on local known bacterial risks. If in doubt regarding antibiotic choice it is wise to seek the opinion of an infectious diseases clinician. For the majority of wounds a single dose of antibiotic is indicated, but in the presence of significant contamination or in lengthy operations a supplementary dose may be indicated. Prolonged prophylactic use of antibiotics has not been proven to reduce the risk of SSI and is associated with an increased risk of development of antibiotic-resistant bacteria.

Intraoperative management

Skin preparation

To minimise contamination of the wound from skin flora, an antiseptic skin preparation is used.

A solution of chlorhexidine in alcohol is more effective in reducing SSI than aqueous solutions. Care must be taken to prevent pooling of alcohol-containing skin preparations especially when diathermy is used to avoid ignition of the flammable solution. Alcoholic solutions should not be used around the eyes or in the external auditory canal to avoid corneal damage or the potential for the alcohol to affect the inner ear.

Choice of wound closure technique

The method of wound management is finally decided at the completion of the operation, taking into account the preoperative risk assessment, the conduct of the surgery and the patient's physiological state. The surgical choices are to manage the wound open, to partially close the wound or, as in most instances, to close all layers of the wound.

In a well patient with a clean or clean contaminated wound, primary wound closure is recommended. This is achieved by closure of any deeper layers of the wound such as the fibrofacial layer of the abdomen with a strong, usually slowly absorbed, non-irritant monofilament suture. In thin patients where no undermining of the wound edges has occurred, the subcutaneous layer does not require any suturing. The skin edges are then opposed accurately, avoiding any gaps using sutures or staples. Both techniques produce comparable results with no significant difference in SSI between continuous or interrupted suture techniques. In general, low tension sutures are more conducive to healing while excessive tension can produce pressure injury to the wound edge. Retention sutures in abdominal wall closure have not been found to prevent wound dehiscence or evisceration or lessen SSI or postoperative wound pain.

For wounds with significant contamination or in patients with major continuing risk factors for SSI, the surgeon may decide to close only the deeper layers of the wound, leaving the superficial layers open to allow free drainage of any inflammatory exudate. A subsequent wound management plan is developed postoperatively based on assessment of the state and progress of the wound. If no signs of infection appear to be developing, the edges of the wound appear healthy and exudation is minimal, delayed primary closure is usually performed. If the wound is slow to progress and separation of the edges occurs, the resulting unhealed wound may be suitable for split skin grafting. This is referred to as healing by tertiary intention.

In patients who are very unstable at the completion of surgery, particularly with abdominal operations, a decision may be made to leave the wound open using a vacuum dressing to control the resulting laparostomy. Patients are transferred to an intensive care unit for resuscitation, including vascular filling, correction of any metabolic or clotting abnormality and warming to normal temperature. The patient is subsequently returned to the operating theatre in 24–48 hours for closure of the wound.

Postoperative management

General patient care

To support wound healing the patient's general condition should be optimised. Adequate fluid resuscitation to maintain wound perfusion, ensuring oxygen saturation is above 95% if possible, avoiding hypothermia and providing nutritional support will ensure the best conditions for wound healing.

Local wound care

The care of the wound will depend on the chosen method of wound healing.

Wounds closed at the end of the operation with the expectation of healing by primary intention require a protective supportive dry dressing which only needs attention for the first few days if there are concerns about the possible onset of infection or if there is soiling or exudation visible. Wounds with well-opposed skin edges undergoing normal healing should achieve re-epithelialisation between the skin edges within 24–48 hours. While it is safe to allow showering once the wound is sealed, most patients prefer a protective dressing over the wound to minimise the chances of abrasion from clothing or inadvertent tension on the wound causing separation of the edges. For these reasons, dressings are usually left intact for 5–7 days, after which the wound may be left open. A number of waterproof dressing are available to allow normal showering during this healing phase. Closed wounds at greater risk of healing problems may benefit from the use of negative pressure wound therapy. These dressing are designed to stay on for 5–7 days. The potential benefits of these dressings are the removal of exudate, reduction in lateral wound tension and a decreased chance of seroma or haematoma formation. The use of these expensive dressing techniques is currently being investigated in randomised controlled trials.

Open surgical wounds require a dressing technique that controls wound discharge, minimises bacterial contamination, provides a moist wound environment and is comfortable for the patient. For small wounds hydroscopic gels covered by a semi-occlusive absorbent layer may be suitable. For larger open wounds negative pressure wound therapy has revolutionised patient and wound care. These devices are utilised until a healthy granulating wound base is achieved, following which skin grafting or vascularised flaps are contemplated to provide permanent epithelial cover.

Wound packing and the frequent use of hypochlorite-soaked dressings are becoming treatments of the past as rapid advances in dressing technology evolve. Chronic slow to heal wounds are best cared for by wound care specialists who possess the skills and understanding necessary to select the most appropriate management plan for these difficult and distressing clinical situations.

Wound follow-up

All surgical wounds should be reviewed in 7–10 days to ensure infection-free healing is occurring. Any signs of infection should prompt action, with antibiotic therapy for mild cellulitis or wound drainage if there are signs of suppuration (pus formation). In small wounds drainage may be accomplished, using an aseptic no-touch technique, by gently opening the wound using artery forceps at the site of swelling. Any fluid drained should be sent for microbiological testing to direct antibiotic therapy if indicated.

SSI surveillance should extend for 30 days for superficial incisional and deep incisional wounds; 90-day follow-up is recommended for surgery involving prostheses. Some deep SSIs may not be clinically apparent for many months or even years following surgery, for example the newly recognised slow-growing mycobacterial infections following surgery involving cardiopulmonary bypass.

Further reading

Harris CL, Kuhnke J, Haley J *et al. Best Practice Recommendations for the Prevention and Management of Surgical Wound Complications.* Canadian Association of Wound Care, 2018. Available at www. woundscanada.ca

MCQs

Select the single correct answer to each question. The correct answers can be found in the Answers section at the end of the book.

1 Regarding antibiotic wound prophylaxis:
   a broad-spectrum antibiotics should be used following wound closure until there are signs of epithelial closure
   b antibiotic prophylaxis must be used prior to closure of all wounds
   c antibiotic prophylaxis should be used when prosthetics are implanted at surgery
   d prophylactic antibiotics should be used for at least 48 hours
   e antibiotic wound prophylaxis should include coverage of anaerobic organisms

2 Which of the following factors has not been proven to delay wound healing?
   a uncontrolled diabetes
   b malnutrition
   c corticosteroids
   d anxiety
   e smoking

3 Wound infection is more common following:
   a the use of a continuous skin closure technique
   b primary closure of contaminated wounds
   c delayed closure of contaminated wounds
   d removal of the sterile wound dressing in less than 5 days
   e the use of sterile saline rather than antiseptic solutions for wound cleansing

7

Nutrition and the surgical patient

William R.G. Perry[1] and Andrew G. Hill[2]

[1] Department of Colorectal Surgery, Oxford University Hospitals NHS Foundation Trust, Oxford, UK
[2] University of Auckland and Middlemore Hospital, Auckland, New Zealand

Introduction

The last 10 years have been exciting times for surgeons. Along with advances in surgical techniques and perioperative care, there has been significant improvement in understanding nutrition and the nutritional management of surgical patients.

Such advances in nutrition have developed in parallel with a growing understanding of metabolic responses to injury and sepsis. This field has been energised by discoveries in molecular biology, including the role of proinflammatory and anti-inflammatory cytokines as biological response modifiers, the putative role of oxygen free radicals, and the identification of other mediators of the inflammatory response. Knowledge of metabolism and expertise in nutrition are now fundamental for all surgeons.

Nutrition features low in the body's homeostatic economy. Its priorities are oxygen delivery, regulation of acid–base balance and maintenance of fluid compartments. Threats to oxygen delivery are dealt with almost instantaneously by changes in minute ventilatory volume, alterations of cardiac output, and improved efficiency of oxygen uptake and extraction by tissues. Acid–base abnormalities take longer to adjust, with both acute buffering and chronic excretion mechanisms. Changes in extracellular and intracellular compartment volumes occur even more slowly.

The body's adjustments to malnutrition are slower still, because they are not immediately life-threatening. Nevertheless, these changes are profound and critical. Nutritional deprivation and inappropriate response to the deprived state are a major cause of morbidity and mortality in the surgical setting, particularly in the context of sepsis and injury.

This chapter explores this paradigm by reviewing body composition, nutritional requirements, malnutrition, response to stress and injury, and nutritional interventions.

Nutrition

Nutritional requirements

There are six components of adequate nutrition: protein, water, energy, electrolytes, minerals and vitamins (Table 7.1). The requirements for these different components vary according to the patient and the clinical condition. Daily energy requirements are approximately 25–30 kcal/kg. This energy is the result of the breakdown of carbohydrates, fats and proteins. Proteins are required for maintenance of normal cellular function and are an essential component of dietary intake. Daily recommended intake is 0.8 g/kg.

Proteins themselves are made up of smaller amino acid units held together by peptide bonds. Amino acids can be divided into essential and non-essential, the latter so-named because we are able to synthesise them ourselves. Correspondingly, we rely on dietary intake of essential amino acids.

Finally, several other elements are required for metabolism and growth. These include water-soluble vitamins (B and C), fat-soluble vitamins (A, D, E and K), and trace elements such as copper, iron, selenium and zinc.

Body composition

The energy stores and body composition of an average 40-year-old man weighing 73 kg are shown in Table 7.2. Of note, women have lower total body water, less muscle mass and higher total body fat. Composition also varies by ethnicity.

Fat can be hydrolysed to free fatty acids and glycerol, representing a high-energy source producing 9.4 kcal of energy per gram (Box 7.1). The body's

Textbook of Surgery, Fourth Edition. Edited by Julian A. Smith, Andrew H. Kaye, Christopher Christophi and Wendy A. Brown.
© 2020 John Wiley & Sons Ltd. Published 2020 by John Wiley & Sons Ltd.

Table 7.1 Nutrition requirements in 25–55 year olds.

Component	Requirement in health	Requirement after major surgery
Protein	1.0–1.5 g/kg	1.5–2.0 g/kg
Water	40 mL/kg	Variable per losses
Energy	40 kcal/kg	40 kcal/kg
Electrolytes	75 mmol sodium	Variable per losses
	15 mmol potassium	
Minerals	15 mEq calcium	Variable per losses
	40 mmol potassium	
	10 mEq magnesium	
Vitamins	B group, C, fat soluble	Additional vitamins may benefit during surgical illness

Table 7.2 Energy stores and body composition in a 40-year-old 73-kg man.

	Mass (kg)	Available energy (kcal)
Water	42	0
Fat	15	110 000
Protein	12	25 000
Glycogen	0.6	2 500
Minerals	3.4	0

Box 7.1 Energy availability

- **Fat** 9.3 kcal/g
- **Glucose** 4.1 kcal/g
- **Protein** 4.1 kcal/g

stores of carbohydrate are low and act as a rapid-response provider of glucose, particularly in stress situations. Of the body protein, 45% is structural and not available for metabolic interchange, while the remaining 55% is circulating proteins or contained in cells. If this protein is lost it leads to loss of function, including muscle weakness and immune deficiency. The ratio of the fat-free mass (total body weight minus fat) to total body water (fat-free body hydration) is remarkably constant in a healthy person, but varies markedly in the unwell patient.

Malnutrition

Malnutrition is the inability to match both metabolic and nutrient requirements. The European Society for Clinical Nutrition and Metabolism (ESPEN) has defined it as either (i) BMI below 18.5 kg/m^2 or (ii) weight loss over 10% (or 5% over 3 months) and reduced BMI (<20 kg/m^2 if <70 years old, <22 kg/m^2 if >70 years old) or a low fat-free mass index (FFMI, <15 kg/m^2 in females and

<17 kg/m^2 in males). Severe malnutrition can be defined as measured weight being greater than 20% less than 'well' weight. Approximately 5% of patients coming to surgery are severely malnourished, and malnutrition is present to varying degrees in up to 50% of patients who have undergone surgery.

Studies of malnourished children, particularly in the context of low- and middle-income countries, have recognised two broad syndromes of malnutrition that can be usefully transposed to the adult surgical setting. The first is marasmus, due to inadequate intake of an otherwise balanced diet (Table 7.3). In the adult this is commonly termed protein–energy malnutrition (PEM). Marasmus can result from anorexia, a decrease in appetite. However, depression, medications, dementia and illness are more common causes in hospitalised patients.

The second entity is kwashiorkor, which results from an inadequate as well as unbalanced diet containing relatively more calories than protein. There is characteristic fluid retention, which may mask the commonly seen and often rapid erosion of muscle and fat stores. In the adult patient, this is often seen with sepsis and after trauma.

It also useful to know of two further subsets of malnutrition, cachexia and sarcopenia. Cachexia is characterised by profound loss of adipose and skeletal muscle mass with associated haematological derangement and deconditioning. It usually results from an interplay of altered metabolism and inflammation. Common causes include metabolic disease, cancer, acquired immunodeficiency syndrome (AIDS) or end-stage organ disease states. Sarcopenia is the loss of muscle mass and quality and manifests as frailty. It is associated with decreased strength, and results from reductions in androgenic hormones, increasing resistance to insulin, decreased exercise and decreased protein intake that is seen with ageing.

Diseases also play an important role in malnutrition syndromes. Gastrointestinal disease can produce

Table 7.3 Comparisons between marasmus and kwashiorkor

	Marasmus	Kwashiorkor
Nutritional defect	Impaired delivery	Impaired utilisation
Protein catabolism	Compensated	Uncompensated
Aetiology	No food	Sepsis
	No appetite	Major trauma
	Gastrointestinal dysfunction	Burns
Metabolic rate	Normal or reduced	Increased
Prognosis if untreated	Months	Weeks
Principles of treatment	Replenish with standard nutrition	Resuscitate and support
	Use simplest available route	Control sepsis
	Treat underlying illnesses, if any	Provide non-standard nutritional regimens
Clinical course	Straightforward	Complicated

obstruction, malabsorption and fistulas resulting in gastrointestinal dysfunction. Inflammatory mediators associated with the inflammatory phlegmon may secondarily lead to PEM and worsen fluid and electrolyte disturbances. AIDS leads to severe cachexia, similar to that seen in cancer. This is probably mediated by cytokines such as tumour necrosis factor (TNF)-α and is complicated by chronic infection and malignancies. In cancer there is a rise in resting energy expenditure and the tumour avidly retains nitrogen as well as operating at a glucose-wasteful, high rate of anaerobic metabolism. Unlike the situation in experimental animal models, these tumour effects are unlikely to explain the degree of cachexia often seen in humans. Cancer-induced anorexia and host cytokine production are probably involved.

Response to stress and injury

In starvation, glycogen is initially broken down to produce glucose in order to maintain brain function. However, glycogen is rapidly exhausted and in marasmus the body undergoes an important change, over several days, to using ketone bodies (keto-adaptation) from fat as brain fuel. This adaptation preserves muscle protein.

In sepsis and trauma, however, this does not occur. Surgery, injury or infection induces a systemic inflammatory response – a complex interplay of proinflammatory and anti-inflammatory responses – and modification of immunological and non-immunological pathways. The metabolic response to systemic inflammation is shown in Figure 7.1. Glycogen, fat and protein are catabolised to increase glucose, free fatty acids and amino acids in the circulation that are integral to the immune response and phases of healing. As a result, there is a decrease of these substrates in the peripheries for maintenance of protein with a resultant loss in muscle mass, which ultimately impacts on functional recovery.

With severe sepsis and in burns, this protein catabolism is even more marked and energy expenditure massively increases, fuelled by intense free fatty acid oxidation. All the while, there is a

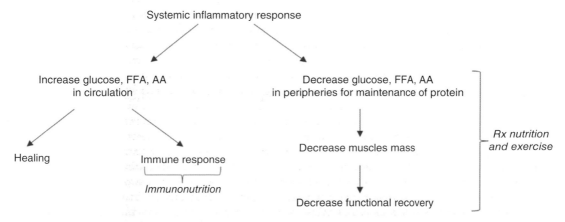

Fig. 7.1 Metabolic response to systemic inflammation. AA, amino acid; FFA, free fatty acid.

blunted systemic inflammatory response which can lead to hypothermia, leucopenia and impaired healing amongst other sequelae.

The body's response to surgery is now known to last well beyond the initial postoperative period. Within a few minutes of beginning an operation the level of counter-regulatory hormones (cortisol, glucagon and catecholamines) rises. In uncomplicated surgery these act only to initiate protein catabolism, as the endocrine response is relatively short-lived (lasting 24–48 hours). However, protein catabolism continues for up to 1 month after major surgery as a result of proinflammatory cytokines such as TNF-α, interleukin (IL)-1, IL-6 and IL-8. These probably act locally, at the site of injury, and indirectly (via the bloodstream and in the central nervous system). Imbalances between proinflammatory and anti-inflammatory cytokines also probably play a role in anorexia, pyrexia, fatigue and fat catabolism.

Consequences of injury and malnutrition

Malnutrition is associated with increased postoperative complications, mortality, increased length of stay and decreased quality of life. It is complicated by immune incompetence and decreased wound healing ability. Protein–energy metabolism may be accompanied by physiological changes such as poor muscle function, manifest as physical weakness and poor respiratory muscle function. Such changes increase postoperative complications such as pneumonia and prolong length of stay. Furthermore, oncological outcomes can also be compromised by poor perioperative nutrition.

Fatigue is a common concomitant of surgical illness and is characterised by prolonged mental and physical exhaustion. After surgery it is most pronounced at 1 week, and slowly improves for up to 3 months. It is worse in the elderly, in patients who were tired prior to surgery and in patients with cancer.

Nutritional assessment

Some 30% of all patients presenting to hospital are malnourished. It is thus important to screen patients to help predict outcomes and enable nutritional intervention. However, there is only one prospectively validated scoring system, the Nutritional Risk Screening (NRS-2002) (Figure 7.2), and no single clinical or laboratory test defines nutritional status (Box 7.2).

The aim of nutritional assessment is to define how much the patient has lost from his or her body stores of protein and fat and, as a corollary, how

> ### Box 7.2 Markers for nutritional assessment
>
> - **A**nthropometric measures: skinfold thickness (biceps, triceps, subscapular), BMI
> - **B**iochemical measures: albumin, lymphocyte count, skin recall antigens
> - **C**linical history
> - **D**ietary history

much remains. Most screening tools therefore address four main principles.

1 What is the patient's current condition? For example, what is their BMI?
2 Is their condition stable? Do they have more than 5% involuntary weight loss over 3 months?
3 Will the condition get worse? Have they recently reduced intake for example?
4 Will the disease process accelerate nutritional deterioration?

Nutritional assessment begins with a careful clinical evaluation. Important features of the history are weight loss greater than 5% during the past 3 months and a change in exercise tolerance. Physical examination may reveal non-healing wounds, oedema and fistulas.

Body composition is assessed by simple clinical tests and a standard blood test. Loss of body fat is often apparent from observations of the patient but is also assessed by palpating the triceps' and biceps' skinfolds. If the dermis can be felt between finger and thumb, then it is likely that the body mass is composed of less than 10% fat.

Protein stores are assessed by observation and palpation of the temporalis, deltoids, suprascapular and infrascapular muscles, the bellies of biceps and triceps and the interossei of the hands. If the tendons are palpable or the bony shoulder girdle is sharply outlined (tendon–bone test), then the patient is likely to have lost more than 30% of total body protein stores.

Plasma albumin levels are of assistance in determining the type of PEM. In kwashiorkor, the albumin may be low, reflecting the expansion of the extracellular fluid space, and this may manifest clinically as pitting oedema. It is a good prognostic indicator, with values less than 30 g/L associated with poorer surgical outcomes. However, it is a poor nutritional marker, since those suffering from starvation may in fact have a normal serum albumin. Furthermore, it is a negative acute-phase protein. As such, albumin values must be interpreted with caution.

Assessment of physiological function is of vital importance because weight loss without evidence

Part A: Initial screening

1. Is BMI <20.5?
2. Has patient lost weight within last 3 months?
3. Has patient had a reduced dietary intake in the last week?
4. Is the patient severely ill? (e.g. in intensive care)

If yes to any of these questions, proceed to Part B. If no, rescreen weekly.

Part B: Final screening

Impaired nutritional status		Severity of disease (= increase requirements)	
Absent **Score 0**	Normal nutritional status	Absent **Score 0**	Normal nutritional requirements
Mild **Score 1**	Wt loss >5% in 3 mths **or** food intake below 50-75% of normal requirement in preceding week	Mild **Score 1**	Hip fracture; Chronic patients, in particular with acute complications: cirrhosis, COPD *Chronic hemodialysis, diabetes, oncology*
Moderate **Score 2**	Wt loss >5% in 2 mths or BMI 18.5–20.5 & impaired general condition **or** food intake 25-60% of normal requirement in preceding week	Moderate **Score 2**	Major abdominal surgery; Stroke *Severe pneumonia, hematologic Malignancy*
Severe **Score 3**	Wt loss >5% in 1 mth (>15% in 3 mths) or BMI <18.5 & impaired general condition **or** food intake 0-25% of normal requirement in preceding week	Severe **Score 3**	Head injury; Bone marrow Transplantation *Intensive care patients (APACHE410).*
Score	+	Score	= **TOTAL SCORE**
Age	*If age >70 add 1 to give "Age-adjusted total score"*		

Score 3+: the patient is nutritionally at-risk and a nutritional care plan is initiated.

Score <3: weekly rescreening of the patient. If the patient e.g. is scheduled for a major operation, a preventive nutritional care plan is considered to avoid the associated risk status.

Diagnoses shown in italics are based on the prototypes for severity of disease:

Score=1: a patient with chronic disease, admitted to hospital due to complications. The patient is weak but out of bed regularly. Protein requirement is increased, but can be covered by oral diet or supplements in most cases.

Score=2: a patient confined to bed due to illness, e.g. following major abdominal surgery. Protein requirement is substantially increased, but can be covered, although artificial feeding is required in many cases.

Score=3: a patient in intensive care with assisted ventilation etc. Protein requirement is increased and cannot be covered even by artificial feeding. Protein breakdown and nitrogen loss can be significantly attenuated.

Fig. 7.2 Nutritional Risk Screening (NRS 2002). Source: Kondrup J, Allison SP, Elia M, Vellas B, Plauth M. ESPEN guidelines for nutrition screening. *Clin Nutr* 2003;22:415–21. Reproduced with permission of Elsevier.

of physiological abnormality is probably of limited consequence. Function is observed while performing a physical examination and then by watching the patient's activity on the ward. Grip strength is assessed, and respiratory muscle strength is assessed by asking the patient to blow hard holding a strip of paper 10 cm from the lips. Severe impairment is present when the paper fails to move.

Metabolic stress will be revealed by history and examination. It is present if the patient has had major surgery or trauma in the preceding week and where there is evidence of sepsis or ongoing inflammation, such as inflammatory bowel disease.

Determining the intensity and type of malnutrition is of great importance in setting nutritional goals. When PEM is severe and affects physiological function, postoperative complications are more common and postoperative stay is prolonged. The identification of metabolic stress is also important: because the extracellular water is expanded, the response to standard nutritional intervention is impaired and the type of malnutrition is predictable.

Perioperative nutrition

Patients often face prolonged preoperative fasting and oral restriction postoperatively. This paradigm has changed with greater understanding of anaesthetic risk profiles and postoperative metabolic requirements respectively. Patients are now encouraged to maintain solid intake up to 6 hours, and clear fluids up to 2 hours, preoperatively. Some surgeons encourage carbohydrate drinks in the preoperative period, although the evidence is mixed. It certainly does not increase the risk of aspiration, and may reduce anxiety and decrease length of stay for those undergoing major surgery.

Postoperatively, early oral nutrition is encouraged, and is a key component in enhanced recovery after surgery (ERAS) programs. ERAS involves a combination of interventions that aim to minimise stress and accelerate return to function. It includes preoperative and postoperative nutrition and fluid balance guidelines, perhaps the most important of which is early implementation of postoperative oral feeding rather than the once traditional 'gut rest'. It was initially developed for colorectal surgery but has now been promoted across several specialties. In fact, its nutritional principles have been adopted in non-operative patients as well. The guidelines for acute pancreatitis published by the International Association of Pancreatology (IAP) and the American Pancreatic Association (APA) include early oral feeding for mild pancreatitis and consideration of tube feeding within 48 hours in severe pancreatitis, a move away from what again used to be the more traditional nil-by-mouth approach.

Indications for nutritional intervention

The principles of nutritional intervention are summarised in Box 7.3. Nutritional intervention is indicated prior to surgery only in severely malnourished patients with physiological impairment. Nutritional support is required in patients who cannot eat, in whom intake is insufficient for their needs, in whom the gastrointestinal tract cannot be used and in those with accelerated losses (Box 7.4).

Enteral nutrition

In circumstances where the gut is functional, enteral nutrition should be preferentially used. Enteral nutrition may be important in maintaining gut barrier function, demonstrated to be of critical

---

> **Box 7.3 Principles of nutritional intervention**
>
> - Preoperative nutrition is indicated in severely malnourished patients.
> - Postoperative early tube feeding within 24 hours should be initiated in those where early oral nutrition cannot be started and in whom oral intake will be inadequate for more than 7 days.
> - Postoperative total parenteral nutrition is provided if a normal intake has not been established within 5–7 days for a depleted patient and 7–10 days for a normal patient.
> - When possible, enteral nutrition is preferred over parenteral nutrition.

> **Box 7.4 Indications for nutritional intervention in surgical patients**
>
> **Indications for preoperative nutrition**
> - Severe malnutrition with physiological impairment
>
> **Indications for total parenteral nutrition**
> - Gut is obstructed
> - Gut is short
> - Gut is fistulated
> - Gut is inflamed
> - Gut cannot cope
>
> **Indications for enteral nutrition**
> - Malnutrition with a functioning gut
> - Postoperative feeding

---

importance in laboratory models. Enteral nutrition is administered by mouth if possible (as high-energy nutritional supplements), but may also be delivered by a fine-bore feeding tube introduced under fluoroscopic control or using an endoscope. Fine tubes can also be placed into the jejunum at surgery and feeding can begin in the recovery room after the operation is complete. If prolonged enteral feeding is anticipated, a gastrostomy should be created, usually via the percutaneous endoscopic route.

Intravenous nutrition

Intravenous nutrition or total parenteral nutrition (TPN) is useful if the gut is obstructed, too short, fistulated, inflamed or simply cannot cope, such as in prolonged postoperative ileus. TPN formulations generally comprise 60–70% dextrose and 10–20% amino acids, with lipid emulsion, vitamins and minerals added as required. It is administered by a dedicated central venous catheter inserted under sterile conditions.

Approximately 50 kcal/kg body weight per day and 0.3 g/kg of nitrogen as amino acids per day is required to achieve gain in body protein. Use of nutritional intervention must be preceded by correction of anaemia, hypoalbuminaemia, fluid and electrolyte abnormalities, and deficits in trace metals. Vitamins must be dealt with by appropriate infusions so that administered nutrients will be used efficiently.

TPN is not without complications. Central venous catheter infection is potentially life-threatening and therefore care must be meticulous. Implementation of the Centers for Disease Control's Checklist for Prevention of Central Line Associated Blood Stream Infections (https://www.cdc.gov/hai/pdfs/bsi/checklist-for-CLABSI.pdf) has seen a significant reduction in infection rates worldwide. TPN has been associated with increased gastrointestinal bacterial translocation, a heightened proinflammatory state and increased pulmonary dysfunction. Overfeeding in particular can lead to respiration difficulties, and excess carbohydrate or fat can lead to fatty liver. Excess protein replacement can lead to elevations in blood urea nitrogen. Long-term TPN users can also suffer from osteoporosis, although the aetiology is unclear.

Immunonutrition

Immunonutrition is the supplementation of nutrients that are thought to impact both immune and inflammatory response to injury. These include arginine, omega-3 fatty acids and glutamine (Table 7.4). Studies investigating the utility of immunonutrition have varied in quality and indeed outcome. Consensus is still building, but it is likely that it may have a role in severely malnourished patients with severe trauma, sepsis, acute respiratory distress syndrome and head and neck cancers.

It should be given for approximately 7 days preoperatively and postoperatively.

Other adjuncts

Epidural anaesthesia blocks much of the early stress response to surgery and this has been postulated to be of critical importance in slowing protein loss. What may be of more importance is the mobility that epidural anaesthesia permits the surgical patient in the immediate postoperative period and the ability of the epidural block to limit postoperative ileus, at least partially due to an opiate-sparing ability.

Non-steroidal anti-inflammatory drugs (NSAIDs) may be important in preventing arachidonic acid-mediated tissue damage, as may nitric oxide inhibition and antioxidants in limiting free oxygen radical damage. These await further evaluation in clinically relevant models.

Minimal access surgical interventions have led, in many cases, to earlier recovery from surgery and faster return to work. When these techniques are combined with other modulators, the improvements in postoperative outcome are likely to be quite profound.

Conclusion

Short-term preoperative nutritional intervention in severely compromised patients decreases postoperative complications. The effect is not nearly as apparent in patients with mild to moderate malnutrition. Postoperative nutritional support is one of the most important developments in modern surgery and has allowed surgeons much greater leeway in the management of surgical complications such as fistulas and bowel obstruction.

Table 7.4 Components of immunonutrition.

	Biological function	Outcome
Arginine Conditional amino acid	Stimulates immune cells, precursor to nitric oxide which may improve microvascular perfusion	May decrease infection, reduce length of stay
Omega-3 fatty acids Polyunsaturated fatty acids, e.g. docosahexaenoic acid (DHA) and eicosapentaenoic acid (EPA)	Maintain cell membranes and modulate inflammatory response	Some evidence of decreased mortality, clinically safe
Glutamine Conditional amino acid, 70% of amino acid mobilised during stress response	Antioxidant, precursor to glutathione providing energy for enterocytes, component of protein synthesis	May decrease infection, reduce length of stay, improve quality of life, improve nitrogen balance, improve sugar control

Further reading

Gustafsson U, Scott M, Hubner M *et al*. Guidelines for perioperative care in elective colorectal surgery: enhanced recovery after surgery (ERAS) society recommendations: 2018. *World J Surg* 2019;43:659–95.

Kondrup J, Allison SP, Elia M, Vellas B, Plauth M. ESPEN guidelines for nutrition screening. *Clin Nutr* 2003;22: 415–21.

Weimann A, Brago M, Carli F *et al*. ESPEN guideline: clinical nutrition in surgery. *Clin Nutr* 2017;36:623–50.

MCQs

Select the single correct answer to each question. The correct answers can be found in the Answers section at the end of the book.

1 Marasmus is characterised by the following characteristics *except*:
   a inadequate intake of an otherwise balanced diet
   b cachexia in the adult
   c fluid retention
   d decreased metabolic rate
   e easy correction with standard nutrition

2 Nutritional markers include the following *except*:
   a skinfold thickness
   b mid-arm muscle circumference
   c total leucocyte count
   d serum albumin
   e skin recall antigens

3 The average requirement for intravenous nutrition per day is:
   a 20 kcal/kg body weight
   b 30 kcal/kg body weight
   c 40 kcal/kg body weight
   d 50 kcal/kg body weight
   e 60 kcal/kg body weight

4 What percentage of patients being admitted to hospital are malnourished?
   a 10%
   b 15%
   c 30%
   d 50%
   e 60%

5 Which of the following is *not* true?
   a perioperative nutrition is only indicated in severely malnourished patients
   b postoperative early tube feeding within 24 hours should be initiated in those where early oral nutrition cannot be started and in whom oral intake will be inadequate for more than 7 days
   c postoperative total parenteral nutrition is provided if a normal intake has not been established within 5–7 days for a depleted patient and 7–10 days for a normal patient
   d when possible, enteral nutrition is preferred over parenteral nutrition

8 Care of the critically ill patient

Jeffrey J. Presneill[1,2], Christopher MacIsaac[2] and John F. Cade[1,2]

[1] University of Melbourne, Melbourne, Victoria, Australia
[2] Intensive Care Unit, Royal Melbourne Hospital, Melbourne, Victoria, Australia

Introduction to critical illness

Intensive care for complex and potentially life-threatening critical illness is currently provided to about 150 000 patients annually across Australia and New Zealand. In Australia, at least 1.7% of acute hospital care episodes involved time in an intensive care unit (ICU), with the average ICU admission almost 4 days in duration, at an average daily cost approaching A$5000.

The concept of ICUs developed over 60 years ago, initially for prolonged mechanical ventilation support. Expanding demand for critical care services has led to there being over 200 ICUs in Australia and New Zealand, with many classified as level 3 or tertiary, meaning hospital facilities capable of supporting patients with complex multisystem organ dysfunction for an indefinite period using methods such as mechanical ventilation, extracorporeal renal support services and invasive cardiovascular monitoring. Such intensive care has permitted many patients to survive hitherto fatal illness or injury, with the interesting consequence that complex pathophysiological responses are now seen which could never have originally been adaptive, which could be helpful, harmful or neutral and which in turn have led to new therapeutic opportunities and challenges.

Overall slightly more than 90% of patients survive admission to ICU in Australia and New Zealand (Figure 8.1). However, an adverse post-ICU syndrome of prolonged physical, cognitive and mental health dysfunction is well described internationally in some survivors of critical illness and their caregivers. A substantial proportion of these declines may be explained by patient age and comorbidities prior to ICU admission rather than the episode of critical illness itself, and recent Australian data suggest ICU survivors experience a quality of life they find acceptable.

A wide variety of comorbidities may adversely influence the prognosis for recovery following critical illness, including ischaemic heart disease, diabetes, peripheral vascular disease, severe chronic obstructive airways disease or malignancy. In the absence of these comorbidities, selected patients of advanced age may benefit from short-term ICU admission. Reliable prediction of patient outcome would greatly assist patient selection, clinical management and resource allocation. Several regression model-based systems for critical illness mortality prediction are in common use internationally. Such models define average effects rather than individual variation, making them suitable for group comparisons but not as arbiters of individual patient care.

Causes of critical illness

The chief categories of causes of critical illness and thus admission to ICU are shown in Figure 8.1. Severe infection remains the most common and concerning problem in the care of seriously ill patients in hospitals worldwide. The rapid diagnosis of sepsis is an urgent medical priority, as early identification and appropriate immediate management in the initial hours after development of sepsis is likely to improve patient outcomes. Severe infection provides an important link between either underlying or complicating illness and serious conditions such as circulatory, respiratory and other organ dysfunction. Some common definitions of infection and related phenomena such as sepsis and septic shock are shown in Box 8.1. Clinically suspected sepsis occurs in approximately 1% of Australian hospital admissions, 10% of ICU admissions, and has a hospital mortality ranging from less than 5% (in the absence of comorbidities and older age) to 20%. Septic shock may have a mortality of approximately 40%, despite early antimicrobial

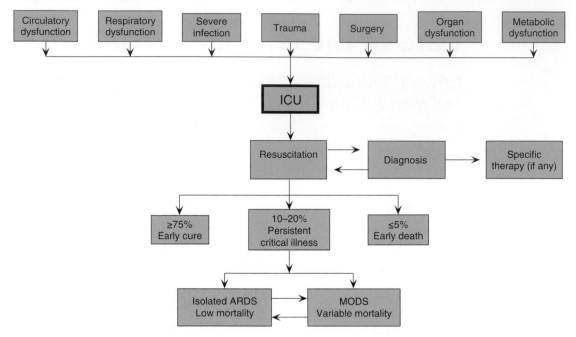

Fig. 8.1 Pathways of critical illness.

therapy and intensive life support; however, delayed recognition of sepsis and administration of relevant antibiotics may substantially worsen patient outcome. Survivors of severe sepsis commonly exhibit a complex post-sepsis immune dysfunction with both innate immune dysregulation and adaptive immune suppression featuring simultaneous inflammatory and anti-inflammatory responses that may persist to hospital discharge after clinical recovery.

An expanding global problem is the continually emerging antibiotic resistance of microorganisms, which challenges the success of the complex and invasive procedures that characterise modern hospital practice. The most commonly isolated organisms are *Staphylococcus aureus*, *Staphylococcus epidermidis*, *Streptococcus pneumoniae*, *Streptococcus pyogenes*, various enterococci, Gram-negative bacilli and *Candida* spp. When sepsis is suspected but the site remains unknown despite an appropriately thorough clinical investigation, potential sources include lungs, urinary tract, abdomen, skin or soft tissue, musculoskeletal system, central nervous system and intravascular devices.

The bodily responses to severe infection may be indistinguishable from those due to non-infective inflammation or indeed to severe injury itself. The systemic response to injury in general is referred to as the systemic inflammatory response syndrome (SIRS; Table 8.1). The definition of SIRS describes a widespread inflammatory response to a variety of clinical insults, not all of which

necessarily involve microbial infection. The constellation of clinical, haematological, and biochemical signs typically found in the presence of infection can often be observed at least transiently in the absence of any identifiable infection, as with pancreatitis, trauma, burns, rhabdomyolysis, necrotic tissue and cardiopulmonary bypass. Patients who are critically ill due to suspected sepsis or septic shock should receive empirical antimicrobial therapy as soon as possible, ideally once cultures of blood and urine samples have been obtained. Attempts are ongoing to develop specific and sensitive diagnostic tests for sepsis using biomarkers such as procalcitonin or numerous others that may improve on the current non-specific clinical signs and long-standing laboratory tools (e.g. white cell count, C-reactive protein) used to diagnose infection.

Over the last 10 years, multiple randomised trials have investigated therapeutic approaches used in the clinical support of patients with sepsis and septic shock. An initial report of improved survival with a protocol-based approach to sepsis management involving a 'bundle' of specified interventions termed early goal-directed therapy (EGDT) was not confirmed by a meta-analysis of individual patient data from three subsequent large multicentre trials testing the EGDT approach.

For those patients with sepsis who remain hypotensive despite adequate fluid resuscitation, two common choices of vasopressor agents used by

Box 8.1 Definitions relevant to the evaluation of sepsis

Infection
A microbial phenomenon characterised by an inflammatory response to the presence of microorganisms or the invasion of normally sterile host tissue by those organisms.

Bacteraemia
The presence of viable bacteria in the blood. Similarly, for other classes of microorganisms including fungi, viruses, parasites and protozoa.

Systemic inflammatory response syndrome (SIRS)
Consists of two or more of the following:
- temperature >38°C or <36°C
- heart rate >90 beats/min
- respiratory rate >20 breaths/min or $Paco_2$ <32 mmHg
- leucocyte count >12 × 10^9/L, <4 × 10^9/L, or >10% immature (band) forms.

Sepsis
Sepsis is life-threatening organ dysfunction caused by a dysregulated host response to infection. It is a syndrome of physiological, pathological and biochemical abnormalities induced by clinically diagnosed infection, where the absence of positive cultures does not exclude the diagnosis. Sepsis is a syndrome without, at present, a validated standard diagnostic test. Any unexplained organ dysfunction should thus raise the possibility of underlying infection. The clinical and biological phenotype of sepsis can be modified by pre-existing acute illness, long-standing comorbidities, medication and interventions. Specific infections may result in local organ dysfunction without generating a dysregulated systemic host response.

For clinical operationalisation, organ dysfunction can be represented by an increase in the sequential (sepsis-related) organ failure assessment (SOFA) score of 2 points or more.

SOFA score
The score summarises (range 0–24) organ system abnormalities, and accounts for clinical interventions. Laboratory variables, namely Pao_2, platelet count, creatinine and bilirubin, are needed for full completion. Organ dysfunction can be identified as an acute change in total SOFA score ≥2 points consequent to the infection. The baseline SOFA score can be assumed to be zero in patients not known to have pre-existing organ dysfunction.

Septic shock
Sepsis with persistent hypotension requiring vasopressors to maintain mean arterial blood pressure ≥65 mmHg and with a serum lactate level >2 mmol/L despite adequate volume resuscitation. Adequate volume resuscitation remains poorly defined. Many studies have specified an intravenous infusion of isotonic fluid, colloid or blood products to restore the effective circulating blood volume. Other studies nominate a volume of 500 mL. Patients who are receiving inotropic or vasopressor agents may not be hypotensive at the time that perfusion abnormalities are measured. Septic shock is a subset of sepsis in which underlying circulatory and cellular/metabolic abnormalities are sufficiently profound to substantially increase mortality.

These designations are based on 2016 international definitions that have deleted the previous term 'severe sepsis', meaning sepsis complicated by organ dysfunction (Singer *et al*. 2016). However, multiple older definitions and terminologies remain in widespread clinical use, including the systemic inflammatory response syndrome, severe sepsis, septic shock and various definitions of organ dysfunction/failure (Abraham *et al*. 2000; Kaukonen *et al*. 2014).

Abraham E, Matthay MA, Dinarello CA *et al*. Consensus conference definitions for sepsis, septic shock, acute lung injury, and acute respiratory distress syndrome: time for a reevaluation. *Crit Care Med* 2000;28:232–5.

Kaukonen KM, Bailey M, Suzuki S, Pilcher D, Bellomo R. Mortality related to severe sepsis and septic shock among critically ill patients in Australia and New Zealand, 2000–2012. *JAMA* 2014;311:1308–16.

Singer M, Deutschman CS, Seymour CW *et al*. The Third International Consensus Definitions for Sepsis and Septic Shock (Sepsis-3). *JAMA* 2016;315:801–10.

intravenous infusion to elevate arterial blood pressure are noradrenaline and vasopressin, which have similar efficacy and toxicity. Beyond appropriate antibiotics, fluid and vasopressor resuscitation and other critical care support, the role of adjunctive glucocorticoids in septic shock has been debated for several decades. In a recent large multicentre randomised trial, hydrocortisone by infusion at 200 mg/day did not influence the risk of death at 90 days (which was the trial primary outcome) overall or in six pre-specified subgroups. Faster resolution of shock, from a median of 4 to 3 days, was noted but this may have been a chance observation. In a separate multicentre trial, the addition of fludro-cortisone to hydrocortisone in severe septic shock was associated with some decrease in the risk of death at 90 days from 49% to 43%, with a relative risk of death in the hydrocortisone-plus-fludrocortisone group of 0.88 (95% confidence interval, 0.78–0.99). It remains to be determined if these contrasting trial results will change clinical practice with respect to adjunctive corticosteroid use in severe infection.

Resuscitation

There is a potential but unproven role for limited pre-hospital fluid administration with permissive hypotension in adult trauma patients with haemorrhagic shock during rapid transport to a suitable surgical facility for definitive haemostasis. In most other circumstances, conventional resuscitation aims to be prompt and complete, with restoration and maintenance of an adequate circulating blood volume (that is, treatment of hypovolaemia). This is a fundamental requirement in all seriously ill patients. Without adequate blood volume expansion, inotropes and other therapies are less likely to be effective and organ function is likely to be compromised. There is no universal ideal resuscitation fluid, although it is reasonable that replacement of losses should usually reflect the major deficit caused by the underlying disease process. Non-blood resuscitation fluids are broadly categorised into crystalloids and colloids. Crystalloids are further described as 'balanced' if their chemical composition, especially their chloride content, approximates extracellular fluid (e.g. Hartmann's, Ringer's and PlasmaLyte solutions). In global clinical practice, the most commonly used crystalloid has been the isotonic but 'unbalanced' 0.9% sodium chloride (so-called normal saline), with 200 million litres per year administered in the USA. However,

the use of 0.9% sodium chloride with its supra-physiological chloride content has been associated with the development of metabolic acidosis and also possibly acute kidney injury. In specific clinical circumstances (e.g. raised intracranial pressure) various hypertonic saline crystalloid solutions (e.g. 3%) are used without strong clinical evidence of improved patient-centred outcomes. Two recent large open label trials have reported a small advantage for balanced salt solutions (lactated Ringer's solution or PlasmaLyte A) compared with normal saline with respect to renal function in hospitalised non-critically ill patients, and also in critically ill patients where balanced crystalloid use was associated with fewer occurrences of a composite adverse outcome (death from any cause, new renal replacement therapy, or persistent renal dysfunction).

The prototypical colloid is human albumin solution (e.g. 4% albumin in saline). Associated with the elevated cost and potentially limited international availability of albumin solutions, several varieties of semi-synthetic colloids were developed, comprising most commonly a form of hydroxyethyl starch (HES), or succinylated gelatin, urea-linked gelatin–polygeline preparations and, least commonly, a dextran solution. While use of saline 0.9% compared with albumin 4% in saline 0.9% in a large randomised trial resulted in equivalent patient outcomes from critical illness, the overall ratio of the volume of albumin 4% to the volume of saline 0.9% administered was approximately 1 : 1.4 to achieve equivalent hemodynamic resuscitation end points, such as mean arterial pressure or heart rate. Potential disadvantages of semi-synthetic colloids compared to crystalloids have been reported. Use of 6% HES as compared with saline in ICU patients was associated with increased need for renal replacement therapy, while in ICU patients with severe sepsis HES was associated with increased mortality compared with the use of the balanced crystalloid Ringer's acetate.

The volume of acute fluid resuscitation required in critically ill patients may be a substantial number of litres. In addition to obvious losses and to anticipated third-space needs, there is often extra volume required due to vasodilatation, capillary leak and blood flow maldistribution. Fluid resuscitation is complete if blood flow is restored (that is, the haemodynamic goal) or if cardiac filling pressures are optimised, whichever is first. If a satisfactory haemodynamic goal has not been achieved despite suitable cardiac filling pressures and thus repair of hypovolaemia, inotrope therapy is required if myocardial contractility is impaired and/or vasopressor therapy is required if blood pressure is inadequate (e.g. in states of low systemic vascular resistance due to vasodilatation). In hyperdynamic vasodilated septic shock, hypotension has been treated for many years by infusion of agents from one or both of two major classes of vasopressors: (i) the sympathomimetic amines/catecholamines such as noradrenaline or (ii) vasopressin or its longer-acting analogue terlipressin. Very recently, a third class of natural vasopressor, angiotensin II, has emerged in preliminary clinical trials after difficulty in its manufacture were eventually solved. While adrenaline is the inotrope of choice specifically for anaphylactic shock, other agents may be used in shock due to myocardial impairment, such as dopamine, or dobutamine often with low-dose noradrenaline, with such choices guided by clinical practice rather than randomised evidence.

Organ dysfunction and severity of illness

Functional assessment of organ damage emphasises a continuum of progressively worsening organ dysfunction rather than an arbitrary dichotomy between normality and organ failure. Thus, the older term 'multiple organ failure' is often replaced by the broader term *multiple organ dysfunction syndrome* (MODS). Except for the acute respiratory distress syndrome (ARDS), which is the pulmonary manifestation of MODS and which has precise (though still arbitrary) definitions set by international consensus, MODS has no universally agreed set of definitions. These definitional difficulties arise primarily because of incomplete understanding of the complex interaction between inflammatory, genetic and potentially other influences underlying the development of MODS, which may be observed following a wide range of human injury, ranging from pancreatitis to severe trauma or most commonly in association with severe infection (septic shock). These complexities are further reflected in the observation that different individuals may have quite different responses to seemingly similar insults.

While criteria for individual organ dysfunction vary, overall patient mortality tends to increase with the number and severity of dysfunctional organ systems present. One widely accepted organ dysfunction score, used alone or in combination with other scores to predict ICU patient outcome within a research or quality assurance context, is the sequential organ failure assessment (SOFA) severity of illness score. This score assesses six organ systems: lungs, blood, liver, kidneys, brain and circulation. With organ system dysfunction values from 0 (normal) to 4 (high degree of dysfunction) based on the worst physiological disturbance in each 24 hours of a patient's admission, the total SOFA score ranges from 0 to 24. Emphasis has shifted in the latest international sepsis and septic shock definitions from SIRS to quantification of organ dysfunction using the SOFA score.

There are numerous other scores measuring the severity of illness, trauma or organ dysfunction that may be used in the study of critical illness or to benchmark ICU performance. Among those more commonly encountered are two versions of the Acute Physiology and Chronic Health Evaluation score (e.g. APACHE II and III), the related Simplified Acute Physiology Score (e.g. SAPS II) and more recently the Australian and New Zealand Risk of Death (ANZROD) model. As already mentioned, all these regression-based outcome prediction models return 'population average' estimates that do not substitute for informed clinical experience in the proper management of individual patients.

The current overall mortality of all patients admitted to ICU in Australia and New Zealand is 8–9%. While development of any substantial organ dysfunction, especially if multiple organ systems are involved (MODS), may increase the probability of ICU or hospital mortality, the incidence of MODS varies greatly with the patient group under consideration. In uncomplicated surgery, it is rare. In serious and complicated surgical conditions, such as trauma, haemorrhage or shock, it may occur in 20%. In uncontrolled sepsis, it may be substantially higher. For patients with organ dysfunction, the time to recovery has been arbitrarily categorised as uncomplicated (<4 days), intermediate (4–14 days) or complicated (>14 days).

The pathogenesis of MODS remains unclear, and several models have been proposed, such as excessive inflammation, a second-hit insult, or a complex disturbance of proinflammatory and anti-inflammatory pathways. Management of MODS continues to be entirely supportive. While available clinical care and resuscitation practices reduce but do not completely prevent its incidence in the patient groups at risk, there is evidence of a slow reduction over time in the mortality risk with MODS that may be related to overall improvements in resuscitation, surgery and critical care support. However, ICU patients who survive severe MODS may have reduced long-term survival compared with those ICU patients who manifest less severe MODS.

Management of the critically ill

The detailed management of the critically ill patient is the subject of a vast literature and of many substantial textbooks. While this management requires clinical experience, the general principles are straightforward, though their implementation can be complex, sophisticated and multidisciplinary.

- Resuscitation and maintenance of an optimal blood volume is just as much a continuing priority as it is an initial goal in the treatment of the critically ill. However, the optimal fluid status of individual patients may be difficult to quantify.
- Treatment of respiratory impairment, together with circulatory management, comprise the twin pillars of life support in ICU. Abnormalities of gas exchange and of pulmonary mechanics are common and are often severe. Specialised and sophisticated mechanical ventilation is the mainstay of respiratory support.
- After initial resuscitation, and while circulatory and respiratory support are in train, early diagnosis and specific therapy (if any) are required.
- Optimal intensive care aims to balance simultaneous resuscitation, appropriate diagnostic algorithms and the provision of definitive management.
- There is much emphasis on the early treatment of sepsis and on the prevention and treatment of complicating infections.
- Metabolic support is essential, because malnutrition may develop rapidly and is a covariable in mortality and because adequate nutrition is required for tissue repair. Enteral nutrition is preferred if technically feasible.
- Renal support may require renal replacement therapy (most commonly with continuous venovenous haemofiltration techniques).
- Psychosocial support is important for both the patient and the family. The patient requires analgesia, anxiolysis, comfort and dignity, and the family requires access, information and support. Humanity of care in ICU extends to end-of-life care in those patients with unsurvivable conditions.
- Intensive care requires continuous patient management by a skilled multidisciplinary team in a specialised environment. Attention to detail is necessary to identify problems and therapeutic opportunities as early as possible. In general, much of the care of the critically ill is founded on complex physiological support which buys time for healing to occur.

Further reading

Bersten AD, Handy J (eds) *Oh's Intensive Care Manual*, 8th edn. Elsevier, 2019.

Kelley MA. Predictive scoring systems in the intensive care unit. *UpToDate*. https://www.uptodate.com/contents/predictive-scoring-systems-in-the-intensive-care-unit (accessed 28 April 2018).

Marino PL. *Marino's The ICU Book*, 4th edn. Philadelphia: Wolters Kluwer Health, 2014.

MCQs

Select the single correct answer to each question. The correct answers can be found in the Answers section at the end of the book.

1 Treatment of critically ill patients in an intensive care unit:
  a increases the cost of care but does not improve the prognosis
  b is associated with an approximately 50% survival rate overall
  c is associated with approximately a 5–10% death rate overall
  d is required for 25% of all hospital patients at some point in their illness
  e is not indicated for any patient over 80 years of age

2 Infection in critical illness is:
  a almost always followed by dysfunction in multiple organ systems
  b only able to be diagnosed in the presence of septic shock
  c rarely associated with septic shock
  d rarely caused by common bacteria
  e often found in the lungs or abdomen

3 The sequential organ failure assessment (SOFA) score:
  a quantifies the overall amount of dysfunction across six organ systems
  b scores above zero nearly always imply the presence of invasive bacterial or fungal infection
  c rarely exceeds zero after cardiopulmonary bypass procedures
  d helps in the clinical differential diagnosis between infection types
  e is based on the worst physiological disturbance in each 8 hours of a patient's admission

4 Intravenous fluid resuscitation of hypotensive, hypovolaemic critically ill patients in hospital should be in most cases:
   a slow and gentle using only colloids
   b rapid and partial using crystalloids only
   c slow and complete using colloids only
   d rapid and complete using crystalloids or colloids or both
   e composed mostly of a solution of 4% albumin

5 Commonly applied critical care organ support involves all of the following *except*:
   a mechanical ventilation for hypercarbia
   b vasopressor infusions for low cardiac output states
   c hemodiafiltration for uraemia
   d platelet transfusion for thrombocytopenia
   e inotropic infusions for low cardiac output states

9 Surgical infection

Marcos V. Perini and Vijayaragavan Muralidharan

University of Melbourne and Austin Health, Melbourne, Victoria, Australia

Introduction

Surgical infection refers to infections that require surgical treatment or those occurring in the aftermath of surgery. They may occur *de novo* in healthy patients or as complications of surgical procedures (postoperative infections). Most postoperative infections do not require surgical intervention. However, it is important for the surgical team to be aware of the prevention, diagnosis and management of such infections after a surgical procedure. Surgical site infection (SSI) should always be considered high amongst the myriad of possible postoperative infections and active management instituted to reduce its morbidity.

Postoperative infections occur in up to 5% of the patients undergoing a surgical procedure. The incidence and severity depends on patient-related (host) risk factors and situational risk factors (surgeon, type of surgery). Some risk factors that cannot be avoided, such as immunosuppressed patients and contaminated emergency procedures, increase the risk of postoperative complications. Some medical conditions are associated with a high risk of postoperative infection. These include malnutrition, diabetes mellitus, obesity, chronic inflammation, previous irradiation, advanced age, steroid therapy, re-operations and coexisting infection remote to the surgical site. Awareness and prevention are the key factors in achieving optimum outcomes, particularly in elective operations.

General principles and detailed evidence-based guidelines for prevention of SSI, central line-associated bloodstream infection and ventilator-associated pneumonia have been published. Attention to detail in postoperative management, with strict adherence to hand hygiene and universal body fluid precautions and avoiding under- and over-resuscitation, central line insertion under suboptimal conditions, early removal of abdominal drains and use of prophylactic antibiotics, are important factors in reducing surgical infections.

Natural barriers to infection

The inflammatory and immune response to a break in the natural barriers in the body starts early after the insult. When natural barriers such as the epithelium of the skin, respiratory system, gastrointestinal tract and urinary system are breached, microorganisms are able to enter tissues locally and start the process of infection. In some circumstances bacteraemia may result in distal spread leading to infective endocarditis, abscesses in solid organs (liver, spleen) and osteomyelitis. The protection afforded against infections by the mechanical barrier (integument, mucosa) is supplemented by the immune system. Impairment of the immune system due to disease (diabetes, cancer, chronic illness), patient factors (advanced age, malnutrition) or direct suppression (chemotherapy, organ transplantation) leads to a blunted and delayed response to infection. This may also result in unusual clinical presentations and uncommon microbes, including infections by commensal organisms. Imbalance of one or more components of these defences may have substantial negative impact on resistance to infection.

The skin is the most extensive physical barrier in the body preventing infections. In addition to the mechanical barrier, local skin flora also play major a role in limiting the population of non-commensal microorganisms. The respiratory system has additional defensive mechanisms against sepsis. In the upper respiratory tract, respiratory mucus traps larger particles and microorganisms while smaller particles arriving in the lower respiratory tract are phagocytosed by pulmonary alveolar macrophages. Impairment of these mechanisms increases the risk of respiratory infections.

Textbook of Surgery, Fourth Edition. Edited by Julian A. Smith, Andrew H. Kaye, Christopher Christophi and Wendy A. Brown.

The pancreato-biliary ductal system, urogenital and distal respiratory tracts do not possess resident microflora in healthy individuals. Microorganisms may be present if these barriers are impaired by disease or if they are introduced from an external source. In contrast the gastrointestinal tract in a normal individual teems with microorganisms, especially in the colon. The highly acidic, low-motility environment of the stomach significantly reduces the concentration of microorganisms entering the stomach from the oropharynx during the initial phases of digestion. This explains the small number of microorganisms present in the gastric mucosa, amounting to approximately 10^2–10^3 colony-forming units (CFU)/mL. Patients receiving proton pump inhibitors have higher number of bacteria likely due to diminished gastric acidity. Microorganisms that are not destroyed in the stomach may proliferate in the small intestine, reaching up to 10^5–10^8 CFU/mL in the terminal ileum.

In the colon, due to its low-level oxygen status, there is a steady growth in the number of anaerobic microorganisms and approximately 10^{11}–10^{12} CFU/g are present in faeces. Large numbers of facultative and strict anaerobes (*Bacteroides* and other species) and several orders of magnitude fewer aerobic microbes (*Escherichia coli* and other Enterobacteriaceae, *Enterococcus* and *Candida* species) are present.

Pathogenesis of infection

When microorganisms enter a sterile environment in the host (e.g. subcutaneous tissue, peritoneal or pleural cavity), a non-specific general inflammatory response is activated by local immune cells (resident macrophages), complement (C) proteins and immunoglobulins (non-specific antibodies). Resident macrophages secrete a wide variety of cytokines that regulate the cellular components of immune response. Macrophage cytokine synthesis is upregulated and includes secretion of tumour necrosis factor (TNF)-α, interleukin (IL)-1, IL-6, IL-8 and interferon (IFN)-γ within the tissue. These are pro-inflammatory cytokines which cause vasodilatation, increased vascular permeability and oedema. These cytokines may sometimes initiate a cascade of inflammatory responses leading to widespread systemic effects described as systemic inflammatory response syndrome (SIRS). Simultaneously, a counter-regulatory response is initiated consisting of anti-inflammatory cytokines (IL-4 and IL-10) in an attempt to limit the extent of the response.

The interaction of microorganisms with the first-line host defences leads to microbial opsonisation (C1q, C3b), phagocytosis, and extracellular and intracellular microbial destruction. The classical and alternate complement pathways are activated both by direct contact with, and by IgM and IgG binding to, surface cell proteins. This releases a number of different complement protein fragments (C3a, C4a and C5a) that enhance vascular permeability. Bacterial cell wall components and a variety of enzymes expelled from leucocyte phagocytic vacuoles during phagocytosis act in this capacity as well.

The simultaneous release of substances chemotactic to polymorphonuclear leucocytes (PMNs) in the bloodstream takes place. These consist of C5a, microbial cell wall peptides containing N-formylmethionine, and macrophage cytokines such as IL-8. This process of host defence recruitment leads to further influx of inflammatory fluid and PMNs into the area of incipient infection, a process that begins within several minutes and may peak within hours or days. The magnitude of the response is related to several factors: (i) the initial number of microorganisms, (ii) the rate of microbial proliferation in relation to containment and killing by host defences, (iii) microbial virulence, and (iv) the potency of host defences.

The inflammatory and immune response leads to signs and symptoms that will depend on the amount of cytokine expression and the geographical area in which they are released (local tissue or bloodstream). Signs of local inflammation include pain (dolor), warmth (calor), redness (rubor) and swelling/oedema (tumor) which may progress locally to abscess formation or spread to cause a systemic response.

Sepsis is defined as the presence of at least two of four SIRS criteria in the setting of confirmed infection (Box 9.1). Severe sepsis is defined as sepsis resulting in tissue hypoperfusion or end-organ

---

Box 9.1 Systemic inflammatory response syndrome (SIRS)

An inflammatory response that may or may not be associated with infection. The presence of two or more of the following criteria, one of which must be abnormal temperature or leucocyte count, defines SIRS:

- Core temperature (measured by rectal, bladder, oral or central probe) >38.5°C or <36°C
- Tachycardia >90 beats/min
- Hyperventilation demonstrated by respiratory rate >20 breaths/min or $P\text{aco}_2$ <32 mm Hg
- White blood cell count >12 × 10^9/L, <4 × 10^9/L, or consisting of >10% immature forms (bands)

dysfunction. Septic shock is defined as sepsis with persistent hypotension despite adequate fluid resuscitation. Sepsis-induced hypotension is defined as a systolic blood pressure lower than 90 mmHg or a mean arterial pressure lower than 70 mmHg.

Surgical site infection

Definition

SSI is the most common complication after surgery with an overall incidence of 2–5%. It is defined as an infection related to an operative procedure that occurs at or near the surgical incision within 30 days of the procedure (or within 90 days if an implant is left in place). Clinical criteria for defining SSI include one or more of the following: (i) purulent exudate draining from a surgical site; (ii) positive fluid culture obtained from a surgical site that was closed primarily; (iii) surgical site that was reopened in the setting of at least one clinical sign of infection and is culture positive or not cultured; and (iv) the surgeon makes the diagnosis of infection. SSIs increase the risk of death by 2–11 times, which is directly related to the infection, and have an overall mortality of 3%. It is estimated that 40–60% of SSIs are preventable.

Classification (Box 9.2)

SSIs can be classified as incisional (in the wound) and organ/space (any part of the anatomy that was opened or manipulated during the operative procedure including anastomotic leaks). The latter account for one-third of SSIs but are responsible for more than 90% of the deaths related to SSI. Wound infections may occur at any time after the procedure and will depend on patient status and aggressiveness of the pathogen. Most wound infections will be clinically evident between 5 and 10 days after surgery.

Pathogens

The most common organisms causing SSI after a clean procedure are skin flora including streptococcal and staphylococcal species. In clean-contaminated procedures, Gram-negative bacilli and enterococci are predominant. When a viscus is entered, the pathogens usually reflect the endogenous flora of the viscus.

Prevention

A number of perioperative preventive measures have been demonstrated to reduce SSI especially in major and complex operations. Preoperative

---

> **Box 9.2 Classification of surgical wounds**
>
> Wound classification is based on the degree of expected contamination during the surgery.
>
> **Clean**
> Uninfected operative wounds in which no inflammation is encountered, and the wound is closed primarily. By definition, a viscus (respiratory, alimentary, genital or urinary tract) is not entered during a clean procedure.
> *Risk of infection*: 1.3–2.9%
>
> **Clean-contaminated**
> A viscus is entered under controlled conditions and without unusual contamination.
> *Risk of infection*: 2.4–7.7%
>
> **Contaminated**
> Open fresh accidental wounds, operations with major breaks in sterile technique, or gross spillage from a viscus.
> *Risk of infection*: 6.4–15.2%
>
> **Dirty**
> Old traumatic wounds with retained devitalised tissue, foreign bodies or faecal contamination.
> *Risk of infection*: 7.1–40%

---

measures include cessation of smoking, nutritional supplementation and good glycaemic control in patients with diabetes. Intraoperative measures include prophylactic antibiotics, appropriate skin hair removal at the surgical site, sound surgical technique, hand hygiene and selective use of drains. More recently, the prophylactic use of intraoperative wound irrigation devices has shown decreased infection rates compared with non-irrigated wounds in the setting of clean-contaminated incisions. Irrigation of the surgical wound has been found to offer benefits by hydrating the tissues, allowing better visualisation and removing contaminated material. These lower the microbiological burden and expedite the healing process. However, no benefits have been seen when antibiotics are added to the irrigation solution. In the postoperative period maintaining normoglycaemia and normothermia are important factors.

Antibiotic prophylaxis

The goal of antimicrobial prophylaxis is to prevent SSI by reducing the burden of microorganisms at the surgical site and to control any bacteraemia that may occur during the operative procedure. Repeat intraoperative doses are warranted for procedures that exceed two half-lives of the drug or for procedures in which there is excessive blood loss (>1500 mL). Patients receiving prophylactic antibiotics 1 or 2 hours before the surgical procedure have less SSIs than patients receiving earlier or later. There is no role for postoperative prophylactic antimicrobial therapy in routine surgery. In selected cases where prophylaxis beyond the period of surgery is considered, discussion with the infectious disease team should be undertaken and prophylaxis extended to no more than 24 hours. A multidisciplinary approach including infectious disease and cardiology teams should be adopted in patients with a prosthetic valve, cardiac pacemaker device or previous infective endocarditis. Staphylococci and β-haemolytic *Streptococcus* species are of prime concern with regard to infective endocarditis. The main oral pathogen associated with this type of infection is *S. viridans*.

Early drain removal

Drains are often used after major elective abdominal operations, emergency surgery and thoracic surgery (pancreas resection, total gastrectomy, oesophagectomy, low anterior resections and cardiothoracic surgery). In elective surgery, drains are used to remove the accumulation of inflammatory fluid and haematoma while identifying surgical complications. Early drain removal policies have been adopted in many institutions in order to expedite recovery and reduce hospital length of stay. Increasingly, the use of drains is being eschewed in many major elective operations based on accumulating evidence (liver resections, colectomies, large hernia repairs, partial gastrectomy and splenectomy).

Wound breakdown

Simple surgical wound infections presenting as cellulitis may be managed with antibiotic therapy. The presence of underlying collections or actual breakdown of part or whole of the wound requires additional intervention. This may be radiological or open surgical drainage of purulent material and mechanical debridement of devitalised tissue. Wounds opened in such a manner are managed by packing and programmed dressing changes supported by antibiotics.

Where more intense and continuous aspiration of the exudate is warranted, negative pressure therapy (NPT) may be applied using vacuum-assisted closure wound management devices. Sealed suction is applied continuously over the infected area in order to aspirate the purulent tissue and to avoid the creation of abscess. NPT optimises blood flow, decreases oedema, facilitates bacterial clearance and improves management of the exudate. It promotes wound contraction to cover the defect and may trigger intracellular signalling that increases cellular proliferation. The clinical usefulness has been demonstrated in treatment of SSI (skin, subcutaneous and muscular infection) and has also been applied in the management of patients not amenable to abdominal closure (laparostomy) in the emergency situation.

Central line-associated bloodstream infection

Central venous catheters (CVCs) are essential to intraoperative and postoperative management of sick patients and in healthy patients undergoing major operations. They are used widely and for prolonged duration in patients in intensive care units (ICUs) for the delivery of vasoactive drugs and hypertonic solutions and for monitoring and management. Central line-associated bloodstream infection (CLABSI) is defined as a bloodstream infection in a patient who had a central line in place within 48 hours before the development of the infection and in whom no other source of infection is found. It is a significant burden on healthcare systems and is associated with increased length of stay in both ICU and the hospital.

The majority (50–70%) of CLABSI cases are thought to be preventable by using current evidence-based guidelines. Hand hygiene has been shown to be a simple and safe method of prevention but some studies show lack of compliance rates of up to 30%. Aseptic technique, involving skin preparation with alcohol-based solution and the use of full barrier precautions (gloves, masks, gowns), are also essentials. Choosing the ideal site of insertion to minimise sepsis is also important. The site with the lowest infection rate for CVC insertion is the subclavian vein, although the internal jugular vein remains the most widely used site. Patients with neutropenia, severe burns, malnutrition and chronic inflammatory conditions are at great risk of CLABSI. Duration of catheterisation, catheter material, insertion conditions and quality of site care also affect the incidence of CLABSI.

The source of infection in CLABSI may include contamination from surrounding skin, contamination of the CVC, colonisation of the CVC from a concomitant bloodstream infection and contamination of the infusions. The skin flora (coagulase-negative staphylococci and *Staphylococcus aureus*) is the most common type of bacteria seen in bloodstream infection.

Treatment involves initially sampling the blood peripherally, changing the catheter with the assistance of a guidewire (if there are no signs of skin infection) and sampling the catheter tip. Broad-spectrum antibiotics should be commenced empirically and modified depending on blood culture results and clinical progress. Patients with positive peripheral blood culture should be treated with long-term antibiotics and change of the CVC.

Intra-abdominal collections

Most SSIs occur in the skin, subcutaneous space and muscle close to the incision. However, organ or space-occupying infections such as intra-abdominal, intrapleural and intracranial (intracavitary) infections are life-threatening events due to delayed diagnosis and the underlying aetiology. These include inflammatory fluid collections and haematomas that subsequently become infected and develop into an internal abscess. Alternatively, there may be leakage of fluid from the cut surface of an organ or an anastomosis which develops into an infected collection. These deep infections may remain occult or manifest with few symptoms, mimicking superficial SSI and possibly delaying diagnosis and initial treatment. Such complications then become evident when major signs of a systemic infection become apparent (e.g. leucocytosis, fever, hypotension, sepsis, elevated lactate and C-reactive protein). Diagnosis often requires radiological evaluation. CT is the most practical choice for intra-abdominal, pelvic and thoracic collections. Affected patients should be resuscitated and broad-spectrum antibiotics commenced based on the most likely pathogens to be found.

Intra-abdominal collections are one of the most common complications that surgeons will face in clinical practice. Treatment depends on the size, cause, underlying medical condition and systemic status of the patient. Small collections (<4 cm) may be treated successfully with systemic antibiotics. Radiologically guided percutaneous aspiration and drainage are indicated for larger localised collections within solid organs or the peritoneal cavity with a high rate of success. For those collections that are not amenable to radiological intervention, those associated with widespread intra-abdominal sepsis and where a surgical procedure is warranted for other reasons, open surgical drainage is performed. This also allows high-volume lavage of the peritoneal cavity. Widespread intra-abdominal sepsis in the postoperative period has a high mortality rate of 25–30%, but may exceed 70% where hospital-acquired pathogens are involved. Such widespread sepsis may require multiple laparotomies to control the source of sepsis and can lead to abdominal compartment syndrome, which may require open abdominal wound management.

Hospital-acquired pneumonia

Hospital acquired pneumonia (HAP) is one that occurs 48 hours or more after admission and did not appear to be incubating at the time of admission. Pneumonia is the leading cause of infectious mortality in hospitalised patients. Surgery and prolonged intubation are the main predisposing factors. Surgical patients who undergo thoracic and upper abdominal surgery, those requiring postoperative mechanical ventilation and those with previous lung conditions are particularly susceptible to pneumonia. The risk of HAP increases 6 to 20-fold in mechanically ventilated patients, denoting that airway intubation itself is a major risk factor for postoperative mortality.

Ventilator-associated pneumonia (VAP) is a subtype of HAP that develops more than 48–72 hours after endotracheal intubation. Risk factors for VAP are listed in Box 9.3. The diagnosis of VAP requires one or more of the following: fever, leucocytosis or leucopenia, purulent sputum, hypoxaemia, or a new or evolving chest radiograph infiltrate. A pathogen does not need to be identified. Defining the aetiology of postoperative pneumonia is difficult, as most patients are unable to produce an adequate sputum sample.

The pathogenesis of HAP and VAP is related to the numbers and virulence of microorganisms entering the lower respiratory tract and the response of the host. The primary route of infection of the lungs is through micro-aspiration of organisms which have colonised the oropharynx.

Box 9.3 Risk factors for VAP

- Acute respiratory distress syndrome
- Advanced age
- Large-volume gastric aspiration
- Blood transfusion
- Immunosuppression
- Organ failure
- Coma
- Chronic obstructive pulmonary disease
- Trauma
- Burns
- Prolonged ventilation

Prevention strategies for intubated patients are well defined and their cost–benefit proven worldwide. The strategy involves (i) elevating the bed head to between 30 and 45°; (ii) actively lightening sedation on a daily basis; (iii) actively assessing the potential to wean or extubate on a daily basis; (iv) avoiding antacids and histamine H$_2$ blockers unless clearly indicated; and (v) prophylaxis of deep vein thrombosis.

The choice of the antibiotic treatment regimen for HAP or VAP should be tailored to the patient's recent antibiotic therapy, resident flora in the hospital/ICU, degree of underlying diseases, severity of illness, available blood and sputum cultures, and risk for multidrug-resistant pathogens. Generally, initial antibiotic treatment for HAP targets *S. aureus*, *Pseudomonas aeruginosa* and Gram-negative bacilli.

Catheter-associated urinary tract infection

Catheter-associated urinary tract infection (CAUTI) is a common hospital-acquired infection. The most important risk factors are the duration of catheterisation followed by errors in catheter insertion and management. Classic symptoms include flank pain, suprapubic discomfort, urinary discoloration and catheter obstruction. However, in the elderly these often present with non-specific findings such as delirium, leucocytosis, malaise or general signs of sepsis. In the presence of CAUTI the urinary catheter should be removed or (if required) replaced, a urine sample acquired for culture, and empirical antibiotic therapy commenced and subsequently tailored based on culture results.

Avoidance of unnecessary catheterisation, use of sterile technique for insertion, and removal as soon as possible are essential in the prevention of CAUTI. There is no role for antibiotic prophylaxis in patients with a urinary catheter.

Pseudomembranous colitis

Pseudomembranous colitis is an inflammation of the colon caused by *Clostridium difficile* overgrowth in the colon. It is characterised by elevated yellow-white plaques that coalesce to form pseudomembranes on the mucosa. It is also known as antibiotic-related colitis due to the relationship to previous use of antibiotics. The most common antibiotics implicated are fluoroquinolones, clindamycin and cephalosporins. Other risk factors associated are recent hospitalisation, age more than 65 years and immunosuppression.

Symptoms of *C. difficile* infection (CDI) are abdominal pain, fever, diarrhoea, blood in the stool and leucocytosis. It is classified as severe and non-severe colitis. Non-severe CDI results in watery diarrhoea (three or more loose stools in 24 hours) with lower abdominal pain and cramping, low-grade fever and leucocytosis ($\leq 15 \times 10^9$ cells/L). Severe CDI presents with diarrhoea, severe lower quadrant or diffuse abdominal pain, abdominal distension, fever, hypovolaemia, lactic acidosis, hypoalbuminaemia and marked leucocytosis ($>15 \times 10^9$ cells/L). Fulminant colitis is a severe episode that is complicated by hypotension, shock, ileus or megacolon.

The diagnosis of CDI is established by a positive stool test for *C. difficile* toxin. Laboratory testing should be pursued only in patients with clinically significant diarrhoea, since testing cannot differentiate CDI from asymptomatic carriage that does not warrant treatment. Radiographic imaging, usually with contrast CT of the abdomen and pelvis, is advised for patients with clinical manifestations of severe illness or fulminant colitis to exclude the presence of toxic megacolon or any condition that requires surgical intervention. Colonoscopy is not needed in patients with classic symptoms, positive laboratory tests and improvement after antibiotic therapy. For non-severe cases oral vancomycin is the initial treatment, with metronidazole as the second choice. Surgical evaluation should be considered for patients with peritoneal signs, severe ileus, toxic megacolon, white blood cell count of 15×10^9/L or more and/or elevated plasma lactate (≥ 2.2 mmol/L). The rational use of antibiotics is the mainstay of prevention of CDI. Faecal microbiota transplantation is currently emerging as an effective therapy for recurrent CDI.

Necrotising fasciitis

Necrotising fasciitis (NF) (Figure 9.1) is a serious and devastating infection that can evolve rapidly without showing any superficial physical evidence of spread. NF is characterised clinically by fulminant tissue destruction, systemic signs of toxicity and high mortality. Risk factors for NF include skin or mucosal breach, traumatic wounds, diabetes and other immunosuppressive conditions. Fournier's gangrene (Figure 9.2) is a subtype of NF originating in the perineal area and spreading through the fascia, leading to extensive muscle necrosis. The diagnosis can sometimes be difficult, so a low threshold

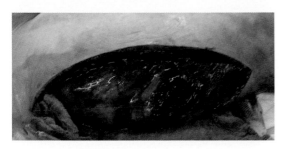

Fig. 9.1 Necrotising fasciitis of the right thigh. Note that the subtle mottling and erythema of the surrounding skin vastly underestimates the underlying muscle necrosis of subcutaneous fat and muscle.

for suspicion of this condition in patients presenting with perineal problems is advised, mainly when they have signs of sepsis and marked leucocytosis.

NF occurs when the bacteria enter the subcutaneous layers in regions with relatively poor blood flow and hypoxia. These conditions delay the immune system response and allow bacterial overgrowth and production of toxins. These toxins cause vasoconstriction and vascular thrombosis of the perforating vessels, increasing hypoxia and tissue necrosis and starting a vicious cycle of hypoxia, necrosis, bacterial growth and more hypoxia. NF may be polymicrobial (type 1) or monomicrobial (type 2). The former is caused by aerobic and anaerobic bacteria, usually occurring in older adults or diabetic patients. Type 2 NF is most commonly caused by group A *Streptococcus* and other β-haemolytic streptococci. It may occur in any age group and in individuals with no underlying comorbidities.

On physical examination, patients may show signs of erythema, oedema extending beyond the visible erythema, severe pain which may be out of proportion to clinical findings, fever, crepitus, and bullae, necrosis or ecchymosis in the skin. Systemic toxicity may be observed. NF usually presents acutely and most commonly involves the extremities, with the lower extremity more commonly involved than upper extremity. It should be suspected in patients with soft tissue infection and signs of systemic illness (fever, haemodynamic instability) in association with crepitus, rapid progression of clinical manifestations and/or severe pain (out of proportion to clinical signs).

The best initial radiological examiation is CT of the affected region. Presence of gas in the tissues is highly specific for NF and surgical exploration should be expedited. The diagnosis of necrotising infection is established via surgical exploration of the soft tissues in the operating room, with physical examination of the skin, subcutaneous tissue, fascial planes and muscle.

Aggressive surgical debridement and broad-spectrum antibiotic therapy accompanied by intensive care for haemodynamic support should be offered promptly. Factors associated with increased mortality include white cell count in excess of 30×10^9/L, creatinine above 177 mmol/L, age over 60 years, *Clostridium* infection, delay of more than 24 hours in surgical intervention, and infection involving head, neck, thorax and abdomen.

Antimicrobial resistance and antibiotic stewardship in surgery

The ever-increasing number of multidrug-resistant microorganisms has been recognised as a grave and emergent threat to global public health (Box 9.4). There is an increasing risk of life-threatening therapeutic failures due to many drug-resistant microbial

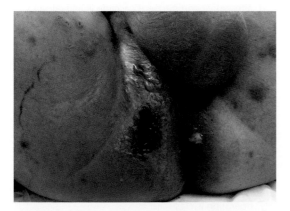

Fig. 9.2 Fournier's gangrene involving the scrotum and right buttock

> **Box 9.4 Serious threats identified by the Centers for Disease Control and Prevention**
>
> - Pan-drug-resistant (PDR) or extended-spectrum drug-resistant (XDR) *Acinetobacter* species
> - Drug-resistant *Campylobacter* species
> - Fluconazole-resistant *Candida* species
> - Extended-spectrum lactamase-producing Enterobacteriaceae (ESBLs)
> - Vancomycin-resistant enterococci (VRE)
> - Multidrug-resistant *Pseudomonas aeruginosa*
> - Drug-resistant non-typhoidal *Salmonella* species
> - Drug-resistant *Salmonella*
> - Meticillin-resistant *Staphylococcus aureus* (MRSA)
> - Drug-resistant *Streptococcus pneumoniae*
> - Total drug-resistant *Mycobacterium tuberculosis*

infections. These result in prolonged hospital stay, higher cost of alternative therapy and increased mortality.

Although much of the effort on responsible antibiotic stewardship has focused on primary care providers, there is a significant opportunity for surgeons to contribute, as antibiotic misuse appears to be quite common. Potential areas for surgical antimicrobial stewardship supported by evidence are as follows.

- Discontinuation of antibiotics after routine elective surgical cases. Prolonged postoperative use does not prevent SSI.
- No role for topical wound site antibiotics when systemic preoperative antibiotic prophylaxis is administered.
- Limited, fixed courses of antibiotics are adequate for treating complex intra-abdominal infections after the source control has been achieved.
- Antibiotics are not required after incision and drainage of superficial skin abscesses and opening of infected superficial SSIs.
- Uncomplicated diverticulitis does not require antibiotic therapy.
- Bacteriuria in patients without frequency, urgency, dysuria or unspecified suprapubic pain (asymptomatic) does not constitute a urinary tract infection and should not be treated with antibiotics.
- Presence of C. *difficile* in stool samples in the absence of clinical symptoms should not be treated with antibiotics.

Summary

Infection is a major cause of surgical morbidity and is multifactorial. Hand washing, universal body fluid precautions and attention to surgical technique are the factors that surgeons may implement to reduce the infection rate. Attention to patient (host) factors that may be improved (nutritional status, anaemia, sarcopenia) prior to surgery, awareness of high-risk patients and strict implementation of perioperative preventive strategies will help reduce the incidence, morbidity and mortality of surgical infections.

Further reading

Adamina M, Kehlet H, Tomlinson GA, Senagore AJ, Delaney CP. Enhanced recovery pathways optimise health outcomes and resource utilization: a meta-analysis of randomised controlled trials in colorectal surgery. *Surgery* 2011;149:830–40.

Leaper DJ, Edmiston CE. World Health Organization: global guidelines for the prevention of surgical site infection. *J Hosp Infect* 2017;95:135–6.

Mazuski JE, Tessier JM, May AK *et al*. The Surgical Infection Society revised guidelines on the management of intra-abdominal infection. *Surg Infect (Larchmt)* 2017;18:1–76.

Rhodes A, Evans LE, Alhazzani W *et al*. Surviving sepsis campaign: international guidelines for management of sepsis and septic shock: 2016. *Intensive Care Med* 2017;43:304–7.

MCQs

Select the single correct answer to each question. The correct answers can be found in the Answers section at the end of the book.

1 Which of the following statements is true?
  a use of alcohol-based solutions on surgical site skin does not change the SSI rate
  b hand wash has poor compliance in most of the studies
  c sterile technique is not warranted to insert a central venous catheter
  d use of prophylactic antibiotics during elective surgery is not necessary
  e for most skin infection, cefazolin-based antibiotics are warranted as they target the Gram-negative skin flora

2 Regarding the immune response to infection, which statement is true?
  a resident inflammatory cells do not play a role in the development of infection
  b proinflammatory cytokines such as IL6- and IL-10 are produced locally
  c anti-inflammatory cytokines are produced in response to infection and can lead to chronic infection when overproduced
  d alternative complement cascade is activated by direct contact with type 2 antigen-presenting cells
  e all of the above are correct

3 Which of the following is a true statement?
  a sepsis may occur in the absence of SIRS
  b surgical infection is diagnosed only when bacterial overgrowth is documented
  c SSI occurs only in the first 7 days after an operation
  d SSI only applies to infections that occur in the skin and subcutaneous tissue
  e intra-abdominal abscess after an abdominal operation is classified as SSI

4 Regarding surgical infections, which of the following is true?

a necrotising fasciitis is called Fournier's gangrene when the infection dissects the deep neck fascia towards the upper mediastinum

b necrotising fasciitis is easily diagnosed with ultrasound scan

c pseudomembranous colitis is an infection characterised by diffuse involvement of the colon

d pseudomembranous colitis is diagnosed by stool samples that are incubated for 24–48 hours and show *Clostridium difficile* overgrowth

e catheter-associated infection is more common when the central line is inserted in the jugular area than the subclavian area

5 Perforated appendicectomy wounds are classified as being:

a clean

b clean-contaminated

c contaminated

d contaminated-dirty

e none

10 Transplantation surgery

Michael A. Fink

University of Melbourne and Austin Health, Melbourne, Victoria, Australia

Introduction

Transplantation is the implantation of an organ, part of an organ or tissue derived from one individual into another individual. The indication is most commonly chronic or acute organ failure, but liver transplantation is also performed for metabolic diseases and some forms of malignancy. Transplantation of all organs has been shown to improve survival and quality of life of recipients. Aspects that have elements common to transplantation of all organs include recipient assessment, organ donation, recipient selection, transplantation surgery, post-transplant management including immunosuppression, and complications.

Recipient assessment

Recipient assessment takes into account the need for transplantation, and thus the natural history of the disease for which transplantation is contemplated, and the expected outcome, or utility of transplantation. Without transplantation, some forms of organ failure can only be managed in a supportive fashion. For example, liver failure is managed by endoscopic surveillance and ligation of oesophageal varices, antibiotics to minimise the development of encephalopathy, and diuretics, ascitic drainage procedures and sometimes transjugular intrahepatic portosystemic shunts (TIPS) to manage ascites. None of these interventions actually reverses the underlying process of liver failure. There is no reliable method of organ support for liver failure. Likewise, respiratory failure can be managed by oxygen therapy, but there is no viable long-term mechanical alternative. On the other hand, in the case of chronic renal failure, organ support is available in the form of haemodialysis and peritoneal dialysis. Ventricular assist devices are available for cardiac failure and are often used as a bridge to transplantation. The artificial pancreas is under development but is not yet used in standard practice.

Assessment of the benefit of transplantation needs to take into account the survival of the potential recipient with and without transplantation. Modelling of survival of patients with organ failure can be helpful in making these assessments. For example, the model for end-stage liver disease (MELD) score, which was originally developed to assess the mortality risk of patients with cirrhosis undergoing TIPS, has been validated as a prognostic indicator for patients with end-stage liver disease on the liver transplant waiting list. It has been shown that the risk of liver transplantation is not justified for patients with a MELD score less than 15, but that the benefit of transplantation increases for patients with increasing MELD scores above this.

Recipient selection should take account of the expected utility of transplantation. Transplantation requires either using the precious resource of deceased donor organs or putting a living donor at risk of morbidity and mortality and therefore it is important that the expected outcome of transplantation justifies this. Potential transplant recipients therefore undergo a process of evaluation that includes assessment of factors that might impact on post-transplant outcomes. This includes assessment of fitness for the transplant operation, such as assessment of cardiac and respiratory function. In addition, psychological and social factors that might impact on post-transplant outcomes, such as adherence to immunosuppression medications, investigations and clinic follow-up, are assessed. The decision to list a patient for transplantation is made in the context of a multidisciplinary assessment. In the setting of acute organ failure, where the patient's life is at imminent risk, the assessment process needs to be undertaken in a more urgent fashion.

Textbook of Surgery, Fourth Edition. Edited by Julian A. Smith, Andrew H. Kaye, Christopher Christophi and Wendy A. Brown.
© 2020 John Wiley & Sons Ltd. Published 2020 by John Wiley & Sons Ltd.

Organ donation

There are two main sources of organs for transplantation: deceased and living donors.

Living donors

The process of living donor transplantation includes careful assessment of the potential living donor. Living organ donation is a unique surgical procedure, in that, unlike other forms of surgery, the person undergoing the procedure is not expected to derive any physical benefit from it, although they might obtain a psychological benefit from the act of giving a precious gift to a loved one that should help to prolong their life and/or improve their quality of life. In this situation, the risk borne by the organ donor is balanced against the expected benefit to the recipient. The process of assessment of a potential living organ donor includes assessment of the quality of the organ, to ensure that there is a strong likelihood of successful transplantation and long-term good graft function, and assessment of the safety of organ donation for the recipient, in terms of both the perioperative risk and long-term risk of morbidity and mortality. Living donor assessment should include independent review by a physician who will not be caring for the transplant recipient and who can therefore advocate on behalf of the donor.

The living donor may be genetically related to the recipient (e.g. parent, sibling, child) or unrelated (e.g. spouse, friend). Some living donor transplantation is performed using the organ of an altruistic, or 'good Samaritan' donor. In this situation, the donor donates their organ to a stranger. Most commonly, living donor transplantation occurs in a simple one-to-one fashion; that is, one donor donates to one recipient. However, in some circumstances, such as ABO incompatibility between donor and recipient, or recipient antibodies against donor antigens, this is not possible. In this situation, 'paired exchange' can be a solution to the problem. The simplest example occurs when donor A is incompatible with recipient A and donor B is incompatible with recipient B. If donor A is compatible with recipient B and donor B is compatible with recipient A, a paired exchange can be undertaken whereby donor A donates an organ to recipient B and donor B donates an organ to recipient A. More complex chains of donation and transplantation involving multiple donor and recipient pairs can be undertaken. These chains will sometimes involve an altruistic donor. The greater the number of potential donors and recipients, the greater the number of transplants that can be performed. Therefore, organising networks of paired exchange across large populations can be beneficial. The Australian Paired Kidney Exchange program oversaw a total of 154 paired kidney transplants across 22 centres throughout Australia to the end of 2015.

Whilst transplantation of all organs (other than heart, for obvious reasons) has been undertaken from living donors, the relative proportion of transplantation undertaken from living donors varies by organ and geographic region. Kidney transplantation is commonly performed using living donor organs. In 2017, 24% of kidney transplants in Australia and 37% of kidney transplants in New Zealand were performed using grafts from living donors. Previously, donor nephrectomy was performed as an open operation, but it is now routinely performed either laparoscopically or retroperitoneoscopically. The steps of donor nephrectomy surgery include surgical access (laparoscopic or retroperitoneoscopic), mobilisation of the renal artery (or arteries) and vein, mobilisation, clipping and transection of the ureter, mobilisation of the kidney, placing the kidney in a bag in preparation for extraction, preparation of the wound for extraction but without opening the peritoneum (e.g. Pfannenstiel incision), securing the renal artery and vein with staples or clips, transecting the renal artery and vein, removal of the kidney, placing the kidney in saline slush, and cannulation of the renal artery and flushing the kidney with a suitable cold preservation solution (e.g. Ross solution, Soltran or histidine–tryptophan–ketoglutarate).

Liver transplantation can be performed by removing a portion of the liver from a living donor. Living donor liver transplantation is relatively uncommon in Australia and New Zealand; between 1985 and 2016, 100 living donor liver transplants were performed in the countries out of a total of 5553 transplants (1.8%). In other parts of the world, particularly Asia, where deceased organ donation rates are lower, living donors are a more frequent source for liver transplantation. Adult-to-child living liver transplantation most commonly involves removal of segments 2 and 3 (usually approximately 25% of liver volume) or the left hemi-liver (segments 2, 3 and 4, usually approximately 40% of liver volume). Adult-to-adult liver transplantation most commonly involved removal of the right hemi-liver. The steps in living donor hepatectomy include surgical access (open or laparoscopic); parenchymal transection, which can be undertaken by cavitron ultrasonic aspirator or a variety of energy devices; securing and transecting the appropriate hepatic artery, portal vein, hepatic duct and hepatic vein; removal of the portion of liver to a saline slush bath; and cannulation of the hepatic artery and portal vein and flushing with a suitable cold preservation solution.

Deceased donors

Deceased organ donation is usually considered in the setting of patients with a severe neurological injury in the intensive care unit (ICU) or emergency department. Between 2014 and 2018 in Australia, 38% of donors died of intracranial (intracerebral or extra-axial, i.e. extradural, subdural or subarachnoid) haemorrhage, 36% from cerebral hypoxia or ischaemia, 16% from traumatic brain injury, 6% from cerebral infarct, 1% from other neurological conditions and 0% from non-neurological conditions.

Work-up for organ donation is a complex multi-step process.

- Information regarding the process is provided to the potential donor's family.
- Assessment for suitability for organ donation is undertaken. This includes obtaining information from the family, the general practitioner and the medical records in order to determine the likely organ quality and to assess risks of transplantation of the donor organs, such as transmission of infection and cancer.
- Death is confirmed (this step may occur later in the process, as outlined in the following section).
- Informed consent for donation is obtained from the donor's family.
- Communication with recipient units regarding organ offers occurs.
- Coordination of the donor procurement operation is undertaken.

There are two main pathways of deceased organ donation: donation after brain death (DBD) and donation after circulatory death (DCD). These pathways are based on the two definitions of death that are enshrined in legislation in all jurisdictions across Australia and New Zealand and most jurisdictions in the rest of the world: the irreversible cessation of all functions of the brain in the person and the irreversible cessation of circulation of blood in the body of the person.

Donation after brain death

In Australia, declaration of brain death requires that a severe brain injury sufficient to cause death has occurred and that other causes of deep coma, such as metabolic, electrolyte and endocrine derangements and sedative drugs, have been excluded. The confirmation of brain death can be made either on clinical grounds or based on imaging. The clinical criteria are:

- the absence of response to noxious stimuli in the cranial nerve distribution and all four limbs and trunk, *and*
- the absence of all the following brainstem reflexes:
  - pupillary light reflex
  - corneal reflex
  - reflex response to pain in the trigeminal nerve distribution
  - vestibulo-ocular reflex
  - gag reflex
  - cough/tracheal reflex *and*
- the absence of respiratory effort on an apnoea test (disconnection of the endotracheal or tracheostomy tube from the ventilator).

The imaging criterion is the demonstration of the absence of intracranial blood flow, which can be assessed by angiography, contrast-enhanced CT or MRI or a nuclear perfusion scan. In all Australian jurisdictions, declaration of brain death requires performance of the assessment by two medical practitioners, although the required experience and training of the doctors varies slightly between jurisdictions.

Donation after circulatory death

In the early days of transplantation, the majority of deceased donor transplants were performed by the DCD (also known as donation after cardiac death and non-heart beating donation) pathway. With the enactment of the legal definition of brain death in the 1980s, DBD became the predominant pathway of deceased organ donation. However, the recognition of the imbalance between supply of suitable deceased donor organs and the demand for these organs and the consequent prolonged period of waiting for transplantation and risk of death on the waiting list has resulted in a resurgence of DCD transplantation in recent years. In 2018 in Australia and New Zealand, 163 of 616 donors (26%) were DCD donors. The rate of DCD donors varied by jurisdiction; Victoria had the highest rate at 33%.

There are several ways that potential DCD donors can present, and these are defined as the Maastricht categories:

1 dead on arrival
2 unsuccessful resuscitation after cardiac arrest outside hospital
3 awaiting cardiac arrest after withdrawal of cardiorespiratory support
4 cardiac arrest in a brain dead donor
5 unexpected cardiac arrest in hospital.

The vast majority of DCD donors in Australia and New Zealand are Maastricht 3 (as outlined in the following discussion), though occasionally Maastricht 4 donation may occur if the donor team is in the donor hospital at the time that the cardiac arrest occurs. Other categories of donors have occurred in some parts of the world (notably Spain).

Organ donation by the DCD pathway occurs in donors with similar underlying brain injury to those who donate via the DBD pathway: stroke, trauma and hypoxia. Occasionally, DCD donation occurs in the setting of other conditions with a poor expected outcome, such as a high spinal cord injury. The patient must be confirmed to have a poor expected outcome. Once consent for donation has been obtained and the organ procurement team has indicated that they are ready to perform the organ procurement procedure, cardiorespiratory support is withdrawn. This usually comprises extubation and cessation of inotropic support. The vital signs are recorded at frequent intervals following withdrawal of cardiorespiratory support. Once circulation has ceased and a sufficient period after this has elapsed to ensure that the process is irreversible, the patient is declared dead and organ donation can occur. The exact time between asystole and certification of death varies between jurisdictions and even between hospitals in some jurisdictions but is usually between 2 and 5 minutes.

The DBD and DCD organ procurement pathways are summarised in Figure 10.1. In DBD donors, there is usually no period of warm ischaemia (unless a cardiac arrest occurs during the procedure). In contrast, in DCD donors, following withdrawal of cardiorespiratory support, there will usually be a period of reduced organ perfusion prior to cardiac arrest. Following this, a period of observation is required, in order to ensure irreversibility of the loss of circulation and then the donor must be transferred to the operating theatre (unless withdrawal has occurred in the operating theatre), the chest and abdomen opened, the relevant vessels cannulated and cold perfusion commenced.

The period of warm ischaemia (whose exact definition varies depending on the organ) can have a detrimental impact on the outcome of transplantation. The kidneys and lungs, which are relatively resilient to this period of hypoxia, can function well, with transplantation outcomes similar to those of DBD transplantation; however, the results of heart and liver transplantation using DCD donation are inferior to those using DBD donation. In addition, not all potential DCD donors progress to circulatory death within the time required for organ donation. In 2018 in Australia, 111 of 265 (42%) intended DCD donors did not proceed to organ donation; 64 of these died outside the required time frame for organ donation. In contrast, only 49 of 400 (11%) of intended DBD donors did not proceed to organ donation. Therefore, any potential donor should be given a period of observation to determine the likelihood of progression to brain death and the DCD pathway used only if it is anticipated that progression to brain death will not occur.

Deceased organ procurement operation

The aims of the deceased donor organ procurement operation are to assess the quality and anatomy of the organs, to replace the blood in the organs with a cold organ preservation solution, to remove the organs from the body without injury to the organs or the vasculature of the organs, to package the organs appropriately and to place them in an appropriate cold (usually ice-filled) transport container. The concept of organ preservation fluids is

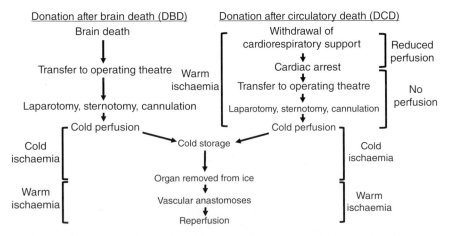

Fig. 10.1 Comparison of the donation after brain death and donation after circulatory death pathways.

that they enable the organ to survive outside the body and without circulation for an extended period (the time varies between organs). Most organ preservation fluids have a composition similar to intracellular fluid, in order to minimise movement of solutes across cell membranes, and also contain energy substrates, buffers and osmotic agents. Some also contain membrane stabilisers and antioxidants. Cooling of the organs both by perfusion with a cold solution and the application of ice saline slush results in reduction of the metabolic requirements that assists the preservation process.

The operation starts out with a time-out procedure that includes confirmation of the information regarding the donor, including the documentation confirming death, the donor blood group and serology, and confirmation of donor identity comparing the donor identification bracelet with the donor documentation. The details in the timing of this process vary slightly between DBD and DCD donor procedures.

For a DBD donor, intravenous broad-spectrum antibiotics and methylprednisolone 1 g are given. The organ procurement teams consist of an abdominal and/or thoracic team. After prepping and draping, a midline laparotomy and median sternotomy are performed. A Cattell–Braasch manoeuvre (complete mobilisation of the bowel from the retroperitoneum) is performed and the aorta and inferior vena cava are exposed. Slings (usually heavy silk ties) are placed around the infrarenal aorta and the inferior vena cava can also be slung. The quality and vascular anatomy of the organs to be procured are assessed. In particular, the porta hepatis is palpated to determine whether there is a replaced (or accessory) right hepatic artery arising from the superior mesenteric artery and the gastrohepatic (lesser) omentum is examined for the presence of a replaced (or accessory) left hepatic artery arising from the left gastric artery. Further dissection may be required, particularly mobilisation of the pancreas if this is to be procured. The crura of the diaphragm are split and divided, exposing the supracoeliac aorta.

The thoracic team undertakes a preliminary dissection. After heparinisation (heparin 300 units/kg i.v.), the aorta and pulmonary artery are cannulated. The infrarenal aorta (and inferior vena cava, if desired) is then cannulated. The superior vena cava is ligated. Decompression of the heart and abdominal organs is ensured by venting the left atrium and inferior vena cava, respectively. Immediately following this, the supracoeliac and ascending aorta are cross-clamped and perfusion of the thoracic and abdominal organs commences.

After cold perfusion, the organs are removed with care to avoid injury to the organs, the vasculature and associated structures (bile duct, ureters, trachea and bronchi).

The organs are placed in a saline slush bath on the donor back table. The organs are assessed for quality and injuries and this information is documented and communicated to the recipient teams. It is preferable to remove the liver and pancreas en bloc, in order to minimise warming of the pancreas, and these organs are separated on the back table. Further perfusion on the back table is performed for the abdominal organs. The organs are triple bagged, labelled and placed on ice in insulated containers ready for subsequent transport to the recipient teams. It is also routine to procure iliac artery and vein grafts for use as extension grafts. These are sent in the transport container with the liver and the pancreas. The chest and abdomen are then closed in routine fashion.

An alternative to this method of organ preservation, which is known as static cold storage, is machine perfusion, which can be hypothermic, subnormothermic or normothermic (at body temperature). In the latter case, oxygenated blood is generally circulated through the organ using pumps and a membrane oxygenator. Machine perfusion can allow (i) assessment of suitability for transplant (whether to use or discard the organ) and (ii) resuscitation of the organ with or without modification of the organ. Machine perfusion systems are becoming commercially available and it is likely that this technology will have an increasingly important role in organ preservation.

Recipient selection

Selection of the appropriate recipient of a donor organ offer is based on the ethical principles of equity, which is characterised by equal distribution of risk and benefit, and therefore fairness, and utility, which in this context is characterised by the best outcome for donated organs. The relative contribution of these principles to recipient selection varies between organs mainly in relation to the risk of waiting list mortality.

For those organs whose failure results in a high risk of waiting list mortality, such as liver, heart and lung, allocation of donor organs is based on the 'sickest first' principle, the primary aim being to rescue those on the waiting list who have the greatest risk of waiting list mortality. Scores that assess the risk of waiting list death, such as MELD score in the case of liver failure, can help inform recipient selection and, indeed, MELD score is used in this capacity in many parts of the world.

In the case of kidney transplantation, in which waiting list mortality is less prominent, utility is a more prominent principle of organ allocation. Aspects of allocation that impact on post-transplant outcome, such as human leucocyte antigen (HLA) matching, play a role. However, patients on the kidney transplant waiting list who have a reduced access to donor organs, such as highly sensitised individuals (those who have multiple HLA antibodies secondary to blood transfusions and previous transplants), are given preferential access to suitable donor organs.

Transplantation surgery

Transplantation surgery can be performed as an orthotopic procedure, in which the organ is removed and replaced with a donor organ in the same position as the original, or as a heterotopic procedure, in which the organ is usually not removed and the donor organ is implanted in a different position to the original. Heart, lung and liver transplantation are usually performed as orthotopic procedures, whilst kidney and pancreas transplantation are performed as heterotopic procedures.

Kidney transplantation involves placing the graft in an extraperitoneal position in the iliac fossa, with anastomosis of the renal artery and vein to the iliac artery and vein, respectively, and of the ureter to the bladder.

Pancreas transplantation is performed by initially anastomosing a donor iliac artery Y graft to the superior mesenteric and splenic arteries and then anastomosing the iliac artery graft to the recipient iliac artery, the portal vein to the iliac vein (in the past, this was often anastomosed to the superior mesenteric vein) and the duodenum to the small bowel to drain the exocrine fluid (in the past this was often anastomosed to the bladder, but the irritant effect of the pancreatic enzymes caused haemorrhagic cystitis). The pancreas is placed in an intraperitoneal position (as is the kidney, which is anastomosed to the opposite iliac vessels) in the case of simultaneous pancreas and kidney transplantation.

Liver transplantation requires anastomosis of the donor inferior vena cava either to a common opening of the recipient left, middle and right hepatic veins (the 'piggyback' approach) or side-to-side to the recipient inferior vena cava. The removal of a segment of recipient vena cava with the liver and two anastomoses of the superior and inferior ends

of the donor vena cava to the recipient vena cava (cava replacement) was previously common but is now rarely performed. Liver transplantation requires the anastomosis of two inflow structures (the portal vein and hepatic artery). The donor bile duct is most commonly anastomosed directly to recipient bile duct, but a Roux-en-Y anastomosis is sometimes required (e.g. in the case of biliary atresia or primary sclerosing cholangitis).

The steps of a transplant operation include the following.

- Back table preparation of the donor organ: removal of extraneous tissue, such as the diaphragm in the case of liver transplantation, and reconstruction of the vasculature, such as anastomosis of an iliac artery Y graft to the superior mesenteric and splenic arteries in the case of pancreas transplantation.
- Induction of anaesthesia.
- Administration of broad-spectrum antibiotics.
- Prepping and draping.
- Surgical access: overwhelmingly by open surgery, although kidney transplantation has been performed laparoscopically and robotically in some centres.
- Removal of the native organ, if appropriate (liver, heart, lung).
- Vascular anastomoses (inflow and outflow).
- Reperfusion: removal of the vascular clamps, allowing blood to perfuse the organ.
- Anastomosis of associated structures, such as the trachea or bronchus, bile duct, duodenum and ureter in the case of lung, liver, pancreas and kidney transplantation, respectively.
- Haemostatic check.
- Closure.

Heart–lung transplantation requires additional steps, including cannulation and commencement of cardiopulmonary bypass, removal of ventricular assist devices if applicable, and weaning of cardiopulmonary bypass and decannulation.

Post-transplant management

The site of initial postoperative management varies with the organ transplanted and the condition of the patient. Heart, lung and liver transplant recipients are routinely initially cared for in the ICU. Organ function may need to be supported postoperatively, such as by intra-aortic balloon pump or haemofiltration, in some cases. Post-transplant management includes elements of postoperative care following any major operation, including analgesia, antibiotics when appropriate, thromboprophylaxis, mobilisation, physiotherapy, introduction of oral diet and discharge planning. In addition, careful ongoing evaluation of graft function is required. This may include assessment of routine parameters such as haemodynamic observations or measurements; organ output, such as bile or urine production; blood tests, such as urea and electrolytes, liver function tests, blood glucose and arterial blood gases; and imaging, such as chest X-ray, echocardiography or Doppler ultrasound to assess the graft vasculature. More invasive investigation, including graft biopsy, may be required if there is concern about graft function.

Immunosuppression

Immunosuppression is required to prevent graft rejection. The first dose is often given intraoperatively during the transplant procedure. The choice and dose of immunosuppression varies depending on the organ transplanted, the immunological compatibility of the donor and recipient and the clinical state of the recipient. Some organs are more immunogenic than others. The intestine, which is accompanied by a large load of donor antigen and immunocompetent cells, is particularly immunogenic. In contrast, the liver tends to be less immunogenic and therefore usually requires less immunosuppression than other organs. The presence of donor-specific antibodies will necessitate higher levels of immunosuppression than would be otherwise necessary. There are also special cases, such as ABO incompatible transplantation, that may require other immunological approaches, such as plasmapheresis and T-cell depletion therapies.

Immunosuppression is generally (at least early post transplant) a combination of medications that target different aspects of the immune response and are therefore synergistic in their effect. Steroids, such as prednisolone, reduce the transcription of inflammatory proteins such as interleukin-2 and tumour necrosis factor α. Side effects include fluid retention, delirium, obesity, hypertension, diabetes mellitus and osteoporosis. Calcineurin inhibitors, such as tacrolimus and ciclosporin, reduce interleukin production and inhibit the replication of T cells. Their side effects include tremor, headache, hypertension, diabetes mellitus, hyperlipidaemia and nephrotoxicity. Antiproliferative drugs, such as mycophenolate mofetil and azathioprine, reduce the production of lymphocytes. They can cause neutropenia. Mycophenolate mofetil also commonly causes gastrointestinal side effects, including bloating and diarrhoea. mTOR (mammalian target of rapamycin) inhibitors, such as sirolimus and everolimus, reduce

the production of T lymphocytes and prevent the transition of B lymphocytes into plasma cells. They have a lower risk of nephrotoxicity than calcineurin inhibitors and therefore can be used in patients with impaired renal function. They also have a degree of antitumour activity. They reduce wound healing and should therefore be changed to an alternative immunosuppressive agent prior to surgery.

Complications of transplantation

Surgical complications

Surgical complications occur most often in the early post-transplant period and include bleeding, vascular complications and complications related to outflow structures (such as the ureter and bile duct). Postoperative monitoring of the patient's observations, wound and blood tests should allow early identification of bleeding. Early return to the operating theatre is generally advisable for anything other than minor bleeding. Potential vascular compromise should be monitored and this generally requires routine use of postoperative Doppler ultrasound. Arterial or venous kinking, torsion or thrombosis will usually result in graft loss unless it is dealt with expeditiously, most commonly by repeat operation. Ureteric or bile duct leakage will generally be detected by change in the drain tube output. Stricture of these structures is most commonly related to ischaemia. Ureteric and biliary anastomotic complications can usually be managed endoscopically, but revision surgery is sometimes required. Lymphocele is a collection of lymphatic fluid that can complicate kidney transplantation. Careful ligation of lymphatics at the time of mobilisation of the iliac vessels in preparation for the vascular anastomoses can help prevent lymphoceles from occurring. Drainage of lymphoceles can be performed percutaneously or by creating a window into the peritoneal cavity.

Rejection

Transplantation involves a complex interplay between the host innate and adaptive immune system and the donor antigens. In addition, donor passenger lymphocytes and dendritic cells often accompany the transplanted organ. Recipient antigen-presenting cells, such as macrophages and dendritic cells, ingest antigenic products of donor cells, process these and present the foreign antigens on the surface in association with the recipient major histocompatibility complex (MHC). MHCs are highly polymorphic and are important in the recognition of self versus non-self and therefore in combating infection and cancer. Class I MHC loci include HLA-A, HLA-B and HLA-C, while class II MHC loci include HLA-DP, HLA-DQ and HLA-DR. Foreign antigens presented in association with the MHC on the surface of antigen-presenting cells bind to the T-cell receptor of CD8-positive (cytotoxic) T cells and CD4-positive (helper) T cells. CD8-positive T cells lyse cells that display the relevant foreign antigen and CD4-positive cells have a variety of actions including the production of CD8-positive cells and activation of B cells. Increasing levels of HLA matching between donor and recipient reduce the risk of rejection in kidney and lung transplantation but is less relevant in liver transplantation. Microchimerism, in which donor lymphocytes become incorporated into the host immune system, and increased numbers of recipient regulatory T cells lead to a greater chance of tolerance, in which the immune response to the transplanted cells is ameliorated and the amount of immunosuppression can be reduced or, in some cases, ceased altogether.

Rejection is classified as cell-mediated or antibody-mediated and acute or chronic. Cell-mediated rejection is the more common pathway and occurs by activation of CD8-positive and CD-4 positive T cells, resulting in secretion of proinflammatory cytokines and cell lysis and apoptosis. Hyperacute antibody-mediated rejection results from the interaction of preformed antibody, such as those produced due to previous blood transfusion or transplantation, with donor HLA and occurs immediately on reperfusion of the organ. This is very rare. Antibody-mediated rejection can also occur later after transplantation due to antibodies that develop in response to damaged endothelial cells and occurs in response to activation of the complement cascade. The hallmark of antibody-mediated rejection is the presence of C4d deposition, which can be identified in allograft biopsies.

Rejection is diagnosed based on identification of allograft dysfunction, such as a rising creatinine in the case of kidney transplantation or rising liver function tests in the case of liver transplantation, and is confirmed by biopsy of the allograft. Treatment is usually a course of intravenous or oral steroids and increase in the dose of the calcineurin inhibitor.

Graft dysfunction

The process of brain death is associated with a 'cytokine storm'. In DCD donors, warm ischaemia occurs. These processes as well as cold storage and then reperfusion in the recipient result in ischaemia reperfusion that can impact on graft function. This is sometimes referred to as 'harvest injury'. Initial poor function or delayed graft function may necessitate supportive measures, such as dialysis in the case of kidney transplantation. Complete early failure of the graft is referred to as primary non-function and urgent re-transplantation of non-renal grafts is required to prevent death.

Chronic transplant dysfunction, which can lead to late graft loss, can occur through incompletely understood complex immunological and non-immunological mechanisms. The pathology of chronic transplant dysfunction varies between different organs and includes interstitial fibrosis and tubular atrophy in the kidney, graft fibrosis and ductopenia in the liver, bronchiolitis obliterans in the lung and arteriosclerosis in the heart.

Infection

Infection can occur by a variety of means. The operation itself can be associated with infection, such as a wound infection or infection of the pleural space or abdomen. There is a risk of transmission of organisms from the donor to the recipient. The commonest of these are viruses, including cytomegalovirus (CMV) and Epstein–Barr virus. Serology for these viruses is routinely tested in the donor and the recipient. In some circumstances, particularly if donor CMV serology is positive and recipient CMV serology is negative, pre-emptive antiviral treatment (valganciclovir) is commenced. In lower risk situations, polymerase chain reaction (PCR) can be used to monitor for the presence of CMV and treatment commenced if the patient becomes PCR positive. Donors are also routinely tested for the presence of antibody and (in Australia) nucleic acid testing (NAT) for hepatitis B virus (HBV), hepatitis C virus (HCV) and HIV. Cases of transmission of these viruses have been reported, but the residual risk of transmission of these viruses from a donor who tests negative with NAT is exceedingly small, even in donor groups at increased risk of infection. Bacteria and fungi can also potentially be transmitted from donor to recipient. Latent infections, particularly viral, can be reactivated in the recipient upon immunosuppression. Finally, the immunosuppressed patient is at increased risk of transmission from other people in the post-transplant period. The risk is highest in the early post-transplant period, because immunosuppression is generally most intensive at that time.

Cancer

The immune system is important in the monitoring of and defence against cancer and therefore it is not surprising that immunosuppression predisposes to the development of cancer. Of patients who have undergone liver transplantation in Australia and New Zealand, 20% have developed *de novo* cancer after transplantation. Skin cancer developed in 13%, including 0.9% of the total transplant population who developed melanoma, and non-skin cancer developed in 7%. Transplanted patients require cancer monitoring, including regular skin checks as well as standard screening as occurs in the general population, prevention, such as sun protection, and treatment as required.

Cardiovascular and cerebrovascular disease

Complications of immunosuppression, such as hypertension, diabetes mellitus, hyperlipidaemia and obesity, contribute to long-term risks of metabolic syndrome, ischaemic heart disease and cerebrovascular disease. Monitoring and treatment of risk factors for these conditions is important in the management of transplant recipients.

Disease recurrence

Some indications for transplantation can recur. For example, in liver transplantation, primary sclerosing cholangitis, hepatocellular carcinoma and viral hepatitis are at risk of recurrence. The risk of recurrent viral hepatitis has been greatly reduced by effective antiviral therapy (resulting in suppression of viral replication in the case of HBV and eradication in the case of direct-acting antiviral therapy for HCV).

Results of transplantation

Kidney transplantation

Kidney transplant outcomes in Australia and New Zealand are reported by the Australia and New Zealand Dialysis and Transplant Registry. In 2017, 1109 kidney transplants were performed in Australia and 187 in New Zealand. The most frequent indications for listing for kidney transplantation in 2017 were glomerulonephritis (42%), diabetic nephropathy (14%) and polycystic disease (12%). Kidney transplantation in Australia and New Zealand has excellent results. In recent years for primary (first) deceased donor grafts, the 1-, 5- and 10-year patient survival rates have been 97%, 90% and 75%, respectively and the 1-, 5- and 10-year graft survival rates have been 94%, 83% and 62%, respectively. Living donor kidney transplantation has results that are superior to deceased donor kidney transplantation. In recent years for primary living donor kidney transplantation, the 1- and 5-year patient survival rates were 99% and 96%, respectively, and the 1- and 5-year graft survival rates were 98% and 90%, respectively.

Liver transplantation

Liver transplantation outcomes in Australia and New Zealand are reported by the Australia and New Zealand Liver Transplant Registry. To 31 December 2016, 5553 liver transplants had been performed in the countries, 1012 in children and 4541 in adults. The commonest indications in children are biliary atresia (54%) and metabolic diseases (14%). The commonest indications in adults are HCV disease (22%), alcoholic liver disease (10%), malignancy, predominantly hepatocellular carcinoma (11%), primary sclerosing cholangitis (10%) and fulminant hepatic failure (9%). It is likely that the indications will evolve over time. In particular, the widespread availability of direct-acting antiviral therapy for HCV is likely to result in a reduction in the proportion of liver transplants performed for this indication and the increasing rate of obesity in the community is likely to result in an increase in the proportion of liver transplants performed for non-alcoholic fatty liver disease (NAFLD). Indeed, the proportion of liver transplants performed for HCV decreased from 28% in 2010–2014 to 19% in 2015–2016 while the proportion of liver transplants performed for NAFLD increased from 6% to 8% over the same period.

Liver transplantation has been a highly successful treatment for selected patients with end-stage liver disease, hepatocellular carcinoma and fulminant hepatic failure. In recent years, the 1-, 5- and 10-year patient and graft survival rates in Australia and New Zealand have been 95%, 86% and 77% and 91%, 82% and 71%, respectively. Patient survival is superior in children compared with adults (10-year patient survival 83% vs. 72%, respectively; P <0.001). The results of split liver transplantation, whereby a deceased donor liver is split into two grafts, generally one for a child and one for an adult, have been excellent. In children, the 5-year graft survival rates for split and whole liver transplantation are 80% and 82%, respectively, and for adults are 75% and 78%, respectively.

Pancreas and pancreatic islet transplantation

Pancreas transplantation can be undertaken as a whole, solid organ transplant or as an islet cell transplant. Whole pancreas transplantation is most commonly (97% of pancreas transplants in Australia and New Zealand) performed simultaneously with kidney transplantation, in the situation of a patient with diabetes mellitus (overwhelmingly type 1) who also has renal failure (most commonly due to diabetes). However, pancreas transplantation can be performed after kidney transplantation or, occasionally, without prior or simultaneous kidney transplantation.

Pancreas transplantation outcomes in Australia and New Zealand are reported by the Australia and New Zealand Islets and Pancreas Transplant Registry. From 1984 to 2018, 866 solid organ pancreas transplants were performed in Australia and New Zealand. In recent years in Australia and New Zealand, the 1- and 5-year patient survival rates following whole organ pancreas transplantation were 97% and 94%, respectively, and the 1- and 5-year death censored graft survival rates were 94% and 88%, respectively.

In islet cell transplantation, the islets of Langerhans are separated from the pancreatic acinar tissue in a complex process of enzymatic digestion. The resuspended islets are then injected percutaneously into the portal vein, following which the islets can engraft in the liver and produce insulin. The main indication for islet transplantation is type 1 diabetes mellitus with hypoglycaemic unawareness, which can be life-threatening, occurring in patients who do not require kidney transplantation. To achieve insulin independence, it may be necessary to perform islet transplantation from more than one donor into a recipient. The best results seem to be achieved in small recipients, who have a low insulin requirement. A total of 116 islet transplants were performed in 58 patients in Australia (there is no program in New Zealand) from 2002 to 2018. Of these, 20 (34%) achieved insulin independence, two patients after a single transplant, 11 after their second transplant and seven after their third transplant.

Intestinal transplantation

Intestinal transplantation is a low-volume procedure performed predominantly for patients with intestinal failure and life-threatening complications of total parenteral nutrition. The major categories of intestinal failure are short gut syndrome and motility disorders. A variety of grafts are used including intestine only, liver–intestine (which includes the pancreas), multivisceral (liver, stomach, pancreas, intestine) and modified multivisceral (the same as multivisceral, but without the stomach). Seven intestinal transplants have been performed at a single centre (Melbourne) between 2010 and 2019 in Australia. The 1- and 5-year patient and graft survival rates are 86%.

Heart transplantation

Heart and lung transplant outcomes in Australia and New Zealand are reported by the Australia and New Zealand Cardiothoracic Organ Transplant Registry. From 1984 to 2018, 2974 heart and 208 heart–lung transplants were performed. The commonest indications were idiopathic dilated cardiomyopathy (42%) and ischaemic heart disease (31%). In 2018, 39% of patients were supported by a ventricular assist device at the time of transplantation and 1% were supported by an intra-aortic balloon pump. In recent years in Australia and New Zealand, the 1-, 5- and 10-year patient survival rates were 89%, 83% and 70%, respectively.

Lung transplantation

From 1984 to 2018, in addition to the 208 heart–lung transplants, 552 single lung and 2749 bilateral lung transplants were performed. The commonest indications were emphysema (29%), cystic fibrosis (23%) and idiopathic pulmonary fibrosis (1%). In recent years in Australia and New Zealand, the 1-, 5- and 10-year patient survival rates for DBD lung transplant were 90%, 66% and 50%, respectively, while the 1-, 5- and 10-year patient survival rates for DCD bilateral lung transplant were 92%, 68% and 61%, respectively (P = NS).

Surgical issues that can arise in transplant recipients

Considering the success of transplantation, many transplant recipients are living in the community and can present with surgical issues. Some of these will be related to the graft, as outlined in the section on complications of transplantation, but others will be independent of the graft. If a patient presents to a healthcare facility with a problem related to the graft, immediate transfer to the transplant centre should be arranged. However, surgical problems that arise independently of the graft are often best dealt with expeditiously at the peripheral centre, although the transplant unit should be contacted to ensure that they are aware of the issue and so that relevant advice, including anatomical information and advice regarding perioperative management of immunosuppression, can be given. Indeed, undue delay in management of an urgent surgical problem can result in a poor outcome.

The variety of emergency surgical issues that occur in transplanted patients is similar to that in the general community. The presentation of emergency surgical issues can differ in immunosuppressed patients compared with the general population in that immunosuppression can mask the symptoms and signs of diseases, particularly those that are infective in nature. In addition, infective processes can have a poorer outcome in immunosuppressed patients.

The preoperative work-up of a transplant patient should occur in similar fashion to any other surgical patient. However, immunosuppression and indications for transplantation mean that there is an increased risk of diabetes mellitus, hyperlipidaemia and cardiovascular disease, including hypertension and ischaemic heart disease, in transplant recipients which will require appropriate preoperative assessment, potentially including cardiological investigations.

There is no evidence to suggest that transplant recipients have bacterial agents that are different to non-immunosuppressed patients and the antibiotic prophylaxis that is appropriate to the case should be used. However, given the predisposition to infection in the immunosuppressed population, prophylactic antibiotics should be given even in clean cases, in which they would not normally be used. The choice of prophylactic antibiotic should be that which would normally be used for the case. As with operations performed in patients who are not immunosuppressed, prophylactic antibiotics should be given prior to skin incision. Although the risk of a perioperative hypotensive crisis in patients who have been on long-term steroid therapy is low (approximately 1%), it is appropriate to provide steroid cover over the perioperative period.

The position of the transplanted organ and vascular grafts may be of importance in some forms of surgery. Transplanted kidneys are generally extraperitoneal and therefore not usually at physical risk in a laparotomy, but transplanted pancreata (and the kidneys in the case of pancreas–kidney transplantation) are intraperitoneal and consideration will need to be given to this fact in planning intraabdominal surgery. The transplant unit will be in a position to provide advice in these circumstances. Conversely, operations involving the abdominal wall of the iliac fossa or groin, iliac vessels or bladder will potentially put a transplanted kidney at risk of physical injury.

Further reading

Alexander S, Hirst K (eds) *41st Annual ANZDATA Report*. Adelaide, Australia: Australia and New Zealand Dialysis and Transplant Registry, 2018. Available at https://www.anzdata.org.au/report/anzdata-41st-annual-report-2018-anzdata/

Forsythe JLR (ed.) *Transplantation*, 5th edn. Philadelphia: Saunders Elsevier, 2014.

Keogh A, Williams T, Pettersson R (eds) *ANZCOTR Report 2018*. Sydney, Australia: Australia and New Zealand Cardiothoracic Organ Transplant Registry, 2018. Available at http://www.anzcotr.org.au/pub/e0cc941a/PDFS/ANZCOTR2018_text.pdf

Lynch SV, Balderson GA (eds) *ANZLT Registry Report 2016*. Brisbane, Australia: Australia and New Zealand Liver Transplant Registry, 2016. Available at https://www3.anzltr.org/wp-content/uploads/Reports/28thReport.pdf

Webster AC, Hedley J, Kelly PJ (eds) *ANZIPTR Report 2017*. Sydney, Australia: Australian and New Zealand Islet and Pancreas Transplant Registry, 2019. Available at http://anziptr.org/wp content/uploads/2019/06/ANZIPTR-Annual-Report-2019.pdf

MCQs

Select the single correct answer to each question. The correct answers can be found in the Answers section at the end of the book.

1 A 48-year-old man is in the intensive care unit after a brainstem stroke. Brainstem reflex testing reveals absence of pain response in the trigeminal distribution and lack of the pupillary, corneal, vestibulo-ocular, gag and cough reflexes. An apnoea test is performed, with disconnection of the endotracheal tube from the ventilator. After 4 minutes, a breath is taken. This patient could become a deceased organ donor if:
  a he had registered as an organ donor
  a his family agrees to proceed
  a donation occurs following a DCD pathway
  b there is a patient urgently awaiting transplantation
  c he has no history of infection or cancer

2 Cell-mediated rejection following liver transplantation:
  a occurs less frequently in the presence of microchimerism
  b occurs more frequently than following transplantation of other organs
  c occurs less frequently than antibody-mediated rejection
  d is characterised by deposition of C4d which can be demonstrated on a liver biopsy
  e does not usually require modification of immunosuppression

3 In Australia and New Zealand, living donor kidney transplantation:
  a is performed most commonly for diabetic nephropathy
  b accounts for approximately 10% of all kidney transplants
  c has results that are slightly inferior to deceased donor kidney transplantation
  d can only be performed between donors and recipients who have a close personal or genetic relationship
  e has a 5-year graft survival of approximately 90%

4 A 52-year-old brain-dead potential donor is known to be a man who has sex with men. Transplantation of organs from this donor:
  a cannot occur under any circumstances
  b can be considered if the donor serology is negative
  c can be considered if the donor nucleic acid testing is negative
  d can occur if condoms had been used during sexual intercourse
  e can occur without the need for further testing

11 Principles of surgical oncology

G. Bruce Mann[1,2] *and Robert J.S. Thomas*[1]

[1] University of Melbourne, Melbourne, Victoria, Australia
[2] Victorian Comprehensive Cancer Centre, Melbourne, Victoria, Australia

Introduction

Surgical oncology focuses on the surgical management of tumours, especially cancerous tumours. Surgical oncology embraces cancer care in a multi-disciplinary framework, internationally recognised as the standard of care for patients with cancer. This relies on coordination of surgery with medical and radiation oncologists, diagnostic specialties such as pathology and radiology, together with input from cancer nurses, allied health disciplines and palliative care specialists.

Surgical resection of cancers remains the cornerstone of treatment for many types of cancer. Historically, surgery was the only effective form of cancer treatment, but developments in radiation therapy and systemic therapies mean that optimal outcomes require multidisciplinary treatment planning and delivery in a team-based approach.

Surgery plays various key roles in cancer care. Determining what role surgery has in a particular situation depends on accurate definition of the problem via preoperative staging investigations and multidisciplinary treatment planning. It is sometimes needed for diagnosis, is effective for various premalignant conditions or *in situ* malignancies and is a central part of treatment for most localised malignancies. Its role in metastatic disease is limited, most often used when surgery can provide effective palliation by either treating or preventing a specific local problem.

Communication with the patient and family, the obtaining of informed consent and the careful, honest, realistic but where possible optimistic explanation of the results of surgery are all matters of high importance to all surgical practice. However, the ability to talk sympathetically to cancer patients and their families is particularly important in the field of surgical oncology.

Clinical trials are required to evaluate new treatments and treatment combinations. There has been a huge amount of basic cancer research that continues to provide new insights. Translating these basic findings into clinically meaningful management is a major challenge and is a key aspect of the discipline of surgical oncology.

Multidisciplinary care

All clinical disciplines involved in cancer care must understand the principles and practical consequences of the treatment offered by surgeons, radiation oncologists, medical oncologists and the allied health disciplines in order to be able to work in a team to care for cancer patients.

Radiation oncology

Radiation therapy may be delivered alone with curative intent in some cancers, as an adjuvant therapy to reduce the risk of recurrence in many situations, and frequently as a palliative treatment, for example of painful bony metastases in breast and prostate cancer. Effective symptom relief is often achieved with the use of radiation therapy.

Radiation oncology involves the use of ionising radiation to selectively kill tumour cells. Radiation kills living cells by both direct DNA damage and the formation of free oxygen radicals in the cells. Free radical formation is the predominant effect and depends on the level of oxygenation of the tissue.

Ionising radiation is usually delivered to tumours as external beam therapy, generated by linear accelerators. When a linear accelerator is used to supply external beam therapy to a tumour, the patient goes through a series of planning exercises to accurately delineate the tumour and direct the radiation as

Textbook of Surgery, Fourth Edition. Edited by Julian A. Smith, Andrew H. Kaye, Christopher Christophi and Wendy A. Brown.
© 2020 John Wiley & Sons Ltd. Published 2020 by John Wiley & Sons Ltd.

accurately as possible to the tumour to minimise the impact on normal tissues.

An alternative method of administration of radiation is by using a local radiation source applied close to the tumour. This is known as brachytherapy. It is a highly effective form of therapy in tumours such as cervical cancer, other gynaecological cancers and prostate cancer.

Both normal and neoplastic cells are affected by radiation, so the dose which can be given in any situation is limited by the tolerance of the surrounding normal tissues. Tissues particularly at risk include the bone marrow and gastrointestinal tract, which contain rapidly dividing cells. The spinal cord is also at risk as it does not have repair mechanisms able to manage radiation-induced injury.

Normal tissues can recover from radiation provided the dose is not extreme, while malignant cells repair such damage less well. Fractionation of radiation, splitting the total dose into multiple daily low doses, allows normal tissues to recover better between doses than cancerous cells or tissues, allowing better selectivity of the impact of radiation.

Medical oncology

While surgery and radiotherapy are 'local' treatments – they have their impact by treating the tissues that are removed or radiated – many cancers have disseminated around the body at the time of diagnosis. 'Systemic' treatments are needed to address these, and it is improvements in systemic therapy of cancers that have had the biggest impact on outcomes over the last 20 years.

Medical oncologists use a variety of agents to modify tumour growth. Many of these are cytotoxic chemotherapy drugs that are toxic to dividing cells; others are endocrine therapies that target the cellular pathways related to hormones (tamoxifen and the aromatase inhibitors in breast cancer are the best examples of these), while others are 'biological' therapies that have been developed to modify some aspect of cellular function or to modify the immune response to a cancer.

Some cancers can be cured with systemic therapy alone. Many lymphomas and other haematological cancers, and some testicular tumours are such examples. However, these are the exceptions and for most solid tumours systemic treatment alone produces a limited or partial response.

Many randomised controlled clinical trials have demonstrated a survival benefit from the use of chemotherapy and other systemic therapies when given as either neoadjuvant (preoperatively) or adjuvant (postoperative) therapy. Adjuvant therapy is treatment given in the absence of known disseminated disease in order to reduce the risk of subsequent emergence of metastatic disease. Breast cancer and colon cancer are two cancers where landmark clinical trials have demonstrated significant improvement in survival with the use of adjuvant systemic therapy. Subsequently, effective adjuvant systemic therapy has become available for a wide variety of cancers.

In cases of disseminated disease where cure is not generally possible, systemic therapy usually forms the basis of treatment, with surgery and radiotherapy used to address specific problems.

Supportive care

The holistic approach to the care of the cancer patient encompasses a range of supportive and coordinating services through the treatment phases. This is often delivered by a range of nursing and allied health professionals. Psychosocial support includes investigation and treatment of cancer patients by suitably trained nursing staff, social workers, psychologists and psychiatrists. Each discipline can offer some support depending on the problem faced by the cancer patient. A nurse coordinator often aids in the management of the patient. The use of such professionals has been shown to improve outcomes for cancer patients.

Survivorship

Survivorship is a concept that has become prominent over recent years. As the incidence of cancer has increased along with the ageing population, and cure rates for common cancers have increased, there is an increasing number of people who have apparently been cured but are left with uncertainty regarding the chance that the cancer will recur, and may be suffering morbidity from the cancer and/or its treatment. These issues should be directly addressed at the end of active treatment, where patients are ready to move to a long-term follow-up phase of care. General practitioners and other primary care practitioners are well placed to manage many of these issues.

Palliative care

Modern palliative care programs are part of the services offered to cancer patients in whom cure is not possible. These services include ambulatory and hospice programs for management of the end stages of life when attempts to cure or actively treat the cancer have ceased. Physical and psychological symptom control is an important part of modern multidisciplinary care. Palliative care physicians also help in pain control and symptom control in the earlier stages of the illness and thus broaden their influence in the journey of the patient with cancer. Early involvement of palliative care has been shown to improve both the quality and also the length of life of many cancer patients.

Principles of surgery for malignant disease

The principles involve screening and diagnosis, assessment of the patient, staging of the extent of cancer, decisions about treatment by the multidisciplinary team, principles of operative surgical oncology, rehabilitation and follow-up. Each of these will be dealt with in turn.

Screening and diagnosis of malignant disease

Screening

Randomised controlled trials of population screening have shown survival benefit in a number of diseases. For screening to be effective, the test must be able to detect a common cancer at a stage where treatment is more effective than treatment given when a cancer becomes symptomatic. The test must be sensitive, specific and acceptable to the public.

The most effective screening program has been cervical screening where, since its introduction, there has been a substantial fall in mortality from cervical cancer in all age groups. Recently, the Pap smear is being replaced by an assay for human papillomavirus (HPV), and this should dramatically improve the already very good outcomes. Similar less dramatic effects are seen with breast cancer screening by mammography and colon cancer screening using faecal occult blood testing and follow-up colonoscopy.

Population screening for prostate cancer using prostate-specific antigen (PSA) testing remains controversial due to the potential morbidity of prostate cancer treatment, and the inability to distinguish indolent from aggressive cancers. As these problems are addressed, evidence around an optimal approach to prostate cancer screening is likely to emerge.

Diagnosis

A tissue diagnosis is essential prior to the creation of a management plan for a cancer patient. The consequences of many cancer treatments are so severe that only rarely can treatment be commenced without a pathological diagnosis. Tissue is obtained by fine-needle aspiration, core biopsy or excisional biopsy.

Percutaneous biopsy

Fine-needle aspiration cytology and core biopsy can be done on an outpatient basis and provides a rapid diagnosis of accessible lesions such as breast lumps, head and neck lymph nodes and thyroid swellings. Ultrasound guidance for the biopsy needle is necessary and commonly used; CT or MRI guidance may also be used. Endoscopic biopsy is the basis of most diagnoses of upper and lower gastrointestinal cancers and lung cancer.

All these techniques rely on the expertise of the pathologist to make a definite diagnosis on the basis of either the cytological or histological characteristics of the tumour, supplemented by a variety of immunohistochemical assays to accurately define the tissue of origin and assess its likely natural history and response to particular treatments.

Excisional biopsy

Where a local mass or skin lesion can be completely excised without significant morbidity, excisional biopsy is the treatment of choice, removing the problem at the same time as making the diagnosis. This technique is commonly used for skin lesions, particularly suspected squamous cell carcinoma, basal cell carcinoma and melanoma.

Sometimes excisional biopsy (or incisional, where not all the lesion is removed) of a deeper lesion is required when attempts to reach a diagnosis in a less invasive manner have failed or are too dangerous, or when the lesion should be removed for cosmetic or other reasons.

Assessment of the patient

An important early part of the assessment of a patient with cancer is to determine health and fitness and ability to tolerate various treatments with acceptable risk of complications. Many cancer treatments are demanding on the physical and psychological resources of the patient. An idea of the 'health' of the patient can be gained from a simple clinical assessment, the Eastern Cooperative Oncology Group (ECOG) performance status, with more complex assessments needed prior to more intense treatments.

Staging of malignant disease

Accurate staging of the extent of disease is of great importance in formulating a treatment plan. Clinical stage is that defined by clinical examination and imaging of the patient. High-quality imaging has led to improved accuracy of clinical staging. Pathological staging is that defined after excisional surgery.

The most commonly used staging system is the TNM (tumour, nodes, metastases) system. The AJCC (American Joint Committee on Cancer) defines the TNM staging for all cancers. Suffixes to the T, N and M indicate the size of the tumour and extent of nodal disease or metastases. For example, T2N1M0 indicates the stage of a tumour, for example carcinoma of the colon where the tumour has spread into the muscularis propria but not through the wall of the colon (T2) and where there are adjacent lymph nodes involved (N1) but no metastases detected (M0). Combinations of T and N stages are grouped into overall stages with similar prognoses, ranging from stage 0, indicating premalignant disease (e.g. ductal carcinoma *in situ* of the breast) to stage IV, indicating metastatic disease. The staging system varies dramatically according to the primary site of the tumour.

Recommendations about treatment: the multidisciplinary meeting

Armed with information about the diagnosis of the cancer, the extent of the disease and the fitness of the patient, recommendations and decisions can be made about the most appropriate treatment program. Consultation with a multidisciplinary team may occur prior to surgery; however, if the decision regarding surgery is straightforward, the multidisciplinary meeting may occur after surgery when full pathological information is available. However, many cancers may benefit from down-staging with radiotherapy or chemotherapy prior to surgery, and early multidisciplinary consultations are important to facilitate this process.

Principles of operative surgical oncology

The technical issues in surgical oncology are no different from other surgical interventions. Open surgery, laparoscopic surgery, robotic surgery, ablative interventions and other technical interventions all have a place in modern surgical oncology. However, some important oncological principles exist which must be followed by the surgeon for a satisfactory outcome.

Definition of curative surgery

So-called curative surgery generally involves an apparent total excision of the tumour. The primary tumour and the associated lymph node drainage fields are often excised where nodal involvement is known, suspected or reasonably likely.

A measure of the adequacy of the oncological surgical operation is demonstrated by the findings on pathological examination of the specimen. Standards exist for ensuring the adequacy of the surgical excision to be assessed in many tumours. The operative specimens need to be correctly orientated by the surgeon to allow the pathologist to carefully examine and interpret the specimen. The key issues are usually:

- the precise histopathology of the cancer, including relevant tumour markers
- whether the margins of the specimen removed are clear of tumour
- the total number of lymph nodes excised and the number of involved nodes.

A major focus of modern cancer surgery has been the preservation of function. Improved surgical techniques and effective use of multidisciplinary treatment has resulted in diminished morbidity of major cancer surgery. Examples of this include larynx-preserving treatment for head and neck cancer, limb-sparing surgery for soft tissue sarcoma and sphincter-sparing treatment for rectal cancer.

Margins of surgical excision

The degree to which normal tissues should be removed with the primary tumour is a subject constantly being researched. A universal rule is not possible to formulate. The principle of complete local excision with an adequate margin is paramount in surgical oncology and many trials have helped clarify what 'adequate' means. It varies significantly according to the cancer, its natural history and the availability of effective adjuvant therapies.

Lymph node resection

Traditionally, the draining lymph nodes from a primary tumour were excised with the cancer. The main benefit of this removal is improved prognostic information, which may affect the decisions regarding postoperative adjuvant therapy. In some situations there may be a local control or survival benefit from removal of early-involved lymph nodes.

The extent of lymph node surgery has reduced over recent decades. This is partly due to the recognition that prophylactic excision of uninvolved nodes does not provide a survival advantage to the patient and exposes the patient to increased morbidity from the node removal. It is also due to the introduction of lymphatic mapping and sentinel node biopsy, where the first draining lymph node can be identified and removed, giving prognostic information without a great risk of morbidity, and allowing better informed decisions regarding further nodal surgery.

Palliative surgery

Palliative surgery aims to improve quality of life by either preventing or avoiding some symptom-producing consequence of the tumour by resection or bypass. This is done even though a cure is known to be impossible. Examples include the following.

- In the case of pyloric obstruction from an advanced cancer of the stomach, a gastrojejunostomy may provide good palliation of vomiting.
- Resection of a bleeding cancer of the colon is justified even in the presence of metastases.

Many other examples exist. 'Tailoring' this type of surgery to the needs of the patient without undue morbidity is an important role for an oncological surgeon.

Follow-up of patient after initial treatment program

A program of follow-up is required for cancer patients after their initial treatment. This is for two main reasons. The first is to monitor and investigate when appropriate to detect recurrent disease. In general, early diagnosis of symptomatic recurrence is appropriate, as it allows the most effective palliative treatment. Whether imaging to detect asymptomatic recurrent disease is appropriate depends on whether there is treatment for the recurrence that is more effective in the asymptomatic phase. Early detection of liver metastases after colorectal cancer treatment is appropriate, as cure may be possible when appropriately staged patients with liver metastases are successfully resected. On the other hand, detection of asymptomatic breast cancer metastases has not been shown to be beneficial, and therefore routine surveillance CT and bone scans are not done. However, screening for asymptomatic new primary cancers is performed.

The second reason for follow-up is that it provides an opportunity to identify and manage side effects of the disease and its treatment and to support the patient psychologically. Increasingly, it is recognised that severe psychological morbidity may exist in cancer patients who have been treated, even if the cancer is apparently cured. This has led to a developing interest in the concept of survivorship – understanding the needs of the 'cured' cancer patient. Psychosocial support is essential for many cancer patients and is best delivered in the setting of multidisciplinary care.

Clinical trials and research

Clinical research is essential for evaluating new and previously untested treatments. Surgeons are involved in a number of ways:

- Provision of tissue for tissue banking. This is a fast-growing program throughout the world. The provision of fresh tissues for genetic studies is of paramount importance to the understanding of malignant disease. Collection of accurate clinical data to accompany the tissue is valuable.
- Surgeons design, implement and run clinical trials to assess new surgical approaches to cancer. The recruiter for randomised clinical trials must have equipoise in relation to the arms of the study and be able to assure the patient that there is no reason why he or she should not enter the trial, as current knowledge does not suggest that one or other arm is clearly 'better'.

Conclusion

The surgeon operating on cancer patients in the twenty-first century must have a deep understanding of the malignant process, be prepared to work as part of a team and offer multidisciplinary care, communicate well, operate with a high level of skill, help the patient rehabilitate from the treatment and finally be involved in the advancing area of surgical science as applied to cancer care.

Further reading

Cancer Australia. All about multidisciplinary care. https://canceraustralia.gov.au/clinical-best-practice/multidisciplinary-care/all-about-multidisciplinary-care

Feig BW (ed.) *The MD Anderson Surgical Oncology Handbook*, 6th edn. Philadelphia: Wolters Kluwer, 2019.

Morita SY, Balch CM, Klimberg VS, Pawlik TM, Posner MC, Tanabe KK (eds) *Textbook of Complex General Surgical Oncology*. New York: McGraw-Hill Education, 2018.

MCQs

Select the single correct answer to each question. The correct answers can be found in the Answers section at the end of the book.

1 Screening for malignant disease is *not* effective in which of the following situations?
   a where a tumour is detected at a stage where it can be cured by treatment

   b screening is undertaken on an individual patient basis

   c there is high public acceptance of the process

   d specificity of screening is high

   e sensitivity of screening is high

2 Which of the following statements in relation to regional lymph node dissection at the time of primary tumour excision is *incorrect*?

   a allows more accurate tumour staging

   b allows provision of appropriate prognosis to the patient

   c can be undertaken with little morbidity

   d allows appropriate adjuvant treatment to be undertaken

   e may confer a survival advantage

3 What is adjuvant therapy in the setting of cancer treatment?

   a treatment given to relieve symptoms of the disease

   b treatment given if a cancer cannot be resected

   c treatment given in the absence of known disease to reduce the risk of recurrence

   d treatment of non-cancer conditions in patients with cancer

   e treatment that has few side effects

4 What are the objectives of ongoing consultations once cancer therapy has been delivered?

   a to check for the presence of local recurrences

   b to assess for late effects of anticancer treatment

   c to check for evidence of distance recurrence

   d to provide supportive care

   e all of the above

12 Introduction to the operating theatre

*Andrew Danks[1], Alan C. Saunder[2]
and Julian A. Smith[3]*

[1,2,3] Monash University, Victoria, Australia; [1] Department of Neurosurgery, [2] Surgery and
Interventional Services Program, and [3] Department of Cardiothoracic Surgery, Monash Health,
Clayton, Victoria, Australia

> Surgery has been made safe for the patient; let us
> now make the patient safe for surgery.
>
> *Lord Moynihan of Leeds (1865–1936)*

Introduction

The operating theatre is a complex clinical environment where the care of the surgical patient is facilitated by the coordination and coalescence of many crucial factors. Depending on the healthcare facility that the operating theatre is in, the operating theatre deals with a broad spectrum of procedures, from the very simple to extraordinarily complex, multi-team, high-technology operations, in both planned and emergency situations. In order to facilitate this, there is effectively an inner sanctum or immediate direct operating team that includes the patient, surgeon, surgical assistants, anaesthetists, nursing staff and theatre technicians (i.e. those in the operating theatre).

Supporting the direct operating team, there is a complex network outside the operating theatre but essential to the conduct and successful completion of safe surgery. This network includes the central sterile and supply department (CSSD), the ward staff preparing the patient for surgery and caring for the patient postoperatively, the suppliers of essential equipment, imaging resources and pathology back-up, as well as hospital administrators.

From the patient's perspective there is a feeling of approach–avoidance ambivalence. The 'approach' element is the patient's need to have their clinical problem rectified, whilst the 'avoidance' reflects the normal fear of the unknown, possible pain, complications and even mortality. This ambivalence over whether one should or should not proceed is based rationally on the perceived risks and benefits of the operation, but the influence of multiple emotional and experiential factors may be more powerful for many people. These aspects may be optimised by a caring and expert assessment and professional behaviours by the preoperative team.

From the surgical team's perspective, there is the opportunity to work together to rectify the surgical problem that the patient is suffering from. Specifically, for surgeons there is the opportunity to practise and employ the full array of skills that they have developed during their training, such as those described by the Royal Australasian College of Surgeons (RACS) competencies (see Box 12.1).

From the anaesthetist's point of view, there is the challenge of safely inducing, maintaining and awaking the patient from anaesthesia by applying the pharmaco-physiological knowledge and skills that they possess.

Nursing staff are involved in both the anaesthetic and surgical teams. Their specialised skills and training are vital to the smooth conduct of all operative procedures.

The theatre technical staff are crucial for safe patient transport, positioning and ensuring that all appropriate equipment is available and safely functional for the planned procedure.

All these groups must work together as a team, each bringing their unique skill sets together in a coordinated, collaborative and respectful way to facilitate the patient's care. Appropriate and effective professional behaviour is essential for creating and maintaining a functional team. Respect for each member of the theatre team is invaluable and the common courtesy of saying 'please' and 'thank you' is a powerful factor in enhancing respect and

Textbook of Surgery, Fourth Edition. Edited by Julian A. Smith, Andrew H. Kaye, Christopher Christophi and Wendy A. Brown.
© 2020 John Wiley & Sons Ltd. Published 2020 by John Wiley & Sons Ltd.

developing trust in each other. Despite this, emotions may run high under the pressure of surgery. This may lead to behaviours which may in turn be counterproductive rather than improving a tense situation. Appropriate training may help practitioners to adapt to these challenges more effectively.

The operating theatre is an excellent venue for teaching and training in all professional disciplines. It is important that students and junior staff have access to this environment to develop their understanding of surgery and anaesthesia. However, there needs to be careful supervision in order to maintain patient safety. Ultimately, the safety of the patient is of paramount importance throughout any visit to the operating theatre.

In this chapter, we consider an overview of each component that contributes to the patient's journey in the operating theatre under the broad headings of the operating theatre and the direct patient care team, followed by the important role of the indirect support staff and systems to support care in the operating theatre.

The operating theatre (the 'inner sanctum')

The fundamental goal of the modern operating theatre is the establishment of a safe and appropriate environment for effective and safe surgery. Surgery is potentially very dangerous. Key dangers include excessive bleeding, damage to vital organs, failure to achieve the goals of the operation, poor wound healing, surgical site infection (SSI) or other infections, venous thromboembolism, fluid imbalance and other concerns.

A central concept is the creation of a *sterile field* to provide the safest access to the part of the body to be operated upon in such a way that the risk of SSI is minimised. It must be the focus of all contributors to the inner sanctum that an appropriate sterile field is established, protected and maintained

during any operative procedure. The creation and maintenance of a sterile field is discussed in this section, which also describes important factors relating to each member of the inner sanctum that enhance the chance of a satisfactory outcome from the planned surgery. Professional communication and the important issue of occupational safety for the theatre team are also covered.

As a general point, it is ideal to have a separate preparation room for the scrub team to set up the instruments on sterile trolleys, and another separate room for the preparation of the patient for anaesthesia.

Patient

Patient preparation is essential to safe surgery (see also Chapter 1). There are many aspects to this. The first step is the establishment of the correct diagnosis or diagnostic possibilities, and the choice of the correct operative strategy. During this process, a therapeutic relationship must be established between the surgeon and/or the surgical team and the patient (and their relatives). Special tests or preparations may be required to clarify the diagnosis and to further assess the condition. The patient's overall medical condition must be assessed and optimised. Some patients may not be fit enough for the first-line surgical option, so alternatives may need to be considered.

Once the surgical plan has been established, it is necessary that the patient understands the diagnosis and its implications, the risks and benefits of the planned procedure, and alternative treatments including non-operative options. It is important that this information is conveyed in their usual language with appropriate support available. This process is termed achieving *informed consent*. Consent must be clearly documented, both for legal reasons and to facilitate safe 'time-out' procedures (see section Surgeon). In the elective situation, it is necessary that this consent is achieved prior to attendance at the operating theatre. In truly urgent situations, consent may be waived if it is genuinely in the patient's best interest. However, it is always best that the patient and relatives understand as much as possible, even in an emergency. The comprehensive approach to gaining an informed consent can be achieved by describing the planned procedure, its goals and expected outcome, and embellishing it along the lines of the mnemonic SCAR:

S   Side effects
C   Complications
A   Alternatives
R   Risks

A patient information brochure for the specific operation (Figure 12.1) may be an invaluable aid to

ROYAL AUSTRALASIAN COLLEGE OF SURGEONS
THE AUSTRALIAN AND NEW ZEALAND SOCIETY OF CARDIAC AND THORACIC SURGEONS

CORONARY ARTERY BYPASS GRAFT SURGERY
A guide for patients

The Coronary Arteries

As the work of pumping blood requires a lot of energy, the heart has its own source of blood to distribute oxygen and nutrients throughout the heart muscle.

Blood is pumped to the heart muscle through the two main coronary arteries (left coronary artery and right coronary artery) that branch from the aorta and run over the surface of the heart, as shown in the illustration (right).

The left coronary artery and the right coronary artery give rise to many other smaller branches that carry blood deep into the heart muscle.

Coronary Artery Disease

As people age, the walls of coronary arteries often develop deposits of a fatty substance called plaque. This process is called coronary artery disease or atherosclerosis. If enough plaque is formed, blood flow through the artery will decrease significantly. Low blood flow through one or more coronary arteries can lead to recurrent chest pains (angina).

A heart attack occurs when blood flow in a coronary artery stops due to a clot that forms over the plaque. This can result in permanent damage to the heart.

Coronary Artery Bypass Grafts

When a coronary artery becomes too narrowed with plaque, it can be treated surgically by using another blood vessel to deliver blood beyond the narrowing. Such a vessel is called a graft. The procedure is called coronary artery bypass graft (CABG) surgery.

CABG surgery is an effective treatment that has been performed in millions of patients over the past 40 years. It has become a common procedure and is the most common heart surgery performed in Australia, New Zealand and other Western countries.

Outcomes for this operation in Australia and New Zealand are among the best in the world.

By restoring good blood flow to the heart, CABG surgery can stop or ease angina, improve exercise capability, and prolong life.

Improvements in surgical methods, anaesthesia and care after surgery have allowed treatment of older and sicker patients who previously would not have been eligible for a CABG procedure.

Illustration of heart showing Aorta, Right coronary artery, Left coronary artery

THE PROCESS OF CORONARY ARTERY DISEASE (ATHEROSCLEROSIS)

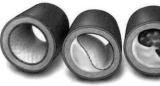

In a normal coronary artery, the inside surface is smooth.

Plaque has developed inside this coronary artery.

The coronary artery is totally blocked with plaque and a blood clot.

Common Grafts

The use of one to six grafts is common. More grafts may be required in some patients.

Grafts may be arteries or veins. The most common grafts are:

- internal thoracic (mammary) arteries from the chest wall
- radial artery from the forearm
- saphenous vein from the leg.

See page three for more information about the types of grafts.

TALK TO YOUR HEART SURGEON

This pamphlet is intended to provide you with general information. It is not a substitute for advice from your heart surgeon and does not contain all the known facts about CABG surgery or every possible complication.

It is important that you have enough information about the surgery to enable you to compare the benefits and risks. If you are not sure about the benefits, risks and limitations of treatment, the terms used in this pamphlet, or anything else, ask your surgeon.

Read all the information in this pamphlet, and save it for reference. Technical terms are used that may require further explanation by your surgeon. Write down questions you want to ask, and discuss them with your surgeon. You are encouraged to fully discuss with your surgeon:

- the surgery to be done and why
- the alternatives to surgery
- the outcome you can expect.

This pamphlet should only be used in consultation with your surgeon.

IMPORTANT: Fill in all details on the sticker below.

DEAR SURGEON: When you discuss this pamphlet with your patient, remove this sticker and put it on the patient's medical history or card. This will remind you and the patient that this pamphlet has been provided. Some surgeons ask their patients to sign the sticker to confirm receipt of the pamphlet.

TREATMENT INFORMATION PAMPHLET

PROCEDURE:...

PATIENT'S NAME:...

DOCTOR'S NAME:...

EDITION NUMBER:.......DATE: (day)..............(month)...........(year)..........

Edition number: 3

Consumer and carer feedback: To provide feedback about this pamphlet, send comments to: feedback@mitec.com.au or by post to Mi-tec, PO Box 24, Camberwell, VIC, 3124, Australia

Fig. 12.1 Sample pages from a patient information brochure for coronary artery bypass grafting.

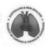

ROYAL AUSTRALASIAN COLLEGE OF SURGEONS

THE AUSTRALIAN AND NEW ZEALAND SOCIETY OF CARDIAC AND THORACIC SURGEONS

Possible Complications of CABG Surgery

As with all surgical procedures, CABG does have risks, despite the highest standards of practice. While your surgeon makes every attempt to minimise risks, complications can occur. Some may have permanent effects.

It is not usual for a surgeon to outline every possible or rare complication of the operation. However, it is important you have enough information to fully weigh up the benefits and risks of surgery. Most people having surgery will not have a complication, but if you have concerns about possible side effects, discuss them with your surgeon.

The following possible complications are listed to inform and not to alarm. There may be others that are not listed.

General risks of surgery

● All surgery has a risk of infection, which can occur some days or weeks after the operation. Infection can usually be treated effectively with antibiotics.

● A blood clot may form in a deep vein, most often in the leg or thigh (deep venous thrombosis). This can be life threatening and requires treatment.

● Most incisions heal well, but a few people develop raised or widened scars. Wound infection or areas of movement increase the risk of adverse scarring.

Specific risks of CABG surgery

● The mortality in Australia and New Zealand is about one or two patients per 100 CABG procedures. However, the risk of not having the surgery can be associated with a higher risk of dying. The risk of death or serious complications increases with increasing age, other serious illnesses, heart damage, urgency of operation, and recurrent surgery.

● The risk of stroke or a cerebrovascular accident increases significantly with age and disease of the aorta, but is an uncommon complication. The effects of stroke may be temporary and resolve over a few days, or may be permanent and include:

■ loss of feeling or sensation in a part of the body
■ speech difficulty
■ visual disturbances
■ paralysis of one side of the body or arm or leg (the paralysis may be complete or partial).

Most people with stroke related to

CABG surgery will require some degree of rehabilitation.

● Treatment of infections of the breastbone usually require re-hospitalisation, prolonged administration of antibiotics and often surgery.

● Uncommonly, the incision in the breastbone may not heal normally. This is more likely following protracted coughing after surgery. In some cases, the wire sutures in the breastbone may pull out. Some patients may need to have further surgery to repair the breastbone. This complication can also be caused by infection of the breastbone.

● This is the most common complication. About five patients in 100 require further surgery to control excessive blood loss. In most cases, this resolves well with no further adverse effects.

● The most common arrhythmia (irregular heart beats) postoperatively is atrial fibrillation. It can affect up to one in three patients in the first week. It is usually treated with medication. Occasional extra beats are common and not a cause for concern. Uncommonly, a serious irregular rhythm can occur and may need an electrical shock to correct. If you feel palpitations after you go home, tell your cardiologist. If palpitations do not subside after a few minutes or if you are feeling unwell or dizzy, call an ambulance.

● A graft may not successfully bypass a narrowing or blockage. The graft may become blocked with a blood clot, leading to a heart attack after surgery.

● Even if a graft does not fail, occasionally heart damage or a heart attack can occur.

● It is common for patients to have some anxiety and loss of confidence related to their heart and general health. This usually improves during the weeks following surgery.

● Removal of the radial artery may cause temporary sensations of numbness and tingling at the back of the thumb near the wrist. Hand function is not affected.

● Removal of the saphenous vein may cause swelling and aching of the legs. Special stockings may reduce the swelling. Small nerves near the vein may be injured, resulting in decreased sensation or skin numbness in the affected leg.

Some patients report that they have more pain and discomfort from the leg wound than the chest wound.

● Many patients have some impairment of short-term memory, difficulty with concentration and reading, and visual blurring. As such symptoms usually occur during the first few weeks, driving is not allowed for four to six weeks after CABG. It not unusual for six to nine months to pass before symptoms resolve completely.

● Persistent pain from the healing breastbone and ribs may occur.

● Other risks: Although uncommon, numerous other risks of CABG surgery exist, including:

■ temporary or permanent kidney failure
■ respiratory failure and the need for a tracheostomy
■ blood infection
■ permanent pacemaker due to changes in heart rhythm
■ accumulation of fluid around the heart and in lung cavities that may require further drainage
■ accumulation of air in the chest (pneumothorax), requiring temporary tube drainage.

● Graft occlusion: Over several years, one or more grafts may become occluded. Coronary artery disease may progress in grafted or ungrafted arteries. Reoperation may be necessary.

REPORT TO MEDICAL STAFF

Tell medical staff at once if you develop any of the following after discharge:

■ fever (more than 38°C) or chills
■ bleeding from the surgical area
■ wound that drains for more than a day
■ increasing pain or redness of a wound
■ any concerns you may have about the surgery.

YOUR SURGEON

Edition number: 3   29/April/2015   Mi-tec Medical Publishing© +61 3 9888 6262   Facsimile +61 3 9888 6465   e-mail: orders@mitec.com.au   online orders: www.mitec.com.au

Fig. 12.1 (Continued)

the consent process. This can help the patient and their family to understand and discuss the forthcoming operative treatment. It may also be valuable in providing some standardisation of the discussion process, and in avoiding the omission of important information.

For planned elective procedures, the patient's comorbidities should be identified and corrected as much as possible so that the patient's general condition is optimised prior to surgery. A simple example of this is the cessation of smoking, ideally for a minimum of 4 weeks prior to the operation, which has been shown to significantly reduce postoperative complications and may lead to the patient stopping smoking altogether. Another critical issue is the management of antithrombotic and antiplatelet agents perioperatively. A targeted history is required to identify these and other health issues that may have an impact on the planned surgery and its conduct.

Careful synthesis of the operative candidate's health and readiness for surgery can be amplified by appropriate investigations, especially in the older patient (>70 years), such as urinalysis, full blood examination, electrocardiogram (ECG), electrolytes, chest X-ray and so on. Subsequently, preoperative assessment may involve other specialties such as cardiologists, diabetic specialists, nephrologists and our allied health colleagues, for example physiotherapists to help with breathing exercises preoperatively. The concept of training the patient to be ready for elective surgery is becoming more popular, so-called 'prehabilitation' that helps to prepare the patient both physically and mentally for the forthcoming operative procedure.

Operating theatre equipment and technical support

Modern surgery frequently requires specific specialised equipment. Good planning and communication is essential in order that the right equipment is available in good working order for the right patient at the right time. This may be challenging to coordinate in busy operating suites where similar procedures are occurring simultaneously, placing conflicting demands on certain pieces of specialised equipment. Awareness of what is required for any particular operation and coordination of theatre lists are important for minimising such conflicts.

There are certain key items common to all theatres, such as operating lights, anaesthetic machines, gas supplies, operating tables, suction, electrocautery and theatre trolleys. Specific items are required for specialty surgery, including simple items such

as a hand table for surgery of this region or a tourniquet for many orthopaedic limb operations, through to more complex devices such as cardiopulmonary bypass machines for cardiac surgery, the ultrasonic surgical aspirator for hepatic and neurosurgical resections, and operating microscopes for the most delicate work.

The value of experienced well-trained theatre technicians cannot be underestimated in contributing to the care of the patient from the perspective of equipment provision. They also play a key role in transferring and positioning the patient for surgery. Patients may be placed in a variety of positions to facilitate their surgery. The theatre technician's knowledge of how to do this well is crucial for the welfare of both the patient and the operating team. Many patients are operated on in the supine position. However, prone, lateral and lithotomy positions are required for certain surgeries, whilst specialised head frames are required for intracranial procedures. Specialised operating tables and add-on components allow for patient positions to be achieved safely, and even allow for changes or adjustment of position intraoperatively. There is a real expertise required to do this. The final responsibility for patient position remains with the surgeon, so careful overview of this aspect is required.

One of the critical aspects of positioning is the avoidance of pressure and traction injuries. Certain pressure points need particular attention, such as the heels in the supine position or the condyles of the ankle in the lateral position. The ulnar nerve posterior to the medial epicondyle of the elbow is particularly vulnerable to pressure, which may result in a disabling tardy ulnar palsy. Likewise, pressure on the head of the fibula may damage the lateral peroneal nerve.

An increasing challenge in this domain is the management of morbidly obese patients who require surgery. Special equipment such as hover mats may be required to move these patients safely without risk to the theatre personnel, as well as specially designed bariatric operating tables to safely cope with the loads involved.

Anaesthetists and anaesthetic care (see also Chapter 3)

Modern anaesthesia is a beautiful blend of knowledge of human physiology and complex pharmacology and its interaction with a complex spectrum of pathology and the challenges created by the surgical procedure. Chapter 3 deals with many aspects of how anaesthetists assess and manage this complex myriad of challenges. Underlying this are essential principles of teamwork within the operating theatre where the anaesthetist is vital.

Once again, excellent communication is fundamental in achieving exemplary teamwork during the patient's journey through theatre. This commences with a thorough assessment of the patient's suitability for operation and the associated risks. This may be summarised in the universal American Society of Anesthesiologists (ASA) scoring system. Flowing on from this is the concept of the patient's potential frailty as judged by their physiological status and whether the planned procedure may indeed be futile. The anaesthetist can make significant contributions to the detailed discussions with the patient, their family, the surgical team and other interested parties about proceeding with surgery, and how this may be done as safely as possible.

Each operating theatre will have an anaesthetic machine with appropriate monitoring equipment, and an anaesthetic trolley with drugs and other equipment. Typically, expiratory carbon dioxide and tissue oxygen saturation (pulse oximetry) are monitored as well as the ECG and normal observations. Temperature monitoring and warming blankets are also important as intraoperative hypothermia has been linked with increased infection rates, as well as slow wakening from anaesthesia.

Drugs of addiction need to be managed specifically to meet legal requirements, so they are securely stored outside the actual operating theatre. Another key role of the anaesthetists intraoperatively is the administration of prophylactic medications, such as antibiotics and thromboprophylaxis as well as therapeutic agents such as heparin or blood products for cardiac and vascular surgeries. The lines of communication between the anaesthetic and surgical teams are critical to the smooth administration of such agents.

Surgical (scrub) and scout (circulating) nurse

For the vast majority of operative procedures, a minimum of two surgical nurses are required. Both are specially trained to work within the theatre environment and must have an exceptional understanding of sterility and the process of establishing a sterile field. The surgical or *scrub* nurse scrubs, gowns and gloves according to the established standards and is in charge of the instruments and disposable items that will be used for the planned operation. The *scout* or circulating nurse is also a trained scrub nurse who opens and provides all the equipment in a sterile fashion to the scrub nurse. The two nurses work as a team within the operating room and require quarantined time and space to do their essential work.

As well as ensuring that all equipment and instruments are sterile and working for the forthcoming operation, the scout and scrub 'count in' all instruments and disposable items before the operation and 'count out' the same items as the operation concludes. It is important that interruptions be minimised during this process, as this is one of the key safety checks of all operative procedures. Obviously, the numbers must match in all categories. An incorrect count at the conclusion of the operation warns the team that an object from the scrub nurse's original count may be still in the patient. This must necessitate a recount, and a search of the operative field and surrounds. If the count is still not correct, the patient must be either re-explored or imaged radiologically to exclude the possibility of a retained instrument or device before they leave the theatre. Once again, good communication is the key to ensuring excellent patient safety.

An easy way to summarise the method for the nursing staff to be maximally effective is to practise the PAP principles of Proper Preparation, Astute Anticipation, and Professional Participation.

An experienced scrub nurse who is well prepared, anticipating the next step in the operation and participating by timely smooth delivery of instruments to the surgical team greatly enhances the efficiency of the procedure and thereby facilitates safe surgery. The scout is his or her supply line for whatever is needed in the sterile field and must adopt a similar attitude of anticipation and participation.

One of the benefits of this approach is the smooth and efficient exchange of instruments and equipment between the surgical team and the scrub nurse. For non-sharps instruments, if the surgeon is clear in his or her request of what is required next, then the scrub nurse should be able to place it in the correct way into the surgeon's hand without the surgeon having to look away from the operative field. Sharp instruments should not be passed hand to hand, but in an appropriate container such that the surgeon picks up the sharp item and after use returns it to the container (Figure 12.2), in order to minimise the risk of injuries.

Surgeon

The surgeon is responsible for the decision to operate, and the preoperative, operative and postoperative management of the patient. This requires many skills, summarised by the nine RACS competencies (Box 12.1). Whilst many tasks are delegated to others, the surgeon is responsible for the overall outcome of the patient and must at all times be an advocate for that patient. Additionally, the surgeon and the anaesthetist are the most highly trained members of the team. At law, the senior doctors are held accountable, in whole or in part, for all aspects of the operation. Therefore, the surgeon must act as leader of the cohesive operative team, in partnership with the anaesthetist.

The surgeon, whether in training and being supervised by a more senior colleague or a specialist, fully trained surgeon, must be able to take charge of the operating team for the commencement and safe conduct of the operation. There are

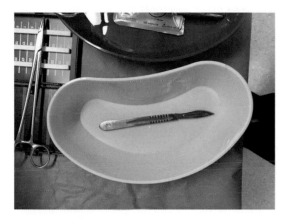

Fig. 12.2 Scalpel in a plastic bowl in readiness for passing to the surgeon.

many ways and idiosyncrasies about how this may occur, which will reflect cultural and societal norms, as well as individual differences in style. In twenty-first century Australia, a collegiate and relatively democratic style is generally optimal in engaging all staff in the team.

An important step in team engagement and a critical element in patient safety is the preoperative *team time-out* (TTO). This is now internationally recognised under the banner of the World Health Organization (WHO) checklist (Figure 12.3). This must be overseen by the operating surgeon. At the simplest level, this aims to ensure that the correct part of the correct patient is to undergo the correct operation at the right time. However, the process extends beyond this to encompass review of critical elements of patient assessment and theatre equipment. Anticipated critical events are anticipated and discussed.

All team members in the inner sanctum of the operating team must participate in the TTO. If any member has concerns, they must feel empowered to voice those concerns with the rest of the team before proceeding to start the operation. Ideally, in order to involve the patient in this crucial step, the TTO should be completed with the patient awake, wherever possible.

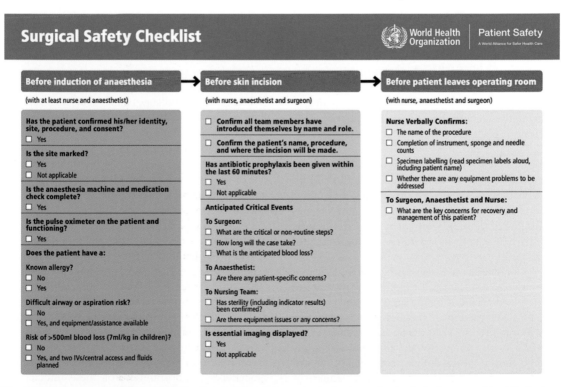

Fig. 12.3 WHO Surgical Safety Checklist. Source: https://www.who.int/patientsafety/topics/safe-surgery/checklist/en/. Reproduced with permission of WHO.

Surgical assistant

Surgical assisting can be one of the most challenging and yet one of the most rewarding activities for medical students, surgical aspirants and trainees. It is also part of the role for senior surgeons mentoring trainees during their training. It is an art of sorts and requires undivided attention to the operation as well as a mindset of 'What can I do to make this operation as straightforward as possible for the operating surgeon?' If the assistant is new to theatre or has not seen the operation before, this can be very difficult, especially if the procedure is not going well (e.g. unexpected bleeding). Timely appropriate questioning can help assisting to be a most rewarding educational experience.

Retraction may be a challenging task for the inexperienced assistant. The goal is to display the anatomy in the best possible way for the surgeon. It is best to maintain the retractor position to the best of one's ability until it is adjusted by the surgeon. Remember that excessive force may cause trauma to the tissues of the patient. It is important to follow the operation, as the required retraction does change as the operation evolves and of course will ultimately be dispensed with as the operation concludes.

Other assisting activities, such as cutting sutures and deploying electrocautery and suction, should be done at the direction of the operating surgeon. In general, dissecting scissors are not used to cut sutures. It is important to develop the habit of cutting with the tips of the scissors to reduce the risk of cutting a vital structure deep to the suture.

Electrocautery involves closure of bleeding points by heat from an electrical current. Monopolar diathermy involves the flow of current from the instrument to the surrounding tissues, then back to the machine via a return plate. Typically, the surgeon will grasp the bleeding point with the tips of a forceps and will ask the assistant to touch the monopolar probe to the forceps and activate the current via a switch. Generally, this contact is best made high on the surgeon's instrument, avoiding the surgeon's line of sight. It is important to listen carefully about when to stop in order to prevent charring of the tissues.

Bipolar diathermy involves the electrical current flowing between the tips of special forceps applied to the bleeding point by the surgeon. The assistant may be asked to activate the circuit via a pedal and may be required to keep the tips moist by application of a small volume of fluid. The goal is to apply enough fluid to allow boiling at the tips of the forceps, avoiding charring or flooding by under- or over-application.

Suction must be done carefully, as excessive suction may traumatise the tissues and cause bleeding or damage to a vital structure. Start gently and listen to the instructions provided. The assistant must avoid blocking the light illuminating the surgical field or obscuring the surgeon's line of sight to the operative field at all times.

It is essential to avoid breaking sterility at any time. Hands should be kept above the waist and below the shoulders, out in front at all times, while avoiding contact with anything non-sterile. If this occurs accidentally, the person responsible should immediately own up and avoid touching the sterile field until the loss of sterility can be rectified.

As one gains more experience, better anticipation and initiative develop. Opportunities to become more 'surgical' readily present themselves to those who continue to show interest in the safe conduct of operative procedures. Preparation of one's skills at workshops and practice of these at quiet times are important in readying oneself for opportunities that may arise to take an important role in surgery. Another important role of the more experienced assistant is that of the co-pilot, supporting and backing up the primary surgeon.

The medical student in the operating suite

Clearly, the work that goes on in the operating suite is central to the care of the surgical patient. Therefore, it is essential that students attend the operating suite to witness a range of surgeries. This is also an excellent environment to learn about sterile practice.

There are challenges in achieving access. Regrettably, there is a relationship between the number of personnel in an operating room and infection rates. Therefore, many theatres will limit the number of observers in the operating room to one or two at any one time. However, most surgical units perform many surgeries per week, so there are always opportunities to observe.

In order to gain a patient-centred understanding of surgery, it is essential that the student understands the patient's illness and indications for surgery before attending. It is necessary to read the notes, and to meet the patient preoperatively. A proper history and examination should be performed. Medical students must be mindful of the nursing and other staff needing to prepare the patient and also to be respectful of the patient and their anxiety about the forthcoming procedure. Nonetheless, opportunities for these interactions are available for the careful and patient student.

Verbal consent for observation should sought from the patient preoperatively.

In the operating theatre, it is necessary to introduce oneself to the surgical team, and request permission to observe the procedure. A balance needs to be found between being involved as closely as possible, whilst not interfering with the safe and efficient conduct of the procedure. Respect for the sterility and safety of the procedure is paramount at all times. It is wise to be prepared to present the patient's clinical details to one's senior colleagues if requested.

Creation and maintenance of a sterile field

The creation and maintenance of a sterile zone for the operation is a fundamental tenet of modern surgery as previously noted. This section covers preoperative preparation, surgical scrubbing, gowning and gloving, skin preparation, draping and protection of the sterile field. These principles apply to all types of wound (see Chapter 6) but may need to be adapted to the particular circumstances.

Preoperative preparation

In some surgical procedures (e.g. cardiac, neurological and prosthetic joint replacement surgeries), the patient's skin flora are a major cause of SSI. The skin cannot be completely sterilised because of the complex adnexal structures (sweat glands, hair follicles and sebaceous glands) and the complex microbiome that inhabits the skin. Normal commensals include potential 'weak' pathogens such as *Propionibacterium*, *Corynebacterium* and *Staphylococcus epidermidis*, whilst colonisation with *Staphylococcus aureus* may occur in up to 25% of normal individuals. Colonisation with multiple serious pathogens is common in hospitalised patients, especially when they are sick, receiving antibiotics or have diseases or ulceration of the skin.

Therefore, it is necessary to achieve the maximal possible reduction in the burden of pathogenic skin flora in the immediate preoperative period. The patient may be asked to use an appropriate skin decontaminant before coming to the operating theatre. The patient's operative area must *not* be shaved before arriving in theatre, as this practice has been proven to increase the risk of postoperative infection.

In many forms of surgery, preoperative carriage of *Staphylococcus aureus* in the nose, groin or other areas is a common risk factor for SSI. In many services, screening for this pathogen is undertaken and clearance programs instituted preoperatively for the colonised patients.

In surgery of the large bowel, a major cause of postoperative SSI is related to contamination from the bowel flora. Preparation of the bowel with strong osmotic aperients may reduce infection rates. Sometimes, for certain common procedures (e.g. hysterectomy or colectomy) a so-called bundle of care is initiated as a protocol-driven way of minimising SSI by commencing preoperative risk reduction strategies and continued appropriate strategies through the operation and into the postoperative period.

Once intravenous access has been achieved by the anaesthetist, appropriate antibiotic prophylaxis is administered as per guidelines. It has been demonstrated that it is optimal that this be given at least 30 minutes before skin incision so that adequate antibiotic levels are achieved at the incision site. It is critical that excessive antibiotic use and duration be avoided to minimise the risk of antibiotic resistance developing in the bacteria in the hospital environment. After the patient is positioned as per surgical requirements, the planned operative field and surrounding skin is clipped, not shaved, in readiness for the operation.

Theatre dress code and hand hygiene

Staff may carry pathogens picked up from other patients or from the hospital environment including some with high levels of antibiotic resistance. It is important that appropriate clean theatre attire be donned by all staff before entering the operating suite, and that this be changed when they return to theatre from other environments. It is important that hand hygiene be performed before entering and leaving the individual theatre, and whenever contamination might occur. Each institution will develop specific hand hygiene and dress codes for the theatre environment.

The operating theatre

The operating theatre must be an extremely clean environment, with appropriate surfaces that provide a high level of cleanliness and specific cleaning protocols to ensure that this is maintained. The room must be large enough to accommodate all the personnel and equipment and to allow sufficient space to create an ideal sterile field. Modern standards dictate that the airflow is controlled and specifically filtered to a high standard to minimise bacterial contamination by this route. Some theatres have laminar flow to optimise this further.

Skin preparation

In theatre, the surgeon has a choice between four common skin preparation solutions, as well as some less common alternatives. The principal options are aqueous preparations of chlorhexidine or iodine (typically povidine iodine), or solutions of each of these agents in alcohol (typically 70% ethanol in water). All these options achieve substantial reductions in bacterial counts on the treated skin surface. Studies demonstrate a greater effect on pathogenic species than the normal flora. The alcohol-based preparations achieve greater reductions over a shorter time period. However, the organisms tend to reappear over time, and can be cultured from the wound in increasing numbers as the operation proceeds. Phage typing has demonstrated that organisms present on the skin preoperatively are commonly the cause of postoperative infections.

There is a theoretical benefit to chlorhexidine over iodine, as chlorhexidine is still bactericidal in the dry state. Iodine-based preparations are no longer active once they dry. Iodine is also inactivated by blood, whereas chlorhexidine is not. In general, infection rates have been demonstrated to be about 50% lower in patients receiving either of these alcoholic skin preparations, as compared with the aqueous solutions. Another advantage to alcoholic iodine is that it dries the skin and thereby improves the adhesion of adhesive plastic drapes, which facilitates this style of draping.

There are time constants involved in the bactericidal effects of these preparations. Typically, at least 5 minutes of contact with the wet solution is required to achieve optimal decontamination of the skin with the alcoholic preparations. Some authorities advise preparation for as long as 20 minutes for aqueous preparations, but this is often deemed to be impractical.

Unfortunately, there are serious limitations and dangers associated with alcoholic skin preparations. These are real dangers that have caused serious harm to patients. The authors are aware of specific cases of each of the problems listed here. For this reason, many hospitals have removed these solutions from the formulary despite their proven benefits in infection prevention.

- There is a risk of fire if pools of the solution are left under the patient allowing alcoholic vapours to rise and be ignited by sparks from electrical cautery.
- If an alcoholic skin preparation is left on the skin in a liquid state (in pools or even just a film under plastic) during an operation, then serious chemical burns may result. Full-thickness burns have been reported. Indeed, many cases of so-called iodine allergy are actually chemical burns because a plastic drape has been placed over wet alcoholic iodine preparation, keeping it in a liquid state on the skin.
- Alcoholic preparations must not be used on mucous membranes, open wounds or recent incisions as chemical burns will result, even from limited exposure.
- If an alcoholic preparation is allowed to enter the eye, then blindness is likely to result because of damage to the cornea. Therefore, the surgeon who uses these alcoholic skin preparations is assuming a serious but manageable responsibility.

Fortunately, the aqueous skin preparations may be used safely without these concerns. They are clearly the preparation of choice for eye surgery, operations involving the mucous membranes or open wounds, or for re-operations. They may also be required for teams that cannot manage the responsibility of alcoholic preparations.

Surgical scrub

All surgical staff need to perform a surgical scrub before gowning and gloving for the procedure. The process is akin to the skin preparation of the patient. Each operating theatre will have its own protocols for this. The first scrub of the day should ensure a high level of cleanliness of the hands and forearms including the fingernails and up to the elbows. The appropriate antiseptic must then be applied to these regions for the correct time period. Common antiseptics are chlorhexidine 4% or povidone iodine 10% diluted in tap water. Generally, the first scrub should be for 5 minutes, with 3-minute scrubs for subsequent cases, unless significant contamination has occurred. Alcohol-based scrub solutions achieve a lower bacterial count than water-based solutions in shorter time periods and are therefore preferable; 90 seconds is an acceptable scrub time for these agents.

Gowning and gloving

Meticulous technique and practice are required to effectively utilise the closed technique as shown in Figure 12.4. Double gloving is widely recommended to reduce the risk of bacterial contamination from the hands of the staff through micropores or tears in the gloves. This practice also reduces the risk and severity of needlestick injuries to staff members.

(a)

(b)   (c)

(d)   (e)

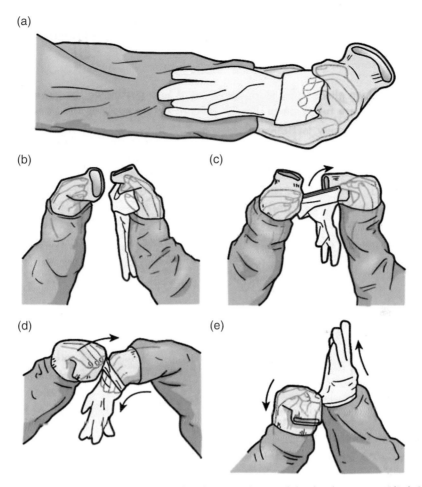

Fig. 12.4 Closed gloving where the hands remain within the gown sleeves whilst the gloves are applied. Source: Sullivan EM. Surgery. In: Ballweg R, Sullivan EM, Brown D, Vetrosky DT. *Physician Assistant: A Guide to Clinical Practice*, 5th edn. Philadelphia: Elsevier Saunders, 2013:356–409. Reproduced with permission of Elsevier.

Surgical drapes

After adequate skin preparation of a wider zone than the anticipated operative field, surgical drapes are applied to define the operative component of the sterile field and to cover the surrounding area. Sometimes these are extensive enough to exclude the non-sterile part of the operating theatre. The drapes are performing a true barrier function, so they need to be resistant to fluid strike-through and be robust enough to not tear easily but also flexible enough to conform to the idiosyncrasies of the human body. Most modern drapes are disposable as opposed to the old-fashioned linen drapes. The surgical drapes are usually attached by an adhesive backing but care must be exercised in their removal, especially in the elderly and infirm due to the possibility of fragile skin, which may tear readily. This includes the adhesive films which are often deployed for many surgeries as an extra protective layer after skin preparation and draping has been completed.

Preservation of the sterile field

Once the sterile field is established, it should not be left unattended. Scrubbed staff should stay close to the sterile field and movements by non-scrubbed staff kept to a minimum whilst surgery is in progress. This includes traffic in and out of the theatre. There should be an ethos of respect to the patient that the sterile zone created for their operative treatment is a sacrosanct zone. Indeed, it is important that any breach of the sterile zone is dealt with and rectified immediately.

With the establishment of the sterile field for the anaesthetised patient, and with all the essential staff and equipment ready, the operation can commence. Every member of the team confirms that they are ready to go and the scalpel is passed to the surgeon in the appropriate way. During the operation, noise should be kept to a low level as clear communication within the surgical team is key to safe surgery. The surgical team must be focused on the task at hand. Some surgeons use background music to enhance the ambience of the theatre and optimise their performance, but there is a risk that this may act as a distraction or inhibit good communication.

Occupational safety in the operating theatre

It is essential that everyone in an operating theatre is aware of the potential occupational hazards and aspires to minimise their impact. The most concerning hazard is the potential for exposure to bodily fluids, especially blood with the resultant risk of blood-borne infections. The potential risks include contracting HIV/AIDS or various forms of viral hepatitis. The prevention of penetrating injuries by careful attention to safe handling practices of sharp instruments is fundamental to reducing this risk of transmission. Personal protective equipment, such as appropriate eyewear, gowns, gloves and masks, are of considerable benefit.

There are also potential risks from X-ray radiation during intraoperative radiography, which must be prevented by the use of protective lead clothing and lead shielding. Lasers may cause eye damage, so specific precautions are required when this technology is employed.

The commonest cause of workplace injuries in the operating suite are the physical forces involved in the handling of the unconscious patient. Injuries to the lumbar and cervical spine may result. It is important that there is proper planning and personnel resourcing for patient movement and positioning. Four people are typically required for the physical work of rolling a patient to the prone position, as well as two people to handle the head and the feet respectively, and the anaesthetist must also be free to manage the airway during patient movement.

Operative recording and information transfer

Accurate recording of the anaesthetic, the operative findings and the procedure performed are essential for the care of the patient, audit of surgical activity and coding. There are different systems to do this, but accuracy and detail must be achieved. The example in Figure 12.5 highlights the basic dataset required for an accurate surgical operation note.

Furthermore, clear postoperative orders must be documented to communicate clearly to the staff

involved in the aftercare, both immediately in the recovery room and subsequently on the ward. This includes such information such as the frequency of observations, reportable observations using medical emergency team (MET) criteria, fasting status, fluid management, oxygen administration, wound care management, patient positioning, postoperative test ordering and allied health management. These orders must be enhanced by appropriate protocols prepared to underpin the teamwork between the surgical and postoperative teams.

One critical element is the transmission of information about the patient's general medical condition, preoperative assessment of this, and routine medications. Errors of omission involving the patient's essential medications may be a significant source of postoperative mishap.

The outer network (supporting the inner sanctum)

Holding bay and recovery room

Most operating suites will have a holding bay where patients can be held prior to entering the operating theatre proper. This is an appropriate environment for a preoperative check to ensure identity, site and side of surgery, allergies and a number of other basic checks.

The recovery room is a specialised environment staffed by specially trained nursing staff who are skilled in managing patients emerging from anaesthesia. The first hour after surgery is a risky time, when significant medical and surgical issues may arise. Skilled observation by a nurse committed one-on-one to the individual patient plays a crucial role in shepherding the patient through this challenging phase. In some hospitals, a high proportion of patients are admitted to an intensive care environment for the first 12–24 hours at least, but this is substantially more expensive and is not the common practice in Australia.

Central sterile and supply department

The provision of working instruments that are properly sterilised is one of the most basic requirements of modern safe surgery. The CSSD is often adjacent to operating theatres, and generally shares a linked management structure. It must be efficient and function at a very high standard.

After being used, non-disposable surgical instruments must undergo prompt initial cleaning to remove contaminants before they dry and harden. This may be performed by the scrub team or in the

NSN 7540-00-634-4156

MEDICAL RECORD	**OPERATION REPORT**

PREOPERATIVE DIAGNOSIS

SURGEON	FIRST ASSISTANT	SECOND ASSISTANT	
ANESTHETIST	ANESTHETIC		TIME BEGAN:
			TIME ENDED:
CIRCULATING NURSE	SCRUB NURSE	TIME OPERATION BEGAN	TIME OPERATION COM-PLETED

OPERATIVE DIAGNOSES

DRAINS *(Kind and number)*	SPONGE COUNT VERIFIED

MATERIAL FORWARDED TO LABORATORY FOR EXAMINATION

OPERATION PERFORMED

DESCRIPTION OF OPERATION *(Type(s) of suture used, gross findings, etc.)*	PROSTHETIC DEVICES *(Lot no.)*	DATE OF OPERATION

SIGNATURE OF SURGEON	DATE

PATIENT'S IDENTIFICATION *(For typed or written entries give: Name - last, first, middle; grade; date hospital or medical facility)*	REGISTER/I.D. NO.	WARD NO.

OPERATION REPORT
Medical Record

STANDARD FORM 516 (REV. 5-83)
Prescribed by GSA/ICMR
FIRMR (41 CFR) 201-45.505

Fig. 12.5 Example of an operation note template. Source: https://www.gsa.gov/Forms/TrackForm/33055. Reproduced with permission of General Services Administration.

CSSD. A further clean and inspection under magnification then takes place in the CSSD. Once the instruments are clean and confirmed to be in good working order they are sterilised, which is the process that kills all forms of life, whether done chemically or physically. Modern standards are more stringent than previously in order to kill prions such as CJD, as well as the standard bacteria, viruses and fungi.

Typically, the instruments are assembled as sets, defined in a standard way for a variety of standard procedures. The sets of instruments are wrapped and labelled, sterility indicators incorporated and an expiry date determined. Sterilisation is then performed. Stringent quality control is routine in this process. Appropriate storage is required until the set is used. When instruments are brought to the theatre, it is essential to check that the packaging is intact and dry and that the expiry date and the sterility indicator status are acceptable. This safety check of the instruments during set-up is one of the critical roles of the scout and scrub nurses.

Ward nursing staff

The ward staff, whether in a day surgical facility or an inpatient ward, have a comprehensive checklist to run through to ensure that patients are ready to go to the operating theatre. This includes the fasting status of the patient, allergy alerts, definition of the planned operation and consent. Rigorous processes are essential, which may be challenging in urgent situations. Conducting these checks in a highly professional manner is important to avoid error, and to reassure the patient and their family, who are likely to be anxious at that time. The postoperative care on the ward must be a real team effort as it is a truly multidisciplinary activity. The complexity varies greatly depending on the nature of the surgery and the patient's illness. Once again, the key aspect is good professional skills in all personnel and good communication in both written and verbal formats. Accurate and clear postoperative orders and agreed protocols for patient care set the agenda. Regular review, and repeated communication between medical and nursing teams must continue through the postoperative phase.

Imaging, radiography and pathology

Many operations are planned on the basis of a series of preoperative images, which may range from plain X-rays to MRI scans, angiograms or nuclear medicine studies. For the safe performance of the operation on the correct part of the correct patient, it is essential that there is a system in place that allows secure and reliable access to imaging for the patient.

In addition, intraoperative radiology using image intensification (Figure 12.6) is critical to many operative procedures. Examples include cholecystectomy with intraoperative cholangiography, cardiac pacemaker insertion, spinal surgery and many orthopaedic procedures. It is essential that there be clear systems of planning and communication to ensure the availability of staff and equipment for

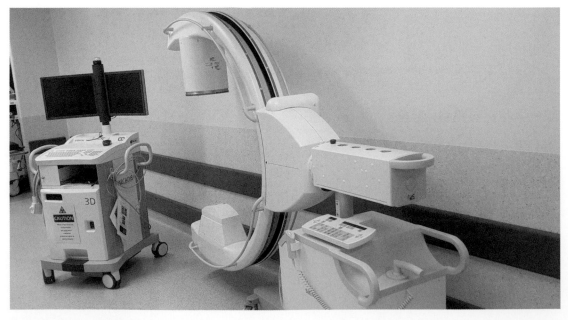

Fig. 12.6 Image intensifier system used in the operating theatre.

these procedures. Everyone in the operating theatre must take appropriate radiation precautions and wear the protection as stipulated for their own protection. Similar organisation and appropriate precautions must also be taken with the use of radioisotopes, such as in the procedure of sentinel node biopsy.

Intraoperative histopathology is sometimes required to assist with making a diagnosis or determining if the resection margin around a tumour is adequate or not. Expert pathological support and the necessary communication intraoperatively to manage and discuss the specimen may be critical to the patient's outcome. Again, preoperative planning and organisation are required to ensure the availability of this resource.

The back-up of blood bank for blood and blood products may be critical in many operations. Furthermore, intraoperative monitoring of the patient's biochemical, haematological, coagulation and blood gas parameters is important in many complex and prolonged procedures. There is an increasing trend towards so-called point-of-care testing to simplify much of this and provide immediate information about the patient's status, effectively in real time. This facilitates enhanced patient safety.

Hospital administration

Organising for a patient to have an operation is a complex undertaking and requires robust secure systems and many personnel. To open and staff a theatre with no extras costs about A$1000/hour; adding extra complex equipment increases the costs dramatically. The role of hospital and surgical department administration in securing and confirming funding, and managing all this cannot be underestimated.

The introduction of new procedures, devices and techniques requires a clear governance process overseen by the hospital administration, as it is ultimately accountable for patient welfare. It is essential that the health service administration works with the operating theatre teams to maximise the value for the funding dollar. Quality assurance must occur through audit of patient outcomes, as well as case reviews at morbidity and mortality meetings. Variations in care and outcomes require governance mechanisms to assure everyone, but especially patients and their families, that the highest standards of surgical care are being pursued and maintained. The monitoring of SSI rates is a prime but simple example of measuring how well a system of surgical care is functioning and being maintained.

Conclusion

Operating theatres are complex systems involving many staff and sophisticated equipment. The maintenance of the highest standards of performance at all levels is crucial to the ultimate goal of safe patient care in the operating theatre environment. Underpinning the culture of safety must be excellent communication at all times by all the participants, both within the immediate operating theatre team but also the supporting network.

Further reading

Cochran A, Braga R (eds) *Introduction to the Operating Room*. New York: McGraw-Hill, 2017.
Fuller JK (ed.) *Surgical Technology: Principles and Practice*, 7th edn. St. Louis, MO: Elsevier, 2017.
Woodhead K, Fudge L (eds) *Manual of Perioperative Care: An Essential Guide*. Oxford: Wiley Blackwell, 2012.

MCQs

Select the single correct answer to each question. The correct answers can be found in the Answers section at the end of the book.

1 John is a normal 19-year-old man who presents to the emergency department with right iliac fossa pain, and a temperature of 37.5°C. He looks mildly unwell. The surgical diagnosis is acute appendicitis and appendicectomy is advised. Regarding consent:
  a consent is not necessary because this is an emergency
  b full surgical consent is obtained from John in the emergency department, with proper discussion of possible complications, alternate treatment options, etc.
  c it is not necessary to disclose who will be doing the operation because he is a public patient
  d full surgical consent should be obtained from his parents, with proper discussion of possible complications, alternate treatment options, etc. because he is under 21 years of age
  e full surgical consent is obtained from John when he arrives in theatre, with proper discussion of possible complications, alternate treatment options, etc.

2 The most important aim of the surgical team time-out is:
  a financial consent and checking of insurance status

b building teamwork and common goals within the broader surgical team

c checking that the patient is fit for surgery and anaesthesia

d checking contact details of the next of kin

e verifying the correct patient and procedure with identification of the site and side of surgery

3 The risks of aqueous povidine iodine skin preparations include:

a fire

b chemical burns of the skin

c blindness

d wound infection

e none of the above

4 You have just closed the wound after a long and challenging open craniotomy for removal of a large meningioma. The scrub nurse informs you that there is a surgical patty missing. What is the optimal response?

a inform the nurse that you checked for patties before closing so it is not possible that one could have been left inside; you then proceed to place dressings and ask the anaesthetist to wake the patient

b pause and take a short break while the nurse performs a repeat count to see if an error may have occurred, and then undertake a search of all possible places where a patty could be hidden

c open the wound immediately to look for the missing patty

d request an image intensifier to take an X-ray to see if the missing patty can be seen in the wound

e close the wound and take the patient for an urgent CT scan, keeping them under anaesthesia to allow return to theatre to find the missing patty if it can be seen inside the head

5 The most common cause of surgical site infection in clean elective orthopaedic surgery in a modern operating theatre is:

a the organisms present in the nostrils of the surgical team

b the organisms present on the hands of the surgical team

c the organisms present on the anaesthetists

d the organisms present on the skin of the patient prior to surgery

e the organisms present on the surgical instruments or prostheses

6 It is possible to sterilise which of the following:

a the patient's skin where the surgical wound will be incised

b the surgical assistant

c the surgical instruments

d the hands of the surgeon provided that they glove correctly

e all of the above

13 Emergency general surgery

Benjamin N.J. Thomson[1,2] and Rose Shakerian[2]

[1] University of Melbourne, Melbourne, Victoria, Australia
[2] Royal Melbourne Hospital, Melbourne, Victoria, Australia

Introduction

In Victoria, Australia, during the year 2010–2011, 24% of all surgical admissions were emergency surgical admissions. In some of the large metropolitan hospitals the emergency surgery caseload can be as high as 38%. This increase in emergency surgery workload is not limited to Australia, with similar proportions and increases reported in Europe and the USA.

Emergency general surgery admissions account for over 50% of total admissions in general surgery departments in public hospitals in Australia. In the year 2015–2016, the Royal Melbourne Hospital Department of General Surgical Specialties admitted 7298 patients, with 4936 (68%) emergency general surgery and trauma admissions. An emergency general surgery patient is defined by the American Association for the Surgery of Trauma (AAST) as 'any patient requiring an emergency surgical evaluation for disease within the realm of general surgery'. It has been estimated that emergencies in general surgery account for 80–90% of general surgical deaths. Furthermore, complication rates in emergency surgery exceed those of a similar elective procedure by twofold to fourfold.

Traditional models of emergency general surgery care

Individual general surgical units who manage both elective and emergency surgery patients without dedicated resources characterised the traditional model of care for emergency general surgery patients. These resources included dedicated surgical staff, wards and theatre access. Emergency admissions were managed by general surgical units on a rotating on-call roster. This would result in patients being admitted to subspecialty units where some surgeons would not routinely manage abdominal conditions. The emergency work was in competition with elective surgery and endoscopy lists, as well as outpatient services. Surgical trainees in consultation with the on-call consultant most frequently led the traditional model.

Emergency general surgery models

The main features of emergency general surgical models of care include the separation of elective and emergency work, consultant-led care, robust handover and trainee supervision. The model is specific to each hospital and depends on the patient volume, case mix, complexity and available resources. Consultant-led care is also a critical component, allowing for proven benefits of improved patient care, teaching and better utilisation of radiological investigations. Various names exist for the models, including emergency general surgery (EGS) services, acute care surgery (ACS) units and acute surgical units (ASUs). The on-call period for each consultant surgeon may be 24 hours up to 7 days.

The first specialised emergency surgical units were designed for trauma care and started at the Birmingham Accident Hospital in the UK in 1947. In the USA the first shock trauma centers opened in Chicago and Baltimore in 1966. Meta-analysis of the comparison of patient care before and after the formation of trauma centres and systems demonstrated a 15% reduction in mortality.

The concept of consultant-led care for emergency general surgical patients originated in the UK, following the National Confidential Enquiry in Patient Outcome and Death (NCEPOD) that demonstrated poor outcomes for emergency surgery patients undergoing operative procedures by junior surgical staff. This in part led to the development of ASUs in the UK.

Textbook of Surgery, Fourth Edition. Edited by Julian A. Smith, Andrew H. Kaye, Christopher Christophi and Wendy A. Brown.
© 2020 John Wiley & Sons Ltd. Published 2020 by John Wiley & Sons Ltd.

In Australia, trauma centers have been the mainstay of trauma care since the late 1990s. The redesign of emergency general surgery services was led by a number of bodies that included the relevant state departments of health, the Royal Australasian College of Surgeons and General Surgeons Australia. The impact of subspecialty training has also been problematic because it has often limited the exposure to emergency surgery, with many surgeons consequently believing that they lack the required skills to manage acute general surgical admissions.

There have been many studies from the USA, Europe, Australia and New Zealand that report significant improvements in the care of emergency general surgical patients, with a reduction in mortality, morbidity, length of stay, time to surgery, emergency department length of stay and out-of-hours theatre. From a workforce perspective, the impact has included increased access to training opportunities for surgical trainees, increased consultant supervision in theatre, a reduction in on-call commitments and a reduction in workload.

Emergency general surgical disorders

The majority of emergency general surgical admissions are for abdominal complaints (Table 13.1). In comparison to elective surgical admissions, emergency general surgical patients are older with higher rates of comorbidities, such as hypertension, dyslipidaemia, type 2 diabetes mellitus and renal impairment.

Not all emergency general surgical procedures require surgical intervention. The commonest surgical intervention remains appendicectomy and along with cholecystectomy, laparotomy and perianal surgery these four surgical groups account for more than 50% of surgical interventions (Table 13.2). The overall 30-day mortality for emergency general surgery patients is around 4%, with an increasing mortality rate with age.

Laparotomy is a common general surgical operation accounting for 12.5% of surgical procedures at the Royal Melbourne Hospital. In the UK, 30 000–50 000 laparotomies are performed per year. It carries a significant risk of morbidity and mortality. The initial Emergency Laparotomy Network

Table 13.2 Common emergency general surgical operations*.

Procedure	Percentage
Appendicectomy	29.7
Cholecystectomy	13.2
Laparotomy	12.5
Perianal abscess/pilonidal abscess/anal fistula	10.1
Wound debridement/soft tissue abscess	8.4
Hernia repair	4.7
Other	21.3

* These data relate to 1804 emergency general surgical operations over a 2-year period at the Royal Melbourne Hospital.

Table 13.1 Emergency general surgical admissions*.

Admission diagnosis	Percentage	Chapters
Non-specific abdominal pain	12.5	68
Acute appendicitis	11.9	28
Biliary disease	8.1	19
Perianal/pilonidal disease	4.9	34
Constipation	4.9	63
Acute pancreatitis	4.7	22
Diverticular disease/diverticulitis	4.3	30
Intestinal obstruction	4.0	26, 31, 32
Gastritis/colitis/gastroenteritis	3.7	16, 29
Skin and soft tissue infection	3.4	46
Gastrointestinal bleeding	2.8	16, 17, 65, 66
Gynaecological	2.1	68
Hernia	1.9	43
Urological	1.0	59
Other	32.9	

* These data relate to 4468 admissions to the Royal Melbourne Hospital over a 2-year period, with corresponding references to other chapters in this book.

prospective study of 1853 patients reported a 30-day mortality of 14.9%, whilst the American College of Surgeons National Surgical Quality Improvement Program (NSQIP) database of 37 553 patients reported a 30-day mortality of 14% during 2005–2009. The various surgical pathologies necessitating surgery are wide-ranging and include peptic ulcer disease, diverticulitis, small bowel obstruction, large bowel obstruction and trauma.

Non-specific abdominal pain comprises the majority of general surgical emergency admissions, accounting for 13–40% of admissions in the UK. The diagnosis is made after appropriate assessment and investigation of a patient, with a diagnosis unable to be reached in a small percentage. The majority of patients will settle within 2 weeks of onset of pain.

Causes of abdominal pain that may be missed include intra-abdominal malignancy and, in particular, colon cancer. Other diagnoses include irritable bowel syndrome, viral infections, gastroenteritis and acute gynaecological conditions such as pelvic inflammatory disease and ovarian cysts. Far less frequently, medical conditions such as myocardial infarction, diabetic ketoacidosis and pneumonia may present with abdominal pain.

Abdominal wall pain is also a common cause for abdominal pain due to iatrogenic nerve injuries, occult hernias, myofascial pain syndromes, rib pathology, nerve root pain or rectus sheath haematoma.

Further reading

General Surgeons Australia (GSA). 12 Point Plan for Emergency General Surgery. GSA, Melbourne, Australia, 2010. Available at https://www.generalsurgeons.com.au/media/files/Publications/PLN%202010-09-19%20GSA%2012%20Point%20Plan.pdf

Paterson-Brown S, Paterson HM (eds) *A Companion to Specialist Surgical Practice: Core Topics in General and Emergency Surgery*, 6th edn. Edinburgh: Elsevier, 2019.

Shakerian R, Thomson BN, Gorelik A, Hayes IP, Skandarajah AR. Outcomes in emergency general surgery following the introduction of a consultant-led unit. *Br J Surg* 2015;102:1726–32.

MCQs

Select the single correct answer to each question. The correct answers can be found in the Answers section at the end of the book.

1 Emergency general surgical patients:
   a have a lower rate of morbidity compared with elective general surgical admissions
   b have a higher mortality rate compared with elective general surgical admissions
   c only account for a small proportion of admissions
   d can be adequately managed without specialised emergency general surgical units
   e all of the above

2 Common emergency general surgical procedures include:
   a appendicectomy
   b laparotomy
   c abscess drainage
   d cholecystectomy
   e all of the above

3 Non-specific abdominal pain is:
   a a failure to make a diagnosis
   b usually caused by appendicitis
   c the commonest reason for admission to an emergency general surgical unit
   d best treated with opiate analgesia
   e usually leads to a chronic abdominal pain syndrome

Section 2
Upper Gastrointestinal Surgery

14 Gastro-oesophageal reflux disease and hiatus hernias

Paul Burton and Geraldine J. Ooi

Monash University and Alfred Health, Melbourne, Victoria, Australia

Introduction

Gastro-oesophageal reflux disease (GORD) is defined as 'symptoms or complications resulting from the reflux of gastric contents into the oesophagus or beyond, into the oral cavity (including larynx) or lung'.[1] GORD is one the most common diseases in Western societies. It is responsible for substantial symptoms, impairment in quality of life, results in significant healthcare costs as well as lost work time and is an important risk factor for oesophageal adenocarcinoma.

It is important to note that some reflux of gastric contents into the oesophagus probably occurs intermittently in everyone, particularly after eating. When this occurs excessively and there is damage to the mucosa and/or significant symptoms develop, it is referred to as GORD. Around 10–15% of the population have significant symptoms and many more have intermittent symptoms.

In practical terms it is when we become aware of it, usually because of symptoms of burning retrosternal pain (heartburn) and/or regurgitation of contents into the mouth or excessive, intense salivation (water brash) that we call the condition GORD and think of it as a medical disorder.

Another important point is to differentiate a hiatus hernia from GORD, although these terms are frequently confused. Certain types of hiatus hernia promote reflux. However, the presence of a hiatus hernia is by no means representative of reflux disease. Additionally, hiatus hernias can cause problems, sometimes severe, that are not related to reflux.

Surgical anatomy and physiology

The oesophagus is an approximately 25-cm long muscular tube that runs from the upper oesophageal sphincter, passing through the thoracic cavity, then via the oesophageal hiatus in the diaphragm to intersect the gastric cardia. Above the intersection with the cardia, the intrinsic lower oesophageal sphincter (LOS), a thickening of oesophageal circular smooth muscle, protects the lower oesophagus from reflux.

The LOS can actually be thought of as a complex. The smooth muscle component is reinforced by the diaphragmatic crura, hiatal canal and phreno-oesophageal ligament. These components work synergistically to provide an optimal barrier to reflux. The intrinsic LOS remains tonically contracted, preventing reflux. When food is swallowed it opens in a coordinated fashion to allow the food bolus into the stomach.

Aetiology/pathogenesis of GORD

The precise reasons why gastro-oesophageal reflux develops is unknown, but it certainly appears to be a disease associated with the western lifestyle, and most clinicians believe that overeating, obesity, alcohol and smoking are important factors.

The pathophysiology of reflux predominantly relates to events known as transient lower oesophageal sphincter relaxations. Several times every hour the LOS relaxes, allowing the stomach to vent air. This is not consciously controlled and people are

---

[1] Vakil N, van Zanten SV, Kahrilas P, Dent J, Jones R. The Montreal definition and classification of gastroesophageal reflux disease: a global evidence-based consensus. *Am J Gastroenterol* 2006;101:1900–20.

---

unaware of this happening. Reflux of gastric juice into the oesophagus can occur during these relaxations. Another factor that favours reflux is separation of the LOS from the crural diaphragm as in a sliding hiatus hernia. Weakness of the intrinsic LOS can also occur, reducing the barrier function of the sphincter.

Other specific factors that may influence reflux include increased intra-abdominal pressure (pregnancy or central obesity). Reflux occurs after meals because there is hypersecretion of acid and a thin layer of concentrated acid appears immediately beneath the oesophago-gastric junction. A delay in gastric emptying may also be a factor in increasing reflux.

Surgical pathology

Most patients with GORD have normal oesophageal mucosa. In severe forms of the disease mucosal erosions can occur. Erosive oesophagitis is thought to be primarily due to the low pH of gastric fluid contacting oesophageal mucosa. It is also likely at times that bile and other enzymes contribute to the mucosal injury.

Oesophagitis is graded according to the Los Angeles classification (grade A, B, C and D), with A representing the presence of damage of the least severity and D representing disease of the highest severity. Figure 14.1 shows an example of erosive oesophagitis.

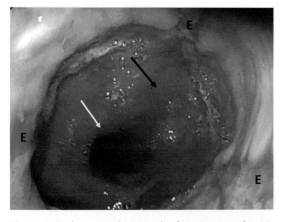

Fig. 14.1 Endoscopic photograph of erosive oesophagitis in the lower oesophagus. The black arrow indicates gastric mucosa projecting above the level of the diaphragm as a sliding (type I) hiatus hernia. The white arrow indicates the diaphragm. Regions of erosive oesophagitis (LA grade A) can be seen, where the pale oesophageal mucosa has been eroded due to reflux (E).

Complications of gastro-oesophageal reflux

Chronic irritation of the lower oesophageal mucosa due to refluxed gastric juice can lead to severe problems. Prior to widespread availability of powerful acid-suppressing medication, significant complications were far more common.

Severe oesophagitis and oesophageal ulcers represent an advanced form of reflux and can result in chronic blood loss and anaemia. If reflux is severe and long-standing, the inflammatory process and healing is associated with the development of fibrous tissue. If enough fibrous tissue forms, like any scar it will contract, leading to narrowing of the oesophageal lumen. Patients can have dysphagia as a result.

Spillover of refluxate can be aspirated via the larynx into the lungs. This can result in chronic cough, lung infection and even lung abscess in extreme cases. This is usually associated with specific situations where there is a large volume of reflux and impaired protective reflexes.

Barrett's oesophagus

In a small proportion of patients, the oesophageal mucosa responds to reflux by replacing the squamous mucosa with columnar mucosa, a process known as intestinal metaplasia or Barrett's oesophagus. The significance of Barrett's oesophagus relates to its status as a premalignant condition, thought to be the precursor of oesophageal adenocarcinoma.

Obesity and reflux

Obesity is a significant risk factor for reflux. Increased intra-abdominal fat raises intra-abdominal pressure, thereby favouring reflux due to an increased pressure gradient between the intra-abdominal stomach and intrathoracic oesophagus. Obesity independently increases transient LOS relaxations. Given the epidemic of obesity, there are not surprisingly many obese patients with GORD.

Hiatus hernias

A hiatus hernia is present where there is projection of the stomach more than 2 cm into the mediastinum, above the diaphragm. In the normal situation there is 2–3 cm of oesophagus within the abdominal cavity.

Hiatus hernias are subdivided into three different types.
- *Type I hiatus hernias* are the most common and often asymptomatic. These hernias are present when the LOS is located greater than 2 cm above the diaphragm. They are also called sliding hernias, because the LOS has slid vertically up above the diaphragm. This predisposes to reflux by disrupting the coordinated effect of the LOS complex. Additionally, it creates a positive pressure gradient from the higher pressure intra-abdominal stomach to the lower pressure intrathoracic LOS, favouring reflux.
- *Type II hiatus hernias* occur when the LOS remains within the abdomen and the greater curve of the stomach 'rolls up' into the mediastinum through the oesophageal hiatus. This type of hernia is called para-oesophageal, as the hernia occurs alongside the oesophagus. These hernias can sometimes be huge and involve virtually all the stomach. Other organs such as the transverse colon and spleen can be present in very large hiatus hernias. Figure 14.2 shows a CT image of a type II hiatus hernia.
- *Type III hiatus hernias* are mixed hernias, with components of both sliding and para-oesophageal hernia (Figure 14.3). Most hernias, where there is a significant portion of the stomach in the mediastinum, are type III rather than type II, as the LOS has migrated upwards slightly rather than staying fixed within the abdomen.

Common symptoms of para-oesophageal hernias include pain and discomfort after meals, probably associated with intermittent twisting and partial obstruction of the stomach. Patients can have some reflux symptoms, but that is usually not the major problem. Despite their size, para-oesophageal hiatus hernias are occasionally asymptomatic. If the hernia is asymptomatic, then it seems reasonable to leave it, instructing the patient to seek urgent medical attention if pain and/or vomiting should develop.

Stasis and possibly mechanical trauma in the intrathoracic stomach can result in chronic blood loss due to linear erosions of the stomach at the level of the diaphragm, known as Cameron's ulcers. Patients sometimes present as an acute emergency, with obstruction of the hernia, where the stomach twists and patients are unable to eat because the stomach has twisted. In extreme cases of obstruction, the stomach can occlude its own blood supply, becoming strangulated.

Clinical presentation of GORD

The majority of patients with GORD present with heartburn, a sensation of retrosternal burning pain, usually occurring after eating, with particular foods (spicy, rich or fatty food as well as chocolate, wine or caffeine) more likely to provoke symptoms.

(a) (b)

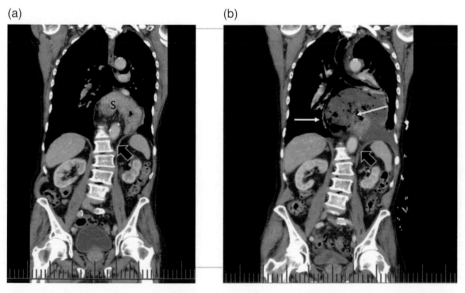

Fig. 14.2 Large type II hiatus hernia. Coronal CT scans of the same patient taken 4 weeks apart. (a) A large uncomplicated hiatus hernia can be seen, with almost all the stomach (S) in the mediastinum, above the diaphragm (thick arrow). (b) The hernia has become obstructed and grossly distended, with substantial food residue within the stomach (yellow arrow). Gas is also noted in the gastric wall (white arrow). This patient required emergency surgery and a total gastrectomy to remove the infarcted stomach.

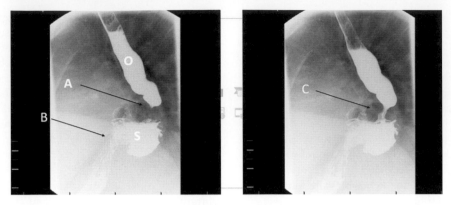

Fig. 14.3 Barium swallow demonstrating a type III hiatus hernia (mixed sliding and para-oesophageal components). The images are in the lateral projection. The oesophagus (O) can be seen above the diaphragm. The lower oesophageal sphincter (A) is seen above the diaphragm and the stomach (S) has 'rolled up' into the mediastinum. Barium (B) can be seen flowing into the stomach below the diaphragm. In the second frame (*right*), the lower oesophageal sphincter is relaxing to allow barium to pass into the stomach (C).

Symptoms are typically episodic and may wax and wane over many years. Often, over a period of 6–8 weeks symptoms are significant then may gradually recede.

Symptoms of reflux can usually be classified into typical symptoms (those that have a high likelihood of association with reflux) and atypical (those that have a lower likelihood of association with reflux). Typical symptoms can be further divided into irritant and volume symptoms. Irritant symptoms are primarily heartburn. Volume symptoms include regurgitation of liquid or semi-digested food in a passive manner, which may occur on exertion or when leaning forward. Nocturnal regurgitation can be particularly troublesome and frightening for patients as they may awake choking.

Atypical symptoms include chest pain, dyspepsia, epigastric pain, nausea, bloating and belching as well as extra-oesophageal manifestations such as chronic cough, a hoarse voice or sore throat. These symptoms may or may not be attributable to reflux.

Investigation of GORD

The great majority of patients with reflux either never go to the doctor with their problem, or are relatively simply treated with medication and changes to their lifestyle.

Which patients should be investigated further? Patients with typical heartburn that can be treated easily do not require further investigation. Some symptoms are so-called alarm symptoms and when a patient presents with dysphagia, haematemesis, weight loss or anaemia, urgent investigation with endoscopy is usually required.

Endoscopy should be considered in patients with symptoms that persist despite compliance with 4–8 weeks of twice-daily proton-pump inhibitor (PPI) therapy. If patients respond appropriately to acid suppressive therapy and do not manifest alarm symptoms, endoscopic evaluation is not deemed necessary, except for men older than 50 years with chronic symptoms (>5 years) and additional risk factors, such as nocturnal reflux, elevated body mass index, tobacco use and family history of Barrett's oesophagus or oesophageal adenocarcinoma.

If erosive oesophagitis is found, further investigation is not usually warranted. If the patient has a normal oesophagus on endoscopy, then 24-hour pH monitoring can be performed to obtain a more specific assessment and diagnosis of reflux.

Oesophageal manometry

Oesophageal manometry is performed to evaluate the function of the oesophagus. In particular, the strength and coordination of peristalsis and the tone and relaxation of the LOS are measured. Surgeons very frequently perform manometry prior to anti-reflux surgery to exclude a significant problem with contraction of the oesophageal muscle that may impact surgery or to establish an alternative diagnosis such as achalasia.

Manometry is often performed prior to 24-hour pH monitoring to determine the location of the LOS and thereby guide placement of the pH probe. Oesophageal manometry involves placement of a thin tube, via the nose, into the oesophagus and thence into the top of the stomach. Pressure measurements can then be taken

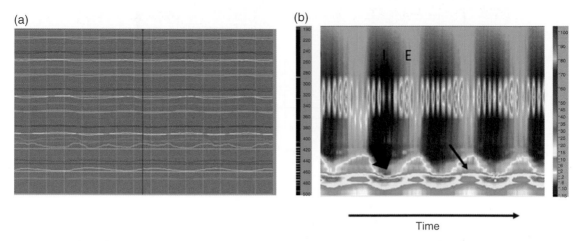

Fig. 14.4 High-resolution manometry trace displayed as a line plot (a) and spatiotemporal plot (b). This manometry plot was taken from a patient in quiet respiration, aiming to assess the function of the lower oesophageal sphincter over several respiratory cycles. The line plot displays a series of pressure measurements over time. Each line represents data from a single pressure sensor. Data presented in this way is very difficult to interpret. In the spatiotemporal plot, distance from the nares is on the *y*-axis, time on the *x*-axis and different pressures are represented by different colours (scale on right of image). The respiratory cycle can be seen, with deeper blue (I) representing lower intrathoracic pressure during inspiration and lighter blue expiration (E). The yellow and pink colours around a depth of 46–48 cm represent the lower oesophageal sphincter and diaphragm. The thick black arrow indicates high pressure at the diaphragm due to inspiration and the thin arrow the intrinsic lower oesophageal sphincter pressure during expiration.

along the tube, which has a series of pressure sensors along its length.

Figure 14.4 demonstrates an oesophageal manometry plot in the resting phase. Manometry data are displayed as a spatiotemporal colour plot, where pressure, time and depth data (distance from the nose) are displayed. The spatiotemporal plot is similar to a topographical map, where colours may represent different heights of terrain. As often 30–40 sensors (more than 16 sensors represents high-resolution manometry) are placed on the manometry catheter, it is very difficult to interpret the data collectively if they are displayed as individual line traces. Spatiotemporal presentation of data allows an overview to be obtained at a glance. Computerised algorithms aid greatly in the interpretation of high-resolution oesophageal manometry.

Twenty-four-hour pH monitoring

Twenty-four-hour pH monitoring (now usually also incorporating impedance monitoring) is considered the gold standard for assessing and quantifying GORD. This is because it provides an objective measure of the amount of reflux and the pattern of reflux over a 24-hour period. Additionally, when patients experience symptoms, they can be recorded and it can then be determined whether that symptom correlated with a reflux event. The information

provided from 24-hour pH monitoring is very important in making treatment decisions, particularly if surgery is being considered.

This test involves passage of a fine tube through the nose into the oesophagus (with the sensor located in the oesophagus, 5 cm above the top of the LOS). The sensor detects changes in pH and, more frequently now, flow of fluid can be measured using changes in impedance (resistance) along the tube. The sensor remains in place for 24 hours.

In most laboratories, over 24 hours, the normal value for percentage time spent with pH below 4 in the oesophagus is 4% or less. If more than 50% of reported symptoms are correlated with a period of oesophageal acid exposure (pH <4), the symptoms are considered to be due to reflux and a diagnosis of GORD made. A 24-hour pH trace is shown in Figure 14.5.

Imaging investigations

Barium swallow is a simple investigation but has a limited role in simple reflux, although it is an accurate means of assessing hiatus hernias. Radiopaque barium is swallowed, and the outline of the oesophagus can be identified using fluoroscopy. Figure 14.3 shows a barium swallow of a type II hiatus hernia.

Computed topography (see Figure 14.2) provides better anatomical delineation, particularly of large hiatus hernias. This allows quantification of the

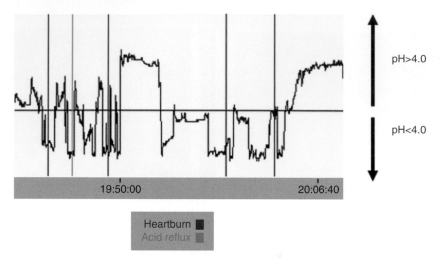

Fig. 14.5 Recording from a 24-hour pH monitoring test. The line trace is a simple graph over time, in this case a 25-minute period. It represents a continuous measure of pH, 5 cm above the top of the lower oesophageal sphincter. In this snapshot the horizontal line represents a pH of 4. A series of dips in pH below this level represent reflux events. Importantly, the red and blue coloured vertical lines represent reported symptoms by the patient (heartburn and acid reflux). Symptoms closely correlated with dips in pH to less than 4, suggesting that reflux is responsible for the symptoms.

extent of stomach or other organs herniating into the mediastinum and aids in operative planning.

Nuclear scintigraphy is a functional test that involves the patient consuming a radiolabelled semi-solid meal such as porridge. The presence of reflux can be seen over several hours and gastric emptying assessed (as delayed gastric emptying can be a precipitating factor of GORD).

Upper gastrointestinal endoscopy

Upper gastrointestinal endoscopy involves passage of a flexible tube via the mouth into the oesophagus and stomach. Images are then transmitted to a screen, frequently in high definition. Endoscopy has the advantage of being able to visualise the mucosa (see Figure 14.1) and inspect for changes of reflux oesophagitis as well as identify other mucosal problems such as Barrett's oesophagus. Endoscopy is usually performed in a sedated patient or under local anaesthesia. It allows direct sampling of the mucosa with biopsies.

Treatment of gastro-oesophageal reflux

As many people experience reflux, initial advice would usually centre around lifestyle change. Changes advocated include improvement in diet, avoiding trigger foods, not eating immediately prior to going to bed, obtaining regular exercise or modest weight loss, smoking cessation and reduction in alcohol intake.

A range of medications are commonly used to treat GORD and many are available over the counter without a prescription. These medications are more likely to be effective in improving irritant symptoms of reflux such as heartburn. The three most common categories of medication are antacids, histamine H_2 receptor antagonists and PPIs.

Antacids are essentially buffers that aim to coat the lining of the oesophagus and stomach, thereby protecting the mucosa. They have rapid onset and offset of action. Antacids contain specific compounds such as calcium carbonate.

Histamine H_2 receptor antagonists are effective acid-suppressing medications. These work via inhibition of histamine at H_2 receptors, thereby reducing gastric acid secretion. They have a rapid onset of action and may work particularly well overnight.

PPIs are the most powerful acid-suppressing medications available. They work by blocking the parietal cell proton pump (H^+/K^+ exchange pump), preventing secretion of H^+ ions into the gastric lumen. Very effective acid suppression is achieved. These medications have a slower onset of action and should be taken daily to maintain acid suppression.

The advantage of drug therapy is its simplicity and efficacy. In severe GORD, medication may be required long term and there are potentially adverse effects of taking medications for many years. If volume or atypical symptoms are the major problem, medications are less effective because they do not stop gastro-oesophageal reflux occurring.

Surgery

Surgery is a generally safe and highly effective treatment for chronic GORD. It is usually considered in patients with more severe disease, affecting health and disrupting quality of life. Indications for surgery include non-response to lifestyle change or medication, volume symptoms, breakthrough symptoms despite maximal medical therapy and patient reluctance to take medications longer term.

Fundoplication

This is generally a simple laparoscopic procedure with a hospital stay of one to two nights. In a fundoplication any hiatus hernia (even small) is repaired with sutures. The fundus of the stomach is then wrapped around the lower oesophagus. Effectively, this creates a one-way valve. Physiologically, the LOS resting pressure increases and transient LOS relaxations are eliminated. Importantly, surgery almost completely stops reflux, rather than just reducing symptoms which is achieved with medication.

Over 90% of patients are extremely satisfied with the results of surgery and would be willing to do it again. Recent data suggest that 20 years following surgery most patients have achieved and sustained an excellent outcome from surgery.

Patients undergoing laparoscopic fundoplication should also be aware that there are (uncommon) perioperative risks, including infections, bleeding splenic injury and oesophageal perforation. There is an approximately 2% conversion rate to open operation because of difficulties that may be encountered during the laparoscopic procedure.

Complications specific to fundoplication are usually related to dysphagia, which occurs if the procedure is made too 'tight'. In some patients, the wrap seems to break down with time and the incidence of recurrent reflux is about 15% over many years. It is possible to undertake further surgery in such circumstances, although it is usually more difficult the second time around.

Postoperative management is relatively standard, with oral fluids being commenced immediately, and a soft diet introduced when the patient can tolerate it. Patients are advised to refrain from anything that raises their intra-abdominal pressure to high levels (such as heavy lifting) for about 8 weeks, to allow the hiatus to adequately seal with fibrous tissue.

Hiatus hernia repair

This operation is very similar to a fundoplication, but is used to treat a type II or III hiatus hernia and is usually a more significant undertaking. The major problem is breakdown of the phreno-oesophageal ligament and widening of the oesophageal hiatus. The operation aims to reposition the stomach within the abdominal cavity. Additionally, the oesophageal hiatus needs to be repaired and reduced to a normal size to prevent recurrent herniation. Repair can be performed with sutures or mesh.

Bariatric surgery in patients with GORD

Obesity and reflux are closely associated, and therefore performing a procedure that can control reflux and achieve substantial weight loss has considerable attraction. There are several bariatric surgery options available: Roux-en-Y gastric bypass (RYGB), gastric banding and sleeve gastrectomy. RYGB is a highly effective and durable option that effectively controls reflux. Laparoscopic adjustable gastric banding (LAGB) is an effective anti-reflux procedure; however, in situations where there is dilatation above the LAGB, reflux may develop. Sleeve gastrectomy is the most commonly performed bariatric surgical procedure but is considered to have a higher incidence of reflux following surgery.

Further reading

Engstrom C, Cai W, Irvine T *et al.* Twenty years of experience with laparoscopic anti-reflux surgery. *Br J Surg* 2012;99:1415–21.

Keung C, Hebbard G. The management of gastro-oesophageal reflux disease. *Aust Prescr* 2016;39:6–10. Full text free online at www.australianprescriber.com

Mikami DJ, Murayama KM. Physiology and pathogenesis of gastroesophageal reflux disease. *Surg Clin North Am* 2015;95:515–25.

MCQs

Select the single correct answer to each question. The correct answers can be found in the Answers section at the end of the book.

1 Which of the following is *not* considered an alarm symptom requiring urgent investigation in a patient presenting with reflux symptoms?
   a large hiatus hernia
   b dysphagia
   c haematemesis
   d weight loss
   e anaemia

2 Initial assessment and management of a patient with suspected GORD should *not* include:

   a history and examination

   b endoscopy

   c lifestyle advice

   d evaluation of risk for oesophageal cancer

   e consideration of treatment with medication

3 Which of the following is true concerning hiatus hernias?

   a patients with sliding hiatus hernias generally have reflux

   b bariatric surgery should not be performed in a patient with a large hiatus hernia

   c very few patients have type II hiatus hernias

   d oesophageal manometry and pH testing are required prior to operative repair of types II and III hiatus hernias

   e Barrett's oesophagus is commonly associated with a hiatus hernia

15 Tumours of the oesophagus

Ahmad Aly[1,2] and Jonathan Foo[2]

[1] University of Melbourne, Melbourne, Victoria, Australia
[2] Austin Health, Melbourne, Victoria, Australia

Types of tumour

Benign

Benign oesophageal tumours are rare and account for less than 1% of all oesophageal neoplasms. Leiomyomas account for two-thirds of these and arise from the muscularis propria or muscularis mucosa. These smooth muscle tumours are often solitary, indolent and with an intact overlying mucosa. There are only rare case reports that describe progression to leiomyosarcoma.

Small leiomyomas are often asymptomatic and found on routine imaging or endoscopy. As they increase in size or have an annular configuration they may cause dysphagia. If symptomatic or large (>5 cm) excision should be considered. Rather than a formal oesophageal resection, these firm and well-encapsulated masses can often be surgically enucleated via either an open or minimally invasive approach. On occasion, leiomyomas may be very large and necessitate formal resection such as oesophagectomy (Figure 15.1).

Other rarer entities include schwannomas, epithelial polyps, haemangiomas, granular cell tumours and duplication cysts. While gastrointestinal stromal tumours are found in the oesophagus, their presence in the oeosphagus is rare in comparison with other parts of the gastrointestinal system.

Malignant

Oesophageal cancer is the ninth most common cancer worldwide; in Australia around 1400 people per year are diagnosed with oesophageal cancer. The survival outcomes are poor in comparison with other types of cancer and only 16–27% of all patients survive 5 years from the initial diagnosis. The common histological subtypes are adenocarcinoma and squamous cell carcinoma. Rarer subtypes include adenosquamous carcinoma, neuroendocrine carcinomas, melanomas, lymphomas, sarcomas, small cell carcinomas and adenoid cystic carcinoma.

The prevalence of squamous cell carcinoma and adenocarcinoma depends on the prevailing risk factors in differing regions of the world. Geographically, squamous cell carcinoma has a 50- to 100-fold greater incidence in high-risk areas compared with the rest of the world. For example, in Henan Province, China the incidence rate is over 160 per 100 000 compared with 2–3 per 100 000 in North America, Australia and Europe. While the most predominant histological subtype worldwide is squamous cell carcinoma, adenocarcinoma is much more common in the western world and is increasing in incidence, for example in the USA the incidence has increased from 3.6 per million in 1973 to 25.6 per million in 2006.

Geographical differences and changing distribution over time relate to changes in risk factors (Box 15.1). Patients with other aerodigestive malignancies have a 5–8% risk of developing synchronous or metachronous oesophageal squamous tumours, probably because of exposure to the same environmental carcinogens and the phenomenon of 'field change'. While smoking and alcohol induce chronic oesophageal inflammation, this plays a much smaller role in the aetiology of adenocarcinoma compared with squamous cell carcinoma.

Instead obesity, particularly with an intra-abdominal distribution of fat and the associated gastro-oesophageal reflux-induced acid and bile injury to the distal oeosphagus, is a more prominent risk factor. The injured oesophageal tissue adapts, via an unknown mechanism, by changing from normal stratified squamous epithelium to metaplastic columnar epithelium with characteristic goblet cells. Known as Barrett's oeosphagus, this change to intestinal metaplasia is thought to be a precursor to the dysplasia–cancer sequence of

Textbook of Surgery, Fourth Edition. Edited by Julian A. Smith, Andrew H. Kaye, Christopher Christophi and Wendy A. Brown.
© 2020 John Wiley & Sons Ltd. Published 2020 by John Wiley & Sons Ltd.

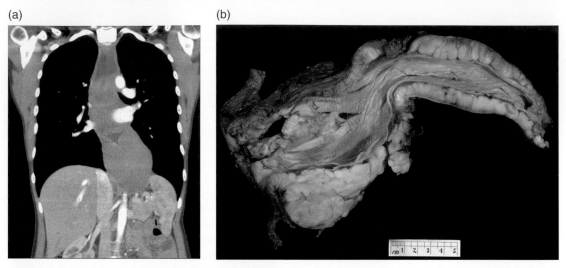

Fig. 15.1 (a) Large oesophageal leiomyoma on coronal CT and (b) resected specimen.

Box 15.1 Risk factors for squamous cell carcinoma and adenocarcinoma of the oesophagus

Squamous cell carcinoma
Smoking
Alcohol
Diet rich in nitrosamines
Deficiency in trace elements
Caustic injury
Low socioeconomic status
Achalasia
Hereditary tylosis
Plummer–Vinson syndrome

Adenocarcinoma
Barrett's oeosphagus
Obesity
GORD
High dietary fat
Male sex
Smoking

Another factor proposed as being involved in the epidemiology of oesophageal cancer may be the increasing prevalence of *Helicobacter pylori* infection. Since *Helicobacter pylori* induces gastritis and decreased acid secretion, this may in turn reduce acid reflux, and hence Barrett's oesophagus and cancer. The treatment of Barrett's oeosphagus is primarily through the use of proton-pump inhibitors (PPIs) to reduce acid reflux. There is no evidence for a difference in the incidence of adenocarcinoma in Barrett's oesophagus between patients who are treated with a PPI or anti-reflux surgery.

Anatomy and clinical features

The oeosphagus extends from the cricopharyngeus muscle in the neck, which is typically 15 cm from the upper incisor teeth, to the gastro-oesophageal junction. The oeosphagus is divided into a cervical, thoracic and abdominal component. The upper third of the thoracic oesophagus begins at the thoracic inlet and extends to the tracheal bifurcation at 24 cm. The middle third extends from 24 to 32 cm and the distal oesophagus from 32 cm to the diaphragm. The abdominal oeosphagus is a short length of 2 cm as it enters the gastro-oesophageal junction (usually 40 cm from the incisors). Anatomically, adenocarcinoma commonly involves the lower oeosphagus and gastric cardia rather than the upper and middle thoracic oesophagus in which squamous cell carcinoma is more common. Since the bulk of adenocarcinomas occur in the distal third and near the gastro-oesophageal junction, tumours in proximity to the gastro-oesophageal junction are categorised using the Siewert

adenocarcinoma. While most people with Barrett's oesophagus do not progress to oesophageal adenocarcinoma, further cellular injury from reflux may then lead to low-grade dysplasia, high-grade dysplasia and ultimately oesophageal adenocarcinoma. The risk of cancer progression is estimated to be 1 per 100 patient-years and surveillance endoscopy with biopsy should be considered in these patients. Recent developments suggest that molecular biomarkers may be employed to identify patients at increased risk of progression to oesophageal adenocarcinoma.

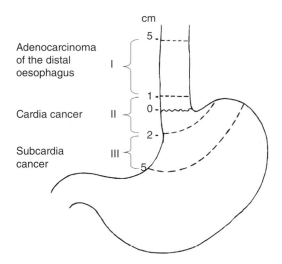

Fig. 15.2 Classification of adenocarcinomas around the gastro-oesophageal junction. Subcardial tumours (Siewert III) are staged with the stomach cancer TMN.

classification to differentiate between gastric and oesophageal tumours and to guide limits of resection (Figure 15.2).

Around the oeosphagus there is a rich submucosal lymphatic system that drains the mucosal lymphatics. Lymphatic metastases may spread longitudinally along this plexus to the regional lymph nodes all the way to the neck and abdomen or through the muscularis mucosa into the thoracic duct and venous system. Tumours may be found incidentally on imaging or endoscopy, diagnosed during surveillance endoscopy or present with symptoms.

Most patients are older than 50 years, with a male predominance. Early oesophageal cancer is often identified incidentally on surveillance endoscopy for Barrett's oeosphagus or the presence of only non-specific symptoms. In contrast, the presence of specific symptoms is usually an ominous indicator of at least locally advanced disease. Progressive dysphagia is common and the patient describes difficulty in swallowing solid food and eventually liquids. The site of the 'hold-up' sensation has only a modest correspondence to the location of the tumour; it is usually located above, but not below, the actual site of obstruction.

Other symptoms include odynophagia, melaena, regurgitation, substernal pain and weight loss. Acute gastrointestinal haemorrhage is more commonly associated with adenocarcinoma than squamous cell cancer and in rare cases this can be a herald bleed from an aorto-oesophageal fistula. Aspiration from an aero-oesophageal fistula, symptomatic para-neoplastic syndromes and vocal change from involvement of the recurrent laryngeal nerve are less common.

Diagnosis/staging

Initial upper gastrointestinal endoscopy provides a histological diagnosis and assesses the tumour's anatomical dimensions. The tumour must then be staged accurately to dictate appropriate management and provide prognosis. Oesophageal tumours are staged using the eighth edition of the American Joint Committee on Cancer (AJCC) TMN staging system (Table 15.1) published in 2018. Typical staging investigations include a combination of upper gastrointestinal endoscopy, computerised tomography (CT), endoscopic ultrasound and positron emission tomography (PET). CT of the chest, abdomen and pelvis is often the first study performed and provides information about potential resectability and/or presence of metastatic disease. Endoscopic ultrasound is a useful complement to detail T staging and mediastinal lymphadenopathy where it may affect treatment choice.

Table 15.1 American Joint Committee on Cancer TMN Classification for Oesophageal Cancer, 8th edition.

T category	
TX	Tumour cannot be assessed
T0	No evidence of primary tumour
Tis	High-grade dysplasia, defined as malignant cells confined by the basement membrane
T1	Tumour invades the lamina propria, muscularis mucosae or submucosa
T1a	Tumour invades the lamina propria or muscularis mucosae
T1b	Tumour invades the submucosa
T2	Tumour invades the muscularis propria
T3	Tumour invades adventitia
T4	Tumour invades adjacent structures
T4a	Tumour invades the pleura, pericardium, azygos vein, diaphragm, or peritoneum
T4b	Tumour invades other adjacent structures, such as aorta, vertebral body or trachea
N category	
NX	Regional lymph nodes cannot be assessed
N0	No regional lymph node metastasis
N1	Metastasis in 1–2 regional lymph nodes
N2	Metastasis in 3–6 regional lymph nodes
N3	Metastasis in 7 or more regional lymph nodes
M category	
M0	No distant metastasis
M1	Distant metastasis

T, tumour; N, node; M, metastases.

Fluorodeoxyglucose PET with integrated CT is also conducted in the initial staging work-up to further corroborate CT findings or identify distant metastatic disease not initially identified on CT.

Further investigations such as staging laparoscopy (particularly for adenocarcinoma), thoracoscopy, bronchoscopy, endoscopic bronchial ultrasound and neck ultrasound-guided fine needle aspiration should be considered depending on whether resection is offered or initial staging investigations are insufficient for accurate staging.

Staging investigations complement each other. No single investigation is sufficient and the sequence of investigations depends on each patient and the institution's oncological multidisciplinary team.

Principles of treatment

Once the tumour is accurately staged, the patient and tumour factors are normally reviewed at a cancer multidisciplinary meeting (Figure 15.3). With the complexity of staging investigations and treatment decisions, the multidisciplinary meeting provides subspecialty review and a pivotal point to offer multidisciplinary consensus on therapy for the individual patient. In over one-third of cases the diagnostic and staging information or treatment plan may be altered after review by the multidisciplinary meeting.

Early-stage disease (defined as stage I/node negative) may be considered for surgery alone since 5-year survival is 80% or greater. In selected cases, endoscopic resection may be considered for early

cancer (T1a) but this does not allow nodal assessment, which is important for prognosis and decisions about adjuvant therapy. Locally advanced disease (stage II/III) is considered for multimodal therapy while metastatic disease is treated with palliative intent. Without a screening program, oesophageal cancers in western countries are normally diagnosed when they are symptomatic and, by inference, either locally advanced or metastatic.

Neoadjuvant therapy is used in locally advanced disease and may involve either chemotherapy or chemoradiotherapy. While previously there has been controversy about whether surgery alone should be offered, a Cochrane review has demonstrated a 19% relative increase in survival post neoadjuvant chemotherapy at 5 years. The choice of chemotherapy or chemoradiotherapy depends on histological subtype and unit preference. The role of interval PET imaging and biomarkers to assess tumour response has the potential to tailor neoadjuvant therapy to the individual.

Following the publication of the CROSS trial in 2012 (chemoradiotherapy comprising carboplatin and paclitaxel with concurrent radiotherapy of 41.4 Gy in 23 fractions) and the MAGIC trial in 2006 (chemotherapy comprising epirubicin, cisplatin and 5-fluorouracil in three preoperative and three postoperative cycles), it has become widely accepted that locally advanced tumours are best treated with a multimodal approach since surgery alone has a 5-year survival of less than 20%. Neoadjuvant therapy in the form of either chemotherapy alone or chemoradiotherapy may be offered and then surgical resection is undertaken.

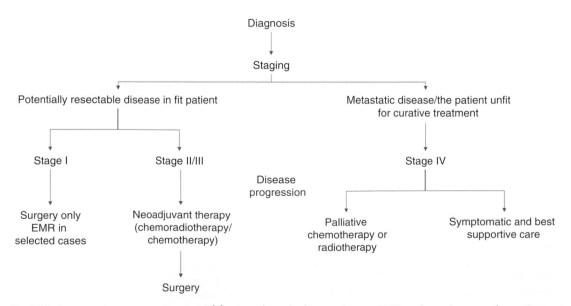

Fig. 15.3 An example management protocol for oesophageal adenocarcinoma. EMR, endoscopic mucosal resection.

Definitive chemoradiotherapy with resulting higher doses of radiotherapy is favoured in upper oesophageal squamous cell cancers or in resectable disease where surgery cannot be performed in a comorbid or elderly patient.

Surgical

Contraindications to surgery include distant visceral or nodal metastases and direct infiltration of the tracheo-bronchial tree or aorta. There is no role for palliative oesophagectomy. Instead, the goals of surgical resection are to completely resect the tumour with an adequate margin and an adequate lymphadenectomy of the representative nodal stations. Most surgeons will perform a lymphadenectomy of the upper abdomen and mediastinum, which is known as a two-field dissection. A three-field dissection (incorporating the cervical nodes) is sometimes considered in some centres for squamous cell carcinoma.

Careful selection is required to achieve the goals of surgery because a curative resection may involve two or all three of the cervical, thoracic or abdominal compartments. Potential surgical candidates should have a careful risk assessment, especially with regard to their cardiopulmonary status because of the high postoperative morbidity of oesophagectomy.

There are three archetypal procedures for thoracic and gastro-oesophageal junction tumours: a two-stage subtotal oesophagectomy (Figure 15.4a), a three-stage subtotal oesophagectomy (Figure 15.4b) and a transhiatal oesophagectomy. While the three differ in the manner of resection, all three preferentially use the stomach as the conduit to replace the resected oesophagus via the posterior mediastinum. If this route is unavailable because of previous surgery or sepsis, then the retrosternal and subcutaneous routes are possible alternatives.

Ivor Lewis oesophagectomy (two-phase oesophagectomy)

This operation was named after the eminent Welsh surgeon Ivor Lewis who in 1945 published his novel approach to the oesophagus via the right chest, where by simply dividing the azygos vein the oesophagus would be exposed for dissection.

It is commonly performed for tumours of the lower third of the oesophagus and Siewert I tumours. A laparotomy is first performed to mobilise the stomach on its right gastric and right gastroepiploic arterial pedicles. A lymphadenectomy is performed at the coeliac trunk to skeletonise the common hepatic and root of the splenic artery and the left gastric artery is ligated at its origin. Our preference is to also perform a pyroclastic to improve gastric drainage and for a feeding jejunostomy tube to be inserted.

The supine patient is then repositioned for a right posterolateral thoracotomy. This allows the exposure required to perform a radical en-bloc resection and lymphadenectomy. Once the tumour specimen is exenterated then the stomach is delivered via the diaphragmatic hiatus into the chest. The stomach is fashioned into a tube, mobilised up to sit mainly in the thoracic cavity to reduce the risk of reflux and an oesophago-gastric anastomosis is performed high in the thoracic cavity (Figure 15.5).

Mckeown's procedure (three-stage subtotal oesophagectomy)

This operation is commonly performed for tumours that involve the upper to middle thoracic oesophagus and involves a cervical oesophago-gastric anastomosis. A right thoracotomy is first performed to mobilise the thoracic oesophagus. The patient is then placed in a supine position and both a left cervical incision and a laparotomy are performed. The stomach is fashioned into a conduit and brought up through the posterior mediastinum into the neck where an anastomosis is performed.

Transhiatal oesophagectomy

This procedure involves the 'shelling out' of the oesophagus by a surgeon's hand via the diaphragmatic hiatus and neck without a thoracotomy. The stomach is brought up into the neck to fashion a cervical oesophago-gastric anastomosis. In experienced hands this partially blind procedure is safe, with similar perioperative mortality rates. However, the operation is controversial as an oncological procedure since extensive thoracic lymphadenectomy is not formally performed.

Laparoscopic, thoracoscopic and robotic approaches

The anatomical boundaries of the oesophagus mean that open procedures expose the patient to lengthy incisions in the chest and abdomen. Increasingly, high-volume centres have introduced minimally invasive oesophagectomies to minimise the impact of multi-compartment surgery, such as degree of blood loss and time spent in intensive care and in hospital. Large-volume case series in these centres demonstrate comparable cancer outcomes with open surgery but careful case selection is still required.

While there are several approaches for oesophageal resection, the stomach remains the preferred

(a)

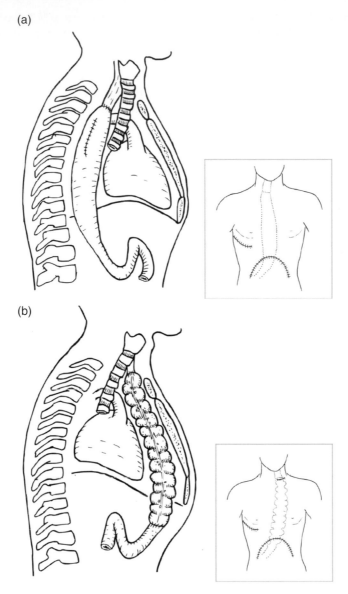

(b)

Fig. 15.4 (a) Ivor Lewis oesophagectomy with an intrathoracic oesophago-gastric anastomosis. (b) Three-stage oesophagectomy. In this example, a colonic interposition is depicted in the retrosternal route with an anastomosis in the neck.

conduit for oesophageal reconstruction because it is relatively robust and only a single anastomosis is required. The lesser curvature of the stomach is largely excised, but the right gastroepiploic artery and right gastric artery are preserved. The high point of the fundus is used to anastomose the oesophagus to the isoperistaltic stomach. Should the gastric conduit fail or the stomach is a non-viable option, then the colon or jejunum can be fashioned into a conduit.

Tumours of the cervical oesophagus require resection of the hypopharynx and the larynx as well as the oeosphagus. These often require a multidisciplinary approach with a head and neck surgical unit. Typically, these tumours are squamous cell type and the survival outcomes of treatment with chemoradiation are similar to those of surgery. For this reason, and because of the extensive nature of surgery, many of these patients are treated with definitive chemoradiotherapy.

Historically, an oesophagectomy was regarded as a highly morbid procedure with a significant mortality rate. Perioperative mortality has improved and now in major centres this is considerably less than 5%. The dramatic reduction in mortality is due to increasing referrals to specialised units

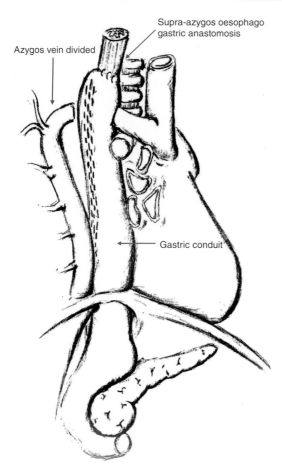

Azygos vein divided

Supra-azygos oesophago
gastric anastomosis

Gastric conduit

Fig. 15.5 Two-stage oesophagectomy, with the stomach
in the posterior mediastinum.

in tertiary-level hospitals, careful patient selection, multidisciplinary consensus for management, enhanced recovery programs and improved postoperative management.

The use of early mobilisation, careful fluid balance, early nutritional support and adequate thoracic analgesia has served to reduce complications and the ensuing morbidity and mortality. Unfortunately, there remains a significant risk of complication following oesophagectomy which entails surgery in at least the thoracic and abdominal compartments.

Complications of surgery

Complications exist in all surgeries. Oesophageal resections have a high risk of morbidity with the extensive en-bloc dissection in both abdominal and thoracic cavities. Postoperative complications may be categorised into general medical or procedure-specific complications (Box 15.2).

Box 15.2 Complications after oesophagectomy

Medical

Cardiac
Atrial arrhythmia*
Myocardial infarction
Cardiac failure

Pulmonary
Atelectasis*
Pneumothorax
Bronchopneumonia with or without aspiration*
Sputum retention*
Pleural effusion*
Pulmonary embolism
Respiratory failure

Other medical†
Renal failure
Hepatic failure
Stroke

Surgical
Intraoperative or postoperative haemorrhage
Tracheobronchial tree injury
Recurrent laryngeal nerve injury
Anastomotic leakage
Gangrene of conduit
Intrathoracic gastric outlet obstruction or gastric stasis
Herniation of bowel through diaphragmatic hiatus
Chylothorax
Empyema
Wound infection

Note that surgical complications are technique- and operator-dependent, thus incidences can vary

* Relatively common occurrence

† Should all be uncommon

Multi-compartment surgery increases the likelihood of typical post-surgical conditions such as pulmonary, cardiac and renal complications. Pain, fluid balance, blood loss and pre-existing cardiorespiratory risk factors can all potentiate the risk of these complications, which can occur in 30–40% of all patients. On occasion, complications such as a unilateral pleural effusion or atrial fibrillation are subtle signs of more significant complications such as an anastomotic leak and a high index of suspicion is required to intervene early. Specific early oesophagectomy complications include anastomotic and conduit leaks, chyle leaks and laryngeal nerve injuries.

Historically, the anastomotic leak rate has been 20–30% but in recent times the incidence of this has fallen to less than 5% in major units. Leaks may occur because of excessive conduit tension, poor vascularity, faulty surgical technique or patient factors such as malnutrition or underlying vascular disease. These are diagnosed with cross-sectional imaging, fluoroscopy and upper gastrointestinal endoscopy. Early anastomotic leaks often within 72 hours may be investigated with surgical exploration, whilst late leaks are typically managed with aggressive non-operative management. Whether early or late, nutritional support and control/drainage of mediastinal and thoracic sepsis are critical components.

The thoracic duct enters the thoracic cavity through the aortic opening between the aorta and azygous vein. It is divided as part of the en-bloc resection for an oesophagectomy. Occasionally, the secured duct may leak or there is aberrant anatomy resulting in a chylothorax. The chyle losses are rich in free fatty acids and immune complexes, which can swiftly result in malnutrition. High-volume losses require surgical exploration whilst losses of less than about 500 mL may be treated with a medium-chain triglyceride enteral diet. Resistant leaks may require a lymphangiogram with embolisation or shunting procedures.

Laryngeal nerve palsies can occur during an oesophagectomy. The long looping path of the recurrent laryngeal vagus nerve is vulnerable to injury in the upper thorax and in particular during the cervical mobilisation of a three-stage oesophagectomy.

The postoperative complications of oesophagectomy may quickly become life-threatening. Often subtle signs and biochemical aberrations are present in a physiologically well patient. A high index of suspicion, early investigation and treatment are required to minimise the rapid physiological deterioration with chest or abdominal sepsis.

Symptomatic treatment

The majority of patients in western countries present with stage IV disease, with dysphagia and significant weight loss. While there are other symptoms, dysphagia from malignant obstruction is extremely debilitating. With careful patient selection, dilatation and the endoscopic placement of a self-expanding metal oesophageal stent provide symptomatic relief and a normal route for nutrition (Figure 15.6).

Palliative radiotherapy can be delivered via brachytherapy or external beam. Brachytherapy is an alternative in dysphagia and external beam therapy can be useful with symptomatic bleeding or pain.

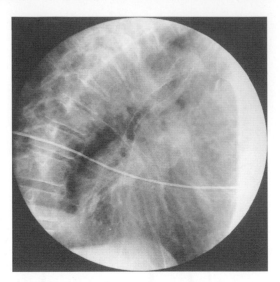

Fig. 15.6 Self-expanding metallic oesophageal stent *in situ*.

Argon-beam plasma coagulation and laser treatments such as the neodymium yttrium–aluminium–garnet (Nd:YAG) laser are less frequently used with the popularity of stents, although they can be considered when a stent cannot be deployed, such as in the cervical oesophagus. Less common palliative treatments also include photodynamic therapy and the injection of intralesional alcohol.

Prognosis

The survival from oesophageal cancer remains poor in comparison with other cancers, with an overall survival of 8–16% at 5 years. Two-thirds of patients are not suitable for resection and with palliative management they have a median survival of 8 months. The remaining one-third of patients have potentially curative disease at the time of diagnosis. Care should be delivered with a multidisciplinary approach in specialised centres. Since survival is so dependent on stage, early detection and accurate staging is crucial for delivering optimal treatment.

Further reading

Cunningham D, Allum WH, Stenning SP *et al*. Perioperative chemotherapy versus surgery alone for resectable gastroesophageal cancer. *N Engl J Med* 2006;55:11–20.

Rice TW, Patil DT, Blackstone EH. 8th edition AJCC/UICC staging of cancers of the esophagus and esophagogastric junction: application to clinical practice. *Ann Cardiothorac Surg* 2017;6:119–30.

Ronellenfitsch U, Schwarzbach M, Hofheinz R *et al.* Perioperative chemo(radio)therapy versus primary surgery for resectable adenocarcinoma of the stomach, gastroesophageal junction, and lower esophagus. *Cochrane Database Syst Rev* 2013;(5):CD008107.

van Hagen P, Hulshof MC, van Lanschot JJ *et al.* Preoperative chemoradiotherapy for esophageal or junctional cancer. *N Engl J Med* 2012;366:2074–84.

MCQs

Select the single correct answer to each question. The correct answers can be found in the Answers section at the end of the book.

1 For patients suffering from oesophageal cancer, which of the following symptoms indicates the *worst* prognosis?
   a hoarseness of voice
   b weight loss of more than 10% of usual body weight
   c dysphagia to solid and semi-solid food
   d regurgitation of swallowed food
   e odynophagia

2 A 75-year-old man complains of progressive dysphagia for 2 months. He has lost 4.5 kg in weight and can only tolerate a liquid diet. Oesophageal cancer is suspected. Which of the following investigations is most likely to detect evidence of distant metastases from his cancer?
   a upper endoscopy

   b endoscopic ultrasonography
   c positron emission tomography
   d ultrasound with or without fine-needle aspiration of neck
   e CT scan

3 Which of the following is the most likely risk factor for development of a squamous cell cancer of the oesophagus?
   a smoking
   b alcohol intake
   c obesity
   d history of cancer of the larynx
   e achalasia

4 The most common benign tumour of the oesophagus is:
   a adenosquamous carcinoma
   b fibrovascular polyp
   c leiomyoma
   d haemangioma
   e neurofibroma

5 The diagnosis of chylous leak after oesophagectomy is *not* helped by:
   a analysis of chylomicrons in the chest tube output
   b lymphangiogram
   c milk challenge
   d Gastrografin contrast swallow
   e test for triglyceride in chest tube output

16 Peptic ulcer disease

Paul A. Cashin[1] and S.C. Sydney Chung[2]

[1] Monash University and Monash Health, Melbourne, Victoria, Australia
[2] Chinese University of Hong Kong and Union Hospital, Hong Kong

Introduction

Peptic ulcer is a common condition. Each year, peptic ulcer disease (PUD) affects approximately 4 million people worldwide; 2–10% of these ulcers will perforate. The incidence and severity of PUD has been decreasing in the western world and has now reached a stable incidence. However, as a result of the widespread use of freely available non-steroidal anti-inflammatory drugs (NSAIDs), the incidence of ulcer disease in the elderly is increasing in many parts of the world. Complications of the disease such as perforation and bleeding can be quite catastrophic.

Aetiology

Peptic ulcers occur when the balance between acid secretion and the natural defence mechanism of the mucosa is disturbed. Classical sites for peptic ulcers are the first part of the duodenum, the angula incisura and the antrum/pre-pyloric region of the stomach, the lower end of the oesophagus in patients with gastro-oesophageal reflux, along the edges of a gastroenterostomy (marginal ulcers), and inside a Meckel's diverticulum if there is ectopic gastric mucosa.

Whilst acid hypersecretion has traditionally been thought to be the most important factor in the causation of ulcers, in particular duodenal ulcers, this is now known not to be the case. The classical example of the effect of increased acid production is the infrequently seen Zollinger–Ellison syndrome. Uncontrolled gastrin production by pancreatic or duodenal adenoma causes maximal stimulation of the parietal cell mass, producing massive amounts of acid and resulting in a particularly aggressive form of PUD.

The most common and important aetiological factor is *Helicobacter pylori*, a Gram-negative organism that resides in the mucus layer of the antrum, and is the real culprit in the majority of cases. *Helicobacter pylori* remains one of the most common bacterial infections in the world. In the upper gastrointestinal tract it is considered a hostile commensal. Its global presence in humans is estimated to be up to 50%. Chronic infection with *H. pylori* is a major aetiological factor in PUD. Individuals colonised with *H. pylori* have a sevenfold increase in the risk of developing PUD. The organism is found in more than 90% of patients with duodenal ulcers and more than 80% of patients with gastric ulcers. Antibiotic eradication of the bacterium heals the ulcer and prevents recurrence. Such a discovery has completely revolutionised the understanding of the pathogenesis and management of peptic ulcers.

Other associated factors have been implicated in the co-aetiology of PUD. These include age (the old in developed countries and the young in developing countries), NSAID ingestion, smoking, genetic factors, and those with multiple endocrine neoplasia (MEN)-1. Many of these act by amplifying the effect of *H. pylori* on the gastric epithelium or by leading to pathological acid hypersecretion (MEN-1/gastrinoma in association with this).

Mucosal defence against acid–pepsin digestion consists of the mucous layer on the mucosa, which serves as a barrier between the lumen and the epithelial surface, the secretion of bicarbonate and the rapid turnover of mucosal cells. Other factors can acutely damage this barrier, such as reflux of bile into the stomach and by mucosal ischaemia. These are additional factors that can weaken the mucosal defence and contribute to the development of ulcers. 'Stress' ulcers are common in severely ill patients, particularly those treated in intensive care units, when not receiving prophylactic acid suppression. Cushing's ulcers and Curling's ulcers are stress ulcers occurring after head injuries and severe burns, respectively. These ulcers are caused by increased acid production in stressed patients, and

Textbook of Surgery, Fourth Edition. Edited by Julian A. Smith, Andrew H. Kaye, Christopher Christophi and Wendy A. Brown.
© 2020 John Wiley & Sons Ltd. Published 2020 by John Wiley & Sons Ltd.

mucosal ischaemia as a result of splanchnic hypoperfusion.

Duodenal ulcer

Practically all duodenal ulcers occur in the first and second parts of the duodenum, being most common in the duodenal bulb. This part of the duodenum is in the direct path of the acid contents of the stomach. Alkaline pancreatic juice and bile, which enter the duodenum in the second part, have not yet had an opportunity to neutralise the gastric acid. Duodenal ulcers are more common than gastric ulcers. They tend to occur in younger patients and are more common in men than women. There is also a genetic predisposition; the disease is more common in family members of index cases, patients with blood group O, non-secretors of blood group antigens in the saliva, and those with high circulating pepsinogen.

Clinical features

The cardinal symptom of duodenal ulcer is pain. The pain is typically localised to the epigastrium, is dull or burning in character, starts several hours after a meal, wakes the patient at night and is relieved by food or antacids. Nausea, bloating and vomiting may be present during an acute exacerbation but are not prominent features. In contrast to patients with non-ulcer dyspepsia, ulcer patients localise the pain to the epigastrium with one finger. Apart from mild tenderness in the epigastrium, patients with uncomplicated ulcer disease do not have physical signs.

The course of duodenal ulcer disease is one of relapses and remissions. The patient complains of episodes of severe pain lasting for weeks, interspersed by months of remission, the pattern repeating itself over several years. The disease may burn itself out after 10–15 years.

Diagnosis

It is difficult to clinically differentiate duodenal ulcer from other causes of upper abdominal pain (gastric ulcer, acute gastritis, non-ulcer dyspepsia, reflux oesophagitis, gastric cancer, gallstones) with confidence on clinical grounds alone. Upper gastrointestinal endoscopy is the most accurate diagnostic method, and essential to the diagnosis. The oesophagus, stomach and the first and second part of the duodenum can be clearly seen, and ulcers biopsied using this technique.

Helicobacter pylori can be demonstrated by serology, by the urea breath test, or in antral biopsies using microscopy or the rapid urease test. The detection of *H. pylori* proteins and antigens in faecal specimens has also been used. Culture of organisms is difficult and rarely performed in clinical practice. Serology detects past as well as current infection and is simple to conduct as only a drop of blood is necessary. The accuracy of the commercially available test kits has improved but their validity must be confirmed for each country as there are geographical differences in the genetic make-up of the bacterium. Serology cannot be reliably used to assess the success of eradication therapy, as antibody levels can remain raised for prolonged periods even after successful eradication.

In the urea breath test, urea labelled with a non-radioactive (^{13}C) or radioactive (^{14}C) carbon isotope is given by mouth. *Helicobacter* produces urease, which splits the urea into ammonia and carbon dioxide. If ^{13}C or ^{14}C is detected in the exhaled breath, the presence of *Helicobacter* is confirmed. The urea breath test is a reliable non-invasive way of confirming the success of eradication therapy, but care must be used when attempting to use it as a primary diagnostic modality as associated gastric diseases such as gastric cancer may be missed. For this reason, endoscopic examination and biopsy remains the most important test.

In patients who have undergone endoscopy, a convenient test is the rapid urease test. Antral biopsies are embedded in a gel containing urea and an indicator dye (neutral red). The ammonia produced as a result of urease is alkaline and changes the indicator dye to a red colour. This gives a rapid result, often within an hour, and is cheaper than histology. The use of proton pump inhibitors (PPIs) such as omeprazole lead to a suppression of organism numbers in the gastric mucosa. This can lead to false-negative results in patients undergoing the urea breath test, urease test and even histology. It is recommended that patients on PPIs have these ceased at least 2 weeks prior to urea breath testing or, if testing is to be performed at endoscopy, that biopsies are taken for histology from both antrum and body of stomach to increase the yield.

Treatment

The aim of treatment is to alleviate the ulcer pain, to heal the ulcer, to prevent recurrence and to forestall complications. With powerful acid-inhibiting drugs (PPIs) and effective regimens to eradicate *Helicobacter*, these aims can be achieved by medical therapy in the great majority of patients. Apart from giving up smoking and avoiding, if possible, ulcerogenic drugs, lifestyle modification such as a change in diet or avoidance of stress is not necessary. Such changes are difficult to make and there is little evidence that they accelerate ulcer healing. Nowadays, elective surgery for uncomplicated ulcer disease is rarely, if ever, indicated. Nearly all ulcer surgery is performed as an emergency procedure for complications.

Commonly used drugs

Antacids
Antacids may be in tablet or liquid form. They are either magnesium based (liable to cause diarrhoea) or aluminium based (may cause constipation). Antacids give rapid temporary relief of ulcer pain but do not heal ulcers unless taken in very high doses. This is not recommended.

Histamine H₂ receptor antagonists
Antagonists of the histamine H_2 receptor (H_2 blockers) were the first group of drugs to be marketed that effectively block gastric acid secretion. Examples are cimetidine, ranitidine and famotidine. Relief of pain occurs after a few days and up to 90% of ulcers heal after a 6-week course. Once the drug is stopped, however, acid production returns to normal and ulcer recurrence is highly likely.

Proton pump inhibitors
PPIs such as omeprazole, esomeprazole, pantoprazole and lansoprazole lead to near complete inhibition of gastric acid production. Symptomatic relief and ulcer healing is even more impressive than with H_2 blockers. However, once the drug is stopped ulcer recurrence is common. PPIs have been shown to both prevent and heal ulcers associated with NSAID use. For this reason, they are used as prophylaxis in acutely ill patients to prevent 'stress' ulceration, particularly in the intensive care setting. PPIs are now first-line treatment for PUD, in conjunction with *H. pylori* eradication.

Sucralfate
Sucralfate is a drug that is not absorbed but exerts its action by physically covering the ulcer base. Ulcer healing rates are similar to those with H_2 blockers.

Eradication of Helicobacter pylori
Antibiotic eradication of *H. pylori* is now the cornerstone of ulcer treatment, coupled with PPI therapy. It is also the main reason why elective surgery for PUD is now very rare. The bacteria dwell in, and are protected by, the mucous layer of the gastric pits and are difficult to eradicate. Multiple drugs need to be administered simultaneously. Effective combinations should result in eradication in more than 90% of patients if patient compliance is satisfactory. Examples of such combinations are 1–2 weeks of triple therapy using a PPI, clarithromycin and amoxicillin. Side effects, especially gastrointestinal upsets, are common. Combinations of a PPI and two other antibiotics can be used if allergy issues arise. These combinations have become first-line therapy in most countries.

In some countries, *H. pylori* has begun to exhibit significant resistance and cause issues with both failure of treatment and in recurrent disease. Recurrence may be partly socioeconomic with repeated infections but may be partly the result of treatment leaving resistant organisms in the upper gastrointestinal tract. Improper and uncontrolled use of antibiotics is also a major problem in some countries, with a potential impact worldwide. In patients with recurrent or non-responsive infections, antimicrobial resistance should be investigated.

The addition of PPIs to the antibiotics improves the eradication rate by maintaining a gastric pH close to or above 6 and may also help to reduce the development of resistance.

Surgery

The classical operations for non-emergency duodenal ulcer disease are designed to reduce gastric acid production (Table 16.1). Nowadays their use is almost entirely confined to the management of ulcer complications (non-healing or obstruction) or not done at all. Essentially one can remove the acid-producing part of the stomach or sever the vagus nerve, which controls acid secretion. With so many

Table 16.1 Operations for duodenal ulcers.

	Mortality (%)	Side effects	Recurrence rate (%)
Pólya's gastrectomy	2–5	+++	5
Vagotomy and drainage	1	+	5–10
Highly selective vagotomy	<0.5	±	15
Vagotomy and antrectomy	2–5	++	1

of these operations having been performed in the past, it remains important to understand them.

Billroth II gastrectomy

Acid is secreted by parietal cells in the body and the fundus of the stomach. In order to ensure adequate reduction of acid output, at least two-thirds of the stomach needs to be resected. Patients who have had this operation are unable to tolerate large meals. Weight loss, malnutrition and anaemia are common unless actively managed. The rapid entry of food into the intestine leads to 'dumping' syndromes – the patient feels faint or unwell after a meal. This may be due to transudation of fluid in response to an osmotic load in the gut (early dumping, occurring 10 minutes after a meal) or rapid absorption of glucose, leading to insulin release and rebound hypoglycaemia (late dumping, occurring 2–3 hours after a meal). Although rare these functional complications can be distressing and difficult to manage.

Truncal vagotomy and drainage

Gastric acid production may also be decreased by dividing the vagus nerve, thus removing the nervous stimulation of the parietal cell mass. If the whole vagal trunk is cut, delay in gastric emptying occurs in a significant number of patients because the motor supply to the antrum is also severed. A drainage operation, either a pyloroplasty or gastroenterostomy, is necessary. These operations are relatively easy to perform and are useful in emergency situations. Between 5 and 10% of patients complain of diarrhoea, due to rapid transit of food through the gut.

Highly selective vagotomy

This operation aims to divide the vagal fibres supplying the parietal cell mass but leave the innervation of the antrum (the nerve of Latarget) intact. The operation is technically demanding and time-consuming. Side effects are almost non-existent but the recurrence rate is higher than in other procedures.

Vagotomy and antrectomy

In this operation the vagal trunks are divided to remove the vagal stimulation of acid production and the antrum is resected to remove the source of gastrin, another potent stimulator of gastric acid secretion. Continuity of the gastrointestinal tract is restored by Roux-en-Y gastrojejunal anastomosis. The main attraction of this operation is the very low ulcer recurrence rate.

Most operations for duodenal ulcer disease are done in an emergency setting for complications of

the disease and are described in a subsequent section.

Gastric ulcer

Gastric ulcers are less common than duodenal ulcers. They affect the older age group. Gastric ulcers are more common in patients from lower socioeconomic groups. NSAIDs are a common cause of gastric ulcers as is *H. pylori* infection. In patients with non-healing gastric ulcers, malignancy or a gastrinoma should be considered.

Clinical features

As in duodenal ulceration the usual presentation is epigastric pain. The pain is typically exacerbated by food. Nausea, unremitting pain and weight loss are common. Any clinical differentiation from duodenal ulcer and gastric cancer is unreliable.

Diagnosis

All suspected gastric ulcers must be investigated by endoscopy and biopsy. Biopsy is essential as gastric cancer is common and sometimes difficult to differentiate from benign ulceration.

Double-contrast barium meal X-ray examinations were extensively used in the past and were often inaccurate and misleading. Nowadays they are largely confined to history.

As seen through the endoscope a benign gastric ulcer has smooth regular margins. The most common site is the angular incisura, followed by the lesser curvature and the antrum. An ulcer seen outside these locations should raise the suspicion of malignancy, although all gastric ulcers can be malignant or benign. Malignant ulcers are often irregular with raised, rolled-up edges. With potent acid suppression, even malignant ulcers may completely heal over temporarily, leaving an area of mucosal irregularity. All gastric ulcers must be subjected to multiple biopsies. After a course of eradication therapy, repeat endoscopy to assess healing and repeat biopsy are mandatory. This is usually performed 6–12 weeks after completion of pharmacological treatment.

Treatment

Although acid output is normal or low in patients with gastric ulcers, ulcer pain is controlled and the ulcer heals with acid suppression. PPIs are the medications of choice. Because gastric ulcers are often larger than duodenal ulcers they generally take longer to heal. Greater than 80% of gastric ulcers are associated with positive *H. pylori* on urease testing or seen at biopsy. Eradication of the bacterium is indicated in all patients to reduce the recurrence rate. Other gastric ulcers are caused by NSAIDs, but these medications are so frequently used in the community that it is not indicated to simply cease these drugs. Full treatment with PPIs, *H. pylori* eradication and re-endoscopy is still best practice. If it is not possible for the patient to stop taking an NSAID, a PPI taken concurrently confers a degree of protection.

Gastric cancer may masquerade as a gastric ulcer. If complete healing of the ulcer is not achieved with two courses of medical therapy, surgical resection of the ulcer may be considered. However, repeat biopsies will usually provide the answer, often aided by endoscopic ultrasound in a non-healing ulcer. Pre-resection diagnosis allows the patient with gastric cancer to receive optimum cancer care with neoadjuvant chemotherapy/radiotherapy to achieve maximum cure rates.

Non-healing benign ulcers should be investigated for Zollinger–Ellison syndrome (see the last section in this chapter). Poor medication compliance should also be considered and these patients often have low serum gastrin levels, consistent with them not taking their PPIs.

The aim of surgical treatment for benign disease is to resect the ulcer-bearing part of the stomach. The operation of choice for gastric ulcers is Billroth II style gastrectomy, in which the distal half of the stomach is removed and intestinal continuity restored with a Roux-en-Y gastrojejunostomy. In patients where it is medically indicated not to perform major resectional surgery, for example age and comorbidities, or the ulcer is in the proximal stomach, local excision of the actual benign ulcer has reasonable results, coupled with ongoing PPI therapy.

Complications of ulcer disease

Complications of duodenal ulcers include bleeding, perforation and gastric outlet obstruction.

Bleeding

Peptic ulcer bleeds occur when the ulcer erodes a vessel in the ulcer base. Classical textbook cases of posterior duodenal ulcers eroding the gastroduodenal artery and gastric ulcers eroding the left gastric artery are rarely seen in the modern era. Most cases of ulcer bleeding result from erosion of medium-sized arteries in the submucosa.

Peptic ulcer bleeding is the most common cause of upper gastrointestinal haemorrhage and is a frequent cause of emergency hospital admission. The mortality is up to 10% and has remained constant despite advances in diagnosis and treatment. This is due to an increase in the number of elderly people presenting with this condition.

About 85% of bleeding ulcers stop bleeding spontaneously and do not require specific measures to stop the haemorrhage. The mortality in those who continue to bleed or develop rebleeding while in hospital is 10-fold higher. The likelihood of rebleeding may be predicted on clinical grounds and the appearance of the ulcer on endoscopy. Haematemesis and shock on admission suggest a large initial bleed and are associated with a higher risk of recurrent haemorrhage. Ulcers with stigmata of recent haemorrhage, such as a visible vessel or an adherent blood clot seen on endoscopy, are also more likely to rebleed but, if possible, treated endoscopically they are less likely to rebleed. On the other hand, if a clean-based ulcer is seen on endoscopy the risk of rebleeding is very low. Larger ulcers are more likely to rebleed. The risk of rebleeding decreases with time after the initial bleed. If rebleeding does not occur within the first 72 hours on PPI treatment, it is unlikely to occur. Higher acute transfusion requirements correlate with higher rebleeding risk.

Clinical features

The patient may vomit fresh blood and clots (indicating torrential bleeding) or coffee-ground material (acid haematin resulting from the action of gastric acid on haemoglobin). More commonly the patient passes melaena (semi-liquid tarry black stool with a characteristic sickly smell). The consistency and colour of the melaena may give some clue to the rapidity of the bleeding: the redder and less well formed the stool, the brisker the haemorrhage. There may be a background of long-standing PUD, and history of another episode of bleeding in the past. In 30% of patients there is a history of recent intake of NSAIDs or aspirin. The patient may complain of dizziness or faint on getting up from a supine position or demonstrate a postural drop in their blood pressure indicating hypovolaemia in association with the bleed.

Patients are sometimes diagnosed with rectal bleeding if transit is quick enough and the bleeding significant. All patients with semi-altered blood on rectal examination should be considered for gastroscopy first to rule out a rapid transit upper gastrointestinal bleed.

Apart from melaena on rectal examination, patients with a mild to moderate amount of blood loss show little abnormality on examination. Tachycardia, sweaty palms, hypotension, anxiety and agitation are signs of shock and call for urgent blood volume replacement. Abdominal pain is an unusual feature.

Treatment

Resuscitation

All patients who have had a significant gastrointestinal bleed within the past 48 hours should be admitted to hospital. Two large-bore intravenous cannulas should be inserted and blood drawn for baseline tests and cross-matching. In the acute stage, the haemoglobin level is a poor guide to the need for transfusion as haemodilution may not have occurred. The decision to replace the blood volume by plasma expanders or blood should be based on signs of hypovolaemia and the rapidity of the bleeding. In elderly patients with poor cardiac reserve, or in patients with massive bleeding, monitoring central venous pressure by a central venous line gives a more accurate indication of the amount of fluids needed.

Identify the bleeding point

If facilities allow, all patients admitted with upper gastrointestinal haemorrhage should undergo endoscopy within 24 hours of admission. Patients who vomit fresh blood or are in shock may have ongoing massive blood loss and should undergo endoscopy once they are resuscitated. An accurate diagnosis forms the basis of logical treatment, and the precise location of bleeding is of paramount importance should surgery be needed to control bleeding.

Control bleeding

Ulcer bleeding stops spontaneously in about 80% of patients. Only a small percentage require specific measures to stop bleeding. In recent years endoscopic procedures have become the first-line method of controlling ulcer bleeding. The most popular methods are injection therapy using adrenaline solution and/or sclerosants, such as polidocanol, absolute alcohol or ethanolamine; contact thermal methods, such as the heater probe or multipolar electrocoagulation; or direct endoscopic clipping of a visible vessel in the base of the ulcer. Not infrequently, multiple methods need to be used to achieve control at gastroscopy. Endoscopic haemostasis should be applied for ulcers with active

bleeding or stigmata of recent haemorrhage predictive of high risks of rebleeding. In the modern era, rebleeding is usually again treated endoscopically.

If immediate control cannot be achieved, in both gastric and duodenal ulcers, in a setting where it is available, radiological embolisation of the bleeding vessel can control the bleeding or delay the need for acute surgical intervention. All these interventions require a multidisciplinary team approach.

If none of these means is able to control the bleeding, surgery needs to be considered with at least the advantage of almost always knowing the site of bleeding in the upper gastrointestinal tract. Direct suture of the bleeding vessel via a duodenotomy in bleeding duodenal ulcers is the treatment of choice in this case. In bleeding gastric ulcers, local excision of the ulcer should be considered to obtain a definitive biopsy. Rarely is an antrectomy or vagotomy required given the effectiveness of PPI therapy and *H. pylori* eradication therapy.

Perforation

Perforation occurs when the ulcer erodes through the full thickness of the gut wall. Gastric and duodenal contents spill into the peritoneal cavity causing sudden acute pain and then generalised peritonitis. The most frequent site of perforation is the anterior wall of the first part of the duodenum. Males outnumber females in a ratio of 9 : 1. The incidence of ulcer perforation in the elderly is increasing because of the increased use of NSAIDs. Often there are few prodromal ulcer symptoms.

Clinical features

The patient presents with sudden onset of severe abdominal pain. The onset of pain is so sudden that the patient can often accurately pinpoint the exact moment when the perforation occurred. Approximately 10% of patients have no preceding history of classic ulcer symptoms. Meticulous history is important in terms of identifying risk factors and comorbidities such as cirrhosis and portal hypertension, immunological diseases requiring steroid therapy and renal failure. The physical signs in the abdomen are dramatic. There is generalised tenderness, guarding and rebound tenderness. The abdominal muscles are held rigid, giving the classical board-like rigidity. Abdominal respiratory movements and bowel sounds are often absent. The percussion note over the liver may be resonant because of free intraperitoneal air. In patients in whom the perforations are sealed off by adjacent organs the signs may be localised to the epigastrium. In other cases, the spillage from the perforation may track down the right paracolic gutter, resulting in maximal tenderness in the right iliac fossa. This is the so-called right paracolic gutter syndrome, and may be mistaken for acute appendicitis. Similar tracking may occur down the left side of the abdomen to mimic perforated diverticulitis.

Investigations

A plain chest radiograph with the patient in the erect position shows free gas under the diaphragm in 80% of cases. Large volumes of subphrenic free gas are more indicative of a perforated ulcer, whereas small volumes may suggest a colonic perforation but this is not diagnostic as peptic ulcers may be walled off by omentum leading to small volumes of gas.

The presence of free gas on plain X-ray is generally sufficient information to proceed to definitive surgical treatment. Further investigation with contrast CT scanning may be required if the diagnosis is not clear.

Treatment

Once an acute abdomen has been recognised or the diagnosis is made, the patient should be given parenteral opiates for pain relief, intravenous fluids and antibiotics should be administered and a nasogastric tube passed as soon as possible to decompress the stomach to avoid ongoing contamination. Unless there is clear evidence that the ulcer has been sealed off, an operation should be performed without delay. In young patients with localised signs, trials of conservative management with intravenous antibiotics, nasogastric drainage and contrast X-ray to confirm sealing of the ulcer within 24 hours have been successful in some studies.

The operation of choice for a perforated *duodenal ulcer* is a simple patch repair. A piece of well-vascularised omentum is sutured over the perforation to plug it (Figure 16.1). This is followed by a thorough lavage of the peritoneal cavity with copious amounts of warm saline to remove all the exudate and food particles. An intraperitoneal drain tube may be inserted in the vicinity of the repair. In most cases this is now done with laparoscopic surgery, avoiding a painful wound.

For a perforated *gastric ulcer*, the preferred repair is done by excising the ulcer, thereby obtaining a biopsy to rule out a malignant ulcer, and primarily

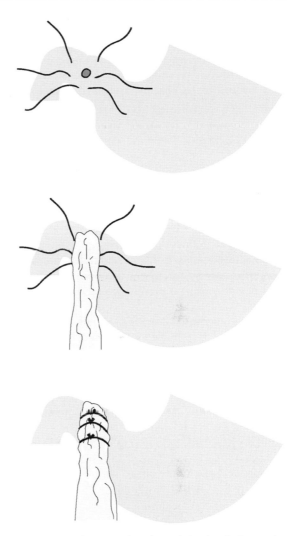

Fig. 16.1 Patch repair of perforated duodenal ulcer with a vascularised omental plug.

closing the defect. The closure of the defect in the stomach does not narrow the lumen and healing is usually excellent with the well-vascularised stomach.

The discovery that PUD can be cured by eradication of *H. pylori* has diminished the enthusiasm for definitive surgery at the same time as the patch repair and it is now rarely performed. For patients known to be *Helicobacter* negative, an ulcer-curing operation (e.g. Billroth II gastrectomy or Pólya gastrectomy) may be considered if there has been a long history of troublesome ulcer disease with complications, provided that the condition of the patient is good and the degree of contamination of the abdomen not too severe.

Obstruction

Long-standing duodenal or pre-pyloric ulcers may cause gastric outlet obstruction. It may be due either to fibrosis resulting from chronic ulceration and healing or to oedema associated with acute ulceration.

Clinical features

The cardinal symptom is repeated vomiting of undigested food that is not stained with bile. A history of long-term PUD is frequent, as is long-term NSAID use. There may be weight loss and dehydration. In more indolent forms there may be early postprandial fullness and bloating. Abdominal examination shows a dilated distended stomach. Succussion splash (splashing noise on rocking the patient's abdomen) is present several hours after a meal.

The inability to take fluids by mouth and vomiting of gastric juice lead to severe fluid and electrolyte problems. The patient rapidly becomes dehydrated and salt depleted. Loss of acid and chloride ions in the gastric juice result in hypochloraemic alkalosis. There may be a large deficit of total body potassium. Because of the severe sodium depletion, the distal renal tubules secrete potassium and hydrogen ions in exchange for sodium ions in the glomerular filtrate. The urine is therefore acidic in severe cases of gastric outlet obstruction, although the patient is alkalotic. This is the so-called paradoxical aciduria.

A gastric cancer in the antrum or the pyloric canal causing obstruction may present in an identical manner.

Treatment

Fluid and electrolyte losses should be replaced by infusion of normal saline. Large amounts of potassium are likely to be required. Administration of potassium supplements should be guided by estimation of the serum level and acid–base balance. It should only commence when renal failure is excluded. Correction of alkalosis is not necessary. Once the fluid and electrolyte deficiencies are corrected the body's homeostatic mechanisms will restore the acid–base balance.

The stomach should be decompressed with a nasogastric tube. Food particles may block the tube, requiring gentle gastric irrigation. Intravenous PPIs are administered. Once the stomach is decompressed, an endoscopy should be carried out to confirm the diagnosis and to exclude malignancy. If the obstruction is due to oedema around an active ulcer, such measures may restore patency. In the majority of cases, operative management is required. Modern treatment involves a surgical antrectomy and a Roux-en-Y reconstruction. In the less fit a gastroenterostomy alone may bypass the obstruction but does not address the ulceration. In elderly patients unfit for surgery, dilatation of the stenotic area using a balloon catheter under endoscopic guidance may be considered.

Zollinger–Ellison syndrome

This is a rare disease accounting for less than 1% of PUD and is caused by over-production of gastrin by G-cell tumours of the pancreas or duodenum. This is most often associated with the gastrin-secreting neuroendocrine tumor gastrinoma. Maximal gastrin stimulation of the parietal cells leads to intractable peptic ulcerations. The majority (90%) of gastrinomas occur within the 'gastrinoma triangle' bounded by the cystic duct and bile duct, the junction of the head and neck of the pancreas, and the second and third parts of the duodenum. Two-thirds of all gastrinomas occur outside the pancreas. Approximately 50% of gastrinomas are malignant and up to one-third have liver metastases; 10% of patients with Zollinger–Ellison syndrome have multiple lesions of the pancreas rather than discrete tumours.

Clinical features

The diagnosis should be suspected when peptic ulcers occur at unusual sites, such as the second part of the duodenum or the jejunum, or ulcers recur after adequate surgery. One-third of patients have watery diarrhoea due to high gastric output. Dehydration and acid–base or electrolyte imbalance may occur.

Diagnosis

Gastrin can be measured by radioimmunoassay. The diagnosis is confirmed by demonstrating a high fasting gastrin level. This may be confounded by high-dose PPIs, which also elevate gastrin levels but usually not to the level of a gastrinoma. Nuclear medicine studies and MRI are helpful in localising these tumors in the gastrinoma triangle.

Treatment

The aim of treatment of Zollinger–Ellison syndrome is twofold:

- to control the high gastric acid output and sever the ulcer diathesis
- to treat the gastrinoma.

In the past a total gastrectomy was recommended to remove gastric acid production. Nowadays, the ulcer diathesis can usually be controlled by a high dose of PPI. If a single discrete tumour can be identified in the pancreas or the duodenum, surgical excision is the treatment of choice.

Further reading

Cirocchi R, Soreide K, Di Saverio S *et al*. Meta-analysis of perioperative outcomes of acute laparoscopic vs open repair of perforated gastroduodenal ulcers. *J Trauma Acute Care Surg* 2018;85:417–25.

Debraekeleer A, Remaut H. Future perspective for potential *Helicobacter pylori* eradication therapies. *Future Microbiol* 2018;13:671 87.

Lagoo J, Pappas TN, Perez A. A relic or still relevant: the narrowing role for vagotomy in the treatment of peptic ulcer disease. *Am J Surg* 2014;207;120–6,

Malmi H, Kautiainen I I, Virta LJ, Färkkilä N, Koskenpato J, Färkkilä MA. Incidence and complications of peptic ulcer disease requiring hospitalisation have markedly decreased in Finland. *Aliment Pharmacol Ther* 2014;39:496–506.

Smith RS, Sundaramurthy SR, Croagh D. Laparoscopic versus open repair of perforated peptic ulcer: A retrospective cohort study. *Asian J Endosc Surg* 2019;12:139–44.

Spiliopoulos S, Inchingolo R, Lucatelli P *et al*. Transcatheter arterial embolization for bleeding peptic ulcers: a multicenter study. *Cardiovasc Intervent Radiol* 2018;41:1333–9.

MCQs

Select the single correct answer to each question. The correct answers can be found in the Answers section at the end of the book.

1 With a perforation of a duodenal ulcer which occurred 6 hours ago, which of the following features is *least* likely to be present?
   a generalised abdominal tenderness and guarding
   b the bowel sounds are hyperactive
   c percussion over the liver may demonstrate resonance
   d the respiration is shallow and the abdominal muscles are held rigid
   e plain radiograph shows free gas under the diaphragm

2 Which of the following factors is most likely to be associated with a significant risk of rebleeding from a duodenal ulcer?
   a no further bleeding within 72 hours of the initial bleed
   b a clean based ulcer seen on endoscopy
   c age less than 50 years
   d a visible vessel with adherent clot seen on endoscopy
   e the patient is female

3 Which of the following is the treatment of choice for a perforated duodenal ulcer in a 56-year-old man with a strong history of ulcer disease and signs of peritonitis after 12 hours?
   a conservative management with nasogastric suction and intravenous fluids
   b vagotomy and pyloroplasty
   c omental patch repair and peritoneal lavage
   d highly selective vagotomy
   e partial gastrectomy

17 Gastric neoplasms

John Spillane

University of Melbourne and Division of Cancer Surgery, Peter MacCallum Cancer Centre, Melbourne, Victoria, Australia

Gastric adenocarcinoma

Gastric cancer is the fourth most common cancer and the second most common cause of cancer-related deaths worldwide. It is a tumour that in the western world is often diagnosed late, with almost 50% of patients having locally advanced or metastatic disease at the time of diagnosis. High-incidence areas occur in eastern Asia, particularly Korea and Japan, as well as central and eastern Europe. It is more common in men. Over the last 40 years the worldwide incidence of gastric cancer has been decreasing with an associated fall in the mortality. The majority of the fall has been associated with tumours within the middle and distal stomach as well as tumours involving the entire stomach. The incidence of proximal gastric cancer has remained unchanged, making up approximately 30% of all gastric cancers. Gastric cancers can be classified anatomically into gastro-oesophageal junction tumours and true gastric cancers. Symptoms include dyspepsia, upper abdominal pain, anorexia and in more advanced stages weight loss, vomiting and anaemia.

Epidemiology

Risk factors in areas with high incidence are thought to be due to a combination of poor nutrition, sanitation, obesity, smoking and alcohol consumption. Diet, particularly foods that are salted, smoked, pickled or preserved foods rich in salt and nitrites, increase the risk of gastric cancer. *Helicobacter pylori* is also directly associated with the development of gastric cancer; particular strains, for example those positive for cytoxin-associated gene (*cagA*) and vacuolating cytotoxin gene (*vacA*), are implicated. In western countries, approximately 60% of *H. pylori* are *cagA* positive but in Japan almost 90% of strains are positive. Epstein–Barr virus has been detected in gastric cancers although its role in pathogenesis is unclear.

Approximately 10% of gastric cancers are hereditary, with 30–40% of hereditary diffuse gastric cancer due to a germline mutation in the E-cadherin *CDH1* gene. This was initially diagnosed in New Zealand Maori families with a high penetrance (70–80%) and a lifetime risk of approximately 67% in men and 83% in women, who also have an increased risk of breast cancer (mostly lobular) of 20–40%. It is recommended that at-risk patients over the age of 20 years with a *CDH1* mutation or patients of any age with a positive biopsy have a total gastrectomy. Patient under the age of 20 or over the age of 20 and who have declined prophylactic surgery should be placed in an endoscopic surveillance program.

Gastric cancer is also associated with other genetic conditions, such as hereditary non-polyposis colorectal cancer syndrome and, less commonly, with familial adenomatous polyposis coli and Li–Fraumeni and Peutz–Jeghers syndromes.

Histology

The majority of gastric cancers are adenocarcinomas. The remainder are a mixture of lymphomas, gastrointestinal stromal tumours and uncommon malignancies such as neuroendocrine tumours.

Adenocarcinomas are divided histologically using the Lauren classification into two main types, diffuse and intestinal, plus mixed and indeterminate. Another classification is the World Health Organization (WHO) system, which defines tumours based on the histological pattern (tubular, papillary, mucinous, poorly cohesive and rare).

Staging

The eighth edition of the American Joint Committee on Cancer (AJCC) staging system has defined tumours crossing the oesophago-gastric junction (OGJ) with their epicentre in the proximal 2 cm of

Textbook of Surgery, Fourth Edition. Edited by Julian A. Smith, Andrew H. Kaye, Christopher Christophi and Wendy A. Brown.
© 2020 John Wiley & Sons Ltd. Published 2020 by John Wiley & Sons Ltd.

the stomach as oesophageal cancers. Cancers crossing the OGJ with the epicentre in the proximal 2–5 cm of the stomach are stomach cancers.

Staging is based on the T (tumour), N (node) and M (metastases) system and is now subdivided into different categories. Clinical staging (cTNM) is a clinical assessment of the patient usually with staging investigations completed but no pathological specimen. Pathological staging (pTNM) occurs after assessment of the pathological specimen. Assessment post neoadjuvant therapy and pathological specimen analysis is now termed ypTNM. This assesses the response of the cancer to therapy and assesses if viable tumour cells are still present within the resected stomach and lymph nodes. Depending on which system is used, the stage of the tumour can be different (Table 17.1). Staging correlates with survival and varies according to which of the three systems are used.

T staging is based on the depth of penetration of the primary tumour (Table 17.2). Gastric cancer has a higher incidence of metastasis to lymph nodes, which increases with advancing T stage (T1a, ~3%; T1b, ~20%; T2, ~40%; T3, 50–60%; T4, ~70%).

Regional lymph nodes

Regional nodes are defined as perigastric nodes along the greater and lesser curvature, and the supra- and infra-pyloric and right and left pericardial regions, plus regional nodes along the left gastric, coeliac, common hepatic and splenic arteries, the hilum and hepatoduodenal nodes. The Japanese Research Society categorises this into 16 lymph node stations, six perigastric and 10 regional stations. Lymph node resections are then designated D1 (removing only perigastric nodes) or D2 (including D1 nodes plus the other regional nodes). Routine removal of the spleen is no longer performed as it increases the morbidity without improving survival, although is still resected in selected cases. Nodes around the porta hepatis or adjacent to the aorta are classified as D3. A D2 lymphadenectomy is considered the standard of care

Table 17.1 AJCC staging system for gastric cancer (8th edition) including clinical staging (cTNM), pathology staging (pTNM) and post-neoadjuvant therapy (ypTNM).

T	N	M	cTNM	pTNM	ypTNM
Tis	N0	M0	0	0	
T1	N0	M0	I	IA	I
T1	N1	M0	IIA	IB	I
T2	N0	M0	I	IB	I
T1	N2	M0	IIA	IIA	II
T2	N1	M0	IIA	IIA	II
T3	N0	M0	IIB	IIA	II
T1	N3a	M0	IIA	IIB	II
T2	N2	M0	IIA	IIB	II
T3	N1	M0	III	IIB	II
T4a	N0	M0	IIB	IIB	II
T2	N3a	M0	IIA	IIIA	III
T3	N2	M0	III	IIIA	III
T4a	N1	M0	III	IIIA	III
T4a	N2	M0	III	IIIA	III
T4b	N0	M0	IVA	IIIA	III
T1	N3b	M0	IIA	IIIB	II
T2	N3b	M0	IIA	IIIB	III
T3	N3a	M0	III	IIIB	III
T4a	N3a	M0	III	IIIB	III
T4b	N1	M0	IVA	IIIB	III
T4b	N2	M0	IVA	IIIB	III
T3	N3b	M0	III	IIIC	III
T4a	N3b	M0	III	IIIC	III
T4b	N3a	M0	IVA	IIIC	III
T4b	N3b	M0	IVA	IIIC	III
Any T	Any N	M1	IVB	IV	IV

Table 17.2 Definition of gastric TNM staging.

T stage

TX	Primary tumour not assessable
T0	No primary tumour
Tis	Intraepithelial tumour without invasion of lamina propria
T1a	Invasion of lamina propria or muscularis mucosae
T1b	Invasion of submucosa
T2	Invasion of muscularis propria
T3	Invasion of subserosal connective tissue without invasion of visceral peritoneum or adjacent structures
T4a	Invasion of serosa/visceral peritoneum
T4b	Invasion of adjacent organs/structures

N stage

NX	Regional lymph nodes unable to be assessed
N0	No regional metastatic nodes
N1	1 or 2 positive regional nodes
N2	3–6 positive regional nodes
N3	7 or more positive regional nodes
N3a	7–15 positive regional nodes
N3b	16 or more positive regional nodes

M stage

M0	No distant metastases
M1	Distant metastases

Box 17.1 Paris classification of microscopic morphology of early gastric cancer

Type 0-I	Protruded type (0-Ip, pedunculated or 0-Is, sessile)
Type 0-IIa	Superficial and elevated type
Type 0-IIb	Flat type
Type 0-IIc	Superficial and depressed type
Type 0-III	Excavated type

---

throughout most of the world. At least 16 lymph nodes must be assessed pathologically, with the removal of more than 30 nodes felt to be desirable. Nodal involvement outside these areas is considered metastatic disease. The nodal staging is based on the total number of positive nodes removed (see Box 17.1).

Metastatic sites

The most common sites of metastatic disease are the liver, peritoneum and non-regional lymph nodes. Pulmonary and central nervous system metastases occur but are less common.

Investigation

The diagnosis is made by gastroscopy and biopsy of the tumour. Tumours are further evaluated with endoscopic ultrasound (EUS) which assesses the T and N staging. It can discriminate between superficial (T1–T2) and advanced (T3–T4) tumours as well as assess lymph node positivity.

Computed tomography (CT) can assess nodal and metastatic disease sites. Positron emission tomography (PET) is less useful because signet ring tumours and poorly differentiated or diffuse adenocarcinomas often lack fluorodeoxyglucose (FDG) uptake that can lead to under-staging of the disease. A diagnostic laparoscopy with peritoneal washings and biopsy of any atypical peritoneal nodules will detect low-grade metastatic disease not assessed by conventional imaging. The risk of peritoneal spread increases with advancing T stage and is highest with T4 and linitis plastica tumours.

Molecular testing for over-expression of human epidermal growth factor receptor (HER2) should be performed. HER2 is a transmembrane tyrosine kinase receptor that regulates cell proliferation and suppresses apoptosis. Approximately 12–20% of gastric adenocarcinomas are HER2 positive.

Early gastric cancer

Early gastric cancer is gastric cancer confined to the mucosa or submucosa (T1) regardless of lymph node status. The microscopic morphology of the lesions is defined by the Paris classification (Box 17.1). More than 65% of cases are type 0-IIc.

In countries with high levels of gastric cancer, screening programs have been introduced. In Japan, approximately 50% of gastric cancers are diagnosed at an early stage compared with approximately 20% in western countries. The frequency of gastric cancer is significantly lower in western countries, making mass screening programs not cost-efficient. However, they can be considered for high-risk groups such as *CDH1* carriers.

The diagnosis of early gastric cancers can be difficult. In addition to conventional endoscopy with white light imaging, chromoendoscopy uses dye-based enhancing agents such as acetic acid and indigo carmine that are sprayed across the surface of suspicious lesions to aid diagnosis and identify the margins of the lesion. Other techniques include narrow-band imaging technology and magnifying endoscopes that allow near-focus imaging of the gastric mucosa and are built into modern gastroscopes.

Surgery

Complete surgical resection with or without neo-adjuvant and adjuvant therapy is still the only curative modality for gastric adenocarcinoma. The type of operation varies depending on the position of the tumour, stage of disease and type of cancer.

Endoscopic therapy

The treatment of early gastric cancer with endoscopic resection has become more common over the last decade. The two main techniques are endoscopic mucosal resection (EMR) and endoscopic submucosal dissection (ESD). EMR involves the separation of mucosa from submucosa by an injection of fluid. A variety of different techniques are then used to resect the mucosa, including injection-assisted, cap-assisted and ligation-assisted techniques. ESD involves resecting the mucosa around the lesion using an electrosurgical knife followed by resection of the submucosa. The advantages of ESD over EMR are a higher en bloc and histological complete resection rate and lower local recurrence. The disadvantage is a higher perforation rate (1–4.5%). Bleeding, both intraoperative and delayed (~15%), is similar between the two methods. Recurrence rate following ESD is up to 1.1%. The 5-year overall survival is 92%.

This technique is used on tumours that are less than 2 cm in diameter, well differentiated and without ulcerative features. Attempts to expand these criteria are being investigated and well-differentiated non-ulcerated tumours of 3 cm or less could be considered for endoscopic resection. This relies on knowing that the risk of lymph node metastases is less than 3% for a T1a tumour. T1b–T4 tumours should undergo standard surgical resection. If complete endoscopic resection is not possible, patients should undergo surgical resection. Ongoing endoscopic follow-up is required due to the risk of metachronous gastric cancer.

Surgical resection

A total gastrectomy is indicated if the tumour involves the entire stomach or proximal stomach or if the patient is a carrier of the *CDH1* mutation. A distal gastrectomy is indicated for tumours in the body or antrum, where a 4–6 cm proximal margin can be obtained and leave a sufficient proximal stomach (minimum of 2 cm margin to the OGJ) for good functional capacity. For a distal gastrectomy the short gastric vessels must be preserved as the other arteries supplying the stomach (left and right gastric, left and right gastroepiploic arcade) will be resected with the surgical specimen. In both cases a reconstruction is performed with the proximal jejunum in a Roux-en-Y fashion or Billroth II anastomosis that can be used for distal gastrectomies. Complications include anastomotic leakage, fluid collections, abscesses and issues related to ileus, bowel obstructions or poor motility. Late complications include gastritis, oesophagitis, dumping, weight loss, and vitamin B_{12} and folate deficiencies.

There has been increasing use in recent years of minimally invasive surgery, laparoscopic and, more recently, robotic surgery to perform distal and total gastrectomies. The advantages of these approaches are a shorter length of stay, less intraoperative blood loss, decreased pain, less use of intensive care services and quicker return to full function. The lymph node resection numbers are equivalent to open surgery, although the operating time is longer. The morbidity and mortality of laparoscopic surgery is equivalent in most studies to open surgery. Both robotic and laparoscopic gastrectomies have a considerable learning curve, with a significant early conversion rate.

Chemotherapy and radiation therapy

As many patients present with advanced disease at the time of initial diagnosis, combined with the poor overall outcomes, particularly in the West for all but the most early disease, a concerted effort has been made in the last two decades to investigate the benefits of chemotherapy and radiotherapy in the treatment of gastric cancer. Treatments have used combinations of neoadjuvant (treatment prior to surgical resection), adjuvant (commencing after surgical resection) and perioperative (both neoadjuvant and adjuvant) therapies. The type of chemotherapy also varies between studies. This can make data interpretation confusing as to which regimen is best. Additionally, studies within Asia have excellent results but sometimes use treatments that are not available in the West. The following sections summarise general information regarding the use of these therapies, which should be considered for any patient with nodal involvement or stage II–IV.

Neoadjuvant chemotherapy

Neoadjuvant chemotherapy down-stages disease before surgical resection. A number of trials have examined this issue, the largest being MAGIC (Medical Research Council Adjuvant Gastric

Infusional Chemotherapy). This British study used three cycles of neoadjuvant and adjuvant chemotherapy in addition to surgery for patients with stage II or higher disease versus surgery alone. The trial showed a significantly improved overall and progression-free survival for perioperative chemotherapy. However, 34% did not commence postoperative chemotherapy and only 42% received the planned dose. The study included patients with distal oesophageal and gastro-oesophageal junction tumours in addition to gastric cancers and used what is now considered slightly older chemotherapy regimens. However, a meta-analysis of this study and a number of other smaller studies has shown a statistically improved overall and progression-free survival plus R0 resection rates in patients receiving neoadjuvant chemotherapy. Despite the limitations of all these studies, neoadjuvant therapy became one standard of care approach. Ongoing studies are investigating the best type of chemotherapy regimen.

Neoadjuvant chemoradiation

Chemotherapy is known to be radiosensitising – it makes tumour cells more responsive to radiation therapy. However, very few studies have investigated this with regard to gastric cancer and there are no published randomised controlled trials. There have been a number of studies investigating this treatment for oesophageal cancer, and have included patients with gastro-oesophageal junction and gastric cardia tumours. Studies such as CROSS (ChemoRadiotherapy for Oesophageal Cancer followed by Surgery versus Surgery alone) have shown an improved overall survival. Whether this can be extrapolated to gastric cancers is not clear but is the subject of ongoing investigations such as the TOPGEAR trial, an international predominantly western trial that has randomised patients to neoadjuvant chemotherapy or chemoradiotherapy prior to surgery with adjuvant chemotherapy.

Adjuvant chemotherapy

A number of older small studies have investigated adjuvant chemotherapy. They used old chemotherapy regimens that failed to show an improvement in survival. Two recent trials have investigated adjuvant chemotherapy, both conducted in Asia, but it is not clear if the results can be transferred to western populations. Both studies used a D2 gastrectomy as an entry criterion. The Japanese ACTS-GC (Adjuvant Chemotherapy Trial of S1

for gastric cancer) had an improved disease-free and overall survival, although it required patients to use a chemotherapy drug called S-1 which is not available outside of Asia. The CLASSIC (Capecitabine and Oxaliplatin Adjuvant Study in Stomach Cancer) used more conventionally available chemotherapy, again showing an improved disease-free survival and an estimated improved overall survival at the 5-year follow-up analysis. Further studies are ongoing in this area, predominantly in Asia.

Adjuvant chemoradiation

The first trial to show a benefit of adjuvant chemoradiotherapy was the Intergroup 0116 trial, which investigated surgery plus adjuvant chemoradiotherapy versus surgery alone. Although there was an improved overall and disease-free survival, which persisted at 10 years, there were some significant criticisms of the study. The surgery was not controlled, with 36% of patients receiving a D1 resection and only 10% receiving a D2 resection. Only 65% completed the chemoradiotherapy as planned, the majority due to toxicity. However, this study changed the treatment approach for gastric cancer and was adopted in many countries. The Korean ARTIST trial, comparing chemotherapy with chemoradiotherapy following a D2 resection, showed no difference in overall survival at 7 years of follow-up; however, it did show an improvement in sub-analysis of patients who were lymph node positive. A few other smaller trials have shown similar results, namely no survival difference between chemotherapy and chemoradiotherapy. It is not clear if chemoradiotherapy adds a significant benefit to a D2 resection.

Molecular therapy

The ToGA trial (Trastuzumab for Gastric Cancer) showed an improved overall and progression-free survival for HER2-positive advanced gastric cancer treated with trastuzumab plus chemotherapy with no increase in adverse advents. Herceptin-based therapies have now been incorporated into the chemotherapy treatments for patients with gastro-oesophageal junction and gastric cancers that are HER2 positive.

A number of ongoing studies are investigating the use of targeted therapies as well as immune system modulating agents in the treatment of gastric cancer. The results of these trials may significantly alter the management of gastric cancer in the coming years.

Gastrointestinal stromal tumours

Gastrointestinal stromal tumours (GIST) can arise anywhere within the gastrointestinal tract but are most commonly found within the stomach (50–60%). One-third of tumours are asymptomatic with the rest presenting with symptoms related to mass effect such as dysphagia, early satiety, abdominal discomfort, obstruction plus perforation and anaemia. The median age at diagnosis is 60 years, with most having a mutation of *C-Kit* or less commonly *PDGFRA*, succinate dehydrogenase deficiency and *BRAF* mutations.

Up to 50% of patients present with metastatic disease, most commonly to the omentum, peritoneum or liver. It is unusual, except in paediatric cases, to have lymph node metastases. GIST push onto surrounding structures without invading them.

Surgical resection is recommended for primary tumours greater than 2 cm or for smaller tumours that are either symptomatic or increasing in size. Tumours of less than 2 cm often do not progress and can be conservatively managed with follow-up CT scans. Tumours with high-risk features on EUS (irregular borders, ulceration, echogenic foci, heterogeneity and cystic spaces) should be resected. Surgery involves segmental resection of only the tumour to achieve negative resection margins allowing stomach preservation. Recurrence is high, particularly in cases of increased size and high mitotic rate. Intermediate and high-risk tumours are treated with tyrosine kinase inhibitors (imatinib). Current recommendations are for 3 years of adjuvant therapy.

For unresectable or metastatic disease, tyrosine kinase inhibitors can achieve partial response rates of 50% and in stable disease of 30%. It is sometimes possible for tumours to subsequently become surgically resectable. Although response rates are good, drug resistance occurs within 2–2.5 years. Initial treatment is dose escalation with imatinib. If further progression occurs, second-line therapy with sunitinib or third-line therapy with regorafenib can improve progression-free survival.

Gastric neuroendocrine tumours

Gastric neuroendocrine tumours arise from the enterochromaffin-like (ECL) cells located within the gastric fundal mucosa. They are rare but have been increasing in incidence over the last 50 years due to increased use of endoscopy and improved histopathological diagnosis. They comprise 2% of all gastric malignancies.

Gastric neuroendocrine tumours have been classified into well-differentiated (types I–III) and a poorly differentiated neuroendocrine carcinoma (type IV). Tumours are graded according to the number of mitoses per 10 high-power fields and percentage of tumour cells labelling positive for Ki-67 antigen.

These tumours are diagnosed by endoscopy and staged with EUS, CT, FDG and ^{68}Ga DOTA-TATE PET. Serum chromogranin A, which is expressed in secretory granules of the ECL cells, may be elevated and is a useful marker of response to treatment and recurrence.

- *Type I tumours* (70–80%): occur more commonly in women, and are associated with chronic atrophic gastritis, pernicious anaemia, elevated plasma gastrin and low gastric acid levels. They are usually asymptomatic, with small (5–8 mm) frequently multiple lesions found predominantly within the fundus or gastric body. They are usually benign, with a 96% 5-year survival. Histology: grade 1, exhibits mitoses of less than 2 and Ki-67 of less than 3%. Management is conservative, with endoscopic follow-up to detect the rare event of malignant transformation. Surgery is reserved for high-risk cases (six lesions, with three to four lesions larger than 1 cm or one lesion larger than 2 cm).
- *Type II tumours* (5–10%): caused by autologous gastrin secretion from a gastrinoma and associated with the Zollinger–Ellison syndrome, with 92% having multiple endocrine neoplasia type I syndrome. Up to 35% have metastatic disease at diagnosis. The tumours are usually less than 1 cm, have a low pH (<2), and may be multiple and located in the proximal stomach. Histology: grade 2, exhibits mitoses of 2–20 and Ki-67 of 3–20%. Treatment is surgical resection along with the gastrinoma. If the gastrinoma cannot be resected, acid hypersecretion needs controlling with proton pump inhibitors or serotonin antagonists.
- *Type III tumours* (5–25%): occur predominantly in males (~80%), and are usually large solitary tumours (1–2 cm) found in the fundus and body but can occur within the antrum. Histology: grade 3, exhibits mitoses of greater than 24 and Ki-67 of greater than 20%. More than 50% have metastatic disease at the time of diagnosis. Tumours are often poorly differentiated, with a high mitotic rate and Ki-67. They are not associated with hypergastrinaemia.
- *Type IV tumours*: poorly differentiated, also known as anaplastic high-grade neuroendocrine

tumour or small cell carcinoma of the stomach. The tumours are large (>2 cm), solitary and occur throughout the stomach. Approximately one-third have a concurrent gastric adenocarcinoma. There may be a reduced chromogranin A level due to loss of ECL cell secretory function.

Types III and IV are treated with a radical partial or total gastrectomy and an extended lymph node dissection. Metastatic disease is treated with somatostatin analogues or peptide receptor radionuclide therapy with lutetium-177 or yttrium-90 and chemotherapy.

Gastric lymphoma

Gastric lymphoma arises from lymphoid tissue in the lamina propria. It is rare, comprising 3% of gastric tumours and 10% of lymphomas. More than 90% belong to two histological subtypes, low-grade mucosa-associated lymphoid tissue (MALT) lymphoma (40%) and diffuse large B-cell lymphoma (DLBL; 55%). The remainder comprise Burkitt's lymphoma and low-grade non-MALT lymphomas.

Most present with symptoms of epigastric pain, anorexia, weight loss, bleeding and vomiting. B symptoms (fever, night sweats and weight loss) are not common in gastric lymphoma. At endoscopy, multiple superficial and deep biopsies are needed to aid the diagnosis and test for *H. pylori*. Staging is completed with CT, PET, bone marrow biopsies and blood films. Chemotherapy and occasionally radiotherapy are the mainstay of treatment, with surgery for complications (bleeding or perforation). Eradication of *H. pylori* is important in the treatment of MALT but also for DLBL disease. This can result in remission in up to 80% of cases with localised disease.

Further reading

Ajani JA, In H, Sano T *et al*. Stomach. In: Amin MB, Edge SB, Greene FL *et al.* (eds) *AJCC Cancer Staging Manual*, 8th edn. New York: Springer, 2017:203–20.

Olino KL, Tyler DS. Gastric neoplasms. *Surg Clin North Am* 2017;97:xv–xvi.

Van Cutsem E, Sagaert X, Topal B *et al*. Gastric cancer. *Lancet* 2016;388:2654–64.

MCQs

Select the single correct answer to each question. The correct answers can be found in the Answers section at the end of the book.

1 A 55-year-old male has been diagnosed with a T2N1M0 gastric cancer in the upper body of the stomach on staging investigations. Which of the following is the correct management plan?
   a radical total gastrectomy and D2 lymphadenectomy
   b perioperative chemotherapy, total gastrectomy and D2 lymphadenectomy
   c radical distal gastrectomy and adjuvant chemoradiotherapy
   d neoadjuvant chemoradiotherapy then total gastrectomy

2 A 60-year-old female is diagnosed with a GIST tumour in the proximal stomach invading the diaphragm and spleen. Which of the following is the correct management?
   a imatinib
   b radical total gastrectomy
   c resection of proximal stomach, diaphragm and spleen
   d sunitinib

3 A 22-year-old female with *CDH1* mutation had a recent endoscopy with biopsies showing no evidence of gastric cancer. She is reluctant to undergo a prophylactic gastrectomy. The management options include:
   a insist she undergo a total gastrectomy
   b regular endoscopic follow-up
   c treatment with trastuzumab
   d EUS to better assess the stomach

18 Obesity and bariatric surgery

Yazmin Johari[1] and Wendy A. Brown[2]

[1] General Surgery Registrar, Alfred Health, Melbourne, Victoria, Australia
[2] Department of Surgery and Centre for Obesity Research and Education, Monash University and Alfred Health, Melbourne, Victoria, Australia

Introduction

Obesity is a rapidly growing problem in today's society. The prevalence of obesity worldwide has nearly tripled since 1965. According to the World Health Organization (WHO), in 2016 there were over 1.9 billion overweight or obese adults and 41 million overweight or obese children under five. Over two-thirds of adults in the USA are overweight or obese. In 2015, 63% of adults in Australia were considered overweight or obese, compared with 56% in 1995.

The WHO defines overweight and obesity as follows.
- Overweight: body mass index (BMI) greater than or equal to 25 kg/m^2
- Obese class I: BMI 30–34.99 kg/m^2
- Obese class II: BMI 35–39.99 kg/m^2
- Obese class III: BMI greater than or equal to 40 kg/m^2.

The significance of obesity is considerable. It is well known to be closely related to a wide variety of diseases, including type 2 diabetes, heart disease, stroke, cancers, hepatic steatosis, osteoarthritis of the spine and weight-bearing joints, and obstructive sleep apnoea. The American Obesity Association has stated that obesity increases the risk of death by at least 50%, making obesity the second leading cause of preventable death in the USA. In addition to health consequences, the economic impact of obesity is significant. The cost of treatment of obesity and its complications in the USA is over US$200 billion. Furthermore, obesity may lead to other indirect costs, such as absenteeism or loss of productivity at work.

Baiatric surgery and its role in weight loss

Fundamentally, obesity is caused by consumption of energy in excess of expenditure of energy. In theory weight loss should be easy, a simple reversal of the energy equation. In practice it is very hard to achieve. Only 3% of obese persons can lose a substantial amount of weight and keep it off. This is because the body defends its fat mass vigorously, a concept known as the *fat homeostat*. Once an obese person loses weight, hormones that promote hunger are produced, hormones that produce satiety are decreased and the metabolic rate slows down.

Weight loss is a powerful health improvement tool: the loss of just 5% of total body weight leads to impressive improvements in cardiovascular and metabolic health. This means that once an obese person loses weight, they can only consume around 1200 kcal per day to maintain that weight loss for the rest of their life, and they are hungry. Hunger is very difficult to control in the long term, and the characteristics of those persons who do manage to sustain weight loss are that they weigh themselves daily, they severely caloric restrict on days that they have gained even 0.5 kg and they exercise vigorously.

Bariatric surgery refers to surgical management aimed to promote weight loss. All bariatric procedures aim to help a patient control their hunger, allowing them to consume that small amount of 1200 kcal/day and maintain their weight loss. On average, all bariatric procedures enable patients to lose and maintain around 50% of their excess weight, where excess weight is defined as the weight above a BMI of 25 kg/m^2. This translates to around 25–30% total body weight loss, which is much higher than what may be achieved with conservative programs.

Prevalence

It is estimated that 220 000 people underwent bariatric surgery in the USA in 2008. Between 2014 and 2015, 22 700 bariatric surgeries were performed in Australia, compared with 9300 procedures between 2005 and 2006. The number of procedures worldwide has relatively plateaued since 2008, with the

USA being the most prolific, followed by Brazil, France, Mexico, Australia and New Zealand.

The most common procedures performed are:

- sleeve gastrectomy
- laparoscopic adjustable gastric band (LAGB)
- Roux-en-Y gastric bypass (RYGB)
- biliopancreatic diversion with duodenal switch (BPD/DS).

Indications

- BMI of greater than or equal to 40 kg/m^2
- BMI of 35–39.9 kg/m^2 with an obesity-related comorbidity
- BMI of 30–34.9 kg/m^2 with uncontrollable type 2 diabetes mellitus or metabolic syndrome

Contraindications

- Untreated depression or psychosis
- Untreated eating disorder
- Current drug and alcohol abuse
- Severe cardiac disease prohibiting anaesthesia
- Inability to comply with nutritional changes and requirements

Benefits

- Sustained weight loss: bariatric surgery has been proven to be more effective than behavioural or medical management of obesity in morbidly obese patients. In the 10-year prospective controlled Swedish Obese Subjects Study, bariatric surgery successfully reduced patients' weight by 16.1% compared with an increase in weight of 1.6% in the control group who underwent behaviour modification.
- Increased physical function.
- Improvement in medical comorbidities:
  - Type 2 diabetes: better glycaemic control contributes to remission and improvement in distal peripheral neuropathy.
  - Hypertension: improves obesity-related hypertension.
  - Dyslipidaemia: improves lipid profiles with reduction in low-density lipoprotein, triglyceride and total cholesterol, and increase in high-density lipoprotein.
  - Obstructive sleep apnoea: decreased apnoea–hypopnoea index (AHI, the number of apnoea and hypopnoea events per hour of sleep), reduced daytime sleepiness.
  - Joint pain: decreased load on weight-bearing joints such as the spine, hips and knees.
  - Polycystic ovarian syndrome: restored menstrual cycles, lessened hirsutism and hyperandrogenic symptoms, and increased ability to conceive.
- Improvement in psychosocial status: improvement in depression, body image and quality of life.

Mechanisms of weight loss

- Early induction of satiety and sustained satiation: these procedures alter the normal hormonal milieu or change the neural signals to cause early cessation of feeding and sustained satiation so that the person does not seek more than two to three meals per day.
- Malabsorption: procedure decreases the effective absorption of nutrients by shortening the length of functional small bowel, for example in biliopancreatic diversion.
- Combination of restriction and malabsorption, such as RYGB and BPD/DS.

Laparoscopic adjustable gastric band

LAGB is a satiety-inducing procedure whereby a saline-filled adjustable silicone band is placed near the gastro-oesophageal junction to create a small stomach pouch with a capacity of 15–20 mL. The band is then connected to a port that is placed subcutaneously. The port can be easily accessed in the clinic to increase or decrease the amount of saline in the band to adjust the stoma (opening) of the band, thus controlling the food intake (Figure 18.1).

When the band contains the appropriate amount of saline, patients describe feeling satisfied after a small amount of food. They then do not seek further food for several hours as they are not hungry. Typically, patients will eat two to three small meals a day, meaning they are consuming around 1200 kcal/day.

Patient compliance and regular long-term follow-up are vital for monitoring satiety, food intake and weight. This information is used to frequently adjust the amount of saline in the gastric band system to individualise therapy. A multidisciplinary team involving the surgical team, nutritionist and general practitioner is important for providing education about food choice and eating style, band adjustment and monitoring for complications, as the foreign body *in situ* may potentially fail or develop late complications (see Table 18.1).

Advantages

- The expected weight loss (EWL) achieved by LAGB is 50% over 1–2 years, at a rate of 0.5–1.0 kg/week. Results have been demonstrated to be durable beyond 10 years.
- It is a reversible procedure.

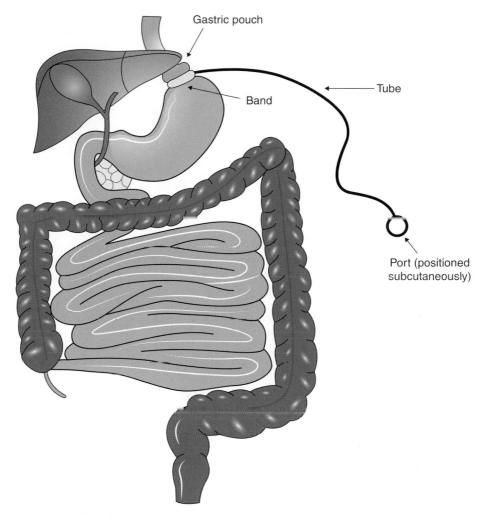

Fig. 18.1 Laparoscopic adjustable gastric band.

- The adjustability of the band offers advantages when addressing various nutritional needs, such as increased nutrient and caloric intake in pregnancy.
- It is a relatively simple procedure, with a lower perioperative complication rate compared with a more involved procedure such as RYGB.
- Several conversion options are available: sleeve gastrectomy, RYGB, BPD/DS.

Disadvantages

- Rate of weight loss is slower (0.5–1.0 kg/ week) compared with sleeve gastrectomy until it stabilises 2 years postoperatively
- Strict follow-up is required to adjust caloric intake and maintain weight loss especially in the first year.
- There is a 10–30% risk of re-operation or revision in 10 years.

Complications

See Table 18.1.

Sleeve gastrectomy

Laparoscopic sleeve gastrectomy is currently the most common procedure in Australia, accounting for 52.5% of total bariatric procedures between 2014 and 2015. It involves removing the fundus and greater curvature of the stomach and reducing stomach volume from 2 L to 100–150 mL. The new tubular stomach is resistant to stretching due to the removal of fundus. It was first described in 1998 as a part of biliopancreatic diversion but is now considered a stand-alone procedure due to its efficacy and minimal invasiveness (Figure 18.2).

Table 18.1 Complications of laparoscopic adjustable gastric band.

	Symptoms/signs	Investigations	Management
Acute			
Acute stomal obstruction			
• Acute postoperative period secondary to postoperative oedema or inadequate removal of perigastric fat	Inability to tolerate oral fluids postoperatively	Barium swallow	Expectant management until oedema reduced May require revisional surgery
• Post-adjustment excessive fluid inserted into the system	Inability to tolerate oral fluids post adjustment	—	Remove excess fluid from port
• Acute food bolus obstruction after eating difficult textured food in excess and too quickly	Vomiting undigested food and saliva	—	Drink carbonated fluids to dislodge the food bolus Remove fluid from the system
Acute band slippage and stomach herniation	Epigastric pain Haematemesis Dehydration Vomiting Unable to tolerate solid food	Abdominal X-ray Barium swallow	Nil orally Remove all fluid from the system Prompt band revision
Port infection (can be associated with band erosion)	Cellulitis/collection over port site	Gastroscopy should be considered to assess gastric integrity in suspected band erosion	Antibiotics Drainage of infective collection Removal with or without replacement of port
Chronic			
Band erosion	Loss of satiety Weight gain Spontaneous port infection	Gastroscopy	Nil orally Intravenous antibiotics Band removal and drainage or omental patch
Chronic band slippage and stomach herniation	Vomiting Regurgitation Volume reflux (especially with recumbency) Inability to tolerate a solid diet	Barium swallow	Remove all fluid from the system May require revisional surgery
Pouch dilatation	Vomiting Regurgitation Volume reflux Weight gain Decreased satiety Increased need for adjustment	Barium swallow	Remove fluid from the system Introduce small amounts of fluid into the system gradually May require revisional surgery
Port flipped	Difficulty in accessing port	Abdominal X-ray	Port revision
Port leaking. Tubing disconnected, kinked or leaked	Decreased satiety Increased need for adjustment	Repeatedly checking the amount of fluid within the system Fluoroscopy	Port/band revision

Advantages

- EWL is approximately 60–66% at 2 years. There are only three series describing results beyond 8 years at this time. All have a weight loss of 50% EWL at the later time points.
- It is technically easier to perform than RYGB or BPD as it does not require multiple anastomoses.
- It does not require strict and close follow-up as for LAGB.

Disadvantages

- Conversion from sleeve gastrectomy usually involves more difficult operation such as RYGB or BPD/DS.
- Gastro-oesophageal reflux: sleeve gastrectomy has been shown to increase pre-existing symptoms of reflux or encourage the development of symptoms of reflux if the patient is asymptomatic preoperatively. There have been recent reports of a 15–20% incidence of de novo Barrett's oesophagus at 5 years post surgery. This procedure is not suitable for patient with pre-existing symptomatic reflux. Preoperative

gastroscopy is recommended for assessing reflux in patients with symptoms of reflux but which remains undiagnosed.
- Weight regain: there are only three studies published beyond 8 years and all report around a 30% conversion rate to RYGB for weight regain or reflux.
- Nutritional problems: patients must be vigilant with multivitamin supplementation. There are case reports of beri-beri in patients who were vomiting after this procedure. There a risk of iron, calcium, B-group vitamin and protein deficiencies (see Table 18.2).

Complications

See Table 18.2.

Roux-en-Y gastric bypass

RYGB, developed with the intention of creating restriction and malabsorption, has been the gold standard of weight loss operations since the 1980s. Alan Wittgrove and Wesley Clark first described the laparoscopic approach in 1994. There has been

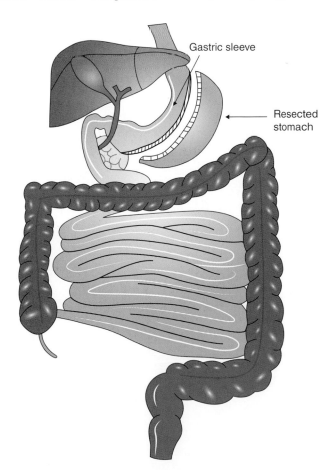

Fig. 18.2 Sleeve gastrectomy.

Table 18.2 Complications of laparoscopic sleeve gastrectomy.

	Symptoms/signs	Investigations	Management
Acute			
Bleeding/haematoma at staple line	Symptoms of blood loss and intra-abdominal bleeding	Full blood examination	May require return to theatre
Gastric leak	Abdominal pain Symptoms of sepsis	Inflammatory markers CT (on-table oral contrast to assess for leak and associated collection) Gastroscopy	Nil orally and parenteral nutrition Intravenous antibiotics Drainage of intra-abdominal collection Endoscopic/ surgical intervention
Chronic			
Gastro-oesophageal reflux disease and Barrett's oesophagus	Heartburn Volume reflux Effortless regurgitation	Barium swallow Gastroscopy	Proton pump inhibitors Conversion to RYGB
Stenosis (commonly at the incisura)	Dysphagia Vomiting Inability to tolerate oral diet	Barium swallow	Endoscopic balloon dilatation Revisional surgery/ conversion to RYGB
Expansion of gastric sleeve	Loss of restriction Weight gain	Barium swallow	Revisional surgery/ conversion to RYGB

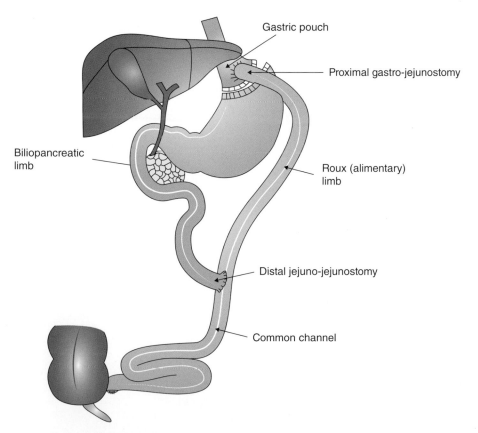

Fig. 18.3 Roux-en-Y gastric bypass.

a gradual decline in its use globally, with the discovery of more minimally invasive options such as sleeve gastrectomy and other bariatric procedures.

It involves creating a small gastric pouch of 15–30 mL isolated from the distal stomach, the jejunum is divided and the distal end attached to the stomach pouch (alimentary or Roux limb), whilst the other end (biliopancreatic limb with output from duodenum, liver and pancreas) is attached to the alimentary limb about 1 m distal to the stomach, so that the remainder of the stomach and duodenum are bypassed. Most nutritional absorption occurs in the common channel.

The small gastric pouch serves to restrict caloric intake. Dividing the small bowel reduces the length of functional small bowel for nutrient absorption (Figure 18.3).

Advantages

- EWL after RYGB at 2 years is around 70% and 50% at 5 years.
- Improves gastro-oesophageal reflux symptoms.

Disadvantages

- It is a more complex procedure with higher intra-operative risk of complications such as anastomosis leak (see Table 18.3).
- It is a permanent procedure.

Table 18.3 Complications of Roux-en-Y gastric bypass.

	Description	Symptoms/signs
Acute		
Anastomotic leak	Can occur at either anastomosis Revision of previous bariatric procedures carries higher risk	Abdominal pain Symptoms of sepsis and vascular compromise
Gastric remnant distension	The blind end pouch becomes distended secondary to distal obstruction or paralytic ileus postoperatively, and may lead to rupture, spillage of gastric content and severe peritonitis	Abdominal pain, hiccups, shoulder pain, abdominal distension, shortness of breath
Internal herniation	Secondary to mesenteric defects that are not closed intraoperatively • Mesenteric defect at jejuno-jejunostomy • Space between the transverse mesocolon and Roux-limb mesentery (Petersen's defect) • Defect in the transverse mesocolon in retrocolic Roux limb (when Roux limb positioned posterior to transverse colon)	Abdominal pain Symptoms of small bowel obstruction
Chronic		
Dumping syndrome	Secondary to rapid transit of food into small bowel	Nausea, diaphoresis, abdominal pain, diarrhoea after high sugar meals
Malnutrition	Occurs due to reduced intake and absorption of micronutrients, particularly iron, calcium, vitamin B_{12}, thiamine, folate	Symptoms of micronutrient deficiencies
Pouch dilatation	Can also occur with dilatation of the anastomosis between gastric pouch and Roux limb	Loss of restriction, weight gain
Anastomosis/ stomal stenosis	Usually occurs at the gastro-jejunal anastomosis typically several weeks after surgery Presents clinically when the stoma narrows to <10 mm in diameter	Vomiting, volume reflux, dysphagia, and inability to tolerate oral intake
Marginal ulcers	Occur commonly near gastro-jejunal anastomosis due to gastric acid injuring the jejunum Can occur in association with gastro-gastric or gastro-colic fistula	Abdominal pain, symptoms of gastrointestinal bleeding, stomal stenosis or perforation
Candy cane Roux syndrome	Occurs due to excessive long blind afferent Roux limb that distends with food Can present as early as 3 months postoperatively or as late as 10 years	Postprandial epigastric pain often relieved by vomiting, reflux, food regurgitation
Cholelithiasis	Secondary to rapid weight loss causing changes in bile constituents Develops in 38% of patients within 6 months postoperatively	Symptoms of biliary colic or other complications of cholelithiasis
Gastro-gastric fistula	Connection between the gastric pouch and the excluded stomach remnant Commonly causes marginal ulcers	Weight gain Symptoms of marginal ulcers

- Revision is complicated and incurs higher operative risk.
- There is a higher risk of nutritional deficiency.

Complications

See Table 18.3.

Biliopancreatic diversion with duodenal switch

BPD/DS is both restrictive and malabsorptive. It involves creating a gastric sleeve and preserving the pylorus. The ileum is then divided with the distal end attached to the remaining stomach, creating an alimentary/Roux limb with a short common channel. The proximal ileum, which contains the output from the duodenum, liver and pancreas, is attached to the terminal ileum 50–100 cm away from the ileocaecal valve (Figure 18.4).

This procedure differs from the original biliopancreatic diversion that involves the division of the duodenum from the pylorus and removal of the pylorus. This is to avoid the complication of stasis and lowers the incidence of anastomostic ulcers and diarrhoea.

Because of its technical difficulty and risks, BPD/DS is relatively uncommon, accounting for 1% of bariatric procedures performed in the USA and only 0.2% in Australia in 2017.

Advantages

- Rapid and substantial weight loss: EWL at 2 years is 70–80%.

Disadvantages

- This is a more complex procedure with higher mortality and intraoperative and postoperative risks such as anastomosis leak.
- Malnutrition: protein malnutrition, anaemia, metabolic bone disease, fat-soluble vitamin deficiency.

Conclusions

Bariatric surgery plays a key role in the treatment of obesity. It has been shown to be an effective adjunct in achieving and maintaining substantial

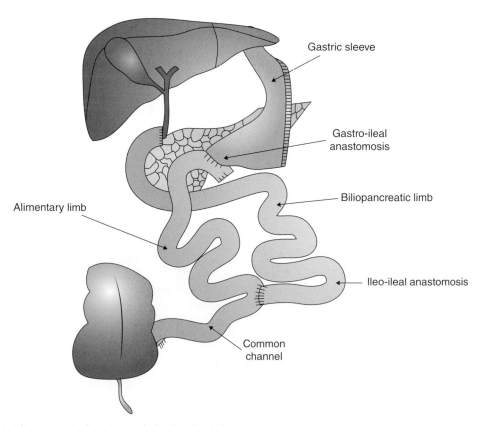

Fig. 18.4 Biliopancreatic diversion with duodenal switch.

Gastric sleeve

Gastro-ileal anastomosis

Biliopancreatic limb

Alimentary limb

Ileo-ileal anastomosis

Common channel

weight loss, as well as treating obesity-related disease. Whilst procedures differ in their weight loss trajectories, by 5 years it appears that weight loss is similar for all procedures. Patient selection and compliance with follow-up and dietary recommendations are crucial in the success of these procedures.

Severe complications from bariatric surgery are uncommon, but high suspicion is warranted when patients with a history of bariatric surgery present to the clinic or emergency department. Long-term follow-up is pertinent for ensuring the success of surgery, maintaining adequate nutrition and monitoring for complications as these may present many years after the initial operation.

Further reading

O'Brien PE. Bariatric surgery: mechanism, indications, and outcomes. *J Gastroenterol Hepatol* 2010;25:1358–65.

O'Brien PE, Dixon JB, Brown W. Obesity is a surgical disease: overview of obesity and bariatric surgery. *ANZ J Surg* 2004;74:200–4.

Sjostrom L, Lindroos A, Peltonen M *et al*. Lifestyle, diabetes, and cardiovascular risk factors 10 years after bariatric surgery. *N Engl J Med* 2004;351:2683–93.

Telem D, Greenstein AJ, Wolfe B. Late complications of bariatric surgery operations. https://www.uptodate.com/contents/late-complications-of-bariatric-surgical-operations?search=bariatric%20surgery&source=search_result&selectedTitle=12~150&usage_type=default&display_rank=12 (accessed 9 February 2018).

MCQs

Select the single correct answer to each question. The correct answers can be found in the Answers section at the end of the book.

1 Which of the following procedures is most likely to increase gastro-oesophageal reflux?
  a Roux-en-Y gastric bypass
  b sleeve gastrectomy
  c biliopancreatic diversion with duodenal switch
  d laparoscopic adjustable gastric band
  e all of the above

2 Which of the following is *not* a contraindication for bariatric surgery?
  a severe cardiac disease
  b untreated major depressive disorder
  c inability to comply with nutritional changes and requirements
  d obstructive sleep apnoea
  e current alcohol dependence

3 Lucy underwent a bariatric procedure that involves dividing the jejunum and attaching the distal end to a small gastric pouch that is disconnected from the remaining stomach. Which procedure did she have done?
  a Roux-en-Y gastric bypass
  b sleeve gastrectomy
  c biliopancreatic diversion with duodenal switch
  d laparoscopic adjustable gastric band
  e jejunoileal bypass

4 Jon presented to the emergency department 5 days after laparoscopic sleeve gastrectomy. He has not been quite well since, with epigastric pain, nausea, intermittent fevers and chills, and is unable to tolerate much oral intake. What investigation would be most helpful in the emergency department to diagnose his problem?
  a gastroscopy
  b barium swallow
  c computed tomography
  d abdominal ultrasound
  e magnetic resonance cholangiopancreatography

5 Sookyung underwent laparoscopic adjustable gastric banding 6 months ago and was doing well with regular small increments of saline inserted into her band system up to 7 mL. At her 6-month outpatient review, she had a further 0.5 mL of saline inserted into her band, but 2 hours later she noticed she was unable to tolerate her smoothie. What is the most likely cause of Sookyung's problem?
  a acute prolapse of proximal stomach
  b acute stomal obstruction from excessive fluid in system
  c band erosion
  d port leaking
  e acute food bolus obstruction

Section 3
Hepatopancreaticobiliary Surgery

19 Gallstones

Arthur J. Richardson

University of Sydney and Westmead Hospital, Sydney, New South Wales, Australia

Incidence: an overview

In most western countries, and certainly in Australia, gallstones are the most frequent gastrointestinal surgical cause for admission to hospital. In Australia, the gallbladder is the most frequently removed organ and approximately 50 000 cholecystectomies are done each year.

The incidence of gallstones varies widely depending on the demographic group. In Australia, the incidence of gallstones is estimated to be 10–15% and most of these patients are asymptomatic. In comparison, the incidence of gallstones amongst black sub-Saharan Africans is less than 5%. In Asian populations, the incidence may be lower (5–10%) but as more Asians are exposed to high-fat western diets this incidence is on the increase. The incidence of gallstones amongst the indigenous peoples of Chile is 49% in women and 12% in men, whereas the indigenous peoples in North America may have the highest reported rates with up to 29% of men and 64% of women developing gallstones. Gallstones are the chief risk factor for the development of gallbladder cancer. This is important: gallbladder cancer is rare in western countries (less than two cases per 100 000 population per year) but more common in Chile (15.6 cases per 100 000 women per year).

Importantly, the incidence of gallstones increases with age and this is a significant issue, especially in western countries with ageing populations. In particular, gallstones are much more frequent over the age of 40. A British autopsy study showed that the incidence of gallstones in women aged 50–59 years was 24% and this increased to 30% in the ninth decade. The same study showed that amongst men the incidence increased from 18% in those aged 50–59 years to 29% in the ninth decade.

Types

Gallstones are essentially crystals that develop in the gallbladder; however, in some circumstances they may develop outside the gallbladder, primarily in the bile duct. In 80% of cases in western countries the gallstones will be cholesterol or mixed stones which contain calcium. Pigmented stones are black or brown in colour. Black stones are generally associated with haemolytic conditions and are small and composed predominantly of calcium bilirubinate and mucin glycoproteins. Brown stones are more commonly seen in Asian populations and are associated with parasitic or bacterial infections. Unlike black stones they more commonly form in the biliary passages.

Bile production and the enterohepatic circulation

Bile acids are formed by two pathways. The classic pathway occurs only in the liver as it requires the enzyme cholesterol 7α-hydroxylase (CYP7A1), which is found in the hepatocytes, to hydroxylate a sterol nucleus. The alternate pathway occurs in extrahepatic tissue such as the kidney, macrophages and vascular endothelium where the enzyme oxysterol 7α-hydroxylase oxidises cholesterol to oxysterols, which are then transported to the liver where the primary bile acids, cholic and deoxycholic acid, are formed. In healthy individuals without liver disease the alternate pathway only contributes 10% of overall bile acid synthesis.

After the bile acids are synthesised in the liver they are conjugated with either glycine (75%) or taurine (25%) and are then secreted into the bile ducts and stored in the gallbladder where

Textbook of Surgery, Fourth Edition. Edited by Julian A. Smith, Andrew H. Kaye, Christopher Christophi and Wendy A. Brown.
© 2020 John Wiley & Sons Ltd. Published 2020 by John Wiley & Sons Ltd.

concentration of the bile occurs. When a meal is eaten the gallbladder is stimulated by cholecysto-kinin (CCK) and the gallbladder empties 70–80% of its contents into the bile duct and subsequently into the duodenum and small bowel. Once in the intestine the bile forms micelles and is responsible for digesting fats, fat-soluble vitamins and some drugs. It is thought that the primary cause of cho-lesterol gallstones is the presence of cholesterol-supersaturated bile, which is lithogenic. This lithogenicity may be modified by factors within the bile such as excess cholesterol, changes in the bil-iary and bowel microbiome, low bile salt levels, abnormal lipid transport, mucus secretion and impaired gallbladder emptying. The production of bile acids is the main pathway for the excretion of cholesterol, accounting for about 50% of daily excretion. In a healthy adult the liver produces 600–750 mL of bile per day.

Once primary bile acids are secreted into the bowel, some are deconjugated to secondary bile acids by intestinal bacteria. In the ileum some of the secondary bile acids are reabsorbed passively, whereas the conjugated bile acids are reabsorbed by an active transport system. In most individuals 95% of bile acids are reabsorbed in the ileum and transported back to the liver and only 5% are excreted via the large bowel. If there is increased secretion via the large bowel, due to a variety of causes such as ileal resection, previous cholecystec-tomy, inflammatory bowel disease or radiation therapy, this may be associated with the develop-ment of chronic diarrhoea.

Risk factors

In the majority of patients who develop gallstones the causes are multifactorial. However, there are many factors that predispose to gallstones that are modifi-able. The causes of gallstones include the following.
- *Age*: as previously noted the incidence of gall-stones increase with age.
- *Gender*: females are at least twice as likely to develop gallstones as men, at least up to meno-pause. This is probably related to both endoge-nous oestrogen and the oral contraceptive.
- *Pregnancy*: this is an independent risk factor for the development of gallstones. It is common for women to develop symptoms during pregnancy and this is because of increased oestrogen secre-tion, which results in increased biliary sludge for-mation. This may resolve after childbirth but may result in definitive persistent gallstones in about 5% of women.

- *Obesity and dietary factors*: obese individuals have a higher risk of gallstones compared with lean individuals. It has been estimated that the relative risk of gallstones is increased by a factor of at least two in both men and women who are obese. Morbidly obese women (BMI >32 kg/m²) have an even higher risk of gallstone formation with an age-adjusted relative risk of 6. A diet which leads to increased obesity increases the risk of gallstone formation. It does appear that any diet which is high in fats and cholesterol increases the risk of gallstone formation. Conversely, the risk of gallstones may be reduced by a low-fat diet, legumes and a moderate intake of alcohol. Certainly, it does appear that some ethnic groups who have a low risk of gallstone formation such as Native Americans may form gallstones at an increased rate with exposure to a western diet, which is usually low in fibre and high in refined carbohydrates and fat. Rapid weight loss is also associated with an increased risk of gallstone formation.
- *Genetic predisposition*: gallstones often run in families, with an increased risk of gallstone for-mation related to family history.
- *Ethnicity*: as noted earlier, the incidence of gall-stone formation varies for different ethnic groups.
- *Total parenteral nutrition (TPN)* is a known risk factor for cholelithiasis. It was recognised some time ago that seriously ill patients in intensive care on TPN were at increased risk of acalculous cholecystitis. However, more recently it has been recognised that many of these patients do in fact have microlithiasis. It has been shown that for seriously ill patients in intensive care that biliary sludge may appear after a few days of fasting. Biliary sludge will appear ultrasonographically after 4 weeks of TPN in up to 50% of patients and this may increase the longer the TPN is con-tinued. After cessation of TPN many instances of microlithiasis will resolve rather than progress to gallstone formation. The mechanism of gallstone formation may be related to ileal atrophy due to TPN.
- *Haemolytic diseases*: particularly in sickle cell disease, hereditary spherocytosis and hereditary elliptocytosis where there is chronic haemolysis, this leads to increased bilirubin secretion with the formation of black pigment gallstones.
- *Other chronic diseases*: ileal Crohn's disease is asso-ciated with an increased incidence of gallstones. Likewise, cystic fibrosis is associated with an increased prevalence of gallstones. Cirrhosis is associated with an increased prevalence of

gallstone formation. Spinal cord injury is associated with a significant increase in the risk of formation of gallstones possibly due to gallbladder stasis.

- *Drugs*: those which may increase the risk of gallstone formation include thiazide diuretics, ceftriaxone and octreotide. Conversely, statins may decrease the risk of gallstone formation.

Presentation

Biliary colic and acute cholecystitis

It is estimated that 10–15% of the population in Australia and the USA will have gallstones. However, most people with gallstones are asymptomatic. It is estimated that each year 2–4% of people with gallstones will develop symptoms and, generally, once symptoms develop they will continue, although this is unpredictable and may be modified by a change in diet and other factors. Most patients who develop symptoms related to gallstones will develop biliary colic. This usually manifests as epigastric and right upper quadrant pain that may radiate to the back and often follows a fatty meal. This is often associated with nausea or vomiting and there may be a history of fatty food intolerance. The pain may vary from relatively mild to excruciating. The pain is caused by a stone lodging in the outlet of the gallbladder and the pain may resolve suddenly with dislodgement of the stone.

If the stone does not dislodge, the blockage of the gallbladder outlet or cystic duct causes increased pressure within the gallbladder. The bile is then forced into the wall of the gallbladder, resulting in oedema and inflammation. As the pressure increases this causes venous ischaemia, which can lead ultimately to necrosis of the wall of the gallbladder if the process is not arrested. Pathophysiologically, this can result in an empyema of the gallbladder where the gallbladder is full of pus or indeed perforates. This infection may result in translocation of bacteria, resulting in bacteraemia or indeed septicaemia. The most common organisms involved in this process are Gram-negative organisms such as *Escherichia coli*, *Klebsiella* or *Pseudomonas*. Other organisms that may be present include *Clostridium*, *Staphylococcus* or *Salmonella*.

Acute cholecystitis is associated with persistent right upper quadrant pain and tenderness. Nausea or vomiting is frequently present and the patients are often febrile. Murphy's sign, when an examiner notes that a patient stops breathing due to pain over the inflamed gallbladder, is helpful in diagnosing acute cholecystitis but its absence does not exclude it (Table 19.1). The severity of acute

Table 19.1 Tokyo diagnostic criteria for acute cholecystitis.

A Local signs of inflammation, etc.
  1 Murphy's sign
  2 RUQ mass/pain/tenderness
B Systemic signs of inflammation, etc.
  1 Fever
  2 Elevated CRP
  3 Elevated WBC count
C Imaging findings
  Imaging findings characteristic of acute cholecystitis
Definite diagnosis
  1 One item in A and one item in B are positive
  2 C confirms the diagnosis when acute cholecystitis is suspected clinically

CRP, C-reactive protein; RUQ, right upper quadrant; WBC, white blood cell count.
Source: Yokoe M, Takada T, Strasberg SM *et al*. New diagnostic criteria and severity assessment of acute cholecystitis in revised Tokyo Guidelines. *J Hepatobiliary Sci* 2012;19:578–85. © 2012 Japanese Society of Hepato-Biliary-Pancreatic Surgery. Reproduced with permission of John Wiley and Sons.

cholecystitis is highly variable and influences the choice of treatment. The Tokyo guidelines are an attempt to grade the severity of acute cholecystitis and are widely used by clinicians (Table 19.2).

Gallstone pancreatitis

Gallstones are the most common cause of pancreatitis in western countries and account for 60–70% of cases. In the majority the pancreatitis is mild and self-limiting. It may be severe in 20% and in such cases mortality may approach 20–30%. Gallstone pancreatitis is increasing in incidence in western countries and has an estimated incidence of about 40 per 100 000 population per year. It is most common in women in their sixties.

Although the association between gallstones and pancreatitis was first described in the nineteenth century, the mechanism was not well understood. It is now believed that a stone passing through the sphincter of Oddi causes irritation, oedema and temporary obstruction to the pancreatic duct, resulting in outflow obstruction to the pancreatic duct and a raised intraluminal pressure. This causes a cascade of biochemical reactions that result in release of pancreatic enzymes and oedema of the pancreas resulting in inflammation. If the process continues unabated this results in further inflammation, release of inflammatory cytokines and a systemic inflammatory response syndrome (SIRS). The severity of the pancreatitis is unpredictable but

Table 19.2 Tokyo guidelines for severity of acute cholecystitis.

Grade III (severe) acute cholecystitis
Associated with dysfunction of any of the following organs/systems:
- Cardiovascular dysfunction: hypotension requiring treatment with dopamine ≥5 µg/kg per min or any dose of noradrenaline
- Neurological dysfunction: decreased level of consciousness
- Respiratory dysfunction: Pao_2/Fio_2 ratio <300
- Renal dysfunction: oliguria, creatinine >2.0 mg/dL
- Hepatic dysfunction: PT-INR >1.5
- Haematological dysfunction: platelet count <100 × 10^9/L

Grade II (moderate) acute cholecystitis
Associated with any of the following conditions:
- Elevated white cell count >18 × 10^9/L
- Palpable tender mass in right upper quadrant
- Duration of complaints >72 hours
- Marked local inflammation (gangrenous cholecystitis, pericholecystic abscess, hepatic abscess, biliary peritonitis, emphysematous cholecystitis)

Grade I (mild) acute cholecystitis
Does not meet the criteria of grade II or grade III acute cholecystitis. Grade I can also be defined as acute cholecystitis in a healthy patient with no organ dysfunction and mild inflammatory changes in the gallbladder, making cholecystectomy a safe and low-risk operative procedure

PT-INR, prothrombin-international normalised ratio.
Source: Yokoe M, Takada T, Strasberg SM et al. New diagnostic criteria and severity assessment of acute cholecystitis in revised Tokyo Guidelines. J Hepatobiliary Sci 2012;19:578–85. © 2012 *Japanese Society of Hepato-Biliary-Pancreatic Surgery*. Reproduced with permission of John Wiley and Sons.

Table 19.3 Causes of acute cholangitis.

Cholelithiasis
Benign biliary stricture
Congenital factors
Postoperative factors (damaged bile duct, strictured choledojejunostomy, etc.)
Inflammatory factors (oriental cholangitis, etc.)
Malignant occlusion
  Bile duct tumour
  Gallbladder tumour
  Ampullary tumour
  Pancreatic tumour
  Duodenal tumour
Pancreatitis
Entry of parasites into the bile ducts
External pressure including Mirizzi syndrome and Lemmel syndrome
Fibrosis of the papilla
Duodenal diverticulum
Blood clot (haemobilia)
Sump syndrome after biliary enteric anastomosis
Iatrogenic factors

it may be that increased time of obstruction of the pancreatic duct is associated with more severe cases.

Risk factors for gallstone pancreatitis include multiple small stones and a dilated cystic duct. Gallstones are found in the faeces of up to 90% of patients with gallstone pancreatitis. A minority of patients with choledocholithiasis develop gallstone pancreatitis. Of those patients with symptomatic gallstones, the annual risk of developing gallstone pancreatitis is about 1%.

Choledocholithiais and jaundice

Gallstones present in the biliary tracts are common. The elderly are at highest risk and jaundice or abnormal liver function tests may be the presentation. Up to 20% of patients with gallstones may present in this way. It may or may not be associated with pancreatitis or cholangitis.

Cholangitis

Cholangitis was first described by Charcot in 1887 and was termed 'hepatic fever'. Charcot's triad consists of fever accompanied by rigors, jaundice and right upper quadrant abdominal pain. It can be defined as acute inflammation and infection in the biliary tract. It requires elevated bile duct pressure usually due to some form of obstruction and the presence of increased bacteria in the bile duct. The causes of cholangitis are summarised in Table 19.3.

Cholangitis is a medical emergency that requires prompt treatment. The mortality may approach 10% overall and is higher in elderly patients with significant comorbidities. Charcot's triad as diagnostic criteria for cholangitis is not adequate. Although the specificity is probably greater than 90%, the sensitivity is low at about 25%. As such, the Tokyo guidelines are a better method of diagnosis in acute cholangitis and these are set out in Table 19.4. Likewise, there is a severity assessment (Table 19.5).

Fistulisation of gallstones into the bowel

This is uncommon but may be seen rarely but more commonly in elderly patients. A large gallstone may obstruct the bowel if this occurs. The obstruction will more commonly occur at the ileo-caecal valve (Barnard's syndrome) but may occasionally obstruct the duodenum (Bouveret's syndrome).

Table 19.4 Diagnostic criteria for acute cholangitis.

A Systemic inflammation
   A-1 Fever and/or shaking chills
   A-2 Laboratory data: evidence of inflammatory
       response
B Cholestasis
   B-1 Jaundice
   B-2 Laboratory data: abnormal liver function tests
C Imaging
   C-1 Biliary dilatation
   C-2 Evidence of the aetiology on imaging (stricture,
       stone, stent, etc.)

Suspected diagnosis: one item in A plus one item in
either B or C
Definite diagnosis: one item in A, one item in B and
one item in C

Definitions

A-2 Abnormal white blood cell counts, increase in
     serum CRP levels, and other changes indicating
     inflammation
B-2 Increased serum ALP, GTP (GGT), AST and ALT
     levels

Other factors which are helpful in diagnosis of acute
cholangitis include abdominal pain (RUQ or upper
abdominal) and a history of biliary disease such as
gallstones, previous biliary procedures and placement
of a biliary stent. In acute hepatitis, marked systematic
inflammatory response is observed infrequently.
Virological and serological tests are required when
differential diagnosis is difficult

Thresholds

A-1 Fever: temperature >38°C
A-2 Evidence of inflammatory response: white cell
     count <4 or >10 × 10^9/L, CRP >5 mg/L
B-1 Jaundice: bilirubin >2× normal limit
B-2 Abnormal liver function tests
     ALP >2× upper limit of normal
     GTP >2× upper limit of normal
     AST >2× upper limit of normal
     ALT >2× upper limit of normal

ALP, alkaline phosphatase; ALT, alanine
aminotransferase; AST, aspartate aminotransferase;
CRP, C-reactive protein; GTP (GGT),
γ-glutamyltransferase; RUQ, right upper quadrant.
Source: Kiriyama S, et al. New diagnostic criteria and
severity assessment of acute cholangitis in revised
Tokyo Guidelines. J Hepatobiliary Pancreat Sci.
2012;19:548–56. © 2012 *Japanese Society of
Hepato-Biliary-Pancreatic Surgery*. Reproduced with
permission of John Wiley and Sons.

Table 19.5 Severity assessment criteria for acute
cholangitis.

Grade III (severe) acute cholangitis
Defined as acute cholangitis associated with the onset
of dysfunction in at least one of any of the following
organs/systems:
- Cardiovascular dysfunction: hypotension requiring
  dopamine >5 µg/kg per min, or any dose of
  noradrenaline
- Neurological dysfunction: disturbance of
  consciousness
- Respiratory dysfunction: Pao_2/Fio_2 ratio <300
- Renal dysfunction: oliguria, serum creatinine >2 mg/dL
- Hepatic dysfunction: PT INR >1.5
- Haematological dysfunction: platelet count <100 × 10^9/L

Grade II (moderate) acute cholangitis
Associated with any two of the following conditions:
- Abnormal WBC count: >12 × 10^9/L, <4 × 10^9/L
- High fever: ≥39°C
- Age: >75 years old
- Hyperbilirubinaemia: total bilirubin >5 mg/dL
- Hypoalbuminaemia: <STD ×0.7

Grade I (mild) acute cholangitis
Grade I acute cholangitis does not meet the criteria of
grade III (severe) or grade II (moderate) acute
cholangitis at initial diagnosis

Notes
Early diagnosis, early biliary drainage and/or treatment
for aetiology, and antimicrobial administration are
fundamental treatments for acute cholangitis classified
not only as grade III (severe) and grade II (moderate)
but also grade I (mild). Therefore, it is recommended
that patients with acute cholangitis who do not
respond to the initial medical treatment (general
supportive care and antimicrobial therapy) undergo
early biliary drainage or treatment for aetiology

PT-INR, prothrombin-international normalised ratio;
STD, lower limit of normal; WBC, white blood cell count.
Source: Kiriyama S, et al. New diagnostic criteria and
severity assessment of acute cholangitis in revised
Tokyo Guidelines. J Hepatobiliary Pancreat Sci.
2012;19:548–56. © 2012 *Japanese Society of
Hepato-Biliary-Pancreatic Surgery*. Reproduced with
permission of John Wiley and Sons.

significant risk factor for gallbladder cancer, with more
than 75% of patients having gallstones. The relative
risk of gallstones causing gallbladder cancer is 4.9.

Diagnosis

Gallbladder cancer

Gallbladder cancer is rare in western countries but
highly lethal. In Australia the incidence is less than 2
per 100 000 population per year. Gallstones are a

Baseline haematological and biochemical investigations

Elective investigation of a patient with gallstones
should include a routine full blood count,

electrolytes and liver function tests. Up to 10% of patients who present electively may have choledocholithiasis, the presence of which may be suggested by abnormal liver function tests. If there is a history of jaundice it is important to determine bilirubin and alkaline phosphatase concentrations and INR (international normalised ratio). In the patient who presents acutely with abdominal pain, measurement of C-reactive protein to estimate the degree of inflammation is helpful and amylase and lipase levels should be done to exclude pancreatitis.

Plain abdominal X-ray

This has limited usefulness. Only 15% of gallstones will have enough calcium to be seen on a plain abdominal X-ray.

Ultrasound

This is the investigation of choice for gallstones and avoids ionising radiation, which is particularly important in young people. Good-quality ultrasonography has a sensitivity and specificity in excess of 95% in uncomplicated cases. Obesity, previous surgery and bowel gas may impede the accuracy of the test in diagnosing gallstones. The stones are shown by a bright echogenic appearance with posterior shadowing (Figure 19.1). Ultrasound has variable accuracy in diagnosing choledocholithiasis, with a sensitivity of 50–80% but a specificity of over 90%.

Ultrasound is also useful in diagnosing cholecystitis by demonstrating tenderness over the gallbladder associated with thickening of the gallbladder wall (>4 mm) and sometimes fluid collections. It is accurate in demonstrating masses or polyps within the gallbladder and will show if there is abnormal biliary dilatation (>7 mm).

Abdominal CT

An abdominal CT scan is not recommended in the routine diagnosis of gallstones. It may have a place in imaging for severe complicated cholecystitis but has a lower sensitivity and specificity for diagnosing gallstones in the gallbladder than ultrasound. It also carries the risk of exposure to ionising radiation and a higher cost than ultrasound. Abdominal CT scanning in the diagnosis of choledocholithiasis has a sensitivity of 60–80% with a specificity in excess of 95%. CT cholangiography is infrequently performed because of the risk of allergic reactions but does increase the sensitivity for the diagnosis of choledocholithiasis to 85–95% and the specificity to 88–98%.

Endoscopic ultrasound

In Australia, this technique is becoming more widely available and although not a first-line investigation for the diagnosis of gallbladder gallstones is very accurate. In the diagnosis of choledocholithiasis it is even more accurate, with a sensitivity reported as 89–94% and a specificity of about 95%. The disadvantage is that it requires specialised equipment and training and cannot be done on an outpatient basis. It is most useful in patients where the diagnosis is uncertain.

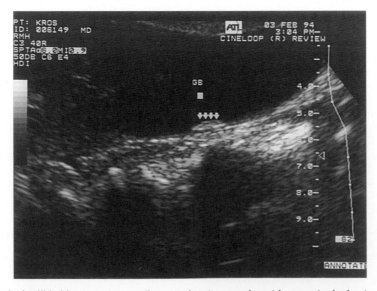

Fig. 19.1 Ultrasound of gallbladder containing gallstones, showing an echo with acoustic shadowing.

Magnetic resonance imaging cholangiopancreatography

Magnetic resonance cholangiopancreatography is the diagnostic modality of choice for choledocholithiasis. It does not involve ionising radiation. The disadvantages of the modality relate to its cost, limited availability, patient claustrophobia and previous procedures such as pacemakers which may contraindicate it. However, the technique is highly accurate in diagnosing choledocholithiasis, with a sensitivity of 92–94% and a specificity of 99%.

Endoscopic retrograde cholangiopancreatography

Endoscopic retrograde cholangiopancreatography (ERCP) is uncommonly used as a diagnostic test and is a therapeutic tool to clear the bile duct of stones. There are rare but serious complications, such as bleeding, bowel perforation and pancreatitis.

Laparoscopic ultrasound

This is sometimes used at the time of laparoscopic cholecystectomy to diagnose common bile duct stones.

Technetium-labelled hepato-iminodiacetic acid

This test has little use in the diagnosis of gallstones but may be useful in diagnosing acute cholecystitis or chronic acalculous cholecystitis.

Treatment

Asymptomatic gallstones

There is little evidence to justify treating asymptomatic gallstones. Likewise, there is little evidence that lifestyle modifications will lower the risk of developing symptoms related to gallstones if they are found incidentally. There are situations where a discussion with a patient with asymptomatic gallstones is important. For example, in a patient who requires a heart transplant where the risk of biliary sepsis is significant, where a patient is going to spend a significant period in a remote area such as Antarctica or with a patient whose ethnic group has a high risk of gallbladder cancer. There may also be occasional circumstances where a patient has to undergo surgery for another reason and it may be reasonable to consider removal of the gallbladder at the same time.

Symptomatic gallstones

Non-operative measures

Some patients are able to control their symptoms for a significant period of time with a low-fat diet. Unfortunately, most patients find that they are unable to stay on the diet and recurrence of symptoms is common. There are a variety of herbal and naturopathic treatments and diets which are reputed to dissolve gallstones or alleviate symptoms but there is little evidence to support this approach.

Dissolution therapy with ursodeoxycholic has been shown to have a low rate of cure, with only 27% of patients exhibiting dissolution of stones after treatment and a high rate of recurrence.

Extracorporeal shock wave therapy (lithotripsy) is highly successful for renal tract stones and has also been tried for gallstones. One of the major issues is that breaking up gallstones results in multiple small stones that may be more likely to pass into the biliary tract and cause pancreatitis and other complications. Lithotripsy may cause dissolution of stones in up to 55% of patients but more than 40% of patients will develop recurrent gallstones within 4 years. This treatment is also limited by expense and availability.

Cholecystectomy

Removal of the gallbladder in patients who are fit for surgery is the treatment of choice in symptomatic gallstones. This is usually performed by a laparoscopic (keyhole) technique due to shorter length of hospital stay, less pain, shorter return to work and better cosmesis. It usually involves four or five small incisions of 1 cm in length. The majority of elective procedures can be done with an overnight stay, although there is now good evidence that a majority of elective procedures can be done as day-only admissions. In many centres in Australia the procedure is accompanied by an operative cholangiogram to check the anatomy and exclude choledocholithiasis.

In elective cases, the 30-day mortality is under 0.5% and the majority of patients will have recovered fully within 2 weeks. However, there are risks associated with the procedure, including infection, need to convert to an open procedure (normally <2%), bile leaks, pneumonia and deep venous thrombosis. The most feared risk is a bile duct injury (BDI). This will usually be a result of misidentification of the anatomy. When laparoscopic cholecystectomy was introduced there was an increase in the incidence of this complication. This risk now appears to have stabilised and a major transection of the bile duct probably occurs at a rate of about one in 800–1000 cases in Australia. Emergency procedures carry a higher risk of complications. An emergency laparoscopic cholecystectomy can be an extremely difficult procedure due to the difficulty in identifying the anatomy. Occasionally, it may be impossible to perform a complete cholecystectomy and the surgeon may consider a cholecystostomy where the gallbladder is drained or a subtotal cholecystectomy. In the acute situation where the patient is extremely ill and not fit for operation, a percutaneous cholecystostomy performed radiologically may be an option to allow the condition to settle followed by a laparoscopic cholecystectomy when the patient has recovered.

Most patients will not notice significant digestive problems after removal of the gallbladder. A small proportion will develop fatty food intolerance that may be quite individualistic and there is also an incidence of bile-salt-induced diarrhoea.

Timing of surgery

In the patient who does not require hospital admission for biliary colic the procedure can be planned electively. However, this does depend on the resources available. If the procedure is likely to be delayed for some months, then there is a high likelihood of re-presentation to the hospital and a higher risk of prolonged hospital stay and other complications.

In the patient who presents with acute cholecystitis and requires hospital admission for intravenous antibiotics, the timing of surgery is controversial. The concern is that earlier surgery in this group may be associated with a higher risk of conversion to an open procedure and an increased risk of BDI and other complications. However, there is now good evidence from meta-analyses that early operation is associated with a more rapid recovery with no increase in complications than delayed operation after the cholecystitis has settled.

Likewise, in the patient who presents with acute pancreatitis related to gallstones the timing of surgery is controversial. There is an argument that some delay in removing the gallbladder is appropriate because there is a risk that the pancreatitis may worsen, particularly in the first 48 hours. This is a clinical decision as to when operation should be performed and there is a move to performing cholecystectomy on the index admission depending on resources available. In any case removal of the

gallbladder within 4 weeks is regarded as best practice to avoid the risk of repeated episodes in the patient with mild uncomplicated pancreatitis.

Burden of disease on Australian society

In Australia, approximately 50 000 laparoscopic cholecystectomies are performed each year. It is one of the most common surgical procedures performed in Australia and represents a significant expenditure of public resources. The demand for the procedure appears to be on the increase. Patient outcomes indicate wide variability in the cost, hospital stay and complications and there is no evidence that this situation is different in other western countries. A recent study in private hospitals in Australia showed that 98% of patients stayed at least one night in hospital, despite evidence that a majority can be done as true day cases. Furthermore, amongst 320 surgeons who performed five or more procedures per year the total hospital cost varied from A$4543 to A$21 419, with an average cost of A$7235. The average 30-day readmission rate was 7.8%. This suggests that for a common procedure, there are significant variations in outcome and cost and that there is a substantial opportunity for efficiency gains and savings.

Further reading

Cremer A, Arvanitakis M. Diagnosis and management of bile stone disease and its complications. *Minerva Gastroenterol Dietol* 2016;62:103–29.

Gurusamy KS, Davidson BR. Gallstones. *BMJ* 2014;348: g2669.

Knab LM, Boller AM, Mahvi DM. Cholecystitis. *Surg Clin North Am* 2014;94:455–70.

Mayumi T, Okamoto K, Takada T *et al.* Tokyo Guidelines 2018: management bundles for acute cholangitis and cholecystitis. *J Hepatobiliary Pancreat Sci* 2018;25: 96–100.

Miura F, Okamoto K, Takada T *et al.* Tokyo Guidelines 2018: initial management of acute biliary infection and flowchart for acute cholangitis. *J Hepatobiliary Pancreat Sci* 2018;25:31–40.

Portincasa P, Di Ciaula A, de Bari O, Garruti G, Palmieri VO, Wang DQ. Management of gallstones and its related complications. *Expert Rev Gastroenterol Hepatol* 2016;10:93–112.

Royal Australasian College of Surgeons and Medibank. Surgical Variance Report 2017 General Surgery. Available at https://www.surgeons.org/media/25242159/surgical-variance-report-2017-general-surgery.pdf

Shabanzadeh DM, Sorensen LT, Jorgensen T. Determinants for gallstone formation: a new data cohort study and a systematic review with meta-analysis. *Scand J Gastroenterol* 2016;51:1239–48.

MCQs

Select the single correct answer to each question. The correct answers can be found in the Answers section at the end of the book.

1 An 80-year-old woman presents with biliary pain and stones are seen in the gallbladder on ultrasound. The probability of the pain being due to a stone in the common bile duct is approximately:
   a 5%
   b 10%
   c 20%
   d 30%
   e 50%

2 A 73-year-old man presents with cholangitis. He has had no previous abdominal operation. The definitive treatment should be:
   a cholecystectomy and choledocholithotomy
   b ERCP and sphincterotomy with stone extraction
   c antibiotic therapy followed by laparoscopic cholecystectomy
   d choledocholithotomy
   e ERCP, sphincterotomy with stone extraction and later consideration of cholecystectomy

3 Which of the following is the appropriate investigation in a patient presenting with a recent episode of right upper quadrant pain and a normal physical examination?
   a abdominal CT scan
   b ERCP
   c plain X-ray of the abdomen
   d upper abdominal ultrasound
   e cholescintigraphy

20 Malignant diseases of the hepatobiliary system

Thomas J. Hugh[1] and Nigel B. Jamieson[2]

[1] University of Sydney and Royal North Shore Hospital, Sydney, New South Wales, Australia
[2] University of Glasgow and Glasgow Royal Infirmary, Glasgow, UK

Introduction

The most common primary malignant tumours arise from either hepatocytes (hepatocellular cancer) or the epithelial cells of the bile duct (cholangiocarcinoma). Secondary tumours (liver metastases) can spread from many different primary tumour types.

Assessment of liver function preoperatively (Box 20.1)

Preoperative assessment of liver function is important for determining the risk of hepatic failure and mortality after liver resection. Conventional laboratory testing (liver function tests, platelet count, coagulation studies) should reflect the extent of underlying liver function. Unfortunately, these tests alone have a low sensitivity for predicting the risk of remnant liver dysfunction following a major resection and need to be considered preoperatively in the context of organ imaging studies.

In patients with primary malignant liver tumours, the presence of underlying chronic liver disease may limit the extent of hepatic resection. In patients with colorectal liver metastases a particular hazard is the possible effect of prior systemic chemotherapy, which may cause either steato-hepatitis or sinusoidal dilatation, both of which increase morbidity after resection.

Clinical risk scores are based on selected clinical symptoms and conventional test results and provide an assessment of whole liver function. The Child–Pugh score has been the gold standard for decades but does not discriminate well between mild and moderate liver dysfunction. Similarly, the model for end-stage liver disease (MELD) score is mostly only helpful in patients with severe liver disease.

Dynamic quantitative liver function assessment tests have been used to predict the safe limits of the extent of hepatic parenchymal resection. The most frequently employed modality in patients with primary liver tumours is the indocyanine green retention test. This can be done using a simple non-invasive pulse dye densitometry measurement (a bedside test).

Sophisticated computed tomography (CT) with three-dimensional reconstruction helps measure the likely functional liver remnant (FLR) volume after resection. In general, an FLR of 25% or more is considered safe in patients with preoperative normal liver function, whereas a value in excess of 30–40% is necessary in patients with underlying liver disease. Portal vein embolisation may be used preoperatively to stimulate liver hypertrophy.

Emerging important tools of liver function assessment before liver resection include molecular imaging techniques using either ^{99m}Tc-diethylenetriaminepentaacetic acid (DTPA)-galactosyl human serum albumin or ^{99m}Tc-mebrofenin hepatobiliary scintigraphy. These tests may be used to provide an indication of functional hepatocyte mass and are particularly helpful if done in conjunction with CT volumetry.

Ultrasound

Ultrasound is a widely available, cheap and non-invasive investigation. The detection of space-occupying lesions in the liver, porta hepatis or pancreas is dependent on body habitus and may be affected by the amount of surrounding intestinal gas.

Endoscopic retrograde cholangiopancreatography

Endoscopic injection of contrast directly into the bile ducts is an accurate method of demonstrating biliary obstruction and determining cause. Endoscopic retrograde cholangiopancreatography (ERCP) can be combined with cytological brushings or biopsy for diagnosis, as well as insertion of plastic or partially covered self-expanding metal stents for temporary or permanent relief of malignant biliary obstruction. Before requesting an ERCP for potential hilar or intrahepatic ductal obstruction, it is important to consider the risk and management options in the likely event of contamination of the obstructed liver segments.

Percutaneous transhepatic cholangiography

Radiological injection of contrast directly into the intrahepatic bile ducts may be preferable to ERCP in some circumstances to relieve jaundice without contaminating obstructed liver segments. In fact, it may be the only option when the ampulla is inaccessible endoscopically due to a large distal cholangiocarcinoma or when there has been previous foregut surgery. Complex interventional techniques including biliary stricture dilatation, stent placement or 'rendezvous' procedures in conjunction with an endoscopic approach may provide temporary or permanent palliation for malignant tumours.

Computed tomography

CT scans play a critical role in the diagnosis, staging and characterisation of primary and secondary liver tumours. In most cases, the diagnosis can be made without the need for tissue sampling confirmation. This modality is readily available and can be performed with faster scan times than magnetic resonance imaging (MRI). Generally, it is well tolerated especially by elderly patients or those with multiple morbidities who often have difficulty cooperating with the breath-hold requirements of an MRI scan. Contrast-enhanced multidetector CT provides fast, high-quality, thin-section imaging of both intrahepatic and extrahepatic disease.

The characteristic feature of hepatocellular carcinoma (HCC) is late arterial enhancement with relative washout compared with the liver parenchyma during the venous or delayed phases. In contrast, liver metastases are typically hypo-attenuating during the non-contrast phase, and enhance less than surrounding liver following contrast. In the presence of hepatic steatosis, liver metastases may be iso-attenuating or even slightly hyper-attenuating. The enhancement pattern is typically peripheral, and while there may be central filling in during the portal venous phase, the contrast usually washes out in the delayed phase. Some primary tumours produce hyper-enhancing (hypervascular) liver metastases including renal cell, thyroid and neuroendocrine tumours.

CT cholangiography

CT after intravenous drip infusion of Biliscopin (meglumine iotroxate) provides non-invasive visualisation of the biliary tree by excretion of contrast into bile. It may help evaluate the extent of involvement of the biliary tree by a malignant tumour (Figure 20.1). This modality cannot be used in patients with an iodinated-contrast hypersensitivity, and is ineffective and hazardous in those with a serum bilirubin level above 30 mmol/L.

Magnetic resonance imaging

MRI provides useful imaging of the liver without exposure to radiation. There have been rapid advances in MRI technology over the past decade and this modality is emerging as a critical investigation for diagnosing and staging malignant hepatobiliary tumours. Use of the hepatobiliary-specific contrast agent Gd-EOB-DTPA (Primovist) produces

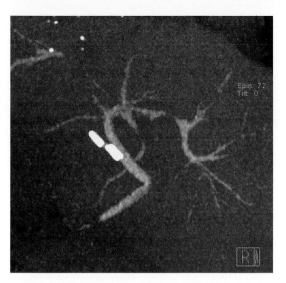

Fig. 20.1 CT cholangiogram of a malignant biliary stricture in the left duct due to an iCCA.

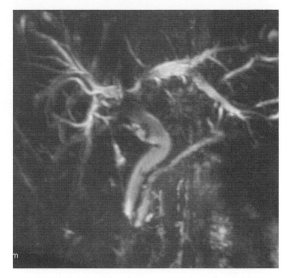

Fig. 20.2 Magnetic resonance cholangiogram of a benign biliary stricture mimicking a Klatskin tumour.

both dynamic and liver-specific images and is more sensitive than MRI without contrast or with non-specific contrast agents. Advantages of MRI over CT include the capacity to evaluate a greater variety of tissue properties, including fat content, restriction of diffusion and T2-weighted signalling, all of which improve lesion detection and characterisation. However, disadvantages include the limited availability of this modality in some countries, slower scan times compared with CT, and poor tolerance in some patients because of claustrophobia and the need for prolonged breath-holding.

The characteristic diagnostic features of HCC on Gd-EOB-DTPA enhanced MRI are arterial phase hyper-enhancement followed by portal venous or delayed phase washout. In contrast, liver metastases typically demonstrate a peripheral rim enhancement and lack of central enhancement in the dynamic phase, especially when central tumour necrosis is present. During the hepatobiliary phase, liver metastases usually become hypointense.

Magnetic resonance cholangiopancreatography

Magnetic resonance cholangiopancreatography (MRCP) enables rapid non-invasive evaluation of both the biliary and pancreatic ducts without the use of intravenous contrast agents. Significant improvements in spatial and temporal resolution over the past decade make MRCP an ideal non-invasive investigation of the intrahepatic and extra-hepatic biliary tree in patients with malignant biliary tumours. This modality is used instead of CT cholangiography in patients with elevated serum bilirubin levels secondary to obstruction (Figure 20.2).

CT or MRI for investigating malignant hepatobiliary tumours?

There have been many comparative studies of the two techniques over the past 20 years with demonstrated advantages and disadvantages for each modality. In practical terms, both modalities may be necessary and helpful but ultimately the decision to perform one over the other will depend on institutional preferences, specific patient needs and accessibility. In general, CT scans are more widely available, and possibly need less expertise to perform and to interpret than MRI scans. MRI is certainly more prone to artefacts than CT, and detailed and specialised interpretation of the images may not be available outside of specialist centres.

In relation to HCC, both modalities have similar sensitivity and specificity when considered on a per-patient basis, and most clinical practice guidelines recommend either multiphase CT and MRI with extracellular contrast agents as the first-line investigation for diagnosis and staging. However, MRI may have superior per-lesion sensitivity in differentiating tumour from non-tumour tissue, particularly in patients with chronic liver disease. As with all malignant hepatobiliary tumours both techniques are limited in detecting lesions of less than 10 mm in diameter.

In patients with perihilar cholangiocarcinoma, both multiphase CT and Gd-EOB-DTPA enhanced MRI (including MRCP) yield similar staging accuracy. To determine resectability it is critical to obtain detailed imaging of the porta hepatis to examine the extent of disease spread along the biliary tree and into adjacent vascular structures. This can be achieved with three-dimensional computer-assisted reconstruction of the portal structures obtained from a standard multiphase CT scan with the aid of commercially available software. However, MRI may have an advantage over CT because of better soft-tissue contrast resolution, which is particularly helpful for evaluation of infiltrating tumours and peripheral ductal involvement.

Numerous clinical guidelines recommend that a multiphase CT scan of the chest and abdomen as well as an MRI scan should be done at the beginning of the management process in all patients with colorectal liver metastases. Contrast-enhanced MRI is certainly better than CT for detecting lesions of less than 10 mm and when there is known steatosis. It is also more sensitive than CT for detecting residual disease in the post-chemotherapy liver.

Positron emission tomography

Positron emission tomography with fluorodeoxyglucose (FDG-PET) is widely used in clinical oncology. In patients with colorectal liver metastases, this investigation may identify otherwise radiologically occult disease beyond the liver, thereby improving selection of patients for resection. Although a recent meta-analysis of retrospective data did not show any improvement in disease-free or overall survival in patients with colorectal liver metastases, most clinical guidelines recommend routine use in the assessment of patients with potentially resectable disease. There should be a 3–4 week delay between the end of chemotherapy and the PET/CT examination to prevent false-negative findings.

In contrast, the sensitivity of FDG-PET in primary malignant tumours is low because of wide variations in glucose 6-phosphatase activity in the liver. Accordingly, this investigation is not commonly used for the diagnosis and staging of patients with either HCC or cholangiocarcinoma outside of high-volume specialist centres.

Role of percutaneous biopsy for malignant hepatobiliary tumours

Percutaneous biopsy should not be done in patients with possible malignant hepatobiliary tumours who might be suitable for a potentially curative resection. This is because of the risk of needle track seeding after transperitoneal procedures and the potential negative impact of this on survival. In most cases modern multimodal imaging can make the diagnosis without the need for tissue confirmation. When there is doubt, referral for a specialist hepatobiliary opinion is preferable to biopsy. Of course, there are some situations in patients who are eligible for resection where a tissue diagnosis is needed to help guide neoadjuvant treatment. This can be done percutaneously under radiological guidance or alternatively as a controlled core needle biopsy under laparoscopic vision.

Primary malignant tumours (Box 20.2)

Cholangiocarcinoma

Cholangiocarcinoma (CCA) is a relatively rare tumour but the second most common primary hepatobiliary malignancy after HCC. The overall incidence rate is 0.4–4 per 100 000, and in 2013 Australia had an incidence rate of 2.9 per 100 000. The disease is more prevalent in certain parts of Southeast Asia such as northeast Thailand where rates in men are as high as 96 per 100 000. Overall men are more frequently affected than women, and most cases occur over the age of 65 years. Over the past three decades there has been a steady increase in the incidence of CCA in western populations, although the reasons for this are unknown.

Cholangiocarcinoma is anatomically classified as intrahepatic (iCCA, 10–15%), perihilar (pCCA, 50–70%, Klatskin tumour) and distal (dCCA, 20–30%). Inflammation and cholestasis are known to be key factors in carcinogenesis but there are

---

Box 20.2 Classification of malignant hepatobiliary tumours

Primary
Hepatocellular origin
   Hepatocellular cancer
   Hepatoblastoma
Biliary origin
   Cholangiocarcinoma
   Gallbladder carcinoma
   Biliary cystadenocarcinoma
Other rare tumours
   Haemangiosarcoma
   Hepatic epithelioid haemangioendothelioma
   Primary hepatic lymphoma
   Primary hepatic neuroendocrine tumours

Secondary
Liver metastases

Box 20.3 Risk factors for cholangiocarcinoma

Definite
Primary sclerosing cholangitis
Biliary parasites (*Opisthorchis viverrini, Clonorchis sinensis*)
Hepatolithiasis
Caroli's disease
Choledochal cysts (types I and IV)
Exposure to the radiocontrast agent Thorotrast

Possible
Cirrhosis
Diabetes mellitus
Obesity
Chronic hepatitis B/C infection
Excessive alcohol intake (>80 g/day)

distinct genetic mutational changes associated with each of the different tumour locations (Box 20.3). Whole-genome expression profiling has confirmed activation of pathways driving proliferation (e.g. EGF, K-Ras, AKT/mTOR/PI3K and MET), angiogenesis (e.g. vascular endothelial growth factor receptor) and inflammation (e.g. interleukin 6). Morphologically, these tumours are classified as mass-forming, periductal-infiltrating or intraductal papillary. Most iCCAs are mass-forming while pCCAs and dCCAs are typically periductal-infiltrating. Histopathologically, up to 95% of CCAs are adenocarcinomas.

The clinical presentation of CCA depends on the location of the tumour and varies from an incidental finding or vague abdominal symptoms for intrahepatic mass-forming tumours to painless obstructive jaundice for extrahepatic tumours. Often, local invasion into surrounding blood vessels and nerves is found at presentation, and in the case of iCCAs tumour growth may infiltrate extensively into adjacent liver parenchyma. Vascular compression or occlusion occurs in advanced disease and may contribute to segmental or hemilobar liver atrophy.

Several staging systems for CCA have been proposed but the most widely adopted is the American Joint Committee on Cancer/Union for International Cancer Control (AJCC/UICC) system. This has shown stage-survival correlation for the different tumour types but is limited by the need to include histology to determine T and N status.

Serum tumour markers such as carcinoembryonic antigen (CEA) and CA19-9 are often used in patients with cholangiocarcinoma.

Management

The prognosis following diagnosis of CCA depends on the location and stage of the tumour as well as patient comorbidity. Overall, iCCAs have a worse prognosis than cancers in extrahepatic sites (pCCA and dCCA). Median survival for unresectable tumours is 5–12 months, and palliative chemoradiotherapy can provide a modest survival advantage over best supportive care. In Australia in 2014, the overall 5-year relative survival after diagnosis of CCA was 19%. Only radical resection offers the chance of cure. However, the extent of lymphovascular spread and the ability to achieve an R0 margin clearance are critical factors impacting long-term outcome.

Contraindications to resection include bilateral multifocal disease, distant metastases and comorbidities that outweigh the operative risks. Regional lymph node metastases are not an absolute contraindication to resection, although N1 disease is an independent prognostic factor for a poor outcome.

After adequate staging and concluding that the tumour can be resected, it is important to thoroughly assess for any comorbidity that might limit a major surgical procedure. Depending on the size and stage of the disease, these operations can be a formidable undertaking due to local infiltration of adjacent structures and the frequency of underlying chronic liver disease. A preoperative cardiac and respiratory assessment is often helpful. Relief of jaundice, control of sepsis, minimisation of alcohol intake and strict diabetic control in the weeks leading up to the operation are also important.

Treatment options

Intrahepatic cholangiocarcinoma
Although resection is usually only possible in less than 30% of cases, this can result in a median survival of up to 39 months and a 5-year survival rate of up to 40%. Adjuvant chemoradiotherapy after resection does not improve outcomes. Systemic chemotherapy and/or best supportive care may be offered to patients with unresectable iCCA or to those who are unable to tolerate a major resection. However, the results are often disappointing in relation to toxicity, oncological benefit and overall survival. Other palliative treatment options for liver-only or liver-dominant disease include locoregional treatments such as radiofrequency ablation (RFA) or microwave ablation (MWA), transarterial chemoembolisation (TACE) or selective internal radiation therapy (SIRT).

Perihilar cholangiocarcinoma (Klatskin tumour)

A multidisciplinary approach and multimodal treatment is needed for this complex disease. Biliary drainage for hilar CCA may be warranted and can be done by either ERCP or percutaneous transhepatic cholangiography, and the choice is usually institution dependent.

Resection offers the only chance of long-term survival for pCCA. This involves removal of the extrahepatic bile duct in conjunction with a hepatectomy and radical porta hepatis lymphadenectomy. Concomitant vascular resection increases the potential for morbidity but may be necessary to achieve a negative (R0) resection margin. In contrast to portal vein resection, hepatic artery excision causes more morbidity and does not improve long-term survival. Overall morbidity and mortality rates after major resection are 40–70% and 5–15%, respectively. The 5-year survival after resection of a Klatskin tumour ranges from 10 to 40%. Patients with primary sclerosing cholangitis complicated by pCCA should be considered for liver transplantation if they meet the appropriate criteria.

Surgical palliation in the form of cholecystectomy and biliary–enteric anastomosis for biliary drainage is sometimes undertaken but is associated with increased morbidity and mortality compared with endoscopic management. Other palliative treatment options include stereotactic radiotherapy and photodynamic therapy.

Distal cholangiocarcinoma

Cancer of the distal common bile duct (dCCA) often presents clinically just like a pancreatic cancer. When imaging and endoscopic findings demonstrate locoregional disease only, patients with an adequate performance status should be offered pancreaticoduodenectomy. Median survival after a potentially curative resection is approximately 24 months, with 5-year survival rates ranging from 20 to 40% depending on the extent of disease. As with hilar tumours, placement of a covered metal biliary stent by ERCP provides excellent relief of jaundice in most patients.

Palliative systemic chemotherapy for unresectable or metastatic disease is usually based on gemcitabine and cisplatin. Unfortunately, median survival is usually less than 12 months in most patients.

Gallbladder cancer

Gallbladder cancer is rare, with a worldwide variation in incidence of 1–25 per 100 000. The prominent geographic variation correlates with the prevalence of gallstones. High rates are seen in South America (Chile, Ecuador and Bolivia) and in northern India, Pakistan, Japan and Korea. The most important risk factor for the development of gallbladder cancer is gallstones but the presence of primary sclerosing cholangitis or an anomalous pancreatobiliary junction also increase the risk.

Gallbladder cancer occurs mostly in patients over 50 years old and there is a marked female preponderance in the order of 6 : 1. It is found in the fundus of the gallbladder in approximately 60% of cases. Adenocarcinoma accounts for 98% of cases but other rarer variants include papillary, mucinous, squamous and adenosquamous subtypes. A range of genetic alterations have been implicated, including oncogene activation, tumour suppressor gene inhibition, microsatellite instability and methylation of gene promoter areas.

The three most common ways that gallbladder cancer may present are as follows:

- an unsuspected discovery at the time of cholecystectomy for presumed benign disease
- incidentally at histopathology after routine cholecystectomy
- less commonly with abdominal symptoms due to advanced disease.

The presence of abdominal pain, a mass, weight loss or jaundice are ominous signs usually indicating either local invasion or metastatic spread. Most of these patients have unresectable disease. The clinical presentation may be like benign gallbladder disease and the radiological findings may be confused with acute or chronic cholecystitis. A preoperative diagnosis of Mirizzi syndrome (extrinsic compression of the extrahepatic bile duct due to pressure and inflammatory change from an impacted stone in the neck of the gallbladder) proves to be due to a cancer of the gallbladder in a small proportion of patients.

Diagnosis and staging

Transabdominal ultrasound allows accurate assessment of the features of a gallbladder polyp, including size and depth of invasion. Dynamic contrast-enhanced CT of the abdomen and chest document the extent of local and distant spread. For large tumours, Gd-EOB-DTPA (Primovist)-enhanced MRI may provide additional evaluation of possible involvement of the biliary tree or infiltration into liver parenchyma. Lymph node metastases from gallbladder cancer are not easily detected by either CT or MRI. ^{18}F-FDG-PET, if available, may identify distant occult disease, which would preclude radical surgical intervention.

Diagnostic laparoscopy to identify peritoneal dissemination may be helpful in patients with radiologically detected advanced tumours. In patients with an incidental gallbladder cancer found at histopathology after laparoscopic cholecystectomy, repeat staging laparoscopy before undertaking a radical resection may exclude disseminated disease. However, the yield from laparoscopy is generally low except in patients with poorly differentiated, large cancers or when there has been a positive resection margin.

The histopathology report from the original cholecystectomy should be carefully reviewed for the exact tumour location, the depth of invasion and the extent of lymphovascular spread. The presence of involved resection margins will determine the need for radical resection of adjacent structures including the bile duct.

Serum tumour markers such as CEA and CA19-9 may be elevated and will help confirm the diagnosis in patients with suspicious gallbladder polyps. However, the sensitivity and specificity of these tests is too low to warrant routine use for screening purposes.

The most common staging system for gallbladder cancer is the AJCC/UICC TNM staging system. This identifies five different stages depending on the extent of disease and incorporates histological information about T and N status. In Japan, where gallbladder cancer is relatively common, the Japanese Society of Biliary Surgery staging system is more often used. This system differs slightly by expanding on both the T and N stage definitions. It may provide slightly better prognostication after resection compared with the AJCC/UICC system, especially in patients with more advanced disease. Incorporation of the histological subtype and grade of the gallbladder cancer has been advocated to improve the prognostic value of these staging systems further.

Management

The prognosis for patients with gallbladder cancer depends on the location and stage of the tumour as well as patient comorbidity. The lack of a submucosa in the gallbladder wall and the proximity to the liver predisposes this malignancy to direct spread into the adjacent hepatic segments (4 and 5), the bile duct and nearby abdominal viscera. Lymphatic dissemination occurs commonly, and the cystic and peri-choledochal lymph nodes are often the initial site of spread. However, the number of involved nodes rather than the location is most predictive of long-term outcome, and this in turn is influenced by the depth of invasion of the primary tumour.

Gallbladder cancer is the most aggressive of the biliary tract cancers and has the shortest median overall survival duration. Complete resection offers the only chance of cure but unfortunately recurrence rates are high. Positive resection margins, lymph node metastasis and poorly differentiated tumours are independent risk factors for poor prognosis after 'curative' resection. Laparoscopic cholecystectomy is contraindicated when gallbladder cancer is known or suspected preoperatively unless there is clear radiological evidence of localised mucosal disease only.

Incidentally discovered gallbladder cancer following cholecystectomy

Cholecystectomy alone is sufficient treatment for tumours confined to the mucosa (Tis) or lamina propria (T1a). Surgical options for tumours that invade the muscular layer of the gallbladder ($\geq$T1b) are more controversial. Although there is ongoing debate, a consensus statement of experts in 2014 recommended en-bloc resection of adjacent liver (Couinaud segments 4b and 5) and complete portal lymphadenectomy for patients with T1b tumours (Figure 20.3). Regional lymph node metastases (N1 or N2) are found in 18–60% of patients with T2 tumours (invasion of the muscularis layer of the gallbladder). Accordingly, there is consensus that these patients should undergo similar radical resection to reduce the risk of local and distant recurrence.

Resection of the extrahepatic bile duct should only be undertaken when there is direct extension or microscopic involvement of the cystic duct margin. Addition of a biliary anastomosis in the presence of non-dilated ducts is associated with a significant risk of bile leak and stenosis. Similarly, port-site excision should not be carried out routinely as this is not associated with improved long-term outcome.

The 5-year survival rates in patients with T1b–2 cancers range from 10 to 60% after cholecystectomy alone compared with 59–90% following more radical resection. Given the propensity for recurrence after R0 resection of T2–4 disease in N1 gallbladder cancer, patients with nodal metastases should be considered for adjuvant systemic chemotherapy and/or chemoradiotherapy.

Treatment of patients with a large gallbladder mass due to malignancy may also involve a radical resection, but this often provides only marginal benefit particularly in the presence of jaundice.

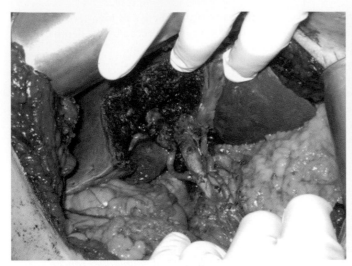 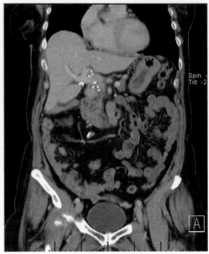

Fig. 20.3 Gallbladder cancer (T2bN0M0) immediately after resection and at 4 years follow-up.

Instead, staging laparoscopy may be warranted to exclude disseminated disease, which might prevent an unhelpful resection. Direct invasion of either the duodenum or colon does not necessarily indicate nodal involvement and in carefully selected patients en-bloc resection may still be appropriate.

Several Japanese groups have reported the feasibility of radical resection for advanced gallbladder cancer including the addition of extended hepatectomy or pancreaticoduodenectomy, with acceptable morbidity and mortality and an apparent improvement in patient survival. The 5-year survival rates vary from 29 to 87% but this is at the expense of significant morbidity (40–50%) and mortality (up to 60%). It is worth stating that these results come out of highly experienced centres and may not necessarily be transferable to non-Japanese centres. In most western series, radical treatment of locally advanced tumours by resection of adjacent organs, extended hepatectomy or vascular reconstruction has not been associated with prolonged disease-free or overall survival, and so this cannot be recommended. Instead, these patients should be considered for clinical trials of neoadjuvant chemotherapy.

Laparoscopic, robotic-assisted and total robotic radical resection of gallbladder cancer have been performed at specialised centres. Small cases series have reported safety and feasibility outcome data for T1b, T2 and even T3 tumours that are equivalent to outcomes following an open procedure. However, there are significant technical challenges related to the adequacy of the lymphadenectomy and the difficulty of a bile duct reconstruction that will need to be overcome before these approaches are adopted more widely. For now, these procedures are likely to be limited to a few specialist centres.

Many patients present with advanced disease and are therefore not resectable and have a poor prognosis. Palliative options include biliary drainage (endoscopic or by surgical bypass), systemic chemotherapy and radiotherapy. Gemcitabine alone or in combination with 5-fluorouracil (5-FU), capecitabine or cisplatin is well tolerated in most patients and provides marginal improvement in survival compared with best supportive care.

Hepatocellular carcinoma

Hepatocellular carcinoma is a malignant tumour of hepatocytes that often arises in the context of end-stage chronic inflammation (cirrhosis). It is the most common primary liver tumour (worldwide age-standardised rate is 15.3 per 100 000), and the fifth most common malignancy in men and the ninth in women. For both sexes, HCC is the second highest cause of cancer-related deaths. It occurs more often in men than women, and the incidence rates peak after age 60 years. There are significant variations of disease burden across the world, with the highest age-standardised rates per 100 000 occurring in underdeveloped regions in eastern Asia (31.9), Southeast Asia (22.2), western Africa (16.4) and Melanesia (14.8). In 2012 the age-standardised rate per 100 000 in Australia/New Zealand was 6.4. Incidence and mortality rates are rising in some western countries, which traditionally have had a low disease burden. Although the reasons for this are not fully understood, it may be due to a combination of factors including changing migration patterns, an increased prevalence of hepatitis

C infection from intravenous drug abuse, and because of rising rates of obesity and type 2 diabetes. A curative treatment for hepatitis C has been available since 2013 and although this reduces the risk of developing HCC, the risks are not eliminated and these patients require ongoing surveillance.

HCC is a complex disease with multiple possible aetiologies. The main risks are chronic hepatitis B virus (HBV) infection, chronic hepatitis C virus (HCV) infection and dietary exposure to the carcinogen aflatoxin B1. Other risks include non-alcoholic fatty liver disease, alcohol-induced cirrhosis, obesity, dietary iron overload, metabolic disorders such as antitrypsin deficiency, and inherited conditions such as haemochromatosis and Wilson's disease. However, approximately 15–20% of patients in 'western' countries have no obvious predisposing risk factors.

Various underlying gene and protein expression patterns have been described in hepatocellular cancer. These include point mutations of the c-*KRAS* gene, co-amplification of the cyclin D1 gene, mutation of the β-catenin gene, reduction of expression of p21WAF/Cip1 and p16, and increased expression of transforming growth factor (TGF)-β and DNA methyltransferase (DNMT1) mRNA.

The clinical presentation of HCC varies depending on whether patients are in a high- or low-risk group. In those with compensated chronic liver disease, most liver cancers are detected during screening or surveillance. A progressively rising serum AFP level should raise suspicion of a new hepatocellular cancer. Malignant change should also be suspected when there is a sudden deterioration in liver function. Frequently, this is due to either hepatic or portal vein thrombosis. Spontaneous rupture of HCC occasionally occurs in patients with large exophytic tumours, and this is associated with significant risk of mortality from peritonitis and shock. In patients with no risks for chronic liver disease, mild to moderate abdominal pain, weight loss, early satiety or a palpable mass in the upper abdomen are the most frequent presentations. These symptoms often signify locally advanced disease.

The overall prognosis after a diagnosis of HCC is poor, with a median survival of approximately 3–5 months for untreated symptomatic patients. Outcome is dependent on the tumour biology, the stage of the disease, the patient's underlying comorbidity and liver function, and optimal therapy. The fibrolamellar variant that usually occurs in non-cirrhotic young adults is less aggressive than more common subtypes, and prolonged survival may be possible even in advanced disease.

Diagnosis

Several different imaging modalities including ultrasound, CT and MRI may be used to either evaluate patients with chronic liver disease or diagnose and characterise a suspected HCC. Screening programs in high-risk patients usually involve 6-monthly ultrasound scans. The addition of serum alpha-fetoprotein (AFP) levels improves the sensitivity of these programs for detecting small tumours and worldwide this has led to a decrease in late-stage presentations.

Dynamic, multiphase, contrast-enhanced CT or MRI is the current standard for the imaging diagnosis of HCC. The use of hepatobiliary contrast agents and the inclusion of diffusion-weighted sequences during MRI have improved detection rates and may be particularly helpful in differentiating regenerative nodules from early HCC. Except in specific circumstances these imaging modalities have largely replaced tissue biopsy for the diagnosis of HCC. Chest CT is important to assess for metastatic disease, particularly before undertaking radical surgical intervention.

The yield from routine diagnostic laparoscopy prior to undertaking resection of HCC is low except in patients with cirrhosis, multifocal tumours and radiological evidence of major vascular invasion.

Staging and predictive models

Several clinical models focus on the impact of the underlying liver function. These include the Child–Pugh classification, the MELD score and the albumin–bilirubin (ALBI) grading system.

Child–Pugh grade A patients do well following surgical intervention, but the classification is not particularly helpful for predicting outcomes in more advanced disease. The MELD score is helpful in cirrhotic patients only, and is derived from three laboratory values (international normalised ratio, serum total bilirubin and serum creatinine). Patients with a MELD score of 10 or less are suitable for surgical intervention. Those with a score of 10–15 have a moderate risk of complications, while patients with a MELD score above 15 should not undergo surgical intervention. The ALBI grade is based on assessment of the serum albumin and bilirubin and can be used in patients with or without cirrhosis. This may be a better prognostic discriminator for early-stage disease than either the Child–Pugh classification or the MELD score.

Other clinical decision models combine liver function parameters with markers of disease biology (e.g. size, number of tumours, the presence of vascular invasion). The two most commonly used are the Barcelona Clinic Liver Cancer (BCLC) staging system and the Cancer of the Liver Italian Program (CLIP) score.

The two main staging systems that include a histopathological assessment of disease are the AJCC/UICC staging system (8th edition) and the Japan Integrated Staging (JIS) score. The AJCC/UICC staging system is the most commonly used classification in patients who undergo resection or transplantation. However, the JIS score is simpler to use and may be better at discriminating outcome in early HCC. Of all the histopathological factors, the most consistently identified predictor of poor long-term survival after both resection and liver transplantation is the presence of microvascular invasion (MVI). This is difficult to determine preoperatively and while several clinical predictive models have been proposed none of these have been widely validated.

Management

Hepatocellular carcinoma is a complex disease that is best managed within a multidisciplinary environment. Management of the chronic liver disease is just as important in many of these patients as management of the HCC. Curative intent treatments should be offered to all eligible patients with early-stage disease. Although patients with more advanced disease may still be offered curative treatment, this will depend on the tumour staging and the underlying liver reserve.

Early-stage HCC is defined both clinically and pathologically, and this leads to difficulty interpreting the literature regarding treatment algorithms. Clinically, early-stage HCC usually refers to tumours of 3 cm or less in size and three or fewer in number, and with underlying good liver reserve (Child–Pugh A). Some groups classify tumours of 2 cm or less as 'very' early stage disease. Confusingly, tumours described by the Milan criteria (which includes solitary lesions up to 5 cm) are also sometimes considered early-stage HCC.

There is ongoing controversy about the best management of patients with early-stage tumours (≤2 cm). Several meta-analyses of both non-randomised and randomised studies have concluded that percutaneous RFA may be inferior to liver resection, but that MWA may have an advantage when comparing overall and recurrence-free survival. Regardless, both ablation techniques are less invasive and associated with fewer complications and shorter hospitalisation than liver resection.

Therefore, ablation is the preferred option for patients with underlying liver dysfunction (Child–Pugh B–C). Of course, RFA or MWA are only possible for tumours that are anatomically accessible and not adjacent to major vascular or biliary structures. A reasonable approach in patients with early-stage HCC and good liver reserve is to offer upfront percutaneous ablation followed by close post-treatment radiological surveillance. If local recurrence does occur, the tumour and surrounding ablated area can then be resected.

Although liver transplantation is associated with significant perioperative risk and requires long-term immunosuppression, it is appealing because it eliminates the tumour and underlying chronic liver disease, as well as the risk of new intrahepatic cancers. Overall, liver transplantation provides the best long-term survival for early-stage HCC compared with other treatment options. Only patients aged under 70 years are considered, and selection is determined by the Milan criteria (one lesion <5 cm or up to three lesions, each <3 cm, no extrahepatic disease, and no evidence of gross vascular invasion). The 5-year overall survival rates after liver transplantation for HCC range from 52 to 81%. Selection beyond the Milan criteria has been advocated (one lesion <6.5 cm or up to three lesions, each <4 cm with a cumulative diameter <8 cm) to treat patients with more advanced tumours. Critics of this more liberal approach argue this is associated with higher rates of post-transplant recurrence and lower long-term survival. Patients may be offered locoregional therapy such as ablation or TACE while waiting for their liver transplant.

Living-donor liver transplantation (LDLT) has theoretical advantages of shorter waiting times, higher-quality grafts and shorter ischaemic times compared with traditional deceased donor liver transplantation. Disadvantages include the potential for perioperative risks in the donors, and ongoing concerns that this approach may increase recurrence rates in recipients. Generally, the criteria for transplantation for HCC are more liberal for 'eastern' countries than 'western' countries. This may be because LDLT is performed more often than deceased donor transplantation because of a shortage of deceased donor organs. Worldwide, HCC accounts for approximately 20–40% of liver transplantations, although in Australia and New Zealand the figure is closer to 10%.

Many patients with early-stage HCC and good liver reserve are treated by liver resection because of the shortage of donors for liver transplantation. Specialist surgical expertise is now widely available in most countries, and a potentially curative liver resection results in comparable 5-year and 10-year survival outcomes to liver transplantation. Unfortunately, only 10–40% of patients with HCC are suitable for resection at the time of diagnosis. In the absence of underlying parenchymal disease, up to 65–75% of the liver can be resected provided that vascular inflow/outflow and biliary drainage are maintained. Minor resections can be undertaken in patients with early Child B disease without portal hypertension, but this is often associated with significant morbidity.

Complications after hepatectomy are common, with morbidity rates of 31–50%. Reported 5-year overall survival rates after liver resection range from 37 to 61%, while 5-year disease-free survival rates range from 23 to 32%. Unfortunately, recurrence occurs commonly and to date there are no universally accepted adjuvant treatments to reduce this risk. Variables most frequently found to predict long-term outcome include tumour size, tumour number and severity of the underlying liver disease. Other important prognostic factors are untreated HBV and HCV infection, and the histological finding of MVI in the tumour specimen. To reduce recurrence and improve survival TACE is sometimes used as neoadjuvant therapy in patients with resectable HCC. However, a recent systematic review of the literature concluded that this does not improve disease-free survival.

To date, laparoscopic resection of HCC has mostly involved minor resections. This approach is associated with less blood loss and transfusion requirements, less overall morbidity and a shorter length of stay compared with open resections. Importantly, there appears to be no difference in short- or long-term oncological outcomes. Laparoscopic and robotic major liver resections for HCC have also been done and early reports suggest that oncological outcomes are also comparable with open techniques.

Intermediate or advanced stage HCC

Unfortunately, more than 50% of all HCCs are diagnosed at an intermediate or advanced stage, and in those who do not satisfy the Milan criteria the only hope of cure is liver resection. These patients have a high risk of recurrence, and outcomes following resection must be weighed against the lack of other potentially curative options. Certainly, long-term disease-free survival is possible in some patients, even those with large (>10 cm) or multinodular tumours (Figures 20.4

and 20.5). Careful preoperative assessment is required to determine adequate remnant liver reserve and to exclude the presence of extrahepatic disease. In general, liver resection is contraindicated in patients with extensively multifocal or bilateral tumours, or when there is involvement of the main portal vein or the inferior vena cava.

Palliative options for patients with inoperable disease include locoregional therapy such as TACE or SIRT. Although these patients may have improved quality of life and survival compared with best supportive treatment, overall they have a poor prognosis with a median survival of only 11–20 months. TACE is the best option for patients with large or multifocal HCC without macrovascular invasion or extrahepatic metastasis. Objective tumour responses are achieved in 35–50% of patients, and TACE can be repeated if necessary depending on tumour response and the patient's underlying liver reserve.

Oral administration of the multi-kinase inhibitor sorafenib may also prolong survival in patients with advanced-stage HCC who are unsuitable for either resection or locoregional treatment. SIRT does not provide a survival advantage over sorafenib but may be associated with better tumour response rates and less side effects.

Ruptured HCC

Spontaneous rupture of HCC is a rare and life-threatening complication. The exact mechanism of rupture is not fully understood, and while this complication can happen anywhere in the liver it occurs most frequently in large exophytic tumours. Urgent fluid resuscitation is required, and subsequent transarterial embolisation (TAE) for haemostasis has a high success rate (53–100%). Overall 30-day mortality rates after TAE are lower than after urgent open surgical haemostasis. Furthermore, emergency liver resection is also associated with poor long-term outcomes because the tumour stage and functional liver reserve are unknown, and disseminated malignant cells increase the risk of peritoneal and distant metastases. Tumour re-rupture after TAE has an extremely poor prognosis.

In patients who remain stable after the initial TAE, laparoscopy and washout of the haemoperitoneum several days later may speed up recovery from the inevitable ileus that follows such a catastrophic event. Most groups advocate re-imaging later to reassess the role of a staged liver resection in patients who have non-progressive disease.

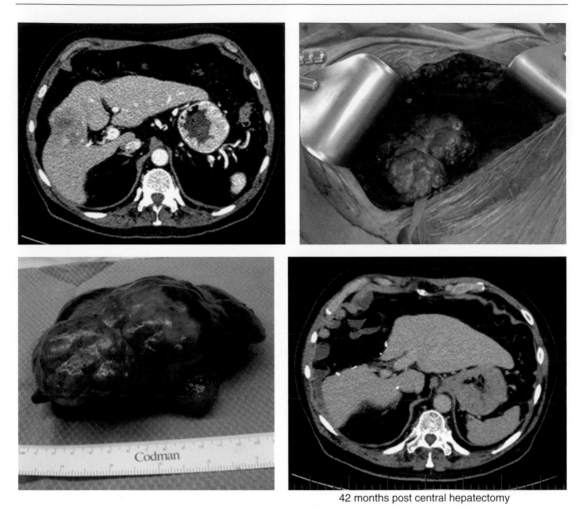

42 months post central hepatectomy

Fig. 20.4 Large central hepatocellular carcinoma secondary to haemochromatosis in a patient with Child–Pugh A disease.

Secondary tumours (liver metastases)

Liver metastases are a major cause of death in advanced malignant disease. Untreated metastases are associated with short survival especially when derived from oesophageal, stomach, pancreas or breast primary neoplasms. The most common primary sites for liver metastases are, in order of frequency, the bronchus, breast, colon and rectum, and uterus. The predilection for metastases to develop in the liver is because of direct portal venous blood flow from the intra-abdominal viscera. However, other biological factors are also involved given that tumours such as melanoma, breast and testicular carcinoma which have no portal venous drainage also spread frequently to this site. Management decisions in patients with liver metastases are difficult and relatively undefined except in those with colorectal liver metastases.

Colorectal liver metastases

Colorectal cancer is the third most common cancer worldwide and ranks as the second leading cause of cancer-related deaths in developed countries. In patients who undergo preoperative imaging, liver metastases are found in 35% of newly diagnosed patients and another 8–30% of patients develop metastatic spread to the liver during subsequent follow-up. Synchronous colorectal liver metastases (CRLM) are detected at or before the diagnosis of the primary cancer; metachronous CRLM are detected at any time 3 months after the diagnosis of the primary cancer. The exact cut-off for diagnosing metachronous CRLM is arbitrary (and controversial) and depends on the thoroughness of investigations at the original presentation.

Following the introduction of effective chemotherapeutic agents in the mid 1990s (oxaliplatin and irinotecan) and targeted biological agents in

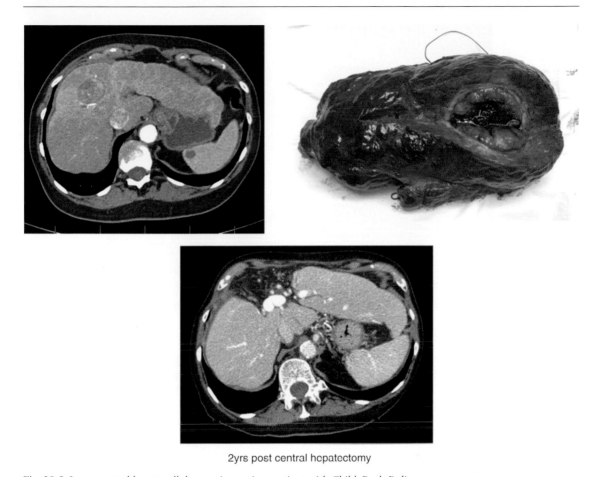

2yrs post central hepatectomy

Fig. 20.5 Large central hepatocellular carcinoma in a patient with Child–Pugh B disease.

the late 2000s (bevacizumab and cetuximab), there have been dramatic improvements in outcomes for patients with CRLM. Treatment strategies are evolving rapidly because of the development of new therapeutic agents and improvements in our understanding of the molecular heterogeneity of colorectal cancer. Ideally, patients should be managed in a multidisciplinary environment which includes surgeons, medical and radiation oncologists, radiologists and nuclear medicine physicians. At present, it is not routine to have geneticists and molecular scientists involved in multidisciplinary team discussions, although this may be helpful and necessary as personalised treatment options become more readily available.

Investigations

Contrast-enhanced abdominal/pelvic and thoracic CT is the investigation of first choice. A second modality such as ultrasound or MRI should be used when further clarification is needed. Gd-EOB-DTPA enhanced MRI is more sensitive than CT for detecting liver metastases under 10 mm in diameter

and for excluding residual disease in the post-chemotherapy liver (Figure 20.6). PET/CT scans detect extrahepatic disease including local recurrence at the site of the primary tumour excision. Although numerous clinical guidelines recommend routine PET/CT for all patients with CRLM, there is ongoing debate about the value of this investigation. Meta-analyses demonstrate that PET findings can alter management decisions in up to 24% of patients but this is mainly in patients at high risk of extrahepatic disease. Ideally, PET/CT should not be done within 6–8 weeks after completion of chemotherapy to avoid false-positive results. However, this may not always be practical.

Elevated levels of serum carcinoembryonic antigen (CEA) may be used to support the diagnosis and to monitor progress after treatment.

Staging

The original Dukes staging system for colorectal cancer does not include a classification for liver metastases and therefore is not applicable. The AJCC TNM system designates patients with CRLM

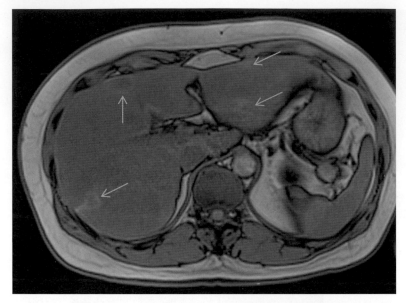

Fig. 20.6 MRI scan showing multifocal colorectal liver metastases (arrows) not seen on CT.

as stage IV disease. This is further subdivided into STAGE IVa (spread to the liver only), stage IVb (spread to more than one distant organ) or stage IVc (spread to distant parts of the peritoneum).

Clinical risk models

Several clinical risk scoring systems have been developed that stratify patient prognosis based on preoperatively identifiable clinicopathological factors. Variables that consistently relate to survival include the number and size of liver metastases, the nodal status of the primary tumour and the preoperative serum CEA level. Externally validated systems include the Nordlinger score, MSKCC score, Basingstoke index, Iwatsuki score and Mayo scoring system. Although these stratification systems help predict overall survival, they do not accurately select patients who might benefit from adjuvant treatment. This is likely to be improved by incorporation of proteomic and genomic biomarkers into the models (e.g. *KRAS* and *BRAF* mutation status).

Chemotherapy and biologics in the management of patients with CRLM
(Box 20.4)

Adjuvant chemotherapy is considered standard of care for patients with high-risk primary colorectal cancers without distant metastases. Although chemotherapy is frequently given, the evidence for a benefit in patients with resectable liver metastases

Box 20.4 Treatment options for patients with colorectal liver metastases

Systemic treatment
   Chemotherapy (5-FU, oxaliplatin, irinotecan)
   Biologics (cetuximab, panitumumab, bevacizumab)
Liver resection
Liver ablation (microwave ablation, radiofrequency ablation, cryotherapy)
Regional arterial treatments
   Irinotecan DC-beads
   Selective internal radiation therapy
   Direct chemotherapy infusion (5-FU, oxaliplatin)
Stereotactic body radiation therapy
Best supportive care

(other than in 'high-risk' disease) is not strong. Regardless, the pros and cons of systemic treatment must be discussed in detail and this is time-consuming and can be confusing for the patient with newly diagnosed CRLM.

At the initial diagnosis, it is important to determine whether the liver metastases are resectable, potentially resectable or not resectable, and if patients are fit for surgical intervention. In practical terms this provides a guide for the use of systemic treatment, although there are numerous other factors that contribute to this decision.

In patients with otherwise 'low-risk' resectable liver metastases, and where an R0 resection margin (microscopically clear) can be achieved, upfront liver resection or preoperative chemotherapy followed by resection are equally appropriate treatment options. Treatment usually consists of a doublet regimen of 5-FU and oxaliplatin limited to six cycles (FOLFOX). Overall 5-year survival rates of 48–51% are equivalent for these two approaches. Adjuvant therapy post liver resection is not routine but may be warranted based on pathological assessment of the resected specimen.

In contrast, patients with resectable but 'high-risk' liver metastases (e.g. multiple or large metastases, synchronous disease, suspicion of low-volume extrahepatic disease) should be offered perioperative doublet chemotherapy (FOLFOX) for 3 months before and after liver resection. This may or may not be combined with monoclonal antibody therapy (either bevacizumab or cetuximab depending on *KRAS* status). More aggressive triplet regimens combining 5-FU, oxaliplatin and irinotecan (FOLFOXIRI) have been advocated but this requires careful selection of patients because of the toxicity of this treatment.

Patients with potentially resectable CRLM may be down-staged with aggressive systemic treatment. The best combination in this situation is unknown and is the subject of ongoing study. In patients with *KRAS* wild-type disease, doublet chemotherapy plus an anti-EGFR (epidermal growth factor receptor) antibody may be the best option, although triplet therapy (FOLFOXIRI) plus bevacizumab (a vascular endothelial growth factor inhibitor) may also be considered. In patients with *RAS*-mutant disease, a cytotoxic doublet plus bevacizumab or FOLFOXIRI plus bevacizumab is recommended. Maximum response is usually seen after 12–16 weeks of treatment. These patients need to be re-evaluated regularly to identify non-responders and to prevent over-treatment of patients who respond and then become candidates for liver resection.

Some patients achieve a complete radiological response after treatment and this poses a clinical dilemma about whether to resect or watch these original sites of tumour in the liver. Despite evidence that up to 40% of these treated tumours have pathological evidence of microscopic residual disease, most surgeons prefer a watch-and-wait approach rather than performing a blind resection of the tumour site based on the original imaging.

Patients with non-resectable CRLM and who are unlikely ever to be offered liver resection because of local factors or extrahepatic metastases may be considered for locoregional treatments combined with systemic therapy. Locoregional treatments include thermal ablation (RFA or MWA), TACE (with DC beads), SIRT using yttrium-90 radiolabelled particles, or stereotactic body radiation therapy.

Biomarkers and molecular signatures in CRLM

Colorectal cancer is a heterogeneous disease associated with multiple different gene mutations. Assessment for *KRAS* and *BRAF* mutations is now routine before treatment with EGFR-targeted monoclonal antibodies (cetuximab or panitumumab). Only patients with *KRAS* wild-type disease should be offered these therapies. However, there is mounting evidence that 'expanded RAS' analysis may be needed to identify tumour subtypes with varying response rates due to different codon mutations.

Recently, a classification was proposed that identified four molecular genotypes of tumour associated with distinct prognoses:
- CMS1 (immunogenic and hypermutated)
- CMS2 (epithelial, marked WNT and MYC signalling activation, best prognosis)
- CMS3 (metabolic dysregulation)
- CMS4 (mesenchymal features, worst prognosis).

These classifications represent a breakthrough in our understanding of the underlying molecular mechanisms of this disease and may help individualise treatment regimens including the role of hepatectomy. Numerous new biomarkers are emerging but are not yet in routine clinical practice. Ideally, these will enhance further our ability to predict response to treatment.

Liver resection: postoperative outcomes and long-term survival

Resection offers the best chance of cure for patients with isolated CRLM. The first step in a multidisciplinary team-managed treatment strategy is to determine whether the patient has resectable disease, and whether they are fit enough to undergo an operation. Classical indications for liver resection are based on the number and size of the metastases and whether there is extrahepatic disease or not. More recently, there is consensus that all patients should be considered for potentially curative resection if there is enough liver remnant and adequate vascular inflow/outflow and biliary drainage can be obtained. This radical surgical approach has resulted in a shift of thinking towards the contraindications rather than the indications for liver resection (Figure 20.7).

Refinements of surgical technique have contributed to the increased safety of liver resection over the past two decades. These include the use of low central venous pressure anaesthesia, intermittent portal inflow occlusion (Pringle manoeuvre), precise tumour localisation using intraoperative ultrasound, and improved transection instruments

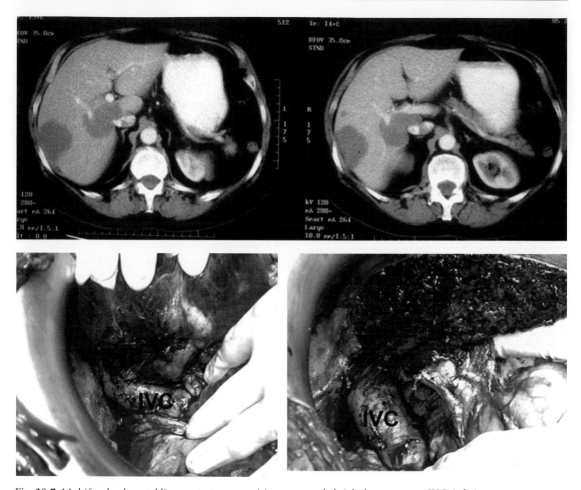

Fig. 20.7 Multifocal colorectal liver metastases requiring an extended right hepatectomy. IVC, inferior vena cava.

including the Cavitron ultrasonic surgical aspirator (CUSA), stapling devices and energy-based surgical vessel sealing tools.

Major morbidity after liver resection (defined as a complication of Clavien–Dindo grades III or IV) occurs in up to 20% of patients and depends on the extent of resection. Specific complications of liver resection include post-hepatectomy liver failure, bile leakage, haemorrhage and intra-abdominal sepsis.

Laparoscopic operations are associated with less overall morbidity, lower transfusion rates and shorter length of hospital stay than open procedures. Furthermore, several meta-analyses have shown that oncological outcomes are not compromised by a laparoscopic approach and in fact may allow patients to return to adjuvant treatment faster than after an open procedure.

There is growing interest in robotics for the management of patients with liver metastases because of the advantages of three-dimensional imaging and multi-degree operative freedom. Robotic liver

resection may be particularly beneficial in apical and dorsal segment resections which are difficult to resect laparoscopically. To date most reports involve small case series undertaken by highly specialised units. Barriers to more widespread adoption include limited access to robots in many hospitals, higher costs compared with open or laparoscopic approaches, and lack of a suitable robotic liver-dissecting device.

Overall, in-hospital and 90-day mortality rates after liver resection are usually less than 5%. Regardless of the approach, patients with advanced age, comorbid disease and who undergo synchronous hepatic and colon resection have the highest procedure-related mortality following major liver resection.

After liver resection, overall 5-year survival rates range from 25 to 63% (mean 40%) and 5-year disease-free survival rates range from 4 to 47% (mean 25%). Overall 10-year survival rates as high as 36% have been reported in some series.

Strategies to increase resection rates

Upfront liver resection is feasible in only 15–25% of patients, although systemic chemotherapy is effective in down-staging some patients with initially unresectable disease. There are several other options that are used in clinical practice in conjunction with chemotherapy to expand the number of patients who might undergo a potentially curative liver resection. These include portal vein embolisation to cause hypertrophy of the proposed remnant liver, thermoablation combined with liver resection, two-stage hepatectomy, extreme liver surgery including resection of the vena cava, and the ALPPS (associating liver partition and portal vein ligation for staged hepatectomy) procedure. Although promising, this latter technique is associated with significant perioperative risks and therefore has not been widely adopted.

Synchronous resection

The surgical approach in patients who present with synchronous CRLM can be challenging and often depends on whether the primary tumour is symptomatic or not. Options include simultaneous resection of the primary and liver metastases or a staged resection. The staged approach can be either the primary first (classic) or the liver first (reverse approach). Systematic review of the literature shows no significant difference in outcomes between these approaches. An obvious advantage of a synchronous bowel and liver operation for the patient is the need for only one anaesthetic. A general rule of thumb to avoid the risk of complications is that a simultaneous operation should be avoided if both the bowel and liver procedures are major resections.

Surveillance after liver resection

Following a potentially curative liver resection patients usually undergo regular surveillance as they may be considered for a second potentially curative resection if recurrence occurs. Although there is no universal consensus, a reasonable approach to surveillance advocated in several clinical guidelines includes:
- CEA testing every 3–6 months for 2 years, then every 6 months for 3 years
- chest/abdomen and pelvis CT scan every 6 months for 2 years, then every 12 months up to a total of 5 years

- colonoscopy 12 months after liver resection; if no adenomatous polyps are identified, repeat every 3–5 years; if advanced adenomatous polyps are identified, repeat in 1 year.

Non-colorectal hepatic metastases
(Box 20.5)

Improvements in the perioperative mortality and morbidity of major hepatic resection have led to a more liberal application of this procedure for metastatic disease other than from colorectal cancer. However, most reports of resection for non-colorectal metastases involve relatively small numbers of patients and hence firm conclusions are difficult to make. The biological behaviour of the primary tumours is usually so different that it is often not appropriate to group these cases together for survival analysis.

The timing of onset and the total burden of the liver metastases, along with any patient comorbidity, must be evaluated through multidisciplinary discussion. Systemic chemotherapy, ablative therapies or locoregional chemoembolisation may be used in selected patients, sometimes in conjunction with liver resection.

Certain primary tumours, including ovarian, gastric and pancreas, have a predilection for peritoneal metastases and therefore laparoscopy is an important part of the staging process before considering liver resection.

Box 20.5 Non-colorectal hepatic metastases that may be suitable for resection

Definite
Neuroendocrine tumours
Melanoma
Renal cell carcinoma
Bladder carcinoma
Sarcoma
Endometrial carcinoma

Possible
Breast carcinoma
Thyroid carcinoma
Ovarian
Gastrointestinal stromal tumours
Pancreaticoduodenal carcinoma
Oesophagogastric carcinoma
Squamous cell carcinoma

Further reading

Dhir M, Sasson AR. Surgical management of liver metastases from colorectal cancer. *J Oncol Pract* 2016;12:33–9.

Guinney J, Dienstmann R, Wang X *et al*. The consensus molecular subtypes of colorectal cancer. *Nat Med* 2015;21:1350–6.

Kitisin K, Packlam V, Steel J *et al*. Presentation and outcomes of hepatocellular carcinoma patients at a western centre. *HPB (Oxford)* 2011;13:712–22.

Saha SK, Zhu AX, Fuchs CS, Brooks GA. Forty-year trends in cholangiocarcinoma incidence in the US: intrahepatic disease on the rise. *The Oncologist* 2016;21:594–9.

Soares KC, Kamel I, Cosgrove DP, Herman JM, Pawlik TM. Hilar cholangiocarcinoma: diagnosis, treatment options, and management. *Hepatobiliary Surg Nutr* 2014;3:18–34.

Van Cutsem E, Cervantes A, Adam R *et al*. ESMO consensus guidelines for the management of patients with metastatic colorectal cancer. *Ann Oncol* 2016;27:1386–422.

MCQs

Select the single correct answer to each question. The correct answers can be found in the Answers section at the end of the book.

1 Cholangiocarcinoma is most commonly found:
   a in the periphery of the liver
   b in the gallbladder
   c at the biliary confluence (Klatskin tumour)
   d in the distal bile duct
   e in the duodenum

2 Primary sclerosing cholangitis is *not* associated with:
   a inflammatory bowel disease
   b carcinoma of the bile duct
   c gallstones
   d multifocal biliary strictures
   e hepatocellular carcinoma

3 Which of the following does *not* cause primary hepatocellular carcinoma?
   a alcohol
   b haemochromatosis
   c hepatitis B virus
   d steroids
   e gallstones

4 Which of the following is *not* a treatment for liver metastases?
   a arterial chemoembolisation
   b ablation
   c laparoscopic resection
   d open resection
   e portal venous chemoembolisation

5 The most aggressive biliary tumour with the shortest overall survival rate is:
   a gallbladder cancer
   b biliary cystadenoma
   c hepatocellular cancer
   d Caroli's disease
   e distal cholangiocarcinoma (dCCA)

21 Liver infections

Vijayaragavan Muralidharan, Marcos V. Perini and Christopher Christophi

University of Melbourne and Austin Health, Melbourne, Victoria, Australia

Introduction

Liver infections are broadly classified based on the infecting agent as viral, bacterial or parasitic infections. Viral aetiology includes targeted infection of the liver by hepatitis viruses or secondary involvement of the liver during systemic viral infections such as cytomegalovirus (CMV), Epstein–Barr virus (EBV), herpes simplex virus (HSV) and human immunodeficiency virus (HIV). Bacterial infections manifest as pyogenic abscesses. Parasitic infestations include invasive amoebiasis, hydatid disease and liver fluke disease. Surgical intervention forms part of the management strategy (Box 21.1) for bacterial and parasitic infections, which will be the focus of this chapter.

Bacterial and parasitic infections of the liver universally originate at a distal site, spread to the liver by blood, biliary tree or direct extension and may manifest local as well as systemic signs and symptoms. Diagnosis is based on a combination of clinical presentation and microbiology, heavily supported by imaging.

Bacterial infections

Pyogenic abscess

The introduction of modern antibiotic therapy has progressively reduced the mortality from pyogenic liver abscess to 5–10%. The epidemiology has also shifted from the young male (20–30 years) with a liver abscess complicating an intra-abdominal infection to the elderly (60–70 years) diabetic male with previous history of biliopancreatic pathology, biliary instrumentation or colonic disease.

Aetiology

Classically, pyogenic liver abscess may arise by ascending infection from the biliary tract, haematogenous spread via the portal vein and hepatic artery or by direct extension from adjacent site of sepsis.

- *Ascending biliary tract* infections are responsible for 30–50% of patients presenting with pyogenic abscess. The resultant cholangitis leads to liver abscesses, which are frequently multiple. This is usually associated with biliary obstruction due to choledocholithiasis and benign and malignant strictures. Biliary reflux secondary to biliary bypass or endoscopic sphincterotomy and iatrogenic instrumentation by endoscopic retrograde cholangiopancreatography (ERCP) or percutaneous transhepatic procedures (percutaneous transhepatic cholangiography/percutaneous transhepatic biliary drainage) are less common causes of liver abscess.
- *Portal vein bacteraemia/pyaemia* is also a common cause for pyogenic abscess. Complicated diverticular disease, appendicitis, peritonitis and pancreatitis may cause portal vein pyaemia. Occult colorectal neoplasia should be suspected in patients diagnosed with pyogenic liver abscess, particularly due to *Klebsiella pneumoniae* and in the absence of any obvious underlying hepatobiliary disease.
- *Hepatic artery* seeding may occur in septicaemia from any cause and account for 5–15% of pyogenic liver abscesses. Common causes include bacterial endocarditis, pneumonia and intravenous drug abuse.
- *Other causes* of liver abscess include complicated blunt or penetrating liver trauma by direct extension from adjacent septic conditions such as empyema of the gallbladder.

Textbook of Surgery, Fourth Edition. Edited by Julian A. Smith, Andrew H. Kaye, Christopher Christophi and Wendy A. Brown.

Box 21.1 Management strategy

Source control
Identifying the point of origin of the infection and treating it to prevent recurrent or persistent infections

Local control
Managing the local effects within the liver by a combination of pharmacology, interventional radiology and surgery

Systemic control
Treatment of the systemic effects of the disease and control of the disease elsewhere in the body

---

- *Cryptogenic liver abscess* describes the situation where no cause is identified, which comprise up to 25% of the cases.

The infecting organism varies according to the site of entry. In biliary or portal vein sepsis, the organisms are enteric and usually polymicrobial. *Staphylococcus aureus* is evident in 20% of cases and is confirmed predominantly from haematogenous spread.

Clinical presentation and diagnosis

The most common presenting symptoms include pyrexia and rigours associated with right upper quadrant pain, general malaise, anorexia and weight loss. In the elderly the systemic manifestations may be blunted. Examination may reveal tender hepatomegaly. Occasionally, hypotension and cardiovascular collapse may be the presenting symptoms.

Abscess rupture is a rare complication (around 3% in some series) and is associated with diameter of more than 6 cm and a background of cirrhosis. Pyogenic liver abscesses most commonly involve the right lobe of the liver, possibly due to its larger mass and greater blood supply than the left.

Investigation

Liver function tests may show hyperbilirubinaemia and raised alkaline phosphatase and transaminase levels. Blood cultures are frequently positive. A leucocytosis is usually evident. A reactive pleural effusion may be present in about 50% of cases and the chest X-ray may show an elevated hemidiaphragm. Blood cultures are positive in up to 50% of cases and serology for *Entamoeba histolytica* and hydatid disease tested where appropriate.

The initial diagnosis is usually made with a diagnostic abdominal ultrasound searching for biliary pathology. Cross-sectional imaging with contrast-enhanced computed tomography (CT) will define the size, number and anatomical location of the liver abscesses. It will also delineate the presence of gas, level of parenchymal necrosis, hepatic and portal vein distortion or thrombosis and establish a baseline for future reassessments. Contrast-enhanced magnetic resonance imaging (MRI) has the distinct advantage of imaging the biliary tree using magnetic resonance cholangiopancreatography (MRCP) sequence for an underlying aetiology while also being superior in differentiating liver tumours and cysts. It also allows assessment of liver parenchymal disease and may help differentiate amoebic from pyogenic abscesses.

Determining the underlying aetiology may require biliary imaging by MRCP, CT intravenous cholangiogram, echocardiogram or colonoscopy based on clinical suspicion.

Treatment

Therapeutic principles based on systemic, local and source control include resuscitation, analgesia, appropriate antibiotic therapy, abscess drainage and eradication of the underlying cause.

General measures include resuscitation according to the Surviving Sepsis Campaign guidelines in order to maintain blood pressure and tissue perfusion. Symptomatic measures include a regimen of analgesics, temperature control and nutritional support.

Antimicrobial therapy is dependent on the underlying cause. Biliary or enteric causes involve microbial cover against Gram-negative and anaerobic organisms. Haematogenous causes require antibiotic cover against staphylococcal organisms. Administration of antibiotics is usually prolonged over several weeks to eradicate infection and avoid recurrence. This usually includes 2–3 weeks of intravenous antibiotics that may be changed to oral administration for another 3–4 weeks to complete a total of 4–6 weeks of antibiotics. Broad-spectrum antibiotics (piperacillin/tazobactam, carbapenems or second-generation cephalosporin with metronidazole) should be started as soon as blood cultures are taken and later on tailored in accordance with clinical progress and microbiology results.

Local control of the liver abscess is achieved by a step-up program commencing with antibiotic therapy for small abscesses, especially if widespread and multiple. Ultrasound- or CT-guided aspiration is useful in unilocular abscesses of less than 5 cm diameter. In 50% of such cases a repeat aspirate will be required.

Abscesses lager than 5 cm and those failing aspiration may be treated by percutaneous catheter drainage. Large, complex, multilocular abscesses may require a multidisciplinary approach between radiologists, infectious disease experts, endoscopists and surgeons. Open or laparoscopic surgical drainage or resection of the affected liver lobe is a last resort to remove dead material not amenable to retrieval with catheter drainage and is rarely indicated.

Parasitic infections

Amoebic liver abscess

Aetiology
Amoebic infestation is caused by the organism *Entamoeba histolytica*. It is rare in Australia but endemic in many areas of the tropics such as India and other parts of Asia. Faeco-oral transmission occurs by passage of cysts in the stool, the cysts contaminating food or water sources due to poor hygienic practices and being ingested. The organism penetrates the mucosa of the gastrointestinal tract to gain access to the liver via the portal venous system. The resultant abscess has an 'anchovy paste' appearance and may be secondarily infected, usually by enteric organisms. Amoebic liver abscess is the most common extra-intestinal manifestation of amoebiasis. Risk factors include malnutrition, depressed immunity and low socioeconomic status. Complications of amoebic abscess include rupture into the peritoneal cavity or hollow viscus such as colon or stomach. Rarely there may be pleuro-pulmonary involvement.

Clinical features
The onset of the disease may be sudden or gradual. For individuals returning from an endemic area, the clinical presentation typically occurs within 8–20 weeks (median 12 weeks). Right upper quadrant pain sometimes radiating to the right shoulder, associated with general malaise and weight loss, are the most common symptoms on presentation. Pyrexia and sweating occurs in about 60% of patients. Concurrent diarrhoea is present in less than one-third of patients, although some patients report a history of dysentery within the previous few months. Signs may include tender hepatomegaly and, occasionally, jaundice. Intra-abdominal rupture may occur in up to 5% of cases. Other rare complications include hepatic vein and inferior vena cava thrombosis; these have been attributed to mechanical compression and inflammation associated with a large abscess.

Investigation
Full blood examination may show leucocytosis and eosinophilia. Liver biochemistry is frequently deranged and shows a hepatocellular pattern of injury. Amoebic serology and stool cultures are usually positive. Approximately 99% of patients with amoebic liver abscess develop detectable antibodies, but serologic testing may be negative in the first 7 days. In endemic areas, up to 35% of uninfected individuals have anti-amoebic antibodies due to previous infection with *E. histolytica*. Therefore, negative serology is helpful for exclusion of disease, but positive serology cannot distinguish between acute and previous infection. Ultrasound with needle aspiration and culture confirm the diagnosis.

Treatment
Symptomatic measures include analgesics and attention to nutrition and hydration. Antimicrobial therapy is the mainstay of treatment, with metronidazole being the antibiotic of choice (500–750 mg orally three times daily for 10 days). The cure rate with this therapy is over 90%. Shorter duration of metronidazole is not generally recommended. Metronidazole is well absorbed from the gastrointestinal tract. Intravenous therapy offers no significant advantage as long as the patient can take oral medications and has no major defect in small bowel absorption. Needle aspiration under ultrasound or CT guidance or insertion of a pigtail catheter are not routinely required but may be warranted if the cyst appears to be at imminent risk of rupture especially if present in the left lobe, if there is clinical deterioration or lack of response to empirical therapy, or if exclusion of alternative diagnoses is needed. Mortality rate from uncomplicated amoebic abscess is less than 1%.

Hydatid disease

Hydatid disease is caused by infection with the metacestode stage of the tapeworm *Echinococcus*, which belongs to the family Taeniidae. Six species of *Echinococcus* produce infection in humans; *E. granulosus* and *E. multilocularis* are the most common, causing cystic echinococcosis and alveolar echinococcosis, respectively. *Echinococcus vogeli* and *E. oligarthrus* cause polycystic echinococcosis and are rarely seen. Two new species, *E. felidis and E. shiquicus*, have been identified recently though little is documented of their impact on humans.

Echinococcus granulosus

Pathology
Dogs and other canids are definitive hosts while ungulates are intermediate hosts. The human is an aberrant intermediate host in this disease. The ova are ingested by humans from the faeces of tapeworm-infected dogs. Dogs are usually infected by

feeding of offal of infected sheep. The ova reach the stomach of the human, where they hatch, penetrate the wall of the intestine and pass to the liver by the portal vein. Others may pass from the liver into the lung, brain or other organs. The liver is affected in approximately two-thirds of patients, the lungs in approximately 25%, and other organs including the brain, muscle, kidneys, bone, heart and pancreas in a small proportion of patients. Single-organ involvement occurs in around 80% of patients with *E. granulosus* infection, and only one cyst is observed in more than 70% of cases. When reaching the liver parenchyma, development of the cyst occurs. These cysts exhibit a slow growth pattern, typically increasing in diameter at a rate of 1–5 cm per year. Infection usually occurs in childhood but only becomes apparent in adulthood.

The cyst has a characteristic appearance. The capsule or exocyst is composed of compressed host tissue. The endocyst includes the laminated membrane from the parasite, which contains the germinal layer and scolices. The cyst is fluid-filled and contains brood capsules. The natural history of hydatid cysts is that of slow progressive growth. Apart from local compressive effects, rupture may occur into the biliary tree causing pain, obstructive jaundice, cholangitis or even pancreatitis. Rupture into the peritoneal or thoracic cavity may also occur in addition to haematogenous spread to other organs such as lung, bone, brain and spleen. The cysts may become secondarily infected.

Clinical presentation

Hydatids are often asymptomatic and are detected as incidental findings on radiological investigations for other conditions. Common symptoms include right upper quadrant pain, jaundice, pruritus and pyrexia. A persistent cough may indicate pulmonary involvement. Mass effect by the cyst may cause biliary obstruction, compression of the portal vein or inferior vena cava and rarely result in Budd–Chiari syndrome, cholestasis or portal hypertension.

Rupture into the abdominal cavity leads to pain with peritonitis. It may result in acute hypersensitivity reactions, including anaphylaxis, due to the antigenic material present in the fluid, which triggers an immunological reaction.

Rupture into the pleural cavity results in pulmonary hydatidosis or bronchial fistula. Lung involvement in hydatidosis may manifest with cough (50–60%), chest pain (50–90%), dyspnoea and haemoptysis (10–20%). When the lungs are involved by direct extension, 60% involve the right lung, especially the lower lobes. Lung involvement occurs more commonly in children.

Investigations

Liver function tests may show either an obstructive or hepatocellular pattern. Full blood examination may reveal a leucocytosis or eosinophilia. There are numerous serological tests available. Hydatid cyst fluid antigen B (AgB) and antigen 5 (Ag5) from *E. granulosus* are the most specific antigens for the immunodiagnosis of cystic echinococcosis. The most sensitive and specific test is immunoelectrophoresis, which is not only diagnostic but an indicator of response to treatment. The current enzyme-linked immunosorbent assay (ELISA) for antigen has a sensitivity of 85–89%, with some degree of cross-reactivity for other cestode or helminthic infections.

Ultrasound is an excellent cost-effective modality for examining cystic lesions of the liver and the World Health Organization (WHO) has classified them according to number, size and the presence of daughter cysts, endocysts and calcification (Box 21.2). CT provides better anatomical characterisation of cystic lesions and their relation to the hepatic vasculature and biliary anatomy and is useful for preoperative evaluation and planning. It also shows extrahepatic disease (lung) and has accuracy in visualising the cystic matrix. MRI/MRCP can be helpful in assessing the presence of biliary communication or bronchobiliary fistulas.

ERCP or MRCP may be specifically indicated where biliary involvement is suspected. The presence of heavy calcification in the wall of the cyst is an indicator of a dead/inactive cyst.

Treatment

Medical treatment is mandatory to mitigate symptoms and prevent progression of the disease and the development of secondary infections. Parasite

---

Box 21.2 WHO classification of cystic echinococcosis

CE1	Unilocular simple cysts with liquid content often with the CE1-specific 'double line' sign
CE2	Multivesicular multiseptated cysts
CE3a	Cysts with liquid content and CE3a-specific detached endocyst
CE3b	Unilocular cyst with daughter cysts inside a mucinous solid cyst matrix
CE4	Heterogeneous solid cysts with degenerative CE4-specific canalicular structure of cyst content
CE5	Cysts with degenerative content and heavily calcified wall

eradication is a long-term achievement. Treatment may be medical, percutaneous or surgical and is dependent on the stage of the cyst based on the WHO classification.

CONSERVATIVE

Asymptomatic CE4 and CE5 cysts, which are deep in the parenchyma, require no treatment. Complications are rare but patients need regular follow-up.

MEDICAL

Medical therapy alone may be used in small CE1–CE3a (<5 cm) cysts and is successful in 30–50% of cases. Drug therapy may be used alone or in conjunction with surgical procedures. Mebendazole or albendazole may be used in patients with hydatid disease who are regarded as poor risk for surgery or with widely disseminated disease. Albendazole gives excellent bioavailability and concentration in the cyst at a dose of 10–15 mg/kg daily. It may also be delivered by percutaneous injection under ultrasound localisation directly into the cyst. These drugs may be administered either before or after definitive surgery to minimise the risk of recurrence. Prolonged courses over 3–6 months are recommended. These drugs may be toxic to the liver and bone marrow and require careful monitoring.

PERCUTANEOUS TREATMENTS

This involves drainage of the cysts and destruction of the germinal layer under ultrasound guidance. It involves puncture of the cyst, aspiration of the content, injection of a protoscolicidal agent (95% ethanol, 20% saline) and re-aspiration of fluid (or PAIR). This is used in larger CE1 and CE3a cysts (>5 cm), in patients unable to undergo surgery or where recurrence occurs after surgery. When applied for CE2 and CE3b cysts there is a high recurrence rate. It is contraindicated in superficial cysts, those that are inactive or heavily calcified and in the presence of biliary communication.

SURGERY

The principles of surgical management include (i) complete neutralisation and removal of the parasite components, including the germinal membrane, scolices and brood capsules; (ii) prevention of contamination or spillage to prevent anaphylaxis or recurrence; and (iii) management of the residual cavity. Surgery is the first choice for large CE2–CE3b cysts or those that are superficial with a risk of rupture (Figure 21.1).

Procedures may be radical, including liver resection with total excision of the cyst or pericystectomy.

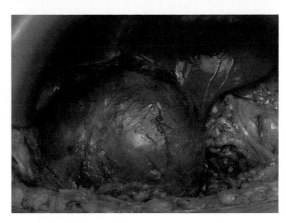

Fig. 21.1 Hydatid liver lesion arising from the left lobe of liver.

Liver resection is rarely indicated and is suitable for peripheral or pedunculated cysts.

More commonly used is the conservative option of de-roofing of the cyst (endocystectomy). Scolicidal agents are frequently injected into the cyst prior to manipulation to destroy active components and prevent recurrence if spillage occurs. Commonly used agents include cetrimide or hypertonic saline. The contents of the cyst are then evacuated. The residual cavity may be filled with saline and closed (capittonage) or obliterated by an omental pedicle, especially in infected cysts. Biliary communications may need to be closed and bile duct explored to remove hydatids causing biliary obstruction.

Alveolar echinococcosis

Pathology

This is a rare condition caused by *E. multilocularis*, whose life cycle is different from that of *E. granulosus*. Natural hosts include foxes, rodents, dogs and cats. It is endemic in the northern hemisphere, especially Japan, China and central Europe. Humans are an unusual and intermediate host. It is a progressive, destructive disease. Death results from liver parenchymal destruction and liver failure. The disease may extend to the brain and lung and may be associated with severe myositis. Vesicles invade the host liver tissue by extension of the germinal layer, which remains in an active proliferative state.

Clinical features

Early symptoms are usually non-specific and vague. The most common initial presentation is mild right upper quadrant pain. Tender hepatomegaly or a mass may be present. As the disease progresses, jaundice, ascites and hepatic insufficiency occur. In the early stages, a high index of suspicion in endemic areas is required. Differential diagnosis includes hepatoma, tuberculosis, haemangioma or focal nodular hyperplasia.

Investigation

Radiological investigations such as ultrasound, CT and MRI may provide additional information. Serology may be inconclusive in the early stages of the disease but may subsequently confirm the underlying process. Occasionally, laparoscopy and biopsy may be required. Even at operation, the accuracy of diagnosis is only 50%.

Treatment

The only known definitive cure for *E. multilocularis* is liver resection. Transplantation has been performed in selected patients but long-term outcome is uncertain. Albendazole, although unable to eliminate the parasite, may slow progression of the disease and should be administered on an indefinite basis in conjunction with surgery.

Liver fluke disease

Infestations of clinical importance include those by *Fasciola hepatica* and *Clonorchis sinensis*. These parasites are trematodes and undergo both sexual (definitive host) and asexual (intermediate host) reproduction.

Fasciola hepatica

Pathology

This is prevalent all over the world and commonly seen in Europe, South America, Africa and the Caribbean. It is known as the common sheep fluke and is found in sheep- and cattle-rearing countries. The parasite inhabits the gallbladder and bile ducts and passes ova in the stool. Humans are incidental hosts, especially those eating raw vegetables. Cysts are ingested from vegetables and subsequently penetrate the intestinal wall. They then migrate by the transperitoneal route and invade the liver capsule and enter the biliary system, where they may be mistaken for gallstones.

Clinical features

Patients may be asymptomatic or present with acute or chronic symptoms. Acute symptoms include sudden onset of right upper quadrant pain, pyrexia or cholangitis and symptoms of allergic reactions. Hepatosplenomegaly may be present. Chronic symptoms include intermittent biliary colic, cholecystitis, jaundice, anaemia and hypoproteinaemia.

Investigation

Full blood examination may show eosinophilia. Liver function tests show features consistent with cholestasis. Stools are examined for the presence of ova. Specific serological testing usually confirms the diagnosis.

Treatment

The condition is treated with albendazole, praziquantel or bithional. Cholecystectomy and exploration of the common bile duct by ERCP may be necessary.

Clonorchis sinensis

Pathology

Clonorchis sinensis is a flatworm that inhabits the biliary tree. Cysts from infected fish are ingested and migrate from the duodenum into the bile ducts. Ova are excreted from the stools. The intermediate host is a snail, which completes the life cycle by infecting fish. Humans are infected by eating raw fish.

The biliary epithelium becomes inflamed from constant irritation, leading to cholangitis, ductal fibrosis, biliary strictures and stone formation. There is a high incidence of cholangiocarcinoma.

Clinical features

The classic symptom associated with *Clonorchis* infestation is recurrent pyogenic cholangitis. There are recurrent attacks of right upper quadrant pain, jaundice and pyrexia. Examination may reveal tender hepatomegaly and splenomegaly if portal hypertension exists.

Investigation

Imaging of the biliary tree by MRI or ERCP is essential for delineating the distribution of stones and strictures. Ova are demonstrated in faeces or duodenal aspirate.

Treatment

The drug of choice is praziquantel. Surgery is indicated if stones or strictures are present.

Biliary ascariasis

Pathology

The roundworm *Ascaris lumbricoides* is endemic in tropical and subtropical areas. The worms inhabit the small intestine and enter the common bile duct by the duodenal ampulla of Vater.

Clinical features

They induce mechanical obstruction of the biliary tree. Cholangitis, empyema of the gallbladder and multiple liver abscesses may occur as a result of secondary infection.

Investigation

Stool examination commonly demonstrates the presence of worms. Ultrasound is highly accurate in delineating the worms in the biliary tree.

Treatment

Non-operative management is successful. Mebendazole and pyrantel palmoate are used over 3 days. ERCP may be required for patients with cholangitis and biliary stones.

Further reading

Mezhir JJ, Fong Y, Jacks LM *et al*. Current management of pyogenic liver abscess: surgery is now second-line treatment. *J Am Coll Surg* 2010;210:975–83.

Nunnari G, Pinzone MR, Gruttadauria S *et al*. Hepatic echinococcosis: clinical and therapeutic aspects. *World J Gastroenterol* 2012;18:1448–58.

Pang TC, Fung T, Samra J, Hugh TJ, Smith RC. Pyogenic liver abscess: an audit of 10 years' experience. *World J Gastroenterol* 2011;17:1622–30.

Stojkovic M, Rosenberger K, Kauczor HU, Junghanss T, Hosch W. Diagnosing and staging of cystic echinococcosis: how do CT and MRI perform in comparison to ultrasound? *PLoS Negl Trop Dis* 2012;6(10):e1880.

Xia J, Jiang SC, Peng HJ. Association between liver fluke infection and hepatobiliary pathological changes: a systematic review and meta-analysis. *PLoS One* 2015;10(7):e0132673.

MCQs

Select the single correct answer to each question. The correct answers can be found in the Answers section at the end of the book.

1 Regarding pyogenic liver abscesses, which one of the following is true?
   a mortality rate is high even with drainage
   b *Staphylococcus aureus* is the most common pathogen
   c they are usually incidental findings in patients with abdominal pain
   d drainage of the abscess and appropriate antibiotic therapy are the mainstay of management
   e laparoscopy is the less invasive approach for the treatment of liver abscess

2 Regarding amoebic liver abscesses, which one of the following is *false*?
   a poor sanitary hygiene is the most determinant factor
   b mainstay of treatment is intralesional antimicrobial therapy
   c for asymptomatic small abscesses, oral antibiotics can achieve high rates of cure
   d presence of positive serology and a cystic liver lesion are the two main diagnostic criteria in the diagnosis of amoebic liver abscess
   e amoebic liver abscess can be drained by percutaneous technique

3 Regarding hydatid disease, which one of the following is *incorrect*?
   a the human is an end host, which breaks the development cycle of the parasite
   b initial infection occurs through the alimentary tract and is asymptomatic
   c the natural history of a hydatid cyst in the human is one of slow progressive growth
   d rupture of a hydatid cyst is a common event
   e most symptoms are related to pressure effects on the liver and surrounding organs

4 Which one of the following statements regarding the management of hydatid cysts is *false*?
   a extremely small cysts may be managed conservatively provided they are followed up to monitor growth
   b medical management is successful in the vast majority of cases
   c medical therapy is usually used to supplement surgical intervention
   d the most common surgical technique is that of evacuation of the contents and de-roofing of the cyst and the placement of an omental patch in the cavity
   e prevention of spillage of the contents into the peritoneal cavity is of critical importance

5 You are at the emergency department and have been called to give a second opinion in a young patient with right upper abdominal pain, fever and

a history of recent travel to India. He presented with fever, chills and rigors. On examination his heart rate is 110 and blood pressure 90/60 mmHg. His white cells are elevated and liver function tests are slight deranged. Ultraound was done and a cystic liver lesion in the right lobe measuring 10 cm was seen. What is your initial management?

a call a surgeon to evaluate the patient

b ask for a CT scan to better assess the liver lesion

c request blood culture and wait for the results to start antibiotics

d treat the pain, resuscitate the patient and start broad-spectrum antibiotics

e transfer the patient to the intensive care unit to be better assessed

6 In outpatient clinic, you are called by a colleague to give an opinion on a liver MRCP scan requested for a middle-aged man presenting with vague abdominal pain for months. The MRCP scan is shown below. What is the main diagnosis?

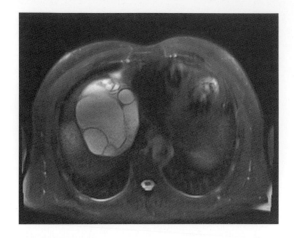

a liver haemangioma

b liver cancer

c cholecystitis

d hydatid liver lesion

e normal liver

22 Pancreatitis

Peter S. Russell[1] and John A. Windsor[1,2]

[1] Department of Surgery, University of Auckland
[2] Auckland City Hospital, Auckland, New Zealand

Introduction

Until recently pancreatitis has been considered two distinct diseases, acute pancreatitis and chronic pancreatitis. Now they are considered part of a continuum, which also includes recurrent acute pancreatitis. Acute pancreatitis is one of the most common acute gastrointestinal presentations. It usually resolves but when severe is associated with a significant risk of mortality. Chronic pancreatitis is progressive and one of the most painful diseases. When severe it is associated with malnutrition and diabetes. Although there is no specific treatment for either disease, important advances in management have resulted in improved outcomes.

Acute pancreatitis

Acute pancreatitis is an acute inflammatory disorder characterised by oedema and, when severe, necrosis of the pancreas. It is a protean disease with a wide range of severity and a highly variable course, ranging from mild self-limiting disease to critical illness involving infected pancreatic necrosis, multiple organ failure and mortality. Acute pancreatitis is divided into two types; interstitial oedematous pancreatitis and necrotising pancreatitis. The former involves acute inflammation of the pancreatic parenchyma and peripancreatic tissues without recognisable necrosis and usually resolves within a week or two. The latter is characterised by inflammation associated with pancreatic and/or peripancreatic necrosis. Necrotising pancreatitis is seen in about 5–10% of cases, is more variable in its course and is almost always more severe. The traditional view is that acute pancreatitis completely resolves with no morphological, functional or symptomatic sequelae. However, necrotising pancreatitis can leave significant scarring, strictures and impairment of exocrine and endocrine pancreatic function.

There are two recognised phases in the course of this dynamic disease. In the early phase, lasting around a week, systemic disturbances to the patient are a result of the host response to pancreatic inflammation. This inflammation triggers cytokine cascades that drive the systemic inflammatory response syndrome (SIRS) and can result in early organ failure. The later phase occurs only in patients with more severe pancreatitis and is characterised by persistent organ failure, usually secondary to infected necrosis.

The incidence of acute pancreatitis is estimated to be 13–45 per 100 000 and is increasing in most developed nations. The incidence and aetiology vary with country, age and gender. Gallstone-induced pancreatitis is more common in females and patients presenting in the sixth decade, while alcohol-induced pancreatitis is more common in males and patients in the third or fourth decades.

Aetiology and pathogenesis

There are many recognised causes of acute pancreatitis with the two most common being gallstones and alcohol, which combined account for approximately 80% of presentations. Other causes include hyperlipidaemia, iatrogenic, trauma, gene mutations, tumours and hypercalcaemia. Drugs can also cause acute pancreatitis, including thiazide diuretics, frusemide, oestrogen replacement therapy, steroids, chemotherapy and immunosuppression. If a cause cannot be determined after a systematic search, it is considered to be idiopathic acute pancreatitis.

The pancreas produces digestive enzymes (e.g. amylase, lipase) that break down the complex structure of carbohydrates, lipids, proteins and nucleic acids into simple molecules such as amino acids and glucose for absorption in the small

Textbook of Surgery, Fourth Edition. Edited by Julian A. Smith, Andrew H. Kaye, Christopher Christophi and Wendy A. Brown.
© 2020 John Wiley & Sons Ltd. Published 2020 by John Wiley & Sons Ltd.

intestine. These enzymes are stored in membrane-lined zymogen granules in acinar cells. Several mechanisms have evolved to prevent their premature activation, including synthesis as inactive precursors (zymogens), secretion into an alkaline fluid that dilutes the inactivated enzymes, activation in the duodenum separate from the site of production, and presence of trypsin inhibitors within the pancreas. Acute pancreatitis occurs when these physiological protective mechanisms break down, causing acinar cell injury and local inflammation.

The exact means by which gallstones cause acute pancreatitis has not yet been proven. Previous suggestions include gallstones impacting at the sphincter of Oddi causing reflux of bile into the pancreatic duct, or the passage of a gallstone causing transient incompetence of the sphincter allowing reflux of duodenal fluid. A third possibility, perhaps the most likely, is that a gallstone obstructing the pancreatic duct, leading to ductal hypertension, causes disruption of the minor ducts and extravasation of pancreatic juice back into the less alkaline interstitium of the pancreas, thus promoting intra-pancreatic enzyme activation. Other causes of duct obstruction such as pancreatic neoplasm may cause pancreatitis via the same mechanism. Alcohol can also lead to ductal hypertension due to deposition of protein plugs that can obstruct small pancreatic ducts.

Other causes of acute pancreatitis are due to direct injury to the acinar, ductal or stellate cells. Alcohol is metabolised by acinar cells via oxidative and non-oxidative pathways. It, and its metabolites, can damage all three cell types by a variety of mechanisms, such as increasing intracellular levels of digestive enzymes and decreasing zymogen granule stability. Pancreatic cells can also be damaged by surgical procedures including biopsy, bile duct exploration, distal gastrectomy and splenectomy. Endoscopic retrograde cholangiopancreatography (ERCP) is by far the most frequent iatrogenic cause, where acute pancreatitis occurs after about 5–10% of procedures.

The most common mutation leading to hereditary pancreatitis is in the cationic trypsinogen gene (*PRSS1*). This leads to premature activation of trypsinogen to trypsin as well as abnormalities of ductal secretion, leading to acute pancreatitis. This mutation has an autosomal dominant mode of inheritance but other mutations leading to hereditary pancreatitis may have an autosomal recessive mode.

Despite the diverse aetiologies, evidence suggests that each causative mechanism results in a single precipitating event common to all – the premature activation of trypsinogen to its active form trypsin. This in turn activates other proenzymes such as prophospholipase, proelastase and prekallikrein, the latter activating the clotting and complement systems. The resultant inflammation and small-vessel thromboses further damage the acinar cells and amplify the autodigestion caused by the digestive enzymes.

The severity of acute pancreatitis is generally determined by the events that occur after trypsin activation and initial acinar cell injury. Activated macrophages release cytokines that mediate both local and systemic inflammation. On a local level, these mediators can lead to haemorrhage, oedema and microthrombi. Fluid can collect in and around the pancreas, which may compress the bile duct causing obstructive jaundice, or the duodenum causing vomiting.

When failure of the pancreatic microcirculation is severe, it will result in pancreatic and peripancreatic hypoperfusion and necrosis. If this becomes infected, which usually occurs at least 2 weeks following the onset of illness, disease severity will increase and can lead to organ failure. In roughly half of cases the infection is enteric in origin (e.g. bacterial translocation from the adjacent colon, or lymphogenous spread via mesenteric lymph), with extrapancreatic infections (e.g. pneumonia, bacteraemia) being another major source. Calcium can also be deposited in these areas of necrosis and result in a fall in serum calcium.

On a systemic level, pancreatic inflammation has the potential to lead to systemic inflammation and multiorgan failure, which is the major determinant of severity and mortality. The mechanism leading to systemic inflammation is still to be fully elucidated but involves the recruitment and activation of neutrophils and macrophages releasing multiple cytokines and chemokines. It appears these proinflammatory mediators, travelling via mesenteric lymph, bypass the liver and directly contribute to dysfunction of the lungs (acute respiratory distress syndrome), heart (ventricular dysfunction) and kidney (acute tubular necrosis). In the acute setting, local and systemic inflammation, along with oedema and fluid collections, lead to hypovolaemia and hypotension.

Surgical pathology and complications

The pancreas in acute pancreatitis can vary from swollen and inflamed through to necrotic, infected or haemorrhagic. Complications of acute pancreatitis are divided into local and systemic. The local complications have been redefined by the Revised

Table 22.1 Definitions of local complications of acute pancreatitis based on CT morphology.

Content	Acute (<4 weeks, no defined wall)		Chronic (<4 weeks, defined wall)	
	No infection	Infection	No infection	Infection
Fluid	APFC	Infected APFC	Pseudocyst	Infected pseudocyst
Solid ± fluid	ANC	Infected ANC	WON	Infected WON

APFC, acute peripancreatic fluid collection; ANC, acute necrotic collection; WON, walled-off necrosis.
Source: modified from Escott ABJ, Phillips AJ, Windsor JA. Part B: Locoregional pathophysiology in acute pancreatitis: pancreas and intestine. In: Adams DB, Cotton PB, Zyromski N, Windsor JA (eds) *Pancreatitis: Medical and Surgical Management*. Oxford: Wiley Blackwell, 2017. Reproduced with permission of John Wiley & Sons.

Atlanta Classification in 2012, and are classified according to chronicity, content and infection (Table 22.1 and Figure 22.1). They include acute peripancreatic fluid collection (APFC), pancreatic pseudocyst, acute necrotic collection (ANC) and walled-off necrosis (WON), all of which can be either infected or sterile. An APFC is peripancreatic fluid associated with interstitial oedematous pancreatitis with no necrosis. It is differentiated from a pseudocyst because it occurs within 4 weeks of onset of symptoms and has no defined wall. A pseudocyst is an encapsulated fluid collection with a defined inflammatory wall that develops after 4 weeks. It is not a true cyst because the wall is not lined by epithelial cells. An ANC occurs within 4 weeks and contains variable amounts of both fluid and necrosis with no definable wall. This is differentiated from WON that occurs after 4 weeks and does have a defined inflammatory wall. Other possible local complications include gastric outlet dysfunction, splenic and portal vein thrombosis, paralytic ileus and colonic necrosis.

Systemic complications include new-onset organ failure, as well as exacerbation of a pre-existing comorbidity, such as coronary artery disease or chronic lung disease. Organ failure is defined as either transient (resolves within 48 hours) or persistent (persists beyond 48 hours) and requires a score of 2 or more for at least one of the three major organ systems (respiratory, cardiovascular and renal) using the modified Marshall scoring system (Table 22.2).

The presence of local and systemic complications determines the severity of pancreatitis and subsequently guides the management. The Revised Atlanta Classification defines severity as mild (absence of local and systemic complications), moderately severe (transient organ failure or local or systemic complications in the absence of persistent organ failure) and severe (characterised by persistent organ failure). An alternative is the Determinant-based Classification that defines severity as mild (no (peri)pancreatic necrosis or organ failure), moderate (sterile necrosis and/or transient organ failure), severe (infected necrosis or persistent organ failure) and critical (infected necrosis and persistent organ failure). Both these international multidisciplinary classification systems are validated, though differences indicate that further refinement will be necessary.

Clinical presentation

Acute pancreatitis most often presents with the sudden onset of severe and persistent epigastric pain that radiates to the middle of the back. Nausea and vomiting may also be present. It is important to determine the presence of any known aetiological risk factors, including gallstones, alcohol consumption or recent procedures such as ERCP.

Examination will vary depending on the severity of the attack, but may reveal a patient distressed from severe pain. In some cases the patient may present with hypotension, tachycardia and tachypnoea. The abdomen will be tender in the epigastrium, possibly with guarding but usually without peritonism. Other findings will be based on the later development of complications such as a palpable mass from a fluid collection or distension due to a developing ileus. Rarely, flank ecchymosis (Grey Turner's sign) or periumbilical ecchymosis (Cullen's sign) will be present, which results from haemorrhagic fluid tracking from the retroperitoneum.

Investigation

The diagnosis of acute pancreatitis requires two of the following three features: (i) abdominal pain consistent with acute pancreatitis; (ii) serum lipase or amylase at least three times greater than the upper limit of normal; and (iii) characteristic findings of acute pancreatitis on contrast-enhanced computed tomography (CT) or magnetic resonance imaging (MRI).

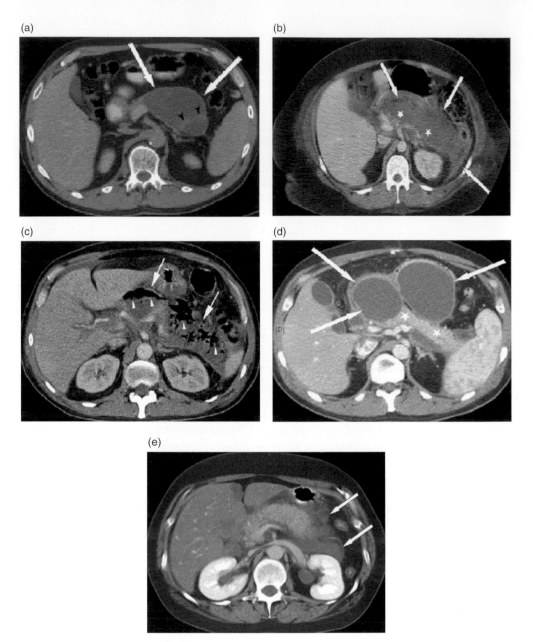

Fig. 22.1 CT scans of various complications of acute pancreatitis. (a) A 38-year-old woman with acute interstitial oedematous pancreatitis and acute peripancreatic fluid collection (APFC) in the left anterior pararenal space (white arrows showing the borders of the APFC). The pancreas enhances completely, is thickened and has a heterogeneous appearance due to oedema. APFC has fluid density without an encapsulating wall. (b) Patient with acute necrotising pancreatitis and acute necrotic collection (ANC): there is extensive parenchymal necrosis (white stars) of the body and tail of the pancreas. Heterogeneous collections are seen in the pancreatic and peripancreatic tissues (white arrows pointing at the borders of the ANC) of the left anterior pararenal space. (c) A 47-year-old man with acute necrotising pancreatitis complicated by infected pancreatic necrosis. There is a heterogeneous ANC in the pancreatic and peripancreatic area (white arrows pointing at the borders of the ANC) with presence of gas bubbles (white arrowheads), usually a pathognomonic sign of infection of the necrosis (infected necrosis). (d) A 40-year-old man with two pseudocysts in the lesser sac 6 weeks after an episode of acute interstitial pancreatitis on CT. Note the round to oval, low-attenuated, homogeneous fluid collections with a well defined enhancing rim (white arrows pointing at the borders of the pseudocysts), but absence of areas of greater attenuation indicative of non-liquid components. White stars denote normal enhancing pancreas. (e) Patient with walled-off necrosis (WON). A heterogeneous, fully encapsulated collection is noted in the pancreatic and peripancreatic area. Non-liquid components of high attenuation (black arrowheads) in the collection are noted. The collection has a thin, well-defined and enhancing wall (thick white arrows). Source: modified from Banks PA, Bollen TL, Dervenis C *et al.* Classification of acute pancreatitis – 2012: revision of the Atlanta classification and definitions by international consensus. *Gut* 2013;62:102–11. Reproduced with permission of SAGE Publications.

Table 22.2 Modified Marshall scoring system for organ dysfunction: a score of 2 or more in any system defines the presence of organ failure.

Organ system	Score				
	0	1	2	3	4
Respiratory (Pao_2/Fio_2)	>400	301–400	201–300	101–200	≤101
Renal*					
Serum creatinine (µmol/L)	≤134	134–169	170–310	311–439	>439
Serum creatinine (mg/dL)	<1.4	1.4–1.8	1.9–3.6	3.6–4.9	>4.9
Cardiovascular: systolic blood pressure (mmHg)[†]	>90	<90, fluid responsive	<90, not fluid responsive	<90, pH <7.3	<90, pH <7.2

For non-ventilated patients, the Fio_2 can be estimated from:

Supplemental oxygen (L/min)	Fio_2 (%)
Room air	21
2	25
4	30
6–8	40
9–10	50

* A score for patients with pre-existing chronic renal failure depends on the extent of further deterioration of baseline renal function. No formal correction exists for a baseline serum creatinine ≥134 µmol/L or ≥1.4 mg/dL.
[†] Off inotropic support.
Source: modified from Banks PA, Bollen TL, Dervenis C *et al.* Classification of acute pancreatitis – 2012: revision of the Atlanta classification and definitions by international consensus. *Gut* 2013;62:102–11. Reproduced with permission of SAGE Publications.

The diagnosis is most often confirmed by elevated serum levels of the enzymes lipase or amylase, which are released into the bloodstream from the damaged pancreas. However, hyperamylasaemia cannot be relied on alone as it can also occur from other conditions including parotitis, renal failure, small bowel obstruction and perforated duodenal ulcer. At times serum amylase may be completely normal, as in the presence of extensive necrosis. Usually serum amylase increases almost immediately with symptom onset and peaks within several hours. Both amylase and lipase are rapidly cleared from the serum by the kidneys and so the peak is often short-lived and serum amylase returns to normal after 3–7 days. Serum lipase is now preferred because of a slower return to normal. Urinary levels of amylase or lipase, which peak and fall later, can also be measured and may be more sensitive than serum levels.

Elevations of pancreatic enzymes, while useful in diagnosing pancreatitis, are not useful in predicting or determining the severity of acute pancreatitis. There have been numerous prognostic systems validated in trials, such as the commonly used modified Glasgow criteria and Ranson's criteria, which rely on clinical and biochemical parameters scored over the first 48 hours of admission. Although prognostic scoring systems attempt to predict the severity,

their accuracy is often only 70–80% for actual severity (as per the Revised Atlanta Classification). Current guidelines recommend that the prediction of severe acute pancreatitis is best with the presence of two or more SIRS criteria (temperature >38 or <36°C; heart rate >90 beats/min; respiratory rate >20 breaths/min or $Paco_2$ <32 mmHg; white cell count >12 × 10^9/L, <4 × 10^9/L or >10% bands). Other prognostic markers in common use include blood urea nitrogen (BUN), the Bedside Index for Severity in Acute Pancreatitis (BISAP) score and C-reactive protein (CRP). Despite the limitations of accuracy in applying predictors to individual patients, prognostication on admission is important as it allows early identification of those with more severe disease who might require transfer to an intensive care unit (ICU) or tertiary hospital.

Contrast-enhanced CT may be important in the diagnosis, but there is no routine role within the first 5–7 days of admission. It is not better at predicting severe disease than other approaches, but is very important for the diagnosis of local complications, including the extent of necrosis when suspected. If using CT to determine the extent of necrosis, it is best to wait at least 5 days from the onset of illness to determine the full extent. MRI is superior to contrast-enhanced CT in detecting any solid content within collections. Ultrasonography is used to determine any evidence of gallstones. If choledocholithiasis is suspected, it is usually confirmed by magnetic resonance cholangiopancreatography (MRCP) before ERCP, unless the patient has overt cholangitis, cholestasis and a dilated duct on ultrasonography.

Treatment

All patients with suspected acute pancreatitis should be admitted to hospital. Management then varies depending on the severity of the attack. Patients with mild pancreatitis have a less than 1% risk of mortality and usually stay in hospital for less than a week. At the other end of the spectrum, patients with critical disease have a mortality rate above 40% and may require many weeks or months of intensive multidisciplinary treatment. The essential aspects of management are accurate diagnosis, appropriate triage based on predicted severity, high-quality supportive care, detection and treatment of local complications, and treatment of the underlying cause.

Supportive care

As there is currently no specific treatment for inflammation of the pancreas, management focuses on good supportive care. For patients with evidence of organ dysfunction or failure it is important for them to be managed in an ICU setting. Supportive care in acute pancreatitis centres on pain management, fluid resuscitation and nutritional support.

Pain is the cardinal symptom of acute pancreatitis and rapid and effective analgesia (non-steroidal anti-inflammatory or opioid, administered intravenously) should be given early. Fluid resuscitation is the most important intervention in the early management, especially if the patient presents with haemodynamic instability or hypotension. Fluid should be given as a balanced crystalloid solution (lactated Ringer's being preferred) aiming to restore normal blood volume, blood pressure and urine output. Evidence suggests that aggressive fluid resuscitation is associated with increased risk and that the aim should be normalising haematocrit over 48 hours. Historically, the patient was made 'nil by mouth' on admission to hospital, but this is no longer required. Acute pancreatitis is a highly catabolic state associated with rapid nutrient depletion and there is good evidence that nutritional support, implemented from early in the disease (after volume repletion), is important in determining a favourable outcome. In mild pancreatitis the patient can be allowed to drink and eat *ad libitum*. If the acute pancreatitis is more severe, it has been shown that enteral nutrition (via nasogastric or nasojejunal tube) is superior to parenteral nutrition or no nutrition. This is because gut rest is associated with villous atrophy, gut barrier failure, bacterial overgrowth and subsequent bacterial translocation, which can drive systemic inflammation and multiple organ dysfunction. On rare occasions it is necessary to give parenteral nutrition if the nutrition goals are not being met due to feeding intolerance (e.g. ileus). This may be combined with trophic enteral feeding at a reduced rate to maintain enterocyte health and mucosal barrier function.

Prophylactic antibiotics, aiming to prevent the development of infected necrosis, should be avoided, as it has been shown they are ineffective and can lead to antibiotic resistance and fungal infection. However, patients with suspected or confirmed infected complications should be started on intravenous antibiotics. A carbapenem (e.g. imipenem) or a quinolone and metronidazole can be used empirically until bacterial sensitivities are known.

Managing local complications

Local complications are suspected if there is no clinical improvement or deterioration on serial clinical examinations and elevated inflammatory markers. Contrast-enhanced CT is performed to diagnose any local complication, such as necrosis or a fluid collection. The decision to intervene is based on the patient's clinical status and response to supportive care, not on the CT findings per se. In the acute setting, intervention is usually reserved for an infected fluid collection or infected necrosis in a patient not responding to antibiotics. Infection is diagnosed on contrast-enhanced CT with the presence of extraluminal air within the suspected area, or rarely by positive microbial culture from a fine-needle aspirate. If possible, any treatment of a local complication, including infected necrosis, is delayed to allow the lesion to become walled off (encapsulated) and therefore safer to treat. If intervention becomes necessary, a 'step-up' approach is used, with percutaneous or endoscopic drainage first, followed by percutaneous or endoscopic debridement (depending on location and topography of the collection) if required. Open surgery to drain and debride the area is rarely required, but may be indicated for abdominal compartment syndrome or if non-occlusive mesenteric ischaemia is suspected.

Treatment of the cause

Patients with predicted severe gallstone-associated pancreatitis may benefit from early ERCP (within 24–48 hours of admission) but only if there is clear evidence of cholangitis. This is because ERCP may exacerbate pancreatitis in the acute setting and this risk needs to be weighed against any potential benefit. Patients with cholestasis without cholangitis may need delayed ERCP for this reason. Cholestasis may resolve spontaneously after the passage of a stone into the duodenum. All patients with gallstone-associated pancreatitis should have a cholecystectomy following recovery from an attack of acute pancreatitis in order to prevent repeated attacks. Those with mild to moderate acute pancreatitis should have the cholecystectomy before discharge. Timing of cholecystectomy is more challenging for severe disease, and is usually delayed unless surgery is required for other reasons. Patients with alcohol-associated pancreatitis should embrace abstinence to avoid further episodes, and often require extensive community support to achieve this. Hyperlipidaemia usually requires treatment with a statin and dietary advice. In the rare instances of sphincter of Oddi dysfunction, division of the sphincter is sometimes associated with a good response, but this is controversial.

Chronic pancreatitis

Chronic pancreatitis is an incurable, irreversible condition characterised by fibrosis and chronic inflammation. It is variable in presentation and aetiology, and very difficult to treat successfully. The prevalence ranges from 5 to 40 per 100 000 population, with considerable geographic variation, and the incidence has been increasing over the past 50 years.

Aetiology and pathogenesis

Chronic pancreatitis most often follows recurrent acute pancreatitis, and therefore has a similar range of aetiologies. The most common cause in developed countries is alcohol abuse, as these patients are more likely to have repeated acute attacks, as opposed to patients with gallstone-related acute pancreatitis where cholecystectomy offers complete cure. Recent evidence shows that smoking is a very important risk factor, often combined with excess alcohol. Other causes include genetic mutations, which account for up to 25% of patients, longstanding obstruction of the duct by a neoplasm or calculi, autoimmune pancreatitis, nutritional causes

(tropical pancreatitis) and distal pancreatitis resulting from trauma. As with acute pancreatitis, a relatively significant number of patients have no discernible cause found after extensive investigation and are deemed to have idiopathic chronic pancreatitis. This patient group is now smaller as more genetic mutations are found and implicated in the aetiology.

All forms of chronic pancreatitis are associated with the development of fibrosis, caused by the activation of pancreatic stellate cells. These cells are activated by proinflammatory cytokines and other proliferative factors, which are released in response to pancreatic injury. Once activated, stellate cells transform into myofibroblast-like cells, proliferate, secrete collagen and transform the extracellular matrix, resulting in fibrosis and eventually acinar cell loss.

The pathogenesis of chronic pancreatitis varies depending on the cause. One common mechanism, especially prevalent in alcohol abuse, is the development of calcific pancreatic stones or concretions. It has been shown that alcohol reduces the secretion of a potent inhibitor of calcium carbonate crystal formation. These concretions can cause mechanical damage to the ductal epithelium or cause obstruction of the distal ductal network. Another mechanism leading to chronic pancreatitis is compression or occlusion of the proximal ductal system (for example, by tumour, gallstone, post-traumatic scar or pancreas divisum). This can result in diffuse fibrosis, dilated main and secondary pancreatic ducts, and acinar atrophy.

Surgical pathology and complications

In chronic pancreatitis the pancreas is characterised by fibrosis and atrophy, often with parenchymal and ductal calcifications. There is a variable amount of duct dilation, strictures and ductal epithelial dysplasia. In severe advanced chronic pancreatitis, broad coalescing areas of fibrosis replace acinar tissue and there is a reduction in the size of islet tissue.

Atrophy and destruction of pancreatic parenchyma can eventually result in exocrine and endocrine dysfunction, leading to both malabsorption and diabetes respectively. Because of chronic inflammation and epithelial dysplasia there is an increased risk of developing pancreatic adenocarcinoma, which is progressive and cumulative relative to the duration of the disease. Pseudocyst development is more common compared with acute pancreatitis and is caused by a pancreatic duct leak and subsequent extravasation of pancreatic juice and encapsulation. If the extravasation of pancreatic juice does not form a pseudocyst it can drain feely into the peritoneal cavity, causing pancreatic ascites, or rarely into the thoracic cavity, causing a pancreatic pleural effusion.

Clinical presentation

Epigastric pain that radiates through to the back is the most common symptom of chronic pancreatitis. It is usually steady and lasts for hours or days. Patients will often be unable to find a position of comfort and sit or lie with their hips flexed. Pain is usually recurring, and exacerbations may be brought on by eating or alcohol or may occur without any precipitating cause. Anorexia, nausea and vomiting are all common associated symptoms. Generally, as the disease progresses pain may become less of a feature and symptoms of malabsorption (e.g. steatorrhoea, weight loss) and diabetes become more prominent. Frank malabsorption, evidenced by steatorrhoea, is indicative of advanced disease and pancreatic exocrine function that has fallen below 10% of normal. Because untreated malabsorption is associated with long-term adverse effects such as malnutrition and osteoporosis, there is a trend towards early enzyme supplementation before overt symptoms develop.

Investigation

Diagnosis is based on clinical presentation, laboratory investigation of pancreatic function and imaging. Unlike acute pancreatitis, serum levels of lipase and amylase are seldom helpful in the diagnosis. Pancreatic function can be assessed in a variety of ways. Exocrine function can be measured directly via aspiration of pancreatic juice but is more often measured indirectly. Common methods include the measurement of faecal fat content, or of faecal levels of chymotrypsin and elastase. As well as standard tests for diabetes (e.g. HbA1c), endocrine function can be assessed by the pancreatic polypeptide response to a test meal. When severe, chronic pancreatitis is associated with a blunted or absent pancreatic polypeptide response to feeding.

A plain abdominal X-ray may reveal a calcified pancreas and CT may show calcification, duct dilatation and cystic disease. MRCP is a sensitive radiological test for the diagnosis of chronic pancreatitis and may show duct dilatation, stricture formations and calculi. ERCP is also valuable, but invasive. Overall, however, endoscopic ultrasound (EUS) is the preferred imaging for diagnosis as it offers high-resolution images of the pancreatic parenchyma, ductal systems, cystic lesions and calcific changes and, importantly, is highly reliable in ruling out pancreatic carcinoma through EUS-guided fine-needle aspiration for cytology.

Treatment

There is no specific proven treatment for chronic pancreatitis, with care focusing on symptom management and treatment of complications. The long-term outlook is generally poor, with 10- and 20-year survival rates approximately 70% and 45%, respectively, compared with 93% and 65% for patients without pancreatitis. Survival declines even further for patients with alcoholic chronic pancreatitis who continue to abuse alcohol. It is therefore essential that these patients abstain from alcohol in order to improve both their symptoms and survival rate.

Autoimmune pancreatitis is a rare subset of chronic pancreatitis that responds to steroid therapy. Plasma IgG4 may be elevated and other organs affected. This diagnosis should always be considered, particularly before embarking on invasive interventions.

Effective analgesia is required for the pain, which often requires oral opioids. Care should be taken, as it is common for these patients to become opioid dependent, and all alternative strategies should be explored, including cognitive behavioural therapy. Attempts to alleviate pain with anti-secretory therapy (e.g. octreotide, a somatostatin analogue) has had mixed success. The development of central sensitisation in patients with chronic pancreatitis is associated with a worse response to endoscopic or surgical intervention and these patients should be under the care of a pain specialist. Those with pancreatic exocrine insufficiency will need pancreatic enzyme replacement therapy, which not only reverses the malabsorption but also prevents secondary complications such as metabolic bone disease from inadequate absorption of fat-soluble vitamins. Patients with diabetes will likely require treatment with insulin.

Endoscopic therapies can also be utilised to manage symptoms and complications when indicated, especially in those not fit for surgery. Pancreatic duct decompression (via surgical or endoscopic approach) is the only therapy shown to delay or prevent the progression of chronic obstructive pancreatitis (a subset of patients with chronic pancreatitis). Endoscopic therapies (via ERCP) include pancreatic duct stenting, which is used to treat proximal pancreatic duct stenosis, endoscopic stone removal, and sphincterotomy for conditions such as pancreas divisum.

Operative management

Surgery is the most effective treatment for pain, although it is common practice to offer endoscopic treatment first. It has been shown that surgery is much less effective if there is a delay of more than 3 years, opioid dependence has occurred and if five or more endoscopic treatments have been given. Patients who require a drainage procedure to relieve an obstructed duct are best treated with a Frey procedure, which involves a Roux-en-Y pancreatico-jejunostomy and 'coring out' of the head of the pancreas. If there is an inflammatory mass, and when pancreatic cancer is suspected, then pancreatic resection is indicated. Patients with multiple strictures might also require pancreatic resection. Other pancreatic resections are more extensive and include a pancreaticoduodenectomy (Whipple procedure) or duodenum-preserving pancreatic head resection (Beger procedure). Recurrence of pain does occur, but overall there is significant benefit with an improvement in the quality of life following surgery.

Total pancreatectomy is also possible, and is now being offered with islet autotransplantation to reduce the severity of diabetes. This is now being considered for patients with a genetic basis for the chronic pancreatitis and before advanced disease occurs.

Further reading

Adams DB, Cotton PB, Zyromski N, Windsor JA (eds) *Pancreatitis: Medical and Surgical Management*. Oxford: Wiley Blackwell, 2017.

Banks PA, Bollen TL, Dervenis C *et al*. Classification of acute pancreatitis – 2012: revision of the Atlanta classification and definitions by international consensus. *Gut* 2013;62:102–11.

Beger HG, Warshaw A, Hruban R *et al.* (eds) *The Pancreas: an Integrated Textbook of Basic Science, Medicine, and Surgery*, 3rd edn. Oxford: Wiley Blackwell, 2018.

Crockett SD, Wani S, Gardner TB, Falck-Ytter Y, Barkun AN. American Gastroenterological Association Institute guideline on initial management of acute pancreatitis. *Gastroenterology* 2018;154:1096–101.

MCQs

Select the single correct answer to each question. The correct answers can be found in the Answers section at the end of the book.

1 There are many recognised causes of chronic pancreatitis but the most common is:
a gallstones
b gene mutations
c smoking
d alcohol
e gallstones and alcohol equally

2 Which of the following findings would classify the patient as having actual severe acute pancreatitis?
a Glasgow score of 4 after 48 hours in hospital
b creatinine of 175 μmol/L that has risen from a normal value and persists at that level for 3 days
c presence of pancreatic necrosis on contrast-enhanced CT scan
d heart rate of 112 and temperature of 38.5°C on admission to hospital
e all of the above

3 Alcohol can cause pancreatitis by:
a increasing the rate of conversion of inactive trypsinogen to the active form trypsin
b obstruction of small pancreatic ducts leading to ductal hypertension
c increasing formation of calcium concretions in the pancreatic duct
d increasing instability of zymogen granules
e all of the above

4 Which of the following is the most important initial step in management of an unwell patient with acute pancreatitis?
a administer strong analgesia via an intravenous line
b ensure the patient is given intravenous crystalloid fluid
c determine the predicted severity by calculating the Glasgow score
d commence broad-spectrum antibiotics intravenously
e arrange an urgent ERCP if the patient has a fever with rigours, cholestatic liver function tests and tenderness in the right upper quadrant

5 Chronic pancreatitis most often presents with:
a weight loss
b steatorrhoea
c diabetes mellitus
d fractures
e recurrent epigastric pain

6 Regarding surgery in acute pancreatitis, which of the following statements is true?
a a patient with mild uncomplicated gallstone pancreatitis should have a cholecystectomy booked as an outpatient to occur within 3 months from discharge
b a patient with infected necrosis found on contrast-enhanced CT, which was performed for

a temperature, should have minimally invasive surgery to debride the area within the next 24 hours

c a patient with an infected fluid collection found on contrast-enhanced CT who has been on antibiotics for 48 hours and is developing new

renal impairment and shortness of breath should have radiologically guided drainage within the next 24 hours

d all of the above

e none of the above

23 Pancreatic tumours

David Burnett[1] and Mehrdad Nikfarjam[2]

[1] John Hunter Hospital, Newcastle, New South Wales, Australia
[2] University of Melbourne and Austin Health, Melbourne, Victoria, Australia

Introduction

In 2017, pancreatic cancer was the 10th most common cancer in Australia, but the fifth leading cause of cancer death. The estimated individual Australian's risk of being diagnosed with pancreatic cancer is 1 in 57 (male) and 1 in 73 (female), at a median age of 70 years. The 5-year survival of patients after diagnosis is only 9.8%. Based on large US registry data (Surveillance, Epidemiology, and End Results Program or SEER), 52% of pancreatic cancer patients have metastatic disease at presentation (Figure 23.1). More than 85% of pancreatic tumours are adenocarcinoma (exocrine) tumours, with the remainder made up of neuroendocrine, lymphoma and premalignant/benign lesions. Unfortunately, despite radical surgery and dramatic progress in the survival of other solid organ tumours around the world, there has been little improvement in pancreatic adenocarcinoma survival for more than 40 years.

Aetiology/risk factors

The incidence of pancreatic cancer increases with age and is most frequently diagnosed in the 65–74 age bracket. Tobacco smoking is the oldest and strongest known risk factor which, proportional to exposure, doubles an individual's risk. It is felt that smoking alone contributes to around one-quarter of cases. There is a slight preponderance for males, although it is possible that differential smoking rates between genders may account for this difference. Diabetes mellitus increases the risk of pancreatic cancer by approximately twofold. Abdominal obesity also increases the risk of pancreatic cancer by approximately one-fifth. There may also be elevated risk from occupational exposure to benzene or organochlorines.

While moderate alcohol intake does not appear to be directly associated with pancreatic cancer, heavy alcohol intake (eight or more standard drinks per day for 6–8 years) can lead to chronic pancreatitis. Chronic pancreatitis has a cumulative association with malignant transformation of about 1.7% at 10 years in the best study to date. Less than one in twenty cases of pancreatic cancer are preceded by chronic pancreatitis.

Approximately 10–15% with pancreatic cancers are thought to be familial in origin. Most of these patients have two or more close relatives affected by pancreatic cancer, but without a known specific genetic defect. However, there are certain inherited cancer syndromes associated with pancreatic cancer, including *BRCA1*, *BRCA2*, Lynch syndrome, familial atypical multiple mole melanoma (FAMMM) syndrome and Peutz–Jeghers syndrome.

Molecular pathogenesis

There are three main morphological pathways to pancreatic adenocarcinoma: pancreatic ductal intraepithelial neoplasia (PanIN) (Figure 23.2), conversion of intraductal papillary mucinous neoplasm (IPMN), and malignant mucinous cystic neoplasm (MCN). On a cellular level, there are multiple stepwise epigenetic pathways to carcinogenesis. It is felt that loss of heterozygosity (i.e. loss of a normal gene on one chromosome, leaving a faulty chromosome on the other to act homozygously) leads to the loss of pathways associated with normal cell division. The most common genetic mutations in pancreatic cancer include the proto-oncogene *KRAS* (which prescribes a component of a growth factor receptor), occurring in over 90% of cases, and loss of the tumour suppressor genes *p16*, *CDKN2A* and *p53* (inactivated in 50–75% of pancreatic cancer).

The precise cell of origin is unknown. The expression of acinar, ductal and islet cell markers

Textbook of Surgery, Fourth Edition. Edited by Julian A. Smith, Andrew H. Kaye, Christopher Christophi and Wendy A. Brown.

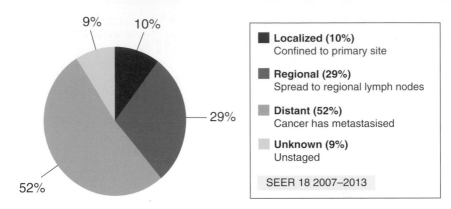

Fig. 23.1 Surveillance, Epidemiology and End Result Program (SEER) database: percentage of cases by stage. Source: https://seer.cancer.gov/. Reproduced with permission of National Institutes of Health (NIH).

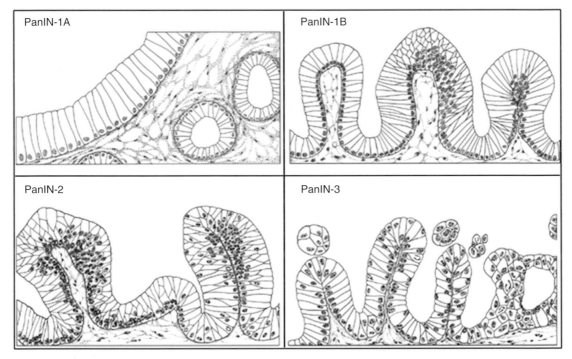

Fig. 23.2 Pancreatic intraepithelial neoplasia progression from early changes (PanIN-1) to carcinoma *in situ* (PanIN-3): PanIN-1A (flat), PanIN-1B (papillary), PanIN-2 (papillary with nuclear changes), and PanIN-3 (severely atypical with mitoses, luminal necrosis and budding structures). Source: images from Johns Hopkins website, http://pds17.pathology.jhmi.edu/N/n.web?EP=N&URL=/MCGI/SEND^WEBUTLTY(12774)/982334336minal necrosis. Reproduced with permission of Johns Hopkins University.

has been described in pancreatic ductal adenocarcinoma. *KRAS* mutation activation is an early change that controls cell division, accumulation and apoptosis. The accumulation of genetic changes over time within the duct epithelium leads to intraepithelial dysplasia, which subsequently transitions into invasive cancer.

Primary pancreatic adenocarcinoma can also arise from an IPMN, which are premalignant cystic tumours involving either the side-branch, main pancreatic duct or both. In contrast to sporadic adenocarcinoma, invasive IPMN, particularly the colloidal histological subtype, has a better overall 5-year survival, up to 70% in some series. This compares to an overall 20–25% postoperative 5-year survival reported for pancreatic ductal adenocarcinoma.

The third pathway to cancer is MCNs. The precursor lesions do not communicate with the main pancreatic duct, are characterised by an ovarian-like stroma and have a variable benign/premalignant period prior to transition to cancer.

Clinical presentation

Three-quarters of pancreatic cancers occur in the pancreatic head. The classical presentation of jaundice and weight loss is present in only about half of patients at diagnosis. Importantly, one in four patients with pancreatic cancer have symptoms associated with another upper gastrointestinal pathology for up to 6 months prior to diagnosis, and 15% of patients present to medical services early for symptoms later attributed to pancreatic cancer. Up to 80% of cancer patients have hyperglycaemia or diabetes at the time of presentation. A diagnosis of pancreatic cancer should be entertained in patients with new-onset diabetes without clear risk factors for diabetes. It is thought that some cancers may produce factors such as islet amyloid polypeptide that can lead to impaired glucose tolerance. Vague abdominal or back pain is often present many months before diagnosis and may be a symptom of perineural invasion. Because of the lack of jaundice, body and tail lesions often present at a more advanced stage.

Investigations

Laboratory tests

Routine measurement of liver function, full blood count, electrolytes, urea and creatinine are performed. Carbohydrate antigen (CA)19-9, a Lewis (a) blood group antigen secreted by pancreatic cancer cells, is elevated in 90% of patients. A small percentage of the population are lacking the enzyme fucosyltransferase, which prevents secretion and elevation of CA19-9. These people are said to be Lewis antigen negative. High levels (>1000 U/mL) are more likely to be associated with metastatic disease. Benign conditions (particularly jaundice, cirrhosis, cholangitis) can also elevate serum CA19-9 so it is important that the baseline measure is taken without cholangitis/biliary obstruction. The greatest utilisation of CA19-9 levels are in serial observation over time, such as monitoring for recurrence following surgery or assessing response to chemotherapy.

Imaging

Multidetector computed tomography (MDCT), with fine (1-mm slice) resolution, is the standard of care for pancreatic imaging in patients being assessed for surgical resection. Pancreatic adenocarcinoma is usually (90%) hypo-attenuating compared with the normal enhancing parenchyma. Indirect signs such as dilation of the common bile duct and/or pancreatic duct can help in cases where the tumour is iso-attenuating within the parenchyma (10%). Multiple sequences through arterial, portal venous and delayed imaging define the relationship between the tumour and the major vessels (superior mesenteric vein/portal vein, superior mesenteric artery and hepatic artery). It provides excellent specificity and sensitivity for both diagnosis and the presence of vascular invasion, though it can overstate resectability in up to one-quarter of cases. CT may not detect small peritoneal nodules or small liver metastases which preclude cure.

Magnetic resonance imaging (MRI) combined with magnetic resonance cholangiopancreatography (MRCP) is rarely required for staging of pancreatic adenocarcinoma. It can be utilised in cases of MDCT contrast allergy, for further delineation of isodense lesions on CT and to differentiate between tumour and focal fatty infiltration of the pancreas. MRI combined with liver-specific contrast is useful for characterisation of indeterminate liver lesions detected by other imaging modalities. MRI/MRCP is commonly used for assessment of cystic pancreatic lesions and follow-up of IPMN and can delineate the relationship between cyst and pancreatic duct, as well as identify solid components.

[18]F-Fluorodeoxyglucose positron emission tomography (FDG-PET) has an emerging role in the assessment of pancreatic cancer. FDG-PET has a sensitivity of up to 71% in adenocarcinoma. The presence of acute pancreatitis can lead to intense uptake of FDG in benign parenchyma, and thus false-negatives should be considered. FDG-PET can change management in up to one-quarter of cases, but currently lacks the special resolution of MDCT and is an adjunct to other imaging modalities. The ability to monitor treatment effect (including in the neoadjuvant setting) has increased its utility.

Endoscopic ultrasound (EUS), although invasive, boasts the highest sensitivity for the diagnosis of small pancreatic adenocarcinoma (99% vs. 55% for MDCT). A high negative predictive value means that it is useful for confirming tumour diagnosis of iso-attenuating lesions noted on MDCT and for identifying tumours in the setting of concurrent pancreatitis. The ability to biopsy tumours with a fine-needle aspirate can confirm the diagnosis, and is essential prior to the initiation of chemotherapy, particularly in the neoadjuvant setting.

Disease staging

Where disease is localised and the patient is being considered for surgery, involvement of major blood vessels on imaging defines resectability, according to the National Comprehensive Cancer Network (NCCN) guidelines. In general, localised tumours which may abut (≤180°) but do not encase (>180°) the superior mesenteric vein/portal vein (SMV/PV) or cause vein contour irregularity are considered *resectable*. Tumours which encase the SMV/PV (>180° or impingement) or cause vein contour irregularity or abut (≤180°) the surrounding arteries are *borderline resectable*, and neoadjuvant therapy may be considered. Reconstruction of the SMV/PV must be technically feasible to proceed. Encasement (>180°) of the superior mesenteric artery (SMA), coeliac axis or hepatic artery designates a tumour as *locally advanced* (unresectable) and palliative treatment options should be considered.

Tumours that are resected are assessed pathologically using the American Joint Committee on Cancer (AJCC) TNM system (Box 23.1), which accounts for tumour size, lymph nodes involved and the presence of metastatic disease. Stage I/II disease includes potentially resectable tumours, while stage III disease is locally advanced and is any T4 tumour with or without nodal involvement. Stage IV disease is defined by distant metastases.

Box 23.1 TNM staging system

Tumour

Tx	Unable to assess primary tumour
T0	No evidence of primary tumour
Tis	Carcinoma *in situ*
T1	Tumour ≤2 cm in greatest dimension, limited to pancreas
T2	Tumour >2 cm in greatest dimension, limited to pancreas
T3	Tumour extending beyond pancreas but without involvement of coeliac or superior mesenteric artery
T4	Tumour involving coeliac or superior mesenteric artery (unresectable primary)

Nodes

NX	Unable to assess regional lymph nodes
N0	No regional lymph node involvement
N1	Regional lymph node involvement

Metastasis

M0	No distant metastasis
M1	Distant metastasis

Surgical management

Curative intent

Approximately 20% of patients are resectable in the first instance, and a further 30% are locally advanced. With advances in neoadjuvant chemotherapy with or without radiotherapy the number of resectable patients may increase. Even with radical surgery, there is only a 20–25% chance of cure, with an overall median survival of 22–24 months. Small tumours (<25 mm) with one or fewer lymph nodes may do better, with a median survival of 70 months in one series. This compares with an average survival of 9–14.8 months in non-operative patients receiving palliative chemotherapy with gemcitabine/nanoparticle albumin bound (nab)-paclitaxel.

The type of surgery performed to remove a pancreatic cancer is guided by its location. In cases of cancers within the head of the pancreas, a pancreaticoduodenectomy is most commonly performed. Also known as a Whipple procedure (Figure 23.3), the head of the pancreas is transected at the level of the SMV/PV confluence. It is removed en bloc with the duodenum, common bile duct, gallbladder and peripancreatic lymphatics. The SMA is skeletonised and detached from the uncinate process of the pancreas. Clear surgical margins (R0 resection) are critical for maximising chance of cure and increasing length of disease-free postoperative survival. Hence en-bloc venous resection of the SMV/PV branches should be performed where necessary to obtain clear margins. Arterial resection is rarely indicated and should generally be limited to clinical trials. The involvement of perineural infiltration around SMA, hepatic artery or coeliac axis often represents aggressive systemic disease. Arterial resection and/or reconstruction of a short length of hepatic artery or accessory hepatic vessels has been performed in extraordinary or rare circumstances, particularly if neoadjuvant therapy results in a very favourable response. The decision whether to perform classical pancreaticoduodenectomy (Whipple procedure) or pylorus-preserving pancreaticoduodenectomy is controversial. A 2016 Cochrane review failed to demonstrate any difference between the two approaches.

The most feared complication after Whipple pancreaticoduodenectomy is clinically relevant postoperative pancreatic fistula (CR-POPF). Risk factors include a soft pancreas, narrow pancreatic duct (without chronic obstruction) and significant blood loss during the resection. With these factors present, the risk of CR-POPF can be as high as

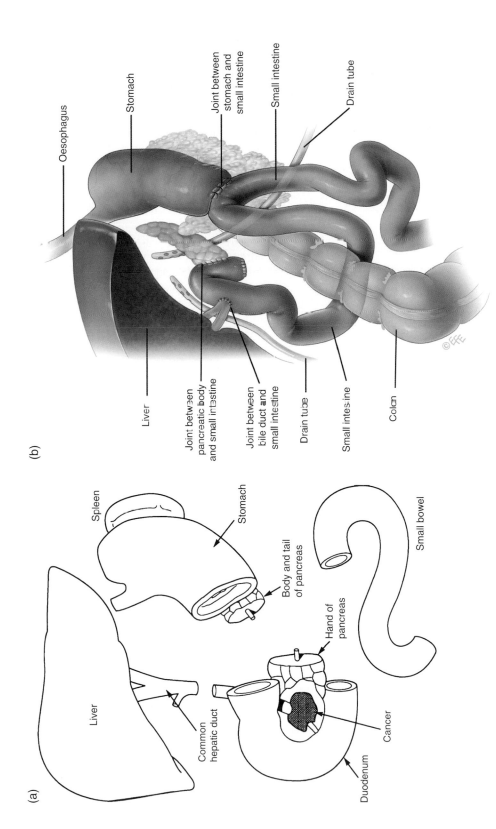

Fig. 23.3 (a) Pancreaticoduodenectomy consists of partial gastrectomy, partial pancreatectomy, and excision of the distal bile duct and all of the duodenum. (b) Reconstruction after pancreaticoduodenectomy.

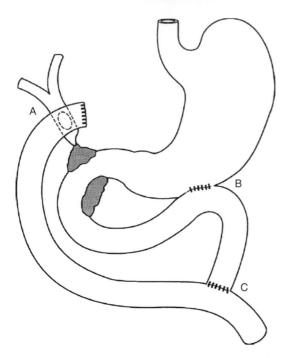

Fig. 23.4 Palliative bypass of the bile duct and stomach in a patient with a non-resectable pancreatic cancer. (A) Choledochojejunostomy, (B) gastroenterostomy, (C) entero-enterosotomy.

25%. Other complications include exocrine pancreatic failure, worsening diabetes, impaired gastric emptying or 'dumping syndrome'.

Pancreatic cancer in the body and tail is more likely to present late due to the absence of jaundice, and are thus less likely to be resectable. Where cure is possible, resection of the body and tail of the pancreas, including the spleen and its associated vessels, using a technique referred to as radical anterior modular pancreatosplenectomy (RAMPS procedure) is the standard of care for malignant tumours, and offers the best lymph node yield. Laparoscopic distal pancreatectomy (often with preservation of the splenic vessels) is appropriate for benign pathology.

Palliative intent

Priorities of palliative management are to resolve symptomatic jaundice and prevent gastric outlet obstruction. Depending on the presence/burden of metastatic disease, endoscopic options can allow stenting of the bile duct or the duodenum or both. If a reasonable life expectancy is predicted, surgical bypass (hepaticojejunostomy and gastrojejunostomy) provides the most reliable relief of symptoms (Figure 23.4).

Chemotherapy for pancreatic adenocarcinoma

Neoadjuvant chemotherapy

The use of chemotherapy in a neoadjuvant setting for pancreatic cancer remains controversial but is increasing around the world. Because of the current lack of level 1 evidence, there is significant variation in practice regionally, and it is uncertain which group of patients will benefit most. Proponents of this approach argue for an increased likelihood of completing a full course of treatment and an increased complete resection (R0) rate. R0 resection gives the best chance of long-term survival for patients with pancreatic cancer. Undertaking neoadjuvant therapy does necessitate a tissue diagnosis (usually via EUS) and decompressive biliary stenting. Initial reports suggest approximately one-third of borderline-resectable patients can be down-staged to become resectable after neoadjuvant chemotherapy, while 3–5% of patients can expect a complete pathological response (no viable tumour left).

FOLFIRINOX (combination therapy comprising oxaliplatin, leucovorin, fluorouracil and irinotecan) has been utilised successfully in the neoadjuvant setting even for locally advanced tumours. A 61% R0 resection rate was achieved as opposed to 46% for gemcitabine and radiation. An average decrease in size from 3.6 to 2.2 cm was noted, with a median decrease in CA19-9 from 169 to 16 U/mL. In the largest dataset to date, equivalent outcomes were noted between a FOLFIRINOX locally advanced/borderline-resectable group and the comparison group containing upfront resectable tumours. Additionally, a 3-year survival of 28% in the FOLFIRINOX group compares favourably with 23% in those receiving neoadjuvant gemcitabine/radiotherapy. Nab-paclitaxel and gemcitabine have also been used in this setting and about one-third of patients have shown some tumour regression on pathological analysis.

Regardless of the regimen chosen, the degree of tumour response achieved when considering resection can be difficult to assess. Desmoplasia from tumour regression can appear similar on cross-sectional imaging to residual tumour. Reduction in tumour marker (CA19-9) levels and decrease in avidity on FDG-PET imaging further aids in prediction of tumour response to therapy. Some authors recommend surgical exploration with intraoperative pathological examination of periarteriolar tissues using frozen section histology if the serum CA19-9 halves during the course of neoadjuvant therapy.

Preoperative chemotherapy does not seem to increase complication rates; indeed the CR-POPF rate may be decreased due to a firmer pancreas with decreased enzymatic secretions. The combination of radiotherapy with chemotherapy may add up to 10% to the rate of resectability, but at the cost of a more technically difficult operation. With data available to date, postoperative complication rates appear similar to those who have not had radiotherapy.

Adjuvant chemotherapy

Patients who have undergone upfront resection for pancreatic adenocarcinoma will be considered for adjuvant chemotherapy. However, not all patients are suitable and serious complications (e.g. pancreatic fistula) reduce the likelihood of completing chemotherapy. In fact, only around half of patients actually complete the full course of chemotherapy treatment following resection.

Currently, combination adjuvant chemotherapy with gemcitabine and capecitabine is standard care, achieving a 5-year survival of 29% in the ESPAC-4 trial. Median postoperative survival is 28 months following resection with such a regimen, but in patients with R0 resection the median survival approaches 40 months. The addition of radiotherapy may reduce local recurrence rates, particularly in microscopically incomplete (R1) resection, though data on overall survival is less convincing. More recently, the use of FOLFIRINOX chemotherapy in the adjuvant setting has shown further survival improvements.

For those patients unable to tolerate combination therapy due to frailty, surgical complication or comorbidities, single-agent gemcitabine still offers significant benefit and is (for the most part) well tolerated.

Palliative chemotherapy

More than half of patients have metastatic disease at presentation. In the 2011 ACCORD study, FOLFIRINOX chemotherapy showed the most promise for metastatic pancreatic cancer, increasing survival from 6.8 to 11 months. Unfortunately, this comes at the cost of significant treatment-related side effects, and not all patients with metastatic disease are suitable for such an aggressive approach.

Nab-paclitaxel has also been combined with gemcitabine for a modest increase in survival compared with gemcitabine alone (9 vs. 6.6 months). Overall, less than one-third of patients have significant response to palliative chemotherapy.

Pancreatic neuroendocrine tumours

Pancreatic neuroendocrine tumours (PNETs) are most easily divided into functional and non-functional tumours, based on syndromes of hormone secretion. Overall, 60–90% of tumours are non-functional. PNETs are not infrequently seen in a number of hereditary conditions, including multiple endocrine neoplasia type 1 (MEN-1) syndrome, von Hippel–Lindau syndrome, neurofibromatosis type 1 and tuberous sclerosis.

In terms of the functional tumours, the consensus is to divide them into three groups: insulinomas, gastrinomas and rare functional tumours. Functional and well-differentiated neuroendocrine tumours are best visualised on gallium-68 DOTA-TATE PET. The radioisotope has an affinity for somatostatin receptors. In contrast, high-grade neuroendocrine carcinomas may lose some of their neuroendocrine differentiation but may be visible on FDG-PET imaging. The tumour marker chromogranin A is positive in approximately 70% of cases. Low and moderately differentiated tumours tend to have an indolent course, with long median survival intervals.

Functional tumours

Insulinoma

Insulinomas are commonly described with the 'rule of 10', as they are less than 10% malignant, 10% associated with MEN-1 and 10% extrapancreatic. They represent 1–2% of pancreatic tumours and can be found anywhere in the pancreas. They present classically with Whipple's triad of fasting hypoglycaemia, symptoms of hypoglycaemia (diaphoresis, tremors and decreased level of consciousness) and immediate relief with glucose. However, 18% can present with postprandial hypoglycaemia alone. Diagnosis is based on a supervised fast, with measurement of fasting insulin, C-peptide and proinsulin. Around two-thirds can be seen on CT, with a higher sensitivity with the addition of MRI. They are hypervascular, with arterial-phase contrast enhancement when compared with normal pancreatic parenchyma. EUS is often required, with sensitivities approaching 100% in some series. Invasive testing, such as arterial calcium stimulation with hepatic venous sampling, can be helpful to confirm the location of isodense tumours or identify the active lesion in the case of multiple tumours such as MEN-1. Primary lesions are often very symptomatic and should almost always be excised. Enucleation for tumours of less than 2 cm, located away from the main pancreatic duct, is a valid treatment option in selected cases, given the low rate of malignancy and metastatic lymph node spread.

Gastrinoma

Zollinger–Ellison syndrome is the presence of multiple peptic ulcers driven by hypersecretion of gastrin leading to over-production of gastric acid. Gastrinomas are usually located within a triangle marked by the junction between the cystic duct and common duct, the junction between the second and third part of duodenum, and the neck of the pancreas. Gastrinomas can be hard to visualise on conventional imaging, are often within the duodenal wall and at least half of them are malignant. Gastrinomas can be very difficult to image preoperatively on conventional imaging or endoscopy. Current recommendations support surgical exploration up to and including pancreaticoduodenectomy for patients with Zollinger–Ellison syndrome without MEN-1 syndrome. In contrast, gastrinomas are present in up to half of patients with MEN-1, are often multiple and tumours under 2 cm rarely metastasise. Metastatic gastrinoma is a cause of premature death in up to 40% of patients with MEN-1 syndrome.

Rare functional tumour syndromes have been described as per their hormonal products, including VIPoma, glucagonoma and somatostatinoma. Localised functional tumours should be resected where technically feasible in a fit patient.

Non-functional

Non-functional tumours are described pathologically in terms of size, histological grade and degree of proliferation (marked by the Ki-67 index). It is uncommon for tumours smaller than 1 cm to metastasise and non-functional tumours of this size are often best observed with serial imaging follow-up. At a diameter of 2 cm, up to 48% may have nodal metastases. However, despite the common presence of lymph node metastases, patients with an isolated PNET of less than 2 cm may have an excellent chance, with 15-year survival of up to 100%. In metastatic disease, the extent of liver metastases correlates with survival, with an overall 10-year survival of 30% in patients with liver metastases.

In a fit patient, primary neuroendocrine tumours greater than 2 cm should be resected in the first instance. The management of non-functional tumours measuring between 1 and 2 cm is more controversial and is guided by the patient's age,

fitness for surgery and nuclear imaging findings. When a major pancreatic resection is required, early data suggest that initial observation is a safe strategy for PNETs under 2 cm.

The management of metastatic disease should be within a multidisciplinary setting and depends on the function and proliferation rate (grade) of the tumour. Low-grade, non-functional, widespread metastatic disease has excellent long-term survival characteristics with somatostatin analogues. The aim for any surgical approach should be R0 resection. Resectable liver-only metastases should have surgery, with a 5-year survival of 60–70% compared with 30% for medical therapy alone. Liver-directed therapy, such as selective internal radiation therapy (SIRT) and drug-eluting beads, has a role in unresectable disease. For metastatic insulinoma and in cases of carcinoid syndrome, improvement in symptomatology has been reported with debulking procedures. Carcinoid syndrome comprises the symptoms of flushing and diarrhoea and, less frequently, heart failure and bronchoconstriction. It is the result of vasoactive substances, including serotonin, released from neuroendocrine tumours into the systemic circulation. Usually these substances undergo hepatic degradation, but in cases of high-volume liver metastases, the liver's ability to metabolise these substances is overcome and they escape into the systemic circulation.

The role of liver transplant for metastatic neuroendocrine tumours is very controversial, given that excellent long-term survival is achievable with liver-directed therapy and hormonal control. Peptide receptor radionuclide therapy targeting the somatostatin receptor is an experimental second-line treatment with promising early results for well-differentiated tumours.

Neuroendocrine carcinoma (high proliferative index, Ki67 >20%) tends to be more aggressive and visible on standard FDG-PET imaging. Metastatic high-grade neuroendocrine carcinomas are unlikely to benefit from resection or hormonal treatment and often require systemic cytotoxic chemotherapy.

Rare malignant disease

Primary pancreatic lymphoma is rare, comprising 0.5% of pancreatic tumours. Management is systemic chemotherapy rather than resection. Metastases to the pancreas are rare, though a small number of cancers like melanoma, renal cell carcinoma and small cell lung cancer do occasionally metastasise in isolation to pancreas. There is a role for resection of isolated renal cell carcinoma metastasis, though improvements in chemotherapy have diminished the role in the other two.

Solid pseudopapillary neoplasms are rare indolent tumours affecting predominantly young women, with a preponderance to local invasion but infrequent metastasis. Resection offers a 95% 5-year survival for localised disease. High survival rates have also been described in cases of liver-only metastases treated by surgery or liver-directed chemotherapy.

Cystic lesions of the pancreas

Intraductal papillary mucinous neoplasm

The incidence of premalignant pancreatic tumours such as IPMN has increased by more than 14 times over the last 20 years. This is partly due to the increasing use of cross-sectional imaging for other indications, particularly CT. Benign cystic lesions have been found in up to 25% of autopsy specimens in a Japanese study, which raises the question of whether the increasing incidence truly represents the discovery of clinically significant disease.

The cystic appearance of IPMN is related to ductal obstruction and subsequent dilatation. There are two classifications, main duct (MD)-IPMN (50–90% risk of malignant transformation) and side-branch (SB)-IPMN (best retrospective data suggest 3–5% risk of malignancy at 5 years from diagnosis). A main pancreatic duct of 1 cm or more strongly suggests MD-IPMN, whereas the presence of a mucinous cyst communicating with the pancreatic duct without main duct dilatation suggests SB-IPMN. Most cases are asymptomatic, but acute pancreatitis is occasionally the presenting symptom, caused by partial mucous obstruction of the pancreatic duct.

The current recommendations are for resection of all MD-IPMNs and resection of SB-IPMNs greater than 3 cm, or with main duct dilatation above 7 mm with or without nodular components. Recommended surveillance (consensus guidelines) is for annual MRI/MRCP to identify early changes in small lesions.

Mucinous cystic neoplasms

In contrast, MCNs are macrocystic and have a significant risk of malignant transformation. They occur (almost) exclusively in females and are more common in the body and tail of the pancreas. Features of malignancy include size over 3 cm, wall thickening, or solid components. Histological examination of MCNs reveals an ovarian-type stroma, and the lesions may even represent ectopic ovarian tissue. MCNs should be resected in fit patients.

Serous cystadenoma

A truly benign cystic neoplasm is the serous cystadenoma, usually found in women. These microcystic tumours classically demonstrate a 'starburst' appearance on cross-sectional imaging and are found most commonly in the pancreatic head. This lesion is usually incidental and requires no further investigation or management.

Diagnosis

The diagnosis of IPMN over other cystic neoplasms is based on communication with the pancreatic duct, best seen initially on MRCP or invasively at ERCP. With regard to the diagnosis of MCN compared with other cystic lesions, EUS gives superior spatial resolution for microcystic changes, internal septations and nodularity. Fine-needle aspiration allows cyst fluid analysis. A cyst fluid carcinoembryonic antigen (CEA) level above 800 ng/mL strongly suggests mucinous pathology. In contrast, high levels of cyst fluid amylase suggest communication with the pancreatic duct, seen commonly in pancreatic pseudocyst and IPMN.

Further reading

Brugge WR, Lauwers GY, Sahani D, Fernandez-del Castillo C, Warshaw AL. Cystic neoplasms of the pancreas. *N Engl J Med* 2004;351:1218–26.

Crippa S, Capurso G, Cammà C, Fave GD, Castillo CF, Falconi M. Risk of pancreatic malignancy and mortality in branch-duct IPMNs undergoing surveillance: a systematic review and meta-analysis. *Dig Liver Dis* 2016;48:473–9.

Kamisawa T, Wood LD, Itoi T, Takaori K. Pancreatic cancer. *Lancet* 2016;388:73–85.

Lewis A, Li D, Williams J, Singh G. Pancreatic neuroendocrine tumors: state-of-the-art diagnosis and management. *Oncology* 2017;31:e1–e12.

MCQs

Select the single correct answer to each question. The correct answers can be found in the Answers section at the end of the book.

1 The most specific symptom associated with pancreatic adenocarcinoma is:
   a weight loss
   b painless jaundice
   c epigastric pain
   d right upper quadrant pain, jaundice and fever
   e back pain relieved by leaning forwards

2 Which of the following cystic neoplasms are found almost exclusively in women?
a serous cystadenoma
b mucinous cystadenoma
c intraductal papillary mucinous neoplasm
d pancreatic pseudocyst
e pancreatic gastrinoma

3 Which factor is most important in deciding whether a pancreatic adenocarcinoma is resectable?
a tumour size
b tumour invasion of the portal vein
c metastatic disease
d enlarged peripancreatic lymph nodes
e serum CA19-9 levels

4 Palpable gallbladder in the absence of pain is most likely associated with:
a gallstones
b hilar cholangiocarcinoma
c gallbladder carcinoma
d pancreatic adenocarcinoma
e chronic pancreatitis

5 Which of the following statements is *false* regarding intraductal papillary mucinous neoplasms (IPMNs)?
a very commonly seen in autopsy series
b main duct IPMN has a higher risk of malignancy than side-branch IPMN
c most patients present with symptoms of acute pancreatitis
d small side-branch IPMN without nodules is usually followed up by serial cross-sectional imaging
e usually have high CEA and amylase levels in cyst fluid aspirate

24 Portal hypertension and surgery on the patient with cirrhosis

Michael A. Fink

University of Melbourne and Austin Health, Melbourne, Victoria, Australia

Introduction

Portal hypertension is associated with many of the most severe complications of cirrhosis and consequently with a high risk of morbidity and mortality.

Anatomy

The portal venous system refers to the splanchnic circulation, through which blood from the intestine and associated structures (pancreas, spleen) passes into the liver. The superior mesenteric vein, which drains the small intestine and colon as far as the splenic flexure, joins the splenic vein behind the neck of the pancreas and continues as the portal vein into the hilum of the liver, where it divides into the right portal vein, which has a short extrahepatic course, and the left portal vein, which has a longer extrahepatic course. The left and right portal veins subsequently ramify within the liver to supply the liver segments. The inferior mesenteric vein, which drains the left colon and rectum, most commonly enters the splenic vein behind the body of the pancreas, but can enter the confluence of the superior mesenteric vein and splenic vein. The right gastroepiploic vein drains into the superior mesenteric vein. The left gastroepiploic vein and short gastric veins drain into the splenic vein. The left gastric vein (sometimes called the coronary vein) and right gastric vein drain into the portal vein. Anastomoses between the portal and systemic venous systems are found around the lower oesophagus, the rectum and anal canal, the umbilicus, the bare area of the liver and the retroperitoneum. These are of importance in the presentations of portal hypertension.

Pathophysiology

The aetiology of portal hypertension can be classified as prehepatic, intrahepatic and posthepatic. Prehepatic portal hypertension is usually due to thrombosis involving the portal venous system. Examples of prehepatic causes of portal hypertension include pancreatitis, prothrombotic states and umbilical sepsis in neonates. The commonest category of portal hypertension in developed countries is intrahepatic and is caused by cirrhosis. Cirrhosis causes increased resistance to portal venous flow, resulting in increased portal venous pressure. Activation of stellate cells and myofibroblasts also occurs, with resulting increase in secretion of vasoactive agents that can increase portal venous flow. Posthepatic portal hypertension is caused by Budd–Chiari syndrome, in which a prothrombotic state results in thrombosis of the hepatic veins, or right heart failure.

Presentation

Patients with portal hypertension can remain asymptomatic or present with ascites, bleeding or hepatic encephalopathy. Ascites can lead to abdominal discomfort, the development of hernias, particularly umbilical, and spontaneous bacterial peritonitis. The latter results from the translocation of gut bacteria into ascites and has a significant risk of mortality. Portal hypertensive bleeding results from the formation of portosystemic anastomoses. Increased resistance within the portal venous system results in preferential flow through these anastomoses as a path of least resistance. The umbilical vein can dilate significantly in portal hypertension

Textbook of Surgery, Fourth Edition. Edited by Julian A. Smith, Andrew H. Kaye, Christopher Christophi and Wendy A. Brown.
© 2020 John Wiley & Sons Ltd. Published 2020 by John Wiley & Sons Ltd.

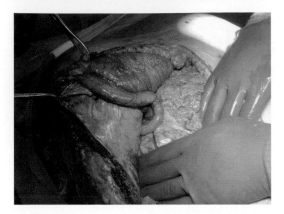

Fig. 24.1 Large recanalised umbilical vein due to cirrhosis.

(Figure 24.1), with decompression through the periumbilical veins, leading to the clinical sign of caput medusae. Anastomoses between the coronary vein and oesophageal veins leads to the development of oesophageal varices. Erosion of the mucosa overlying oesophageal varices can lead to torrential life-threatening haemorrhage. Bleeding can also occur due to gastric varices, portal hypertensive gastropathy, rectal varices and, rarely, retroperitoneal varices.

Diagnosis

The patient with portal hypertension may have a known diagnosis of cirrhosis or other causes of portal hypertension, such as pancreatitis or a prothrombotic state. Symptoms due to cirrhosis such as jaundice and lethargy may be present. The patient may present with symptoms of portal hypertension itself, such as abdominal distension, gastrointestinal bleeding or encephalopathy.

Examination should be focused on detecting the signs of chronic liver disease, liver failure and portal hypertension. The general appearance of the patient may give clues to the diagnosis. In particular, there may be drowsiness or confusion due to hepatic encephalopathy, jaundice or muscle wasting, which is often particularly evident around the shoulders. The hands should be examined for clubbing, leuconychia and palmar erythema. Dupuytren's contracture may be present in a patient with a history of alcoholism. A hepatic flap or fetor hepaticus may be evident in cases of liver failure. Parotidomegaly may occur in cases of alcoholic cirrhosis. Sparsity of chest hair and gynaecomastia may be present in males with cirrhosis. On inspection of the abdomen, caput medusae and abdominal distension may be evident. The liver may be

large (particularly in cases of cholestatic liver disease, such as primary sclerosing cholangitis), normal in size or small. The liver edge is likely to be firm and nodular in cases of cirrhosis. Splenomegaly, if present, strongly supports the diagnosis of portal hypertension, but the absence of a palpable spleen does not exclude the diagnosis. Shifting dullness will be present if there is a significant quantity of ascites. Testicular atrophy may be present.

Significant portal hypertension is usually accompanied by thrombocytopenia. The aetiology was thought to be sequestration of platelets in the enlarged spleen. However, it is likely that reduced production of thrombopoietin by the liver and increased destruction of platelets are also of importance.

Imaging may reveal evidence of cirrhosis, splenomegaly, varices, which are often most evident in the left upper quadrant and around the oesophagus, thrombosis involving the portal venous system, hepatic vein thrombosis or ascites. Oesophageal varices may be evident on upper gastrointestinal endoscopy.

The diagnosis is confirmed by demonstrating elevation of the hepatic venous pressure gradient, calculated as the hepatic venous wedge pressure minus the hepatic venous pressure. Hepatic venous wedge pressure is measured by using a balloon catheter to occlude the hepatic vein and the resulting pressure measurement indicates the pressure within the hepatic sinusoids, which in cirrhosis is equivalent to portal venous pressure. A hepatic venous pressure gradient of 5 mmHg or more indicates portal hypertension and is clinically relevant when it is 10 mmHg or more.

Ascites

The mainstay of treatment of ascites is medical therapy. Ascites can often be controlled with diuretic therapy, usually a combination of spironolactone and frusemide. Fluid and salt restriction are also appropriate. Symptomatic ascites that is resistant to diuretic therapy may require paracentesis, whereby a cannula is inserted percutaneously into the peritoneal cavity to drain ascites. Care should be taken during insertion to avoid injury to the bowel, liver and spleen and this is aided by using an ultrasound-guided technique. Ascites should be drained slowly and intravenous concentrated albumin given during paracentesis to avoid haemodynamic instability. For patients requiring frequent paracentesis, transjugular intrahepatic portosystemic shunt (TIPS) may be required (Figure 24.2). TIPS is a percutaneous radiological procedure that

(a)

(b)

(c)

(d)

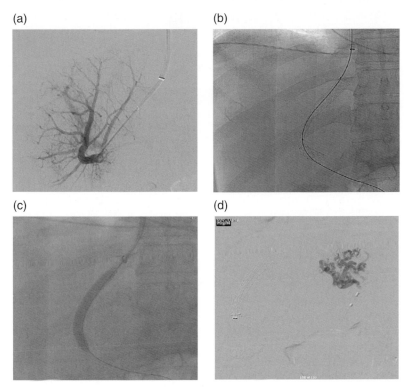

Fig. 24.2 Transjugular intrahepatic portosystemic shunt procedure. (a) Puncture of the right portal vein via the hepatic vein (the middle hepatic vein in this case) with portal venogram. (b) Deployment of metal stent between the middle hepatic vein and left portal vein. (c) Balloon dilatation of the stent. (d) Final position of the stent. The catheter was passed into the oesophageal varices, which are displayed in the venogram (variceal sclerotherapy and embolisation were subsequently performed in this case).

creates a low resistance channel between the portal and systemic venous systems, most commonly between the right portal vein and right hepatic vein, resulting in decompression of the portal venous system and thus amelioration or resolution of the complications of portal hypertension.

The potential complications of TIPS include technical failure, encephalopathy, bleeding, cardiac arrhythmias, haemolytic anaemia and stent stenosis. Encephalopathy in this situation is due to metabolites from the portal venous system bypassing the liver, which would normally remove toxins before they can enter the systemic circulation. The risk factors for encephalopathy complicating TIPS procedures include a high degree of shunting, advanced age, increased severity of liver failure and the presence of encephalopathy before TIPS was performed. Bleeding can occur at the puncture site in the neck or can occasionally occur as a perihepatic haematoma. Recurrent portal hypertension following TIPS can occur as a result of thrombosis of the TIPS stent, kinking or retraction of the stent, pseudointimal hyperplasia or the development of right heart failure. Long-term patency of the TIPS

stent can be attained with revision percutaneous procedures as required.

Surgery, including portosystemic shunt surgery and peritoneo-venous shunt surgery, has been performed, but has limited success and has largely been replaced by TIPS procedures.

Bleeding

Multiple interventions have been developed for the prevention and management of variceal bleeding complicating portal hypertension and the management of this problem has evolved over time. The recommended approach to primary prophylaxis, management of bleeding varices and secondary prophylaxis is shown in Figure 24.3. Patients with cirrhosis should undergo endoscopic surveillance to detect oesophageal varices. Primary prophylaxis (prevention of bleeding from varices) is undertaken with a non-selective beta-blocker or endoscopic variceal banding.

The patient with bleeding varices should be resuscitated immediately. In addition to the

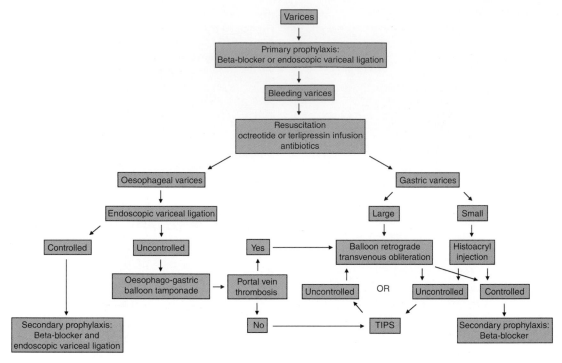

Fig. 24.3 Recommended approach to primary prophylaxis, management of bleeding varices and secondary prophylaxis.

insertion of two large-bore intravenous cannulas and commencement of blood transfusion, reversal of coagulopathy, including the use of Prothrombinex and fresh frozen plasma, may be required. A vaso-active agent (terlipressin or octreotide infusion) and broad-spectrum prophylactic antibiotics should be commenced. Emergency endoscopy is performed and bleeding oesophageal varices are banded. If oesophageal varices are not controlled by endo-scopic variceal ligation, balloon tamponade may be required. If the portal vein is patent, TIPS should be performed. If portal vein thrombosis is present in the patient with bleeding oesophageal varices refractory to endoscopic therapy, balloon-occluded retrograde transvenous obliteration (BRTO) is indi-cated. This procedure is performed by accessing the varices via a spontaneous portosystemic shunt, such as a gastrorenal shunt, occluding the outflow of the varix and injecting a sclerosing agent.

Small bleeding gastric varices are managed by endoscopic injection of histoacryl glue. If this is unsuccessful, TIPS is required. Large bleeding gas-tric varices can be managed by either BRTO or TIPS. Failure to control bleeding with BRTO neces-sitates TIPS and vice versa.

Secondary prophylaxis (prevention of rebleed-ing) is undertaken with a combination of a non-selective beta-blocker and endoscopic variceal banding for oesophageal varices and a beta-blocker for gastric varices.

Surgical procedures for portal hypertension are now very rarely required. The procedures that were developed included shunt procedures and devascu-larisation procedures. Shunt surgery includes the creation of non-selective, selective and partial shunts. Non-selective shunts divert all the portal flow away from the liver and are effective in reduc-ing the portocaval pressure gradient, but have a sig-nificant risk of hepatic encephalopathy, since there is no first-pass detoxification of the portal blood by the liver, and can also accelerate the progression of liver failure, since the liver will now lack the trophic influence of portal venous inflow. Non-selective shunts were used for active portal hypertensive bleeding, medically intractable ascites, anatomical incompatibility with a distal spleno-renal shunt and bleeding stomal varices. Examples of non-selective shunts are end-to-side portocaval shunt, side-to-side portocaval shunt, large diameter interposition portocaval shunt, interposition mesocaval shunt and side-to-side spleno-renal shunt.

Selective shunts preserve portal perfusion to the liver, resulting in a lower risk of encephalopathy and liver failure but a higher risk of portal vein thrombosis. Non-selective shunts require a splenic vein of at least 6 mm diameter and proximity of the splenic and renal veins and portal flow towards the liver (hepatopedal). The usual indication was portal hypertension with absent or medically controlled ascites. Active variceal bleeding is a contraindication. The commonest selective shunt was the distal spleno-renal (Warren shunt), which was performed by mobilising and transecting the splenic vein close to its insertion into the superior mesenteric/portal vein junction and anastomosing the splenic vein end-to-side to the left renal vein and dividing the coronary vein. This diverts the portal venous blood in the left upper quadrant through the shunt into the systemic circulation. Another example of a selective shunt is the left gastric-caval (Inokuchi) shunt.

Partial shunts were designed to incompletely decompress the entire portal venous system, whilst maintaining portal perfusion of the liver. This was achieved by using a small-diameter (8–10 mm) shunt. They were associated with a lower rate of postoperative encephalopathy and liver failure compared with non-selective shunts. Requirements for a partial shunt include compensated (Child–Pugh A or B) cirrhosis, a patent portal vein and preferably no previous surgery in the right upper quadrant. Examples of partial shunts are small-diameter portocaval, mesocaval and mesorenal interposition shunts and the small-diameter side-to-side portocaval shunt.

Devascularisation procedures involve devascularisation of the lower oesophagus over a variable extent (generally 5 cm) and stomach (usually sparing the stomach distal to the incisura), usually accompanied by splenectomy and sometimes by oesophageal transection. These operations are to some extent simpler than shunt procedures and were therefore suited to less specialised centres and in developing countries. They have a lower rate of encephalopathy than shunt procedures, but a higher rate of rebleeding. When accompanied by oesophageal transection, there is a risk of stricture and leak. The indications include an unshuntable patient, such as one with diffuse splanchnic venous thrombosis, recurrent bleeding after shunt surgery and massive splenomegaly with pressure symptoms or hypersplenism. Examples of devascularisation include the Sigura procedure (which is performed via the chest and abdomen) and the modified Sigura procedure (which is performed via the abdomen only and includes excision of the fundus).

Liver transplantation results in surgical correction of portal hypertension and is the treatment of choice for appropriately selected patients with end-stage liver disease (see Chapter 10). It results in decompression of varices, resolution of ascites and encephalopathy, and reversal of the sarcopenic effects of liver failure. In potential liver transplant candidates, the management of portal hypertension should take account of technical factors that might impact on transplantation surgery. For example, the placement of the stent in performing a TIPS procedure has to be carefully planned to ensure the safe removal of the stent at the time of transplantation.

Hepatic encephalopathy

Hepatic encephalopathy is a neuropsychiatric complication of portal hypertension that can result in symptoms ranging from subtle disturbance of mood to confusion to coma. This condition occurs as a result of resistance to portal venous flow in the liver and portosystemic shunts that divert neuroactive peptides into the systemic circulation rather than through the liver, where they would normally be detoxified. Ammonia accumulates in the circulation and can cause cerebral oedema and alterations in astrocyte mitochondrial function, although it is likely that cytokines and other agents contribute.

Strategies that reduce production and absorption of ammonia in the intestine, such as lactulose and antibiotics including rifaximin, are used to reduce the severity of hepatic encephalopathy.

Surgery on the patient with cirrhosis

There are several principles in considering surgical intervention in the patient with cirrhosis. Firstly, one should determine whether the operation is really indicated. The balance of risks and benefits in the presence of cirrhosis is skewed because of the increased risks of surgery, including increased risks of bleeding and decompensation of liver function and therefore an increased perioperative mortality risk. Liver function should be assessed. The Child–Pugh score is a measure of liver function that helps to predict the risk of morbidity and mortality in patients with cirrhosis who require surgery (Table 24.1). Liver function can also be quantified by the model for end-stage liver disease (MELD) score. The MELD score is calculated as:

$$9.57 \times \log_e (\text{creatinine,mg / dL}) + 3.78 \times \log_e (\text{bilirubin,mg / dL}) + 11.2 \times \log_e (\text{INR}) + 6.43$$

rounded to the nearest integer. Online calculators are available to calculate these scores. Both Child–Pugh and MELD scores have been shown to be

Table 24.1 Calculation of Child–Pugh score.

Score	1	2	3
Bilirubin (µmol/L)	<34	34–51	>51
Albumin (g/L)	>35	28–35	<28
INR	<1.7	1.7–2.2	>2.2
Ascites	Absent	Slight	Moderate
Encephalopathy	None	Grade 1 or 2	Grade 3 or 4

Patients with a Child–Pugh score of 5 or 6 are class A, those with a Child–Pugh score of 7–9 are class B and those with a Child–Pugh score ≥10 are class C.

Table 24.2 The 90-day mortality following abdominal surgery in patients with cirrhosis.

Variable	90-day mortality (%)
Child–Pugh class	
A	12
B	24
C	70
MELD score	
6–9	12
10–19	29
20–29	75
30–40	91

Source: modified from Neeff HP, Streule GC, Drognitz O *et al*. Early mortality and long-term survival after abdominal surgery in patients with liver cirrhosis. *Surgery* 2014;155:623–32. Reproduced with permission of Elsevier.

predictive of perioperative mortality for a variety of surgical procedures (see Table 24.2). Secondly, non-surgical alternatives should be contemplated for management of the problem. For example, endoscopic stenting should be considered as an alternative to resection or bypass and conservative management of gallstones should be considered as an alternative to cholecystectomy. Thirdly, consideration should be given to transferring the patient to a hepato-pancreato-biliary or transplant unit. However, conditions requiring emergency surgical management should be dealt with locally, as delay in arranging transfer could result in deterioration in the patient's condition. Fourthly, if surgery is to be performed, attention to appropriate preoperative preparation is required. Consultation with a hepatologist is recommended. Preoperative management may include hydration and possibly commencement of a terlipression infusion to reverse the impact of hepatorenal syndrome, reversal of coagulopathy as well as the standard preparation normally required for the patient's surgical condition. Blood should be cross-matched. Platelets and coagulation factors, such as fresh frozen plasma and cryoprecipitate, may be required intraoperatively. Thromboelastography, which enables point-of-care assessment of clot formation and thrombolysis, can be used in addition to standard coagulation tests to guide management of coagulation. The intraoperative management of the patient with cirrhosis requires experienced anaesthetic and surgical teams.

Cholecystectomy

For the patient with cirrhosis requiring cholecystectomy, the basic approach is similar to that in the patient without cirrhosis, although there are some details which require attention. The Hasson port should be placed in an infraumbilical position to minimise the risk of bleeding from the umbilical vein and adjacent veins. Care should be taken when retracting the gallbladder, since a tear at the edge of the gallbladder fossa can cause bleeding that is extremely difficult to control. If there are varices in Calot's triangle, subtotal cholecystectomy, dividing the neck of the gallbladder, can be performed (Figure 24.4). In addition, the gallbladder wall can be left on the liver to prevent bleeding from the gallbladder fossa. Placement of a subhepatic drain is recommended in such cases.

Umbilical hernia

Umbilical hernia commonly occurs in patients with cirrhosis, particularly in the presence of ascites. Umbilical hernia repair can be performed safely, even in patients with decompensated cirrhosis. The mortality rate (1%) and recurrence rate (3%) are acceptable, although the morbidity (26%) is higher than in patients without cirrhosis. The morbidity is higher for emergency than elective surgery and therefore it is preferable to manage umbilical hernia electively if possible. The sac should be left intact if possible or closed in watertight fashion if this is not possible. Mesh repair is recommended. Meticulous haemostasis is required. The subcutaneous space should be drained.

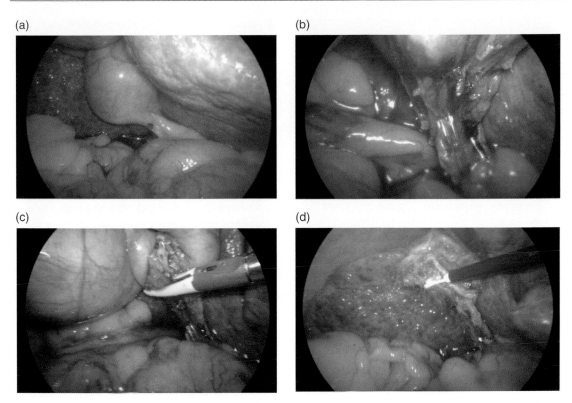

Fig. 24.4 Subtotal cholecystectomy in a patient with frequent biliary colic and compensated cirrhosis. (a) Gallbladder and cirrhotic liver. (b) The cystic duct has been clipped and divided. Varices can be seen around the cystic artery. (c) Subtotal cholecystectomy, starting with transection through the neck of the gallbladder, performed with Ligasure, leaving gallbladder wall on liver. (d) Mucosa of residual gallbladder ablated with argon beam coagulator.

Bowel resection

Bowel resection is generally performed in similar fashion to that in the non-cirrhotic patient. As with any operation in a patient with cirrhosis, care is required to ensure adequate haemostasis during entry into the abdomen and during mobilisation. The use of the Ligasure and argon beam coagulator can assist with this. If the procedure is being performed for an indication other than cancer, the mesentery should be divided close to the bowel. Care should be taken to ensure haemostasis when dividing the mesentery, such as by performing suture ligation. Proctectomy should be avoided in the patient with cirrhosis. For example, a patient with ulcerative colitis and primary sclerosing cholangitis can be managed with total colectomy, if required, with proctectomy deferred until after liver transplantation.

Liver resection

Liver resection may be required in the patient with hepatocellular carcinoma complicating cirrhosis. Decompensated cirrhosis is a contraindication to liver resection. Small (<3 cm) tumours that are not subcapsular or close to portal structures can be treated with percutaneous radiofrequency or microwave ablation with similar results to resection. Laparoscopic resection can be performed with reduced perioperative morbidity and length of hospital stay in comparison with open resection. The minimum future liver remnant required for safe liver resection in the presence of cirrhosis is generally considered to be 40% of the preoperative non-tumour liver volume.

Further reading

Bloom S, Kemp W, Lubel J. Portal hypertension: pathophysiology, diagnosis and management. *Intern Med J* 2015;45:16–26.

Hew S, Yu W, Robson S *et al*. Safety and effectiveness of umbilical hernia repair in patients with cirrhosis. *Hernia* 2018;22:759–65.

Neeff HP, Streule GC, Drognitz O *et al*. Early mortality and long-term survival after abdominal surgery in patients with liver cirrhosis. *Surgery* 2014;155:623–32.

MCQs

Select the single correct answer to each question. The correct answers can be found in the Answers section at the end of the book.

1 Clinically significant portal hypertension:
   a occurs with a hepatic venous pressure gradient of 5–9 mmHg
   b occurs as a result of decompression of the systemic venous system through the portal venous system
   c frequently results in bleeding from the caput medusae
   d requires endoscopic evaluation of the oesophagus
   e is a contraindication to diuretic therapy for ascites

2 Large bleeding gastric varices in the presence of portal vein thrombosis should be managed with:
   a endoscopic variceal ligation
   b endoscopic histoacryl glue injection
   c balloon retrograde transvenous obliteration
   d transjugular intrahepatic portosystemic shunt
   e distal spleno-renal shunt

3 A patient with hepatitis C virus cirrhosis has a bilirubin of 30 µmol/L, albumin of 33 g/L, INR of 1.4, slight ascites and no encephalopathy. Which of the following describes the patient's Child–Pugh status?
   a class A
   b class B
   c class C
   d cannot be calculated without knowing the creatinine
   e cannot be calculated without knowing the platelet count

4 A 67-year-old woman presents with a large painful umbilical hernia that is not reducible. She has a history of alcoholic cirrhosis complicated by ascites and has a Child–Pugh score of 12. Repair of the hernia:
   a should be performed
   b should be deferred until she is abstinent from alcohol
   c should not be performed because of the high risk of perioperative mortality
   d should be performed without mesh because of the risk of infection
   e should be deferred until the time of liver transplantation

Section 4
Lower Gastrointestinal Surgery

25 Principles of colorectal and small bowel surgery

Ian Hayes

University of Melbourne and Colorectal Surgery Unit, Royal Melbourne Hospital, Melbourne, Victoria, Australia

Introduction

Surgical procedures for small and large bowel pathology involve major operations, often in acutely ill patients with pre-existing medical problems. The physiological impact of abdominal surgery is significant, even in previously healthy patients. Postoperative complications develop out of sight, in the closed cavity of the abdomen and it can be difficult to determine if the patient's physiological alterations are just the expected changes of the recovery process or the first manifestations of a major complication. An understanding of the preoperative preparation, of the principles underlying the operative procedures and of the issues specific to postoperative care is relevant to any doctor involved with these patients.

Preoperative preparation

As for any major surgical procedure, the patient's general medical fitness is important. The majority of patients having major abdominal surgery are older and will have medical comorbidity. The surgeon must be familiar with the patient's pre-existing medical conditions. The decision as to which, if indeed any, operation is appropriate for the patient is based on an understanding of his or her ability to withstand the operation and anaesthetic; to heal the tissues that have been operated on; and, importantly in abdominal surgery, to withstand the physiological challenges of the recovery process.

A separate consideration is the issue of optimising, rather than just assessing, medical fitness. Conditions such as aortic stenosis and reversible myocardial ischaemia may require intervention prior to abdominal surgery. Tachyarrhythmias may require rate control, diabetic control may need to be improved

and hypertension stabilised. Cigarette smoking should cease, alcohol use decrease, the obese should lose weight, and nutritional supplements should be considered for the undernourished.

Anticoagulant use and antiplatelet agents need to be carefully considered. Good haemostasis is very important in bowel surgery. A haematoma in the mesentery can contribute to anastomotic leak, and bleeding into the peritoneal cavity can be very significant as there is nothing to tamponade it. Anticoagulants and antiplatelet agents should be ceased if this is medically safe. If it is not medically safe to cease these agents, then irreversible agents need to be converted to reversible agents and/or long-acting agents converted to short-acting. For example, anticoagulants for low-risk atrial fibrillation can often be ceased for several weeks, whilst anticoagulants used with a mechanical mitral valve repair may need to be converted to short-acting agents and only withheld for the immediate perioperative period.

Patients receiving chemotherapy for cancer or immunosuppressants for inflammatory bowel disease may be able to have surgery scheduled during a medication-free interval. Alternatively, the surgical plan may need to change in anticipation of poor wound healing, creating a stoma for instance rather than a higher-risk anastomosis.

In emergency cases or cancer procedures, there may not be enough time available to optimise all the medical conditions of the patient; nevertheless, the surgical plan should still be based on the patient's underlying fitness.

Who will require a stoma?

A stoma may be created proximally to protect an anastomosis or it may be created instead of an anastomosis (e.g. Hartmann's procedure).

The following conditions make stoma creation more likely.

- Bowel quality factors: chronic radiation change, acute colitis, faecal peritonitis, ischaemia or obstruction may create poor local conditions for the formation of an anastomosis and mean that a stoma is a safer option.
- Patient factors: malnutrition, immunosuppression, haemodynamic instability or multiorgan failure could mean that an anastomosis is likely to have poor healing and make a stoma a safer choice.
- Deep pelvic anastomosis: most patients with ileo-anal pouch or ultra-low anterior resection will receive a temporary defunctioning loop ileostomy to divert the faecal flow away from the anastomosis during the first 3 months to facilitate healing.
- Low rectal cancer: if an adequate distal clearance margin cannot be obtained, the patient is likely to receive an abdomino-perineal excision with permanent colostomy. Patients with rectal cancer less than 5 cm from the anal verge have a high likelihood of permanent colostomy.
- Anticipated faecal incontinence: a restorative resection will generally not be performed in patients who have pre-existing poor sphincter function, as the loss of colonic length with resection is likely to worsen incontinence.
- Irresectable disease (e.g. advanced cancer): a proximal defunctioning stoma may be required due to obstruction or perforation. In this case the area of disease has not been resected and the stoma is used as a temporising manoeuvre or for palliation.

Preoperative planning of stoma site is very important and stoma therapy nurses play a crucial role in education, planning and management. The stoma must be sited away from incisions, bony prominences, skin creases and give due attention to position of clothing. Stomas are also discussed in Chapter 26).

Mechanical bowel preparation

Mechanical cleansing of the bowel prior to colorectal surgery is not an absolute prerequisite but many surgeons prefer to operate with the bowel prepared. There is good evidence that it is safe to perform colonic anastomosis without bowel preparation. Full preparation of the colon remains a requirement for colonoscopy. For rectal resections, at the very least a preoperative enema is required to remove stool mass from the rectum to facilitate use of a circular stapler that will be inserted through the anus.

Bowel preparations can be divided into two types, hyperosmolar and iso-osmolar.

- Hyperosmolar preparations are usually phosphate or sulphate salt solutions taken orally as a relatively small-volume drink. The bowel is cleaned by their powerful osmotic effect. Although patients often prefer these small-volume formulations, they can cause fluid and electrolyte disturbances in medically frail patients.
- Iso-osmolar preparations are usually polyethylene glycol-based. These involve drinking several litres of fluid but with minimal risk of systemic fluid and electrolyte shifts because the solution remains in the bowel lumen without exerting an osmotic effect. Paradoxically, these high-volume solutions are safe for patients with renal and cardiac failure who may be on oral fluid restriction.

Bowel preparation will require the patient to be restricted to just clear fluids by mouth on the day before the procedure. This generally decreases caloric intake and will have implications for diabetes management.

Preoperative investigations

Operative planning is highly dependent on preoperative imaging. Colonoscopy is the principal means of viewing the colorectal and distal ileal mucosa, but to view the surrounding extraluminal tissues requires a three-dimensional imaging technique such as CT or MRI.

Colonoscopy is performed for most patients having colorectal or ileal resection. In addition to allowing biopsy and visualisation of the mucosal disease being considered for resection, a complete preoperative colonoscopy excludes other unexpected tumours or major polyps. It can also be used to insert submucosal marker dye at the site of a lesion to allow the area to be found from the serosal surface at operation. It can be very helpful to have repeated confirmation of the exact position of a lesion, especially the distance from the anal verge and the amount of normal bowel distal to the lesion that will remain after resection. If conditions prevent complete colonoscopy, CT colonography is a useful method of imaging the mucosa.

CT is an important part of cancer staging but also gives information about the relationship of the area of interest to surrounding structures such as ureter, iliac vessels and duodenum. Magnetic resonance enterography is used in the assessment of small bowel Crohn's disease.

Routine blood tests will be required for patients having major surgery.

Conceptualising the anastomosis as a 'graft'

It seems obvious to state that surgery on small and large bowel usually involves removal of a segment of bowel and anastomosis of the two ends. However, to achieve this the two ends of bowel, especially if colon is involved, will need to be mobilised quite a long distance from their previous anatomical sites, whilst preserving an intact blood supply. In many ways, such an anastomosis is similar to a vascularised pedicle graft in plastic and reconstructive surgery, except that the graft is no longer visible to the surgeon once the abdomen is closed and any leakage from the suture line is potentially life-threatening. Continuing with this analogy, maintaining a well-perfused graft requires that the patient has a good cardiac output, adequate blood pressure and haemoglobin, and be well oxygenated and nourished. Thus, for patients having major surgery of the lower gastrointestinal tract, it is important that their general physiological state be kept as normal as possible, during and after the operation, to optimise perfusion of the pedicle graft that forms their bowel anastomosis.

Colon: significance of blood supply

The colon has three main vascular pedicles: the ileocolic vessels supplying right colon; middle colic vessels supplying transverse colon; and inferior mesenteric (IM) vessels supplying left colon. Connecting these pedicles are the marginal vessels which run in the mesentery, parallel and close to the colonic wall. The multiple vascular arcades of the small bowel mesentery, which ensure a rich blood supply, are not present in the colonic mesentery.

Most colon cancer operations involve resecting the tumour-containing segment of large bowel, its mesentery and associated vascular pedicle. The vascular pedicle contains the lymph nodes to which the tumour is likely to metastasise and its resection achieves lymphatic clearance. However, this interrupts the blood flow to the bowel and creates an ischaemic segment of colon. Exactly how much colon is made ischaemic will depend on the collateral flow along the marginal vessels coming from adjacent vascular pedicles. This is the reason why resection of a relatively small cancer involves removal of a much larger segment of large bowel than might have been expected. For instance, in ultra-low anterior resection to treat a rectal cancer,

the IM pedicle is ligated. This creates an ischaemic segment of sigmoid, possibly extending as far as the descending colon. In this operation, the sigmoid and most of the rectum are resected. This means that the remaining viable, proximal end of descending colon will need to be mobilised from its normal position in the mid abdomen down to the deepest part of the pelvis to create an anastomosis near the anorectal junction. An important technical point is that the blood supply will need to travel a considerable distance from its origin at the middle colic artery, along a small-calibre marginal vessel. It is vital that the marginal vessel is not damaged during dissection.

Occasionally, colonic vascular pedicles are divided, not for oncological reasons but to increase mobility of a segment of bowel. Dividing the IM vessels close to their origin near the aorta creates much more mobility of the left colon than dividing distal branches of these vessels close to the bowel wall. In a non-cancer operation, such as resection of sigmoid diverticular disease, this may allow creation of an anastomosis with less tension.

Rectal anatomy: mesorectum

The surgical anatomy of the rectum has some differences to the rest of the large bowel. The colon can be regarded as a tube-like hollow organ, with a veil of mesentery and blood supply suspended from its posterior aspect. In early fetal development, the rectum starts as a similar tube with a posterior mesentery and blood supply derived from the IM vessels. With growth, the rectum is elongated down into the pelvis but its main vascular pedicle remains in position proximally. The usual configuration of a posteriorly situated mesentery now changes to wrap around the posterolateral aspects of both sides of the rectum, forming the mesorectum. The mesorectum attenuates at the distal rectum and terminates near the anorectal junction (Figure 25.1). The significance of the mesorectum is that it contains the lymphatic drainage of the rectum and thus needs to be removed as an intact package in rectal cancer surgery. Furthermore, the dissection plane just outside the fascia encompassing the mesorectum is relatively bloodless. Total mesorectal excision refers to a surgical technique that carefully follows this plane to allow oncologically complete resection of rectal cancer while minimising damage to the autonomic nerves of the pelvis and limiting blood loss.

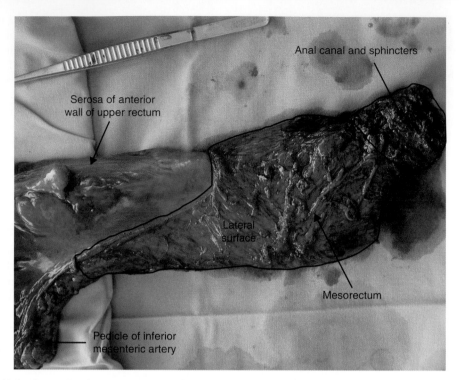

Fig. 25.1 Abdomino-perineal excision specimen showing rectum and anal canal. The blood supply is from the inferior mesenteric artery pedicle which curves downwards into the mesorectum. The mesorectal 'package' can be seen to wrap around the lower rectum, contour to fill the hollow of the sacrum and attenuate at the anorectal junction.

Achieving colon mobility: embryological basis

To reconstruct the colon and rectum after resection requires mobilisation of the remaining proximal and distal segments. The length of bowel resected with some operations can be greater than 60 cm, which leaves a significant distance to bridge between the ends. Although much of the colon is tethered to the retroperitoneum, it is possible to restore the colon to its mobile, early embryological, midline position by appropriate division of adhesions while preserving vascular supply.

The whole gastrointestinal tract starts as a midline organ *in utero* with its mesentery and blood supply coming from the aorta posteriorly. From the 10th week of life onwards, the gut undergoes an anticlockwise 270° rotation to occupy its final position. This leaves the colon overlying the duodenum, with lateral adhesions on the right and left side keeping it in a fixed, mostly retroperitoneal, position. Dividing these embryological adhesions (zygoses) and straightening out the acute angles of the splenic and hepatic flexures creates considerable length of mobile bowel.

Anastomoses

Anastomoses can be classified by their configuration (end-to-end, end-to-side, side-to-side) or technique (hand-sewn or stapled). Usually, anastomoses of the lower rectum are stapled due to the access difficulties of hand-sewing deep in the pelvis. For all other anastomoses, technique is largely based on surgeon preference and there is little difference in outcome among the various types.

Configuration

- End-to-end is the most intuitive way to approximate two segments of bowel. Difficulties may arise, however, if there is discrepancy between the luminal diameter of the two ends (e.g. end of ileum to rectum). Furthermore, because the blood supply is derived from vessels which run at 90° to the direction of the bowel lumen, the end of the bowel segment may be the least vascularised.
- End-to-side or side-to-side generally ensures a well-vascularised anastomosis but each requires plenty of mobility to align the bowel in this fashion.

Method

Suturing

This can be done by multiple methods, with multiple different suture materials. What is required of any method of securing an anastomosis is that the two ends of bowel are approximated and held together until reasonably strong wound healing with native tissue is achieved. Most commonly, a single layer of interrupted sutures is used. The sutures must exert sufficient tension to create an airtight seal but not be so tight as to cause tissue ischaemia.

Staplers

There are three types: linear staplers, linear cutting staplers and circular staplers. Stapling devices are loaded with multiple small titanium staples that are deployed in rows.

- Linear staplers simply fire a linear double row of staples to close off one end of a bowel segment (e.g. proximal end of rectal stump in Hartmann's procedure).
- Linear cutting staplers fire two parallel double rows of staples and automatically cut between them. These are the typical staplers used to join the two lumens of a side-to-side anastomosis. The term 'functional end-to-end anastomosis' usually refers to a type of side-to-side configuration performed with two separate firings of a linear cutting stapler. The two ends are joined like the legs of a pair of trousers.
- Circular staplers are inserted into the bowel lumen and fire a circular double row of staples to join two ends of bowel. These instruments consist of two parts: a circular anvil which is secured to the open end of the proximal bowel and the main part introduced though the anus. Docking of these components brings the two ends of bowel together, after which the staple line is fired and two 'doughnuts' of redundant tissue from each end are produced. Most commonly, this type of anastomosis is performed though a rectal stump previously stapled off with a linear stapler; the resulting join is referred to as a double-stapled anastomosis.

Surgical approach

Traditionally, surgery of the small and large bowel has been performed through a vertical midline laparotomy. In appropriate cases, the right colon or sigmoid can be treated using shorter transverse or oblique muscle-splitting incisions.

Laparoscopic surgery is now the preferred approach when possible. It is important to understand that the intra-abdominal component of laparoscopic surgery is very similar to what is done during open surgery. In general, the bowel mobilisation and division of vascular pedicles are performed laparoscopically; the mobilised bowel is brought up to the surface using a short umbilical or suprapubic incision; and the diseased area is resected and the anastomosis formed at the surface.

Dense adhesions from previous surgery, complex tumours and complex Crohn's disease may favour open laparotomy over a laparoscopic approach.

Operative issues relevant to postoperative care

The detail of the conditions encountered during the procedure informs the postoperative care. For example, extensive division of intraperitoneal adhesions, with associated tissue trauma and prolonged bowel handling, is likely to result in a prolonged postoperative ileus. It also has a risk of unseen injury to the bowel wall and subsequent leakage. Extensive intraoperative bleeding can result in ongoing bleeding. Intraoperative spillage of enteric contents can cause postoperative infection, collections and ileus.

The anatomical site of the bowel resection also alerts the surgical team to potential complications resulting from damage to other organs. The caecum is close to the right ureter and the sigmoid is close to the left. Mobilisation of the right colon can injure the duodenum; the spleen and the pancreatic tail are at risk of injury during splenic flexure mobilisation. Nerve damage from pelvic dissection can produce urinary retention or incontinence.

Postoperative care

Operations on the large and small bowel cause significant changes to the patient's physiological state. It is important to become familiar with the usual patterns of these physiological changes and to note that all physiological parameters improve quite quickly during a routine recovery process (Box 25.1). What is important to recognise is deviation from the expected pattern and to distinguish between the normal recovery process and the warning signs of complications.

> **Box 25.1 Expected postoperative changes**
>
> Abdominal pain
> Abdominal tenderness near the wound
> Decreased mobility
> Ileus (anorexia, nausea, abdominal distension, constipation)
> Atelectasis
> Low urine output
> Mild fever
> Mild tachycardia
> Blood tests: increased C-reactive protein; decreased potassium, haemoglobin, albumin

With any deviation in the patient's course from the expected pattern, the treating doctors must ask themselves whether this could be a manifestation of an intra-abdominal complication. The most serious of these will be gut ischaemia or anastomotic leak. These catastrophic complications are uncommon but may start insidiously and escalate to sepsis, peritonitis and multiorgan failure. Thus, a single abnormality in a patient who is progressing well should be examined but is unlikely to represent a major complication. An example of this is a raised temperature of 38.1°C in a patient who is otherwise progressing well. However, the finding of a fever in a patient with prolonged ileus, escalating abdominal pain and tachycardia is much more concerning.

A further important issue is that all postoperative complications must be treated proactively. A chest infection arising from postoperative atelectasis may not seem to have implications for the bowel recovery but if the patient becomes systemically unwell from this, perfusion of the anastomosis may be compromised and could result in anastomotic leak.

In simplistic terms, the patient must be kept well to maximise the likelihood of the anastomosis healing. If the patient becomes unwell postoperatively, the clinician must also be alert to the possibility that this could be the first sign of an intra-abdominal complication.

Enhanced recovery after surgery

Enhanced recovery after surgery (ERAS) programs usual consist of a series of 15–20 interventions designed to accelerate recovery after lower gastrointestinal surgery and decrease the rate of complications. Individually, the treatments do not always have a strong evidence base to support their use, but used together they have been shown to improve postoperative outcomes. The regimens used vary between hospitals and continue to evolve over time.

Protocols are instituted preoperatively, intraoperatively and postoperatively.
- Preoperative interventions include decreased fasting and careful preoperative counselling.
- Intraoperative interventions include the use of minimally invasive surgical techniques, restricted use of intravenous fluids, use of short-acting anaesthetic agents and decreased opioid use.
- Postoperative interventions include early mobilisation and early feeding, minimisation of opioid and intravenous fluid use, avoiding routine nasogastric tubes and drains, and early removal of urinary catheters.

Even in hospitals which do not formally use these programs, there has been a general acceptance that bowel preparation is not mandatory, that the period of preoperative fasting can be shortened, that restricting intravenous fluid use is safe and that low urine output, of itself, does not need to be aggressively corrected. Early mobilisation after gastrointestinal surgery and early feeding are safe. Setting expectations for early discharge is beneficial for the patient and the health system.

Further reading

Heald RJ. The 'Holy Plane' of rectal surgery. *J R Soc Med* 1988;81:503–8.

Kiran RP, Murray AC, Chiuzan C, Estrada D, Forde K. Combined preoperative mechanical bowel preparation with oral antibiotics significantly reduces surgical site infection, anastomotic leak and ileus after colorectal surgery. *Ann Surg* 2015;262:416–25.

Ljungqvist O, Scott M, Fearon KC. Enhanced recovery after surgery: a review. *JAMA Surg* 2017;152:292–8.

MCQs

Select the single correct answer to each question. The correct answers can be found in the Answers section at the end of the book.

1 Which of the following statements regarding right hemicolectomy for cancer is *incorrect*?
  a a defunctioning loop ileostomy is usually required
  b the ileocolic vessels are ligated and divided close to their origin to maximise the number of draining lymph nodes removed
  c the junction of the second and third parts of the duodenum could be injured during mobilisation of the right colon
  d it is safe to perform an anastomosis for right hemicolectomy without mechanical bowel preparation
  e the anastomosis can be stapled or sutured

2 Which of the following statements regarding a defunctioning loop ileostomy is *incorrect*?
 a it is likely to be required if an ultra-low anterior resection has been performed
 b it diverts the faecal flow away from a distal anastomosis to enhance healing
 c it is used to protect the anastomosis in an abdomino-perineal resection
 d it may be created proximal to a right hemicolectomy anastomosis if the surgeon felt the anastomosis to be at higher risk of leak than usual
 e it has two openings

3 Following a laparotomy for colon resection, which of the following statements is *incorrect*?
 a the patient is likely to experience pain when attempting to sit out of bed
 b a urine output of less than 1 mL/kg per hour should be treated with diuretics

 c most patients are not hungry
 d the pain from the abdominal wound can lead to splinting of the diaphragm and atelectasis
 e new-onset rapid atrial fibrillation at day 4 could be precipitated by an intra-abdominal problem

4 Which of the following statements regarding enhanced recovery after surgery (ERAS) programs is *incorrect*? ERAS programs
 a encourage the use of longer-acting anaesthetic agents for convenience and better pain control
 b do not require the patient to have passed flatus postoperatively before starting oral intake
 c encourage early mobilisation postoperatively
 d encourage the avoidance of routine use of surgical drains and nasogastric tubes
 e have been shown to result in earlier patient discharge

26 Physiology of small and large bowel: alterations due to surgery and disease

Jacob McCormick[1,2] and Ian Hayes[1,3]

[1] Colorectal Surgery Unit, Royal Melbourne Hospital
[2] Peter MacCallum Cancer Centre, Melbourne, Victoria, Australia
[3] Department of Surgery, University of Melbourne, Parkville, Victoria, Australia

Introduction

The small and large bowel are responsible for absorption of fluid and nutrients. Obstruction of the bowel or loss of functional absorptive capacity through surgical resection, injury or disease may cause severe derangements in circulating volume, electrolytes and nutrition. An understanding of the normal physiology of bowel function and an ability to anticipate the likely results of resection and disease are important for the care of gastrointestinal surgery patients. Patients with established intestinal failure or short bowel syndrome are uncommon but have prolonged and repeated hospital stays. Much more common are patients with prolonged ileus after abdominal surgery who require management of their short-term issues of fluid and nutritional support.

Fluid volume

The length of the small bowel can vary between 3 and 8 m. Over 8 L of fluid per day circulates through the lumen of the gastrointestinal tract but only about 200 mL is excreted in faeces. The most rapid small bowel transit occurs in the jejunum (the name means 'empty').

Approximately 3 L/day are ingested as fluid and food but this does not represent the largest component of gut fluid. The gastrointestinal tract produces an additional 0.5 L of saliva, 2 L of gastric secretions, 1.5 L of pancreatico-biliary secretions and approximately 3 L of small bowel fluid each day. A total of 7 L of fluid passes through the duodenojejunal junction daily but due to the significant reabsorptive capacity of the small bowel, only 1 L of fluid arrives in the caecum. Thus, as described in Chapter 27 on small bowel obstruction, if reabsorption is impaired very large volumes of fluid can be sequestered in the lumen of the small bowel (Box 26.1).

Electrolytes

Sodium and nutrients are absorbed actively through the bowel mucosa, whereas absorption of water is a passive process. Gastric juice contains about half the sodium concentration of extracellular fluid (ECF) but bile, pancreatic juice and small bowel fluid have a sodium concentration similar to that of ECF. Gastric juice has a high acid content, pancreatic juice is rich in bicarbonate and small bowel fluid has a high potassium concentration. In general, if intravenous fluid is required to compensate for loss of small bowel content, it will need to have a sodium concentration similar to that of ECF (e.g. 0.9% normal saline or Hartmann's solution). Vomiting, or loss via nasogastric tube, of pure gastric secretions (as in cases of gastric outlet obstruction) can produce hypochloraemic alkalosis, while excessive loss of pancreatic juice (from proximal small bowel obstruction) can produce acidosis.

Nutrients

The three classes of macronutrients – protein, carbohydrate and fat – are absorbed through the bowel. Most protein absorption occurs in the first 100 cm of the jejunum. Lipids and carbohydrates

Box 26.1 Gut fluid volumes produced per day

Ingested: 3 L
Saliva: 0.5 L
Gastric secretion: 2 L
Pancreatico-biliary secretion: 1.5 L
Small bowel secretion: 3 L

are absorbed in the jejunum and ileum. The ileum has some very specific additional functions, including absorption of bile salts and vitamin B$_{12}$. The colon has some nutritional function with absorption of medium-chain triglycerides and complex carbohydrates.

Overall, the proximal jejunum is probably the most important area for nutrition. Some patients can manage with as little as 35 cm of jejunum if it is anastomosed to an intact ileum or 60 cm if the residual jejunum is anastomosed to intact colon, but at least 150 cm of jejunum is required if there is an end-jejunostomy. The gut has a great capacity for adaptation and for increasing its absorption but this can take up to 2 years to achieve.

Stomas

Stoma is the Greek word for 'mouth' and refers to creating an opening of the bowel to the external environment through the abdominal wall. The output is collected in an appliance (stoma bag) that is attached to the skin with specially formulated glue (stomahesive). Depending on the type of output, the appliance can either be emptied or changed.

Whilst modern management of stomas is quite straightforward and patients can lead a normal lifestyle with few restrictions, having a stoma is an alteration of body image. Colorectal surgeons try to avoid creating stomas unless there is no safe or practical alternative. The reasons for creating a stoma are covered in Chapter 25.

In the presence of distal obstruction, there needs to be a means of escape for mucus created by the segment of bowel between the stoma and the obstruction. This requires either a loop stoma or a separate mucous fistula.

Principles of stoma construction

Ileostomy

This type of stoma produces a high-volume output of liquid small bowel fluid that is very corrosive to the skin. To minimise skin damage, the inner lining of the end of the ileostomy is everted back over itself for 2–4 cm to create a raised spout (Brook ileostomy) (Figure 26.1). An ileostomy is usually sited in the right iliac fossa. The output should be less than 1 L/day of fluid with porridge-like consistency. In the first few weeks following construction, the luminal diameter of an ileostomy can be quite narrow and thus at risk of obstruction due to a bolus of undigested food. For this reason, patients with ileostomy are advised to avoid foods which may be poorly digested, including sweet corn, peas, dried fruits and nuts. Generally, patients with an ileostomy created from terminal ileum have no nutritional problems.

When a stoma is created from more-proximal small bowel, the volume of output can be much higher, thus creating a potential need for supplemental fluid administration.

Colostomy

Stomas created from colon have a lower-volume output than small bowel stomas and the faecal material is less irritant to skin, and thus they are sutured without an elevated spout. Most end-colostomies utilise descending or sigmoid colon and are sited in the left iliac fossa. The output is very similar to normal faeces. Colostomies involving transverse or right colon are avoided because they produce high volumes of thick fluid which smells more offensive than ileostomy fluid (Box 26.2).

Loop stomas

Loop stomas are easier to construct and do not require a laparotomy to close. However, they are often bulkier and less easy to fit an appliance to.

End stomas

End stomas are usually the best construction.

Short-gut syndrome

Definition

Short-gut syndrome is loss of bowel mass due to resection, congenital defects or disease and is usually defined as a residual length of small bowel of less than 200 cm. Short-gut syndrome may occur due to disease, surgical resection or enterocutaneous fistulas. It may be transient, with the ability to reconstruct intestinal continuity at a later date, or

(a)

(b)

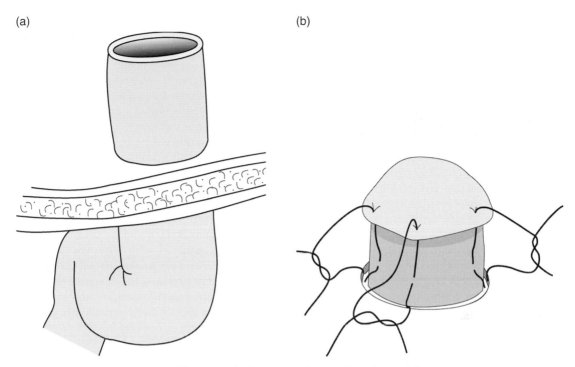

Fig. 26.1 (a) Construction of an end-ileostomy. (b) Eversion and maturation of an end-ileostomy.

Box 26.2 Complications of stomas

High-volume output (requiring fluid and electrolyte support)
Stenosis
Food bolus obstruction (ileostomies)
Hernia
Prolapse
Skin excoriation

permanent. The exact amount of bowel required to survive, independent of supports, varies between patients, with younger patients able to adapt more easily. Many patients with short-gut syndrome achieve adequate nutrition with the aid of oral supplements or intermittent injections (such as vitamin B_{12} with the loss of terminal ileum). A subset of short-gut patients develop intestinal failure. This is defined as inability to meet nutritional needs with oral intake alone and requiring parenteral nutrition. As already discussed, the relationship between remaining gut length and function is determined by the region of bowel remaining and the presence or not of a stoma. The remaining bowel adapts over a period of 6–24 months, so the need for parenteral nutrition may not be lifelong. Adaptive changes include cellular hyperplasia, increase in villous height and crypt depth, intestinal lengthening (slightly) and dilatation to increase the surface area

available for absorption. Transit time is lengthened, and the activity of brush-border enzymes and the bowel's absorptive capacity are increased. These adaptive changes occur as a result of enteral feeding and are not seen in patients solely fed parenterally. Thus, it is important to re-establish enteral feeding as early as is practical. The 5-year survival data for short-gut syndrome is difficult to interpret as it is clouded by the cause of the short gut (often neoplasia or thromboembolic events) but appears to be in the region of 70–80%.

Management

Initially in the perioperative period after extensive bowel resection, the major issues relate to electrolyte and fluid replacement due to ileus, sequestration of fluid, diarrhoea or high-output stoma. Clinical examination, chart assessment and biochemical analysis of serum electrolytes will guide fluid replacement and maintenance. Enteral intake should be commenced early if possible.

In the longer term, patients are encouraged to increase their oral intake to 1.5–2 times their previous intake, as this greater intake will somewhat counteract their relative malabsorption. Feeding should be continuous throughout the day and not limited to three meals a day. Often high-calorie enteral nutrition drinks supplement the diet.

Diarrhoea and high-output stomas cause electrolyte imbalance and are some of the major impediments to quality of life in patients with short-gut syndrome. Opiates are the mainstay of treatment for the control of diarrhoea. Loperamide is commonly used and may require very high dosage. Codeine may be added, but it has the possible side effects of nausea (which in turn reduces oral intake) and sedation. Octreotide (a somatostatin analogue) should be limited to patients with high-volume diarrhoea refractory to other treatment modalities, as it may increase the risk of biliary disease (to which these patients are already predisposed) and decrease gut adaptation. Water (without added electrolytes), particularly in large volumes, may paradoxically result in greater net loss of liquid as the body attempts to equilibrate sodium concentrations between plasma and the bowel lumen. This dehydration stimulates more thirst and leads to a vicious cycle of further water intake, further enteric fluid secretion and worsening of dehydration. Oral rehydration solution, a balanced salt and glucose solution, helps to overcome this.

Nutritional requirements

The baseline adult energy requirement is 20 kcal/kg per day of non-protein energy, 30% of which should be fat and 70% carbohydrate. The adult protein requirement is 1.5 g/kg per day. These requirements are modified by sex, height, weight and disease process. For instance, in severe sepsis requirements increase 45%. Protein losses and requirement can be very high with enterocutaneous fistula.

Total parenteral nutrition

In cases of gut failure, nutrition may be administered parenterally as total parenteral nutrition (TPN). The fluid is hyperosmolar and must be administered via a central venous cannula to a high-flow central vein. The contents of a typical daily 2-L bag of TPN are carbohydrate, 800 mL as a 50% dextrose solution; lipid, 500 mL as a 10% solution; and amino acids, 700 mL as a 10% solution. Carbohydrate and protein each provide 4 kcal/g of energy, while lipid provides 9 kcal/g. Thus, the major macronutrient requirements are delivered with nearly 3000 kcal of energy.

Long-term complications of short-gut syndrome

Long-term complications in short-gut syndrome pertain to absorption problems. Osteomalacia and osteoporosis (with overall decrease in bone mass) is seen in up to 84% of patients on parenteral nutrition, thought largely to be due to a reduction in the absorption of vitamins, particularly vitamin D. Normally, reabsorption of bile salts occurs in the terminal ileum. Short-gut patients have frequently had their terminal ileum resected or their bowel diverted proximally with a stoma. As a result, bile salt depletion is a common occurrence. This, along with reduced gallbladder emptying and the use of octreotide, serve to promote gallstone formation. Some studies have shown the prevalence of gallstones in this population to approach 100%. Bile salt depletion reduces the body's ability to absorb fats, which in turn leads to deficiency of the fat-soluble vitamins A, D, E and K. Kidney stones are common in patients with short-gut syndrome. These may be calcium oxalate (in patients with an intact colon) or uric acid (in patients with a high-output stoma). Hepatic steatosis and cholestasis may be seen in up to 50% of patients with short gut fed parenterally.

The role of the colon

A functioning colon is an important factor in the management of short-gut syndrome. The presence of a colon allows water and electrolytes to be absorbed against a concentration gradient. Bacteria in the colon ferment polysaccharides to short-chain fatty acids which may then be absorbed. Excess monosaccharides or oligosaccharides may cause D-lactic acidosis via abnormal bacterial colonisation of the colon (humans create the L-isomer). D-lactic acidosis may cause ataxia, blurred vision, ophthalmoplegia and nystagmus. Humans do not metabolise the D-isomer. Treatment is with broad-spectrum antibiotics and changing the diet to one that is high in polysaccharides. Patients who do not have a colon require a diet that is iso-osmolar (300 mosmol/kg) and has a sodium concentration of about 100 mmol/L.

Enteric fistula

An enteric fistula is an abnormal communication between a loop of bowel and another epithelial-lined surface. The anatomical classification of this condition names the fistula according to the organs involved. The high-pressure organ from which the fistula arises is named first, followed by the organ to which it travels (e.g. colovesical, enterocutaneous).

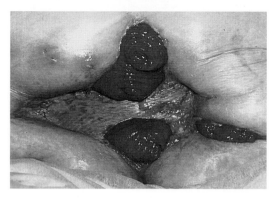

Fig. 26.2 Entero-atmospheric fistula showing large skin defect and multiple fistulating loops of small bowel.

- An enterocutaneous fistula is an abnormal communication between a loop of bowel and the skin. Large-diameter fistulas, where bowel mucosa is visible, are generally referred to as entero-atmospheric fistulas and these are unlikely to heal spontaneously (Figure 26.2).
- An entero-enteric fistula is a communication between two loops of bowel that results in enteric contents bypassing a segment of bowel. They may be created surgically (e.g. to bypass a strictured or obstructed segment of bowel) or occur as a result of inflammatory bowel disease. There is loss of absorptive capacity as enteric contents do not pass through the bypassed segment.

Enterocutaneous fistulas are typically accompanied by intra-abdominal sepsis; 75–85% are iatrogenic in origin and most occur after surgery for inflammatory bowel disease, cancer or adhesiolysis. The original operation is likely to have damaged a segment of bowel which has then leaked. Rather than leading to generalised peritonitis, the leak has partially walled off and eventually fistulated to the surface. Other causes include percutaneous drainage of an abscess (e.g. appendicitis, diverticulitis) or foreign-body erosion (e.g. mesh hernia repair).

A small number of enterocutaneous fistulas may close with conservative management, especially if there is low-volume output with a long narrow tract. If spontaneous closure is to occur, it will be within the first 6 weeks. Fistulas associated with Crohn's disease, previous radiation, downstream obstruction, complete anastomotic dehiscence, ongoing intra-abdominal sepsis, malnutrition, foreign body or diseased bowel are unlikely to heal spontaneously.

The mortality rate for enterocutaneous fistula is up to 10%. In addition to this high rate of mortality, enterocutaneous fistulas are a significant source of morbidity. Patients with enterocutaneous fistulas require diligent care, as they are at risk of recurrent bouts of sepsis (both local and systemic). Line sepsis is not uncommon.

Malnutrition is potentially a major issue due to losses from the fistula tract and loss of absorptive capacity of bypassed segments. High-volume fistulas, defined as more than 200 mL per 24 hours, may require supplementation with parenteral nutrition or intravenous fluids (particularly if proximally located in the small bowel).

The acronym SNAP is a useful mnemonic for the management of patients with intestinal fistulas.

- **S** is for control of sepsis and appropriate skin care. Fistulas are unlikely to heal in the presence of sepsis and the patient may deteriorate clinically if sepsis is left untreated. This may require antibiotics and/or a drainage procedure. Skin care is crucial. Leaking small bowel fluid from an enterocutaneous fistula severely damages skin. Uncontrolled output is very unpleasant for the patient and socially isolating. All the skills of experienced stoma therapy nurses will be required to help with these patients. Usually the best way to control the fluid is to use individually tailored stoma-type appliances.
- **N** is for nutrition. This often requires a combination of enteral and parenteral nutrition.
- **A** is for anatomy. It is important to define the anatomy as clearly as possible prior to re-operative surgery.
- **P** is for planning definitive repair.

Re-operative surgery is difficult within 100 days of the primary procedure due to inflammation and dense adhesions. There is a definite risk of creating more fistulas. Early re-operation should be avoided unless the patient is clinically deteriorating and there is no alternative option (e.g. worsening sepsis, bowel ischaemia). There is some evidence that suggests better outcomes are achieved by waiting at least 6 months before attempting further surgery and by resecting the fistula rather than attempting to repair it. Surgery should ideally be performed in a major centre that has expertise in hostile abdominal surgery and the support of a nutrition service.

Further reading

Bleier JIS, Hedrick T. Metabolic support of the enterocutaneous fistula patient. *Clin Colon Rectal Surg* 2010;23:142–8.

Carroll RE, Benedetti E, Schowalter JP, Buchman AL. Management and complications of short bowel syndrome: an updated review. *Curr Gastroenterol Rep* 2016;18:40.

Nightingale JD. The medical management of intestinal failure: methods to reduce the severity. *Proc Nutr Soc* 2003;63:703–10.

Polk TM, Schwab CW. Metabolic and nutritional support of the enterocutaneous fistula patient: a three-phase approach. *World J Surg* 2012;36:524–33.

MCQs

Select the single correct answer to each question. The correct answers can be found in the Answers section at the end of the book.

1 Which of the following is *not* an adaptation that occurs in the small bowel in the setting of short-gut syndrome?
   a cellular hyperplasia
   b increase in villous height and crypt depth
   c intestinal lengthening and dilatation
   d reduction in transit time
   e increased activity of brush-border enzymes

2 Which of the following is *not* a factor associated with non-healing of an enterocutaneous fistula?
   a sepsis
   b Crohn's disease
   c distal obstruction of the alimentary canal
   d foreign body
   e low output

3 Which of the following statements is *not* correct with regard to intestinal fistulas?
   a require careful planning prior to operation
   b have a mortality rate up to 10%
   c may heal spontaneously
   d should be repaired not resected
   e are often iatrogenic in origin

4 Which of the following is *not* a long-term complication of short-gut syndrome?
   a decrease in bone mass
   b bile salt depletion
   c kidney stones
   d obesity
   e malnutrition

27 Small bowel obstruction and ischaemia

Ian Hayes and the late Joe J. Tjandra

Colorectal Surgery Unit, Royal Melbourne Hospital and Department of Surgery,
University of Melbourne, Parkville, Victoria, Australia

Introduction

There is significant overlap between the clinical manifestations of small bowel obstruction (SBO) and acute ischaemia of the small intestine. It is the danger of developing secondary ischaemia in an obstructed segment of small bowel that makes SBO a serious condition, which sometimes requires emergency surgery. On the other hand, many cases of SBO due to adhesions can be managed non-operatively. It is crucial that clinicians can confidently diagnose SBO and recognise features suggestive of ischaemia.

Small bowel obstruction

Aetiology

The most common causes of SBO in western society are adhesions and hernia (Box 27.1). In considering the possible causes of this condition, a helpful framework can be to divide the causes into the following groups:
- extramural (e.g. adhesions)
- mural (e.g. stricture, malignancy)
- intraluminal (e.g. food bolus obstruction at new ileostomy).

Pathophysiology

Several litres of enteric fluid circulate through the small bowel each day. Obstruction leads to decreased absorption of this fluid, distension of the bowel and vomiting. This in turn leads to hypovolaemia and electrolyte depletion. Whilst a certain degree of extrinsic compression from a narrow-necked hernia or a dense adhesion band will cause obstruction by occluding the lumen, any further increase in compressive force may compromise the blood supply to that segment of bowel. Venous return may be impaired at a relatively low compressive force; this increases oedema, further limiting blood flow. Tissue perfusion of the bowel is counteracted by increased wall tension due to distension, and thus cellular ischaemia is produced. Hypovolaemia may further impair tissue perfusion. These factors can combine to create a vicious cycle of ischaemia, necrosis, perforation and ultimately multiorgan failure (Figure 27.1).

Symptoms

The characteristic symptoms of SBO are listed in Box 27.2. The order of appearance and the prominence of these symptoms are affected by how distal the obstruction is. The pain is characteristically periumbilical, reflecting the embryological innervation of the small bowel. The colicky quality is due to stimulation of stretch receptors with waves of opposed peristalsis. Pain becoming constant and more localised suggests that the patient may be developing inflammation of the parietal peritoneum due to ischaemia of the underlying small bowel.

Vomiting due to SBO is usually bile-stained (green) because the obstruction is distal to the second part of the duodenum where bile flows into the gut. Prolonged obstruction or distal obstruction leads to thick brown feculent vomitus due to bacterial overgrowth in a static column of enteric fluid.

The degree of distension is related to how distal the obstruction point is. Proximal SBO may be associated with relatively little abdominal distension.

Constipation may be a late feature. Strong peristalsis may cause the colon to empty for some hours after the onset of SBO.

Clinical examination findings

The patient is often in moderate abdominal discomfort, nauseated and dehydrated. The abdomen is distended, tympanitic and bowel sounds are high-pitched. Note should be made of previous abdominal incisions and a careful examination performed to exclude hernias. A key concept is that the presence of peritonism suggests ischaemia. In the case of a strangulated hernia, the hernial mass is likely to be tender and irreducible. There may be redness in the overlying skin if the bowel is ischaemic. When the necrotic tissue is confined to the hernial sac, examination of the rest of the abdomen may be normal despite a strangulated hernia.

Investigations

Plain abdominal X-ray is a useful screening test for SBO. Typical findings are dilated small bowel (>2 cm diameter), centrally located and with characteristic spiral valvulae conniventes. The finding of more than five air–fluid levels in distended small bowel on an erect X-ray is diagnostic of SBO but a supine X-ray showing distended small bowel is also useful. CT scan of abdomen and pelvis showing dilated small bowel with a transition point at the site of obstruction is a diagnostic feature of mechanical SBO. CT may give additional information about the cause of the obstruction and suggest features of ischaemia. The radiological diagnosis is strengthened if it can be demonstrated that there is failure of transit of contrast administered orally or via nasogastric tube. However, in the setting of very dilated bowel or distal obstruction, the contrast may become too dilute in the static column of fluid to be of diagnostic value. Furthermore, if the CT scan is performed too soon after administration of luminal contrast, the contrast will not have progressed to the site of obstruction.

Gastrografin follow-through, involving repeat plain X-rays over a time sequence to monitor the progress of luminal Gastrografin contrast, has an important diagnostic role in helping to distinguish ileus from mechanical obstruction. This test can also confirm ongoing complete obstruction after an attempt at conservative treatment of

> **Box 27.1 Causes of small bowel obstruction (in order of frequency)**
>
> - Adhesions
> - Hernia
> - Neoplasm: primary or secondary
> - Strictures: Crohn's disease, fibrosis following ischaemia, chronic radiation changes
> - Volvulus
> - Bezoar/food bolus
> - Gallstone ileus

> **Box 27.2 Characteristic symptoms of small bowel obstruction**
>
> - Crampy abdominal pain
> - Nausea and vomiting
> - Abdominal distension
> - Constipation

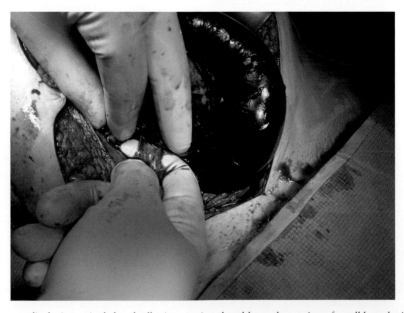

Fig. 27.1 Laparotomy displaying a single band adhesion causing closed-loop obstruction of small bowel with ischaemia.

adhesion-related SBO. The finding of complete obstruction contributes to the decision to operate.

Blood tests may show impaired renal function and hypokalaemia if the patient is dehydrated and vomiting. Raised white cell count and metabolic acidosis suggest ischaemia.

Treatment

Patients with SBO are usually dehydrated and need intravenous fluid resuscitation and electrolyte replacement. Insertion of a nasogastric tube decompresses the stomach and upper small bowel, improving patient comfort and relieving vomiting. When patients have adhesion-related obstruction, this decompression may be enough to release the obstructed segment. Adhesional SBO usually resolves within several days. Failure to resolve means that nutritional support with total parenteral nutrition will need to be considered and surgical intervention may now be required.

Surgery for SBO is challenging. Entry to the abdomen carries the risk of damaging oedematous dilated loops of bowel. Surgery to divide adhesions may, of course, create further adhesions in the future. Laparoscopic surgery for SBO is sometimes possible but open laparotomy is usually safer.

Patients who have not had previous major abdominal surgery (virgin abdomen) are less likely to have adhesions causing their obstruction and will generally require operative treatment. Patients with SBO due to a hernia or who have peritonitis require urgent surgery.

Differential diagnosis

Often the diagnosis of SBO rests on the basis of a plain abdominal X-ray in the setting of abdominal pain and vomiting. Gastroenteritis can be associated with multiple air–fluid levels on a plain X-ray but in non-dilated small bowel. The presence of diarrhoea in this setting makes obstruction less likely. Ileus, either postoperative or secondary to other acute intra-abdominal pathology, may display dilated small bowel on a plain X-ray but the characteristic transition point of mechanical obstruction will be absent on CT. Acute ischaemia of the small bowel may also be associated with dilation of the bowel on imaging.

Small bowel malignancy

Primary cancers of the small bowel are much rarer than colorectal malignancy, accounting for less than 2% of gastrointestinal malignancies

> ### Box 27.3 Primary tumours of the small bowel
>
> - Adenocarcinoma
> - Lymphoma
> - Neuroendocrine tumours (carcinoid)
> - Gastrointestinal stromal tumours (GIST)

(Box 27.3). These tumours can present with non-specific symptoms and are occasionally incidental diagnoses on imaging. They can also present urgently with complications of bleeding, obstruction or perforation. However, it should be noted that the most common cause of malignant SBO is intraperitoneal metastatic spread of other tumours such as ovarian or colorectal cancer.

Metastases from malignant melanoma and breast cancer can form deposits within the wall of the small bowel mimicking a primary small bowel tumour.

Adenocarcinoma of the small bowel

The risk of developing adenocarcinoma of the jejunum and ileum is increased in patients with Crohn's disease, coeliac disease and Peutz-Jeghers syndrome. Patients with familial adenomatous polyposis, Lynch syndrome and sporadic colorectal cancer also have an elevated risk of small bowel cancer. Treatment is similar to that of colorectal cancer except that extensive lymphadenectomy is more difficult to achieve than in the colon.

Small bowel lymphoma

Small bowel lymphoma is associated with coeliac disease and HIV. Most are B-cell non-Hodgkin's lymphomas. Surgical resection is frequently required for definitive diagnosis; in early-stage, localised, low-grade disease this may be definitive treatment. More advanced disease will require chemotherapy postoperatively.

Neuroendocrine tumours of the small bowel

Neuroendocrine tumours (previous called carcinoid tumours) arise in the enterochromaffin cells in the wall of the bowel. Most originate in the appendix and about one-third are multifocal. These tumours are slow-growing and the primary tumour usually remains small. Nodal metastases in the mesentery can produce large masses and a dense desmoplastic reaction which can even lead to ischaemia of the small bowel. The tumours release vasoactive amines, including serotonin, which are metabolised by the liver. However, once the tumour has metastasised to the liver, carcinoid syndrome may occur. This syndrome is characterised by diarrhoea, facial flushing, tachycardia and bronchospasm, and can lead to right heart failure. Carcinoid crisis can be precipitated by general anaesthesia and this is an important consideration when operating on these patients. Carcinoid syndrome is treated with somatostatin analogues.

Diagnosis of neuroendocrine tumours may often be an incidental finding after appendicectomy. Biochemical tests include chromogranin A level and urinary levels of 5-hydroxyindoleacetic acid (5-HIAA). CT may reveal the characteristic desmoplastic reaction in the mesentery and liver metastases. Gallium-68 DODA-TATE positron emission tomography (PET)/CT is the most specific imaging modality.

Surgical treatment involves resection of the primary tumour and involved mesentery. Appropriately sited liver metastases are resectable.

Gastrointestinal stromal tumours

These tumours arise from the interstitial cells of the muscularis propria. The majority have been found to have mutation in the *KIT* oncogene, thus allowing successful treatment with tyrosine-kinase inhibitor drugs such as imatinib. Tumours less than 2 cm in diameter are very low risk and can simply be monitored. Larger tumours require surgical excision but not extensive lymphadenectomy. The decision about adjuvant therapy with imatinib is based on tumour size, mitotic index and history of tumour perforation.

Acute small bowel ischaemia

Secondary ischaemia in the presence of obstruction has been discussed. Primary acute ischaemia of the small bowel can be due to:
- embolism
- arterial thrombosis
- venous thrombosis
- severe hypoperfusion.

Embolism to the superior mesenteric arterial tree is usually of cardiac origin, due to atrial fibrillation or post-infarct cardiac mural thrombus and is the most common cause of primary acute ischaemia. Arterial thrombosis occurs in patients with pre-existing atherosclerotic stenosis at the origin of the superior mesenteric artery. Venous thrombosis can occur in patients with hypercoagulable states. Ischaemia due to hypoperfusion can occur with

> **Box 27.4 Warning signs for the possibility of acute ischaemia**
>
> - Pain out of proportion to signs (early)
> - Peritonism in the setting of dilated bowel on X-ray (late)
> - New history of atrial fibrillation
> - High white cell count
> - High lactate
> - Metabolic acidosis
> - Thickened, non-perfused bowel on CT

non-occluded main vessels in patients in the intensive care unit (ICU) or after major trauma.

Clinical features

The diagnosis of acute small bowel ischaemia is notoriously difficult in the early phase and it may be too late once the condition becomes clinically obvious (Box 27.4). Patients are usually elderly, with significant comorbidities. The new onset of atrial fibrillation preceding abdominal pain is important to note, as is a history of peripheral vascular disease. In an anaesthetised ICU patient, the only diagnostic feature may be the new onset of unexplained metabolic acidosis.

The pain with ischaemic gut is constant, central and characteristically described as being out of proportion to signs. Initial abdominal examination may be normal. As bowel ischaemia and necrosis progress, acute inflammatory changes will lead to peritonitis. Ischaemia leads to breakdown of normal mucosal defences and bacterial translocation to the portal venous system. The patient may be tachypnoeic as a result of respiratory compensation for metabolic acidosis. Systemic sepsis and multiorgan dysfunction soon follow. An elderly patient with severe abdominal pain, who 'looks sick' but initially has few abdominal signs, should alert the clinician to the possibility of acute small bowel ischaemia or 'dead gut'.

Investigations

Blood tests may reveal a high white cell count with a neutrophilia often greater than 20×10^9/L. Elevated serum lactate is a frequent but non-specific finding. Arterial blood gas measurement can be used to confirm metabolic acidosis. Plain X-ray may show dilated small bowel, mucosal thickening with 'thumb-printing' or gas in the bowel wall (pneumatosis intestinalis) as a late sign. Catheter angiography is highly sensitive and specific but is usually a secondary investigation in the rare subgroup of patients suitable for revascularisation. CT with arterial phase contrast can reveal an arterial occlusion with an associated non-perfused segment of bowel. However, CT does not always confirm the diagnosis and exploratory laparotomy may be required on the basis of clinical suspicion in a patient who lacks definitive imaging but is deteriorating physiologically.

Treatment

Acute ischaemia of the small bowel carries a very high mortality. Treatment may require several laparotomies and ICU support and the patient may be left with a permanent stoma or long-term bowel dysfunction. In patients who are elderly and frail or who have dementia, it is appropriate to discuss with the patient and family the issue of setting limits to treatment and possibly just focusing on good palliation, before embarking on what may be a complex surgical course with a poor outcome.

Initial resuscitation will require intravenous fluids and broad-spectrum antibiotics. In most cases, bowel ischaemia will have reached an irreversible level before surgery. Usually the ischaemic segment is not salvageable. Thus the purpose of the operation is to resect the non-viable bowel before systemic sepsis and multiorgan failure occur, and to hopefully reverse the processes of sepsis and multiorgan failure if they have already commenced.

In those uncommon cases where bowel viability has not reached an irreversible level, it may be possible to perform revascularisation of the mesentery and salvage the bowel. Revascularisation can be performed by interventional radiology, open surgery or by combined techniques. Embolectomy, thrombectomy, bypass or stenting may be required.

When bowel is resected for ischaemia, primary re-anastomosis is sometimes appropriate when there is only a short ischaemic segment and the patient is physiologically stable. Frequently, a second-look laparotomy is planned to assess that there has been no further ischaemia prior to re-anastomosis. In some cases, too much bowel is necrotic to be compatible with survival. Unfortunately, all that can be done in such cases is to close the laparotomy incision without resection and palliate the patient.

Ischaemic colitis

This is a very different condition to full-thickness ischaemia of the bowel or 'dead gut'. In the condition of ischaemic colitis, there is acute mucosal ischaemia, usually involving a segment of the colon near the splenic flexure. This position is a watershed of blood supply between the middle colic and inferior mesenteric arteries. Because the muscle of the bowel wall remains viable, the cascade of necrosis and subsequent multiorgan failure associated with full-thickness ischaemia does not occur. As the ischaemic mucosa sheds, bleeding occurs from the underlying submucosa. Patients are generally older and present with left-sided abdominal pain, rectal bleeding, localised peritonism and a high white cell count. The combination of left-sided abdominal pain and rectal bleeding strongly suggests the diagnosis. The bleeding is rarely heavy and the symptoms usually settle within several days. Occasionally the area can develop a fibrous stricture in the following months and this can lead to obstructive symptoms. There is rarely evidence of underlying arterial stenosis as a cause.

Further reading

Chen SC, Lin FY, Lee PH, Yu SC, Wang SM, Chang KJ. Water-soluble contrast study predicts the need for early surgery in adhesive small bowel obstruction. *Br J Surg* 1998;85:1692–5.

Ellis H, Moran BJ, Thompson JN *et al*. Adhesion-related hospital readmission after abdominal and pelvic surgery: a retrospective cohort study. *Lancet* 1999;353:1476–8.

Harpreets S. Radiological evaluation of bowel ischaemia. *Radiol Clin North Am* 2015;53:1241–54.

Reynolds I, Healy P, McNamara DA. Malignant tumours of the small intestine. *The Surgeon* 2014;12:263–70.

MCQs

Select the single correct answer to each question. The correct answers can be found in the Answers section at the end of the book.

1 Three days after a myocardial infarction with cardiogenic shock, a 75-year-old man develops abdominal pain and distension. The abdomen is slightly tender with reduced bowel sounds. A plain abdominal X-ray shows distended small bowel without fluid levels. Blood tests reveal a metabolic acidosis. The most likely diagnosis is:
   a perforated peptic ulcer
   b mesenteric ischaemia
   c pseudo-obstruction of the colon
   d acute pancreatitis
   e diverticulitis

2 Investigations in a patient with acute small bowel obstruction may include the following *except*:
   a supine and erect abdominal radiographs

b blood urea and electrolyte estimation
c Gastrografin small bowel follow-through
d technetium-labelled iminodiacetic acid (HIDA) scan
e computed tomography of the abdomen

3 Which of the following statements regarding neuroendocrine tumours of the small and large bowel is *incorrect*?
a generally slow-growing
b most often found in the appendix
c responsive to treatment with tyrosine-kinase inhibitors
d not at risk of carcinoid syndrome without liver metastases
e characterised by intense mesenteric desmoplastic changes on CT

4 Which of the following features of small bowel obstruction is *incorrect*?
a colicky periumbilical pain due to stimulation of stretch receptors relating to the midgut
b vomiting of clear, yellow, bile-stained fluid
c minimal abdominal distension if the obstruction is proximal
d possible bowel action some hours after the onset of pain
e vomiting of brown feculent fluid if obstruction is distal

28 The appendix and Meckel's diverticulum

Rose Shakerian[1] and the late Joe J. Tjandra[1,2]

[1] Royal Melbourne Hospital, Melbourne, Victoria, Australia
[2] University of Melbourne, Melbourne, Victoria, Australia

Acute appendicitis

Acute appendicitis is the most common intra-abdominal surgical condition that requires operative intervention. It has an incidence of 7–12% in the adult population, occurring most frequently in the second and third decades of life.

Surgical pathology

With acute appendicitis, organisms invade the wall of the appendix and are lodged in the submucosa. Eventually, the full thickness of the wall is involved by acute inflammation and becomes swollen and reddened. With delay in diagnosis, the appendix becomes distended, especially if there is obstruction of the lumen. Venous stasis and then arterial occlusion result in gangrene at the tip of the appendix where the blood supply is precarious, or at the site of obstruction in the appendix because of pressure necrosis. Perforation may follow and can be localised by the greater omentum and loops of small bowel or may become generalised with diffuse contamination of the peritoneal cavity.

Clinical features

Symptoms

Abdominal pain

The nature of the pain may be highly variable. The most common initial presentation is a periumbilical gnawing pain that migrates within a few hours to the right iliac fossa. There may be a preceding period of anorexia, nausea and vomiting that lasts 12–24 hours. The usual sequence is anorexia, followed by central abdominal pain, then vomiting and finally pain in the right iliac fossa.

The initial periumbilical pain is due to obstruction and inflammation of the appendix and is mediated through the visceral pain fibres as a midgut pain. When appendicitis becomes transmural, the serosa of the appendix and the parietal peritoneum are involved, causing a localised pain mediated through the somatic pain fibres in the right iliac fossa.

Atypical presentations may be due to the location of the inflamed appendix. These include pain in the right upper quadrant from a long appendix or a right loin pain from a retrocaecal appendix. Patients presenting with peritonitis from perforated appendicitis have generalised abdominal pain.

Diarrhoea

This is an atypical or non-specific feature in acute appendicitis. Diarrhoea and tenesmus are most likely in the presence of an inflamed pelvic appendix irritating the rectal wall or a retroileal appendix irritating the terminal ileum. Severe and persistent diarrhoea is more likely to be due to gastroenteritis or inflammatory bowel disease.

Signs

General

With more advanced inflammation, the patient may look unwell. Moderate fever and tachycardia may be present and reflect the underlying infective process.

Local

Tenderness over the site of the appendix is the most important sign of appendicitis. The tenderness

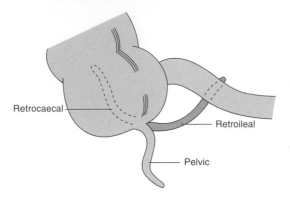

Fig. 28.1 The various positions of the appendix.

is localised and persistent and is classically at McBurney's point (one-third of the way from the anterior superior iliac spine to the umbilicus), although it may vary depending on the location of the appendix (Figure 28.1). Tenderness may be minimal early in the course of the illness and hard to elicit in the obese or if the appendix is retrocaecal.

Local muscular rigidity in the right iliac fossa is produced by inflammation of the parietal peritoneum overlying the appendix. Subtle rigidity can be detected by gently moving the palpating hand toward the area of maximal pain in the right iliac fossa while talking with the patient. This helps to differentiate true rigidity or guarding from voluntary spasm associated with nervousness. It is also helpful to ask the patient to cough or to sit up while watching the patient's facial expression; a grimace further suggests the presence of local peritonitis.

With local peritonitis, palpation in the left lower quadrant may cause pain in the right lower quadrant (Rovsing's sign). Signs of local peritonitis may be minimal in patients with retrocaecal or pelvic appendicitis. The psoas sign – pain caused by the extension of the right hip to stretch the psoas muscle – is generally present in retrocaecal appendicitis. Pelvic appendicitis is often difficult to differentiate from pelvic inflammatory disease but is usually associated with a right-sided tenderness on rectal examination.

Patients who present late with appendicitis may have generalised tenderness and rigidity, indicating perforation and peritonitis. Rebound tenderness indicates peritoneal inflammation and is best elicited by percussion. The delayed presentation of a tender, inflammatory appendiceal mass may occur in the right iliac fossa after three or more days.

Box 28.1 Investigations in suspected appendicitis

- Leucocytosis is usual in the range of $11–17 \times 10^9$/L with a neutrophilia.
- Elevated serum C-reactive protein (CRP) >10 mg/L combined with leucocytosis is indicative of an inflammatory/infective process.
- Urinalysis by ward test and microscopy is useful in order to rule out urinary tract infection, in addition to exclusion of pregnancy. However, pyuria may occur due to irritation of the bladder or ureter by an inflamed appendix.
- Plain abdominal X-ray is not recommended in the diagnostic work-up of appendicitis.
- Ultrasound may show a thick-walled appendix with a dilated lumen. The sensitivity and specificity for appendicitis using ultrasound are 85 and 90%, respectively. However, its greatest value is to rule out gynaecological pathology.
- Computed tomography (CT) has a higher diagnostic accuracy than ultrasound, with a sensitivity of 95% and specificity of 96%. Intravenous and oral contrast administration is recommended for diagnosis of appendicitis. It allows percutaneous drainage of a localised peri-appendiceal abscess and is useful in the evaluation of older patients as well as those with atypical pain.

Investigations

Investigations that are useful in the diagnosis of suspected appendicitis are given in Box 28.1.

Differential diagnosis

Diagnosis of appendicitis is particularly difficult with a retrocaecal appendix. The pain is not as severe as that associated with abdominal or pelvic appendicitis and it does not always localise to the right iliac fossa. The pain vaguely localises to the right side of the abdomen and rarely to the right flank or right upper quadrant. In neglected cases, a retrocaecal abscess develops as a result of perforation of the appendix.

Diagnosis in the elderly is often delayed because of late and less typical presentation. The incidence of perforation is therefore higher. In patients aged over 40 years, underlying malignancy needs to be considered and excluded.

During pregnancy, the appendix may be displaced cephalad by the gravid uterus. In the second trimester of pregnancy, the appendix is displaced upwards to the right upper flank. Appendicitis may be confused with pyelonephritis, as pyuria is common during pregnancy. Owing to abdominal laxity, the abdominal findings are also less acute. Mild leucocytosis is also a normal physiological response in pregnancy.

Mesenteric adenitis

About 5% of patients undergoing an appendicectomy for 'acute appendicitis' are found to have mesenteric adenitis. The patient has clinical features similar to those of appendicitis, but the appendix is normal and there are several enlarged lymph nodes in the mesentery of the terminal ileum.

The condition is most common in children. Some have a history of a recent sore throat together with a high fever. There is no muscle rigidity on presentation. The cause of the illness is obscure but is self-limiting, with spontaneous improvement over 24–36 hours. Ultrasound is recommended to make the diagnosis and exclude appendicitis in this patient population.

Gynaecological conditions

Mittelschmerz pain occurs at mid-menstrual cycle from the rupture of a follicle at ovulation. Fever is uncommon and most patients have had previous painful ovulation.

In pelvic inflammatory disease, including salpingitis and tubo-ovarian abscess, there is a longer duration of symptoms, higher fever, greater leucocytosis and more pelvic pain. Gonococcal and chlamydial infection are the most common causes. Careful gynaecological history and examination are helpful.

Torsion of a fallopian tube and torsion or haemorrhage of an ovarian cyst tend to present with pain of sudden onset. Pelvic examination and ultrasound will help with the diagnosis.

Ectopic pregnancy needs to be excluded early in any patient presenting with abdominal or pelvic pain, with or without abnormal vaginal bleeding. A positive pregnancy test (urine or serum) in the absence of an intrauterine pregnancy on ultrasound is highly suggestive of an ectopic pregnancy.

Urological conditions

Urinary tract infection presents with urinary symptoms and rigors. Lack of abdominal rigidity and presence of pus and organisms in the urine indicate the diagnosis. Right ureteric colic may cause confusion but the radiation of pain and haematuria should give the diagnosis.

Other conditions

Bacterial or viral gastroenteritis causes vomiting, profuse diarrhoea and diffuse abdominal pain without localised tenderness. Diarrhoea associated with appendicitis is rarely prolonged or severe. Non-specific ileitis may be secondary to *Yersinia* or *Campylobacter* infection.

Perforated caecal carcinoma with a pericolic abscess may mimic appendicitis, but the patients are usually elderly.

Acute cholecystitis may be confused with a high retrocaecal appendicitis.

Diverticulitis of a long redundant sigmoid colon lying on the right of midline may cause confusion. Rarely, a solitary caecal diverticulum becomes inflamed; this is usually seen in Asian patients.

Meckel's diverticulitis is rare and the diagnosis is usually made at surgery.

Management

If the diagnosis is clear, an appendicectomy is performed. If the diagnosis is suspected but not definite, a period of observation (usually in hospital) is appropriate. Over the following 12–24 hours, the nature of the illness should clarify itself.

Acute appendicitis is routinely managed with combination of intravenous antibiotics and surgery. Clinically stable patients with computed tomography (CT) diagnosis of uncomplicated appendicitis (absence of faecalith and perforation) can be managed conservatively with intravenous antibiotics only. Approximately 20% of these patients fail conservative management and can re-present with ongoing abdominal pain, requiring surgical intervention.

Laparoscopic appendicectomy has replaced open surgery as the operative approach of choice. The benefits of laparoscopic surgery include smaller skin incisions, reduced postoperative pain, earlier discharge and resumption of normal activities. Additionally, where the diagnosis is unclear despite a period of observation, a laparoscopic approach enables assessment of the intra-abdominal organs and exclusion of gynaecological conditions such as pelvic inflammatory disease.

Alternatively, an appendicectomy can be performed as an open procedure. A skin crease incision is made over the point of maximal tenderness in the right iliac fossa. Under anaesthesia, a mass may be palpable. The external and internal oblique muscles are split. The caecum is identified and the appendix is traced at its base on the posteromedial aspect. The mesoappendix is ligated and divided. The base of the appendix is ligated and transected. The appendix stump may be inverted using a purse-string in the caecum, although there is no firm evidence to suggest that this is necessary. All patients should receive prophylactic antibiotics administered preoperatively, usually in the form of a second- or third-generation cephalosporin and metronidazole. When there is severe sepsis, a full course of 5 days of therapy is recommended.

Patients presenting late may have a right iliac fossa mass. A CT scan is performed to determine whether it is an abscess or a phlegmon. If an abscess is present, it is drained percutaneously under CT guidance. This obviates the need for surgery in most cases in patients with active sepsis. An appendiceal phlegmon is treated with bowel rest and intravenous antibiotics. Non-operative therapy is successful in 85% of cases and most patients are sent home after 7–10 days.

Interval appendicectomy is no longer advocated as routine treatment for appendiceal phlegmon. In patients older than 40 years, a follow-up colonoscopy is recommended to exclude underlying malignancy. Otherwise in the absence of clinically significant symptoms, no further investigations or follow-up is required.

Meckel's diverticulum

Meckel's diverticulum is a congenital condition that arises from failure of embryonic obliteration of the omphalo-mesenteric duct connecting the fetal gut to the yolk sac. As distinct from other small bowel diverticula, Meckel's diverticulum is antimesenteric, contains all coats of the bowel and has its own blood supply (Figure 28.2). It is present in 2% of the population and is commonly within 1 m of the ileocaecal valve. In 20% of cases, the mucosa contains heterotopic epithelium of gastric, colonic or pancreatic origin. Symptomatic cases are usually males.

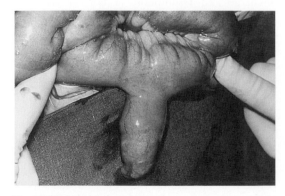

Fig. 28.2 Meckel's diverticulum.

Clinical syndromes

Bleeding peptic ulceration adjacent to ectopic gastric epithelium is found. This usually occurs in young patients.

Small bowel obstruction due to intussusception may occur. The apex of intussusception is usually the inflamed heterotopic tissue at the mouth of the diverticulum. Obstruction of the small bowel may also be caused by the presence of a band between the apex of the diverticulum and the umbilicus, causing kinking or volvulus.

Meckel's diverticulitis is usually due to lodgement of enteroliths or a sharp foreign body in the diverticulum or narrowing of the mouth of the diverticulum. The clinical features are similar to those of appendicitis. Perforation may occur, causing generalised peritonitis.

Gastric heterotopia may cause peptic ulcer-like symptoms, with meal-related pain around the umbilicus because of its midgut location.

Diagnosis

Meckel's diverticulum is more likely to be discovered incidentally during abdominal surgery for another condition. Where it is believed to be the cause of gastrointestinal bleeding, particularly in younger patients, a Meckel's scan should be performed. This is a nuclear medicine study in which technetium-99m pertechnetate is used intravenously to localise heterotopic gastric mucosa in Meckel's diverticulum. Another useful investigation tool is CT angiography which can detect active signs of bleeding that may be difficult to detect with other techniques.

When the clinical presentation is due to obstructive or inflammatory complications of Meckel's diverticulum, CT of the abdomen with oral and intravenous contrast can be helpful in making the diagnosis.

Treatment

Complicated or symptomatic Meckel's diverticulum should be treated with resection of the segment of the small bowel containing the diverticulum.

Incidental Meckel's diverticulum found at laparotomy is usually left alone because most remain asymptomatic. Any band to the umbilicus or other viscus is divided. Resection is considered in children younger than 2 years; with the presence of palpable heterotopia (especially in males); and with evidence of prior Meckel's diverticulitis, such as adhesions.

Further reading

Kotha VK, Khandelwal A, Saboo SS *et al*. Radiologist's perspective for the Meckel's diverticulum and its complications. *Br J Radiol* 2014;87(1037):20130743.

Lamb P. Acute conditions of the small bowel and appendix. In: Paterson-Brown S (ed.) *Core Topics in General and Emergency Surgery*, 5th edn. Edinburgh: Saunders Elsevier, 2014.

Poon SHT, Lee JWY, Ng KM *et al*. The current management of acute uncomplicated appendicitis: should there be a change in paradigm? A systematic review of the literatures and analysis of treatment performance. *World J Emerg Surg* 2017;12:46.

Sauerland S, Jaschinski T, Neugebauer EA. Laparoscopic versus open surgery for suspected appendicitis. *Cochrane Database Syst Rev* 2010;(10):CD001546.

MCQs

Select the single correct answer to each question. The correct answers can be found in the Answers section at the end of the book.

1 Right iliac fossa pain and nausea in a 62-year-old woman may be due to the following except:
   a acute appendicitis
   b caecal cancer
   c urinary tract infection
   d Mittelschmerz pain
   e sigmoid diverticulitis

2 Which of the following statements about sepsis associated with appendicectomy for acute appendicitis is *incorrect*?
   a may present with a pelvic abscess
   b may present as a wound infection
   c is reduced by prophylactic perioperative antibiotics
   d is increased by laparoscopic rather than open appendicectomy
   e is most often associated with anaerobic bacteria

3 Which of the following statements about Meckel's diverticulum is *incorrect*?
   a may cause small bowel obstruction due to intussusception
   b may be located in the mesenteric border of the small bowel
   c may present with meal-related central abdominal pain
   d may present with melaena and a normal upper gastrointestinal endoscopy
   e may be diagnosed with technetium-99m pertechnetate scan in some cases

4 Which of the following statements concerning acute appendicitis is *incorrect*?
   a the diagnosis can be made based on history and clinical examination alone, in the appropriate patient
   b elevated CRP and white cell count can be indicative of the condition
   c plain abdominal X-ray is a standard investigation tool
   d in patients aged over 40, CT scan is recommended to exclude underlying malignancy
   e urinalysis should be routinely performed

29 Inflammatory bowel disease

Susan Shedda[1], Britt Christensen[2] and the late Joe J. Tjandra[1,3]

[1] Department of Surgery, Royal Melbourne Hospital, Melbourne, Victoria, Australia
[2] Inflammatory Bowel Disease Unit, Department of Gastroenterology, Royal Melbourne Hospital, Melbourne, Victoria, Australia
[3] University of Melbourne, Melbourne, Victoria, Australia

Introduction

Inflammatory bowel disease comprises a group of inflammatory diseases of unknown aetiology which vary in distribution from the colon and rectum alone in ulcerative colitis to any part of the gastrointestinal tract in the case of Crohn's disease. These conditions can have a wide spectrum of disease activity. Their treatment requires a multidisciplinary approach where both medical treatment and surgery interplay to maximise the outcome for patients.

Ulcerative colitis

Ulcerative colitis occurs most commonly in temperate climates and in Caucasians. It is rare in Africa and the East. Ulcerative colitis is about two to three times more common than Crohn's disease, although the incidence of Crohn's disease is increasing. The disease is usually diagnosed between 15 and 45 years of age. The aetiology of ulcerative colitis is uncertain, although familial clusters occur and some, as yet unknown, environmental factors may be relevant.

Pathology

Ulcerative colitis is a mucosal disease that almost invariably affects the rectum and spreads proximally in a continuous manner. Inflammation is limited to the mucosa except in fulminant cases, where transmural changes may occur. The mucosa is congested and friable, with varying degrees of ulceration. Microscopy shows diffuse infiltration of acute and chronic inflammatory cells limited to the mucosa. The glandular structure is distorted, with goblet cell depletion and crypt abscesses. In chronic quiescent phases, the glands may be shortened and atrophic, although the endoscopic appearances may be relatively normal.

In severe disease the differentiation between ulcerative colitis and Crohn's disease is difficult. In fulminant cases, the colitis is transmural, with deep ulceration and fissures. The histopathology can be confusingly similar to that of Crohn's disease. In some cases, diagnosis is made only after the rectum is removed or when Crohn's disease appears in the small bowel or the perianal region. Sometimes, the diagnosis remains uncertain and is labelled as 'indeterminate colitis'.

Colitis and dysplasia

Long-standing colitis (whether Crohn's or ulcerative colitis) may be associated with dysplasia of the epithelium. The incidence of dysplasia in longstanding total colitis is probably around 5–10%. The risk for cancer in colitis increases with the extent and duration of the disease. For pancolitis, the risk for cancer is 3% at 10 years, rising by 1–2% per year thereafter. Colonoscopic surveillance with multiple biopsies is generally commenced after 7 years of disease in patients with disease beyond the sigmoid, at 2-year intervals.

The risk of cancer rises significantly with the presence of a dysplasia-associated mass lesion (a plaque or large polyp) or stricture. The tumours are more likely to be multiple and more likely to occur in the right or transverse colon. Carcinoma in ulcerative colitis may occur in flat mucosa and may not be easily visible on colonoscopy. This fact provides a strong argument for routine use of biopsy.

Biopsy specimens are taken from specific lesions and from random sites of the colon. The risk of cancer in patients with left-sided colitis is much lower but rises sharply after 25–30 years of disease.

Clinical features

The clinical features depend on the severity and extent of colitis and have a natural history of periods of exacerbation and remission (Box 29.1). Extra-intestinal manifestations are listed in Box 29.2.

The most common presentation is bloody diar-rhoea in an otherwise fit patient. Patients with proctosigmoiditis may complain of tenesmus as well. More severe disease with extensive colonic involvement may cause severe diarrhoea with abdominal cramps and urgency at stool. Endoscopy shows a confluent proctitis with mucosal friability, contact bleeding, ulceration and granularity.

Acute toxic colitis

Toxic colitis and toxic megacolon are part of the spectrum of severe ulcerative colitis and are more common in patients with pancolitis. While acute fulminating colitis usually occurs as an acute exacerbation of pre-existing ulcerative colitis, it can present as the first manifestation of colitis.

Acute toxic colitis is characterised by the abrupt onset of bloody diarrhoea, urgency, anorexia and abdominal cramps. Patients are often ill with severe anaemia and dehydration. A patient is regarded as 'toxic' when, in addition to severe colitis, there is evidence of at least two of the following:
- tachycardia above 100 beats/min
- temperature above 38.6°C
- leucocytosis more than 10.5×10^9/L
- hypoalbuminaemia below 3.0 g/dL.

Other features commonly present include stool frequency of more than nine per day, abdominal distension, tenderness, mental changes, electrolyte disturbances (hyponatraemia, hypokalaemia) and alkalosis.

Abdominal distension often indicates colonic dilatation, and tenderness suggests impending perforation or ischaemia. Toxic dilatation or megacolon is usually defined as a diameter exceeding 6 cm in the transverse colon on plain abdominal X-ray. Signs of septicaemia may be masked by using steroids.

Investigations

Colonoscopy

Characteristic appearances include an erythematous mucosa with contact bleeding. The normal vascular pattern is lost and there may be blood and pus in the lumen. Biopsies are taken to establish the extent of the disease and the presence of dysplasia. A full colonoscopy may not be performed in acute colitis because of the risk of perforation.

General investigations

General investigations include full blood examination, C-reactive protein (CRP) and liver function test.

Box 29.1 Spectrum of ulcerative colitis

- Proctitis
- Proctosigmoiditis
- Acute ulcerative colitis
- Chronic ulcerative colitis
- Relapsing chronic ulcerative colitis
- Complicated ulcerative colitis
  - o Toxic colitis/toxic megacolon
  - o Perforation
  - o Haemorrhage
  - o Dysplasia/carcinoma
- Extra-intestinal manifestations

Box 29.2 Extra-intestinal manifestations of ulcerative colitis

Present with active disease
- Skin: erythema nodosum, pyoderma gangrenosum
- Mucous membranes: aphthous ulcers of mouth and vagina
- Eyes: iritis
- Joints: flitting arthralgia/arthritis of large joints

Present independent of disease activity
- Joints: sacroiliitis, ankylosing spondylitis
- Hepatobiliary: chronic active hepatitis, cirrhosis, sclerosing cholangitis

---

Therapy for chronic ulcerative colitis

Before initiating therapy for ulcerative colitis, assessment of disease extent by colonoscopy is required. Disease extent is usually defined by the Montreal System as:
- proctitis (E1, limited to rectum)
- left-sided disease (E2, extending up to the splenic flexure)
- pancolitis (E3, disease beyond the splenic flexure).

There are many therapies available for ulcerative colitis. These can generally be broken down into three major categories: aminosalicylates, immunomodulators and biological agents.

Sulfasalazine and aminosalicylates

Sulfasalazine and the aminosalicylates are commonly used to treat ulcerative colitis and have anti-inflammatory activity by inhibiting the formation of prostaglandins. They are available in both oral and topical forms.

Sulfasalazine is composed of sulfapyridine and 5-aminosalicylate (5-ASA) joined by an azo-bond. 5-ASA is the active therapeutic moiety and acts by inhibiting prostaglandin synthesis. The sulfapyridine alone has no therapeutic effect and is responsible for most of the side effects. A small amount (approximately 20%) is absorbed by the small bowel and most of the sulfasalazine enters the colon, where the azo-bond is cleaved by colonic bacteria. 5-ASA is poorly absorbed from the colon and remains intraluminal, where it exerts the therapeutic effects. Sulfapyridine is absorbed and metabolised by the liver. The 5-aminosalicylates are better tolerated than sulfasalazine and are prescribed when patients demonstrate intolerance to sulfasalazine or allergy to sulfa drugs. There are several formulations of 5-ASA available which have specific formulations and dosage schedules.

For patients with proctitis or proctosigmoiditis, topical therapy is possible and is more effective than treatment with oral aminosalicylates alone. 5-ASA suppositories and/or enemas are given rectally and induce remission in more than 90% of patients with mild to moderate proctitis or proctosigmoiditis. In mild disease confined to the rectum, topical mesalazine given by suppository is the preferred therapy. Suppositories only act in the distal 5–8 cm of the rectum. Enemas and foams are less effective for proctitis because their concentration in the rectum rapidly diminishes.

In patients with more extensive disease, however, foam enemas can treat the mid-sigmoid colon and liquid enemas reach the splenic flexure. In these patients, a combination of a mesalazine suppository and an enema may be more effective. Treatment is required for at least 4–6 weeks intensely, followed by a gradual taper as tolerated. For patients who are more symptomatic, who have disease extending more proximally or who fail to respond to topical therapy, a combination of oral and topical therapy has been found to be more effective than either one alone. Higher doses are used to induce remission and once remission is achieved doses are decreased. After remission, long-term maintenance therapy is encouraged.

Side effects from sulfasalazine are more common than with other aminosalicylates but sulfasalazine is cheaper and may be more effective for joint pains. One-fifth of patients will have side effects to sulfasalazine, which can include dyspepsia, nausea, anorexia and headache. In addition, due to the sulfa component, allergic reactions (rash or fever), haematological side effects (haemolysis or neutropenia) and sperm abnormalities can occur. Sulfasalazine also affects folate absorption, so for females it is important to educate about folate supplementation in regard to pregnancy planning.

If patients are intolerant of sulfasalazine, the aminosalicylate medications can be used. Side effects are rarer and consist usually of headache, diarrhoea and nausea. Aminosalicylates can also rarely exacerbate colitis.

Corticosteroids

If patients remain symptomatic despite maximal doses of aminosalicylates, escalation of therapy with oral corticosteroids can be used to induce remission. This is usually achieved with oral prednisolone at a dose of 40 mg daily for several weeks and slowly weaned over a month or two. Intravenous corticosteroids can be used in more severe disease. Corticosteroids are effective at inducing remission but are not used to maintain remission due to lack of efficacy and significant side effects. Side effects include moon facies, weight gain, mood swings, sleep disturbance, diabetes and increased infection risk with short-term use; and osteoporosis, aseptic necrosis, adrenal suppression and cataracts with long-term use.

Budesonide is a potent corticosteroid that undergoes first-pass metabolism by the liver and therefore is associated with minimal systemic side effects when used enterally. It has been found to be safe, efficacious and well tolerated for inducing remission in patients with mild-to-moderate disease.

Immunomodulators

If patients require more than one course of oral corticosteroids in a year despite optimisation of their oral and topical 5-aminosalicylate therapy or if patients are steroid-dependent, a steroid-sparing agent is necessary.

The thiopurines azathioprine (dose 2–2.5 mg/day) and 6-mercaptopurine (1–1.5 mg/day) are the most commonly used immunomodulators in ulcerative colitis. Before commencing therapy, a genetic test for thiopurine S-methyltransferase (TPMT) activity

Table 29.1 Pre-immune suppression screen.

Testing before immunomodulator	Testing before biologics
Thiopurine S-methyltransferase (TPMT) phenotype or genotype Hepatitis B sAg/cAb Hepatitis C Ab HIV serology Varicella serology	As for immunomodulator Interferon-γ assay for tuberculosis (e.g. QFN-gold) Chest X-ray

should be undertaken, as patients with no activity are at risk of severe myelosuppression, which can result in sepsis and even death. In addition, prior to commencing therapy with an immunomodulator, patients should have a pre-immune suppression screen (Table 29.1) and have their vaccination status assessed and updated. Patients cannot receive live vaccines while on these medications.

Immunomodulators are slow-acting and require at least 3 months of therapy to assess efficacy. They are therefore not ideal agents for inducing remission but are routinely used to maintain remission after induction with corticosteroids. 6-Mercaptopurine is the prodrug of azathioprine and may be better tolerated in patients who suffer from side effects with azathioprine. Both drugs can be optimised with testing of thiopurine metabolite levels.

Although these agents have potentially serious side effects, adverse events associated with lower doses used in treating inflammatory bowel disease are infrequent. Patients can initially experience nausea, vomiting or headaches which often subside. Pancreatitis (3% of patients), leucopenia (2%) and abnormal liver function tests (5%) are the most common more serious side effects that can warrant treatment cessation. These agents increase the risk of non-Hodgkin's lymphoma and non-melanoma skin cancer.

Biological agents

In patients who are steroid-refractory or steroid-dependent despite thiopurines, up-titration to a biological agent is required. There are two major groups currently available, the anti-tumour necrosis factor (TNF) agents (adalimumab and infliximab) and the anti-integrin agent vedolizumab.

Anti-TNF agents: adalimumab, golimumab and infliximab

Anti-TNF agents are fast-acting and effective at inducing remission in patients with moderate to severe ulcerative colitis. Adalimumab is given by

injection every 2 weeks, golimumab by injection every 4 weeks and infliximab is an intravenous infusion. Both have similar efficacy with response rates of approximately 80%. Combination therapy with a thiopurine results in the highest response rates and decreases the risk of anti-drug antibody formation, which can result in loss of response.

These medications are well tolerated but patients require close monitoring. Adverse events include skin injection site reactions or infusion reactions, increased risk of infection, demyelinating disease, heart failure, psoriasis, malignancy or a lupus-like reaction.

Anti-integrin agent: vedolizumab

Vedolizumab acts by blocking the $\alpha_4\beta_7$ integrin, preventing the migration of leucocytes into the gut. It is administered intravenously. It appears to be slower-acting than anti-TNF therapy but still works more quickly than the thiopurines. Its advantage is that it is very safe and is a good option in patients with a previous cancer or any infection risk. Side effects are minimal but include flu-like symptoms, joint pains, headaches and increased sinus infections.

Janus kinase inhibitors: tofacitinib

Tofacitinib is an oral selective janus kinase (JAK) inhibitor. JAKs are enzymes that are involved in activating the body's immune response, and by blocking this tofacitinib may stop the inflammatory process in ulcerative colitis. It is fast-acting and effective at inducing and maintaining remission in patients with moderate to severe ulcerative colitis who have failed other biological therapies or are biological therapy-naive. The most common side effects include diarrhoea, headache, nasopharyngitis and upper respiratory tract infections. It can also increase the risk of infections and malignancy, and because of an increased risk of shingles patients should be vaccinated with the shingles vaccine if possible before initiation.

Surgical management

Indications for surgery

Acute illness

Evidence of free perforation, generalised peritonitis and massive colonic haemorrhage indicates the need for emergency surgery. Surgery is indicated with deterioration of acute colitis (increasing toxicity or colonic dilatation) at any time after initiation of adequate medical management. If the improvement has been minor after 5–7 days of adequate medical management, a long-term remission is unlikely. In these cases, surgery is also recommended in conjunction with management by the gastroenterologist. With adoption of more aggressive resuscitation, a coordinated plan of management and early operative intervention, mortality is less than 3%. In contrast, colonic dilatation complicated by perforation has a mortality of 33%. About half the patients with acute fulminating colitis respond to medical therapy, thereby avoiding emergency surgery.

Chronic illness

The main indication for elective surgery is chronic illness that responds poorly to medical treatment or recurrent acute colitis. The threshold for surgery by gastroenterologists and patients is variable. Sphincter-preserving restorative proctocolectomy may now avoid the presence of a permanent stoma and therefore increase its acceptance. Severe extra-intestinal manifestations are rare indications for surgery.

Cancer risk

Dysplasia is currently the most sensitive marker of premalignancy. The presence of dysplasia from a villous or polypoidal lesion or from a stricture is an indication for prophylactic proctocolectomy. The presence of severe dysplasia from an area of flat mucosa at two separate sites in the colon is also an indication for surgery. The presence of low-grade dysplasia in flat mucosa may require surgery due to concerns regarding the underlying malignancy risk of 1–2%.

Preoperative preparation

The patient and the family are counselled jointly by the gastroenterologist and colorectal surgeon. The need for a stoma is discussed and the stoma site is marked preoperatively. Immunosuppression is minimised and broad-spectrum antibiotic prophylaxis is used. Mechanical bowel preparations may be used for elective surgery but are contraindicated in emergency surgery. Prophylaxis for deep vein thrombosis is prescribed.

Surgical options

Restorative proctocolectomy

Restorative proctocolectomy entails removal of the entire colon and rectum. A J-pouch is constructed using loops of the terminal 40–50 cm of ileum to replace the rectum and is anastomosed to the upper anal canal (Figure 29.1).

The double stapled J-pouch leaves approximately 2 cm of distal rectal mucosa in the anal canal. In certain circumstances, this small amount of mucosa needs to be removed and therefore a mucosectomy and hand-sewn anastomosis between the J-pouch and the proximal anal canal is fashioned.

After consideration of the comorbidities, including degree of immunosuppression and operative

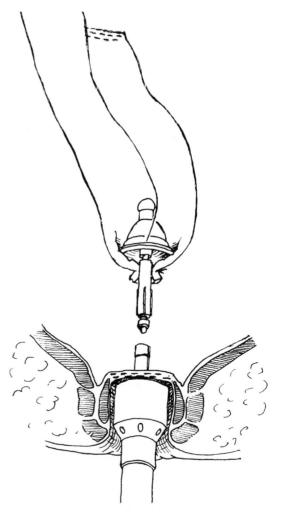

Fig. 29.1 A stapled ileal pouch–anal anastomosis.

conditions, a temporary diverting loop ileostomy is generally performed. The loop ileostomy is then reversed through a small parastomal incision about 3 months later. In selected 'healthier' patients, a diverting stoma may safely be omitted if the surgery proceeds smoothly.

Specific postoperative complications include pelvic sepsis, with or without anastomotic breakdown, adhesive small bowel obstruction and ileostomy-related problems. Overall, 80% recover uneventfully and 20% experience some morbidity.

Functional results following restorative proctocolectomy continue to improve within the first 18 months after surgery. Most patients defecate five to six times daily and will be able to defer defecation without urgency. Few patients suffer severe faecal incontinence, although minor faecal spotting occurs in up to 25% during the day and 40% at night. Some 50% of patients use antidiarrhoeal or bulking agents at least intermittently.

Major failure requiring excision of the pouch occurs in only 2% of patients. The usual causes are persistent pelvic sepsis, unsuspected Crohn's disease or faecal incontinence.

Long-term sequelae of the ileal pouch include 'pouchitis', a syndrome associated with pouch dysfunction. This may manifest as an increase in the number of bowel actions per day or poor emptying of the pouch. It may be associated with endoscopic and histologic evidence of inflammation of the ileal pouch. Treatment of pouchitis is empirical. Most cases respond to ciprofloxacin or metronidazole. Some require long-term low-dose antibiotics to control symptoms. Enemas containing steroid or 5-ASA can be used. In very severe cases, Crohn's disease must be excluded.

Complete proctocolectomy and permanent end-ileostomy

With the advent of restorative surgery, complete proctocolectomy and permanent end-ileostomy is currently indicated only in elderly patients with incontinence, in patients with advanced-stage rectal cancer and in those unwilling to undergo the more complicated restorative proctocolectomy.

Colectomy with ileorectal anastomosis

Colectomy with ileorectal anastomosis is rarely performed because it leaves the rectum with a continuing risk for inflammation and cancer. It might be considered in patients with coexisting severe portal hypertension where rectal dissection is hazardous or in children to allow them to pass through adolescence without a stoma or until conversion to a pouch.

Emergency surgery for severe acute colitis

The optimal operation is subtotal colectomy and end-ileostomy (Figure 29.2) because it avoids a pelvic dissection in an unwell patient and because it allows the later possibility of restorative surgery. Restorative proctocolectomy in the emergency setting is associated with a higher operative morbidity, especially in patients on high-dose steroids, and should be avoided. It would seem perverse to not remove what is often the most diseased segment of bowel, but the aim of surgery in these circumstances is to reduce the inflammatory load or remove the bowel which is perforated. In the acute situation, it is often unclear as to whether the final diagnosis will be ulcerative colitis or Crohn's disease.

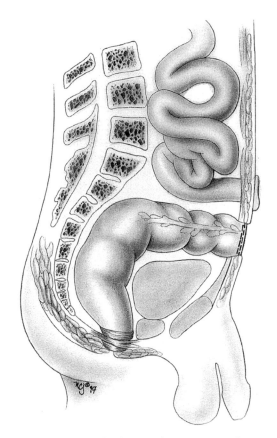

Fig. 29.2 Abdominal colectomy for toxic megacolon. Lateral view showing the end-ileostomy and the implanted rectosigmoid stump. Source: Tjandra JJ. Toxic colitis and perforation. In: Michelassi F, Milsom JW (eds) *Operative Strategies in Inflammatory Bowel Disease*. New York: Springer-Verlag, 1999:239. Reproduced with permission of Springer Nature.

The best method to manage the distal stump is to staple-transect the distal sigmoid colon at a level where it will lie without tension in the subcutaneous plane, at the lower end of the midline incision. This technique avoids a troublesome discharging mucous fistula but allows for discharge of blood and pus through the wound should the distal stump break down. It also allows the rectum to be easily identified at a future laparotomy.

Crohn's disease

In 1932, Crohn and his colleagues described an inflammatory disease of the terminal ileum characterised by ulceration and fibrosis with frequent stenosis and fistula formation. They called it 'regional ileitis'. It was later recognised that a similar inflammatory process could also affect the colon and perianal region. The cause of Crohn's disease remains unknown, although immunological mechanisms play a role in the pathogenesis of mucosal inflammation.

Crohn's disease is a disease of young adults. The age at which Crohn's disease is first diagnosed peaks between 20 and 29 years, with a second smaller peak between the ages of 60 and 80 years.

Pathology

Crohn's disease can affect any part of the gastrointestinal tract. Multiple areas may be involved with intervening areas of normal bowel, referred to as skip areas (Figure 29.3). The mesentery is thickened and the mesenteric fat creeps along the sides of the bowel wall toward the antimesenteric border. This is termed 'fat wrapping'. The disease involves all layers of the bowel wall. Ulcerations range from small shallow aphthous ulcers to deep fissuring ulcers. The fissuring of the mucosa and submucosal oedema can give the bowel a cobblestone appearance with the

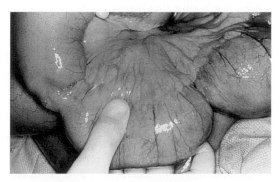

Fig. 29.3 Short strictures of the small bowel separated by normal skip areas.

formation of pseudopolyps. Fistulas and abscesses result from full-thickness penetration of the ulcers. The bowel wall may become thickened with fibrosis, leading to stricture formation.

Perianal Crohn's disease includes large oedematous skin tags, deep fissures, perianal fistulas and abscesses.

The histological appearance varies depending on the severity of the disease, but a lymphocytic infiltrate is usually seen in all layers of the bowel. Non-caseating granulomas are noted in about 50% of surgical specimens.

Crohn's disease and cancer

The risk of gastrointestinal malignancy in Crohn's disease is increased. The small bowel cancers are predominantly adenocarcinomas in the distal small bowel and the tumours have a poor prognosis. Long-standing Crohn's colitis has a similar risk of dysplasia and malignancy as ulcerative colitis.
Clinical manifestations

Patterns of intestinal involvement in Crohn's disease are often separated into three main categories: colonic (25%), ileocolic (40%) and small intestine alone (30%). Duodenal involvement occurs in only about 2%. The symptoms depend on the location of disease.

Extra-intestinal manifestations are similar to those described for ulcerative colitis (see Box 29.2).

Small intestinal Crohn's disease

Clinical features

The most common symptoms of small intestinal Crohn's disease are diarrhoea (90%), abdominal pain (55%), anorexia, nausea and weight loss. Malaise, lassitude and anaemia are frequently present. Most patients present with long-standing symptoms. Some patients present acutely with a complicated episode such as obstruction, inflammatory phlegmon, intra-abdominal abscess or fistula. Occasionally, the initial presentation is with a more acute history of right iliac fossa pain and fever, and a misdiagnosis of acute appendicitis is made. The true diagnosis is revealed only at operation. Careful questioning often reveals a more chronic history that suggests Crohn's disease. Complications of small intestinal Crohn's disease are given in Box 29.3.

Investigations

Computed tomography (CT) or magnetic resonance imaging (MRI) enteroclysis defines the mucosal

Box 29.3 Complications of Crohn's disease

- Obstruction from fibrous stricture or inflammatory oedema
- Fistulas to neighbouring loops of small or large bowel, or to bladder or vagina
- Perforation and intra-abdominal abscesses
- Massive haemorrhage
- Gallstones, especially if the terminal ileum has been resected for the disease. This is due to interruption of the enterohepatic circulation and eventual depletion of bile salts
- Right ureteric involvement from ileocolic phlegmon may lead to a recurrent pyelonephritis or a right hydronephrosis. Renal stones, especially oxalate stones, are common, especially in the presence of steatorrhoea
- Adenocarcinoma of the small bowel, usually in the terminal ileum
- Colonic dysplasia and malignancy

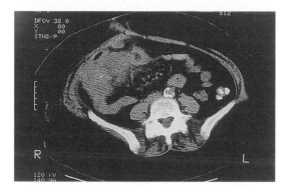

Fig. 29.4 Computed tomography scan showing thick-walled bowel loops in a patient with recurrent Crohn's disease after a prior ileocolic resection.

pattern in detail and therefore demonstrates aphthous ulcers, fissures and mucosal oedema.

Colonoscopy enables a full assessment of the colon. Focal inflammation and granulomas can be seen histologically even when the mucosa is macroscopically normal. Colonoscopy may also allow biopsy of the terminal ileal orifice when the radiological appearances of the terminal ileum are not conclusive.

CT may demonstrate internal fistulas, intra-abdominal abscesses and thickening of the bowel wall (Figure 29.4).

Symptoms in Crohn's disease may be due to active inflammation or obstruction or result from previous surgery or bacterial overgrowth. Laboratory tests including full blood examination, CRP, albumin and faecal calprotectin frequently help to determine disease activity.

Medical management

There is no cure for Crohn's disease and ongoing disease activity can lead to multiple complications including strictures and fistulating disease. It is therefore important to treat inflammation in patients with Crohn's disease.

Aminosalicylates

Aminosalicylate medications have, if any, only minimal efficacy in Crohn's disease. These agents should only be used in patients with very mild disease with no risk of complications. Most expert guidelines do not recommend using these agents.

Corticosteroids

As in ulcerative colitis, corticosteroids are the mainstay of treatment in Crohn's disease for inducing remission. Prednisolone is usually commenced at 40 mg daily and slowly weaned; however, in patients with less severe disease restricted to the terminal ileum and ascending colon, controlled ileal-release budesonide can also be used. Corticosteroids should not be used for maintenance of remission in Crohn's disease due to side effects (see ulcerative colitis section) and lack of efficacy.

Immunomodulators: azathioprine, 6-mercaptopurine and methotrexate

Most patients who have Crohn's disease, unless it is very mild, will require an immunomodulator. As in ulcerative colitis, azathioprine and 6-mercaptopurine are the most commonly prescribed agents and are used in a similar fashion, with the same dosing and monitoring. These agents are slow-acting and response usually takes more than 3 months.

Methotrexate is also an option for patients with Crohn's disease who are intolerant of, or do not respond to, thiopurines. Methotrexate is an antimetabolite medication that is given once weekly. It can take up to 3 months to see a response. To guarantee bioavailability, the recommended dose is 25 mg intramuscularly each week and patients require folic acid supplementation to reduce side effects, which commonly include nausea, vomiting and fatigue. These can be dose-dependent and often improve with time. Methotrexate can also cause bone marrow suppression, opportunistic infections, interstitial pneumonitis and hepatotoxicity. Patients need to avoid excessive alcohol intake, as this can result in cirrhosis. Importantly, methotrexate is teratogenic and results in birth defects so appropriate contraception is required in females, and ideally the medication should be ceased 3 months before conception. It is not safe during breastfeeding.

Biological agents: adalimumab, infliximab, vedolizumab and ustekinumab

In a similar fashion to ulcerative colitis, when patients continue to have symptoms on immunomodulators or if they are steroid-dependent or steroid-refractory, escalation to biological therapy is required. Anti-TNF agents were the first biological agents that became available for Crohn's disease. They are effective at treating moderate-to-severe Crohn's disease. Treatment with an anti-TNF improves quality of life, reduces hospital admissions and surgery. Anti-TNF therapy is also very effective at treating extra-intestinal manifestations of Crohn's disease including joint pains, fistulating disease, erythema nodosum and pyoderma gangrenosum. As in ulcerative colitis, the combination of an immunomodulator and anti-TNF therapy appears to be more efficacious than either therapy alone, although it is associated with increased risk of infection and lymphoma.

Vedolizumab is also an effective therapy for Crohn's disease and is not associated with the malignancy risk or immunosuppression of anti-TNF therapy. However, it is slower-acting than the anti-TNF therapies and requires up to 6 months of therapy for its full effect to be felt. It also appears to be less effective at treating the extra-intestinal manifestations of Crohn's disease.

Ustekinumab is the newest agent recently approved for Crohn's disease. Ustekinumab is a human IgG monoclonal antibody that blocks the activity of interleukin (IL)-12 and IL-23. Clinical trials have demonstrated that ustekinumab is effective at treating moderate-to-severe Crohn's disease. It is a well-tolerated medication that appears to have minimal side effects.

Symptomatic treatment

Treatment of diarrhoea depends on its causation; treatment of active disease has been discussed and bacterial overgrowth is treated with metronidazole. Bile salt-induced diarrhoea following ileal resection is treated with colestyramine. Finally, antidiarrhoeal agents such as codeine phosphate, loperamide and diphenoxylate hydrochloride may have a small role.

Surgical management

Crohn's disease is a diffuse intestinal problem and there is a high incidence of disease recrudescence at various sites. Crohn's disease cannot be cured by surgical excision and a group of patients will require repeated resections with time. Thus, there is a tendency towards more conservative or minimal surgery to minimise the risk of short-bowel syndrome from excessive resections of the small bowel.

Surgery is mainly indicated for:
- stricture-causing obstructive symptoms
- phlegmonous disease not responding to medical therapy
- enterocutaneous or enterovesical fistulas
- intra-abdominal abscesses (most are now drained by percutaneous radiological techniques)
- acute or chronic blood loss (this is a rare indication).

Surgical options

Conservative resection
The severely diseased segment is resected with a 2-cm margin of macroscopically normal bowel on either side. With extensive disease, minor evidence of Crohn's disease at the anastomotic site does not matter. The emphasis should be on preserving bowel length.

The cumulative re-operation rate after the first resection for distal ileal disease is 25% at 5 years after the first operation. Aphthous ulceration on the ileal side of the ileocolic anastomosis is present in almost all patients within 12 months of ileocolic resection. Although recurrent disease after surgery is common, surgery rapidly restores patients with incapacitating obstructing symptoms to good health.

Strictureplasty
In selective cases, strictures of the small bowel may be overcome by strictureplasty without resection. The stricture is incised longitudinally along the antimesenteric border and then sutured transversely as in Heineke–Mikulicz strictureplasty (Figure 29.5) or in a side-to-side bypass as in Finney strictureplasty (Figure 29.6). Strictureplasty can be accomplished with a surgical morbidity similar to that of resection. It relieves obstruction, modifies progression of the disease and allows preservation of functional small bowel.

Enteric fistula and intra-abdominal abscess
Fistula and abscess often coexist. Magnetic resonance enterography is used to evaluate the extent of Crohn's disease in the small bowel and the presence of fistulas. Colonoscopy is performed to rule out severe disease in the colon, and especially the rectum. A CT scan will demonstrate any abscesses that may be appropriately treated by CT-guided percutaneous drainage.

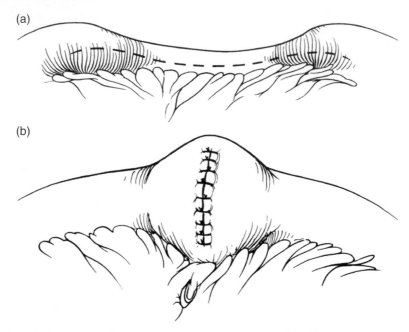

Fig. 29.5 Heineke–Mikulicz strictureplasty. The stricture is (a) incised longitudinally along the antimesenteric border and (b) then sutured transversely.

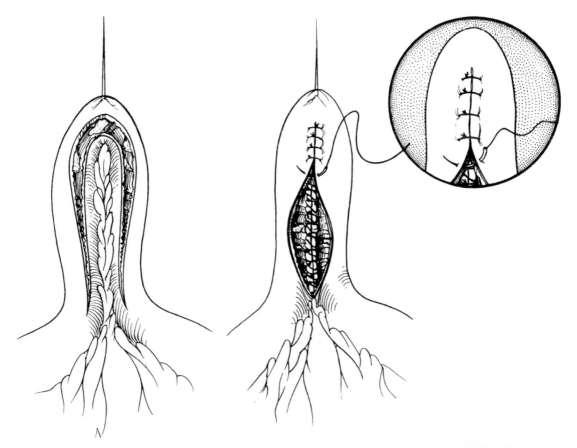

Fig. 29.6 Finney strictureplasty for a longer stricture using a side-to-side bypass. Source: Tjandra JJ, Fazio VW. Strictureplasty in Crohn's disease. In: Cameron JL (ed.) *Current Surgical Therapy*, 4th edn. Philadelphia: Mosby Year Book, 1992:108–13. Reproduced with permission of Springer.

Internal fistulas are often asymptomatic and are identified incidentally at surgery. Ileosigmoid fistulas are usually due to ileal disease. Enterovesical fistulas cause recurrent urinary tract infections and pneumaturia. At operation, the small bowel disease is resected and the viscus that is secondarily involved is closed locally. Following repair of an enterovesical fistula, a Foley catheter is left in the bladder for at least a week.

Enterocutaneous fistula in the early postoperative period is a challenging problem. It arises from anastomotic breakdown or from inadvertent damage to the small bowel that is unrecognised at the time of surgery. Principles of management are discussed in Chapter 26.

Crohn's colitis

Clinical features

Colonic disease presents with bloody diarrhoea, urgency and frequency. Fibrosis and stricture may lead to subacute large bowel obstruction. Fistulation to adjacent viscera can produce colovesical or rectovaginal fistulas. Perianal disease commonly accompanies Crohn's colitis: fleshy anal skin tags, anorectal strictures, relatively painless chronic anal fissures and painful anal canal ulcers with complex perirectal fistulas. The differences between ulcerative colitis and Crohn's colitis are given in Table 29.2.

Surgical management

Emergency surgery

Acute fulminant colitis with toxic dilatation and perforation may occur as in ulcerative colitis. Perforation can occur without toxic dilatation. The procedure of choice is a subtotal colectomy with formation of an end-ileostomy and mucous fistula. Severe colonic bleeding may also necessitate urgent surgery. Subtotal colectomy and ileorectal anastomosis is appropriate if the rectum is relatively free of disease and the patient is fit.

Elective surgery

Segmental colectomy of the involved section of colon may be appropriate for localised disease. Subtotal colectomy and ileorectal anastomosis is indicated in patients with severe diffuse colonic disease and rectal sparing, especially in younger patients. This operation may not be appropriate if there is severe perianal or rectal disease or if the anal sphincters are functionally inadequate. Recurrent disease tends to occur in the pre-anastomotic segment of bowel and is more frequent in patients with a limited resection. Many of these recurrences may be treated medically.

Total proctocolectomy and end-ileostomy is indicated for extensive Crohn's colitis involving the rectum, with or without perianal disease. Sometimes this is performed for severe perianal Crohn's disease. There is a high incidence of delayed perianal wound healing, especially if there is severe perianal Crohn's disease.

Perianal Crohn's disease

More than half the patients with Crohn's disease have anal lesions, especially those with rectal disease.

Medical therapy

Patients with perianal fistulating Crohn's disease have a severe phenotype of Crohn's disease and require aggressive medical therapy.

Treatment of perianal disease is with a multidisciplinary approach between the gastroenterologist and colorectal surgeon. Medical treatment with antibiotics, namely ciprofloxacin or metronidazole,

Table 29.2 Differentiation between ulcerative colitis and Crohn's colitis.

	Ulcerative colitis	Crohn's colitis
Distribution	Continuous	Segmental
Inflammation	Mucosal and submucosal	Transmural
Mucosa	Granular, ulcerated	Cobblestone, patchy inflammation
Involvement of small bowel	No	Common
Complex anal lesions	No	Common
Internal fistula	No	Possible
Granulomas	No	Common
Fibrosis	No	Common
Carcinoma	More common in extensive and long-standing cases	More common in extensive and long-standing cases

improves fistula symptoms and may contribute to healing. Therefore, antibiotics should be used as an adjunctive treatment for active perianal fistulas. Anti-TNF therapy is recommended for anyone with active fistulating perianal disease and results in healing in approximately 50% of patients. Infliximab has the most established evidence and is even more effective when combined with an immunomodulator. Hence, combination therapy with infliximab and an immunomodulator should be used in patients with active perianal fistula where possible.

Surgical therapy

The most common anal lesions are fleshy anal skin tags or anal fissures. These anal fissures are often at atypical sites and cause little pain, unless there is a cavitating ulcer or an associated abscess. Perianal fistulas and abscesses are often multiple and complex. Stricture at the anorectal ring is common as well.

Conservative medical and surgical treatment is the key. The underlying anal sphincter is preserved as much as possible. Many anal lesions are relatively asymptomatic and do not require specific treatment. Proper assessment may demand an examination under anaesthesia, especially in the presence of anorectal stricture and undrained pus. Endoanal ultrasound or MRI facilitates assessment of complex fistulous tracts and abscesses.

Haemorrhoids are common problems but most have few symptoms. Dietary and topical management alone are adequate. In troublesome cases, elastic-band ligation may be performed. A haemorrhoidectomy should be avoided because of the risk of secondary sepsis and fistula formation. Anal surgery for fissure should be avoided whenever possible. Associated abscesses are drained but the anal sphincters must be preserved as much as possible. With more complex fistulous abscesses, a long-term seton through the fistula functions as an effective drain. A tube drain is also effective. If the disease is progressive or fails to respond to adequate local drainage procedures, consideration should be given to faecal diversion, followed by a proctectomy in severe cases.

Further reading

Colonoscopic Surveillance Guidelines: Inflammatory bowel disease. Available at https://wiki.cancer.org.au/australia wiki/images/4/43/Algorithm_for_Colonoscopic_Surveillance_Intervals_-_IBD.pdf#_ga=2.65169134.1343 277047.1518337521-726258687.1518337521

Gionchetti P, Dignass A, Danese S *et al*. Third European Evidence-based Consensus on Diagnosis and Management of Ulcerative Colitis 2016: Part 2: Surgical Management and Special Situations. *J Crohns Colitis* 2017;11:135–49.

Gomollón F, Dignass A, Annese V *et al*. Third European Evidence-based Consensus on the Diagnosis and Management of Crohn's Disease 2016: Part 1: Diagnosis and Medical Management. *J Crohns Colitis* 2017;11:3–25.

Toh JW, Stewart P, Rickard MJ, Leong R, Wang N, Young CJ. Indications and surgical options for small bowel, large bowel and perianal Crohn's disease. *World J Gastroenterol* 2016;22:8892–904.

MCQs

Select the single correct answer to each question. The correct answers can be found in the Answers section at the end of the book.

1 Extra-intestinal manifestations of ulcerative colitis include the following *except*:
   a pyoderma gangrenosum
   b iritis
   c sacroiliitis
   d sclerosing cholangitis
   e eczema

2 Which of the following statements about Crohn's disease is correct?
   a adenocarcinoma of the small bowel never occurs as a complication of Crohn's disease
   b when operative resection is required, the sites of anastomosis should be macroscopically normal
   c strictureplasty does not preserve length of the small bowel
   d haemorrhoidectomy should be performed as early as necessary because severe symptoms are likely
   e inflammation of the colon and rectum cannot be due to Crohn's disease

3 Ulcerative colitis:
   a is a transmural disease that affects both the large and small bowel
   b has a higher risk of colorectal cancer compared to Crohn's disease
   c surveillance for colon cancer is mandatory, starting at diagnosis
   d toxic megacolon exclusively occurs in this disease
   e immunomodulators act within a week of commencement of treatment

4 Indications for restorative proctocolectomy in ulcerative colitis include:
   a toxic megacolon
   b a patient responding to medical therapy after 2 days
   c possible Crohn's-related stricture in the small bowel
   d severe sacroiliitis
   e dysplasia on rectal biopsy

30 Diverticular disease of the colon

Ian Hastie and the late Joe J. Tjandra

University of Melbourne and Royal Melbourne Hospital, Melbourne, Victoria, Australia

Introduction

The term *diverticulum* (pleural, *diverticula*) indicates an abnormal outpouching of the wall of a hollow viscus such as the colon. Colonic diverticula are 'false' diverticula because they only contain mucosa and serosa in their wall. The term *diverticulosis* refers to the presence of diverticula in the bowel wall but without complications or symptoms. Diverticular disease implies that pathophysiological changes and symptoms are arising due to the diverticula. Diverticulosis of the sigmoid colon is associated with a western lifestyle, whilst right-sided diverticulosis is predominantly associated with people of Asian backgrounds. The incidence of diverticulosis increases with age and is identified in over 50% of the population over the age of 60 years, with an increasing incidence in individuals under 40 years. The male to female ratio varies with age, being more predominant in males under 50 years, and in females over this age.

Pathology

Diverticulosis of the colon comprises acquired mucosal herniations protruding through the circular muscle at sites weakened by entry of blood vessels. The incidence appears to be related to the amount of fibre intake in the diet. The over-refined and fibre-deficient diet of western countries produces small hard stools. As the faecal stream is more viscous by the time it reaches the sigmoid colon, hypersegmentation of the colon occurs to generate higher pressures to propel these stools. Diverticula are thus the result of increased intraluminal pressure within the colon. However, this does not readily explain the cause of caecal or pancolonic diverticular disease.

Diverticula penetrate through the circular muscle in four main sites, each relating to penetrating vasa recta (Figure 30.1).

The sigmoid colon affected by diverticulosis appears shortened and thickened. The muscular abnormality is the most important and consistent feature. There is gross thickening of both the longitudinal and circular muscles of the colon, and progressive elastosis of the taeniae coli. This muscular abnormality often precedes the development of diverticulosis and occurs predominantly in the sigmoid colon. The muscle of the sigmoid colon and rectosigmoid is different from that of the more proximal colon, in that it is thicker and more prone to spasm. The colonic mucosa is pleated, with a saccular appearance. Narrowing of the lumen is due to muscular hypertrophy, redundant mucosal folds and pericolic fibrosis.

In classic situations, diverticula with associated muscular hypertrophy occur predominantly on the left side of the colon and are characterised by inflammatory and perforative complications. There appears to be another kind of diverticular disease that is present throughout the entire colon without associated muscle abnormality. This latter group tends to occur in younger patients and may be due to a connective tissue abnormality that allows development of diverticula. Bleeding as a complication is more common in this atypical group. Right-sided diverticulitis with right-sided abdominal pain occurs almost exclusively in the Asian population but whether this is due to genetic or dietary factors remains undetermined.

Microscopically, diverticula have two coats, an inner mucosal and an outer serosal layer. An artery, vein or attenuated muscle may be present close to the neck of the diverticulum. Antimesenteric diverticula do not herniate fully through the circular muscle coat and have a thinned layer of circular muscle in their wall.

Textbook of Surgery, Fourth Edition. Edited by Julian A. Smith, Andrew H. Kaye, Christopher Christophi and Wendy A. Brown.
© 2020 John Wiley & Sons Ltd. Published 2020 by John Wiley & Sons Ltd.

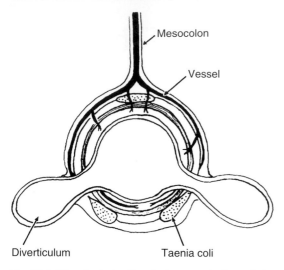

Fig. 30.1 Diverticulosis: diverticula protrude through the circular muscle at the points where the blood vessels penetrate the colonic wall.

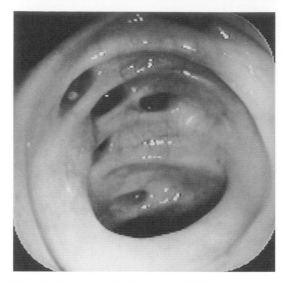

Fig. 30.2 Colonoscopic view of sigmoid diverticula.

Box 30.1 Common complications of diverticulosis

- Acute diverticulitis
- Inflammatory phlegmon
- Pericolic or mesenteric abscess
- Perforation with local or generalised peritonitis
- Fistula
- Diverticular stricture
- Distal large bowel obstruction
- Colonic bleeding

The majority of patients with diverticulosis will remain asymptomatic. Of those with symptomatic diverticular disease, about 30% will develop troublesome complications that may require an operation in their management. The disease tends to pursue a more aggressive course in the young. The likelihood of complications is unrelated to the number of diverticula present. Common complications are listed in Box 30.1.

A diagnostically difficult group involves patients with proven diverticulosis who present with chronic pain but do not have objective evidence of pericolonic inflammation on computed tomography (CT) or other features of complicated diverticular disease. Some of these patients may have concurrent irritable bowel syndrome or other causes of their pain. Treatment of these patients with antibiotics or indeed resection is questionable.

Investigations

Colonoscopy or flexible sigmoidoscopy

Colonoscopy or flexible sigmoidoscopy is most useful in differentiating diverticular disease from carcinoma and has the advantage of allowing tissue to be biopsied (Figure 30.2). Stricturing and angulation may limit the endoscopic evaluation of complicated diverticular disease and necessitate contrast imaging.

CT colonography

CT colonography or 'virtual colonoscopy' allows evaluation of the colonic mucosa as well as the colonic wall and pericolic tissues. The radiation exposure is significantly reduced compared with barium enema. In complex diverticular disease, where complete colonoscopic evaluation may not be not achievable, CT colonography is a reliable alternative.

Acute diverticulitis

Pathology

Approximately 30% of patients with known diverticulosis will develop one or more bouts of diverticulitis. Among patients who require hospitalisation, 20% require an emergency operation. The primary pathogenesis is thought to be related to obstruction at the neck of the diverticulum, giving rise to an inflammatory reaction in the pericolic tissues.

In severe cases, an inflammatory phlegmon will form. Resolution may result in fibrosis. Progression of sepsis can result in perforation, which is often contained locally in the form of an abscess. Pericolic abscesses are usually walled off and, with repeated episodes, the colon may become ensheathed in fibrous tissue and adherent to surrounding structures. Less commonly, free perforation from the diverticulum or the pericolic abscess may ensue, resulting in pelvic or generalised peritonitis. Fistulation to adjacent organs such as bladder, small bowel or vagina may occur.

Clinical features

Acute diverticulitis is associated with constant and protracted pain in the left iliac fossa, with systemic symptoms and fever, leucocytosis and sometimes an abdominal mass. Alteration of bowel habit, with constipation or diarrhoea, may occur. If the inflammatory process involves the bladder, urinary symptoms may be present. In more severe cases, abdominal distension is also present, either secondary to ileus or to partial colonic obstruction. Rectal examination may reveal tenderness in the pelvis and a mass or pelvic collection may be felt. Use of rigid sigmoidoscopy is usually limited because of pain. Differential diagnoses are listed in Box 30.2.

Investigations

CT scanning provides good definition of the extraluminal extent of the disease and is particularly helpful in diagnosing complications such as abscesses and colovesical fistula. The key finding is the presence of diverticula *and* pericolic inflammation. Percutaneous drainage of localised collections of pus can also be performed under CT guidance.

Ultrasound can provide information similar to CT and can facilitate percutaneous drainage of a localised abscess. However, with the extent of gaseous dilatation of the bowel during acute diverticulitis, images from sonography may be limited.

Box 30.2 Differential diagnosis of acute diverticulitis

- Pelvic inflammatory disease
- Appendicitis: when the diverticulitis occurs in the mid-sigmoid area of a redundant colon that lies on the right side of the abdomen
- Crohn's colitis
- Ischaemic colitis
- Perforated colonic carcinoma
- Pyelonephritis

Flexible endoscopy adds little useful information and risks perforating an acutely inflamed bowel. It may have a role if ischaemic colitis, Crohn's colitis or carcinoma is strongly suspected.

CT colonography is generally contraindicated during the acute episode because instillation of the contrast may disrupt a well-contained sepsis. Contrast examination and flexible endoscopy are best deferred for 6 weeks after an acute episode has settled.

Plain abdominal X-ray is rarely helpful because there are no specific features.

Management

Medical management

Mild diverticulitis

Patients with mild symptoms, minimal abdominal signs and minimal features of systemic sepsis can be managed with broad-spectrum oral antibiotics (ciprofloxacin and metronidazole or amoxicillin/lavulinic acid) for 7 days, as outpatients.

Severe diverticulitis

Patients with localised peritonitis need to be hospitalised for resuscitation. The diagnosis is confirmed with CT scanning. Intravenous fluid replacement is provided. A nasogastric tube is only indicated if there is evidence of significant ileus or bowel obstruction. Hospitalised patients are generally given intravenous antibiotics (e.g. cefotaxime and metronidazole) that cover Gram-negative organisms and anaerobes. Adequate analgesia should be prescribed.

Symptoms should begin to subside within 48 hours. If resolution continues, further investigation with colonoscopy is performed 6 weeks later. If medical therapy should fail, a repeat CT scan may be necessary looking for the development of complications such as abscess. Approximately one-fifth of patients with severe diverticulitis will require operation during the first hospital admission, and a further one-fifth radiological drainage in the setting of abscess formation.

For patients with an initial uncomplicated attack of diverticulitis who have responded to medical therapy, 70% will have no recurrence.

Radiological options: percutaneous drainage of diverticular abscesses

With a confined pericolic or pelvic abscess, CT- or ultrasound-guided percutaneous drainage is helpful (Figure 30.3). The drainage catheter is kept patent by regular irrigation with normal saline and kept in place until drainage ceases and the abscess cavity has completely collapsed.

Acute operative management

Indications for operative management during the acute admission include generalised peritonitis and failure of non-operative therapy after 3–5 days. The decision to intervene depends on the severity and extent of peritonism and systemic disturbance.

Laparoscopic lavage

Early laparoscopic intervention with lavage of the inflamed area and drainage of collections is favoured in some centres. Severe cases with faecal peritonitis will still require resection but this technique has a role in purulent peritonitis.

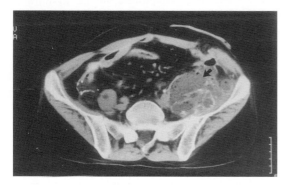

Fig. 30.3 Computed tomography scan showing a localised abscess in the left pelvic region due to complicated diverticulitis.

Hartmann's procedure

Hartmann's procedure (Figure 30.4) involves resecting the diseased segment of colon, stapling off the rectal stump and bringing out the proximal end of colon as an end-colostomy. It has the advantage of removing the septic focus (i.e. phlegmonous or perforated sigmoid colon) and avoids an anastomosis in the presence of gross sepsis and faecal contamination. However, a second-stage operation is necessary after 4–6 months to re-establish intestinal continuity and entails a further laparotomy and bowel mobilisation (and often further resection), with all the attendant risks of colorectal anastomosis.

Hartmann's procedure has evolved as the treatment of choice for patients with faecal peritonitis. It is no longer the treatment of first choice in patients with an abscess, which should be treated primarily by percutaneous drainage.

Resection and primary colorectal anastomosis

Resection and primary colorectal anastomosis has the advantage that the diseased segment is resected and an anastomosis is established. However, in the acute setting, it involves extensive dissection in the presence of intraperitoneal sepsis with the attendant risk of spreading the infective process. When primary anastomosis is performed in cases of severe acute diverticulitis, a proximal diverting ileostomy may be used. Subsequent closure of the diverting ileostomy is more straightforward than the second-stage reversal of Hartmann's procedure. The diverting stoma is generally closed after 2–3 months. A limited Gastrografin enema is performed prior to

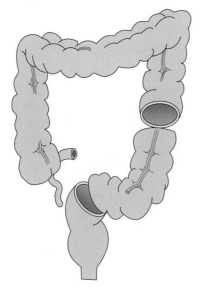
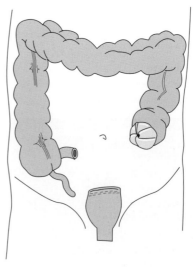

Fig. 30.4 Hartmann's procedure.

closure of the stoma to ensure healing and patency of the colorectal anastomosis.

On-table large bowel irrigation, resection and primary colorectal anastomosis is also another option to avoid a Hartmann's procedure. On-table colonic washout is performed to remove the faecal residue in the otherwise unprepared colon. This manoeuvre is cumbersome and may contaminate the operative field. This technique should be considered only in highly selected situations where the sepsis is confined, with minimal bowel distension and oedema. A proximal diverting ileostomy is often performed in combination with on-table colonic lavage.

Transverse colostomy and drainage

This outdated three-stage procedure involves an initial diverting transverse loop colostomy and tube drainage of the septic area, a subsequent sigmoid resection and, finally, closure of the colostomy. The combined morbidity and mortality of the three stages of operations are high and the procedure is associated with long periods of hospitalisation.

Bleeding diverticular disease

Massive diverticular bleeding probably arises from injury to the vasa recta. The characteristic presentation is that of an otherwise well individual who suddenly passes a large amount of maroon-coloured stool. Characteristically, the bleeding is not associated with significant pain or abdominal tenderness. Bleeding stops spontaneously in about 80% of cases.

Management of massive rectal bleeding is discussed in Chapter 65. Considerable difficulty exists in identifying the source and cause of colonic bleeding, and CT angiography and labelled red cell scan should be considered. In patients with a minor degree of persistent rectal bleeding, the bleeding should not be attributed too readily to the diverticular disease. In many such patients, there is a coexistent carcinoma or polyp of the colon. If diverticular disease is identified confidently as the source of recurrent colonic bleeding, segmental resection is recommended.

Fistula

Fistulas develop from localised perforations to which an adjacent viscus becomes adherent. Eventually the abscess or faeces drains through that viscus.

Colovesical fistula

Most patients are male; presumably the uterus protects the bladder from the colon in females (women who develop colovesical or colovaginal fistulas have often had a hysterectomy). Common symptoms are those of cystitis. There is usually a history of recurrent urinary tract infections that fail to respond to appropriate antibiotic therapy. Faecaluria is diagnostic, as is passage of vegetative matter. Pneumaturia that occurs at the end of voiding is strongly suggestive but gas-forming organisms in the bladder can simulate the condition. Bowel symptoms may be absent.

Flexible sigmoidoscopy will rule out inflammatory bowel disease and may identify the fistula and the presence of diverticula. Barium enema will show the diverticular disease but demonstrates the fistulous communication in only about 50% of cases. Cystoscopy may reveal cystitis and the fistulous opening. Cystograms may demonstrate the fistula in 30% of cases. CT scan or CT colonography can define the extent and degree of pericolic inflammation and may detect air in the bladder that is associated with a colovesical fistula, along with contrast extravasation. Treatment involves separation of the sigmoid colon from the bladder, and sigmoid resection followed by a primary colorectal anastomosis. The opening in the bladder is often not obvious. If an opening in the bladder is seen, it is repaired. The omentum is interposed between the colorectal anastomosis and the bladder.

Other fistulas

Other rarer forms of fistula present with discharge of purulent fluid, flatus or faeces on the abdominal wall (colocutaneous fistula), via the vagina (colovaginal fistula) or with diarrhoea (coloenteric fistula).

Indications for elective operative treatment

Determining factors include the patient's age, general health, and the severity and frequency of the symptoms. Indications for surgery include:
- chronic symptoms despite the use of a high-fibre diet and bulk-forming agents
- recurrent acute diverticulitis
- persistent tender mass
- inability to distinguish colonic lesion from carcinoma or inability to exclude carcinoma
- fistulas.

Elective operations for symptomatic diverticular disease are more commonly recommended in younger patients (<55 years), in those who are immunosuppressed (e.g. after renal transplantation) because of the potential morbidity of further diverticular complications, and in patients with significant radiological abnormalities such as extravasation of contrast or a sigmoid stricture.

The timing of elective operation should ideally be about 12 weeks after the most recent attack of diverticulitis. Only the segment of colon affected by the diverticular inflammatory reaction needs to be removed. In general, this includes the entire sigmoid colon and the rectosigmoid junction. The distal margin of resection must extend below the level of muscular thickening and is usually in the upper rectum (the level at which the teniae coalesce). The proximal extent of transection should include all induration palpable at the junction of the mesocolon with the colon itself and is usually in the descending colon. It is not usually necessary to resect the entire diverticula-bearing proximal colon. A primary colorectal anastomosis is generally utilised. In most cases, a laparoscopic approach is possible, rather than the conventional laparotomy.

Further reading

Angenete E, Bock D, Rosenberg J, Haglind E. Laparoscopic lavage is superior to colon resection for perforated purulent diverticulitis: a meta-analysis. *Int J Colorectal Dis* 2017;32:163–9.

Aydin HN, Remzi FH. Diverticulitis: when and how to operate? *Dig Liver Dis* 2004;36:435–45.

Boynton W, Floch M. New strategies for the management of diverticular disease: insights for the clinician. *Ther Adv Gastroenterol* 2013;6:205–13.

Feingold D, Steele SR. Practice parameters for the treatment of sigmoid diverticulitis. *Dis Colon Rectum* 2014;57:284–94.

MCQs

Select the single correct answer to each question. The correct answers can be found in the Answers section at the end of the book.

1 A 72-year-old woman presents with left iliac fossa pain and is found to have a fever and left iliac fossa peritonism. The most likely diagnosis is:
   a left ureteric calculus
   b tubo-ovarian abscess
   c irritable bowel syndrome
   d acute diverticulitis
   e sigmoid volvulus

2 Diverticulosis of the sigmoid colon is associated with:
   a thickening of the longitudinal but not circular muscle of the colon
   b narrowing of the lumen from mucosal hyperplasia
   c increased intraluminal pressure within the colon
   d high-fibre and high-fat diet
   e a high incidence of anastomotic breakdown in elective surgery

3 Surgical management of perforated diverticular disease with faecal peritonitis includes:
   a preoperative mechanical bowel preparation
   b Hartmann's procedure and sigmoid end-colostomy
   c preoperative barium enema to define the anatomy
   d anterior resection and primary colorectal anastomosis whenever possible
   e preoperative nasogastric feeding to optimise nutrition

4 The complications of sigmoid diverticular disease do *not* include which of the following?
   a sigmoid inflammatory phlegmon
   b colonic bleeding
   c purulent peritonitis
   d colovaginal fistula
   e colon cancer

31 Colorectal cancer

Ian T. Jones and the late Joe J. Tjandra

Department of Surgery, University of Melbourne and Colorectal Surgery Unit, Royal Melbourne Hospital, Melbourne, Victoria, Australia

Introduction

Colorectal cancer (CRC) is the most common internal cancer in the western world. It is the second most common cause of death from cancer and accounts for one in eight of all new cancer diagnoses. However, the prognosis for patients with CRC is superior to that of many other solid tumours, such as lung and pancreas, and Australian cancer statistics reveal that 69% of patients diagnosed with CRC between 2009 and 2013 survived more than 5 years. Even so, CRC accounts for 8.6% of all Australian cancer deaths.

Epidemiology

It is estimated that in 2019, 16 398 new cases of CRC will be diagnosed in Australia, 9069 in males and 7329 in females. The gender difference is largely due to the higher incidence of rectal cancer in males as the incidence of colon cancer is about equal in men and women. These figures are similar on a per-capita basis to other parts of the western world. In the USA, it is estimated that over 145 600 new cases of CRC will be diagnosed in 2018.

The lifetime risk for CRC is 1 in 18 for men and 1 in 24 for women. The peak age of onset is the seventh decade of life (mean age 64 years). CRC is less common in those under 50 years of age (except in individuals with an inherited bowel cancer syndrome).

Aetiology

Whilst most cases of CRC are sporadic, the inherited CRC syndromes such as familial adenomatous polyposis (FAP) and Lynch syndrome have allowed a clearer understanding of the series of cellular genetic mutations that result in the onset of malignancy and these same events are also at play in sporadic or non-inherited cancers.

Two major carcinogenesis sequences have been identified.

- Chromosomal instability (CIN) pathway refers to the traditional adenoma–carcinoma pathway described by Vogelstein in 1990. This pathway accounts for approximately 85% of all CRCs. Progression from benign adenomatous polyps to more dysplastic lesions, invasive cancer and metastases is associated with an aggregation of genetic mutations, the most important of which affects the adenomatous polyposis coli (*APC*) gene. An inherited *APC* mutation is responsible for FAP.
- Microsatellite instability (MSI) pathway is the second major pathway of carcinogenesis and is associated with dysfunction of mismatch repair (MMR) genes that protect the integrity of cellular DNA. An inherited mutation of one or more MMR genes leads to the development of Lynch syndrome.

Whilst inherited CRC syndromes account for perhaps only 5% of all CRCs, family history is a critical factor in CRC. Individual risk for CRC is increased two-and-a-half to three times for those with a first-degree relative with CRC but this increases up to six times when a relative is diagnosed under the age of 55 years.

Epidemiological studies suggest that environmental factors predominate in the causation of most CRCs. A diet rich in fat and meat, and low in fibre, is commonly associated with colorectal cancers. Obesity and alcohol intake are increasingly recognised as major risk factors for CRC (Box 31.1).

Textbook of Surgery, Fourth Edition. Edited by Julian A. Smith, Andrew H. Kaye, Christopher Christophi and Wendy A. Brown.
© 2020 John Wiley & Sons Ltd. Published 2020 by John Wiley & Sons Ltd.

Box 31.1 Risk factors for colorectal cancer

- Environmental factors: fat, red meat, alcohol, obesity
- Adenomatous polyps: most cancers originate within an adenoma
- Family history of CRC
- Genetic syndromes (e.g. FAP)
- Inflammatory bowel disease: ulcerative colitis and Crohn's disease especially when long-standing and extensive
- Irradiation: the risk of rectal cancer is increased following pelvic radiation therapy (e.g. for cancer of the cervix)

Pathology

The outcome of CRC depends on its biological behaviour. The clinicopathological stage (the amount of spread) of the disease is a 'snapshot' in the life of a cancer and provides the most accurate prognostic index at the present time.

Staging

The most common staging method is the Union for International Cancer Control (UICC) TNM classification (Table 31.1), which has largely superseded the traditional Dukes' classification.

Table 31.1 Staging methods for colorectal cancer.

Modified Dukes' staging	
A	Tumour confined to bowel wall
B	Tumour invading through serosa
B_1	Through muscularis propria
B_2	Through serosa or perirectal fat
C	Lymph node involvement
C_1	Apical node not involved
C_2	Apical node involved
UICC TNM staging	
Tumour depth (T)	
T1	Submucosa
T2	Muscularis propria
T3	Subserosa or pericolic tissues
T4	Invade adjacent organs or visceral peritoneum
Nodes (N)	
N0	Nodes not involved
N1	1–3 pericolic nodes involved
N2	≥4 pericolic nodes involved
Metastasis (M)	
M0	No distant metastases
M1	Distant metastases
Stage I	T1–2 N0
Stage II	T3–4 N0
Stage III	T1–4 N1–2
Stage IV	M1

Table 31.2 Prognosis in colorectal cancer: 5-year survival rates (%).

Stage	Colon cancer	Rectal cancer
Dukes' A (stage I)	99	90
Dukes' B (stage II)	80	60
Dukes' C (stage III)	50	40
Distant metastases (stage IV)	<10	<10

Histopathology

Poorly differentiated cancers (including signet ring, mucinous and small cell cancers) have a worse outlook than those that are well to moderately differentiated. Other adverse features include lymphovascular or perineural invasion.

Prognosis

Tumour stage (Table 31.2) is the main determinant of prognosis. Most patients with Dukes' A (stage I) cancers are cured after surgery. Lymph node metastases (Dukes' C, stage III) are a significant adverse prognostic factor. Long-term survival can be achieved after treatment of distant metastases (especially those that are solitary or confined to one organ) but 5-year survival for stage IV disease is low.

Clinical presentation

This varies depending on the primary site and extent of disease.

Caecal and right-sided carcinoma

These account for 20% of all large bowel cancers. Clinical presentations include:
- Iron deficiency anaemia from occult intestinal blood loss
- Small bowel obstruction due to occlusion of the ileocaecal valve
- Palpable mass
- Lethargy, weight loss and hepatomegaly, which may be features of metastatic disease.

Left-sided and sigmoid carcinoma

Half of CRCs arise in the sigmoid colon and rectum. Clinical presentations include:
- Alteration of bowel habit, such as constipation alternating with diarrhoea

- Lower abdominal colic, distension and a desire to defecate
- Passage of altered blood and sometimes mucus in the stool.

Rectal cancer

Unfortunately, the diagnosis is often delayed because symptoms are attributed to haemorrhoids or similar. Rectal examination is essential in all patients with rectal bleeding. Clinical presentations include:
- Rectal bleeding may be dark and mixed with stool or bright and quite separate from the faeces.
- Tenesmus (an urge to use the bowels but with unsatisfied defecation) is common
- Anorectal pain usually indicates locally advanced disease.

Metastatic disease

Liver metastases are asymptomatic in the early stages; hepatomegaly indicates substantial liver involvement. Lung metastases are also usually asymptomatic. Ovarian metastases arise in up to 5% of female CRC patients and are referred to as Krukenberg tumours. Peritoneal spread may produce ascites and carries a poor prognosis.

Clinical assessment

A careful history and physical examination remain the most important assessments with regard to diagnosis, extent of spread and fitness for surgery. For rectal cancer, digital rectal examination and rigid sigmoidoscopy allow an assessment of tumour size and height above the anal verge (critical in determining the appropriate surgical procedure).

Investigations

Colonoscopy

Colonoscopy is the key investigation for the diagnosis of CRC and is used to examine symptomatic patients. It has entirely replaced traditional barium enema.

Computed tomography

Computed tomography (CT) scanning (Figure 31.1) is an essential tool in staging and treatment planning.

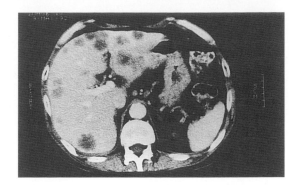

Fig. 31.1 Computed tomography scan of the abdomen showing multiple metastases in both the right and left lobes of the liver.

Magnetic resonance imaging

Magnetic resonance imaging (MRI) is a critical investigation for assessing local spread of rectal cancer, which guides surgeons in performing surgery to remove sites of local spread in continuity with the primary rectal cancer (total mesorectal excision or TME). It also allows selection of patients who might benefit from preoperative neoadjuvant chemoradiotherapy.

Positron emission tomography

Positron emission tomography (PET) is an alternative form of body imaging based on gamma rays emitted by biologically active molecules, usually the glucose analogue fluorodeoxyglucose (FDG). Its particular advantage is its superior sensitivity in the detection of metastatic disease. Its disadvantages include cost and difficulty in differentiating malignancy from other metabolically active conditions such as infection.

Carcinoembryonic antigen

Carcinoembryonic antigen (CEA) is a circulating tumour-associated antigen in CRC. It has little diagnostic value but has a significant role in the follow-up after resection leading to the earlier diagnosis of metastatic disease.

Treatment of colorectal cancer

When CRC is confined to the primary site, surgery with satisfactory resection margins provides the best chance of cure. Quality of surgery, particularly for rectal cancer, has a major impact on cancer outcome. Surgeons performing TME surgery have reduced the dreaded complication of pelvic cancer recurrence from about 30% in the pre-TME era to less than 10%. If unfavourable tumour grade, extramural vascular invasion or metastatic deposits in regional lymph glands are found by histological examination of the cancer (or on preoperative MRI for rectal cancer), surgery can be supplemented by postoperative adjuvant chemotherapy for colon cancer or neoadjuvant (preoperative) chemoradiation for rectal cancer.

The principles of surgery are to remove the segment of bowel containing the cancer, along with a margin of healthy uninvolved bowel in continuity with regional lymph nodes adjacent to the bowel and alongside mesenteric blood vessels. Bowel continuity is restored by constructing an anastomosis between the bowel ends.

Traditional CRC surgery is undertaken through an abdominal wall incision as an open procedure (laparotomy). Increasingly, minimally invasive approaches using laparoscopic-assisted techniques are being used. For colon cancer, oncologic results have been shown to be equivalent to those achieved at open surgery and have the advantage of smaller incisions, less postoperative pain and shorter length of hospital stay. The use of laparoscopic or minimally invasive techniques in rectal cancer is more controversial as large clinical trials have been unable to confirm an equivalent outcome compared with traditional open surgery, possibly due to the adequacy of the TME that can be achieved by minimally invasive techniques.

Preparation for surgery

Bowel preparation

Mechanical bowel preparation with dietary restriction and laxatives similar to those used for colonoscopy are frequently employed.

Antibiotic prophylaxis

Prophylactic antibiotics against aerobic and anaerobic bowel pathogens (usually a cephalosporin and metronidazole) are given on induction of anaesthesia. Such regimens have been shown to substantially reduce the risk of postoperative wound infection.

Prophylaxis for venous thromboembolism

Patients undergoing surgery for CRC carry a significant risk for venous thromboembolism. Mechanical and chemical prophylaxis are given unless contraindications exist.

Surgery for colon cancer

Carcinoma of the caecum or ascending colon

Right hemicolectomy is the standard operation (Figure 31.2). The ileocolic vessels are divided at their origins while maintaining the blood supply to the residual terminal ileum. The right colic vessels and the right branch of the middle colic vessels are also removed. The amount of bowel removed is influenced by the extent of lymphovascular clearance, which in turn is dependent on the site of the primary colon cancer.

Carcinoma of the transverse colon

The blood supply to this area is derived from the middle colic vessels as well as from the right colic vessels. If the cancer is at the hepatic flexure end of the transverse colon, a right hemicolectomy is performed. Lesions of the mid-transverse colon are treated by extended right hemicolectomy, which entails an anastomosis between the terminal ileum and the descending colon. The omentum is removed en bloc with the tumour. A carcinoma at the splenic

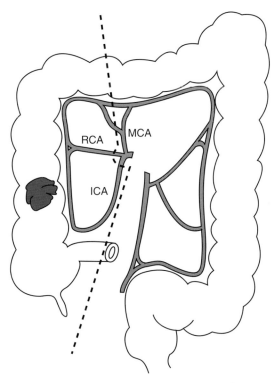

Fig. 31.2 Right hemicolectomy for ascending colon cancer. Dashed line indicates resected material. RCA, right colic artery; MCA, middle colic artery; ICA, ileocolic artery.

flexure can spread to regional lymphatics along the middle colic and left colic arteries. Adequate lymphatic clearance may require subtotal colectomy with an ileosigmoid anastomosis.

Carcinoma of the descending colon

Left hemicolectomy is the operation of choice (Figure 31.3). The inferior mesenteric artery is divided at its origin and the left colic and sigmoid vessels are included in the resection. An anastomosis is performed between the transverse colon and the upper rectum.

Carcinoma of the sigmoid colon

A high anterior resection is favoured, anastomosing the descending colon to the upper rectum. The inferior mesenteric artery is ligated close to the aorta. It is preferable to resect the entire sigmoid colon (which can be affected by diverticular disease) and to anastomose the descending colon to the upper rectum. Most surgeons believe this has a lower incidence of anastomotic leak.

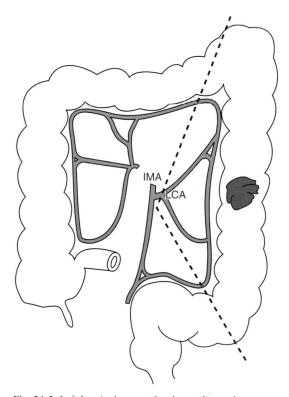

Fig. 31.3 Left hemicolectomy for descending colon cancer. Dashed line indicates resected material. IMA, inferior mesenteric artery; LCA, left colic artery.

Surgery for obstructing colon cancer

This is discussed in Chapter 32.

Surgery for perforated colon cancer

Perforation is less common than obstruction and usually occurs as a result of tumour necrosis. It carries a poor prognosis as the risk of local recurrence is high. Right colon perforations are managed by right hemicolectomy. For left colon perforations, Hartmann's procedure (see Figure 31.7) is generally performed with excision of the perforated bowel. The proximal colon is brought out as an end-colostomy and the distal bowel end oversewn. A primary anastomosis is generally not performed because of the higher leak rate in the presence of sepsis.

Surgery for rectal cancer

Management of rectal cancer is challenging because of the anatomical location of the tumour (particularly in the narrow male pelvis), the greater difficulty in performing low colorectal anastomoses and the potential for pelvic recurrence with inadequate surgery. Rectal cancer surgery is best performed by specialist colorectal surgeons who receive training in TME surgery. Apart from the superior oncologic outcomes with TME, colorectal surgeons have been able to reduce the need for permanent colostomy from around 80% 40 years ago to around 10% in the current era. There is also evidence that TME has a lower incidence of pelvic autonomic nerve injury leading to a lower rate of sexual and bladder dysfunction in men.

Factors influencing choice of operation for rectal cancer

Location of tumour
The height of the lower edge of the cancer above the anal verge is the most important factor in the choice of operation. In general, a tumour less than 5 cm from the anus requires abdominoperineal excision (APE) of the rectum with permanent colostomy, as a restorative anastomosis is usually not possible.

Nature of tumour
A high-grade, poorly differentiated tumour tends to be widely infiltrative and requires wide excision to achieve clear margins. Tethered or fixed tumours are locally advanced and require neoadjuvant chemoradiation with subsequent en bloc excision of any invaded adjacent organs (e.g. prostate or vagina).

Patient factors

The age and medical fitness of the patient and the presence of metastases are important factors in determining the magnitude of the operation. Obesity, male gender and previous pelvic surgery significantly add to the difficulty of rectal cancer surgery.

Anterior resection

Anterior resection (Figure 31.4) is the standard operation for cancers of the rectum. This entails excision of the sigmoid colon and a variable portion of the rectum. The inferior mesenteric artery and vein are divided at the highest possible level to achieve maximal lymph node clearance and to allow mobilisation of the splenic flexure and descending colon so that they reach into the pelvis to enable a tension-free anastomosis between colon and rectum. For mid-to-low rectal cancers, TME removes all the rectal mesentery so that the anastomosis typically lies at the level of the pelvic floor. The level of the anastomosis above the anal verge (determined by the site of the cancer in the rectum) is frequently used to further define anterior

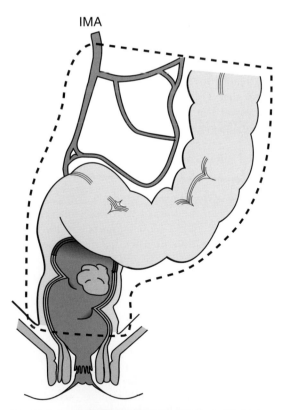

Fig. 31.4 Anterior resection for rectal cancer. Dashed line indicates resected material. IMA, inferior mesenteric artery.

resection as high (anastomosis >10 cm above anal verge), low (6–10 cm) and ultra-low (<6 cm).

The anastomosis is a critical part of the procedure, second only to performance of TME. Traditionally, anastomoses have been constructed by hand suturing techniques but this is technically difficult deep in the pelvis and, in most cases, disposable stapling devices have replaced hand suturing (Figure 31.5). Even in expert hands there is a risk of anastomotic leak (about 2–4%) which is greater for low-lying anastomoses. A proximal loop ileostomy is often used to divert the faecal stream away from the anastomosis to reduce the incidence of leak. When healing is confirmed, the ileostomy can be reversed, usually after 3 months. Bowel function after anterior resection is altered due to loss of the rectal 'reservoir' and low-lying anastomoses may be associated with urgency, increased frequency and clustering of bowel movements.

Abdominoperineal excision of the rectum

APE is required for low-lying rectal cancers (Figure 31.6). The rectum is mobilised down to the pelvic floor through an abdominal incision. The descending colon is divided and brought out as a colostomy. A separate perineal incision is then made to excise the sigmoid colon, distal rectum and anus.

Transanal local excision

Transanal excision of small, early-stage (T1), low-lying rectal cancers may be considered in highly selected cases where cure can be anticipated and where radical rectal excision would otherwise require a permanent colostomy. It can also be considered when age or infirmity of the patient or presence of metastases precludes major resection.

Neoadjuvant chemoradiotherapy

Based on evidence from large clinical trials which have shown reduced local recurrence when neoadjuvant chemoradiation is combined with TME surgery, combined modality treatment is recommended for T3/4 or N1/2 rectal cancers (as demonstrated on MRI). For patients who receive neoadjuvant chemoradiation, as many as 15% will be found to have no viable malignant cells in the surgically removed rectum. This raises the question as to whether surgery can be avoided in these patients. The major problem is that predicting which patients have a complete remission is difficult and potentially puts patients who forgo surgery (so called 'watch and wait') at risk of recurrence.

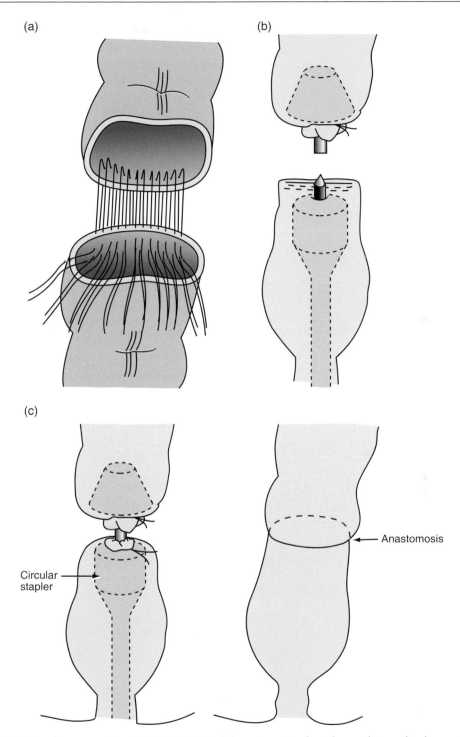

Fig. 31.5 (a) Hand-sewn anastomosis. (b) Double-stapled anastomosis where the rectal stump has been occluded with a linear stapler followed by construction of a colorectal anastomosis with a circular stapler. (c) Single-stapled anastomosis using a circular stapler.

Palliative procedures

Palliative procedures include a low Hartmann's procedure (Figure 31.7) or a diverting stoma only.

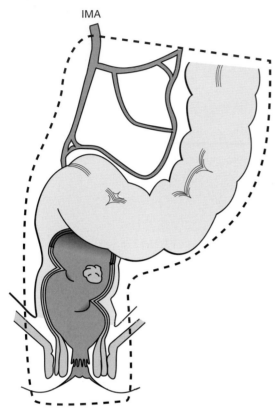

Fig. 31.6 Abdominoperineal excision of the rectum. Dashed line indicates resected material. IMA, inferior mesenteric artery.

Adjuvant therapy

In combination with high-quality cancer surgery, postoperative chemotherapy for node-positive colon cancer (stage III) has been shown in multiple studies to improve overall survival by 10–15%. The usual postoperative regimen consists of 5-fluorouracil, folinic acid and oxaliplatin (FOLFOX) given for a 6-month period.

As already discussed, neoadjuvant chemoradiotherapy has a major role in locally advanced rectal cancer. Perhaps the most influential study was the Dutch trial published in 2001 that evaluated preoperative radiotherapy combined with TME surgery and demonstrated a further significant reduction in pelvic recurrence rates already achieved by TME alone. A subsequent UK study (CR07) confirmed the results of the Dutch trial and also showed a small improvement in disease-free survival.

Treatment of metastatic disease

Treatment for incurable disease should be considered in terms of the possible benefit to be gained from symptom relief against the risk of treatment-associated morbidity in a patient who may have a limited remaining lifespan. In some cases, radical therapy of isolated metastases can achieve long-term survival. The treatment options for metastatic disease are listed in Box 31.2.

Follow-up after treatment for colorectal cancer

The need for follow-up is a source of debate. Follow-up provides reassurance for patients and

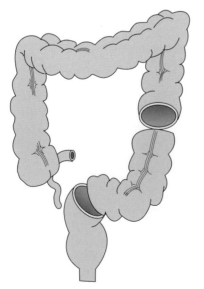
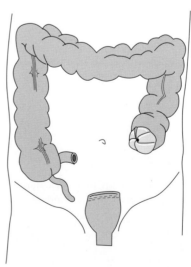

Fig. 31.7 Hartmann's procedure for perforated colon cancer (which can be modified to a lower resection for palliation of rectal cancer).

Box 31.2 Treatment of metastases

Liver
- Resection for single or closely grouped multiple tumours
- Selective internal radiation therapy (SIRT) by targeted hepatic artery injection of radioactive yttrium microspheres
- Chemotherapy
- Radiofrequency ablation

Lung
- Resection by video-assisted thoracoscopic surgical techniques (VATS)

Peritoneum
- Peritonectomy in association with heated intraperitoneal chemotherapy (HIPEC) in selected cases

Small bowel
- Resection
- Bypass

Pelvic/local recurrence
- Pelvic exenteration procedures when distant metastases have been excluded
- Radiotherapy
- Chemotherapy

allows surgical audit of outcomes but is costly and may have a low yield in terms of improved survival. A structured and targeted protocol (by CEA and CT) may detect early onset of recurrent disease, enabling treatment and in some cases long-term cure. Follow-up facilitates colonoscopy, which is recommended every 3–5 years for the detection of metachronous CRC.

Screening for colorectal cancer

Screening is appropriate for cancers that are common and curable, where early detection is accompanied by improved outcome and when it is cost-effective. CRC unquestionably meets these requirements. It is recommended that CRC screening commence at age 50 and continue to an age beyond the peak onset of CRC (e.g. to age 75). The two most common screening modalities are faecal occult blood testing (FOBT) and colonoscopy.

FOBT is recommended screening for most individuals of average risk. In Australia, national CRC screening commenced in 2006 as the National Bowel Cancer Screening Programme (NBCSP). This has been progressively expanded and the aspiration is for all Australians between the ages of 50 and 74 to be offered 2-yearly FOBT by 2020. When FOBT is positive, colonoscopy is required.

For individuals at higher risk of CRC (e.g. those with a family history), colonoscopy is preferred over FOBT because of its greater accuracy.

Colorectal polyps

A polyp is the term used to describe a tissue growth projecting into the bowel lumen. Certain polyps are entirely benign and have limited clinical significance (e.g. inflammatory, lymphoid and lipomatous polyps). Most interest is centred on precancerous adenomas.

Adenoma

An adenoma is a benign neoplasm of the large bowel that is associated with CRC. The most common variety is a tubular adenoma that is usually well-differentiated and pedunculated (Figure 31.8). By contrast, a villous adenoma is less differentiated and usually sessile.

At least 85% of CRCs arise from pre-existing adenomas. The risk of malignancy increases with the size and the histology of the adenoma. Large villous adenomas have the greatest risk (Table 31.3). Carcinoma in polyps smaller than 1 cm in diameter is uncommon. The malignant potential of adenomas is dramatically demonstrated in the inherited polyposis syndrome FAP, where hundreds or thousands of adenomas arise in the colon resulting in early-onset CRC. More recently, the importance of sessile serrated adenomas has been recognised. These are usually sessile polyps found mostly in the right colon.

Most adenomas are asymptomatic and only diagnosed during the investigation of bowel symptoms or by FOBT screening and colonoscopy. Colonoscopy allows therapeutic removal of polyps and a variety of techniques are available, using endoscopic instruments with diathermy to achieve polyp removal (polypectomy) and retrieval (Figure 31.9).

Large polyps may require surgery. Accessible rectal villous adenomas may be treated by transanal excision, which can be improved by the superior visualisation and instrumentation of transanal endoscopic microsurgery (TEMS). For large proximal adenomas, conventional bowel resection is recommended.

For patients who have had multiple or advanced adenomas removed, surveillance by colonoscopy is required because of the high incidence of new adenomas subsequently arising elsewhere in the bowel.

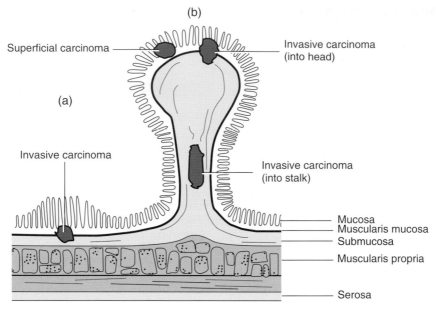

Fig. 31.8 Sessile (a) and pedunculated (b) polyp.

Table 31.3 Relationship of adenoma to invasive carcinoma.

	Incidence of malignancy (%)		
Size	Tubular	Tubulo-villous	Villous
<1 cm	0.3	1.5	2.5
1–2 cm	4	6	6
2–3 cm	7	12	17
>3 cm	11	15	20

Inherited cancer and polyposis syndromes

Familial adenomatous polyposis

FAP is a disorder characterised by autosomal dominant inheritance of a mutation in the tumour-suppressor gene *APC* located on chromosome 5 (5q21) which, when inactivated, results in loss of control over cell proliferation, thus promoting neoplasia. FAP is associated with the formation of multiple colorectal adenomas (Figure 31.10). If left untreated, all FAP patients will develop CRC. Although uncommon, FAP accounts for 0.5% of all CRCs.

Most affected individuals develop polyps by the age of 15 years. Effective management of FAP requires a carefully researched family history and construction of family pedigrees. This and patient education is often best done by dedicated familial cancer clinics.

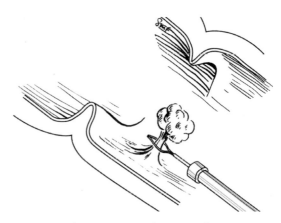

Fig. 31.9 Endoscopic snare polypectomy during colonoscopy.

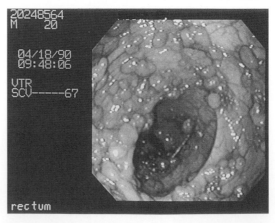

Fig. 31.10 Colonoscopic view of familial adenomatous polyposis.

Bowel symptoms associated with FAP usually indicate the development of cancer. Therefore, it is crucial to diagnose the condition at a pre-symptomatic stage. Endoscopic surveillance is giving way to genetic testing to allow recognition of affected offspring of FAP patients. Those family members who test negative on genetic testing are not at risk for FAP.

Almost all FAP patients have gastroduodenal polyps, and around 5% go on to develop duodenal cancer. Duodenal adenomas at the ampulla of Vater are particularly prone to malignancy. Many duodenal adenomatous polyps can be treated endoscopically but radical surgery including pancreaticoduodenectomy (Whipple procedure) may be necessary in patients with severe duodenal polyposis or cancer.

Several extracolonic manifestations of FAP can arise, including abdominal desmoid tumours that occur in about 10% of patients (Figure 31.11). These are fibroblastic tumours commonly affecting the abdominal wall or small bowel mesentery. They are considered benign because they do not metastasise but can be lethal because of aggressive local growth causing small bowel obstruction and ureteric compression. Treatment of desmoids is difficult, as complete resection is rarely achieved and response to medical therapy is variable. They are not radiosensitive. Brain tumours are also seen in FAP (Turcot's syndrome).

The principal treatment of FAP is prophylactic colectomy timed to occur before the onset of CRC, usually before the age of 20. The surgical options include the following.

- Total colectomy and ileorectal anastomosis (IRA) eliminates colonic polyps. This operation has a low complication rate and good postoperative bowel function and avoids pelvic nerve dysfunction. The retained rectum requires regular surveillance as the risk of rectal cancer is about 15% at 15 years.

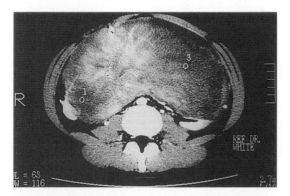

Fig. 31.11 Computed tomography scan of an abdomen showing a large desmoid tumour occupying almost the entire peritoneal cavity.

- Restorative proctocolectomy and ileal pouch–anal anastomosis removes the entire colon and rectum, thus having the major advantage of eliminating CRC risk. Bowel function is preserved by construction of an ileal reservoir joined to the upper anal canal. Surgical complications are higher than for IRA and bowel function is marginally worse.
- Total proctocolectomy and permanent ileostomy is reserved for FAP patients presenting with rectal cancer.

MUTYH-associated polyposis

Mutations in the *MUTYH* gene (chromosome 1) cause defects in base-excision DNA repair that results in a polyposis syndrome with an autosomal recessive pattern of inheritance. Polyps are typically fewer in number and arise later than in FAP. The lifetime risk of CRC is 80% (mostly right-sided) with an average age of onset of 45 years. Treatment is by colectomy and IRA.

Lynch syndrome

Lynch syndrome (LS, previously called hereditary non-polyposis colon cancer) is an inherited autosomal dominant disease arising due to mutations of MMR genes (*MLH1*, *MSH2*, *MSH6* and *PMS2*). It carries a lifetime risk of colon cancer of around 80%. Cancer development is substantially faster than for sporadic CRC. The cardinal features are early age of cancer onset (approximately 44 years), right-sided cancers in 70%, an excess of synchronous and metachronous CRCs and an association with certain extracolonic cancers (endometrial carcinoma, transitional cell carcinoma of the urinary tract, adenocarcinomas of the stomach and small bowel, and other cancers including those of ovaries, pancreas and biliary tract). Polyposis is not a feature of LS, and the incidence of adenomas in LS approximates that of the general population. The colon cancers of LS are more likely to be poorly differentiated and mucinous.

The clinical diagnosis of LS once depended only on family history (Bethesda criteria) but this is imprecise. Suspicion for LS is now guided by immunohistochemistry testing of tumour specimens. Genetic testing can then be initiated to identify a specific MMR gene mutation. As the penetrance of CRC is not 100% (as it is in FAP), prophylactic colectomy is not usually offered. However, annual colonoscopic surveillance is recommended because of the rapid onset of CRC in LS. Total colectomy and IRA is undertaken when colon cancer occurs.

Juvenile polyposis syndrome

Juvenile polyposis syndrome may arise in an auto-somal dominant fashion due to mutations in the tumour suppressor gene *SMAD4 (MADH4)*. It is characterised by hamartomatous (juvenile) polyps in the colon, rectum and small bowel and stomach. The number of polyps is less than seen in FAP and the lifetime risk of colon cancer is 40%. Surveillance by gastroscopy and colonoscopy is commenced at the age of 15 years.

Peutz–Jeghers syndrome

Peutz–Jeghers syndrome (PJS) is due to an autosomal dominant inherited mutation in the tumour-suppressor gene *STK11*. Hamartomatous polyps can occur anywhere in the gastrointestinal tract. Symptoms occur from early teenage years. As the polyps are particularly common in the small bowel, bowel obstruction due to intussusception and gas-trointestinal bleeding are common presentations. Family history, oral mucocutaneous pigmentation and genetic testing aid the diagnosis of PJS. There is a lifetime risk of cancer approaching 85% (over 50% in the gastrointestinal tract). Patients with PJS require surveillance colonoscopy and gastro-duodenoscopy from an early age.

Serrated polyposis syndrome

Serrated polyposis syndrome (formerly called hyperplastic polyposis) is an uncommon polyposis syndrome with the finding of multiple or large serrated polyps in the colon. The inheritance pattern is unknown. There is a definite increase in risk for CRC (especially right-sided cancers) but the actual lifetime risk is uncertain. Individuals with serrated polyposis syndrome require regular colonoscopic surveillance. Colectomy and IRA is recommended for patients with uncontrolled polyposis or colon cancer.

Further reading

Heald RJ, Moran BJ, Ryall RD, Sexton R. Rectal cancer: the Basingstoke experience of total mesorectal excision, 1978–1997. *Arch Surg* 1998;8:894–9.

Kapiteijn E, Marijnen CA, Nagtegaal ID *et al.* Preoperative radiotherapy combined with total mesorectal excision for resectable rectal cancer. *N Engl J Med* 2001;345: 638–46.

Quirke P, Dudley P, Dixon MF, Williams NS. Local recurrence of rectal adenocarcinoma due to inadequate surgical resection. Histopathologic study of lateral tumour spread and surgical excision. *Lancet* 1986;ii(8514):996–9.

Taylor FG, Quirke P, Heald RJ *et al.* Preoperative magnetic resonance imaging assessment of circumferential resection margin predicts disease free survival and local recurrence: 5 year follow up results of the MERCURY study. *J Clin Oncol* 2014;32:34–43.

MCQs

Select the single correct answer to each question. The correct answers can be found in the Answers section at the end of the book.

1 Which of the following is *not* a symptom of caecal cancer?
   a iron deficiency anaemia
   b a palpable mass in the right lower quadrant
   c large bowel obstruction
   d small bowel obstruction
   e liver metastases

2 Which of the following statements regarding FAP is *incorrect*?
   a inheritance is autosomal dominant
   b the condition accounts for 20% of all colorectal cancers
   c most affected individuals develop polyps by the age of 15 years
   d desmoid tumours are an association
   e without colectomy, affected individuals will develop CRC

3 Which of the following proven factors associated with the development of CRC is *incorrect*?
   a long-standing colitis
   b family history of CRC in a parent or sibling
   c recurrent diverticulitis
   d adenomatous polyps
   e pelvic irradiation

4 Which of the following oncologic outcomes for rectal cancer is *incorrect*?
   a improved by preoperative staging by MRI
   b improved by neoadjuvant chemoradiotherapy
   c influenced by surgical technique
   d always improved by early detection of metastases
   e improved by extensive en-bloc resection of surrounding structures adherent to locally advanced tumours

32 Large bowel obstruction

Raaj Chandra

Royal Melbourne Hospital, Melbourne, Victoria, Australia

Introduction

Large bowel obstruction (LBO) needs to be managed as a surgical emergency, although not all cases will need an operation. It can occur anywhere in the colon and rectum due to various causes and has a 100% mortality if left untreated. This is why LBO must be diagnosed and treated promptly with early surgical team referral. Traditionally, LBO has been defined as the absence of flatus or bowel movements for greater than 24 hours associated with abdominal distension, and the visualisation of dilated colon on plain abdominal X-ray. More recently, with modern CT techniques and the use of oral, intravenous and rectal contrast, the diagnosis of LBO has become much easier and more accurate. This chapter discusses the aetiology, clinical features, investigations and treatment of LBO.

Aetiology and pathophysiology

The majority of LBO cases are caused by primary or secondary neoplasms. Just over 50% are caused by colorectal cancers (discussed in Chapter 31). Approximately 10–17% are caused by sigmoid or caecal volvulus. This occurs when the colon twists on its mesentery causing bowel obstruction and is discussed later. Sigmoid volvulus occurs much more commonly than caecal volvulus. A further 10% are attributed to diverticular strictures which result as a complication of diverticular disease. Diverticular strictures may be classified as inflammatory or non-inflammatory. Inflammatory strictures result from an episode of acute diverticulitis, in which the inflammatory process results in transient LBO that resolves as the inflammatory process is treated, usually with antibiotics. Non-inflammatory strictures are more chronic and result after recurrent episodes of diverticulitis. These are more likely to result in

LBO and require surgical treatment. Diverticular disease is discussed in Chapter 30. Strictures from inflammatory bowel disease, including Crohn's disease and ulcerative colitis, as well as strictures caused by radiation and bowel ischaemia are known causes of LBO but are less common. Other uncommon causes include extrinsic tumours, foreign bodies and faecal impaction.

An obstruction in the colon or rectum leads to significant dilatation of the bowel proximal to the obstruction. This leads to a cascade of events including mucosal oedema, venous congestion and reduced arterial flow to the bowel. This increases the mucosal permeability of the colon which progresses to bacterial translocation, the systemic inflammatory response syndrome (SIRS), dehydration and electrolyte abnormalities. Eventually ischaemia progresses to infarction, perforation and soiling of the peritoneal cavity, resulting in generalised peritonitis, multiorgan failure and potentially death.

Clinical features

Patients with LBO commonly present with abdominal pain, distension and absolute constipation or the inability to pass flatus or bowel movements. Nausea and vomiting are less common and usually a late sign, depending on the competency of the ileocaecal valve. For example, if the obstruction is in the rectum, then it may take several days for the proximal colon to distend to a point where perforation is imminent. If the ileocaecal valve is incompetent, then nausea and vomiting may be further delayed since the small intestine will also take time to become distended. Colonic perforation is more likely if the ileocaecal valve is competent since the colon is unable to decompress into the small intestine. The presentation of LBO depends on the underlying aetiology. For example, it is acute in the

Textbook of Surgery, Fourth Edition. Edited by Julian A. Smith, Andrew H. Kaye, Christopher Christophi and Wendy A. Brown.
© 2020 John Wiley & Sons Ltd. Published 2020 by John Wiley & Sons Ltd.

case of sigmoid volvulus but can be more chronic in the case of bowel cancer.

History

When LBO is suspected, the following focused questions will help confirm the diagnosis.
- Is the presentation acute or chronic?
- Is there abdominal pain? If so, is the pain colicky or constant? Obstructive pain is colicky but can progressively become constant if generalised peritonitis develops.
- What is its severity? Pain from LBO is usually severe.
- Are there any aggravating or relieving factors? Any form of bowel obstruction is aggravated by eating food. In the advanced stages of LBO where generalised peritonitis has developed, any form of movement or even coughing will cause severe pain and the patient will much prefer to lie still.
- Vomiting may provide some temporary relief. The contents of the vomitus will be useful. Vomiting from an LBO is commonly described as feculent. It will be foul-smelling and look like faeces, while vomitus from a proximal small bowel obstruction will be bile-stained and green-ish in keeping with small intestinal contents. Other associated symptoms include recent weight loss (a non-specific indicator of malignancy), change in bowel habit, rectal bleeding and passage of mucus. These symptoms should raise the possibility of an underlying colorectal cancer.
- Is there a family history of bowel cancer or inflammatory bowel disease?
- Has the patient had a previous colonoscopy or undertaken the National Bower Cancer Screening Test? It is unlikely that a malignancy is the cause if a colonoscopy has been performed successfully in the preceding 2 years.
- Has the patient had previous abdominal surgery and for what reason? A past history of colorectal cancer would raise the possibility of recurrent or metastatic disease. If a bowel resection has been performed, there could be a stricture at the site of the old anastomosis.

Examination

A detailed examination is very important. On general inspection, signs such as cachexia and pallor may suggest malignancy. Other signs of altered physiology include dry mucous membranes and low urine output, suggestive of dehydration.

Tachycardia, hypotension and fever may also be present. A distended abdomen is an important sign in LBO, although the presence of ascites can also paint the same picture and must be excluded. The presence of shifting dullness on percussion will confirm ascites while percussion over distended colon will remain tympanitic, producing a low-pitched, drum-like sound.
- Is there local or generalised tenderness with signs of peritonism? This includes percussion and rebound tenderness.
- Is there a mass present? This is a sign of advanced disease.
- The absence of bowel sounds raises the suspicion of colonic pseudo-obstruction and can be high-pitched with a mechanical obstruction, although this is an unreliable sign.
- A per rectal examination is mandatory to exclude a rectal tumour or the presence of blood.

Investigations

These patients are often elderly with significantly deranged biochemical markers suggestive of malnutrition, renal failure and multiorgan failure. Classically, patients with bowel ischaemia will have an elevated white cell count and serum lactate and have a metabolic acidosis.

Blood tests

The following blood tests should be performed.
- Full blood count looking for anaemia or an elevated white cell count.
- Electrolytes, urea and creatinine will confirm dehydration and/or renal failure as well as electrolyte disturbances. Renal function should be checked prior to CT with intravenous contrast due to the potential for nephrotoxicity from contrast media.
- Deranged liver function tests can be a sign of multiorgan failure and a low albumin level is a marker of malnutrition. A preoperative level below 30 g/L is a marker of increased perioperative morbidity.
- C-reactive protein is an acute-phase reactant produced in the liver and is raised in the setting of an acute inflammatory process. It is a useful test since it may be markedly elevated despite a normal white cell count.
- A coagulation profile should be performed in all patients who are unwell and potentially requiring surgery. Severely unwell patients regularly become coagulopathic, which needs urgent

correction and control, often concurrent with the operation.

- Serum lactate is a useful test, particularly if bowel ischaemia is a concern. A raised lactate level is a sign of tissue hypoxia.
- An arterial blood gas (if available) is also important. This will give important information on the acid–base status of the patient.
- In the subacute setting, iron studies should be included since preoperative iron infusion (time permitting) has been shown to significantly reduce red blood cell transfusion requirements and length of hospital stay, with higher percentages of normalised haemoglobin levels both at time of discharge as well as at 30 days after surgery.

Imaging

If the patient is unwell with signs of generalised peritonitis, then an erect chest X-ray and plain abdominal films are quick and inexpensive while sufficient to make the diagnosis and exclude perforated viscus requiring immediate laparotomy. The presence of free gas under the diaphragm will confirm the diagnosis of a perforated viscus, while dilated colonic segments proximal to an obstruction with no rectal gas on an abdominal plain film will be suspicious for LBO after correlation with the clinical picture.

In most cases, high-definition CT scanning is the imaging modality of choice (Figure 32.1). The

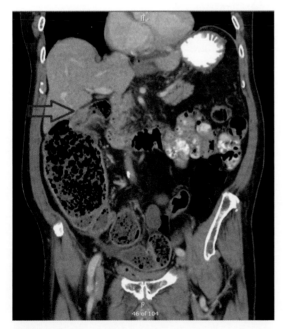

Fig. 32.1 CT scan with intravenous contrast demonstrating an obstructing neoplasm at the hepatic flexure (arrow).

introduction of multidetector CT technology with intravenous contrast medium has made it possible to gather critical information regarding the site of obstruction, aetiology and extent of the lesion as well as associated bowel ischaemia. Multidetector CT is a well-tolerated rapid imaging mode that produces images in one breath-hold. The addition of rectal contrast is very helpful in distinguishing between mechanical distal LBO and pseudo-obstruction. However, in cases where there is a clear transition point separating severely dilated proximal colon and collapsed distal colon, rectal contrast may not be required. If CT is not available or if the results are equivocal, fluoroscopy with contrast enema remains a helpful investigation. The main advantage is that it allows easy distinction between LBO and colonic pseudo-obstruction. It may also be used to confirm a colonic volvulus. Water-soluble iodinated contrast material such as Gastrografin should be used as it is easily absorbed in the peritoneum should there be a perforation.

Treatment

This will depend on the aetiology, site of obstruction and the expertise available at the hospital. It is recommended that, where possible, treatment is under the care of a specialist colorectal surgery unit or, at the very least, a general surgical team. If this service is unavailable, then the patient should be transferred to another centre after initial management is commenced. Figure 32.2 provides an algorithm to help guide surgical management.

Initial management

All patients with suspected LBO should receive appropriate volume resuscitation with intravenous fluids and be offered adequate pain relief. Communication with the anaesthetic team is essential and they should be notified as early as possible after the diagnosis is made so that resuscitation can begin with the correction of biochemical abnormalities well before any planned surgical intervention. A urinary catheter should be inserted so that strict fluid balance information can be obtained. Intravenous broad-spectrum antibiotics may be commenced in the setting of sepsis.

A nasogastric tube should be inserted, particularly in patients who are vomiting with significant abdominal distension. This will help relieve the patient's discomfort and enable decompression of the distended proximal bowel. It is expected that the patient will develop a paralytic ileus after

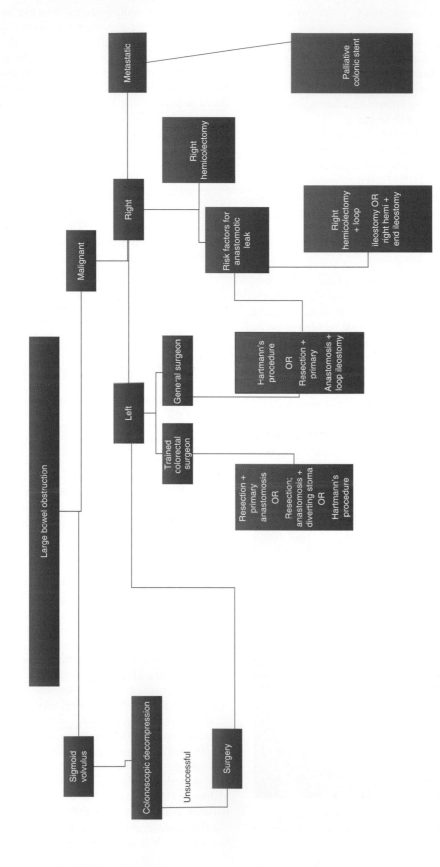

Fig. 32.2 Algorithm for the management of LBO.

surgery, and so the nasogastric tube should remain *in situ* postoperatively until bowel function has returned and nasogastric output reduces to an acceptable level.

Malignant LBO

Right-sided obstruction (proximal to splenic flexure)

A right hemicolectomy with primary anastomosis is the operation of choice, where the distal ileum is anastomosed to the proximal transverse colon after high ligation of the ileocolic vessels close to their origin at the superior mesenteric artery for oncological clearance of the draining lymph nodes. This is known as an oncological resection. If the tumour is closer to the splenic flexure, then an extended right hemicolectomy should be performed with anastomosis of the distal ileum to either the distal transverse colon or the proximal descending colon. In this case both the ileocolic and middle colic vessels should be ligated, divided and all draining lymph nodes removed. If there are significant risk factors for anastomotic leak, then a diverting loop ileostomy may be considered to protect the anastomosis. High-risk patients include those who are malnourished (albumin <30 g/L), have chronic or preoperative renal failure, are immunosuppressed, or have an American Society of Anesthesiologists (ASA) score of III/IV.

Occasionally, a right hemicolectomy with an end-ileostomy and stapling of the colonic stump may be necessary if the patient is very unwell. In this situation, the colonic stump may be brought out and sutured superficial to the rectus sheath as a buried mucous fistula. Thus, if the colonic end leaks, the contamination can be controlled as a wound problem without the more serious complication of intra-abdominal sepsis.

Recommendation: In most cases of right-sided LBO, a right hemicolectomy is the procedure of choice.

Left-sided obstruction (distal to splenic flexure)

There are a number of options when managing left-sided obstruction. Hartmann's procedure is the most commonly performed. This is a surgical resection of the sigmoid colon and part of the upper rectum. The proximal colon is then brought out through the abdominal wall as an end-colostomy. The rectal stump is closed with a stapler and left *in situ*. Other options, particularly when specialist colorectal teams are available, include resection of the affected segment of colon with primary anastomosis, or primary resection with anastomosis and a diverting stoma. Both procedures may include intraoperative colonic lavage with saline. This reduces the amount of faecal matter in the colon, thereby theoretically reducing the risk of anastomotic leak. However, debate continues over whether intraoperative lavage is necessary, or even helps. In all cases, the major arterial supply and draining lymph nodes should be removed for oncological reasons.

In less common circumstances a diverting loop colostomy proximal to the site of obstruction or, rarely, a caecostomy can be formed as a temporising measure to decompress the colon. Proximal diversion is a good option if the obstructing lesion is in the rectum since the management of rectal cancer is different from that of colon cancer in some circumstances (see Chapter 31). In cases of locally advanced rectal cancer, it is better to treat these patients with preoperative chemoradiotherapy since this has been shown to reduce local recurrence rates and helps to down-stage the tumour prior to a curative resection. Therefore, a loop colostomy allows the patient to recover from the effects of the obstruction and provides the opportunity to stage the disease. The patient then undergoes a period of chemoradiation therapy before a definitive resection is performed.

A final option in the management of LBO is the use of colonic stents (Figure 32.3). These can be used for both left- and right-sided obstructions. Their use is beneficial particularly in the setting of metastatic disease when a major operation may be high risk and will not improve the patient's overall survival. As mentioned in the introduction, if left untreated LBO has a 100% mortality. However, with emergency surgery the mortality is still high at 15–20%.

Insertion of a stent provides immediate relief from the obstruction and gives good palliation. It can be performed in an endoscopy suite under light sedation if the patient is too unwell to undergo a general anaesthetic. However, the use of colonic stents is controversial when used as a bridge to surgery if there is no metastatic disease. This is because stents are not without complications, of which the most serious is perforation of the colon. If perforation occurs, this in theory converts a curable cancer into a potentially incurable one due to the spillage of cancer cells into the peritoneal cavity. Colonic stenting should only be performed by experienced endoscopists who have expertise in stenting.

(a)

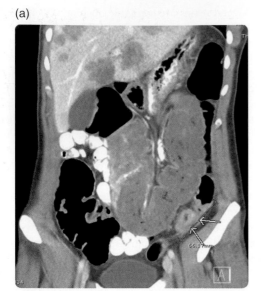

(b)

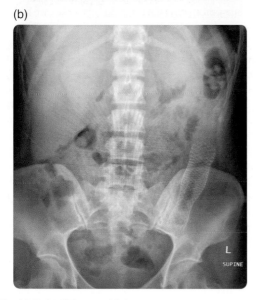

Fig. 32.3 (a) CT scan with intravenous contrast demonstrating an obstructing neoplasm in the sigmoid colon. (b) The obstruction has been relieved with a colonic stent which can be seen on this plain X-ray.

Recommendation: In a patient with significant comorbidities and risk factors, Hartmann's procedure is the operation of choice. Primary resection with anastomosis may be performed but only in expert hands. The use of stenting as a bridge to surgery is not recommended due to the risk of perforation and converting a potentially curable cancer into an incurable one. Stenting as a palliative measure is recommended but only if the expertise is available.

Sigmoid volvulus

Endoscopic reduction is the treatment of choice in the acute setting, with an 80% success rate. A colonoscope is passed via the rectum and the insufflation of gas is able to untwist the colon. The endoscope also allows for decompression of the dilated colon proximal to the obstruction. There is evidence that after a single episode, the rate of recurrence is as high as 50%. Recurrent volvulus is more likely to lead to ischaemic complications and therefore a semi-elective sigmoid resection with primary anastomosis is the treatment of choice once the patient has recovered from the acute episode. This can be performed using a limited left iliac fossa incision due to the length and redundancy of the sigmoid colon, which can be delivered through a small incision. This avoids the need for a midline laparotomy.

Caecal volvulus

Unlike sigmoid volvulus, colonoscopy for caecal volvulus is not recommended. The operation of choice is a right hemicolectomy with primary anastomosis. The right colon is usually very mobile and therefore minimal mobilisation is required. In the past, caecopexy used to be performed, and involved suturing of the untwisted colon to the abdominal wall at multiple points to prevent it from twisting again. This is now not recommended due to its high recurrence rates. Similarly, pexy procedures should not be performed for sigmoid volvulus.

Diverticular and other benign strictures

Stenting or dilatation of 'benign' strictures in the colon is generally discouraged due to the risk of malignancy, (i.e. not resecting a lesion that later proves to be malignant). In the acute setting, these should be treated in a similar fashion to malignant LBO.

Acute colonic pseudo-obstruction (Ogilvie's syndrome)

Acute colonic pseudo-obstruction (ACPO) is a syndrome characterised by a clinical picture suggestive of mechanical obstruction in the absence of any demonstrable evidence of such an obstruction in the intestine. Therefore, it is important that this differential diagnosis is considered in any case of suspected LBO. The colon may become massively dilated. If it is not decompressed, the patient risks perforation, peritonitis and death.

The mortality rate can be as high as 40% when perforation occurs.

ACPO generally develops in hospitalised patients. Studies have documented that as many as 95% of cases of colonic pseudo-obstruction are associated with medical or surgical conditions, the rest being classified as idiopathic. The most commonly associated conditions include trauma, pregnancy, caesarean section, severe infections, and cardiothoracic, pelvic or orthopaedic surgery. These patients are commonly bed bound, have serum electrolyte imbalances and are taking high doses of opiates, all of which have negative effects on colonic motility.

The exact pathophysiology of ACPO is unclear. Current theories continue to suggest the idea of an imbalance in the autonomic nervous system. These theories focus on the increased sympathetic tone (which results in inhibition of colonic motility) and decreased parasympathetic tone (which then also reduces colonic motility), or a combination of both as the cause.

If colonic pseudo-obstruction is suspected, then some form of dynamic contrast imaging study is recommended to exclude a mechanical bowel obstruction. This is essential since the management is different from that of LBO. The mode of imaging study will depend on availability of services and will include either a CT scan of the abdomen and pelvis with rectal contrast, or a contrast enema study using fluoroscopy.

The principles of management for ACPO include the following.
- Correct any underlying biochemical abnormalities.
- Reduce opiate intake.
- Insert a nasogastric tube if the patient is vomiting.
- Insert a rectal tube which can be therapeutic in some cases.
- Consider the use of neostigmine, an acetylcholinesterase inhibitor. Neostigmine inhibits destruction of acetylcholine by acetylcholinesterase, thereby facilitating transmission of impulses across the myoneural junction and enhancing colonic motility. Neostigmine has a significant side-effect profile, particularly cardiovascular and respiratory effects. Cardiovascular complications include arrhythmias and non-specific ECG changes as well as cardiac arrest, syncope and hypotension, particularly when given intravenously. Respiratory complications include increased oral, pharyngeal and bronchial secretions, dyspnoea, respiratory depression/arrest and bronchospasm. Therefore, it is important that neostigmine is administered in an intensive care setting with the availability of cardiac monitoring.
- Colonoscopic decompression can be used as an alternative to neostigmine or if neostigmine fails. It has been shown to be effective in 85% of cases but must be performed by an experienced endoscopist. It is a technically difficult procedure since the bowel is unprepared. Therefore, colonic perforation is a significant possibility. Colonoscopic decompression may need to be repeated several times to achieve full resolution. In the case of bowel perforation, laparotomy and bowel resection with end-ileostomy is usually required. An algorithm for the management of ACPO is shown in Figure 32.4.

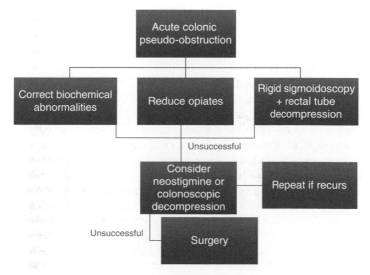

Fig. 32.4 Algorithm for the management of ACPO.

Conclusions

LBO needs to be considered a surgical emergency since it leads to significant morbidity and mortality if not treated promptly. Early surgical team referral is essential. There are many causes of LBO, although colorectal cancer is the commonest. It is imperative that LBO is not mistaken for a colonic pseudo-obstruction since the treatment is different. The treatment of LBO will depend on the location of the obstruction and whether metastatic disease is present. Surgical resection is required in most cases. However, colonic stenting may be used particularly in the setting of metastatic disease. If left untreated, the mortality rate is 100%.

Further reading

Cancer Council Australia. Colorectal Cancer Guidelines Working Party. Clinical practice guidelines for the prevention, early detection and management of colorectal cancer. Available at https://wiki.cancer.org.au/australiawiki/index.php?oldid=173168 (accessed 28 January 2018).

Frago R, Ramirez E, Millan M, Kreisler E, del Valle E, Biondo S. Current management of acute malignant large bowel obstruction: a systematic review. *Am J Surg* 2014;207:127–38.

Saunders MD. Acute colonic pseudo-obstruction. In: Talley NJ, DeVault KR, Wallace MB, Aqel BA, Lindor KD (eds) *Practical Gastroenterology and Hepatology Board Review Toolkit*. Hoboken, NJ: Wiley Blackwell, 2016:343–8.

Yassaie O, Thompson-Fawcett M, Rossaak J. Management of sigmoid volvulus: is early surgery justifiable? *ANZ J Surg* 2013;83:74–8.

MCQs

Select the single correct answer to each question. The correct answers can be found in the Answers section at the end of the book.

1 Which of the following symptoms and signs does *not* commonly present in complete LBO?
   a abdominal pain
   b abdominal distension
   c absolute constipation
   d inability to pass flatus
   e diarrhoea

2 Which of the following is the imaging modality of choice for the diagnosis of LBO?
   a plain abdominal X-ray
   b abdominal ultrasound
   c Gastrografin enema
   d multidetector CT scan of the abdomen and pelvis
   e MRI of the abdomen and pelvis

3 Which of the following is *not* an accepted treatment option in left-sided LBO?
   a Hartmann's procedure
   b chemoradiation therapy
   c colon resection with primary anastomosis
   d colon resection, anastomosis and diverting stoma
   e colonic stenting

4 Which of the following is *not* an acceptable measure to take in the initial management of ACPO?
   a correction of underlying biochemical abnormalities
   b reduce opiate intake
   c administer neostigmine
   d perform colonoscopic decompression
   e perform a laparotomy

33 Perianal disorders I: excluding sepsis

Ian Hayes[1,2] and Susan Shedda[1,3]

[1] Colorectal Surgery Unit, Royal Melbourne Hospital, Melbourne, Victoria, Australia
[2] Department of Surgery, University of Melbourne, Parkville, Victoria, Australia
[3] Royal Women's Hospital, Melbourne, Victoria, Australia

Anatomy and physiology

The anal canal extends from the puborectalis muscle to the anal verge and has a variable length depending on gender. In the male it can be up to 6 cm long, whilst in the female the average length is closer to 2 cm. The anal verge can be identified as the point of transition from hair-bearing to non-hair-bearing skin, visible on inspection of the perineum. The major structures of the anal canal are the sphincter complex, anal glands, columnar and squamous epithelium and the dentate line (Figure 33.1).

The sphincter complex consists of the external and internal sphincter muscles. The external sphincter is the continuation of the puborectalis and is skeletal muscle under voluntary control. It is often divided into three parts but functionally acts as a single unit to provide additional strong contraction when defecation is deferred voluntarily. The internal sphincter is a continuation of the circular muscle layer of the rectum (involuntary, smooth muscle) and is the main muscular component of resting tone (Figure 33.2). The lower part of the anal canal consists of non-hair-bearing squamous epithelium, with the line of transition called the dentate line (Figure 33.3). At this point, the anal glands discharge into the lumen of the anal canal to provide lubricant for the passage of the stool. The proximal part of the anal canal merges with the columnar epithelium of the rectum and is often referred to as the 'transition zone'. In the non-diseased state, the haemorrhoidal complex of blood vessels lies deep to the mucosa at this level.

When stool passes into the distal rectum, it causes reflex relaxation and distension of the internal anal sphincter, allowing the mucosa of the transition zone in the upper anal canal to be exposed to the luminal contents. This rectoanal inhibitory reflex allows for sampling of the contents. If defecation then occurs, there is voluntary relaxation of the external anal sphincter and straightening of the anal canal with relaxation of the puborectalis.

History

Four cardinal symptoms, their details and how they combine, form the basis of diagnosing most perianal conditions:

* pain
* bleeding
* presence of a 'lump'
* discharge.

Pain

The nature of perianal pain can help differentiate perianal conditions. Pain worse with defecation is characteristic of anal fissure. A short history of constantly increasing, severe pain suggests sepsis. Localised pain and a discrete lump suggest perianal haematoma.

Bleeding

Blood from the perianal region is generally bright red, of small volume and not mixed with stools. Bleeding is generally with defecation but blood which stains underclothes strongly suggests a cause that is located external to the sphincter muscles. Blood from haemorrhoids can squirt onto the toilet bowl.

Bleeding and anal pain suggest fissure. Any rectal bleeding should be regarded as an abnormal symptom. It can sometimes be difficult to differentiate bleeding due to an insignificant anal cause from bleeding due to colorectal malignancy. Bleeding

Textbook of Surgery, Fourth Edition. Edited by Julian A. Smith, Andrew H. Kaye, Christopher Christophi and Wendy A. Brown.
© 2020 John Wiley & Sons Ltd. Published 2020 by John Wiley & Sons Ltd.

from colonic lesions may appear bright red even if their location is as far proximal as the descending or sigmoid colon. Colonoscopy to exclude neoplasia should be considered in patients over 40 years of age, those who have a significant family history of bowel cancer, those with other colorectal symptoms such as change in bowel habit, and in all cases where a clear anal cause of the bleeding cannot be identified.

Lump

Patients' description of a perianal lump is often vague because the area is not directly visible. The size and position are relevant, as is the question of whether the lump prolapses (large haemorrhoids and rectal prolapse) and if it needs to be manually reduced back into the anal canal. How long the lump has been present (years for skin tags and warts) and if it is increasing in size should be ascertained.

Discharge

It is important to confirm if the discharge is from the anus itself or from the surrounding perianal skin. Purulent discharge suggests a fistula. Mucous leakage may represent prolapse of haemorrhoids or full-thickness prolapse of the rectum or it may be a manifestation of incontinence due to mild sphincter weakness. Any leakage of mucus or pus onto the perineal skin is very irritating and is an important cause of pruritus ani.

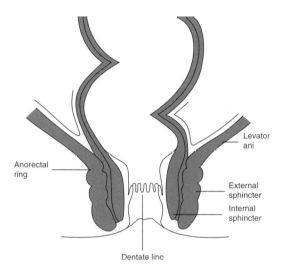

Fig. 33.1 Anatomy of the rectum and anal canal.

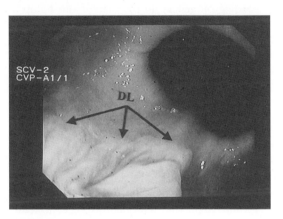

Fig. 33.3 Anal canal. DL, dentate line.

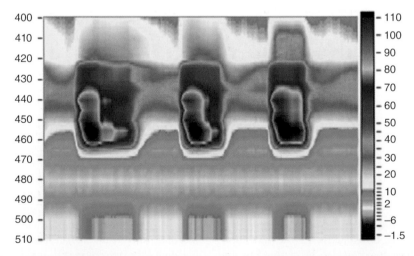

Fig. 33.2 Anal manometry pressure tracing using continuous perfusion catheter. The horizontal axis shows time, the right vertical axis pressure (mmHg). The end of the catheter is in the rectum at the top of the trace. The anal canal is represented by the pink/black horizontal pressure zone and atmospheric pressure is at the bottom of the trace. The three black zones represent three episodes of voluntary contraction of the external sphincter. The baseline pink/orange trace represents resting internal sphincter tone.

Box 33.1 Conditions visible in the perianal region

Perianal skin
- Psoriasis
- Changes of chronic itching
- Fistula
- Abscess
- Hidradenitis
- Warts

Anal verge
- Skin tags
- Perianal haematoma
- Prolapsing haemorrhoids
- Rectal prolapse
- Thrombosed haemorrhoids
- Anal intraepithelial neoplasia (AIN)
- Anal cancer
- Anal fissure

Examination

Many perianal diagnoses are visible without performing an internal examination (Box 33.1). The patient is examined in the left lateral position with good lighting. Patients with chronic anal fissure, intersphincteric abscess or thrombosed haemorrhoids may be too tender to allow digital internal examination without anaesthesia. However, the distal edge of a fissure may be visible externally without causing the patient undue discomfort. If possible, rigid sigmoidoscopy should be part of routine examination for patients with perianal conditions. It should be noted that, in clinical practice, examination with a rigid sigmoidoscope is an examination of the anal canal and rectum, rather than of the sigmoid.

Investigations

Clinical examination alone is sufficient to make a confident diagnosis in most perianal conditions. However, examination under anaesthesia is frequently used as a further investigation when:
- a lesion requires biopsy for histological confirmation
- when the area is too tender to allow clinical examination
- when fistula or sinus tracks need to be probed.

Colonoscopy is a common ancillary investigation in patients with perianal conditions. It can be used to exclude causes of bleeding situated more proximally in the bowel (such as neoplasia) and it is an

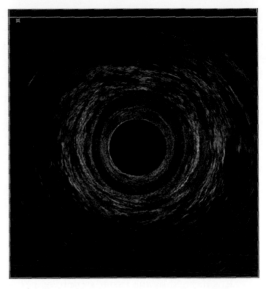

Fig. 33.4 Endoanal ultrasound of the mid-anal canal. The probe is in the lumen, represented by the centre black solid circle. The next grey zone is mucosa with a dense black circle of internal sphincter surrounding this. The broad grey/black striped zone peripheral to this is the external sphincter.

important test if inflammatory bowel disease is suspected.

MRI is used selectively and is helpful in cases of complex fistula or sepsis. MRI is the main imaging mode for perianal neoplasia. CT has limited application for most perianal conditions.

Endoanal ultrasound (Figure 33.4) involves placing an ultrasound probe (the diameter of a finger) into the anal canal. Anaesthesia is not required. This technique provides very good visualisation of the anal sphincters and anal fistulas.

Defecating proctography involves using videofluoroscopy and a rectal contrast medium to observe dynamic movement of the rectum and pelvic floor during defecation. This test is useful in diagnosing occult rectal prolapse and rectocele in patients with symptoms of obstructed defecation.

Blood tests have minimal diagnostic use in most perianal conditions. Information about blood glucose and white cell count (WCC) is relevant in perianal sepsis. C-reactive protein and WCC are useful markers of activity if inflammatory bowel disease (IBD) is suspected. Faecal calprotectin can be used as a screening test for IBD.

In the investigation of faecal incontinence, the function of the internal and external sphincters is tested by measuring resting and squeeze pressure in the anal canal using a manometry catheter. Pudendal nerve function is tested by measuring pudendal nerve terminal motor latency using an electrode placed in the anal canal which stimulates the pudendal nerve and records sphincter contraction. Endoanal ultrasound is used to examine the integrity of the sphincter muscles.

Conditions presenting with pain

Anal fissure

Anal fissure refers to a split in the mucosa of the anal verge causing pain and minor bright-red bleeding. Acute fissure refers to a simple split in the mucosa that heals quickly and rarely requires treatment.

Chronic fissure is the main condition of importance. It is defined by the fissure symptoms persisting for some weeks. The most distressing symptom is severe pain on defecation localised to the site of the fissure. In addition, a less well-defined pelvic pain can persist for hours after defecation, possibly due to spasm in the pelvic floor muscles.

The characteristic clinical findings with a chronic fissure include a sentinel tag at the most distal part, a hypertrophic anal papilla at the proximal extent, and visible white transverse fibres of the underlying internal sphincter muscle at the base. Usually, a chronic fissure is located in the posterior midline of the anal verge but can be located in the anterior midline. Multiple fissures or fissures in lateral positions raise the possibility of underlying IBD.

The initiating cause of anal fissure is uncertain. Relative ischaemia of the base may play a role and there is often a history of passing a hard stool and traumatising the mucosa prior to the onset of symptoms. However, persistence of the fissure is associated with spasm of the smooth muscle of the internal sphincter which, in turn, limits blood supply to the base of the fissure and impairs healing (the bleeding is from the mucosal edges).

Clinical examination is difficult because the area is tender and the anus is tightly closed with sphincter spasm. Usually the lower edge of the fissure can be visualised with gentle separation of the buttocks. Digital rectal examination is not usually possible.

Treatment

Most modes of treatment of chronic fissure are directed towards decreasing the spasm in the internal sphincter muscle. Treatment of constipation, fibre supplements and analgesia are important additions to any regimen. Treatment decisions for this condition involve balancing the severity of the fissure symptoms against the possible risk of sphincter weakness from surgery

In most cases, initial outpatient treatment with 6 weeks of topical 0.2% glyceryl trinitrate (GTN) cream is trialled. GTN acts as a nitric oxide donor causing relaxation of the smooth muscle of the internal sphincter. Its main side effect is headaches and it is effective in approximately 50% of cases. The calcium channel blocking agents diltiazem and nifedipine can be formulated as creams and used topically in a similar manner to GTN but with lower risk of headache.

If topical treatment fails, the next level of intervention often involves botulinum toxin injection into the sphincters, performed under anaesthesia. This is slightly more effective than the topical treatments and has a much lower risk of permanent sphincter impairment than sphincterotomy.

Surgical lateral internal sphincterotomy involves dividing the most distal portion of the internal sphincter. If surgery is performed, the associated sentinel tag and hypertrophic anal papilla can be excised. Any associated fissure/fistula can be de-roofed. Sphincterotomy carries a low risk of long-term incontinence but is by far the most effective treatment for fissure. In general, women have less reserve of sphincter muscle than men and are at risk of previous, or subsequent, obstetric trauma to the pelvic floor. Because of this, sphincterotomy is rarely used as a first treatment in women.

Occasionally, if pain is very severe, the most effective treatment may be to proceed to urgent surgery and perform lateral sphincterotomy or inject botulinum toxin, as appropriate. In this circumstance, the patient may be too tender to allow confirmation of the presence of a fissure preoperatively. Under anaesthesia, the fissure can be confirmed and treated, and other important differential diagnoses, such as intersphincteric abscess, excluded.

Perianal haematoma

Patients with this condition present with fairly sudden onset of a painful hard lump at the anal verge. It is important to note that the lesion is subcutaneous in the perianal skin rather than prolapsing from the anal canal. The lump is dark blue in colour and about the size of a pea. Patients often give a history of straining prior to the onset of the lump. The lesion is due to rupture of a small blood vessel. Because of the dense subcutaneous fibrous bands in the perianal skin, a contained haematoma is formed rather than a spreading bruise.

The natural history is that the lump can be quite painful for several days but gradually resolves.

Occasionally the overlying skin necroses, releasing a small dark haematoma. If the patient is seen in the first day or two, relief of symptoms can be quickly obtained by incising the lesion to release the haematoma. After this period, the haematoma is organising and is less easily released. Most patients can be managed with reassurance about the diagnosis, warm baths and analgesia.

Thrombosed haemorrhoids

Patients with thrombosed haemorrhoids often describe a past history of prolapsing haemorrhoids which have become painful and irreducible following an episode of severe straining (childbirth or severe constipation). The pathological process is that the previously moderately large haemorrhoids become further engorged with blood and oedema, and their increased size results in them becoming partially trapped external to the sphincters. The pain results in sphincter spasm, worsening the situation. The static blood within the haemorrhoids thromboses making them irreducible. On examination, the patient will be in discomfort and have circumferential, large, dark purple-coloured, irreducible haemorrhoids.

The natural history of the condition is that the swelling usually settles over several days. Most patients can be managed conservatively with rest, analgesia and topical application of ice to help reduce the swelling. Urgent haemorrhoidectomy is required if the prolapsed tissue becomes necrotic or infected, or when patients are not improving with conservative treatment. Surgery in this situation is problematic because excising all the haemorrhoidal tissue would remove most of the anal verge skin and mucosa, resulting in long-term stenosis. The solution is to remove the worst of the prolapsed tissue but leave adequate bridges of skin and mucosa, albeit quite swollen, to avoid fibrosis. Generally, patients feel much more comfortable postoperatively.

Perianal sepsis

This is described in Chapter 34.

Conditions presenting with bleeding

Haemorrhoids

Haemorrhoids are a very common condition and usually present with painless, bright red, per rectal bleeding. Patients may also complain of a prolapsing lump, itching (due to mucous leakage) and difficulty with anal hygiene. Clinical examination may reveal externally prolapsed haemorrhoids but often proctoscopy/sigmoidoscopy is required to visualise smaller haemorrhoids. It is important to note that non-prolapsed haemorrhoids are generally too soft to palpate on digital rectal examination. It should also be noted that small haemorrhoids are common and may not always be the source of the bleeding.

The cause of haemorrhoids remains unclear and previously was thought to be due to repeated straining, resulting in engorgement of the haemorrhoidal complex and progressively larger vessels. A more recent hypothesis suggests that haemorrhoids are in fact a prolapse of the anal canal tissue.

Haemorrhoids are graded I–IV depending on whether they are externally visible or not, and if they are manually reducible (Box 33.2). The initial treatment consists of improving the quality of the stool with increasing fibre and water intake. This is usually successful for the lesser grades of haemorrhoid. If this is unsuccessful, then more invasive treatments will be required. The further treatment of haemorrhoids depends on the grade of the haemorrhoid. Rubber-band ligation is reserved for grades I and II, whereas grades III and IV usually require excisional haemorrhoidectomy.

Rubber band ligation is done transanally through a proctoscope and can be performed on a non-anaesthetised patient in an outpatient setting. The mucosa proximal to the area of haemorrhoid is grasped and a narrow-diameter rubber ring placed over it. It is important to note that the band does not encircle the haemorrhoid itself. Generally, the band falls off 2 weeks following the procedure leaving a small ulcerated area that gradually heals by fibrosis. This process draws the haemorrhoidal tissue proximally and may also interfere with the blood supply of the haemorrhoid. The zone where the band is placed should be insensate but it is not uncommon for patients to experience discomfort after the procedure. This is also a risk of secondary haemorrhage when the band sloughs 2 weeks following the procedure.

Box 33.2 Haemorrhoid grades

- Grade I: enlarged internal haemorrhoids that do not prolapse
- Grade II: prolapsing haemorrhoids that spontaneously reduce
- Grade III: prolapsing haemorrhoids that require manual reduction
- Grade IV: irreducible prolapsed haemorrhoids

Haemorrhoidectomy involves surgically excising the redundant haemorrhoidal tissue. This procedure is performed under general or spinal anaesthesia using a variety of surgical techniques but all with similar end results. Patients need to expect discomfort for approximately 2 weeks postoperatively and, because of this, the procedure is reserved for patients with large haemorrhoids causing significant symptoms

Luminal causes of bleeding

This topic has been discussed in the section History. The most important diagnoses which need to be excluded are large polyps, cancer and IBD.

Conditions presenting with lump

Skin tags

These are redundant areas of skin at the anal verge which may have resulted from previously thrombosed haemorrhoids or previous anal fissure. They are more common in patients who have been pregnant and usually increase slowly in size with age. They are usually asymptomatic, although they may cause concern due to cosmesis or difficulty with anal hygiene. Often reassurance is adequate treatment. Surgical excision may be cautiously offered on the understanding that there may be subsequent development of further skin tags and that complete excision may not be possible due to the risk of anal stenosis.

Anal warts

Anal warts are a sexually transmitted infection due to human papillomavirus (HPV), most commonly subtypes 6 and 11. Anal warts may present as nontender lumps that may be itchy or may bleed if larger. They are often multiple, have a distinctive appearance with a 'warty' surface, and can be found in perianal skin and the distal anal canal. The normal skin around a wart may also be infected with HPV which may have spread from other areas of the perineum. Anal intercourse is not required for infection of the anal canal. Importantly, warts may be distributed up to the dentate line inside the anal canal but do not usually progress proximal to this. The macroscopic lumps can be surgically removed but infection remains in the surrounding skin leading to recurrence. Imiquimod is an immune-modifying agent used topically and will act to eradicate HPV but has limited action on large lesions.

Anal cancer/anal intraepithelial neoplasia

Anal intraepithelial neoplasia (AIN) is the precursor to squamous cell carcinoma of the anus. It is caused by neoplastic transformation as a result of HPV infection (usually subtypes 16 and 18). There are three grades of AIN: progression from grade I to III relates to increasing depth of penetration of dysplastic cells into the epithelium. The natural history of AIN in non-immunosuppressed patients remains unclear. Treatment is generally non-operative with close observation, although visible lesions should be excised.

Squamous cell carcinoma (SCC) of the perianal skin most commonly presents with a lump which may cause bleeding, itch and pain. SCC located intra-anally more commonly presents with bleeding. Although most SCCs of the anal canal are located distal to the dentate line, they can be located higher in the anal canal or even in the lower rectum because metaplastic squamous cells can be found in the transitional zone between lower anal squamous and rectal columnar mucosa. On clinical examination, the lesion feels hard, with raised rolled edges and central ulceration (Figure 33.5). Disease external to the anal verge may potentially be excised.

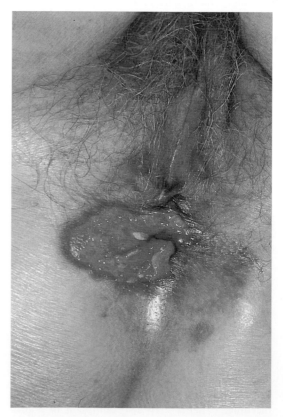

Fig. 33.5 Squamous cell carcinoma of the anal verge.

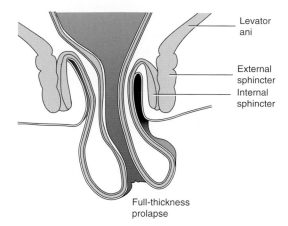

Fig. 33.6 Anatomical features of rectal prolapse.

SCC limited to the anal canal usually requires more aggressive treatment with the modified Nigro protocol consisting of chemoradiation. SCC is sensitive to this regimen and salvage abdominoperineal resection is infrequently required to ensure adequate treatment.

Rectal prolapse

Overt rectal prolapse refers to the full thickness of the rectal wall prolapsing externally through the anal canal (Figure 33.6). Most commonly this is a condition of postmemopausal females and often reflects a generalised weakness of the pelvic floor. The prolapse usually comes out several centimetres during defecation and is manually reduced by the patient. Rectal prolapse interferes with normal sphincter closing and leads to incontinence. The prolapsed mucosa produces leakage of mucus and blood.

Treatment requires surgery. Short-length prolapses in frailer patients usually undergo transanal repair. The Altemeier procedure excises the whole prolapse. The Delorme procedure excises the mucosa and plicates the underlying muscle. Transabdominal procedures involve securing the rectum to the sacrum using mesh or sutures. If constipation has been a major symptom preoperatively, the sigmoid colon may also be resected in a procedure called resection rectopexy.

Internal prolapse of the rectum can produce symptoms of obstructed defecation and solitary rectal ulcer syndrome.

Conditions presenting with discharge

Fistula

See Chapter 34.

Faecal incontinence

Faecal incontinence is a common condition that mainly affects women over the age of 50. The majority of patients will have a history of obstetric difficulties resulting in either direct injury to the sphincter complex or neuronal injury. Other causes include surgical trauma and prolonged straining. The treatment of incontinence is determined by the impact on quality of life rather than the aetiology. It may be classified by the consistency of the faecal loss: flatus, liquid or solid stool. Conservative treatment consists of lifestyle and dietary modification with pelvic floor physiotherapy. These simple measures are often successful in allowing the patient to maintain an acceptable quality of life. Further intervention such as sphincter repair can correct a deficit in the external sphincter. Sacral nerve stimulation is successful (through an unknown mechanism) in approximately 70% of patients who suffer several episodes of solid incontinence a week. This topic is further discussed in Chapter 64.

Further reading

Guerra GR, Kong JC, Bernardi MP *et al.* Salvage surgery for loco-regional failure in anal squamous cell carcinoma. *Dis Colon Rectum* 2018;61:179–86.

MacRae HM, McLeod RS. Comparison of hemorrhoidal treatment modalities. *A meta-analysis. Dis Colon Rectum* 1995;38:687–94.

Mentes BB, Tezcaner T, Yilmaz U, Leventoglu S, Oguz M. Results of lateral internal sphincterotomy for chronic anal fissure with particular reference to quality of life. *Dis Colon Rectum* 2006;49:1045–51.

Senapati A, Gray RG, Middleton LJ *et al.* PROSPER: a randomised comparison of surgical treatments for rectal prolapse. *Colorectal Dis* 2013;15:858–68.

MCQs

Select the single correct answer to each question. The correct answers can be found in the Answers section at the end of the book.

1 Which of the following statements about the anal canal is *incorrect*?
   a the internal sphincter is a continuation of the puborectalis muscle
   b the external sphincter is skeletal muscle and under voluntary control
   c the dentate line separates the zone of squamous mucosa from the more proximal transitional zone containing metaplastic squamous and columnar mucosa

d the haemorrhoidal vessels are located deep to the mucosa proximal to the dentate line

e the anal canal is approximately 4 cm long in males

2 Which of the following statements about investigations for anal disease is *incorrect*?

a defecating proctography can be used to diagnose occult rectal prolapse

b endoanal ultrasound is a useful test for visualising the integrity of the internal and external sphincters

c examination under anaesthesia is an important investigation in delineating anal fistula

d CT scanning has minimal utility in investigating perianal disease

e MRI scanning is contraindicated in the investigation of squamous cell carcinoma of the anal canal

3 Which of the following statements about anal fissure is *incorrect*?

a a chronic anal fissure is usually located posteriorly at the anal verge and has white fibres of the internal sphincter visible at its base

b in the treatment of chronic fissure, glyceryl trinitrate, botulinum toxin and lateral sphincterotomy arc all used to decrease spasm in the internal sphincter muscle

c patients with chronic anal fissure characteristically complain of anal pain with defecation, bright red rectal bleeding and often notice a small lump at the anal verge

d lateral sphincterotomy has been shown to be the most effective treatment for fissures and is usually the operative treatment of first choice for females

e although bleeding is a feature of chronic fissures, ischaemia of the base may contribute to their aetiology

4 Which of the following statements about anal neoplasia is *incorrect*?

a the anal canal is part of the lower gastrointestinal tract and thus the most common anal cancer is adenocarcinoma

b unless the lesion is small and easily excised locally, anal cancer is usually treated with chemoradiotherapy

c once dysplastic epithelial cells have penetrated beyond the epithelium to the submucosa, an area of anal intraepithelial neoplasia becomes a squamous cell carcinoma

d anal intraepithelial neoplasia is associated with HPV subtypes 16 and 18

e anal intraepithelial neoplasia can be difficult to visualise in the perianal skin

34 Perianal disorders II: sepsis

Ian Hayes[1,2] and the late Joe J. Tjandra[1,2]

[1] Colorectal Surgery Unit, Royal Melbourne Hospital, Melbourne, Victoria, Australia
[2] Department of Surgery, University of Melbourne, Parkville, Victoria, Australia

Introduction

Knowledge of the surgical treatment of infections in the perianal region is important. Abscess formation in the perineum causes severe pain, requires urgent surgery, and inadequate treatment can result in progression to dangerous necrotising infections. There is a high rate of subsequent fistula formation, a condition which has challenged surgeons since the time of Hippocrates and continues to do so.

Aetiology: the crypto-glandular hypothesis

The crypto-glandular hypothesis links the various manifestations of abscess and fistula that occur in the perianal region. Anal glands open into the anal canal at the dentate line, which is situated approximately 1.5 cm from the anal verge. The glands reside in the intersphincteric space between the internal sphincter (the innermost cylinder of sphincter muscle) and external sphincter (the outer cylinder of sphincter muscle). In theory, if the opening of the gland into the anal canal becomes blocked, bacteria will proliferate within the gland and an abscess will develop in the intersphincteric space. How that abscess spreads determines how the patient may present clinically and also predicts the anatomy of any subsequent fistula (Figure 34.1).

Perianal abscess

Clinical features

The symptoms of abscess in the perianal region develop over hours to days. A throbbing, unrelenting and increasing pain is the main feature. The patient may notice some fullness in the perianal skin and develop a fever. Clinical examination will usually reveal a patient in considerable discomfort, avoiding sitting or lying on the affected area. There is often moderate cellulitis in the skin and a diffuse, raised, indurated area. The area is very tender but gentle examination may find a fluctuant region at its centre.

Types of abscess (Figure 34.2)

- *Perianal abscess.* Most commonly, the initial abscess tracks inferiorly through the intersphincteric plane to develop a perianal abscess close to the anal verge.
- *Ischiorectal abscess.* If the abscess penetrates the external sphincter, it has the capacity to spread in the large horseshoe-shaped space of the ischiorectal fossa. In this situation, a large abscess, which is more deeply sited than a perianal abscess, can spread peripherally around both sides of the anal canal.
- *Intersphicteric abscess.* Occasionally, the abscess remains localised to the intersphincteric space. An intersphincteric abscess may cause severe pain but without externally visible signs of infection, such as a painful swelling and skin erythema. Usually, there is severe spasm in the sphincter muscles and the patient is too tender to allow digital rectal examination. Similar features may be found with patients experiencing severe symptoms from anal fissure. Failure to consider the diagnosis of intersphincteric abscess may delay treatment and worsen sepsis.
- *Suprasphincteric abscess.* An intersphincteric abscess or an ischiorectal abscess can also track in a cephalad direction to form a suprasphincteric abscess located above the levator muscles.

Investigations

Perianal sepsis is a clinical diagnosis and imaging is usually not required. Blood glucose level should be checked to exclude diabetes as a precipitant.

Textbook of Surgery, Fourth Edition. Edited by Julian A. Smith, Andrew H. Kaye, Christopher Christophi and Wendy A. Brown.
© 2020 John Wiley & Sons Ltd. Published 2020 by John Wiley & Sons Ltd.

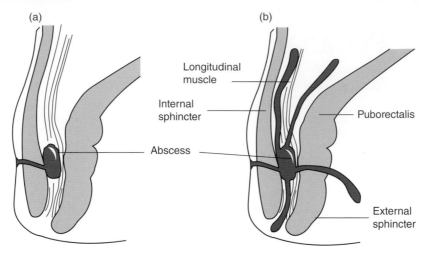

Fig. 34.1 Spread of infection from (a) the primary anal gland abscess to (b) the perianal region.

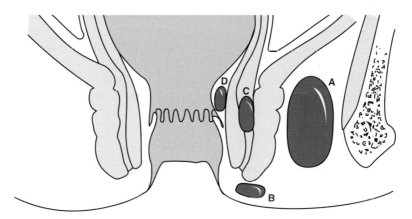

Fig. 34.2 Types of abscess in the perianal region: (A) ischiorectal, (B) perianal, (C) intersphincteric and (D) submucosal.

MRI of the pelvis is the imaging modality most likely to reveal an abscess in unusual cases where there is high suspicion but no clear clinical evidence of a collection. From a practical perspective, the key investigation for patients with suspected sepsis in the perianal region is examination under anaesthesia.

Treatment

In most cases, the clinical diagnosis of perianal sepsis is straightforward and the patient is taken to the operating theatre. Broad-spectrum antibiotic treatment should be initiated early. Under anaesthesia, rigid sigmoidoscopy is done to exclude evidence of underlying malignancy or inflammatory bowel disease. If there is an obvious abscess, an incision is made through the overlying skin down to the abscess cavity. Generally,

pus will be released under pressure. To allow adequate drainage, blunt dissection is used to break down all loculations within the abscess cavity. Sometimes a drain will be left in place for a large or deeply situated cavity. The wound is left open. Adequate drainage of the abscess usually results in rapid improvement in the patient's symptoms.

The finding of severe systemic sepsis and ischaemic tissue is suggestive of Fournier's gangrene, a rapidly progressing, mixed-organism, necrotising infection that may require extensive debridement of dead tissue to gain control of the sepsis. This rare but life-threatening infection can spread upwards along fascial planes to involve the external genitalia and lower abdominal wall.

Patients who have had an abscess in the perianal region have about a 50% chance of developing a fistula.

Anal fistula

A fistula is an abnormal communication between two epithelial-lined cavities. As discussed, perianal sepsis starts with blockage of glands which enter the anal canal at the dentate line. If the sepsis is surgically drained or spontaneously discharges to the skin, a communicating track can arise between the anal canal and the perianal skin, forming a fistula. The course that the fistula track follows is determined by the position of the original abscess.

Clinical features

The main clinical feature of an anal fistula is a 2–3 mm skin opening lined by granulation tissue, discharging a small amount of pus, and located 1–3 cm from the anal verge. The fistula track may be palpable as a subcutaneous chord heading towards the anal verge, especially if the fistula is following a relatively low trans-sphincteric course. The internal opening is not always palpable on digital examination. Internal examination and proctoscopy/rigid sigmoidoscopy help to exclude uncommon, but important, underlying causes such as cancer or inflammatory bowel disease. Digital examination also allows an assessment of the length of the anal canal and strength of the sphincter mechanism, which are important considerations if fistulotomy is planned.

If the openings of multiple fistulas are seen, particularly if associated with oedematous skin tags and fissuring, Crohn's disease should be considered a possible underlying diagnosis (Figure 34.3).

Goodsall's law

Goodsall's law is a rule of thumb which aids in the operative localisation of fistula tracks. It states that fistulas opening into the anterior half of the perianal skin generally follow direct radial tracks to open internally at the dentate line. Thus, a fistula opening to the perianal skin at the 2 o'clock position will be expected to have its internal opening in the anal canal at the 2 o'clock position.

Fistulas opening into the posterior half of the perianal skin also open into the anal canal at the dentate line but follow curved tracks to the 6 o'clock position (posteriorly). A fistula having its external opening in the perianal skin at the 8 o'clock position will usually have an internal opening at the 6 o'clock position (Figure 34.4). (More peripherally located anterior fistulas can originate at the 6 o'clock position.)

Types of fistulas

- *Intersphincteric.* The track starts at the dentate line in the anal canal and runs between the internal and external sphincters, exiting in the perianal skin close to the anal verge. Because relatively little sphincter muscle lies within the confines of

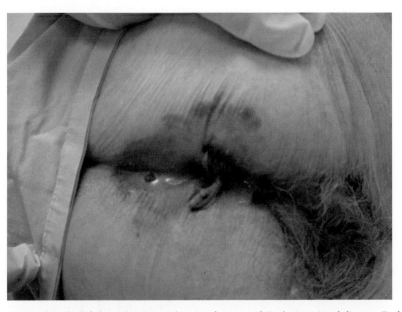

Fig. 34.3 Patient examined in the left-lateral position showing features of Crohn's perianal disease. Red and blue setons are visible and a new fistula opening is seen at the 6 o'clock position (9 o'clock in photograph). There is extensive excoriation of the skin due to irritation from discharge.

the track, this type of fistula is potentially suitable for treatment with fistulotomy without significant risk to continence.

- *Trans-sphincteric.* When the track goes through the external sphincter, the fistula is described as trans-sphincteric. These fistulas can be high or low depending on how much external sphincter muscle is involved. A low trans-sphincteric fistula can be treated with fistulotomy if less than one-third of the sphincter complex is liable to be divided during the surgery.
- *Suprasphincteric.* A suprasphincteric fistula extends superior to the levator muscles. An extensive amount of sphincter muscle is involved, precluding fistulotomy.
- *Extrasphincteric.* An extrasphincteric fistula is a complex fistula starting from an origin higher in the pelvis and *not* from the anal canal. An example is a malignant fistula from an advanced rectal cancer. Treatment requires removal or control of the pelvic source of the sepsis (Figure 34.5).

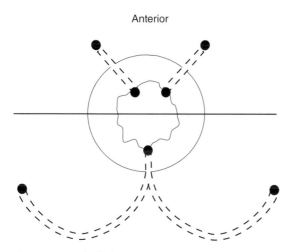

Anterior

Fig. 34.4 Goodsall's law.

Investigations

MRI and endoanal ultrasound are both used to delineate fistulas. MRI delineates the tracks very well, whilst endoanal ultrasound gives very good definition of the sphincters. In many cases, however, much of the relevant information can be deduced by probing the fistula track under anaesthesia.

Treatment

The simplest and most effective treatment for fistula is fistulotomy. This involves dividing the skin and any sphincter muscle included, down to and along the track. This will allow the track to heal from its base by secondary intention. The problem is that most fistulas are trans-sphincteric and some sphincter muscle will need to be divided. Faecal incontinence can result from dividing too much sphincter muscle. As a very general rule, providing there is no pre-existing sphincter damage, the most distal one-third of the sphincter complex can be divided without significant impairment to continence. However, females have shorter sphincters than males and have a risk of previous, or future, sphincter impairment related to childbirth.

If there is concern at operation that a significant amount of sphincter muscle is at risk, then a seton drain (a loop of silastic thread) is inserted (see Figure 34.3). It is more common to insert a seton than perform fistulotomy as a first procedure. Setons are soft and generally well tolerated by patients. This method allows ongoing drainage of the fistula and minimises the risk of further abscess formation. With time, the seton will allow the 'sump' cavity associated with the fistula to decrease in size and become easier to treat. Once a seton has been inserted, the track is easier to delineate with ultrasound or MRI. These tests may reveal that

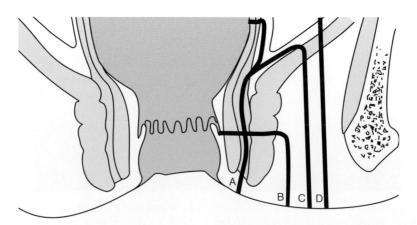

Fig. 34.5 Types of perianal fistula: (A) intersphincteric, (B) trans-sphincteric, (C) suprasphincteric and (D) extrasphincteric.

there is enough reserve of sphincter muscle remaining deep to the fistula track to allow reconsideration of fistulotomy.

Alternatively, a different treatment plan may be required which does not divide sphincter muscle. The options include insertion of tissue glue or fistula plug to seal the track. The fistula track can also be occluded from its internal aspect with a rectal mucosal advancement flap. A low well-defined track track can be approached through the perianal skin, divided and ligated using a LIFT (ligation of intersphincteric fistula track) procedure. All these procedures have a moderately high failure rate.

High complex fistulas pose a major surgical challenge and may require several procedures before resolution. In some cases, a long-term seton may need to remain in place. Occasionally, a defunctioning stoma is required to divert the flow of faeces away from the anus and gain control of the sepsis in a complex fistula.

When a fistula is proving difficult to eradicate, it is important to consider other causes such as missed tracks, inflammatory bowel disease, malignancy, and atypical infections such as tuberculosis and actinomycosis.

Other conditions causing sepsis in the perineal region

Hidradenitis suppurativa

This condition is related to infection of apocrine sweat glands in hair-bearing skin. Characteristically, multiple small sinus openings are seen in affected areas of axillae, groin and perineum (Figure 34.6). With recurrent low-grade infections, scarring develops. Hidradenitis is distinguished from fistula disease by the multiple openings, lack of internal anal

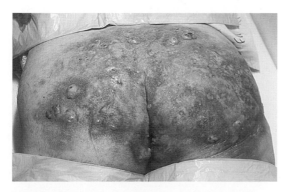

Fig. 34.6 Hidradenitis of the perineum and perianal region.

involvement and the finding of similar disease in other sites separate to the perianal region.

Mild disease may improve with prolonged courses of oral antibiotics. Abscesses may require surgical drainage. Small areas can be surgically excised and primarily closed. The surgical treatment of larger areas can involve significant skin loss and extensive grafting or mobilisation of skin flaps for reconstruction. Occasionally, a diverting stoma may need to be constructed to facilitate hygiene after such major excision and reconstruction. Anti-tumour necrosis factor (TNF)-α inhibitors have been trialled with varying success for control of severe cases of hidradenitis.

Pilonidal sinus

Pilonidal sinus refers to nests of hair located deep to small midline skin openings in the natal cleft. The interdigital region of the hands and the umbilicus can also be involved in this disease. It is hypothesised that the hairs originate from the patient's back and are channelled between the buttocks where they impale the skin, forming the sinuses. The patients are usually hirsute young-adult males. The existence of the nest of hair may not, of itself, produce symptoms apart from occasional minor pressure effects. Problems begin when the sinus opening blocks and infection develops in the cavity, producing an abscess. The pus from the abscess often tracks a short distance laterally to exit in the skin 1–2 cm from the midline. This may allow the pain of the abscess to settle but there is likely to be ongoing discharge of pus and blood from this secondary opening.

Some patients present with an abscess requiring urgent surgical drainage. However, most patients present with chronic discomfort and discharge from the secondary openings of a chronically infected pilonidal sinus.

This condition is usually diagnosed clinically by the characteristic line of small pits in the midline of the natal cleft, with underlying induration and laterally located secondary openings. Occasionally, a pilonidal sinus located very distally in the natal cleft can appear similar to an anal fistula.

Treatment

Non-operative treatment
- If the patient simply has the presence of midline pits but no surrounding induration or symptoms, then treatment is not required.
- Mild cases may improve by permanently removing hair from the back and buttocks.

Operative treatment

- Patients presenting with an abscess require surgical incision and drainage. This will not fix the underlying problem and it is likely that a second procedure will need to be performed electively to remove the diseased area. Removing all the diseased tissue in the setting of an abscess may result in an excessively large wound.
- Patients with significant ongoing symptoms, induration and secondary openings will require surgical excision of the diseased area.
- Bascom's procedure involves a minimalist surgical approach to this condition. The midline pits are individually cored out and a lateral incision is made to excise the hair-filled cavity. This avoids the difficulties of a major wound in the natal cleft but recurrence rate is high.
- Excision and leave open: to clear all the sinus tissue requires quite a deep excision, creating a considerable defect. Leaving the wound open with planned healing by secondary intention is a safe method for dealing with these wounds but may require a prolonged period of dressings.
- Excision and closure: the wound may be primarily closed but this carries a high risk of wound breakdown. Presumably the wound breakdown problems are related to the fact that any leg movement causes strong shearing forces between the sides of the incision; the tissues are under some tension and contamination from perineal flora is highly likely. Furthermore, a midline suture line is a potential site of later hair implantation.
- Karydakis procedure: in an attempt to overcome these issues, this procedure mobilises a thick flap of skin and subcutaneous tissue from one side of the wound and leaves a suture line offset from the midline, creating a skin closure under less tension and avoiding residual midline scar tissue. In cases with large skin defects, rotation flaps, including rhomboid flaps, can be used.

The natal cleft is an unforgiving area for surgery and all surgical procedures for pilonidal sinus carry a risk of recurrent disease and prolonged wound healing. The addition of permanent hair removal from the back and buttocks may help prevent recurrence.

Further reading

Jemec G. Hidradenitis suppurativa. *N Engl J Med* 2102; 366:158–64.

Johnson EK, Gau JU, Armstrong DN. Efficacy of anal fistula plug vs fibrin glue in closure of anorectal fistulas. *Dis Colon Rectum* 2006;49:371–6.

Karydakis GE. New approach to the problem of pilonidal sinus. *Lancet* 1973;ii(7843):1414–15.

Parks AG, Gordon PH, Hardcastle JD. A classification of fistula-in-ano. *Br J Surg* 1976;63:1–12.

MCQs

Select the single correct answer to each question. The correct answers can be found in the Answers section at the end of the book.

1 The preferred treatment of an ischiorectal abscess is:
   a a prolonged course of antibiotics to abort the infection
   b incision and drainage under general anaesthesia
   c warm salt baths
   d fistulotomy
   e defunctioning colostomy

2 The aetiology of anal fistula does *not* include:
   a anal gland infection
   b rectal cancer
   c Crohn's disease
   d actinomycosis
   e levator syndrome

3 Treatment options for anal fistula do *not* include:
   a LIFT procedure, which involves using a silastic cord to gradually occlude the track
   b mucosal advancement flap used to close the internal opening
   c blocking the fistula track with tissue glue
   d long-term placement of a seton
   e fistulotomy if adequate sphincter muscle can be preserved

4 Pilonidal sinus disease:
   a can occur in the natal cleft, the umbilicus and the axillae
   b is characterised by midline pits in the natal cleft and secondary openings laterally
   c frequently results in fistulas to the dentate line of the anal canal
   d usually becomes symptomatic as soon as secondary openings develop
   e is not treated using a fibular free-flap

Section 5
Breast Surgery

35 Breast assessment and benign breast disease

Rajiv V. Dave[1] and G. Bruce Mann[2]

[1] Royal Melbourne Hospital, Melbourne, Victoria, Australia and The Nightingale Centre, Manchester University NHS Foundation Trust, Manchester, UK

[2] Royal Melbourne Hospital and University of Melbourne, Melbourne, Victoria, Australia

Introduction

Management of breast disease has become increasingly specialised. A multidisciplinary, integrated and targeted approach is used, involving oncologic and reconstructive surgeons, radiologists, pathologists, oncologists and breast care nurses. A substantial component of the workload involves advising patients about their personalised risk of breast cancer, differentiating benign breast disease from breast cancer and allaying the patient's anxiety about breast cancer, and maintaining quality of life after diagnosis and treatment.

Anatomy of the adult breast

The main blood supply is via the second perforating branch of the internal mammary and lateral thoracic branches of the axillary artery. Lesser supply is via the thoracoacromial and subscapular arteries. A rich subareolar venous plexus drains via the intercostal, internal mammary and axillary veins.

The distribution of major lymphatics follows the blood supply. About 75% of the lymphatic vessels drain to the lymph nodes in front of and below the axillary vein. Most lymph drains initially to lymph nodes in the lower axilla, while a small amount of lymph drains from the superior aspect of the breast directly to the apical nodes. About 25% of lymph (mainly from the medial half of the breast) drains to the internal mammary nodes in the second, third and fourth intercostal spaces.

Assessment of the patient with a breast lump

Many women attending a breast clinic have a benign breast lump. Assessment of a breast abnormality relies heavily on the 'triple test'. The triple test can be summarised as follows: if an abnormality is clinically benign, radiologically benign and cytologically or histologically benign, then the risk it is malignant is extremely small, and excisional biopsy is not necessary. Adherence to this approach has meant that the number of benign lesions being excised has reduced dramatically. Importantly, if any of the three elements of the triple test is not clearly benign, then further investigation, often with excision of the lesion, is required. The various differential diagnoses for a benign breast lump are discussed later.

In most cases, a thorough history and examination is followed by radiological assessment with or without pathological assessment. It is important in the multidisciplinary management of breast lumps/lesions that all aspects of the triple assessment are considered.

History

A thorough clinical history should be taken, including menstrual, obstetric, family and medication history. A history of presentation of the lump is required, and common concerning symptoms for breast cancer include the following.

- A firm or hard lump with varying degree of fixity to surrounding tissues, overlying skin and underlying pectoral muscles. While pain is an

---

Textbook of Surgery, Fourth Edition. Edited by Julian A. Smith, Andrew H. Kaye, Christopher Christophi and Wendy A. Brown.
© 2020 John Wiley & Sons Ltd. Published 2020 by John Wiley & Sons Ltd.

uncommon symptom, the cancerous lump may have increasing discomfort, especially prior to menstruation.

- Changes to the breast that include distortion, puckering of skin and nipple retraction.
- A blood-stained nipple discharge may arise from an intraductal cancer and is typically unifocal.
- Rarely, distant metastases may be the cause of symptoms such as bone pain, abdominal pain or chest pain and dyspnoea.

Clinical examination

Clinical examination is often normal in screen-detected cancers. Clinical features of benign breast lumps include:

- smooth and mobile (typical for a fibroadenoma, discussed later)
- sudden growth of a smooth lump that can be tense or painful (typical for a breast cyst, discussed later)
- non-specific thickening of breast tissue (often seen in fibrocystic change, discussed later).

Signs of concern for a cancer include the following.

- A lump that is often around 2 cm in diameter when identified, and may be non-specific on examination.
- A larger lump that may be firm to hard, irregular and have skin attachment or distort the breast shape.
- Lymphatic obstruction and 'orange skin' (peau d'orange) appearance, usually seen in more advanced cancers.

- Red and inflamed skin due to lymphatic obstruction seen in inflammatory breast cancer, a rare and aggressive subtype of breast cancer.
- An appearance similar to eczema of the nipple associated with underlying intraductal carcinoma, often with an invasive component (Paget's disease).
- Enlarged and hard axillary and supraclavicular fossae nodes, in keeping with regional (nodal) spread of the breast cancer. Clinical assessment of the axilla is important but inaccurate, and lymph node metastases can only be confirmed or excluded by histological examination.
- Hepatomegaly due to liver metastases (but this is a rare finding).

Investigations in the assessment of possible breast cancer

Assessment of suspicious breast lesions usually involves a combination of mammography, ultrasound and percutaneous needle biopsy. It should be remembered that negative imaging does not completely rule out breast cancer.

Mammography

Mammography has a high level of accuracy in detecting breast cancer and its specificity increases with age. It is generally carried out using digital image acquisition (Figure 35.1a). Tomosynthesis is an advanced form of mammography that utilises lower-dose X-rays and computer-generated reconstructions to create three-dimensional images of the breasts

(a)   (b)

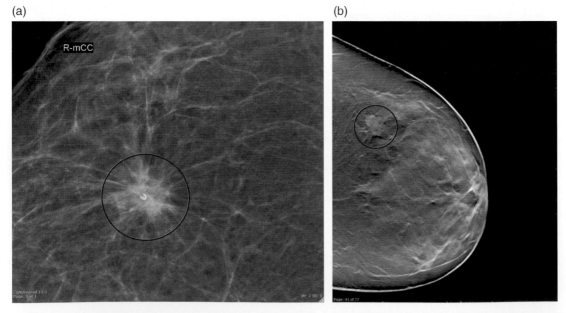

Fig. 35.1 Craniocaudal mammogram (a) and tomosynthesis (b) showing a stellate mass with irregular margins consistent with a breast cancer.

(Figure 35.1b). Suspicious mammographic features include a mass, asymmetry and microcalcification. Mammography detects impalpable cancers and, in clinically palpable cancers, helps assess the extent of the disease and so helps planning of treatment.

Ultrasound

Breast ultrasound is complementary to mammography in assessing breast conditions (Figure 35.2a). Ultrasound has a high sensitivity for breast pathology and also a high negative predictive value. While operator-dependent, ultrasound is most useful in the following circumstances.

- Evaluation of an equivocal lump: many women present to breast clinic after she or her GP finds a possible lump. Ultrasound is useful for distinguishing between a focal abnormality and prominent but normal breast parenchyma.
- Further assessment of an equivocal mammographic abnormality.
- Determining the nature of a definite palpable lump (solid vs. cystic).
- Guiding a percutaneous biopsy.

Breast ultrasound is not generally used for screening of asymptomatic women, but may have a role in adjunctive screening in certain situations such as those with extremely high breast density,

MRI

Breast MRI is a more sensitive test than either mammography or ultrasound, but it is significantly less specific (Figure 35.2b). Thus false negatives are less likely, but false positives are more likely. It is established as a screening test in those at very high risk of cancer, such as carriers of a *BRCA1* or *BRCA2* mutation, and also to screen for an occult primary cancer in the unusual clinical situation where a patient presents with breast cancer in axillary lymph nodes but no apparent primary cancer in the breast.

When used in a patient with a known cancer, breast MRI identifies further unsuspected foci of disease in one or other breast in up to 15% of cases, but it is unclear whether identification of this additional disease is of any benefit.

Percutaneous biopsy

Historically, many breast cancers were diagnosed after excisional biopsy (surgery). This is now uncommon, with a large majority of cancers being diagnosed on percutaneous biopsy.

Core biopsy

Core biopsy, guided by either ultrasound or mammography, is the modality of choice for breast biopsy. It results in histological proof of diagnosis and allows most benign conditions to be diagnosed without the need for surgery. It can distinguish between *in situ* and invasive cancer, and determine the subtype of cancer. It is performed using a 14- or 16-gauge wide-bore needle under local anaesthesia, with larger-gauge vacuum-assisted biopsy techniques also available.

Fine-needle aspiration cytology

Fine-needle aspiration cytology (FNAC) yields cells which may aid in the diagnosis or exclusion of cancer. It is used less frequently than in the past, as it is not possible to distinguish *in situ* from invasive

(a) (b)

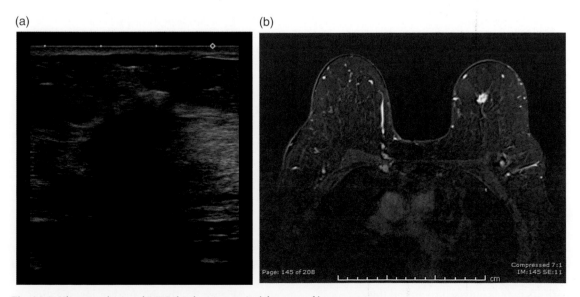

Fig. 35.2 Ultrasound (a) and MRI (b) showing typical features of breast cancer.

cancer. False negatives can occur, although false positives are most unusual. It is most often used to sample lymph nodes that are suspicious on clinical examination and/or ultrasound.

Open surgical (excisional) biopsy

While less common that it once was, this is performed in the following cases:
- if FNAC or core biopsy is inconclusive and there is a clinical suspicion of malignancy
- the patient is anxious and not adequately reassured by standard investigations
- there is a discrete lump and the patient chooses excision.

BENIGN BREAST DISEASE

Many so-called diseases of the breast are actually aberrations of the processes of development, cyclical change and involution. Benign breast disease refers to more severe disorders. In general, there is poor correlation between clinical, pathological and radiological features.

Mastalgia

Mastalgia is a common breast symptom; however, mastalgia does not imply any specific pathological process and the condition is not well understood. Mastalgia can be cyclical, varying with the menstrual cycle, or non-cyclical where there is no such relationship.

Cyclical mastalgia

Cyclical mastalgia is the most common type of breast pain affecting premenopausal women. The median age of presentation is 35 years. The breast discomfort lasts for a varying period prior to menstruation and relief of the pain comes with menstruation. As symptoms of cyclical mastalgia vary with menstrual cycle, there is probably a hormonal basis in the aetiology. However, the precise pathogenesis is poorly understood.

Management

More than 80% of women require no treatment other than reassurance that there is no cancer. The initial treatment is usually advice to stop smoking and a reduction of caffeine intake. Often, inappropriately fitted undergarments may cause pain, and patients may be advised to amend this.

Drug treatments are sometimes used. The initial treatment is usually with evening primrose oil. Natural or treatment-induced remissions are common, but mastalgia does recur. Second-line treatment with low-dose tamoxifen is reserved for severe refractory symptoms.

Non-cyclical mastalgia

The pain has no relationship to the menstrual cycle. It tends to be unilateral, more chronic and sometimes has a well localised 'trigger spot'.

Management

Any primary pathology of the breast and of adjacent structures should be excluded by a careful clinical evaluation and appropriate imaging. Chest wall pain is frequently assessed as being non-cyclical breast pain. This may respond to anti-inflammatory drug treatment. Treatment involves reassurance that there is no underlying pathology but drug treatment is generally unrewarding.

Benign breast lumps

Fibroadenoma

Pathology

Fibroadenoma is a benign breast tumour in premenopausal women, often presenting between 18 and 30 years of age. It consists of fibrous connective tissue stroma and epithelial proliferation, usually with low cellularity. With a benign fibroadenoma, the fibrous stroma has low cellularity. Epithelial hyperplasia may be present but has no prognostic importance. Coarse calcification may also occur later in life and be seen on screening mammography.

Clinical features

Fibroadenoma is smooth and typically very mobile (hence referred to as a 'breast mouse'). Some patients have multiple fibroadenomas at presentation. Others have multiple recurrent fibroadenomas.

Investigations and management

To satisfy the triple test, ultrasound with either FNAC or core biopsy is usually performed (Figure 35.3a). If this confirms a benign fibroadenoma (Figure 35.3b), no further investigation or

(a)

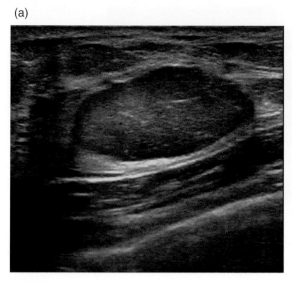

(b)

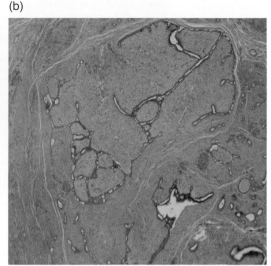

Fig. 35.3 Ultrasound (a) and haematoxylin and eosin (H&E) section (b) of a typical fibroadenoma.

treatment is required. Some women elect to have a fibroadenoma excised, particularly if the lump is prominent and/or tender.

Phyllodes tumour

Pathology

Phyllodes tumour is the name given to a wide spectrum of fibroepithelial lesions that are not clearly benign fibroadenomas. The spectrum extends from benign phyllodes with minimal clinical significance to a malignant soft tissue tumour. Histologically, the fibrous stoma is hypercellular with cellular atypia and mitoses.

Clinical features

Phyllodes tumours occur in premenopausal women and clinically resemble fibroadenomas, but often grow quite rapidly.

Treatment

This entails a complete local excision, avoiding transection of the tumour. Depending on the nature of the tumour, local recurrence may be common; with malignant phyllodes, lung metastases can occur.

Breast cysts

Pathology and incidence

Breast cysts are very common, with up to 10% of women developing a clinical breast cyst during their lifetime. Many women have multiple subclinical breast cysts measuring 2–3 mm identified on

ultrasound and most occur in the perimenopausal age group. The pathogenesis of breast cysts is not clear. The breast cyst may be lined by apocrine or simple cuboidal epithelium.

Clinical features

Breast cysts often appear suddenly and can be quite large. This is because the subclinical flaccid cyst accumulates a small amount of fluid and becomes tense and painful. On clinical examination, the cyst is smooth and firm but not as mobile as a fibroadenoma. The diagnosis of a breast cyst is confirmed by ultrasound and sometimes cyst aspiration (Figure 35.4). Cytological examination of the cyst fluid is not done unless the fluid is evenly blood-stained.

Treatment

Palpable breast cysts are treated by simple aspiration in the consulting room. If a lump persists after aspiration of the cyst, further investigations are required to define the cause of the mass.

Nipple discharge

Clinical features and investigation

Nipple discharge is a common problem and the causes are outlined in Box 35.1. Investigations include mammography and ultrasound occasionally with cytology of the discharge. These investigations are often unrevealing.

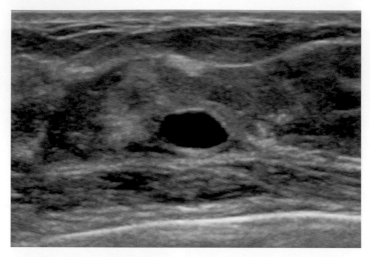

Fig. 35.4 Breast ultrasound showing a well-defined breast cyst.

Box 35.1 Causes of nipple discharge

- Physiological (pregnancy, lactation)
- Duct ectasia
- Galactorrhoea
- Duct papillomas
- Fibrocystic disease
- Carcinoma

Mammary duct ectasia and periductal mastitis

Mammary duct ectasia and periductal mastitis have a diverse clinical spectrum. Nipple discharge in a perimenopausal woman with greenish or brown fluid arising from multiple duct orifices on one or both nipples is the common presentation. The aetiology is unclear but involves the accumulation of secretions in the duct. Especially in smokers, there can be inflammation of the surrounding tissues with infection, a thick nipple discharge and nipple retraction.

Galactorrhoea

Galactorrhoea may be a primary physiological process, occurring during menarche, menopause or secondary to drugs that stimulate dopamine activity. Serum prolactin levels should be requested to investigate for underlying prolactinoma, which may lead to MRI of the pituitary gland.

Intraductal papilloma

Papilloma is the commonest cause of bloody nipple discharge. The discharge may be serous but is often blood-stained and arises from a single duct. Solitary papillomas are benign and do not have malignant potential. The clinical issue is that ductal carcinoma *in situ* (DCIS), a premalignant condition described in Chapter 36, can present with a bloody nipple discharge.

The presence of multiple papilloma is termed 'papillomatosis'. This condition is not often associated with nipple discharge and may develop further away from the nipple.

Management of nipple discharge

Nipple discharge is managed via the usual triple assessment method. Bloody nipple discharge usually requires surgery to exclude serious pathology. Profuse discharge from a single orifice usually requires surgery to make the diagnosis and treat the problem. In most other cases surgery is not required.

Proliferative and non-proliferative conditions of the breast

There exists a spectrum of conditions of the breast often detected on core biopsy of an indeterminate lesion that can be classed as either proliferative or non-proliferative. Commonly, a non-proliferative condition called 'fibrocystic change' is seen on core biopsy of microcalcifications following screening mammography, usually in premenopausal women. It is a benign entity that does not infer an increased risk of developing breast cancer. It may present as a lump, particularly in the upper outer quadrant, and may cause discomfort. The pathophysiology is poorly understood, but it is thought to be due to hormonal influences.

Proliferative conditions of the breast can be classified as either without atypia or as atypical hyperplasia. Radial scars and complex sclerosing lesions are part of the spectrum of the same condition and are distinguished on size criteria (<1 cm and >1 cm, respectively). They appear histologically as a central fibroelastic core from which ducts and lobules radiate circumferentially. Radial scars and complex sclerosing lesions therefore have a stellate appearance on mammography and can mimic breast cancer. There seems to be an association between radial scars and complex sclerosing lesions, but this is controversial.

Atypical ductal hyperplasia (ADH) is a proliferative condition characterised by cellular proliferation (hyperplasia) with atypical epithelium. It is similar histologically to low-grade DCIS (discussed in Chapter 36), but does not meet size criteria (<2 mm) for diagnosis. Thus, excision is usually recommended, and surveillance thereafter, due to the increased risk of breast cancer.

Lobular carcinoma *in situ* (LCIS) and atypical lobular hyperplasia (ALH) are both benign entities characterised by proliferation of cells within a lobule, but may also involve ducts. They are both asymptomatic and mammographically occult, and usually present as an incidental finding. They are a risk factor for breast cancer (LCIS, sevenfold to 11-fold increased risk; ALH, fourfold to fivefold increased risk) but are not premalignant. LCIS and ALH do not usually require radical excision but careful follow-up of the patient.

Some benign breast conditions are a risk for cancer (Box 35.2), although the literature is confusing. The key issue is whether there is any atypical proliferation in the benign breast disease; its presence indicates a significantly increased risk, and more frequent surveillance is appropriate.

Gynaecomastia in males

About one-third of adult males and more than half of normal pubescent boys have some degree of gynaecomastia. Physiological gynaecomastia occurs in the neonate because of circulating maternal sex hormones, at puberty because of a high serum oestradiol to testosterone ratio, and in the elderly because of reduced testosterone production. A common cause of gynaecomastia in young men is due to use of anabolic steroids. Unilateral gynaecomastia, especially in an older man, raises the possibility of breast cancer. This is investigated and managed along similar lines to female breast cancer.

With significant gynaecomastia causing social embarrassment, surgical excision of the breast

---

> ### Box 35.2 Relationship between benign and malignant breast disease
>
> **Increased risk**
> - Atypical ductal hyperplasia
> - Atypical lobular hyperplasia
> - Lobular carcinoma *in situ*
>
> **No increased risk**
> - Cysts
> - Fibroadenoma
> - Duct ectasia
> - Papilloma
> - Epithelial hyperplasia without atypia
> - Sclerosing adenosis
> - Apocrine change
>
> **Uncertain risk**
> - Radial scar without atypia
> - Papillomatosis

---

plaque is recommended. This is done through an incision at the margin of the areola to minimise the cosmetic effect.

Acknowledgement

The authors wish to thank Dr Anand Murugasu, Consultant Histopathologist, Royal Melbourne for assistance with figure 35.3b and Dr Alexandria Taylor, Consultant Radiologist, Royal Melbourne Hospital for assistance with figures 35.1, 35.2, 35.3a and 35.4.

Further reading

Dixon JM (ed.) *ABC of Breast Diseases*, 4th edn. Oxford: Wiley Blackwell, 2012.

Dixon JM (ed.) *Breast Surgery. A Companion to Surgical Practice*, 6th edn. Edinburgh: Elsevier, 2018.

MCQs

Select the single correct answer to each question. The correct answers can be found in the Answers section at the end of the book.

1 A 48-year-old woman presents with thick greenish nipple discharge from both breasts. There is no palpable breast lump, although both nipples are slightly retracted. The patient does not take any medication. Mammogram and ultrasound do not show any evidence of cancer. The most likely diagnosis is:
   a galactorrhoea
   b duct papilloma

c mammary duct ectasia
d fibroadenoma
e lobular carcinoma *in situ*

2 A 57-year-old woman presented with bloody nipple discharge from a single duct. The most likely diagnosis is:
a fibrocystic change
b intraductal papilloma
c ductal carcinoma *in situ*
d mammary duct ectasia
e lobular carcinoma *in situ*

3 Which of the following is *not* a feature of a benign breast lump?
a smooth

b mobile
c tense or painful
d in-drawing of the nipple
e well circumscribed on ultrasound

4 A 36-year-old woman presented to the clinic with a suspicious lump, confirmed on clinical examination. Ultrasound and mammography reveal a benign-appearing mass. What would be the most appropriate course of action?
a discharge from clinic
b repeat imaging in 3 months
c repeat imaging in 3 years
d core biopsy of the lesion
e FNAC of the lesion

36 Malignant breast disease and surgery

Rajiv V. Dave[1] and G. Bruce Mann[2]

[1] Royal Melbourne Hospital, Melbourne, Victoria, Australia and The Nightingale Centre, Manchester University NHS Foundation Trust, Manchester, UK
[2] Royal Melbourne Hospital and University of Melbourne, Melbourne, Victoria, Australia

Introduction

Breast cancer is a heterogeneous disease with a varying propensity for spread. It is now recognised that breast cancer is classified not only by histological type but also by molecular type, and understanding of this tumour biology aids prognostication and treatment decisions.

Although breast cancer is generally slow growing, with pre-invasive phases that may extend over a number of years, some cases are rapidly progressive. Prognosis is usually favourable with early diagnosis and multidisciplinary treatment. However, breast cancer may recur many years after treatment, indicating the need for prolonged monitoring.

Incidence

The incidence of breast cancer rises with age up to age 70, and the lifetime risk by age 85 in an Australian woman is 1 in 8, but is lower in Asian countries. Over the last three decades, the 5-year survival has increased from 72% to around 90% due to a combination of early detection and better treatment.

Risk factors

Most breast cancer is sporadic with no specific identifiable cause. Several interrelated factors are associated with an increased risk of developing breast cancer, which may be broadly classified into modifiable and non-modifiable factors.

Non-modifiable factors

- Gender: breast cancer is about 100 times more common in women than in men.
- Increasing age: breast cancer is very uncommon in women under 30 years of age. The mean age at diagnosis is 60 years.
- Past history of breast cancer: those having had one breast cancer are at higher risk for an entirely new one.
- Family history: most significant if there is breast cancer in first-degree relatives (mother, sister or daughter), especially if they were under 40 years of age when the cancer developed, or if there is a history of bilateral disease.
- Previous history of benign proliferative disease with cellular atypia, i.e. atypical ductal and lobular hyperplasia.
- Other factors, for example nulliparity at 40 years, previous breast irradiation (as part of treatment for conditions such as Hodgkin's disease), younger age at menarche.

Modifiable factors

- Obesity is a risk factor for breast cancer, not only in the primary setting, but also post surgery where weight gain is associated with risk of recurrence.
- Alcohol. it is estimated that alcohol intake is responsible for around 16% of breast cancer cases in Australia.
- Sedentary lifestyle: lack of physical fitness is associated with an increased breast cancer risk.
- Exogenous hormone treatment: the data on the cancer risk with hormone replacement therapy

(HRT) is conflicting. Prolonged use of combined oestrogen/progesterone HRT is definitely associated with an increased incidence of breast cancer. Short duration (<5 years) appears safe, and oestrogen-only HRT (used in women who have had hysterectomy) also appears safe. The risks associated with the oral contraceptive pill (OCP) are low, but recent studies have suggested a small increase in relative risk. The fact that the underlying risk of breast cancer at the age of maximal OCP use is very low means this is not a major concern.

Genetics

Around 5% of cases of breast cancer are due to identifiable genetic mutations. Most of these involve the *BRCA1* or *BRCA2* genes, with smaller numbers due to mutations in the *CDH1*, *ATM*, *TP53* or *PALB2* genes. These cases often, but not always, occur in association with a family history of breast and/or ovarian cancer.

Women of Ashkenazi Jewish ancestry have a risk of inheriting one of three 'founder' mutations present in this group that increases their risk of developing breast cancer. There are other founder mutations in certain communities, but it is the Ashkenazi mutations that are most commonly seen in Australia.

The impact of common minor genetic variations – single nucleotide polymorphisms (SNPs, pronounced 'snips') – is being studied. It has been shown that while the impact of any particular SNP on breast cancer risk is minimal, the overall pattern of SNPs may be significant, and those with multiple higher-risk SNPs may be at a substantially increased risk. This science may be clinically useful in the near future.

Prevention of breast cancer

Modifiable risk factors offer a substantial opportunity to reduce the incidence of breast cancer.

Chemoprevention with tamoxifen for 'high-risk' subjects for 5 years has been shown to result in a 35% reduction in breast cancer development over 15 years. This is not associated with reduced breast cancer mortality, and the side effects of tamoxifen limit uptake of this option.

Prophylactic mastectomy with or without breast reconstruction results in a 95% reduction in the risk of breast cancer development, as complete excision of all the breast ducts is not technically feasible. It is often considered by carriers of genetic mutations, and by some others at high risk.

Screening for breast cancer

Early detection of asymptomatic breast cancer by mammographic screening has been shown to improve survival. Trials of population-based mammographic screening in many countries have confirmed the value of early detection of tumours in reducing breast cancer mortality.

National breast screening programs have been established in many countries. In Australia, women aged 50–75 are invited to screen at 2-year intervals. The program has been successful in reducing mortality from breast cancer by approximately 21–28%, at the current participation rate of 56%. Patients have a two-view mammogram performed and if an abnormality is identified, they are recalled to an assessment clinic. The majority of abnormalities (>90%) detected at screening are benign. The benefits of screening are the reduction in breast cancer mortality and a reduced intensity of treatment, as early detection often allows treatment with less extensive surgery and less chemotherapy.

Screening has also detected an increased number of cases of ductal carcinoma *in situ* (DCIS), many of which may never have become clinically significant. This issue of over-diagnosis and subsequent over-treatment is a harm of screening that some suggest substantially limits the overall benefit of the population-based mammographic screening programs.

Spread of breast cancer

Breast cancer can spread directly via local invasion, through lymphatics or via the bloodstream. In some patients, regional nodal and distant metastases occur rapidly, even if the primary breast cancer is small, while in others (the majority in the current age of screening) the tumour remains apparently localised in the breast at the time of diagnosis.

Local invasion

This occurs by direct infiltration of the breast parenchyma, resulting in the characteristic stellate appearance of breast cancer. Direct invasion of the overlying skin or underlying fascia and muscle can occur but is uncommon. Local invasion of lymphatics and veins indicates a higher likelihood of lymph node involvement and a worse prognosis.

Regional spread

Lymphatic spread to axillary lymph nodes is common with breast cancer. The incidence of axillary nodal metastases is less than 20% in tumours smaller than 2 cm but is more than 50% in tumours larger than 5 cm. The involvement of a high number of nodes (four or more) is associated with a poorer prognosis. Internal mammary lymph nodes lie in the anterior intercostal spaces adjacent to the internal mammary vessels. Spread to the internal mammary nodes or supraclavicular nodes is associated with a poor prognosis.

Distant metastases

The most common sites of disease are the bone, liver and lung. Other sites include the brain, skin and peritoneum. Different subtypes of breast cancer have somewhat different patterns of distant metastasis, but bone metastasis is the most common and the most frequent initial site of distant relapse.

Staging of breast cancer

Staging is the process of classification of cancer according to prognosis. This is complex in breast cancer because of the large number of prognostic variables (Box 36.1) and the heterogeneity of the disease. The most clinically relevant staging system is the American Joint Committee on Cancer (AJCC) TNM classification, which provides an accurate and reproducible assessment and is particularly useful in clinical trials. The AJCC staging system was originally based on T (tumour), N (node) and M (metastasis) criteria, constituting the TNM classification, but this has recently been expanded to include molecular features (Box 36.2).

Staging investigations

Staging investigations are used when there is a significant chance that they would identify metastatic disease, or when the identification of metastatic disease would substantially alter treatment. In general, tests are used if there are clinical symptoms or signs suggestive of metastatic disease (bone pain, shortness of breath, etc.), when the lymph nodes are involved, or when the pathology indicates there is high risk of asymptomatic metastatic disease.

Investigations that are commonly used for breast cancer include:

- full blood examination and liver function tests
- whole body bone scan
- chest and abdominal CT scan.

Positron emission tomography is not routinely used in breast cancer. However, studies have suggested that it may have a place in the future.

Staging investigations are not recommended in situations where the chance of metastasis is very low or where the outcome would not change management, as they have significant false-positive rates and may cause considerable anxiety and follow-up investigations.

Histopathology

Pathological examination (Figures 36.1 and 36.2) is essential in confirming the diagnosis, assessing whether the lesion has been completely excised, providing prognostic information (see Box 36.1) and in determining the most appropriate adjuvant therapy (extra treatments used in the absence of known disease to reduce the risk of a subsequent recurrence).

Breast cancer may be non-invasive (*in situ*) or invasive and can be divided into a number of molecular subtypes with prognostic and treatment implications.

Ductal carcinoma *in situ*

This is a pre-invasive breast cancer and is characterised by proliferation of malignant breast epithelium that is confined to the ducts and which has not invaded through the basement membrane. The entity is often associated with microcalcification on mammography (Figure 36.3) and is usually impalpable. Since the introduction of mammographic screening, DCIS has risen from 2% of breast cancers to around 15%. This condition is premalignant and often multicentric in the breast.

While DCIS may progress to invasive cancer if untreated, not all invasive cancer has a premalignant stage, and not all cases of DCIS will progress. This means that many cases of screen-detected DCIS are examples of over-diagnosis – the

---

Box 36.1 Major prognostic determinants of breast cancer

- Axillary nodal status
- Tumour size
- Histological grade
- Hormone receptor status
- HER2 over-expression
- Ki67

Box 36.2 AJCC staging system for breast cancer

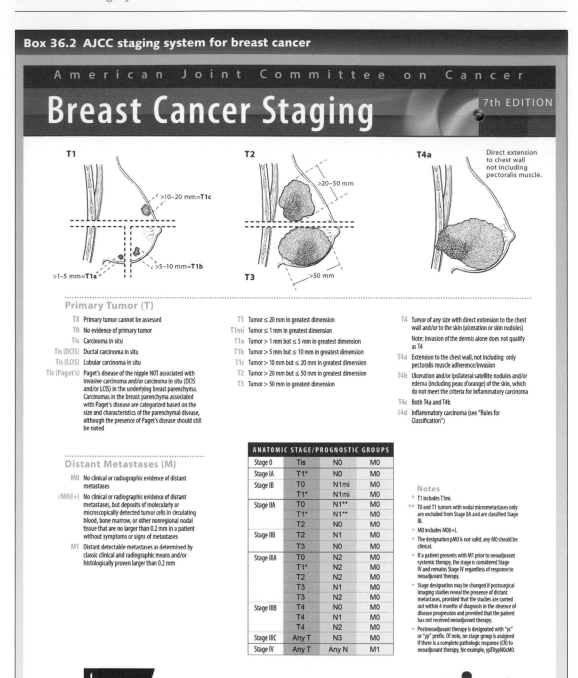

American Joint Committee on Cancer

Breast Cancer Staging

7th EDITION

T1

>10–20 mm=**T1c**

>1–5 mm=**T1a**   >5–10 mm=**T1b**

T2

>20–50 mm

T3

>50 mm

T4a

Direct extension to chest wall not including pectoralis muscle.

Primary Tumor (T)

TX   Primary tumor cannot be assessed

T0   No evidence of primary tumor

Tis   Carcinoma in situ

Tis (DCIS)   Ductal carcinoma in situ

Tis (LCIS)   Lobular carcinoma in situ

Tis (Paget's)   Paget's disease of the nipple NOT associated with invasive carcinoma and/or carcinoma in situ (DCIS and/or LCIS) in the underlying breast parenchyma. Carcinomas in the breast parenchyma associated with Paget's disease are categorized based on the size and characteristics of the parenchymal disease, although the presence of Paget's disease should still be noted

T1   Tumor ≤ 20 mm in greatest dimension

T1mi   Tumor ≤ 1 mm in greatest dimension

T1a   Tumor > 1 mm but ≤ 5 mm in greatest dimension

T1b   Tumor > 5 mm but ≤ 10 mm in greatest dimension

T1c   Tumor > 10 mm but ≤ 20 mm in greatest dimension

T2   Tumor > 20 mm but ≤ 50 mm in greatest dimension

T3   Tumor > 50 mm in greatest dimension

T4   Tumor of any size with direct extension to the chest wall and/or to the skin (ulceration or skin nodules)

Note: Invasion of the dermis alone does not qualify as T4

T4a   Extension to the chest wall, not including only pectoralis muscle adherence/invasion

T4b   Ulceration and/or ipsilateral satellite nodules and/or edema (including peau d'orange) of the skin, which do not meet the criteria for inflammatory carcinoma

T4c   Both T4a and T4b

T4d   Inflammatory carcinoma (see "Rules for Classification")

Distant Metastases (M)

M0   No clinical or radiographic evidence of distant metastases

cM0(i+)   No clinical or radiographic evidence of distant metastases, but deposits of molecularly or microscopically detected tumor cells in circulating blood, bone marrow, or other nonregional nodal tissue that are no larger than 0.2 mm in a patient without symptoms or signs of metastases

M1   Distant detectable metastases as determined by classic clinical and radiographic means and/or histologically proven larger than 0.2 mm

ANATOMIC STAGE/PROGNOSTIC GROUPS		
Stage 0	Tis	N0	M0
Stage IA	T1*	N0	M0
Stage IB	T0	N1mi	M0
	T1*	N1mi	M0
Stage IIA	T0	N1**	M0
	T1*	N1**	M0
	T2	N0	M0
Stage IIB	T2	N1	M0
	T3	N0	M0
Stage IIIA	T0	N2	M0
	T1*	N2	M0
	T2	N2	M0
	T3	N1	M0
	T3	N2	M0
Stage IIIB	T4	N0	M0
	T4	N1	M0
	T4	N2	M0
Stage IIIC	Any T	N3	M0
Stage IV	Any T	Any N	M1

Notes

*   T1 includes T1mi.

**   T0 and T1 tumors with nodal micrometastases only are excluded from Stage IIA and are classified Stage IB.

•   M0 includes M0(i+).

•   The designation pM0 is not valid; any M0 should be clinical.

•   If a patient presents with M1 prior to neoadjuvant systemic therapy, the stage is considered Stage IV and remains Stage IV regardless of response to neoadjuvant therapy.

•   Stage designation may be changed if postsurgical imaging studies reveal the presence of distant metastases, provided that the studies are carried out within 4 months of diagnosis in the absence of disease progression and provided that the patient has not received neoadjuvant therapy.

•   Postneoadjuvant therapy is designated with "yc" or "yp" prefix. Of note, no stage group is assigned if there is a complete pathologic response (CR) to neoadjuvant therapy, for example, ypT0ypN0cM0.

American Cancer Society®

Financial support for AJCC 7th Edition Staging Posters provided by the American Cancer Society

ajcc®

1 of 2

diagnosis of conditions that would never have become clinically significant – and leads to over-treatment. The same may apply to some cases of invasive cancer, and is the subject of ongoing debate around the potential harms of population screening.

Invasive ductal carcinoma

'Invasive' ductal carcinoma refers to cancer which has invaded the basement membrane of the ducts and entered the surrounding tissue. It is classified according to differentiation as grade 1, 2 or 3

American Joint Committee on Cancer

Breast Cancer Staging

7th EDITION

Regional Lymph Nodes (N)

CLINICAL

NX Regional lymph nodes cannot be assessed (for example, previously removed)

N0 No regional lymph node metastases

N1 Metastases to movable ipsilateral level I, II axillary lymph node(s)

N2 Metastases in ipsilateral level I, II axillary lymph nodes that are clinically fixed or matted; or in clinically detected* ipsilateral internal mammary nodes in the absence of clinically evident axillary lymph node metastases

N2a Metastases in ipsilateral level I, II axillary lymph nodes fixed to one another (matted) or to other structures

N2b Metastases only in clinically detected* ipsilateral internal mammary nodes and in the absence of clinically evident level I, II axillary lymph node metastases

N3 Metastases in ipsilateral infraclavicular (level III axillary) lymph node(s) with or without level I, II axillary lymph node involvement; or in clinically detected* ipsilateral internal mammary lymph node(s) with clinically evident level I, II axillary lymph node metastases; or metastases in ipsilateral supraclavicular lymph node(s) with or without axillary or internal mammary lymph node involvement

N3a Metastases in ipsilateral infraclavicular lymph node(s)

N3b Metastases in ipsilateral internal mammary lymph node(s) and axillary lymph node(s)

N3c Metastases in ipsilateral supraclavicular lymph node(s)

Notes

* "Clinically detected" is defined as detected by imaging studies (excluding lymphoscintigraphy) or by clinical examination and having characteristics highly suspicious for malignancy or a presumed pathologic macrometastasis based on fine needle aspiration biopsy with cytologic examination. Confirmation of clinically detected metastatic disease by fine needle aspiration without excision biopsy is designated with an (f) suffix, for example, cN3a(f). Excisional biopsy of a lymph node or biopsy of a sentinel node, in the absence of assignment of a pT, is classified as a clinical N, for example, cN1. Information regarding the confirmation of the nodal status will be designated in site-specific factors as clinical, fine needle aspiration, core biopsy, or sentinel lymph node biopsy. Pathologic classification (pN) is used for excision or sentinel lymph node biopsy only in conjunction with a pathologic T assignment.

PATHOLOGIC (PN)*

pNX Regional lymph nodes cannot be assessed (for example, previously removed, or not removed for pathologic study)

pN0 No regional lymph node metastasis identified histologically

Note: Isolated tumor cell clusters (ITC) are defined as small clusters of cells not greater than 0.2 mm, or single tumor cells, or a cluster of fewer than 200 cells in a single histologic cross-section. ITCs may be detected by routine histology or by immunohistochemical (IHC) methods. Nodes containing only ITCs are excluded from the total positive node count for purposes of N classification but should be included in the total number of nodes evaluated.

pN0(i−) No regional lymph node metastases histologically, negative IHC

pN0(i+) Malignant cells in regional lymph node(s) no greater than 0.2 mm (detected by H&E or IHC including ITC)

pN0(mol−) No regional lymph node metastases histologically, negative molecular findings (RT-PCR)

pN0(mol+) Positive molecular findings (RT-PCR)**, but no regional lymph node metastases detected by histology or IHC

pN1 Micrometastases; or metastases in 1–3 axillary lymph nodes; and/or in internal mammary nodes with metastases detected by sentinel lymph node biopsy but not clinically detected***

pN1mi Micrometastases (greater than 0.2 mm and/or more than 200 cells, but none greater than 2.0 mm)

pN1a Metastases in 1–3 axillary lymph nodes, at least one metastasis greater than 2.0 mm

pN1b Metastases in internal mammary nodes with micrometastases or macrometastases detected by sentinel lymph node biopsy but not clinically detected***

pN1c Metastases in 1–3 axillary lymph nodes and in internal mammary lymph nodes with micrometastases or macrometastases detected by sentinel lymph node biopsy but not clinically detected

pN2 Metastases in 4–9 axillary lymph nodes; or in clinically detected**** internal mammary lymph nodes in the absence of axillary lymph node metastases

pN2a Metastases in 4–9 axillary lymph nodes (at least one tumor deposit greater than 2.0 mm)

pN2b Metastases in clinically detected**** internal mammary lymph nodes in the absence of axillary lymph node metastases

pN3 Metastases in 10 or more axillary lymph nodes; or in infraclavicular (level III axillary) lymph nodes; or in clinically detected**** ipsilateral internal mammary lymph nodes in the presence of one or more positive level I, II axillary lymph nodes; or in more than three axillary lymph nodes and in internal mammary lymph nodes with micrometastases or macrometastases detected by sentinel lymph node biopsy but not clinically detected***; or in ipsilateral supraclavicular lymph nodes

pN3a Metastases in 10 or more axillary lymph nodes (at least one tumor deposit greater than 2.0 mm); or metastases to the infraclavicular (level III axillary lymph) nodes

pN3b Metastases in clinically detected**** ipsilateral internal mammary lymph nodes in the presence of one or more positive axillary lymph nodes; or in more than three axillary lymph nodes and in internal mammary lymph nodes with micrometastases or macrometastases detected by sentinel lymph node biopsy but not clinically detected***

pN3c Metastases in ipsilateral supraclavicular lymph nodes

Notes

* Classification is based on axillary lymph node dissection with or without sentinel lymph node biopsy. Classification based solely on sentinel lymph node biopsy without subsequent axillary lymph node dissection is designated (sn) for "sentinel node," for example, pN0(sn).

** RT-PCR: reverse transcriptase/polymerase chain reaction.

*** "Not clinically detected" is defined as not detected by imaging studies (excluding lymphoscintigraphy) or not detected by clinical examination.

**** "Clinically detected" is defined as detected by imaging studies (excluding lymphoscintigraphy) or by clinical examination and having characteristics highly suspicious for malignancy or a presumed pathologic macrometastasis based on fine needle aspiration biopsy with cytologic examination.

Supraclavicular

High axillary, apical, level III

Halsted's ligament

Mid-axillary, level II

Axillary vein

Low axillary, level I

Pectoralis minor muscle

Internal mammary

pN0(i+)
≤0.2 mm or cluster of fewer than 200 cells

pN1mi
>0.2-2 mm or more than 200 cells

pN1a: 1-3 nodes (at least one tumor deposit >2.0 mm)

pN2a: 4-9 nodes (at least one tumor deposit >2.0 mm)

pN3a: ≥10 nodes (at least one tumor deposit >2.0 mm)

American Cancer Society®

Financial support for AJCC 7th Edition Staging Posters provided by the American Cancer Society

(low, intermediate or high grade). Most invasive ductal carcinomas are of no special type, but several distinct types exist, including papillary, medullary, tubular and mucinous, and these have distinct natural histories.

Invasive lobular carcinoma

Invasive lobular carcinoma is a distinct type of breast cancer that lacks staining for the CDH protein. Classical lobular carcinoma has the histological feature of single files of malignant cells that

(a)

(b)

(c)

(d)

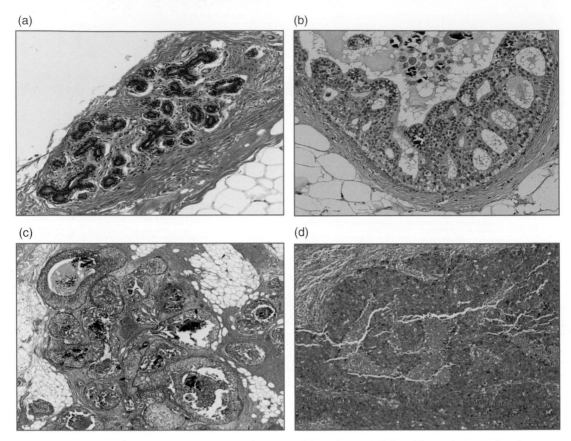

Fig. 36.1 Haematoxlin and eosin (H&E) sections of (a) normal duct, (b) atypical ductal hyperplasia, (c) ductal carcinoma *in situ* and (d) invasive breast carcinoma.

(a)

(b)

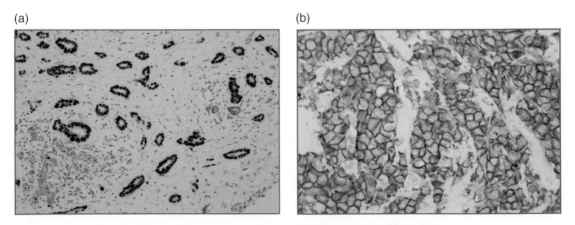

Fig. 36.2 Immunohistochemistry of (a) oestrogen-positive and (b) HER2-positive breast cancer.

diffusely infiltrate the breast tissue (Figure 36.4). It may also be difficult or impossible to see on a mammogram or ultrasound, presenting as a diffuse enlargement of part or all of the breast rather than as a discrete lump.

Molecular subtypes of breast cancer

A major change in breast cancer management has followed the recognition of a range of identifiable molecular subtypes of cancer based on RNA

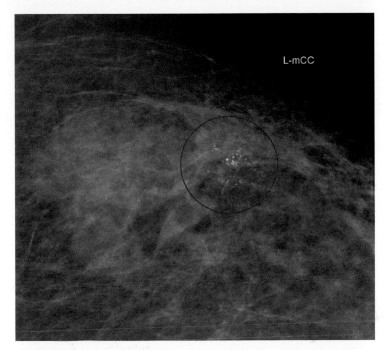

Fig. 36.3 Mammogram showing typical calcification seen in extensive ductal carcinoma *in situ*.

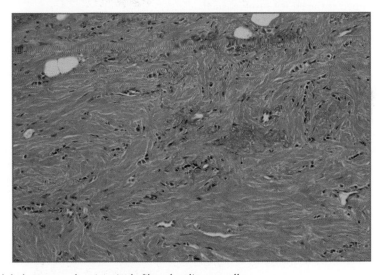

Fig. 36.4 Invasive lobular cancer showing single files of malignant cells.

expression microarrays. Studies have shown that breast cancer can be largely divided into four distinct types based on the patterns of altered gene expression. Various subdivisions of these subtypes is also possible. The different types have different prognoses and treatments. While genetic profiling is not widely practised at present, histological findings and immunohistochemistry provide a cost-effective method of identifying subtypes for treatment purposes. Tumours are classified based on the expression

of oestrogen and progesterone receptors, levels of human epidermal growth factor receptor (HER2), grade and markers of cellular proliferation (Ki67).

Luminal A

Luminal A breast cancer is oestrogen-receptor and progesterone-receptor positive, HER2 negative, and has low Ki-67. It is usually lower grade and proliferates slowly, and has the best prognosis.

Luminal B

Luminal B breast cancer is oestrogen-receptor positive, progesterone-receptor low or negative, HER2 positive/negative with high levels of Ki-67. It is generally higher grade. Luminal B cancers usually grow faster than luminal A cancers and their prognosis is worse.

Triple-negative/basal-like

This cancer is oestrogen-receptor, progesterone-receptor and HER2 negative. It is usually high grade, rapidly proliferative and with a relatively poor prognosis. This type of cancer is more commonly seen in women with *BRCA1* gene mutations.

HER2-enriched

This breast cancer is oestrogen-receptor and progesterone-receptor negative and HER2 positive. It proliferates faster than luminal cancers and though without treatment they have a poor prognosis, they are often successfully treated with targeted therapies aimed at the HER2 protein, such as trastuzumab (Herceptin).

Treatment of breast cancer

The management of breast cancer involves an evidence-based and multidisciplinary approach involving surgeons, radiologists, radiation oncologists, medical oncologists, pathologists and breast care nurses. Management decisions are usually made in a multidisciplinary team meeting, often both before and after surgery. Patient education, counselling and informed consent play an increasing role, and patients may require psychological support, often provided by psychologists specialising in treating those with cancer.

Breast cancer surgery

Until the 1980s, surgery for breast cancer involved total mastectomy and removal of the axillary lymph nodes. A series of randomised trials demonstrated that such radical surgery is not necessary, with similar results being achieved with much less extensive surgery. Breast cancer surgery still involves surgery on both the breast and the draining lymph nodes, and these two components can be considered separately.

Breast conservation surgery

Randomised trials from the 1980s confirmed that breast-conserving surgery, involving complete local excision of the primary breast tumour with a rim of macroscopically and microscopically normal breast tissue on all sides, followed by adjuvant whole-breast radiotherapy, results in equivalent cure rates to total mastectomy. Breast-conserving surgery may be referred to as 'wide local excision', 'lumpectomy' or 'partial mastectomy'. Surgical techniques to improve cosmesis after breast-conserving surgery have allowed more patients to choose breast conservation and to expect improved cosmetic outcomes. Breast conservation surgery is usually followed by radiotherapy to reduce the rate of local recurrence.

Breast conservation surgery and radiotherapy is the standard procedure for patients with breast cancer and is performed on around 70% of all patients. In addition to equivalent survival rates, the cosmetic and psychological results are generally superior to those of mastectomy.

Total mastectomy

This involves complete excision of the breast and nipple with preservation of the underlying pectoral muscles. This is recommended for:
- a cancer that is large relative to the size of the breast
- cancer that involves the nipple or overlying skin (breast conservation surgery might still be possible in selected cases)
- multifocal disease or extensive intraductal carcinoma (DCIS) involving the surgical margins
- those having had prior breast irradiation
- women who harbour a genetic mutation such as *BRCA1* or *BRCA2* who elect to have mastectomy to minimise the risk of further cancers
- women who choose not to have breast conservation.

It is important that the decision for either breast-conserving treatment or total mastectomy is an informed decision by the woman. A minority of fully informed women choose to have total mastectomy, and this is a legitimate decision.

Breast reconstruction

Breast reconstruction should be offered to most women after a total mastectomy. This may be immediate (at the same time as mastectomy) or delayed (after treatment is complete). Reconstruction may be implant-based or autologous (using the patient's own tissue). Autologous options include pedicled flaps, such as the latissimus dorsi flap, and free flaps using microvascular techniques, such as the deep inferior epigastric perforator flap that uses fat and skin from the lower abdomen to reconstruct the breast. There is a significant psychological benefit to immediate reconstruction for many patients, with no evidence to suggest that it worsens oncological outcomes.

Lymph node surgery

For most of the twentieth century, standard surgery for breast cancer included removal of all the axillary lymph nodes – an 'axillary clearance' or 'axillary dissection' – as this is where breast cancer is most likely to be found beyond the breast. The operation effectively removes the lymph nodes, but is associated with substantial morbidity in the form of shoulder dysfunction, numbness and par-aesthesia, and potential lymphoedema of the arm and breast.

Sentinel node biopsy

As the size of cancers became smaller due to population screening, the incidence of nodal involvement reduced, and techniques were developed to identify the key lymph node(s) that receive primary drainage from the cancer, the so-called sentinel node. The sentinel node is usually found in the lower part of the axilla, just deep to the pectoralis major muscle, and is identified via injection of a radioactive colloid and a blue dye. This node is removed in an operation called sentinel node biopsy; if found to be clear of cancer, the likelihood that any other lymph node is involved is very small and further surgery can be safely omitted.

Axillary dissection

Axillary dissection is now reserved for those patients with proven axillary metastatic disease, via either preoperative fine-needle aspiration of suspicious lymph nodes or at sentinel node biopsy. It involves removal of the fatty tissue that lies in the area bounded by the pectoralis major and latissimus dorsi muscles, the lateral chest wall, and the axillary and subclavian veins. This tissue contains somewhere between 10 and 25 lymph nodes, as well as lymphatics and cutaneous nerves.

Adjuvant therapy

Adjuvant therapy refers to anticancer treatments given in the absence of known disease to reduce the chance of disease recurrence. It was first used in breast cancer in the 1980s, and has led to dramatic improvements in outcomes. Adjuvant radiotherapy is used to reduce the risk of residual disease in the breast or regional lymph nodes, while adjuvant systemic therapies are used to reduce the risk of distant recurrence.

Adjuvant radiotherapy

Radiation therapy uses high intensity X-rays as cancer treatment. It takes advantage of the fact that cancer cells tend to be more sensitive to X-rays than normal tissue, so that if radiation is carefully delivered, it can kill cancer cells without significant damage to normal tissue. In breast cancer, it is given as an adjuvant therapy after breast-conserving surgery or sometimes after mastectomy. After breast-conserving surgery for invasive disease it is standard treatment, although some low-risk sub-groups may not benefit. After breast conservation for DCIS it is usually considered, but often not given. After mastectomy for invasive disease, it is recommended when four or more lymph nodes are involved, and considered in cases with less nodal involvement but higher-risk disease. It also has a role in metastatic disease, especially in the bone or brain (this is termed palliative, rather than adjuvant, radiotherapy).

Complications of radiotherapy
The complications following radiotherapy vary with the total dose, the number of fractions and the arrangement of the radiation fields. Recent improvements in delivery techniques have significantly reduced the complications.

Local effects occur in the first 2–6 weeks and include redness, swelling and pain, sometimes with blistering and ulceration of the skin. Discomfort and swelling of the breast occur early and often persist for a number of years. Rib pain and tenderness is common and can be persistent. Lymphoedema of the arm occurs in a small but significant number of patients following surgery and radiotherapy to the axilla.

Cardiac damage particularly in patients with left breast tumours is reported, although modern techniques reduce this. Similarly, radiation-induced cancers occur but are infrequent, and the benefits from radiotherapy usually outweigh the risks.

Adjuvant systemic therapy

Systemic therapy is therapy delivered to treat the whole body. The aim of this is to eradicate micro-metastases in order to ultimately improve survival. Routine use of effective adjuvant systemic therapy has been responsible for a large proportion of the improved outcomes for breast cancer over recent decades. It is used primarily to reduce the risk of distant metastasis and death, but has also been shown to reduce the risk of local recurrence and endocrine therapy has been shown to reduce the risk of new primary breast cancers.

In general, it is recommended that patients with oestrogen receptor-positive cancer receive endocrine treatment, those with receptor-negative cancer chemotherapy, and those with HER2-positive cancer Herceptin and chemotherapy. The most difficult issue is which patients with oestrogen receptor-positive, HER2-negative cancer should receive chemotherapy in addition to endocrine therapy. Several online predictive tools are available when discussing the potential benefit of chemotherapy for an individual patient (e.g. PREDICT in the UK), as well as a number of commercial molecular tests.

Neoadjuvant chemotherapy

Traditionally, treatment of early breast cancer has involved initial surgery, followed by adjuvant therapies of various types to reduce the risk of recurrence. On the basis that adjuvant therapies were targeting the micrometastatic disease that may be destined to cause recurrence, trials were done where chemotherapy was given prior to surgery, so-called neoadjuvant chemotherapy. The hypothesis was that earlier treatment of micrometastatic systemic disease would lead to improved survival. This has not been proven, but it was found that many cases where primary surgery would have involved mastectomy were able to be treated successfully with breast conservation. It was also shown that the response to neoadjuvant chemotherapy was a powerful prognostic factor: those who experienced a so-called pathological complete response (i.e. no residual cancer found at surgery after neoadjuvant chemotherapy) had a far better prognosis than those who did not.

Neoadjuvant chemotherapy is currently considered for large and extensive node-positive cancer, especially those subtypes most likely to be sensitive to chemotherapy, such as the HER-enriched and the triple negative subtypes.

Types of endocrine therapy

Tamoxifen

Tamoxifen was the first widely used endocrine therapy. Five years of tamoxifen reduces the risk of death by around one-third in women with oestrogen receptor-positive tumours. It also reduces the risk of cancer in the contralateral breast, and is also used as chemoprevention. For many years, 5 years of treatment was considered optimal, but recent evidence has shown that extending treatment to 10 years reduces the risk of late recurrences (those occurring between 10 and 15 years). Decisions regarding duration of therapy are a matter of balancing likely benefits with the side effects and potential risks.

Side effects of tamoxifen include hot flushes, vaginal discharge and an increased incidence of endometrial cancer and deep vein thrombosis. This endometrial cancer risk is increased twofold to threefold but still remains low, at less than 1% per year for a 5-year treatment duration, and is generally far outweighed by its beneficial effect. Abnormal vaginal bleeding should be promptly investigated.

Aromatase inhibitors

Whereas in the premenopausal woman, the majority of oestrogen is produced from the ovaries, in the postmenopausal woman this occurs in peripheral fat, muscle and liver. This is facilitated by the enzyme aromatase, which converts androgens into oestrogens by a process called aromatisation. Aromatase inhibitors thus reduce circulating oestrogen levels in postmenopausal women.

Several trials have demonstrated that aromatase inhibitors (anastrozole, letrozole and exemestane) are more effective at reducing the incidence of breast cancer recurrence compared with tamoxifen in postmenopausal women. The side-effect profile of aromatase inhibitors is different to that of tamoxifen, and involves hot flushes and other menopausal symptoms (similar to tamoxifen) but also musculoskeletal symptoms, with arthralgia and myalgias. Reduced oestrogen levels can cause significant gynaecological and urinary side effects with vaginal dryness and urinary incontinence, as well as reduced bone mineral density.

Ovarian function suppression

Ovarian function suppression (OFS) in premenopausal women is associated with improvement in breast cancer outcomes in higher-risk patients. This has been used in trials that show that in lower-risk patients, OFS can be used in place of cytotoxic chemotherapy, while in high-risk patients it can be used in addition to chemotherapy. OFS can be followed with aromatase inhibitors, which are somewhat more effective than tamoxifen, but this combination can lead to significant impacts on the quality of life of a young woman and the balance of effectiveness and side effects can be difficult to achieve.

Supportive care

The manner in which the diagnosis of breast cancer is communicated may have an important impact on the woman's ability to cope with the diagnosis and treatment. There are individual differences in women's views about and need for information, options and support.

Women with breast cancer and their families will need further counselling to allow assimilation of information and should be given repeated opportunities to ask questions. Women with good emotional support from family and friends tend to adjust better to having breast cancer. Doctors, nurses, breast cancer support services and other allied health professionals are all important sources of support.

Follow-up after treatment of early breast cancer

With the multidisciplinary approach in the care for breast cancer, it is important that follow-up is coordinated so that patients are not subjected to an excessive number of visits. The rationale of follow-up is outlined in the following sections. The patient's GP is a key member of the multidisciplinary team, and can safely provide much of the follow-up care in partnership with the hospital-based team.

Detection of local recurrence

The local recurrence rate after breast conservation surgery and radiotherapy or total mastectomy is low. Overall the 5-year rate is below 5%, although late recurrences are possible many years after diagnosis. Most local recurrences are detected on surveillance imaging, although some present as lumps after breast-conserving treatment or mastectomy.

Detection of distant recurrence

The most common sites for distant metastatic disease are the bones, the lungs and the liver. These present with new or different bone or joint pain that does not settle spontaneously; shortness of breath, chest pain or cough; loss of weight or abdominal pain. Brain metastasis can occur, presenting with headache or neurological symptoms.

Follow-up imaging with CT or bone scans in the absence of symptoms is not recommended, as early diagnosis of asymptomatic metastases confers no advantage to the patient. Thus investigations are reserved for those with worrying symptoms.

Breast cancer tends to be slow-growing and may recur many years after apparently successful treatment. Metastatic spread is defined as spread beyond the breast and ipsilateral axillary and/or internal mammary lymph nodes, and is deemed incurable.

Screening for a new breast primary

The risk of a new contralateral breast primary cancer is about 0.5% per year. Annual mammography is recommended, sometimes with ultrasound as well.

Management of treatment-associated toxicities

These include problems after axillary dissection (shoulder stiffness or lymphoedema) or adjuvant radiotherapy (breast and chest-wall pain and tenderness). Women taking tamoxifen or an aromatase inhibitor may have menopausal symptoms, joint pains or gynaecological symptoms that should be addressed. Women on aromatase inhibitors should have their bone density checked and low bone density should be managed.

Psychosocial support

Anxiety and depression are common following diagnosis and treatment. This should be acknowledged. Sometimes referral to a psychologist is appropriate.

Acknowledgement

The authors wish to thank Dr Anand Murugasu, Consultant Histopathologist, Royal Melbourne for assistance with figures 36.1, 36.2 and 36.4 and Dr Alexandria Taylor, Consultant Radiologist, Royal Melbourne Hospital for assistance with figure 36.3.

Further reading

Australian Government, Department of Health. BreastScreen Australia Evaluation Final Report. http://www.cancerscreening.gov.au/internet/screening/publishing.nsf/Content/programme-evaluation

Australian Government, Cancer Australia. https://breast-cancer.canceraustralia.gov.au/treatment/surgery

Dixon JM (ed.) *ABC of Breast Diseases*, 4th edn. Oxford: Wiley Blackwell, 2012.

Dixon JM (ed.) *Breast Surgery. A Companion to Surgical Practice*, 6th edn. Edinburgh: Elsevier, 2018.

MCQs

Select the single correct answer to each question. The correct answers can be found in the Answers section at the end of the book.

1 A 51-year-old woman undergoes a wide local excision and sentinel node biopsy for a 15-mm grade 2 invasive duct cancer, margins clear, nodes negative, oestrogen receptor positive, HER2 positive (amplified). What adjuvant therapy should she be offered?
   a radiotherapy only
   b radiotherapy and endocrine therapy
   c radiotherapy, chemotherapy, targeted anti-HER2 therapy and endocrine therapy
   d chemotherapy, radiotherapy and endocrine therapy
   e chemotherapy only

2 A 39-year-old woman has a 5-cm, grade III breast cancer. Twelve of 16 lymph nodes contain metastases. The oestrogen and progesterone receptor is negative, and the HER2 is negative (non-amplified). There is no evidence of systemic metastases on CT and bone scan. Following a total mastectomy and axillary clearance, the *most likely* follow-up management would be:
   a regular review, with reservation of chemotherapy for recurrent disease
   b adjuvant tamoxifen
   c adjuvant chemotherapy alone
   d adjuvant chemotherapy and post-mastectomy radiotherapy
   e oophorectomy

3 Which of the following statements concerning ductal carcinoma *in situ* (DCIS) is correct?
   a it is usually associated with microcalcification on mammography
   b DCIS is less commonly found in women undergoing routine mammographic screening
   c all DCIS will eventually progress to invasive cancer
   d there is a high risk for lymph node metastasis with the papillary subtype
   e the risk for progression to invasive cancer is smaller than with lobular carcinoma *in situ*

4 Which of the following statements about breast cancer screening is *not* correct?
   a screening has been shown to improve survival
   b screening detects breast cancer at an early stage
   c women are invited to participate from the ages of 50 to 75
   d uptake of screening in Australia is >90%
   e the majority of abnormalities detected on screening mammography are benign

Section 6
Endocrine Surgery

37 Thyroid

Jonathan Serpell

Monash University and Breast, Endocrine and General Surgery Unit, Alfred Health, Melbourne, Victoria, Australia

Introduction

The thyroid gland lies in the anterior triangle of the neck. The thyroid comprises two lateral lobes, an isthmus and a pyramid, schematically represented as a bilobed shield. The function of the follicular cells is to produce, store and release the thyroid hormones thyroxine (T4) and triiodothyronine (T3). The function of the C-cells is to produce the calcium-lowering hormone calcitonin.

Diseases affecting the thyroid gland can generally be grouped into disorders of thyroid function (including hypothyroidism and thyrotoxicosis) or disorders affecting thyroid structure (including nodular goitre and thyroid neoplasms). Disorders of both function and structure may coexist. A goitre refers to enlargement of the thyroid and is a term applicable regardless of the cause of the enlargement. However, from the surgical point of view, a classification of thyroid disease can be considered as comprising the following groups:
- Thyroglossal duct cyst
- Benign thyroid nodules
- Multinodular goitre
- Thyroid cancer
- Thyrotoxicosis
- Thyroiditis.

Disorders of the thyroid gland

Thyroglossal duct cyst

Pathology

Thyroid follicular cells arise from the region of the foramen caecum at the junction of the anterior two-thirds and posterior one-third of the tongue, and during embryological development the gland descends in the midline to the level of the larynx, where it buds laterally. A contribution of neural crest cells arising from the fourth branchial cleft and the ultimobranchial body gives rise to the C-cells of the thyroid as well as to a small projection from the posterolateral surface (the tubercle of Zuckerkandl). As the thyroid gland descends during embryological development, remnants of thyroid tissue may be left behind anywhere along the thyroglossal tract. Occasionally some respiratory epithelium may be included in the remnant, resulting in a thyroglossal duct cyst. A non-cystic benign thyroid nodule, or even thyroid cancer, may also develop anywhere along the tract. Embryological descent may also continue into the anterior mediastinum, giving rise to a thyrothymic thyroid remnant. The junction of the thyroglossal duct tract and the isthmus of the thyroid gland marks the site of the pyramid, a variable-sized projection superiorly of thyroid tissue.

Clinical presentation

Thyroglossal duct cysts usually present in childhood or adolescence but may occur at any age. However, in older patients the possibility of papillary thyroid cancer in a developmental remnant should be considered as an alternative diagnosis to a *de novo* thyroglossal duct cyst. The usual clinical presentation is that of a midline swelling at or just below the level of the hyoid bone, often slightly to one side of the midline. Classically, the swelling elevates with protrusion of the tongue. Inflammation may give rise to an abscess or a fistula.

Investigations

The diagnosis of a thyroglossal duct cyst is usually self-evident on clinical examination. Fine-needle aspiration cytology (FNAC) will confirm the nature of the cyst contents, although this may precipitate inflammation. Cytology will often show colloid,

Textbook of Surgery, Fourth Edition. Edited by Julian A. Smith, Andrew H. Kaye, Christopher Christophi and Wendy A. Brown.
© 2020 John Wiley & Sons Ltd. Published 2020 by John Wiley & Sons Ltd.

cholesterol crystals and benign epithelial cells. Aspiration may be therapeutic as well as diagnostic, with resolution of the cyst. FNAC is important for excluding the uncommon papillary thyroid cancer arising in a thyroglossal duct cyst. Neck ultrasound to confirm the presence of a normal thyroid gland and thyroid function should be undertaken.

Treatment

Treatment is surgical excision through a skin-crease incision. The cyst and the thyroglossal tract must be removed, which involves excision of the mid-portion of the hyoid bone and tracing of the tract to its upper limit. Failure to remove the full extent of the tract will result in recurrence of the cyst or a discharging sinus.

Benign thyroid nodules

Pathology

Between 30 and 40% of clinically solitary thyroid nodules will represent a dominant nodule within an underlying multinodular goitre. Of the remainder, the majority will be benign nodules, comprising simple thyroid cysts, solitary colloid nodules or benign follicular adenoma. Approximately 7% will be a thyroid cancer and a further small group will represent an area of nodularity within thyroiditis (both Hashimoto's and subacute). Apart from rare developmental inclusion thyroid cysts, the majority of thyroid cysts form following haemorrhage into an underlying benign thyroid nodule, which then matures into a thyroid mass consisting of a rim of thyroid tissue and a central liquefied area. Colloid nodules and hyperplastic nodules should be considered part of a similar pathological spectrum.

Clinical presentation

The most common presentation of a single thyroid nodule is that of an asymptomatic swelling in the neck. The characteristic clinical feature of a thyroid nodule is that it elevates on swallowing because the thyroid is enveloped by the pretracheal fascia which attaches to the trachea. This will distinguish a thyroid nodule from a lymph node swelling adjacent to the thyroid which does not elevate on swallowing. Benign thyroid nodules may also present with local pressure symptoms. These include dysphagia from oesophageal pressure, breathlessness or stridor from tracheal pressure, a hoarse voice from pressure on the recurrent laryngeal nerve, or superior vena cava (SVC) obstruction from a large single nodule obstructing the thoracic inlet. A toxic nodule will present with symptoms of thyrotoxicosis. Regional lymphadenopathy should always be sought.

Increasingly thyroid nodules, which may or may not be palpable, are identified incidentally on imaging such as ultrasound, CT, MRI or positron emission tomography undertaken for investigation of other symptoms, for example neck pain and carotid artery studies.

Investigations

Thyroid function tests, including thyroid-stimulating hormone (TSH), free T4 and free T3, should be performed in all patients to exclude subclinical thyrotoxicosis (suppressed TSH will be seen in association with normal free T4 and free T3 levels) or to diagnose a toxic nodule or toxic adenoma.

Ultrasound is routinely performed to establish underlying multinodularity and to characterise the features of the nodule. Features raising an element of suspicion as to the nature of the nodule include solid as opposed to cystic, internal vascularity as opposed to peripheral vascularity, microcalcification, dimensions taller than wide, and irregularity of outline. Further, abnormal lymph nodes may be identified by ultrasound.

FNAC is the definitive investigation, and the possible cytological reports are categorised in Table 37.1. This Bethesda classification is widely used worldwide. FNAC should only be undertaken after exclusion of thyrotoxicosis, as a toxic adenoma

Table 37.1 Bethesda system and cytology diagnostic categories for thyroid cancer.

	Bethesda diagnostic criteria	Risk of malignancy	Recommendations
I	Non-diagnostic/unsatisfactory	1–4%	Repeat fine-needle aspiration
II	Benign	0–3%	Surveillance
III	Atypia or follicular lesion of undetermined significance	5–15%	Surveillance or surgery
IV	Follicular neoplasm or suspected follicular neoplasm	15–30%	Surveillance or surgery
V	Suspicious for malignancy	60–75%	Surgery
VI	Malignant	97–99%	Surgery

may appear concerning on cytology. Further, toxic adenomas are almost always benign. It is important to note that cytology may suggest a follicular neoplasm but cannot differentiate between a benign follicular adenoma and a follicular carcinoma. This diagnosis can only be made by the finding of either capsular or vascular invasion on histology, hence the need for diagnostic hemithyroidectomy in these patients. The likelihood of a follicular lesion on cytology being malignant is up to 30%. FNAC is best performed with ultrasound guidance in order to target the most appropriate part of the nodule and to ensure the nodule of concern is biopsied. An inadequate or non-diagnostic aspirate is not a benign result and should be repeated, as up to 10% of these will be malignant. The exception here is a thyroid cyst on clinical and ultrasound features, where FNAC shows colloid, cyst fluid and degenerate cells only, and where overall the features are consistent with a thyroid cyst, although strictly there is no epithelial material to diagnose a benign thyroid nodule. FNAC may be therapeutic as well as diagnostic for thyroid cysts, and repeated aspiration will result in resolution in at least 50% of cases. FNAC may also show features of thyroiditis, alone or in combination with other cytology. Hashimoto's will show lymphocytes and subacute thyroiditis may show inflammatory cells and giant cells.

The role of nuclear medicine scans is limited to the investigation of patients with thyrotoxicosis or thyroiditis.

Treatment

Asymptomatic thyroid nodules that are benign on FNAC do not generally require treatment. However, follow-up, at least in the short term, is appropriate. Indications for surgery include the presence of obstructive symptoms, thyrotoxicosis, or the finding of malignancy, suspicion of malignancy or atypical or follicular changes on FNAC, and on patient request. The minimal surgical procedure is a hemithyroidectomy, removing all thyroid tissue on the side of the lesion (including isthmus and pyramidal lobe). Thyroxine suppression is ineffective in decreasing the size of single thyroid nodules.

Multinodular goitre

Pathology

Multinodular goitre occurs as the result of repeated cycles of hyperplasia, nodule formation, degeneration and fibrosis occurring throughout the gland. It occurs either in response to iodine deficiency or, in iodine-replete areas, as a result of the intrinsic heterogeneity of TSH receptors. The latter has a high familial incidence. A dominant nodule within a multinodular goitre is most likely to be either a hyperplastic or colloid nodule. However, the incidence of malignancy in a dominant nodule is approximately the same as for a single nodule (7%). Hence, multinodular goitre has a high familial incidence, and is also common in areas where iodine is deficient in the diet.

Clinical presentation

Most multinodular goitres present as an asymptomatic mass in the neck. They may also present with local pressure symptoms to the trachea, oesophagus, recurrent laryngeal nerve or SVC. Clinical retrosternal extension and Pemberton's sign should be assessed, and lymphadenopathy sought. Thyrotoxicosis complicating the goitre is also common, especially in the elderly with large goitres. An otherwise asymptomatic retrosternal multinodular goitre may present incidentally as a mass on a chest X-ray or CT scan.

Investigations

Thyroid function tests, as previously outlined, must be performed on all patients. Ultrasound will document the size of the thyroid lobes and the number and size of nodules, providing a baseline for follow-up, and will also indicate which nodules require FNAC. FNAC of a dominant nodule or nodules aims to exclude malignancy and a CT scan (without intravenous contrast) will assess retrosternal extension or tracheal compression and deviation. Intravenous contrast is avoided because of its iodine content and the possibility it may precipitate iodine-induced thyrotoxicosis. A thyroid nuclear medicine scan is used in a multinodular goitre to assess for a solitary toxic nodule or multiple areas of variable activity.

Treatment

Indications for surgical treatment of a multinodular goitre include the presence of obstructive symptoms, growth of the goitre, thyrotoxicosis, suspicious or malignant changes on FNAC, a strong family history of thyroid cancer, the presence of retrosternal extension, a past history of head and neck irradiation (which increases the risk of malignancy) and patient request. In a young patient with a large multinodular goitre, who is otherwise asymptomatic, thyroidectomy may also be considered for cosmetic reasons. The only effective treatment is surgical excision. If surgery is undertaken, total thyroidectomy is the preferred option, because it removes all tissue likely to cause symptoms and avoids the possibility of later recurrence (which occurs in about 30%). Lifelong thyroxine replacement is required after total thyroidectomy.

Thyroid cancer

Pathology

Thyroid cancer can arise from the follicular cells, the C-cells, or other cells such as lymphocytes or stromal cells, each giving rise to a different form of thyroid cancer. Papillary thyroid cancer (PTC) accounts for about 85% of thyroid cancers, tends to occur in a younger age group (20–40 years), is often multifocal, spreads predominantly to local lymph nodes and has a relatively good prognosis, with 10-year survival rates of at least 90%. Follicular cancer occurs in an older age group (40–60 years), arises as a single tumour, metastasises via the bloodstream and has a worse prognosis than papillary cancer, with 10-year survival rates around 75%. Together, papillary and follicular thyroid cancers are considered differentiated thyroid cancer, and account for the majority of thyroid cancer resulting in the usual overall good prognosis. The incidence of PTC is increasing worldwide at an exponential rate, particularly for tumours less than 4 cm in diameter. Further, there is an increasing recognition of micropapillary thyroid cancer (<1 cm), which is often an incidental pathological finding in a goitre removed for other reasons, usually multinodular goitre. Anaplastic, or undifferentiated, thyroid cancer occurs in the elderly, often presents as a rapidly enlarging diffuse mass, spreads locally and has a very poor prognosis, with 5-year survival rates of less than 1% but is fortunately very rare. Malignancy arising in C-cells gives rise to medullary carcinoma of the thyroid. This tumour secretes calcitonin and may be part of a familial multiple endocrine neoplasia (MEN 2A) syndrome, occurring in association with phaeochromocytoma and hyperparathyroidism. The 10-year survival rate is around 35%. Lymphoma of the thyroid is thought to arise in lymphocytes, often in association with pre-existing Hashimoto's thyroiditis. Follicular-derived thyroid cancer has an association with previous exposure to ionising radiation.

Clinical presentation

Thyroid cancer commonly presents as either a single thyroid nodule or a dominant nodule in a multinodular goitre. It occasionally presents as a metastasis as an abnormal lateral lymph node in the neck, hence the need to undertake FNAC on all abnormal lymph nodes prior to removal. Thyroid cancer may also rarely present as distant metastatic disease, such as bony metastases from follicular cancer, or lymphangitic lung involvement from papillary cancer.

Investigation

Thyroid function tests and neck ultrasound will assess the nodule and possible abnormal lymph nodes. Depending on the presentation, the most useful investigation is FNAC, but CT is of value in determining extent of tumour and lymph node involvement. Serum calcitonin levels may be raised in medullary tumours.

Treatment

Most differentiated thyroid cancer is still treated by total thyroidectomy, with local removal of involved lymph nodes. Following removal of the tumour, patients are classified into those with low-, intermediate- or high-risk tumours on the basis of age, tumour size, lymph node involvement, extrathyroidal extension and distant metastases (Box 37.1).

Subsequent treatment may involve the administration of radioactive iodine (^{131}I) for moderate or higher risk cancers, which allows for both the detection and ablation of metastatic disease. Following total thyroidectomy, thyroxine replacement is required lifelong, and for higher-risk cancers is given in a larger dose to suppress TSH. Low-risk papillary cancer may include young patients, with

---

Box 37.1 Classification of tumours

High risk
Gross extrathyroidal extension, incomplete tumour resection, distance metastases or lymph node >3 cm

Intermediate risk
Aggressive histology, minor extrathyroidal extension, vascular invasion, or more than five involved lymph nodes (0.2–3 cm)

Low risk
Intrathyroidal differentiated thyroid cancer with five or less lymph node micrometastases (<0.2 cm)

tumours less than 4 cm in diameter and with absent extrathyroidal extension or lymph node or distant metastases. In this setting, consideration for treatment by hemithyroidectomy alone is appropriate, although total thyroidectomy is considered an equally appropriate treatment option. For tumours of less than 1 cm (micropapillary PTC) with no other risk factors, hemithyroidectomy alone is considered adequate treatment.

Close follow-up is essential, and further surgery for lymph node recurrences and use of radioiodine usually results in a good prognosis. Newer agents such as tyrosine kinase inhibitors are available for widespread disease, although rarely required.

Medullary thyroid cancer requires total thyroidectomy and a central lymph node dissection, with lateral neck dissection and mediastinal clearance for node-positive patients. Medullary carcinoma does not respond to radioiodine ablation.

Thyroid lymphoma is best diagnosed by multiple core biopsies or occasionally an open incisional biopsy. It is then usually treated by chemotherapy and occasionally radiotherapy. It often responds well to these treatments.

Thyrotoxicosis

Pathology

The causes of thyrotoxicosis include Graves' disease, toxic multinodular goitre (Plummer's disease), toxic follicular adenoma or in the initial stages of thyroiditis (may occur in both Hashimoto's and subacute). Rare causes include a TSH-secreting pituitary tumour or struma ovarii. Graves' disease is an autoimmune condition associated with antibodies to the TSH receptor. Toxic nodular goitre results from autonomous activity in a neoplastic nodule.

Clinical presentation

Thyrotoxicosis presents with symptoms and signs of thyroid overactivity, including tachycardia, heat intolerance, sweating, fine tremor, weight loss and anxiety. In addition, Graves' disease may be associated with exophthalmos, ophthalmoplegia and pretibial myxoedema. Graves' disease typically produces a smooth diffuse goitre, which because of significant blood flow may exhibit a palpable thrill and bruit. Toxic nodules may also present with local pressure or obstruction.

Investigation

The diagnosis of thyrotoxicosis will be confirmed by thyroid function tests, with an elevated free T4 and/or free T3 in association with a suppressed TSH. Clinical examination may indicate the aetiology, demonstrating a diffuse goitre, a multinodular goitre or a single thyroid nodule. Thyroid nuclear scans will confirm the diagnosis (increased activity), as well as the aetiology, and exclude factitious thyrotoxicosis and thyroiditis (absent or reduced activity, respectively). Anti-TSH receptor antibodies are present in Graves' disease and are quantified as a measure of severity and response to medical treatment.

Treatment

Initial treatment is to render the patient euthyroid by administration of antithyroid medications such as carbimazole or propylthiouracil, both of which prevent coupling of iodotyrosine. Patients with Graves' disease are generally treated with medication for 12–18 months. Definitive treatments for Graves' disease include ablation with radioactive iodine, usually reserved for patients over 40 years of age because of the theoretical teratogenic risk, or total thyroidectomy. Graves' disease is treated by surgery if there is relapse following initial medical treatment (about 50% of the time) or non-compliance with such treatment, or if ophthalmopathy is present, in which case radioiodine ablation is contraindicated (as radioiodine may induce worsening ophthalmopathy). Toxic multinodular goitre and toxic adenoma are best treated surgically once the patient is rendered euthyroid by antithyroid medication in order to treat the thyrotoxicosis and remove the goitre.

Thyroiditis

Pathology

Thyroiditis is classified as lymphocytic (Hashimoto's), subacute (de Quervain's), acute (bacterial) or fibrosing (Reidel's). Of these, the two most common are lymphocytic, which is an autoimmune condition often forming part of a spectrum with Graves' disease, and subacute, which is a post-viral phenomenon. The other two are rare.

Clinical presentation

Lymphocytic thyroiditis may present with hyperthyroidism (early phase) or hypothyroidism (late phase), or it may present with a nodular or diffuse goitre. Subacute thyroiditis usually presents with an exquisitely tender, enlarged, firm thyroid gland, with nodularity, often with systemic symptoms of headache, malaise and weight loss. The history is relatively short, usually of several weeks' duration, and the nodularity may sequentially involve different areas of the thyroid. Initial thyrotoxicosis may also be present.

Investigation

Thyroid function tests will determine the level of thyroid activity. A nuclear medicine scan is often diagnostic, showing patchy uptake in lymphocytic thyroiditis and no uptake at all in subacute thyroiditis. The inflammatory markers erythrocyte sedimentation rate (ESR) and C-reactive protein (CRP) will be elevated in subacute thyroiditis but not Hashimoto's. Anti-peroxidase and anti-thyroglobulin antibodies will be elevated in Hashimoto's but not subacute thyroiditis.

Treatment

Subacute thyroiditis usually responds to high-dose steroids and aspirin therapy, although it may take 3–6 months to fully resolve. Lymphocytic thyroiditis may respond to thyroxine suppression. Surgery may be required for lymphocytic thyroiditis with persistent or suspicious nodules, or for pressure symptoms, although surgery may be more difficult because of the solid non-pliable nature of the gland.

Operative management: thyroidectomy

Indications

Thyroidectomy is indicated for relief of local pressure symptoms, for the diagnosis and treatment of thyroid cancer, for the control of thyrotoxicosis or for cosmetic considerations. As previously outlined, thyroidectomy may be total or partial (hemithyroidectomy).

Complications of thyroidectomy

The complications of thyroidectomy include all the general complications of any operation, such as bleeding, wound infection and reaction to the anaesthetic agent. In addition, there are specific complications, including:
- postoperative neck haematoma
- damage to the recurrent laryngeal nerves
- damage to the external branch of the superior laryngeal nerves
- damage to the parathyroid glands.

Postoperative haemorrhage causing a neck haematoma is a major surgical emergency requiring urgent return to theatre and decompression and occurs in 1–2% cases. Enlarging haematoma beneath the strap muscle layer will result in increasing pressure, in turn causing venous and lymphatic obstruction and submucosal oedema of the larynx and trachea, and potential critical airway obstruction. Treatment is urgent release of the pressure by opening the skin and deeper strap muscle layer. Usually there is time to transport the patient to theatre, but occasionally it is more rapidly evolving and will need to be performed on the ward. Hence the need for close observation of the neck postoperatively and a thyroid tray of instruments at the patient's bedside should they be required.

Unilateral recurrent nerve palsy leads to a hoarse voice and is usually temporary, often resolving within weeks but occasionally taking up to 6 months, and occurs in up to 10% of cases. Recurrent laryngeal nerve palsy may be permanent in 1–3% of cases. Voice quality usually improves over time, but occasionally can be improved further by procedures such as vocal cord medialisation. Rarely, bilateral damage may occur and require a tracheostomy because the vocal cords adopt a medial position, causing airway obstruction.

If the external branch of the superior laryngeal nerve is affected (estimated to occur in 10–30%), the patient may lose the ability to sing, shout or project their voice.

Because of postoperative changes and oedema at the site of surgery, up to 80% of patients will experience subtle alteration in their voice quality, in the absence of either recurrent or external laryngeal nerve injury. This change often takes several months to resolve.

Permanent damage to the parathyroid glands will cause permanent hypoparathyroidism and occurs in 1–3% following total thyroidectomy. Temporary hypoparathyroidism causing temporary hypocalcaemia is much more common (usually 8–12% of cases but may be even commoner) and is due to oedema, bruising, devascularisation or inadvertent removal of parathyroid glands. Treatment is short-term administration of oral calcium and/or 1,25-dihydroxyvitamin D for several weeks, but occasionally intravenous calcium is required. These complications are avoided by understanding the surgical anatomy of the thyroid gland (Figure 37.1) and by the technique of capsular dissection, carefully preserving the parathyroid glands and their blood supply and the recurrent laryngeal and external laryngeal nerves. If there is devascularisation of parathyroid glands or inadvertent removal, they should be autotransplanted.

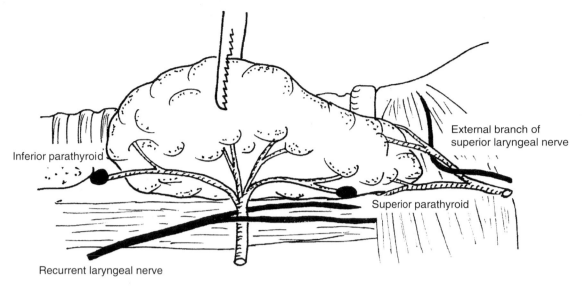

Fig. 37.1 Surgical anatomy of the thyroid gland. The left lobe of the gland is elevated and rotated medially exposing the recurrent laryngeal nerve, the external branch of the superior laryngeal nerve and both parathyroid glands, with their blood supply arising from the inferior thyroid artery.

Further reading

Fundakowski CE, Hales NW, Agrawal N *et al*. Surgical Management of the recurrent laryngeal nerve in thyroidectomy: American Head and Neck Society Consensus Statement. *Head Neck* 2018;40:663–75.

Haugen BR, Alexander EK, Bible KC *et al*. 2015 American Thyroid Association Management Guidelines for adult patients with thyroid nodules and differentiated thyroid cancer: The American Thyroid Association Guidelines Task Force on Thyroid Nodules and Differentiated Thyroid Cancer. *Thyroid* 2016;26:1–133.

Qian SY, Topliss DJ. Thyroid cancer: how to achieve optimal patient outcomes. *Medicine Today* 2017;18:28–35.

Ross DS, Burch HB, Cooper DS *et al*. 2016 American Thyroid Association Guideline for diagnosis and management of hyperthyroidism and other causes of thyrotoxicosis. *Thyroid* 2016;26:1343–421.

MCQs

Select the single correct answer to each question. The correct answers can be found in the Answers section at the end of the book.

1 Thyroid follicular cells arise primarily from:
   a laryngeal cartilage
   b second branchial arch
   c oesophagus
   d base of the tongue
   e neural crest

2 FNAC may diagnose all types of thyroid cancer *except*:
   a follicular thyroid cancer
   b papillary thyroid cancer
   c anaplastic thyroid cancer
   d medullary thyroid cancer
   e metastases from renal cell cancer

3 The type of thyroid cancer with the worst prognosis (5-year survival <1%) is:
   a papillary thyroid cancer
   b follicular thyroid cancer
   c anaplastic thyroid cancer
   d medullary thyroid cancer
   e thyroid lymphoma

4 Thyroiditis presenting following a viral infection with an exquisitely tender, enlarged, firm thyroid gland, and with systemic symptoms of headache and malaise is generally due to:
   a Hashimoto's thyroiditis
   b de Quervain's (subacute) thyroiditis
   c Reidel's thyroiditis
   d acute bacterial thyroiditis
   e non-specific thyroiditis

5 Damage to one recurrent laryngeal nerve during thyroidectomy generally leads to:
   a the need for a tracheostomy
   b inability to sing high notes
   c inability to project the voice to the back of a hall
   d a falsetto voice
   e a hoarse voice

38 Parathyroid

Jonathan Serpell

Monash University and Breast, Endocrine and General Surgery Unit, Alfred Health, Melbourne, Victoria, Australia

Introduction

There are usually four parathyroid glands, two on each side, having a posterolateral relationship to the lateral lobes of the thyroid gland. The two superior parathyroid glands arise from the fourth pharyngeal pouch and ultimobranchial body and migrate medially early in fetal development along with the C-cells to meet the developing thyroid gland. They are generally reasonably constant in position in relation to the lateral lobe or to the tubercle of Zuckerkandl. The two inferior parathyroid glands arise from the third pharyngeal pouch and descend into the anterior neck along with the thymus. Because of their longer course of descent they are more variable in position and may be found in relation to the inferior pole of the thyroid gland, in the thyrothymic tract, or within or adjacent to the thymus, in its cervical or anterior mediastinal components.

Ectopic or supernumerary parathyroid glands are common, being found in over 10% of the population. Ectopic inferior parathyroid glands may be located in a variety of positions, such as within the carotid sheath or as an undescended para-thymus (high in the neck at the level of the submandibular salivary gland) or within the thyroid gland itself. Rare ectopic sites include the pericardium and aorto-pulmonary window. If parathyroid glands enlarge, they may migrate from their original location. Superior parathyroid glands, as they enlarge, often move down along the oesophagus, presumably aided by peristalsis, and can end up in the posterior mediastinum in a para- or retro-oesophageal position. Superior glands tend to move inferiorly and posteriorly, whereas inferior glands move inferiorly and anteriorly.

The course of the recurrent laryngeal nerve acts as a marker to the location of the parathyroid glands, with superior glands usually located posterior to the nerve and above the inferior thyroid artery, whereas inferior glands are located anterior to the nerve and below the inferior thyroid artery. Superior and inferior parathyroid glands take their name from their relationship, either above or below, the inferior thyroid artery.

A normal parathyroid gland weighs 30–35 mg. Both superior and inferior glands derive their primary blood supply from branches of the inferior thyroid artery, although superior glands may receive branches from the superior thyroid artery.

The parathyroid glands secrete parathyroid hormone (PTH), an 84-amino acid peptide with a half-life of about 5 minutes. PTH is rapidly broken down into N-terminal and C-terminal fragments in the reticuloendothelial cells of the liver. PTH acts on bone to mobilise calcium by stimulation of osteoclast activity, leading to bone resorption. PTH also acts on the kidney to increase calcium resorption in the proximal convoluted tubule and inhibit resorption of both phosphate and bicarbonate. An additional renal effect is the production by the proximal tubule of activated 1,25-dihydroxyvitamin D, which results in calcium absorption by the small intestine.

Diseases affecting the parathyroid glands result essentially in disorders of function, either excess or reduced PTH secretion. These include:
- primary hyperparathyroidism
- secondary and tertiary hyperparathyroidism
- hypoparathyroidism.

Disorders of the parathyroid glands

Primary hyperparathyroidism

Pathology

Primary hyperparathyroidism is due to a parathyroid adenoma, usually solitary (85% of cases). It may also be due to parathyroid hyperplasia (up to

Textbook of Surgery, Fourth Edition. Edited by Julian A. Smith, Andrew H. Kaye, Christopher Christophi and Wendy A. Brown.
© 2020 John Wiley & Sons Ltd. Published 2020 by John Wiley & Sons Ltd.

15%) or, rarely, parathyroid carcinoma (<1%). It may occur as a sporadic phenomenon or may be associated with one of the familial endocrine syndromes, including multiple endocrine neoplasia (MEN) 1 and MEN 2A, or familial hyperparathyroidism. Hyperparathyroidism is also associated with a history of previous exposure to ionising radiation to the neck, especially in childhood and adolescent years.

Clinical presentation

Primary hyperparathyroidism occurs predominantly in women, with the highest incidence in the fifth to sixth decades. The commonest presentation is in apparently asymptomatic individuals who are found to have hypercalcaemia during routine blood testing, or who present for routine bone mineral density testing and are found to have osteopenia or osteoporosis. Symptoms specifically associated with primary hyperparathyroidism include neuropsychological manifestations such as tiredness, lethargy and depression, musculoskeletal manifestations such as bone pain and muscle weakness and myalgia, renal stones, abdominal pain from constipation or peptic ulceration, polyuria and polydipsia, leading to their summary description as 'bones, stones, abdominal groans and psychic moans'. However, careful history taking will often elicit evidence of these symptoms in a subtle form, leading many to believe that all patients with primary hyperparathyroidism are in fact symptomatic to some extent, with the corollary that all should be treated. A careful medication history is important, as for example lithium may result in parathyroid hyperplasia, as well as exhibiting renal manifestations.

Investigations

The diagnosis of primary hyperparathyroidism is biochemical and confirmed by the finding of an elevated serum calcium level in association with an inappropriately raised (i.e. non-suppressed) PTH level. Occasionally the PTH may be in the normal range despite the presence of primary hyperparathyroidism but nonetheless still inappropriately elevated. In contradistinction, other secondary causes of hypercalcaemia (e.g. metastatic malignancy) have an elevated serum calcium but a suppressed PTH level. Calcium levels may fluctuate, passing in and out of the normal range, so at least three estimates are required. Further, ionised calcium will be elevated if doubt remains about the diagnosis.

Measurement of 24-hour urinary calcium excretion excludes the rare but confounding genetic autosomal dominant disorder of familial hypocalciuric hypercalcaemia, in which an elevated serum calcium may be associated with a marginally raised PTH level and low urinary calcium excretion. Magnesium and phosphate should be estimated. Vitamin D and serum creatinine are measured to exclude the two common causes of secondary hyperparathyroidism. A bone density study should be undertaken as a baseline to document established osteopenia or osteoporosis and enable assessment of bone remineralisation following treatment.

A careful family history will generally exclude an association with one of the familial endocrine syndromes. If the patient has MEN 1, tumours of the pituitary and pancreatic islet cells need to be excluded, whereas if they are part of a MEN 2A family, serum calcitonin and urinary catecholamines need to be measured to exclude medullary thyroid carcinoma and phaeochromocytoma.

Once a diagnosis of primary hyperparathyroidism has been confirmed, parathyroid localisation studies should be undertaken. The aim of localisation studies is to identify or at least lateralise the site of the parathyroid adenoma to allow a decision to be made as to whether a targeted, focused, unilateral surgical approach is possible. Localisation studies are only undertaken after the diagnosis is clearly established; they should not be done to make the diagnosis of primary hyperparathyroidism. Further, imaging results should not be used to decide whether surgery is indicated, as those who are not localised by imaging remain candidates for surgery. Ultrasound and nuclear medicine scanning are routinely used for localisation. A ^{99m}Tc-sestamibi parathyroid scan using single-photon emission computed tomography (SPECT) will demonstrate uptake in a single parathyroid adenoma in more than 70% of cases, with neck ultrasound providing valuable additional information. If localisation is positive, and the two studies concordant, targeted exploration is possible; this focused approach is also described as a minimally invasive parathyroidectomy. If localisation is not achieved, the patient requires bilateral neck exploration, aiming to identify all four parathyroid glands. The rationale is that without localisation the involved glands are probably smaller, and there may be multiple glands involved due to hyperplasia, hence the need to explore both sides of the neck. Overall, parathyroid imaging is significantly less accurate for those with multi-gland disease.

Rarely, in patients with recurrent primary hyperparathyroidism, other specialised localisation studies are undertaken, including four-dimensional CT scanning (now undertaken by some for initial localisation) and selective venous sampling. However, the radioactivity associated with four-dimensional CT needs to be considered in a younger patient.

At the same time as localisation, neck ultrasound will also assess the thyroid gland for significant abnormalities which may require investigation (thyroid function and cytology of any suspicious nodules) and potential surgery at the same time as the proposed parathyroidectomy. Concomitant thyroid disease is common, found in at least 12% of patients.

Treatment

The only successful treatment for primary hyperparathyroidism is parathyroidectomy. All symptomatic patients should undergo surgery. Other definite indications for surgery are calcium greater than 0.25 mmol/L above normal range regardless of whether symptomatic, evidence of renal involvement (e.g. nephrolithiasis and nephrocalcinosis), osteoporosis and age less than 50 years. There is debate about whether asymptomatic patients may be treated by observation subject to a set of strict criteria; however, there is increasing evidence that even 'asymptomatic' patients obtain significant benefit in relation to improvements in non-specific neuropsychological symptoms following normalisation of serum calcium levels after surgery. As such, most patients, unless there are specific contraindications to surgery, are now offered parathyroidectomy as initial therapy. The likelihood of curing the primary hyperparathyroidism is on the order of 95–98%, with a very low risk of recurrent disease. Further, surgery is probably more cost-effective overall than observation.

Secondary hyperparathyroidism

Pathology

Secondary hyperparathyroidism is the result of prolonged hypocalcaemia and is usually due to chronic kidney disease (CKD), although vitamin D deficiency and gluten-sensitive enteropathy must be excluded as causes. The prolonged hypocalcaemia results in chief cell hyperplasia and PTH secretion. In CKD this appears primarily to be due to difficulty with excretion of phosphate, resulting in hyperphosphataemia and secondary hypocalcaemia. Hyperphoshataemia leads to parathyroid cell

hyperplasia and stimulates PTH secretion. Further, in CKD there is reduced expression of the calcium-sensing receptor in parathyroid cells. Increases in PTH result in osteodystrophy much greater than that normally seen in primary disease. The parathyroid glands initially undergo hyperplasia and then develop nodularity, and the process is often asymmetrical so that some glands will have greater degrees of enlargement than others. Renal osteodystrophy is often a combination of secondary hyperparathyroidism and the disturbed vitamin D metabolism of CKD (osteomalacia). More recently, the role of increasing fibroblast growth factor (FGF)23 levels (which parallel PTH levels) and Klotho deficiency in CKD as biomarkers of osteodystrophy and associated vascular disease has become an area of active ongoing research in secondary hyperparathyroidism.

Clinical features

The osteodystrophy of secondary hyperparathyroidism causes bone, joint and muscle pain and may lead to pathological fractures. There may be deposition of calcium in soft tissues resulting in skin itch and may be associated with severe skin necrosis (calciphylaxis) and conjunctivitis. Ectopic calcification also occurs in blood vessels, heart valves and other organs such as lung and intestines. Neuromuscular and psychiatric symptoms also occur, as well as anaemia and cardiac failure.

Investigations

Secondary hyperparathyroidism is characterised by hypocalcaemia, hyperphosphataemia and an elevated PTH level. Significant bone disease is indicated by elevation of serum alkaline phosphatase. Hypercalcaemia may occur secondary to vitamin D treatment, or development of tertiary hyperparathyroidism. Radiology may demonstrate much grosser changes in the skeleton than is usual in primary hyperparathyroidism in the modern context, with irregular bone density loss and subperiosteal absorption of bone. Classical appearances include 'pepperpot' skull, 'rugger jersey' spine and the less dramatic but more frequent loss of the outer third of clavicle and scalloping of the radial side of the middle phalanges. Metastatic calcification can be seen around vessels and in the capsules of joints.

If surgery is contemplated, localisation with sestamibi scanning is useful to exclude ectopic locations, especially the mediastinum, and ultrasound is necessary to assess the thyroid.

Treatment

Secondary hyperparathyroidism occurs to some degree in all patients with CKD, but especially in those with dialysis-dependent CKD (stage 5 CKD). The symptoms can often be ameliorated by oral calcium-based and other phosphate binders (aimed at reducing intestinal absorption of phosphate), with or without the administration of 1,25-dihydroxyvitamin D (active vitamin D, calcitriol). There has also been considerable interest in extended-hour (nocturnal) dialysis as a mechanism for controlling hyperphosphataemia, as short-hour intermittent dialysis is relatively ineffective at removing phosphate.

Cinacalcet, a calcimimetic, acts as a positive modulator of the calcium sensing receptor located on parathyroid cells. It acts to reduce PTH production from the cells. It has been a major advance in the treatment of secondary hyperparathyroidism but is not always available. Cinacalcet had been shown to reduce the need for parathyroidectomy in 90% of patients.

Although the treatment of secondary hyperparathyroidism is therefore largely medical in nature, some patients will not achieve satisfactory symptom or biochemical control (high phosphate and high PTH). The need for parathyroidectomy has varied in the eras before and after cinacalcet but is about 10% of those on haemodialysis for more than 10 years. With restrictions on the availability of cincalcet, the requirement for parathyroid surgery is likely to increase once more. Indications for surgery include the development of hypercalcaemia because this is likely to lead to metastatic calcification and persistent elevation in alkaline phosphatase, which is an indication of continuing major bone disease. Other indications include inability to control serum phosphorus, calcium and PTH within target ranges; intractable subjective symptoms including itch or bone pain and muscle weakness; ectopic calcification; calciphylaxis; non-availability of cincalcet or when cincalcet does not achieve a satisfactory reduction in PTH level; anaemia resistant to erythropoietin; and dilated cardiomyopathy.

These patients should be treated by parathyroidectomy. The options available include subtotal parathyroidectomy, or total parathyroidectomy with or without parathyroid autotransplantation into the sternocleidomastoid in the neck or brachioradialis in the forearm. Both the subtotal and total procedures should include cervical thymectomy, as rests of parathyroid tissue are common in the thymus. The subtotal procedure aims to leave a 50-mg remnant of what appears the most normal parathyroid tissue, usually of an inferior gland, so if recurrence does occur it will be further away from the recurrent laryngeal nerve at the time of re-exploratory surgery. The subtotal procedure has theoretical advantages for a patient who is likely to receive a renal transplant, in the hope that the remnant will function normally once normal renal function is established. Equally, if transplantation not an option, the total procedure seems sensible. However, studies do not indicate which surgical procedure is preferred, and this is therefore tailored to the individual patient and surgeon's preference.

Tertiary hyperparathyroidism

Tertiary hyperparathyroidism results from the hyperplasia of secondary hyperparathyroidism when the glands become autonomously hyperfunctioning rather than responsive to the original stimulus. Thus, tertiary hyperparathyroidism is a progression of secondary hyperparathyroidism accompanied by spontaneous hypercalcaemia. This is most clearly seen after a successful renal transplant has been performed, where the restoration of normal renal function and the appropriate production of 1,25-dihydroxyvitamin D could be expected to restore normal calcium balance. Most patients should receive active medical treatment in an attempt to avoid end-organ damage and will usually show a return to normal calcium metabolism within a period of 6 months. In the small number of patients whose symptoms are not controlled or in whom the hypercalcaemia persists despite adequate treatment and normal renal function, the glands must be assumed to have developed some degree of autonomy and parathyroidectomy is required. The extent of surgery is dictated by the operative findings, with either subtotal or total parathyroidectomy with cervical thymectomy, and with autotransplantation being undertaken depending on the number of glands involved in this process.

Hypoparathyroidism

Hypoparathyroidism may be due to congenital absence of the parathyroid glands, idiopathic autoimmune failure of the parathyroid glands or, most commonly, surgical removal or damage to the parathyroid glands after total thyroidectomy. Temporary hypoparathyroidism is common (8–12%) after total thyroidectomy, due to oedema, bruising and devascularisation of glands. Temporary hypoparathyroidism is commoner if devascularised parathyroid glands have been autotransplanted during the procedure. Such patients may be asymptomatic or may present with paraesthesiae in the fingertips and toes and around the mouth. This is managed by replacement therapy with oral calcium and/or 1,25-dihydroxyvitamin D awaiting recovery of the autotransplanted glands; this usually is a matter of weeks but can take up to 6 months. Most endocrine surgery units have proactive protocols to manage hypoparathyroidism following total thyroidectomy, and this approach has been shown to aid parathyroid gland recovery, due to a 'splinting' effect, while the parathyroid glands regain their normal function.

Operative management

Parathyroidectomy

Primary hyperparathyroidism

Patients with primary hyperparathyroidism and concordant localisation (sestamibi and ultrasound showing similar localisation to a single site) can undergo minimally invasive parathyroidectomy. Patients with primary hyperparathyroidism where localisation has been unsuccessful may have smaller adenomas or may have multiple gland disease and should undergo bilateral neck exploration parathyroidectomy aiming to identify all four glands in order to assess for a single adenoma or multi-gland disease.

The advantages of minimally invasive parathyroidectomy are unilateral exploration, quicker postoperative recovery and reduced incision length. However, it is important to note that the magnitude of these benefits is small, and most patients still only require an overnight stay with bilateral neck exploration.

The chance of cure is about 95–98% for both surgical approaches. In the small percentage of patients in whom the gland is not detected at the time of primary surgery, it is likely to lie in an ectopic position, such as the pericardium or middle mediastinum, and additional localisation studies such as four-dimensional CT and selective venous sampling will be required prior to considering a second operation.

Secondary hyperparathyroidism

Patients with secondary and tertiary hyperparathyroidism require either subtotal parathyroidectomy or total parathyroidectomy with or without neck or forearm autotransplantation. Both should also have cervical thymectomy. As the stimuli causing secondary hyperparathyroidism affect all glands, the aim of surgery is to identify all glands, and remove the thymus as this contains parathyroid rests of cells. Surgery generally results in a marked and sustained reduction in levels of serum PTH, calcium and phosphorus.

Complications of parathyroidectomy

The complications of parathyroidectomy include all the general complications of any operation, such as bleeding, wound infection and reaction to the anaesthetic agent. In addition, there are specific complications, including:

- damage to the recurrent laryngeal nerves and to the external branch of the superior laryngeal nerves (see Chapter 33)
- failure to locate abnormal parathyroid tissue (discussed previously)
- hypoparathyroidism.

If more than one parathyroid gland is involved, subtotal parathyroidectomy may lead to hypoparathyroidism, which may require short-term administration of oral calcium and 1,25-dihydroxyvitamin D. As in thyroid surgery, devascularised normal parathyroid tissue should be autotransplanted. Thus postoperatively, patients require close observation, evaluating for symptoms of hypocalcaemia and monitoring serum calcium levels.

Cure is defined as normocalcaemia at 6 months. Elevated postoperative calcium levels indicate persistent hyperparathyroidism. Cure followed by recurrence of hypercalcaemia after 6 months indicates recurrent hyperparathyroidism.

Further reading

Norlan O, Wang KC, Tay YK et al. No need to abandon focused parathyroidectomy: a multicenter study of long term outcome after surgery for primary hypoparathyroidism. Ann Surg 2015;261:991–6.

Tominaga Y. Surgical management of secondary and tertiary hyperparathyroidism. In: Randolph GW (ed.) Surgery of the Thyroid and Parathyroid Glands, 2nd edn. Philadelphia: Elsevier Saunders, 2013:639–47.

Wilhelm SM, Wang TS, Ruan DT et al. American Association of Endocrine Surgeons guidelines for definitive management of primary hyperparathyroidism. JAMA Surg 2016;151:959–68.

MCQs

Select the single correct answer to each question. The correct answers can be found in the Answers section at the end of the book.

1 The parathyroid glands arise from:
   a third and fourth branchial pouches
   b base of the tongue
   c first branchial pouch
   d thyroid parenchyma
   e a tracheal diverticulum

2 Parathyroid hormone (PTH) has a half-life of:
   a 7 seconds
   b 5 minutes
   c 1 hour
   d 2 days
   e 5 weeks

3 Primary hyperparathyroidism is due, in 90% of cases, to:
   a metastatic cancer
   b parathyroid cancer
   c parathyroid hyperplasia
   d multiple parathyroid tumours
   e a single parathyroid adenoma

4 The diagnosis of primary hyperparathyroidism is usually confirmed by which of the following biochemical results:
   a raised serum calcium, suppressed PTH
   b raised serum calcium, raised or normal PTH
   c normal serum calcium, raised PTH
   d normal serum calcium, suppressed PTH
   e low serum calcium, raised or normal PTH

5 The most common cause of hypoparathyroidism is:
   a congenital absence of the parathyroids
   b autoimmune parathyroid failure
   c parathyroid cancer
   d surgical removal of the parathyroids at total thyroidectomy
   e acute bacterial infection

39 Tumours of the adrenal gland

Jonathan Serpell

Monash University and Breast, Endocrine and General Surgery Unit, Alfred Health, Melbourne, Victoria, Australia

Introduction

The adrenal glands lie superomedial to the upper poles of both kidneys. Each adrenal gland comprises a medulla and a cortex, and each component has a distinct embryological origin. The adrenal cortex is of mesodermal origin, whereas the adrenal medulla arises from neural crest cells along with the sympathetic ganglia. The adrenal medulla produces catecholamines, including adrenaline, noradrenaline and dopamine, and is under the control of the sympathetic nervous system. The adrenal cortex produces glucocorticoids (cortisol, corticosterone), mineralocorticoids (aldosterone) and the sex steroids oestrogen, testosterone and dehydroepiandrosterone (DHEAS). The adrenal cortex is under the control of adrenocorticotropic hormone (ACTH), a hormone produced by the pituitary gland.

Adrenal and neural crest tumours

Adrenal masses are common, affecting 3–7% of the population. Tumours can arise from both the adrenal cortex and the adrenal medulla as well as from neural crest structures. Tumours of either origin may be benign or malignant, functioning or non-functioning, and solitary or multiple. Adrenal tumours can be considered in the following groups:
- tumours of the adrenal medulla/neural crest (phaeochromocytomas and paragangliomas)
- adrenocortical tumours
- adrenal incidentalomas.

The clinical features and investigation of adrenal tumours are summarised in Table 39.1.

Phaeochromocytoma and paraganglioma

Pathology

Phaeochromocytoma and paraganglioma are tumours arising from the adrenal medulla or neural crest.

Although the classification has been confusing in the past, a consensus is now emerging (Table 39.2). All such tumours are thought to ultimately be of neural crest origin. Adrenal phaeochromocytomas are of sympathetic origin. Extra-adrenal tumours may be of sympathetic origin and are located anywhere from the cervical ganglia to the urinary bladder. They are classified as extra-adrenal phaeochromocytoma, although they have also been labelled as paraganglioma in the past. Extra-adrenal tumours may also be of parasympathetic origin, comprising mainly head and neck tumours such as carotid body tumours. Adrenal phaeochromocytomas are the commonest hormone-secreting adrenal tumour. Extra-adrenal phaeochromocytomas and paragangliomas are rare.

The majority of adrenal phaeochromocytomas are benign and functioning, but between 10 and 20% are malignant. This diagnosis may be difficult to make on histological examination, as with most endocrine tumours, and may not become apparent until the appearance of distant metastases during follow-up. Such tumours have a tendency to grow along the adrenal and renal veins and may extend into the inferior vena cava. Approximately 10% of phaeochromocytomas are bilateral within the adrenal glands.

The majority of extra-adrenal phaeochromocytoma are also functioning, but a greater percentage are malignant compared with adrenal tumours. True paragangliomas only rarely function, and the rate of malignancy is very low.

Phaeochromocytomas and paragangliomas may occur sporadically or in association with a familial disorder such as multiple endocrine neoplasia (MEN) 2A syndrome (comprising medullary carcinoma of the thyroid, phaeochromocytoma and hyperparathyroidism) or von Hippel–Lindau syndrome (retinal, cerebellar, spinal and medullary haemangioblastomas, renal cysts and carcinoma, pancreatic cysts, phaeochromocytoma and papillary cystadenoma of the epididymis).

Textbook of Surgery, Fourth Edition. Edited by Julian A. Smith, Andrew H. Kaye, Christopher Christophi and Wendy A. Brown.
© 2020 John Wiley & Sons Ltd. Published 2020 by John Wiley & Sons Ltd.

Table 39.1 Clinical features and investigations for adrenal tumours.

	Syndrome or tumour	Hormones secreted	Symptoms
Adrenal medullary or neural crest tumours	Phaeochromocytoma Paraganglioma	Adrenaline Noradrenaline Dopamine	Sweating, palpitations, hypertension (intermittent or sustained, and often severe), headache
Adrenocortical tumours	Cushing's syndrome	Glucocorticoids	Central obesity, buffalo hump, abdominal striae, hypertension, proximal muscle weakness, plethoric rounded facies, thin skin, easy bruising, hirsutism
	Conn's syndrome	Aldosterone	Hypertension, hypokalaemia
	Virilising/feminising tumours	Sex steroids	Virilisation in females, feminisation in males
Adrenal incidentaloma	Benign adrenocortical adenomas Adrenal cysts Adrenal lymphomas Schwannomas Myelolipomas Metastases	Non-secreting	Asymptomatic (incidental finding on CT or ultrasound performed for other reasons)

Table 39.2 Classification of adrenal medullary and neural crest tumours.

Origin	Tumour site	Pathology
Sympathetic tissue	Adrenal gland Extra-adrenal	Adrenal phaeochromocytoma Extra-adrenal phaeochromocytoma Zuckerkandl remnant: pre-aortic, below inferior mesenteric artery Filum terminale tumour Urinary bladder tumour Thoracic paravertebral tumour Cervical ganglia tumour
Parasympathetic tissue	Extra-adrenal	Paraganglioma Carotid body tumour Vagal paraganglioma Jugulotympanic paraganglioma Laryngeal paranganglioma Aorticopulmonary paraganglioma

Phaeochromocytomas have been termed the '10% tumour', as roughly 10% are malignant, bilateral, extra-adrenal, extra-abdominal, inherited and occur in children.

Clinical presentation

Phaeochromocytomas present a rare but curable cause of hypertension, with varying combinations of paroxysmal or sustained hypertension (0.5% of patients with hypertension have a phaeochromocytoma), headache, sweating and palpitations. Loss of weight is a common symptom. Up to one-third of cases may be asymptomatic. Some patients present as a hypertensive crisis, or even as sudden death due to a complication such as myocardial infarction or cerebrovascular accident. Paroxysmal hypertension may be precipitated by invasive procedures such as needle biopsy, angiography, CT scanning with intravenous contrast, and general anaesthesia

Investigation

The clinical diagnosis of phaeochromocytoma is confirmed in 99% of cases on the basis of elevated catecholamine levels (adrenaline, noradrenaline, dopamine) or their metabolites – metanephrines – in plasma or in a 24-hour urinary collection. Collections require careful adherence to protocols, and a careful medication history is necessary as

L-dopa and some antidepressants for example interfere with interpretation of results. The catecholamine levels should be elevated greater than twofold, and the estimate repeated to document at least two abnormal levels. Stress-related elevations tend to be marginal and less than twofold. Once a biochemical diagnosis is established, the tumour can usually be localised by CT or MRI. A nuclear medicine scan performed with metaiodobenzylguanidine (MIBG) is useful for confirming the functional status of a tumour, and may detect an extra-adrenal phaeochromocytoma or demonstrate small lesions within the adrenal gland that are not apparent on other forms of imaging, or multifocality. Adrenal phaeochromocytomas are usually at least several centimetres in dimension, and hence are usually readily detected by CT scanning. They tend to be vascular and may have areas of necrosis; as a consequence their appearance on imaging may raise suspicion of malignancy, although the majority are benign.

Treatment

Phaeochromocytoma and paraganglioma are treated by surgical excision. Careful preoperative preparation is required in order to prevent an intraoperative hypertensive crisis, due to the massive release of catecholamine with tumour handling, or profound postoperative hypotension. Unprepared patients will have a significantly constricted intravascular space due to the unopposed action of catecholamines. Hence, following removal of the tumour in an unprepared patient, there will be a dramatic fall in blood pressure requiring intravenous fluids and vasopressors. Preoperative preparation is best undertaken with administration of α-adrenergic blocking agents, such as phenoxybenzamine, usually over several weeks, closely supervised by an endocrinologist. This allows control of blood pressure and expansion of the intravascular space. Fluid loading intraoperatively, as well as the availability of intravenous nitroprusside to lower blood pressure and intravenous noradrenaline to maintain blood pressure, are essential requirements for safe surgical removal.

Adrenocortical tumours

Pathology

These tumours may be non-functioning or may secrete glucocorticoids, aldosterone or the sex steroids. They may occur sporadically, or rarely as part of a hereditary syndrome such as Li–Fraumeni syndrome, Beckwith–Wiedemann syndrome, Carney's complex or MEN 1. The majority of glucocorticoid-producing adrenocortical tumours are benign but up to 20% may be malignant. As with other endocrine tumours, a diagnosis of adrenocortical carcinoma is based on the finding of capsular or vascular invasion, but again may not be made until the later appearance of distant metastases. These tumours may reach a very large size before diagnosis, and as the size increases the risk of malignancy also rises.

Mineralocorticoid-producing adrenal tumours are almost always small (<1 cm) and virtually always benign. Bilateral nodular hyperplasia may be difficult to distinguish from a single aldosterone-producing adenoma.

The majority of sex steroid-producing tumours are malignant at presentation. Adrenocortical carcinomas are rare and 70% are associated with hormonal hypersecretion, the most common being cortisol, but often multiple hormones are produced.

Clinical presentation

Glucocorticoid-producing tumours

Most patients present with features of glucocorticoid excess (Cushing's syndrome). Occasionally a large tumour may present with local symptoms, such as pain or fullness in the flank.

A number of hormone-secreting tumours are diagnosed incidentally on CT or ultrasound scan (adrenal incidentaloma), although many such tumours have now been shown to be associated with subclinical Cushing's syndrome (pre-Cushing's syndrome). This syndrome is associated with hypertension, diabetes, obesity and osteoporosis but without the full biochemical manifestations of Cushing's syndrome. Often all that is demonstrated on investigation is loss of the diurnal rhythm of cortisol secretion and suppression of function of the contralateral gland.

Aldosterone-producing adenomas (Conn's syndrome)

Most of these tumours present during the investigation of hypertension but may be suggested by symptoms such as polyuria, polydipsia and muscle weakness due to the associated hypokalaemia. While hypokalaemia has been used as a screening test for Conn's syndrome in the past, there is increasing evidence that up to 50% of mineralocorticoid-producing tumours may be associated with normal levels of serum potassium.

Sex steroid-producing tumours

Clinical features of these rare tumours will be specific to the type of hormone produced, with either virilisation in females or feminisation in males. Many of these patients also have palpable masses and 50% have metastatic tumour at the time of presentation.

Investigations

Initial screening tests used to diagnose Cushing's syndrome usually involve two of (i) measurement of a spot salivary cortisol, (ii) a 24-hour urinary free cortisol level or (iii) a low-dose dexamethasone suppression test to assess suppression of cortisol overnight. If two of these are normal, Cushing's syndrome is unlikely. If spot salivary cortisol or 24-hour urinary free cortisol is elevated, a low-dose dexamethasone suppression test will usually be undertaken to confirm glucocorticoid excess. Once a diagnosis of Cushing's syndrome is established, further tests are required to establish the aetiology of the excess glucocorticoid production. This may involve measuring serum ACTH, a high-dose dexamethasone suppression test and an abdominal CT scan. The presence of an adrenal tumour as the cause of the glucocorticoid excess, rather than a pituitary tumour (Cushing's disease) or an ectopic ACTH-secreting tumour, can generally be made by measuring plasma ACTH levels and performing abdominal CT. Adrenal tumours producing cortisol will suppress ACTH levels to undetectable or very low levels, whereas Cushing's disease and ectopic ACTH-producing tumours will have elevated ACTH levels. A high-dose dexamethasone suppression test will help distinguish the latter two (ectopic ACTH-producing tumour will not suppress, whereas Cushing's disease will suppress). For adrenal Cushing's, a high-dose dexamethasone suppression test will not suppress the already low ACTH. The rare bilateral nodular adrenal hyperplasia may occasionally be difficult to differentiate from a single small adrenal tumour.

A low serum potassium level will suggest the possibility of an aldosterone-secreting tumour. Measurement of the ratio of plasma renin and plasma aldosterone (PRA ratio) will confirm the diagnosis of hyperaldosteronism, as primary hyperaldosteronism is characterised by low plasma renin activity. A CT scan may detect an adrenal tumour but because many of these tumours are very small, selective adrenal vein sampling for aldosterone may be required to localise the tumour.

Measurement of the sex hormones as well as the 17-ketosteroids will confirm the diagnosis of a sex steroid-producing tumour. These tumours are often large and should be detected on CT scanning.

Elevated DHEAS levels may suggest malignancy, as carcinomas are often deficient in 3-hydroxysteroid dehydrogenase, such deficiency inhibiting conversion of pregnenolone to cortisol and aldosterone but not inhibiting sex hormone production, resulting in their elevation as well as their precursor DHEAS.

Treatment

Surgical excision (adrenalectomy) is the only treatment for an adrenocortical tumour. For large or potentially malignant tumours, wide local excision and local lymph node dissection may be required.

Adrenal incidentalomas

Pathology

Any tumour arising in the adrenal gland can present as an adrenal incidentaloma, including adrenocortical tumours, adrenal medullary tumours, schwannomas, myelolipomas, adrenal cysts, adrenal lymphomas and adrenal metastases from other malignancies, particularly breast cancer. Incidental benign adrenocortical adenomas are common and can be found at post-mortem in up to 10% of the normal population and will be found in about 4% of abdominal CT scans. Metastases are increasingly detected in adrenals on positron emission tomography.

Clinical presentation

By definition, an adrenal incidentaloma will present as an incidental finding, usually on a CT or ultrasound scan. They will not be associated with local symptoms, nor with any of the syndromes of hormonal excess.

Investigation

The tumour will already have been demonstrated by imaging. Hormonal hypersecretion must be excluded by screening tests, including measurement of spot salivary cortisol, 24-hour urinary free cortisol, PRA ratio, adrenal sex steroids, DHEAS, and urinary catecholamines and metanephrines.

Treatment

Incidental adrenal tumours that do not secrete hormones, are not associated with local symptoms and are less than 4 cm in diameter can be treated conservatively, although there are increasing data to suggest that the potential risk for malignancy may require that cut-off to be lower, for example 3 cm. A follow-up CT scan should be performed after 6 months to ensure there is no progressive increase in size, which would suggest malignancy. Large tumours, or those that demonstrate an increase in size, should be removed surgically because of the increased risk of malignancy.

Operative management: adrenalectomy

Adrenalectomy can be performed as an open procedure, as an anterior laparoscopic procedure or as a posterior retroperitoneoscopic procedure. Increasingly, the accepted philosophy is to tailor the surgical approach to the tumour size and clinical situation.

The open approach to the adrenal gland involves (i) an anterior approach (via a midline, transverse or oblique incision) through the peritoneal cavity or (ii) an extraperitoneal approach, either posteriorly through the bed of the 12th rib or posterolaterally or (iii) combined as a thoraco-abdominal procedure. These procedures are now used mainly for very large tumours or those known to be malignant.

Laparoscopic adrenalectomy is associated with reduced postoperative pain allowing the patient to leave hospital after 2 or 3 days, smaller incisions, reduced blood loss and fewer complications. The procedure is ideally suited to small benign adrenal tumours, such as those commonly found in Conn's syndrome, but is also indicated for phaeochromocytoma, including bilateral tumours.

The newer posterior retroperitoneoscopic approach is increasingly used in centres around the world as the preferred technique. It has many of the advantages of the anterior laparoscopic approach, but probably less postoperative pain and shorter postoperative stay, which may be overnight only, and reduced incidence of ileus.

Complications of adrenalectomy include all the general complications of any open abdominal adrenal operation or laparoscopic or retroperitoneoscopic procedure such as bleeding, wound infection and ileus. The particular anaesthetic complications of phaeochromocytoma surgery have already been discussed. Surgery for glucocorticoid-secreting tumours, and occasionally for incidentalomas with subclinical hormone secretion, may potentially lead to a postoperative Addisonian crisis because of suppression of the contralateral adrenal gland. This should be anticipated and prevented by prophylactic steroid administration until the remaining gland recovers, which may take 4–6 weeks.

Further reading

Clark OH, Duh QY, Kebebew E, Gosnell JE, Shen WT (eds) *Textbook of Endocrine Surgery*, 3rd edn. New Delhi: Jaypee Brothers Medical Publishing, 2016:80–93.

Else T, Kim AC, Sabolch A *et al.* Adrenocortical carcinoma. *Endocr Rev* 2014;35:282–326.

MCQs

Select the single correct answer to each question. The correct answers can be found in the Answers section at the end of the book.

1 Adrenal masses occur in:
   a <1% of the population
   b 3–7% of the population
   c 10–20% of the population
   d 40–50% of the population
   e >66% of the population

2 Conn's syndrome is due to a tumour of the adrenal cortex secreting excess:
   a cortisol
   b adrenaline
   c noradrenaline
   d aldosterone
   e sex steroids

3 Paragangliomas arise from:
   a adrenal cortex
   b adrenal medulla
   c carotid bifurcation
   d foregut
   e parasympathetic tissue arising from the neural crest

4 The initial test used to diagnose Cushing's syndrome is measurement of:
   a spot salivary cortisol and 24-hour urinary free cortisol levels
   b serum ACTH
   c serum cortisol after a dexamethasone test
   d plasma renin/aldosterone ratio
   e serum catecholamines

5 Adrenal incidentalomas should be removed when they are:
   a >25 cm
   b >10–15 cm
   c >3–5 cm
   d >1 cm
   e any size at all

Section 7
Head and Neck Surgery

40 Eye injuries and infections

Helen V. Danesh-Meyer

Department of Ophthalmology, School of Medicine, University of Auckland, Auckland, New Zealand

Introduction

Eye injuries can range from the very minor to the catastrophic, resulting in permanent loss of vision or even loss of the eye. Infections can also range from conjunctivitis to serious sight-threatening infections that can cause irreversible damage. A systematic approach to these conditions is necessary so that timely and appropriate treatment can be initiated.

Eye injuries

The aim of the approach to a patient with eye injuries is to identify serious sight-threatening injuries that require immediate action. The most time-critical injury is a chemical injury (see later) in which immediate treatment with irrigation can significantly impact the long-term prognosis. Equally important is identifying the ruptured globe or intraocular foreign body. Therefore, a systematic approach to the history and examination is necessary.

History and examination

A careful history of the cause of the injury should be taken and examination of the eye performed. Specific aspects of the history and examination will assist in determining the severity and nature of the ocular injury.

- *Face*: proptosis may indicate retrobulbar haemorrhage, which is an ocular emergency. If not treated immediately (usually requiring lateral canthotomy and intravenous acetozolamide or mannitol) the ischaemia to the optic nerve and retina may be irreversible.
- *Lids*: check lid movement. Lacerations of the lid tend to increase the risk of having associated ocular injuries.
- *Conjunctiva and sclera*: the white of the eye should be white. Obvious lacerations or haemorrhage may overlay an open globe injury. Dark uveal tissue presenting on the white of the eye (sclera) may suggest an open globe. If a foreign body is suspected, this may be the site of penetration.
- *Cornea*: the cornea should be clear.
- *Anterior chamber*: blood in the anterior chamber (hyphaema) indicates severe blunt trauma or penetrating injury.
- *Pupil*: should be round and respond briskly to light. It is important to check for a relative afferent pupillary defect using the swinging flashlight test.
- *Eye movements*: restriction of motility may suggest orbital fracture, haemorrhage or an open globe injury.

Visual acuity testing

The visual acuity of all patients with an ocular injury must be measured and recorded. Each eye should be tested separately. In instances of chemical burns, the priority is irrigation which should not be delayed under any circumstance.

The visual acuity in ocular trauma is often profoundly impacted. If it is possible, visual acuity should be tested using a Snellen acuity chart. The patient will need to be positioned the appropriate distance from the chart, usually 4 or 6 m, depending of the chart.

- Instruct the patient to read the letters on the chart from the top down. Each line is numbered. The number represents the distance in meters at which a person with normal sight can read the line.
- The last line the patient reads is recorded, e.g. 6/30. The top line represents the distance from the chart, and the bottom line the distance from the chart at which a person with normal sight

Textbook of Surgery, Fourth Edition. Edited by Julian A. Smith, Andrew H. Kaye, Christopher Christophi and Wendy A. Brown.

would read that line. Thus, a measure of 6/30 suggests that the patient reads at 6 m the line a normal person would read at 30 m.

- If no letters on the chart can be seen, bring the chart closer until the top letter can be identified. If this occurs at 2 m the acuity is recorded as 2/60 (the top letter on the chart can be seen by a person with normal sight at 60 m).
- If the top letter cannot be identified at any distance, then wave a hand in front of the eye (with the other eye covered). If the movement is perceived, it is recorded as HM (hand movements).
- If hand movements cannot be seen, shine a light into the eye. If it is seen, this is recorded as LP (light perception). Shine the light into the eye from different directions and instruct the patient to point to the light. If this is performed accurately, the acuity is recorded as 'LP with accurate projection'.
- If a bright light cannot be seen, the acuity is recorded as NLP (no light perception).

Ruptured or open globe

An open globe may result from either blunt or penetrating eye injury. Clinical signs that suggest an open globe include:
- significant visual impairment
- traumatic hyphaema
- large subconjunctival haemorrhage with chemosis
- flat anterior chamber
- 'soft' eye.

Examination

Where suspicion of a perforating injury exists, examine the eye carefully after the instillation of two or three drops of local anaesthetic. Ask the patient to open the eyes. It is important not to force the eye apart or examine the eye under a general anaesthetic.

Immediate treatment

- If an open globe is suspected, cover the eye with a shield made with a device that applies forces to the bony orbit area instead of the eye.
- Do not apply pressure on or manipulate the eye, including ultrasound.
- Do not apply any topical medications.
- Start oral or intravenous antibiotics.
- Schedule an urgent referral to an ophthalmologist.
- Administer tetanus toxoid if indicated.

- Prevent emesis.
- Biplanar radiographs or CT scan of the head may help to identify a metallic intraocular fragment.

Chemical injuries

Both acids and alkalis produce serious damage to the eye. Both penetrate readily into the eye, resulting in corneal opacification and inflammation. Long-term complications include corneal scarring, cataract, retinal detachment and glaucoma. Acids and alkalis also cause thrombosis of the circum-corneal blood vessels that supply nutrients to the cornea, resulting in corneal ischaemia and opacification.

The most important aspect of treatment is irrigation, both at the site of injury and in hospital.

Irrigation

Irrigate the eye immediately with saline for at least 30 minutes. If non-sterile water is the only fluid available, it should be used. Irrigation should not be delayed. If a speculum is available, it is helpful to use this along with topical anaesthetic. The victim should then be transported to specialist care rapidly. Evert the upper and lower lids to ensure that no solid matter is retained behind the lids. After appropriate irrigation, wait 5–10 minutes and use litmus paper to touch the inferior cul-de-sac. Irrigation should be continued until neutral pH is reached.

Once irrigation is completed, fluorescein may be used to assess the cornea for epithelial defects. It is important for the patient to be assessed with a slit-lamp to provide adequate understanding of the extent of the injury. Patients with chemical injuries are usually admitted to hospital for intensive treatment with antibiotics and steroids.

Prognosis

Chemical injuries have a poor prognosis.

Blow-out fracture of the orbit

An object larger than the orbital opening will compress the orbital contents and may produce a blow-out fracture of the orbital floor into the maxillary antrum or, less commonly, of the medial wall into the ethmoidal air cells. These are the thinnest of the orbital walls and are the most likely to be damaged.

Features that suggest a blow-out fracture of the orbit include the following.

- Restricted eye movements, especially upward or lateral gaze. If visual acuity is good in both eyes, the patient will complain of diplopia due to entrapment of the fascia, usually around the inferior rectus muscle in the fracture in the orbital floor (Figure 40.1).
- Hyperaesthesia of cheek and upper lip (distribution of infraorbital nerve).
- Enophthalmos because of prolapse of orbital fat into the antrum.

- There may be pain on attempted vertical eye movements, eyelid swelling and creptitus after nose blowing.

Treatment

The treatment is surgical with release of the entrapped tissues from the fracture site. The appropriate investigation is CT scan of the brain and orbit (axial and coronal views, 3-mm cuts).

(a)

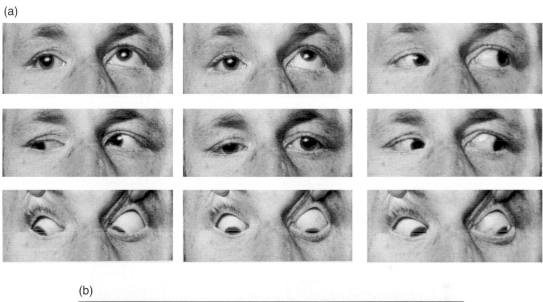

(b)

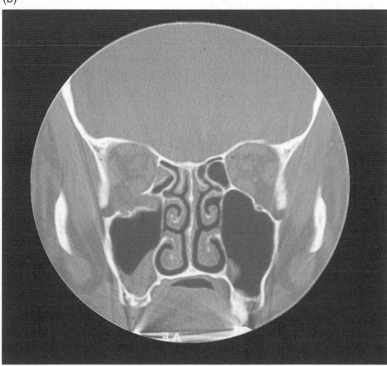

Fig. 40.1 (a) This patient has a blow-out fracture of the right orbit and shows absent elevation in that eye. (b) CT scan of the orbit reveals the blow-out of the floor of the orbit.

Hyphaema

Hyphaema is a haemorrhage into the anterior chamber of the eye (between the cornea and iris). Clinical features include:

- decreased visual acuity
- pupil may not respond to light
- elevated intraocular pressure, which can be estimated by gently palpating the eye and comparing with the other eye.

Where the hyphaema occupies less than three-quarters of the anterior chamber, treat with bed rest and sedation. However, often it may be necessary to lower intraocular pressure with acetazolamide 500 mg initially. The patient must be referred immediately for specialist treatment because a hyphaema may be complicated by intraocular damage, which will not be apparent on presentation.

Traumatic mydriasis

Following a blow on the eye, the iris muscles may be paralysed, producing a fixed dilated pupil, which may recover within a few days. Small tears in the lid margin may involve the sphincter and cause permanent pupil dilatation.

Choroidal rupture

Rupture of the choroid occurs in an arc concentric with the optic nerve. It results in disruption of the overlying nerve fibres and hence produces a permanent visual field defect. If the rupture occurs between the disc and the macula, central vision is permanently lost.

Thermal injuries

Thermal injuries cause burns to the eyelids. The management of the skin burn follows the usual principles, but particular care must be exercised to protect the cornea. Shrinkage of the eyelids in the healing phase puts the cornea at risk from exposure and drying.

Care of the eye

Protect the cornea by the instillation of antibiotic ointment (chloramphenicol) every hour to provide a layer of grease, which delays the evaporation of tears. If this is insufficient to prevent corneal drying, the eyelids must be sutured together (tarsorrhaphy).

Alternatively, cover the eye with transparent plastic film. A piece large enough to cover the orbit reaching from the forehead to the cheek is held in position by applying a layer of Vaseline to the skin around the orbit to which the plastic film adheres.

Corneal abrasion

Corneal abrasions can be very painful. Patients present with sharp pain, photophobia and tearing. The diagnosis is made with the identification of an epithelial defect with fluorescein staining.

Management involves everting the eyelids to ensure that no foreign body is present. Symptoms usually resolve instantaneously with topical anaesthetic drops. Treatment involves antibiotic drops or ointment, a short-acting cycloplegic (for comfort with cyclopentolate 1%, as relaxing the ciliary muscle decreases pain which may be secondary to ciliary spasm) and eye patching (for comfort). Arrange expert ophthalmic assessment if there is any question regarding infection.

Corneal foreign body

The commonest eye injury is probably a foreign body on the cornea. The patient complains of a scratching sensation in the eye, and with good light and magnification the foreign body can usually be seen easily.

If it is not immediately obvious, stain the cornea with fluorescein: moisten a fluorescein strip with local anaesthetic and touch the inner surface of the lower eyelid. Ask the patient to blink to spread the dye and then illuminate with the blue filter in the ophthalmoscope. The site of the foreign body will glow bright green.

The foreign body may be adhering to the deep surface of the upper lid, i.e. a subtarsal foreign body. Evert the upper lid and wipe off the foreign body (Box 40.1).

Corneal foreign body removal

- Lie the patient down.
- Instill local anaesthetic drops: two drops every minute for 3 minutes.

Box 40.1 Tarsal eversion

1 Tell the patient to look down, then grasp the lashes and pull down the upper lid.
2 Push down and back on the upper edge of the tarsal plate.
3 Fold the lid margin up and the tarsal plate rolls over.
4 Hold the lid everted by resting a finger on the lid margin.

- Use a focused bright light to illuminate the eye.
- Lift off the foreign body with a cotton-tipped applicator or needle.
- Instill antibiotic drops and apply an eye pad.

It is helpful to use a magnifying lens to facilitate foreign body removal. However, the ideal environment is to remove the foreign body through a slit-lamp.

Instill antibiotic drops (chloramphenicol) every 2 hours until the cornea heals and the eye is comfortable. If the foreign body is hot, for example from using a grindstone, a rust ring may be left in the cornea after its removal. Instill chloramphenicol ointment in the eye four times daily for 2 or 3 days. The rust ring can then be lifted off with a fine needle.

Eye infections

The main defence mechanisms against infection in the eye are the tears, which contain lysozyme, and the corneal epithelium. Once these are breached, an infection can be established and will progress rapidly.

Extraocular infections

Conjunctivitis

Acute conjunctivitis is common, usually due to a staphylococcus and responds rapidly to the instillation of eye drops every 2 hours. The most commonly used antibiotic is chloramphenicol. Even untreated, most acute conjunctivitis resolves in about 3 days.

Trachoma

Of more concern in rural and under-developed communities is trachoma. This recurrent conjunctivitis is caused by the organism *Chlamydia trachomatis*. The organism replicates intracellularly in the conjunctival epithelium. It is a mild infection but after each attack scarring occurs at the site of the follicles in which the organism replicated. After probably 30 or 40 attacks the scarring becomes serious and causes inversion of eyelashes and subsequent damage to the cornea, causing blindness (Figure 40.2).

The control of trachoma requires attention to the following:

- Surgery to the inverted eyelids
- Antibiotic treatment with azithromycin
- Fly eradication, the commonest vector
- Environmental upgrade.

This is the SAFE strategy devised by the World Health Organization. When trachoma is diagnosed, all members of the family are treated with a single dose of azithromycin. Children and young mothers are most commonly infected.

Intraocular infections

The management of intraocular infection follows the principles of management of any infection:

- identify the organism
- treat it with the appropriate antibiotic.

However, this requires specialist assessment and the patient should be referred to an ophthalmologist as soon as possible.

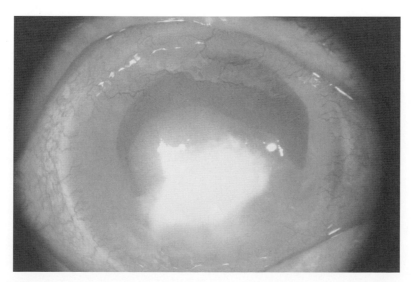

Fig. 40.2 Corneal abscess. The pathological process is visible because of the transparency of ocular structures.

Further reading

Erikitola OO, Shahid SM, Waqar S, Hewick SA. Ocular trauma: classification, management, prognosis. *Br J Hosp Med* 2013;74:C108–11.

Nika B, Wajda B, Calvo C, Durani A (eds) *The Wills Eye Manual: Office and Emergency Room Diagnosis and Treatment of Eye Disease*, 7th edn. Philadelphia: Wolters Kluwer, 2017.

Romaniuk VM. Ocular trauma and other catastrophes. *Emerg Med Clin North Am* 2013;31:399–411.

MCQs

Select the single correct answer to each question. The correct answers can be found in the Answers section at the end of the book.

1 The Snellen visual acuity in a patient is noted to be 6/60 in the right eye and 6/18 in the left eye. Which of the following statements is correct?

  a Snellen acuity in the right eye is better than the left eye

  b the denominator expresses the distance acuity in the tested eye

  c the numerator expresses the near vision in the tested eye

  d Snellen acuity compares a tested eye to a normally seeing eye

2 Which of the following is most likely to be found in a patient with an orbital blow-out fracture?

  a proptosis

  b horizontal diplopia

  c anosmia

  d ptosis

3 The most important aspect of management of chemical burns is:

  a intravenous steroids

  b intensive antibiotic drops

  c intensive irrigation

  d intravenous antibiotics

41 Otorhinolaryngology

Stephen O'Leary[1] and Neil Vallance[2]

[1] University of Melbourne and Royal Victorian Eye and Ear Hospital, Melbourne, Victoria, Australia
[2] Monash University and Department of Otolaryngology, Head and Neck Surgery, Monash Health, Melbourne, Victoria, Australia

Otology

Otologic surgery aims to eradicate aural disease and restore hearing in the ear, or gain surgical access to the skull base. The proximity to the brain, major vessels and the facial nerve demands skill in microsurgery of bone, soft tissues and nerve. Surgical treatment of the hearing apparatus requires a good working knowledge of auditory physiology and pathophysiology.

Surgical anatomy of the ear

The tympanic membrane (TM) and the ossicles (malleus, incus and stapes) collect sound and deliver them to the inner ear (the labyrinth). The space behind the TM is in continuity with a system of air cells extending posteriorly into the mastoid, and together these constitute the middle ear cleft. Aeration of the middle ear cleft is maintained by the eustachian tube (ET), which runs from the nasopharynx to the anterior tympanic cavity (Figure 41.1). The middle ear cleft is lined with respiratory epithelium (mucosa). The external ear canal and external surface of the TM are lined by skin. The facial nerve traverses the middle ear and mastoid.

Chronic otitis media

Chronic otitis media (COM) is an ear disease requiring surgical treatment. It presents as aural discharge with or without hearing loss.

Pathophysiology

Most cases of COM are a consequence of ET dysfunction. The ET's role is to aerate the middle ear cleft (see Figure 41.1). Inadequate aeration of the middle ear leads to negative pressure with respect to the atmosphere behind the eardrum. There is a tendency for the TM to become retracted and the mucosal lining to exude a serous or mucoid discharge. Infection may ensue if bacteria are present in the middle ear cleft, frequently leading to perforation of the TM. In the presence of chronic ET dysfunction, the TM perforation will tend not to heal. An infected discharge follows, associated with chronic changes to the middle ear mucosa (including biofilm) and a low-grade osteitis of the temporal bone.

Indigenous populations, such as the Australian Aborigines or the Inuits in Greenland and Alaska, have a significantly higher prevalence of COM than

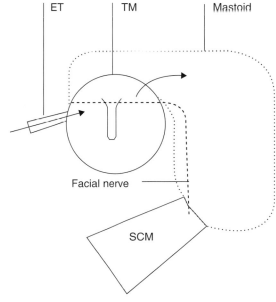

Fig. 41.1 Schematic anatomy of the ear. The sternocleidomastoid muscle attaches to the mastoid tip. The mastoid is a system of air cells within the temporal bone. The arrows depict the flow of air through the eustachian tube into the middle ear and mastoid. ET, eustachian tube; TM, tympanic membrane; SCM, sternocleidomastoid muscle.

Textbook of Surgery, Fourth Edition. Edited by Julian A. Smith, Andrew H. Kaye, Christopher Christophi and Wendy A. Brown.
© 2020 John Wiley & Sons Ltd. Published 2020 by John Wiley & Sons Ltd.

other populations. The reason(s) are not well understood, but contributing factors are thought to include post-nasal colonisation with pathogenic bacteria at a much younger age (often within the first 3 months of life), leading to early onset of otitis media. Socioeconomic disadvantage and overcrowding also contribute.

Cholesteatoma

This is an important manifestation of COM. Acquired cholesteatoma is the invagination of the TM into the middle ear cleft. This occurs where the drum is weakest, usually in its posterosuperior segment. Although causes of cholesteatoma may vary, most often the invagination is secondary to the negative middle ear pressure accompanying ET dysfunction. The invaginated skin continues to desquamate, but the squames become trapped in the retracted pocket of skin. It is at this stage that the retraction pocket is no longer self-cleaning and is, by definition, a cholesteatoma. The desquamated skin within the retraction pocket will usually become infected, with the development of an aural discharge. The cytokines liberated erode surrounding bone, with expansion of the cholesteatoma into the mastoid, the ossicles and/or the labyrinth. Complications of this disease can be serious and include facial nerve palsy, loss of labyrinthine function and intracranial sepsis.

Clinical findings

A history of aural discharge, hearing loss and sometimes otalgia or tinnitus should be expected. Vertigo suggests erosion of the labyrinth and warrants urgent surgical treatment. Non-cholesteatomatous COM is associated with a central perforation of the TM, where the edges of the perforation are visible and bounded by a rim of drum (Figure 41.2a). A marginal perforation is the hallmark of cholesteatoma, where the perforation extends beyond the edge of the drum and 'disappears' behind the posterosuperior wall of the ear canal (Figure 41.2c). The facial nerve should always be examined and the hearing tested clinically and audiometrically. Both ears must be examined. High-resolution CT of the temporal bone helps to define the extent of disease.

Treatment

Cholesteatoma is an absolute indication for surgery, unless the patient is elderly, when regular aural toilet may suffice. COM is a relative indication for

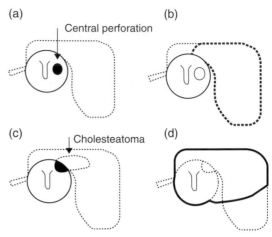

Fig. 41.2 Chronic otitis media and surgical treatment. (a) Chronic otitis media with a central perforation of the tympanic membrane. (b) A canal wall-up mastoidectomy. The mastoid air cells have been removed, as indicated by the thick dashed line. (c) Cholesteatoma presenting as a 'marginal' perforation of the tympanic membrane. The cholesteatoma extends beyond the tympanic membrane into the mastoid. (d) A canal wall-down mastoidectomy. The limits of the mastoid cavity, created by removing the mastoid air cells and taking down the posterior and superior canal walls, is indicated by the thick solid line.

surgery, particularly when medical treatments (such as aural and/or oral antibiotics) and keeping the ear dry have failed to settle recurrent aural discharge. However, the condition of the contralateral ear must be considered. A better hearing ear is a relative contraindication, due to the risk of sensorineural deafness at surgery. Restoration of hearing is a secondary indication for surgery.

The overall aim of surgery is to produce a disease-free and hence non-discharging ear. The surgical principles include the preservation of vital structures, including the facial nerve and inner ear, the eradication of disease and the reconstruction of the TM and hearing. Eradication of disease involves the removal of diseased bone and mucosa, and cholesteatoma if it is present.

The appropriate operative procedure depends on the extent of the disease and the surgeon's preferred operative method, either microscopic or endoscopic. If disease is confined to the middle ear and ET function is only moderately impaired, then grafting the TM (myringoplasty) may be all that is required. If the mastoid is also infected, the classical microscopic approach is exenteration of the mastoid air cell system combined with myringoplasty (a 'canal wall-up' mastoidectomy; Figure 41.2b). The mastoidectomy both removes the disease and reduces the surface area of the middle ear cleft, thus decreasing the work done by a compromised ET. For failed canal wall-up mastoidectomy, especially if there is either persistent ('residual') or recurrent cholesteatoma, a modified radical mastoidectomy is performed. This involves performing a mastoidectomy, removing the posterior and superior (ear) canal walls, and grafting the TM (a 'canal wall-down' mastoidectomy; Figure 41.2d). Following this operation, the mastoid cavity is exteriorised so that it is now part of the external ear and is lined with skin.

The endoscopic approach to surgery for COM provides direct visualisation 'around corners' with angled Hopkins rods, allowing a better view of middle ear structures and more reliable clearance of pockets of cholesteatoma that cannot be seen directly with the microscope. However, unlike microscopic surgery, it has the disadvantage of leaving only one hand free to manipulate surgical instruments. This technique does not require large surgical incisions, so hospitalisation is shorter and recovery may be more comfortable for the patient. It is an option for disease in the middle ear or for cholesteatoma extending as far backwards as the lateral semicircular canal.

Hearing impairment

Pathophysiology

Hearing impairment is classified as either conductive or sensorineural. A conductive loss results from an interruption of sound transmission through the TM and the ossicles. It may arise from an effusion of the middle ear ('glue ear') or a TM perforation. Sound transmission through the ossicular chain may be interrupted if the ossicles are no longer in continuity or if the ossicular chain is fixed. Ossicular discontinuity usually arises from ossicular erosion following COM. The most common cause of ossicular fixation is otosclerosis, where the bone of the labyrinth is abnormal and the stapes footplate becomes fixed to surrounding labyrinthine bone. Sensorineural hearing loss is due to cochlear or, rarely, retrocochlear pathology. The most common causes of sensorineural loss are hereditary, meningitis, ototoxic, trauma and progression of unknown aetiology. In this case, it is thought likely that the hearing loss arises from a combination of environmental exposure(s) and genetic predisposition. A TM perforation will lead to a mild-to-moderate conductive hearing loss (20–30 dB). Ossicular chain discontinuity will lead to an additional 20–30 dB loss. Ossicular chain disruption behind an intact drum leads to a 60-dB hearing loss. A 'mixed' hearing loss has both conductive and sensorineural components.

Treatment

Hearing loss is treated when it impedes an individual's ability to communicate. Surgery is indicated when a hearing aid is not helpful or cannot be worn for medical reasons. For example, occlusion of the external ear canal (by the hearing aid) may cause recurrent otitis externa or persistent aural discharge if there is also a TM perforation. Hearing restoration surgery will also be performed with operations for COM as discussed in the previous section. However, it is usually not possible to reconstruct the ossicular chain if there is a coexistent TM perforation. A better approach is to repair the drum first and perform an ossicular chain reconstruction as a staged procedure. For this reason, ossicular chain reconstruction is usually a second-stage procedure following surgery for COM.

Conductive hearing loss is amenable to surgical treatment. Glue ear may be treated by performing a myringotomy and placing a ventilation tube within the TM. A perforated TM may be grafted (myringoplasty). When the ossicles are disrupted, reconstruction aims to re-establish a stable link between the TM and the stapes footplate. The configuration of the reconstruction depends on which ossicle(s) remain intact. These procedures do not restore anatomical normality, and this is not required to achieve good hearing.

When the middle ear cannot be reconstructed surgically, bone-conducting auditory prostheses are indicated. These devices vibrate the bone behind the ear, and this leads to direct acoustic stimulation of the cochlea. Bone-conducting auditory prostheses have become a preferred method of rehabilitating hearing for children with congenital anomalies of the middle or external ear and are an excellent choice when a hearing aid cannot be worn, or for end-stage COM when ossicular reconstruction is no longer possible.

Cochlear implantation

Severe-to-profound sensorineural hearing loss is characterised by loss of clarity of speech, which is not overcome by the amplification of sound with a hearing aid. Eventually, amplification ceases to aid communication and, under these circumstances, a cochlear implant may be of more benefit. A cochlear implant is also indicated for congenitally deaf children, provided that the operation is performed before the child is 5 years of age. Up until this age a child may learn to comprehend speech with the implant, even though he or she has no previous auditory experience. Children implanted before the age of 3 years may learn to speak. The younger the child at the age of implantation, the better the speech and language outcomes, and it is preferable to implant well before the child's second birthday.

The operation for a cochlear implant involves implanting a prosthesis, the 'receiver–stimulator', which electrically stimulates the auditory nerve within the cochlea. The receiver–stimulator is placed over the parietal bone. Its electrode array passes through the mastoid and middle ear into the cochlea. The receiver–stimulator is entirely subcutaneous. It communicates via a radiofrequency link with an external device called the speech processor. The speech processor translates speech into the pattern of electrical stimulation to be delivered to the auditory nerve.

Cochlear implantation is also considered for unilateral (single-sided) deafness because it is now appreciated that communication in real-life listening conditions, where there is usually competing background noise, is far easier with two working ears rather than one.

Tumours of the ear

The most common type of malignant neoplasm of the ear is a squamous cell carcinoma of the pinna or external ear canal, followed in incidence by melanoma. Symptoms include otalgia, aural discharge or hearing loss if the external ear canal is occluded. Treatment is radical surgical excision and radiotherapy.

Rhinology

Nasal polyps

Nasal polyps are translucent pedunculated swellings arising from nasal and sinus mucosa. They arise from mucosal inflammation, with or without an allergic association, and result in nasal obstruction and discharge. Although these respond (i.e. shrink) in response to oral steroids, they will usually rebound rapidly and surgical excision via an endoscopic approach provides better longer-term control. Nasal polyps have a tendency to recur, so revision surgery is not unusual.

Septal deviation

Deviation of the nasal septum from the midline may be traumatic or congenital. The deviation may involve the cartilaginous or bony septum. It results in turbulence of nasal airflow and hence a sensation of obstruction. Symptomatic septal deviation is treated surgically. The corrective procedure, septoplasty, involves elevating mucosal flaps and removal of the deviated segment of cartilage or bone.

Rhinorrhoea

Rhinorrhea is a clear discharge from the nose. It may arise from allergic rhinitis or be neural in origin when it is termed vasomotor rhinitis. Rarely, a clear discharge from the nose may be cerebrospinal fluid. This is usually post-traumatic and may originate from a breach of the cribriform plate, a paranasal sinus (ethmoid, frontal or sphenoid sinus) or from the middle ear space via the ET. The fluid will test positive for β-transferrin. Surgical repair via an endoscopic approach through the nose or as a combined procedure with neurosurgeons via the anterior cranial fossa will usually be necessary.

Epistaxis

Epistaxis is dealt with in Chapter 77.

Sinusitis

Acute sinusitis is a bacterial infection of the paranasal sinus secondary to obstruction of the sinus ostia. The obstruction is usually due to swelling of the nasal mucosa caused by a virus, but may also follow dental infection or dental work, nasal allergy, facial fractures and barotrauma. It is usually due to aerobic organisms and manifests as facial pain and mucopurulent nasal discharge. Initial medical management requires antibiotics and topical nasal decongestants. Systemic corticosteroids may also be needed to settle a severe attack. Occasionally, drainage of the sinus via an endoscopic antrostomy may be required to remove the pus.

Acute sinusitis can be complicated by spread of the infection through the paper-thin bone (the lamina papyracea) between the ethmoidal sinuses and the orbit. Although this infection is usually extraorbital, it causes proptosis and can if left untreated compromise vision. If there is pus present it must be drained via an endonasal or an external approach, but if less severe intravenous antibiotics may suffice.

Chronic sinusitis may follow poorly treated acute sinusitis or occur in chronic sinus obstruction (e.g. secondary to nasal allergy or polyps). In this situation anaerobic organisms play a significant role. Antibiotic treatment should be tried, but if the infection has been present for more than 3 months functional endoscopic sinus surgery is recommended in order to drain the infection and aerate the sinuses.

Nasal tumours

Benign tumours

Inverted papillomas, squamous papilloma and juvenile angiofibroma may all result in obstruction, sinusitis and bleeding. Diagnosis is made following imaging of the paranasal sinuses (CT or MRI) and, unless a juvenile angiofibroma is suspected, a transnasal biopsy. (Angiofibromas are not biopsied due to a risk of bleeding.) Benign tumours are best treated with surgical excision, performed either transnasally or via an external transfacial approach. Angiofibromas are embolised before surgical excision.

Malignant tumours

Squamous cell carcinoma of the maxillary sinus is the most common paranasal sinus malignancy. The most common cancer of the ethmoid sinus in Australia is adenocarcinoma, which occurs more commonly in people employed in the hardwood industry. Other cancers of the nasal complex include adenoidcystic carcinoma, sinonasal undifferentiated (small cell) carcinoma, transitional carcinoma and malignant melanoma. Diagnosis is made on radiological and histological grounds and treatment involves surgical excision with adjunctive radiation therapy and/or chemotherapy.

Oral cavity, oropharynx and larynx

Tonsil and adenoid disease

The tonsils and adenoids are the commonest areas of infection in the head and neck. They belong to a collection of lymphoid tissue called Waldeyer's ring, which also comprises an aggregate of lymphoid tissue at the base of the tongue called the lingual tonsil and lymphoid tissue around the opening of the ET called the tubal tonsil. The adenoid tissue usually atrophies over the second decade of life and is not a common cause of disease after childhood. Tonsillectomy and adenoidectomy are performed if the tonsils become recurrently infected. In childhood, tonsils and adenoids may become large enough to cause significant obstruction, leading to airway interference and intermittent cessation of breathing overnight (obstructive sleep apnoea). This necessitates removal to re-establish a normal airway and breathing pattern.

Tonsillitis may become complicated by abscess formation in the peritonsillar space, commonly referred to as quinsy. This results in severe pain, toxicity and trismus and usually a large unilateral tonsillar swelling. The abscess must be drained by an incision in the upper half of the tonsil pillar followed by admission to hospital and intravenous antibiotics for several days. In a history of recurrent tonsillitis, this is an indication for a tonsillectomy, usually after the acute abscess has settled down.

Epiglottitis

Epiglottitis is a peculiar and serious disease often affecting children, and occasionally adults. There is acute bacterial inflammation of the epiglottis and supraglottic structures with rapid onset and rapid progression such that the airway may be occluded, with death resulting from acute upper airway obstruction. Intubation in an operating theatre environment is the treatment of choice in both adults and children, with the surgeon standing by to perform urgent surgical access to the airway should intubation fail. After the airway is secure, the problem usually settles rapidly with intravenous antibiotics and, on occasion, steroids. *Haemophilus influenzae* is a common casual organism in the paediatric population. The condition is life-threatening and must be treated urgently.

Benign vocal fold lesions

Vocal nodules are common benign bilateral swellings at the junction of the middle and anterior third of the vocal fold. They result from vocal abuse in children and heavy vocal use and abuse in adults. They may be physiological in heavy voice users, such as singers. There is rarely an indication for surgery as almost all cases will improve or resolve completely with voice therapy and re-education of vocal habits.

Benign cysts and polyps are less common conditions and are usually unilateral and require surgical intervention if the effect on the voice is significant enough for the patient to request intervention. The lesions are removed with microsurgical techniques via a direct laryngoscopy under general anaesthesia.

Reflux commonly causes hoarseness, throat discomfort and a variety of laryngeal conditions resulting from chronic inflammation due to refluxate in the laryngopharynx. Very commonly, heartburn is absent in laryngopharyngeal reflux. The condition responds to anti-reflux measures and medication, including proton pump inhibitors.

Vocal cord paralysis

Loss of vocal fold movement is caused by loss of function of the recurrent laryngeal nerve. The nerve is a branch of the vagus nerve. The left arises in the thorax, looping around the aorta. On the right side it arises higher in the thorax, looping around the right subclavian artery. Both travel in the tracheo-oesophageal groove superiorly to the larynx, where they supply the intrinsic muscles that move the vocal folds. Causes of unilateral paralysis may be tumours of the thyroid or lung or metastatic deposits within mediastinal lymph nodes. Surgical trauma during thyroidectomy may also result in paralysis. However, the commonest cause of paralysis is idiopathic and the commonest nerve affected is the left, probably because of its greater length. The presentation of unilateral paralysis is hoarseness and breathiness. This may improve as the larynx compensates and other muscles assist in phonation. A common misconception is that the intact vocal cord compensates for the palsy, but this is not true, as the functioning vocal fold can never adduct further than the midline. If both vocal folds are paralysed the voice is often normal, but the airway can be severely compromised if the vocal folds both lie well towards the midline. Hence the need to assess vocal fold function prior to thyroidectomy to exclude an asymptomatic old palsy and therefore exercise diligence in protecting the intact nerve.

Diagnosis of the palsy is made by indirect mirror examination or more usually flexible fibre-optic laryngoscopy. A thorough search to exclude tumour, including CT scan from skull base to thorax, must be made. Treatment is required for unilateral palsy if the voice is poor and sufficient time has elapsed (usually 6 months) to exclude spontaneous recovery. Such operations may include medialisation of the vocal fold via laryngeal framework-type surgery or injection of commercially available materials including the patient's own fat lateral to the fold to medialise it. There is no longer any place for Teflon injection of the vocal fold. Bilateral vocal fold paralysis can present as an upper-airway emergency that may require tracheotomy. In the long term, endoscopic laser techniques allow the re-establishment of an airway, often with the preservation of good voice.

Cancer of the head and neck

Cancer of the head and neck is relatively uncommon when compared with the frequency of other, more common tumours such as bowel and breast cancer. Nonetheless, because of the significance of functional impairment and the potential for disfigurement, it is an important management problem. Significant advances have seen improvements in survival and outcomes for patients. These tumours are best treated via a multidisciplinary surgical approach in departments that can make the best use of advances in tumour biology, imaging modalities, radiotherapy and chemotherapy, and conservation and organ preservation techniques. Recent advances in endoscopic laser surgical techniques and transoral robotic surgery have led to an improvement in outcomes and organ preservation for oropharyngeal, laryngeal and hypopharyngeal cancers. Reconstructive techniques and the use of free flaps is well established and continues to provide better outcomes.

Squamous carcinomas of the upper aerodigestive tract

Pathogenesis

Most malignant tumours of the upper aerodigestive tract are squamous cell carcinomas. A significant proportion of these cancers can be attributed to a combination of cigarette and alcohol abuse. Their effects are believed to be synergistic, resulting in widespread changes in the mucosa and the potential for multiple tumours (estimated at 15–20%). Over the last several years human papillomavirus (HPV)-driven cancers have become more common. These cancers are more common in the oropharynx and are usually very responsive to chemoradiotherapy.

Pathology

Most head and neck squamous cancers will metastasise to cervical lymph nodes and this factor bears the most significance in terms of prognosis. It is generally accepted that the survival rate of head and neck cancer is halved when a positive neck node is present. Head and neck cancer surgeons refer to neck nodes in terms of different levels, I through V. Level I comprises the uppermost nodes in the submental and submandibular triangles. Levels II, III and IV correspond to the upper, middle and lower cervical lymph nodes, respectively, and level V represents the nodes in the posterior triangle. On this basis, it is now possible to tailor neck dissection according to the site of primary tumour and the levels of nodes involved. Neck dissections are now almost exclusively of a selective nature rather than the older-style radical neck dissection, which sacrificed the sternomastoid muscle, the internal jugular vein and the accessory nerve. It is rare now to sacrifice the accessory nerve in neck dissection as this often produces significant morbidity, with denervation of the trapezius muscle and resulting shoulder droop. Prognostic variables include the T stage of the primary tumour (Table 41.1) and the N stage of

Table 41.1 Tumour staging in squamous carcinoma.

Regional lymph nodes

Nx	Regional lymph nodes cannot be assessed
N0	No regional lymph node metastasis
N1	Metastasis in a single ipsilateral lymph node, 3 cm or less at greatest dimension
N2a	Metastasis in single ipsilateral lymph node, >3 cm but not more than 6 cm at greatest dimension
N2b	Metastasis in multiple ipsilateral lymph nodes, none more than 6 cm at greatest dimension
N2c	Metastasis in contralateral lymph nodes, none more than 6 cm at greatest dimension
N3	Metastasis in lymph node >6 cm at greatest dimension

Primary tumour

Tx	Primary tumour cannot be assessed
T0	No evidence of primary tumour
Tis	Carcinoma *in situ*
T1	Tumour 2 cm or less at greatest dimension
T2	Tumour >2 cm but not more than 4 cm at greatest dimension
T3	Tumour >4 cm at greatest dimension
T4	Tumour invades adjacent structures

the neck. Usually the greater the T or N stage, the poorer the prognosis. Other poor prognostic factors are the presence of extracapsular spread in cervical lymph nodes; perineural, lymphatic and vascular invasion; and increased depth of tumour invasion. The differentiation of the primary cancer does not appear to have prognostic significance, with the possible exception of the oral tongue.

Clinical presentation and investigation

Clinical presentation is dependent on the anatomical subsite of the disease. In the oral cavity and the oropharynx, for example, common symptoms include a mass or an ulcer with pain and difficulties with speech and swallowing. Painful swallowing (odynophagia) is a serious symptom which indicates the presence of a cancer until otherwise proven. Likewise, pain referred to the ear is a serious symptom. Vocal fold cancers frequently present with hoarseness that does not resolve with adequate treatment after 2 or 3 weeks. Cancers in the hypopharynx may be more subtle in presentation and can reach a significant size before the primary tumour presents problems for the patient. These lesions frequently present with a painless enlarging lump in the neck which represents a metastatic node.

Thorough clinical evaluation is essential to exclude a cancer in a site not readily seen, such as the tongue base or hypopharynx. Thorough endoscopic evaluation and fine-needle aspiration cytology of suspicious nodes (which has not been found to cause recurrent neck disease) should be used to investigate these lesions before open biopsy or surgical removal.

Modern CT and MRI are invaluable for the accurate assessment and staging of head and neck cancer. It is well demonstrated that they are more sensitive than clinical examination in detecting metastatic neck disease. CT scanning is beneficial in the detection of bone disease and spread of laryngeal disease beyond the laryngeal framework. MRI is particularly useful for investigation of the tongue and soft-tissue extension of disease, including involvement of the nerves and brain.

The relatively new technique of positron emission tomography (PET) allows imaging of the metabolic behaviour of the tumour rather than an anatomical mass. However, merging these biological images with CT scans allows a more anatomical perspective.

Guidelines for diagnostic and preoperative work-up of a patient with a suspected head and neck malignancy are given in Box 41.1.

Treatment

The goals of treatment in head and neck cancer are:
- eradication of disease
- preservation or restoration of function, particularly speech and swallowing
- minimal cosmetic deformity.
  The following general points are relevant.
- For early disease, particularly in the larynx, cure rates of radiotherapy and surgery are equivalent.

Box 41.1 Diagnostic and preoperative work-up of the patient with head and neck squamous carcinoma

1 Confirm diagnosis by biopsy of primary lesion and/or fine-needle aspiration cytology of cervical nodes
2 Clinical staging of disease by TNM classification
3 Investigate with CT, MRI or PET for selected cases
4 Endoscopic evaluation under anaesthesia for more accurate staging and to exclude a second primary
5 For cervical node with unknown primary, full endoscopic evaluation and, if no primary found, proceed to open biopsy with frozen section and neck dissection if squamous cell carcinoma confirmed

- Chemotherapy on its own has little role to play in the treatment of squamous cell cancer of the head and neck other than in a palliative sense but is used as an adjunct to the use of radiotherapy.
- The emphasis in treatment is now on organ preservation, particularly with respect to the larynx. There has been a shift away from radical surgery, such as total laryngectomy, to the use of protocols involving chemoradiation for relatively advanced tumours. Partial laryngectomy, particularly with endoscopic laser surgery, often provides organ sparing and successful outcomes. It should be remembered, however, that the preservation of a crippled larynx which does not function and aspirates is a poor outcome.
- The combination of surgery and radiotherapy in advanced disease is superior to single-modality therapy.
- In planning treatment, it is vital to consider general patient factors such as general health and medical condition, fitness for surgery or a challenging course of radiation, and nutritional status, which is often poor in these patients and may need attention before treatment.

Management of the primary tumour

Surgical resection is a better option in the following situations.

- Small tumours where the surgical defect is minimal and functional restoration assured.
- Large tumours with spread beyond the primary site to involve bone or cartilage. These tumours rarely, if ever, respond to radial radiotherapy. Modern reconstructive techniques and the use of free flaps have allowed many of these tumours to be successfully resected and reconstructed in a single-stage procedure. This has allowed a more rapid transition to postoperative radiotherapy, which is essential if all the benefits of multimodality therapy are to be achieved.
- Salvage of lesions unresponsive to or recurrent after radiotherapy. Reconstructive techniques involving free flaps elicit a better blood supply to the area and have allowed improved healing in previously irradiated tissues where the blood supply has been diminished by radiation.
- Endolaryngeal and hypopharyngeal disease is now being successfully treated with endoscopic laser techniques or transoral robotic surgery where previously external partial procedures, and even total laryngectomy, may have been considered.

Radiotherapy is considered for the following situations.

- As a single-modality treatment in early lesions. This was traditionally the case with small tumours of the true vocal fold. Cure rates are excellent, as are functional outcomes. The disadvantage is a 5-week course of therapy. Consequently, laser surgery is tending to replace radiotherapy for these lesions as the outcomes are similar and the treatment involves only a 1- or 2-day stay in hospital.
- In certain advanced hypopharyngeal and laryngeal cancers, where combined radiotherapy and chemotherapy offers organ preservation and good locoregional control without surgery.
- For palliation of recurrent disease or advanced disease not suitable for surgery or organ preservation through chemoradiotherapy.
- Postoperatively and, less commonly, preoperatively in disease where it is felt prudent to use multimodality therapy. Whether radiation is used preoperatively or postoperatively is often determined by the accepted practices in individual cancer treatment units.
- For HPV-driven oropharyngeal cancers in combination with chemotherapy where response rates are often very good.

Radiation is delivered by external beam in dedicated radiotherapy units. Radiation affects both normal tissue and cancer tissue, and the salivary glands and oral mucosa are particularly affected. Dryness is a common post-radiotherapy complaint. The mandible is commonly devascularised following radiotherapy and very prone to osteomyelitis and necrosis, secondary to dental sepsis. Dental consultation and management of the teeth are therefore essential if the jaw is to be involved in the radiotherapy field.

Management of the neck

Metastatic disease in the neck may be obvious or occult at presentation. Secondary neck disease is a significant factor in determining prognosis and, in general, the presence of neck disease lowers the survival by some 50%. Neck disease is often treated by neck dissection unless associated with HPV-driven oropharyngeal cancers, where responses to chemoradiotherapy alone are often very good. Accepted poor prognostic indicators with neck disease include multiple levels of nodes involved or spread of tumour beyond the capsule of the lymph node on pathology assessment. In these instances, postoperative radiotherapy is always used in the neck.

The approach to neck dissection has changed over the years. The mainstay in the past was the so-called radial neck dissection. It is now apparent that similar regional control of disease can be achieved by a more selective approach. These modified or selective neck dissections remove node levels which are most likely to contain metastatic disease from the associated primary. Consequently, fewer than the five levels of nodes are removed and, inherent in this approach, is the preservation of various non-lymphatic tissues, including the spinal accessory nerve, internal jugular vein and sternomastoid muscle. This has led to better functional outcomes with no sacrifice of disease control.

Tumours of the nasal cavity and paranasal sinuses

These are rare tumours. It is worth noting that a significant aetiological factor is wood-dust. People with a long history of wood-dust exposure (cabinet makers, sawmill operators) are usually common among patients diagnosed with ethmoid cancer. This is usually an adenocarcinoma. Efforts have been made to make the woodworking industry aware of this danger.

Presentation depends on the anatomical subsite but, unfortunately, tumours are often very advanced at diagnosis. It is not unusual to find orbital and anterior cranial fossa involvement on CT and MRI scanning.

The usual treatment principle is surgery combined with postoperative radiotherapy. The prognosis of these cancers is poor, usually because of the advanced state of disease at diagnosis and the proximity of the anterior cranial fossa.

Nasopharyngeal carcinoma

Nasopharyngeal cancer is the commonest tumour seen in certain Asian countries (southern China and Southeast Asian countries with Chinese populations). In Hong Kong and China, it accounts for about 20% of all malignancies. In southern China, it comprises approximately 50% of all head and neck cancers.

Pathology

The nasopharynx is the space behind the nasal cavity and above the oropharynx. The mucosa is stratified, ciliated, columnar epithelium, with a large aggregate of lymphoid tissue forming part of Waldeyer's ring.

Nasopharyngeal cancer is classified according to the World Health Organization classification. There are three types.
- Type 1: keratinising squamous carcinoma.
- Type 2: non-keratinising poorly differentiated carcinoma.
- Type 3: undifferentiated carcinoma.

Type 3 is by far the more common subtype in endemic Asian areas. Type 1 is more common in developed countries.

Aetiology

Epstein–Barr virus is implicated in the pathogenesis of nasopharyngeal carcinoma. An elevation of viral titres can precede the onset of disease. Titres are useful as tumour markers following treatment. Genetic markers have also been investigated because of the ethnic predilection of the tumour. An increased incidence is seen in patients with certain major histocompatibility complex (HLA) profiles. The ingestion of preserved foods, especially salted fish, duck eggs and salted mustard green, have also been implicated in nasopharyngeal cancer.

Presentation and management

Nasopharyngeal cancer often presents late and frequently as a lump in the neck. It is a very infiltrative cancer with often very little in the way of mucosal changes. It frequently invades the base of the skull, causing cranial nerve involvement and palsies. It is one of the few cancers of the head and neck with a predilection to distant metastases, with the bone, lung and liver the preferred sites. MRI is the investigation of choice and, universally, radiotherapy with concomitant chemotherapy is the treatment of choice. The tumour is usually radiosensitive and because of the inaccessibility of the site surgery with clear margins is usually not possible. Neck nodes are always irradiated with the primary site.

Further reading

Chan Y, Goddard JC (eds) *KJ Lee's Essential Otolaryngology Head and Neck Surgery*, 11th edn. New York: McGraw Hill Education, 2016.

Probst R, Grevers G, Iro H (eds) *Basic Otorhinolaryngology: A Step by Step Learning Guide*, 2nd edn. Stuttgart: Georg Thieme Verlag, 2018.

Wackym PA, Snow JB (eds) *Ballenger's Otorhinolaryngology Head and Neck Surgery*, 18th edn. Shelton, CT: People's Medical Publishing House, 2016.

MCQs

Select the single correct answer to each question. The correct answers can be found in the Answers section at the end of the book.

1 Which modality of treatment is most useful for nasopharyngeal carcinoma?
   a chemotherapy
   b radiotherapy
   c surgery
   d immunotherapy
   e hormonal therapy

2 Which of the following statements concerning nasopharyngeal carcinoma is *incorrect*?
  a keratinising squamous cell carcinoma is most common in developed countries
  b examination of the nasopharynx is usually positive
  c in 90% of patients, cervical nodes are involved
  d there are known aetiological factors
  e the tumour tends to infiltrate widely

3 Which of the following statements concerning parotid gland tumours is *incorrect*?
  a a cystic lesion in the lower pole is likely to be benign
  b a long-standing tumour that enlarges and becomes painful suggests malignancy
  c bilateral tumours in elderly men are usually benign
  d facial nerve palsy suggests malignant disease
  e needle aspiration cytology of parotid tumours is contraindicated

42 Tumours of the head and neck

Rodney T. Judson

University of Melbourne and Royal Melbourne Hospital, Melbourne, Victoria, Australia

Introduction

The concentration of anatomical structures and the rich traversing lymphatic system, bearing drainage from all parts of the body, explains the diversity of primary and secondary tumours found in the head and neck region. Exposure of the skin to ultraviolet B radiation results in 85–90% of cutaneous carcinomas, the most common human malignancy occurring in the head and neck area. Excluding cutaneous tumours, 90% of head and neck tumours are squamous cell carcinomas arising from the epithelium of the upper aerodigestive tract. These tumours predominantly result from carcinogens released while smoking or chewing tobacco or are secondary to infection with human papillomavirus (HPV). Primary tumours, malignant and benign, can arise from all other structures – glandular, vascular, lymphatic, neural, muscular, bony or connective tissue.

Metastatic tumours to the head and neck are predominantly due to lymphatic spread. Metastatic lymph nodes characteristically firm to hard and matted and which are confined to the upper third of the neck are most commonly the result of tumour spread from a primary squamous carcinoma of the upper aerodigestive tract. Metastatic lymph nodes confined to the lower third of the neck are less commonly from an aerodigestive tract origin and more likely from primary sites such as skin, thyroid or a malignant focus below the clavicle. Rare blood-borne metastases are seen in the parotid gland from colon, kidney, breast and lung and in the thyroid from lung and kidney.

The common mode of presentation of head and neck tumours is that of a painless neck mass or swelling. The approach to solving the problem of a neck swelling is dealt with in detail in Chapter 70.

An understanding of the characteristic features of the common head and neck tumours and of the anatomy of the region should guide the clinician as to the likely diagnosis based on clinical assessment (Table 42.1). However, treatment planning requires a detailed assessment including endoscopy, accurate anatomical localisation with CT or MRI and pathological appraisal utilising the least invasive technique applicable. Fine-needle aspiration cytology, preferably ultrasound guided, provides diagnostic material. Core biopsy or carefully considered open biopsy may be required if cytology is inconclusive.

Characteristics of common tumours

Squamous cell carcinoma

The commonest head and neck malignancy is squamous cell carcinoma (SCC) arising from the upper aerodigestive tract. Full details of this problem are covered in Chapter 41.

Cutaneous squamous cell carcinoma

The lips, forehead and ear are the commonest sites for SCC of the head and neck due to their exposure to sunlight. Lesions vary from an area of crusting through to ulceration and induration. SCC of the upper lip has a higher propensity for lymph node metastasis than SCC arising at other sites. SCC of the temple and ear may metastasise to the pre-auricular intraparotid lymph nodes. Such metastasis may appear some time following successful local excision of the primary tumour. Involvement of the facial nerve from intraparotid metastases carries a very poor prognosis. Metastatic lymph nodes from a cutaneous SCC, like those from an aerodigestive tract origin, often undergo cystic degeneration. Rapid growth, redness of the overlying skin and clinical fluctuance can lead to the mistaken diagnosis of a suppurating lymph node. Thorough clinical assessment, noting the absence of pain and the presence or history of a primary lesion coupled with

Textbook of Surgery, Fourth Edition. Edited by Julian A. Smith, Andrew H. Kaye, Christopher Christophi and Wendy A. Brown.
© 2020 John Wiley & Sons Ltd. Published 2020 by John Wiley & Sons Ltd.

Table 42.1 Tumours of the head and neck.

Tissue of origin	Benign/malignant	Tumour type	Clinical site	Common clinical feature
Upper aerodigestive tract mucosa	Benign	Squamous papilloma	Oral cavity mucosa	Solitary papillary lesion
	Malignant	Carcinoma *in situ*	Oral cavity larynx/pharynx	White or red mucosal patch
		Squamous cell carcinoma	Mucosa of upper aerodigestive tract	Ulcerated infiltrative lesion with raised edges
		Lymphoepithelial carcinoma	Nasopharynx	Ulcerated lesion, frequent nodal metastases, nasal symptoms
Salivary gland	Benign	Pleomorphic adenoma	Parotid commonest	Painless slow-growing firm mass
		Oncocytic tumour (Warthin's tumour)	Parotid grand	Soft to firm, occasionally bilateral, mass
	Malignant	Mucoepidermoid carcinoma	Parotid commonest	Slow-growing firm mass
		Adenoid cystic	Minor salivary glands commonest	Slow-growing submucosal nodule in the upper aerodigestive tract
		Acinic cell tumour	Parotid gland	Slow-growing nodule
		Adenocarcinoma	Minor salivary gland	Submucosal lump
Thyroid	Benign	Follicular adenoma	Thyroid	Slow-growing smooth thyroid nodule
		Hurtle cell adenoma	Thyroid	Slow-growing smooth thyroid nodule
	Malignant	Papillary carcinoma	Thyroid gland ± nodes	Slow-growing nodule; 50% of children have associated nodal metastases
		Follicular carcinoma	Thyroid	Slow-growing smooth thyroid nodule
		Anaplastic carcinoma	Thyroid	Rapidly growing infiltrating mass often arising within a pre-existing goitre
		Medullary carcinoma	Thyroid ± nodes	Firm thyroid nodule, may be associated with multiple endocrine adenoma syndrome
Parathyroid cells	Benign	Parathyroid adenoma	Parathyroid glands (impalpable)	Commonest cause of primary hyperparathyroidism
	Malignant	Parathyroid carcinoma	Parathyroid ± nodes	Progressive hyperparathyroidism, nodule may be palpable
Neuroendocrine	Benign	Paraganglionoma	Carotid body / Glomus jugulare / Glomus intravagale	Mass in region of upper carotid sheath / Occasional symptoms resulting from noradrenaline secretion
	Malignant	Olfactory neuroblastoma	Olfactory mucosa in nasal vault	Bimodal age distribution occurring in adolescents and adults. Epistaxis and nasal obstruction

Tissue	Benign/Malignant	Tumour	Location	Clinical features
Adipose	Benign	Lipoma	Commonest in subcutaneous layer	Mobile superficial soft mass
	Malignant	Liposarcoma	Neck, larynx, pharynx	Rare head and neck tumour. Occurs in elderly patients
Vascular	Benign	Haemangioma	Face, scalp, neck	Seen in childhood. Compressible red to purple mass
		Lymphangioma	Neck	Soft, occasionally translucent neck mass in children
	Malignant	Angiosarcoma	Skin of scalp or face	Ulcerating cutaneous nodule occurring in elderly white males
Fibrous tissue	Benign	Fibromatosis	Commonly in neck	Slow-growing mass in young females
		Dermatofibroma	Skin	Small plaque in skin
	Malignant	Fibrosarcoma	Face, neck, scalp and paranasal sinus	Painless growing mass in adults
		Malignant fibrous histiocytoma	Deep tissues of head and neck	Infiltrating mass in elderly males. Commonest post-irradiation tumour
Neural tissue	Benign	Schwannoma	Cranial nerves VII (rare), VIII, IX, X, XI and XII	Lateral neck mass
		Neurofibroma	Peripheral nerve sheaths	Isolated subcutaneous neck nodule, or multiple nodules and large plexiform benign neuromas in familial neurofibromatosis
	Malignant	Malignant schwannoma	Cranial and cervical nerve roots	Fixed mass, metastases possible
Muscle cell	Malignant	Rhabdomyosarcoma	Orbit, nasal cavity and paranasal sinuses	Commonest soft tissue sarcoma seen in children
Bone	Benign	Osteoma	Bony skeleton of face	Smooth mass occurring in paranasal sinuses, multiple osteomas associated with Gardner's syndrome
	Malignant	Osteosarcoma	Mandible or maxilla	Painless enlarging bony swelling
Skin	Malignant	Squamous cell carcinoma	Sun-exposed skin	Crusting ulcerating lesion
		Basal cell carcinoma	Skin of central face	Translucent nodular lesion. Rarely a deeply ulcerating or erosive lesion
		Malignant melanoma	Skin of face, mucosa of nasal cavity	Pigmented skin lesion or polypoid nasal mass
Lymphoid tissue	Malignant	Lymphoma	Lymphatic tissue, salivary glands, thyroid	Rubbery, discrete, multiple neck nodes
Dental tissue	Benign	Ameloblastoma, Squamous ontogenic tumour, Ondontoma, Ondontogenic fibroma	Usually intra-osseous but may involve the gingiva	Expanding mass arising in association with mandible. Rarely malignant

aspiration cytology, should avert the disaster of inappropriate incisional drainage. Management of cutaneous SCCs involves full clinical assessment of the tumour and draining lymph nodes aided by fine-cut CT scanning if deep tissue or nodal involvement is suspected. Localised small lesions are cured by excision with clear surgical margins. Larger lesions may necessitate extensive surgical resection involving underlying tissues and a planned lymph node clearance. Elaborate reconstructive procedures may be necessary, especially for areas of the face to restore function and attain acceptable cosmesis. Cutaneous SCCs are radiosensitive. Radiotherapy as primary treatment, owing to its protracted treatment time, is reserved for small primary tumours in difficult anatomical sites. Radiotherapy is used as adjuvant therapy postoperatively in the management of advanced infiltrative tumours, especially with multiple lymph node metastases or perineural tumour spread.

Cutaneous basal cell carcinoma

The most common site for basal cell carcinoma of the head and neck is the central face. The most common clinical variant is a translucent nodule made clinically more apparent by stretching of the skin around the lesion. Most tumours run a slow protracted course and nodal metastases are rare. Tumours in areas of embryonal fusion lines may burrow deeply, making surgical clearance difficult. Local surgical excision is the usual form of treatment.

Salivary gland tumours

Salivary tissue is found not only in the three pairs of major salivary glands (parotid, submandibular and sublingual glands) but also in small submucosal glands known as the minor salivary glands, which are scattered throughout the upper aerodigestive tract. The parotid glands are host to a variety of tumours both benign and malignant, primary and secondary.

Anatomy

The parotid glands, so named because of their anatomical proximity to the ear, are the largest salivary glands and produce a high volume of serous saliva. The most important anatomical relationship of the parotid gland is with the facial nerve. This enters the posteromedial aspect of the gland as a single trunk and divides within its substance to emerge at the anterior border as the five main branches. In so doing, the facial nerve, for descriptive purposes, divides the gland into the larger superficial lobe covered by skin, platysma in part and parotid fascia, and the smaller deep lobe, which lies in the parapharyngeal space and through which passes the retromandibular vein and external carotid artery. Saliva drains from the gland via the parotid duct, which crosses the masseter muscle and enters the buccal cavity opposite the upper second molar teeth.

The submandibular glands lie close to the inner aspect of the mandible lying on the mylohyoid muscle. The larger superficial lobe is covered by skin, platysma and deep cervical fascia, with the mandibular branch of the facial nerve crossing its upper border on its way to supplying the depressor anguli oris. The posterior aspect of the submandibular gland is wrapped around the posterior-free border of the mylohyoid muscle, and the deep lobe of the gland passes forward deep to the mylohyoid lying on the hypoglossus muscle. The submandibular duct drains from the deep lobe, running a long course in the floor of the mouth to open at a papilla in the anterior floor of the mouth just lateral to the lingual frenulum. The deep lobe of the gland and the duct are closely related to the lingual nerve, which may be involved in pathological processes and damaged during surgical treatment of the gland. The deep lobe is inferolaterally related to the mylohyoid and supramedially covered only by the oral mucosa in the floor of the mouth, thus being easily assessed clinically by bimanual palpation. Using the gloved left index finger placed in the floor of the mouth and the right fingers applied externally, submandibular glandular swelling may be differentiated from lymph node swellings.

The sublingual glands, predominantly mucus secreting, lie submucosally in the anterior floor of the mouth, supported by the mylohyoid muscles. These glands drain by multiple small ducts opening directly into the floor of the mouth along the sublingual folds and occasionally into the submandibular duct.

Assessment of salivary gland disorders

The diagnosis of salivary pathology can be determined in a high proportion of cases by a thorough history, clinical examination and the judicious use of special tests.

Clinical history

A history of a slowly growing lump suggests a benign tumour. The rapid growth of a lump with the development of pain would strongly suggest a malignant process.

Clinical examination

Clinical examination, including intraoral and manual examination noting the site, size, shape, texture, tenderness, fixation, involvement of surrounding anatomical structures and the state of the regional lymph nodes, should not only define involvement of the salivary gland but also suggest the most likely pathological process. Deep lobe parotid masses may be detected by a diffuse bulge in the root of the soft palate or tonsillar fossa region and also may be palpable manually. Facial nerve function must be assessed with all parotid lesions. Tongue sensation should be tested in the presence of submandibular problems.

Special tests

Computed tomography

Computed tomography (CT) scans are useful for clarifying anatomical detail and detecting impalpable lymph node metastases in suspected malignant processes.

Magnetic resonance imaging

Magnetic resonance imaging (MRI) is indicated if cranial nerve involvement is suspected in malignant processes, especially those involving the parotid gland.

Fine-needle aspiration cytology

Cytological assessment of clinically suspected tumours of the salivary glands produces useful information in treatment planning. This is a safe procedure that is not associated with tumour dissemination or seeding.

Parotid tumours

The parotid gland is not only the commonest site of primary salivary neoplasms but is also affected by a wide variety of infiltrative and inflammatory processes. From a clinical point of view, it is easier to consider the presentation of either diffuse parotid swelling or a mass within the region of the parotid.

Any mass arising within the region of the parotid (i.e. from the zygomatic arch superiorly, the upper neck inferiorly, the anterior border of the masseter anteriorly and the mastoid process posteriorly) should be suspected as arising from within the parotid gland and treated accordingly. An isolated mass within the parotid is most commonly due to a parotid tumour; 80% of all salivary tumours occur within the parotid gland, and approximately 80% of parotid tumours are benign.

Pleomorphic adenoma (mixed salivary tumour)

Approximately 65–75% of mass lesions arising within the parotid gland are benign, slowly growing, firm, smooth, usually asymptomatic tumours called pleomorphic adenoma. It is so named because of its histological appearance of a variable mix of glandular and stromal elements, both of which are thought to arise from myoepithelial cells. While the peak incidence is in the fifth decade with a slight female preponderance, this tumour can occur from childhood to old age. Malignant transformation is uncommon and rarely reported in those tumours present for less than 10 years. While initially a smooth lump, with time multiple bosselations may develop. Rapid growth with pain and facial nerve involvement are the hallmark of advanced malignant change. Given the relentless growth pattern, the chance of malignant change and the inability to differentiate this benign tumour clinically from slow-growing malignant parotid tumours, all parotid tumours are best treated by complete surgical excision.

Usually no preoperative investigation is necessary after establishing that the mass is mobile within the parotid gland. Cytology may help treatment planning by deciding the urgency and timing of surgery. Radiological assessment with CT scanning is only necessary when malignancy is suspected. Treatment consists of excision of the lesion with an intact capsule and preservation of the facial nerve. Incomplete excision or capsular rupture at the time of excision predisposes to local recurrence, which may be multinodular and exceedingly difficult to eradicate. Complete excision is associated with a very low local recurrence rate (usually <2%). The surgical technique involves identification of the main trunk of the facial nerve, which is then traced through the gland while the tumour with the surrounding parotid tissue is excised. This is known as a superficial parotidectomy. For deep tumours, the superficial lobe is excised first. The facial nerve and branches are then fully mobilised to allow removal of the deep lobe, either between or below the facial nerve. With careful surgical technique, the risk of permanent facial damage is low, but some degree of temporary facial weakness due to neuropraxia is not uncommon.

Adenolymphoma (Warthin's tumour)

Approximately 6–10% of parotid masses are due to a benign softer tumour, more commonly found in males and arising in the inferior pole of the parotid, called an adenolymphoma. This tumour is so called because of the dense lymphocytic infiltration. The exact origin of this lesion is uncertain. Approximately 10% of cases are bilateral. The cytological picture is usually diagnostic. Surgical excision in the form of parotidectomy is usually recommended, except in the frail and elderly, in whom clinical observation may be more appropriate.

Malignant parotid tumour

Approximately 15–20% of parotid tumours are malignant. In Australia, the most common malignancy involving the parotid is metastatic SCC from a skin primary arising in the head and neck region. Such tumours tend to spread to intraparotid lymph nodes. These lesions are often characterised by rapid growth due to tumour necrosis producing a cystic lesion within the parotid. Treatment of metastatic SCCs involves parotid resection, often in association with a neck dissection and postoperative radiotherapy. The parotid is uncommonly the site of metastases from other tumours, but kidney, thyroid, lung and breast cancers may all spread to the parotid and mimic primary parotid tumours.

Primary parotid malignancies
MUCOEPIDERMOID CARCINOMA
The most common primary malignancy of the parotid is mucoepidermoid carcinoma, which can occur from childhood onwards, with a peak incidence in the fifth to sixth decades. Approximately 75% of mucoepidermoid carcinomas are of low-grade histological type and present with a slow-growing parotid mass. High-grade tumours have a more rapid growth pattern and a poorer prognosis. Lymph node metastasis is uncommon in low-grade tumours.

ADENOID CYSTIC CARCINOMA
Adenoid cystic carcinoma, formerly known as cylindroma, also presents with a slow-growing asymptomatic parotid mass. These tumours are characterised by early perineural spread and have a propensity for late recurrence, often to bone or lung, even up to 20 years following an apparent cure.

ACINIC CELL TUMOUR
Acinic cell tumour, in which some cells demonstrate differentiation towards acinar cells, was once thought to be a benign adenoma but has been reclassified as a malignant carcinoma with a more common low-grade behaviour. These tumours are more common in females.

MALIGNANT PLEOMORPHIC ADENOMA
Malignant pleomorphic adenoma is a more aggressive tumour that can arise either *de novo* or from a pre-existing pleomorphic tumour.

ADENOCARCINOMA
Adenocarcinoma, otherwise unspecified, may also arise in the parotid and displays a more aggressive growth pattern.

Treatment of malignant parotid tumours
Treatment decisions are based on the biological and histological features of the tumour. Slow-growing, clinically discrete, low-grade lesions are usually cured by complete surgical excision with sparing of the facial nerve. For those tumours demonstrating more aggressive histological features, parotidectomy with facial nerve sparing may be followed by radiotherapy. Clinically aggressive tumours with facial nerve involvement will require radical surgery with sacrifice of the facial nerve and radiotherapy. Primary nerve grafting using the sural nerve if possible is performed. Lymph node dissection is usually only performed for clinically or radiographically detected nodal metastasis.

Submandibular tumours

Unlike the parotid gland, tumours of the submandibular gland are relatively uncommon. However, a higher proportion (approximately 40%) of submandibular tumours are malignant. Pleomorphic adenoma is the most common tumour affecting the gland. As with the parotid, most submandibular tumours present as slow-growing asymptomatic lumps. The diagnosis is usually suspected clinically and based on bimanual palpation. Differentiation from submandibular lymph node pathology can usually be confirmed by aspiration cytology. Submandibular tumours are treated by total gland excision. Malignant lesions with local spread beyond the submandibular gland may require sacrifice of the underlying lingual and hypoglossal nerves followed by radiotherapy to effect a cure.

Sublingual tumours

Primary tumours of the sublingual gland are rare, of which 60% are malignant.

Paraganglionomas

The extra-adrenal paraganglia of neural crest-derived cells can be the site of tumours known as paraganglionomas. These, usually benign, tumours may release neurotransmitters and produce intermittent hypertension and facial flushing. Tumours are named according to the neurovascular structure with which they are associated. The common sites for these uncommon tumours are the carotid body, the jugular bulb and the vagus nerve. Whilst most tumours occur sporadically, 10% represent an autosomal dominant inherited condition often associated with multiple paraganglionomas.

Carotid body tumour

The carotid body paraganglion is a chemoreceptor situated in the adventitia of the carotid bifurcation. Tumours present with a slowly growing, painless, smooth, firm, deep, lateral upper neck mass with limited supero-inferior mobility. Transmitted pulsation may be evident but tumours, although vascular, are not truly pulsatile. The intense contrast enhancement on CT scanning with splaying of the carotid bifurcation and the typical clinical presentation are usually diagnostic. Surgical excision in the sub-adventitial plane with preservation of the carotid vessels is curative for benign small tumours. Occasionally, vascular reconstruction may be necessary for excision of larger and malignant tumours.

Glomus jugulare

Glomus jugulare tumours arise from the jugular bulb at the skull base. These deeply placed tumours are not clinically apparent until their growth impinges on surrounding cranial nerves IX, X, XI and XII or the internal auditory canal. Presenting symptoms include tinnitus, hearing loss and voice and swallowing problems. If bone erosion of the hypotympanum occurs, a vascular mass may be clinically apparent medial to an intact tympanic membrane. A combination of contrast-enhanced CT and MRI should demonstrate the degree of bony erosion and the relationship of the tumour to the surrounding cranial nerves. The optimal treatment of these tumours is unresolved. Complete surgical excision with sparing of the facial and lower cranial nerves may be difficult to achieve. Post-surgical recurrent and persistent disease (7 and 8%, respectively) are usually reported. Radiotherapy leading to tumour fibrosis produces similar imperfect results and carries its own morbidity.

Glomus intravagale

Glomus intravagale tumours arise from the paraganglionic tissue within the perineurium of the vagus nerve. These tumours are usually situated at the level of the inferior vagal ganglion. The usual clinical presentation is that of a neck mass near the origin of the sternocleidomastoid muscle with an associated vocal cord palsy. Multiple cranial nerve neuropathies may develop with progressive tumour growth. Contrast CT scanning demonstrates a vascular tumour within the carotid sheath displacing the vessel anteriorly. Other neural tumours of the vagus nerve form the differential diagnosis. Malignant transformation is commoner with glomus intravagale tumours than other parapharyngeal tumours, with pulmonary metastases present in 20% of cases. Treatment consists of either radiotherapy or surgical excision based on an assessment of tumour size and associated cranial nerve involvement. Although surgical resection necessitates sacrifice of the vagus nerve, more than 50% of cases present with an established vocal cord paralysis.

Neural tumours

Schwannomas

Half of the solitary well-encapsulated tumours arising from the Schwann cells of peripheral nerve sheaths occur within the head and neck. Within the head and neck the common nerves of origin are the acoustic nerve and vagus nerve and, less commonly, from cranial nerves VII, IX, XI and XII. These tumours expand the nerve from which they arise and surgical excision with preservation of the nerve can occasionally be achieved. The clinical presentation is of a slow-growing, painless, deep, lateral neck mass with limited mobility. Neurological signs suggesting the nerve of origin are unusual. Radiological examination demonstrates a well-circumscribed mass with some but not marked contrast enhancement. MRI may demonstrate an associated neural structure suggesting the diagnosis. Tumours arising from a cervical nerve root may extend through the intervertebral foramen, producing a dumb-bell tumour with a cervical and spinal component. Aspiration cytology showing the benign spindle cell pattern is usually inconclusive. Treatment is determined by tumour extent and the clinical picture. Slow-growing small tumours in elderly patients may be observed. Tumours arising peripherally in the neck may be separated from the associated nerve with minimal morbidity. Surgical excision of large tumours or those in surgically less accessible sites or contiguous with important neurological structures such as the brachial plexus is associated with the risk of significant neurological morbidity.

Malignant schwannomas

Less than 5% of schwannonas are malignant. These tumours infiltrate locally, may extend intracranially or intravertebrally and can metastasise to the lungs. Aggressive surgical resection is advocated.

Neurofibromas

Neurofibromas are tumours arising from the peripheral nerve sheaths and present commonly as rubbery, fusiform, subcutaneous nodules. Multiple neurofibromas and plexiform neurofibromas are found along with café-au-lait spots and skeletal, CNS and ocular lesions in the autosomal dominant inherited disorder of neurofibromatosis. Surgical excision, with sacrifice of the associated nerve, is definitive treatment for isolated lesions.

Soft tissue sarcomas

Soft tissue sarcomas are tumours of mesenchymal origin that display a wide spectrum of clinical and biological behaviour. Less than 10% of these uncommon tumours arise in the head and neck. A number of genetic abnormalities have been identified. Many of these clonal aberrations have the potential to be applied to the differential diagnosis, in these, often difficult to categorise tumours. Most tumours present as a painless neck mass. Tumours arising from the tissues of the upper aerodigestive tract or the deep tissue spaces may present with a variety of symptoms such as epistaxis, otalgia, visual disturbance or cranial nerve palsies resulting from local tumour infiltration. A thorough clinical examination including intraoral, neurological and endoscopic examination of the upper aerodigestive tract often forms an impression of the extent of the tumour. Fine-cut CT scanning and MRI allow accurate anatomical assessment. Fine-needle aspiration cytology is simple and safe for accessible tumour and is helpful in differentiating sarcomas from other more common tumours but is usually unhelpful in the precise diagnosis of tumour type and grade. Core needle biopsies, radiologically directed, usually provide adequate tissue for pathological assessment. Tumours are staged according to their size and whether superficial or deep and graded histologically based on differentiation, cellularity, density of the stroma, vascularity and degree of necrosis.

Malignant fibrous histiocytoma

Malignant fibrous histiocytoma is the commonest soft tissue sarcoma in adults. Less than 3% involve the head and neck, with the upper aerodigetive tract being favoured and less commonly neck and salivary glands. The 5-year survival for these aggressive tumours is approximately 50%.

Dermatofibrosarcoma protuberans

Dermatofibrosarcoma protuberans, which accounts for approximately 7–15% of soft tissue sarcomas, usually presents as an elevated, firm, solitary, slow-growing, painless mass in the scalp or neck. Metastases are uncommon and an excellent outcome is achieved if histologically clear margins are obtained following local excision.

Angiosarcoma

Over half of all angiosarcomas present as an ulcerating, nodular or diffuse dermal lesion of the scalp or face in elderly white males. They are uncommon tumours, accounting for only 0.1% of all head and neck tumours.

Rhabdomyosarcoma

Rhabdomyosarcoma is the most common paediatric soft tissue sarcoma. This malignant tumour of striated muscle cell origin arises in the nasal cavity, paranasal sinuses, orbit, nasopharynx and middle ear. Early metastases, both regional and distant, are common. Treatment usually involves chemotherapy and irradiation, with an overall survival of approximately 50%.

Bone tumours

Bone tumours may affect the mandible, maxilla or cervical vertebrae, presenting usually as painless swellings. Tumours are classified according to the matrix produced by the tumour cells into chondrosarcomas if cartilaginous, osteosarcomas if osteoid, and fibrosarcomas if they lack a distinct matrix. Surgical excision with clear margins is associated with survival rates of 40–80% independent of the anatomical sites of origin. Distant metastases are infrequent.

Metastatic tumours

The management of neck metastases is outlined in Chapter 70. An understanding of the pattern of lymphatic drainage should direct the clinician to the likely site of the primary lesion. Primary tumours in the tongue base and the tonsil, occasionally small and hidden within the tissue convolutions, may thwart attempts at detection. Melanoma may also present with metastatic nodes in the absence of a detectable primary lesion, which may be amelanotic or have undergone spontaneous regression. Definitive treatment of the primary tumour and neck metastases arising from SCC of the upper aerodigestive tract may be achieved with radiation often followed by surgery. Palliative radiotherapy may have a role in reducing the local devastating effects of uncontrolled neck disease arising from a distant incurable primary tumour.

Further reading

Ridge JA, Mehra R, Lango MN, Galloway T. Head and neck tumors. CancerNetwork. Available at https://www.cancernetwork.com/cancer-management/head-and-neck-tumors

Shah JP, Patel SG (eds) *Cancer of the Head and Neck*. Hamilton, Ontario: BC Decker, 2001, chapters 13–17.

Thompson LD, Bishop JA (eds) *Head and Neck Pathology*, 3rd edn. Philadelphia: Elsevier, 2018.

MCQs

Select the single correct answer to each question. The correct answers can be found in the Answers section at the end of the book.

1 The commonest tumour of the head and neck area is:
   a pleomorphic tumour of the parotid gland
   b squamous cell carcinoma of the larynx
   c squamous cell carcinoma of the skin
   d basal cell carcinoma of the skin
   e carcinoma of the thyroid gland

2 The most common paediatric soft tissue sarcoma in the head and neck area is:
   a angiosarcoma
   b malignant fibrous histiocytoma
   c dermatofibrosarcoma protuberans
   d rhabdomyosarcoma
   e chondrosarcoma

3 The highest propensity for lymph node metastasis occurs in squamous cell carcinoma of the:
   a ear
   b scalp
   c upper lip
   d nose
   e lower lip

Section 8
Hernias

43 Hernias

Roger Berry[1] and David M.A. Francis[2]

[1] Monash University and Monash Health, Melbourne, Victoria, Australia
[2] Department of Urology, Royal Children's Hospital, Melbourne, Victoria, Australia and
Department of Surgery, Tribhuvan University Teaching Hospital, Kathmandu, Nepal

Introduction

A hernia is an abnormal protrusion of a viscus (or part of a viscus) through a defect either in the containing wall of that viscus or within the cavity in which the viscus is normally situated. The 'wall' refers to the muscle layers of the abdomen or the diaphragm, or the walls of the pelvis. Hernias are either external or internal.

External hernias

External hernias present as an abnormal lump which can be detected by clinical examination of the abdomen or groin; they present externally. The relative occurrence and gender distribution of external abdominal hernias are shown in Tables 43.1 and 43.2.

Internal hernias

Internal hernias are rare and occur when the intestine (the 'viscus') passes beneath a constricting band or through a peritoneal window (the 'defect') within the abdominal cavity, or through the diaphragm or pelvic floor. They present as:
- acute intestinal obstruction, or
- chronic recurrent abdominal pain and vomiting due to incomplete and intermittent intestinal obstruction.

Sites of internal herniation include (i) the paraduodenal and paracaecal fossae, (ii) the lesser sac through the epiploic foramen (foramen of Winslow) or a defect in the transverse mesocolon, (iii) beneath congenital bands or adhesions, (iv) through defects in the small bowel mesentery, (v) between the lateral abdominal walls and intestinal stomas, and (vi) through defects in the diaphragm (hernias of Bochdalek and Morgagni). Treatment consists of surgical reduction of the viscera from the hernial orifice and closure of the defect. If strangulation occurs the compromised viscus has to be resected.

Components of a hernia

Hernias are composed of a sac that protrudes through a defect or hernia orifice and envelops the hernia contents. The sac consists of peritoneum, the parts of which are described as the neck, body and fundus (Figure 43.1). The neck of the sac is situated at the defect. The body is the widest part of the hernial sac, and the fundus is the apex or furthest extremity. Viscera most likely to enter a hernial sac are those normally situated in the region of the defect and those which are mobile, namely the omentum, small intestine and colon. Some hernia contents have been ascribed eponymous names.

Richter's hernia

The sac contains only part of the circumference of the bowel, usually the antimesenteric border (Figure 43.2).

Littré's hernia

A Meckel's diverticulum lies within the hernial sac. Littré's hernia occurs most commonly in a femoral or inguinal hernia (see later section).

Maydl's hernia

The hernial sac contains two loops of intestine (Figure 43.3). The loop of intestine within the abdominal cavity may become obstructed or strangulated, and this may not be recognised unless the hernia contents are inspected and returned to the abdominal cavity ('reduced') completely.

Textbook of Surgery, Fourth Edition. Edited by Julian A. Smith, Andrew H. Kaye, Christopher Christophi and Wendy A. Brown.
© 2020 John Wiley & Sons Ltd. Published 2020 by John Wiley & Sons Ltd.

Table 43.1 Relative occurrence of external abdominal hernias in adults.

Hernia	Percentage
Inguinal	80
Incisional	10
Femoral	5
Umbilical	4
Epigastric	<1
Other	<1

Table 43.2 Sex distribution of abdominal hernias.

	Male (%)	Female (%)
Inguinal hernia	96	45
Femoral hernia	2	39
Umbilical hernia	1	15
Other	1	1

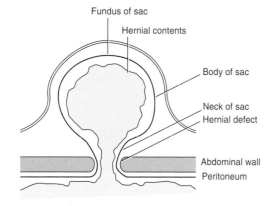

Fig. 43.1 Components of a hernia.

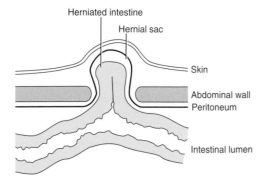

Fig. 43.2 Richter's hernia.

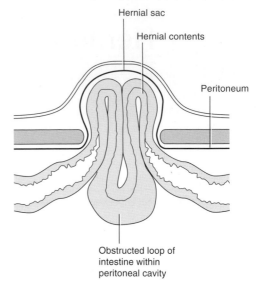

Fig. 43.3 Maydl's hernia.

De Garengeot's hernia

A femoral hernia with the appendix in the hernia sac.

Amyand's hernia

An inguinal hernia in which the hernial sac contains a normal or inflamed appendix.

Predisposing factors

A hernia occurs because of (i) weakness or defect in the abdominal wall and (ii) positive intra-abdominal pressure (IAP), which is often raised, forces the viscus into the defect.

Sites of weakness in the abdominal wall

Weaknesses in the abdominal wall may be due to the following.

- Congenital (i.e. present at birth), for example patent processus vaginalis or canal of Nuck, posterolateral or anterior parasternal diaphragmatic defect, patent umbilical ring in children.
- Where a normal anatomical structure passes through the abdominal wall, for example oesophageal hiatus, umbilical ligament in adults, obturator foramen, sciatic foramen.
- Acquired, for example surgical scar, site of an intestinal stoma, muscle wasting with increasing age, fatty infiltration of tissues because of obesity.

Increased intra-abdominal pressure

Raised IAP stretches the abdominal wall vertically and horizontally, thereby increasing the circumference of any defect. Also, high IAP forces abdominal

Box 43.1 Causes of sudden or sustained increases in intra-abdominal pressure

- Coughing
- Vomiting
- Straining during urination or defecation
- Pregnancy and childbirth
- Occupational heavy lifting or straining, and strenuous muscular exercise
- Obesity
- Ascites
- Continuous ambulatory peritoneal dialysis (CAPD)
- Gross organomegaly

contents through a defect. There are several causes of increased IAP (Box 43.1).

Complications

Most hernias are uncomplicated at presentation. The three important complications of hernias are irreducibility, obstruction and strangulation.

Irreducibility

A hernia is 'irreducible' when the sac cannot be emptied completely of contents. Irreducibility is caused by (i) adhesions between the sac and its contents, (ii) fibrosis leading to narrowing at the neck of the sac, or (iii) a sudden increase in IAP that causes transient stretching of the neck and forceful movement of contents into the sac, which cannot subsequently return to their original location.

Obstruction

A hernia becomes obstructed when the neck is sufficiently narrow to occlude the lumen of the intestine contained within the sac. The contained bowel becomes obstructed by the hernia defect. Obstructed hernias are nearly always irreducible and, if not treated, may become strangulated. Often, there is a history of a sudden increase in IAP that has pushed intestine or other contents into the sac. The patient presents with symptoms and signs of intestinal obstruction (abdominal colic, vomiting, constipation, abdominal distension) (see Chapters 27 and 32), together with a tender irreducible hernia. Identifying an external hernia in patients with intestinal obstruction may alter the operative approach. Obstructed hernias need urgent surgical treatment.

Strangulation

Strangulation occurs when the blood supply of the contents has ceased due to compression at the hernial orifice. Initially, lymphatic and venous channels are obstructed, leading to oedema and venous congestion but with continued arterial inflow. When the tissue pressure equals arterial pressure, arterial flow ceases and tissue necrosis ensues. Strangulation is a serious complication and, if the intestine is involved, leads to peritonitis (see Chapter 68) which can be fatal. A strangulated hernia is both irreducible and obstructed and is very tense and usually exquisitely tender. Erythema of the overlying skin is a late sign. A tense, tender, irreducible hernia implies strangulation and requires urgent surgery.

Principles of treatment

Uncomplicated hernias can be managed conservatively with no treatment or support with a truss, but most will require operative treatment. Complicated hernias always require surgery, often urgently.

No treatment

No treatment may be advised in debilitated patients who are not medically fit for surgery and who have uncomplicated hernias with minimal symptoms. Few patients fall into this category. Most external hernias can be successfully repaired surgically with minimal morbidity. If a patient refuses treatment, then the full implications of this decision must be explained.

Truss or abdominal binder

A truss or some form of hernia support may be used to provide symptomatic relief. After the hernia has been reduced, the truss presses on the hernial orifice to prevent protrusion. However, it frequently does not prevent prolapse of the hernia and simply presses on the hernia contents. They can be uncomfortable to wear.

Reducing raised intra-abdominal pressure

Causes of increased IAP should be corrected. Stopping smoking, investigation and treatment of prostatism and constipation, weight reduction, and effective management of ascites should be attempted where indicated. Changes in occupation and physical exercise also may have to be considered.

Operation

Operation is indicated for all other patients because of symptoms and the risk of complications. Surgery aims to (i) reduce the hernia contents, (ii) excise the sac (herniotomy) in most cases, and (iii) repair and close the defect, either by approximation of adjacent tissues to restore the normal anatomy (herniorrhaphy) or by insertion of additional material (hernioplasty).

Urgent operation

Urgent operation is indicated when obstruction or strangulation is suspected. Resuscitation with intravenous fluids, antibiotics, analgesia and nasogastric aspiration is required before surgery.

Inguinal hernia

Inguinal hernia is the commonest hernia and is approximately 10 times more common in males than females (see Tables 43.1 and 43.2). Two types of inguinal hernia are recognised (Figure 43.4), indirect inguinal hernia (IIH) and direct inguinal hernia (DIH), but they can occur together.

Importance of the integrity of the inguinal canal

The inguinal canal passes through the abdominal wall between the deep (internal) and superficial (external) inguinal rings. It carries the spermatic cord to the scrotum in the male, or the round ligament of the uterus to the labium majora in the female, together with the ilioinguinal nerve. The canal is a site of weakness and therefore potential herniation.

In addition to the presence of a patent processus vaginalis in an IIH, both IIH and DIH result from failure of normal mechanisms that maintain the integrity of the inguinal canal, including the following.

- 'Shutter mechanism' around the deep inguinal ring: during straining, a U-shaped condensation of transversalis fascia which passes under the cord is pulled upward and laterally, closing the deep ring around the cord and increasing the obliquity of the inguinal canal.
- 'Shutter action' of the internal oblique and transversus abdominis muscles: contraction of these muscles draws them downwards so that the inguinal canal tends to close and become more oblique.

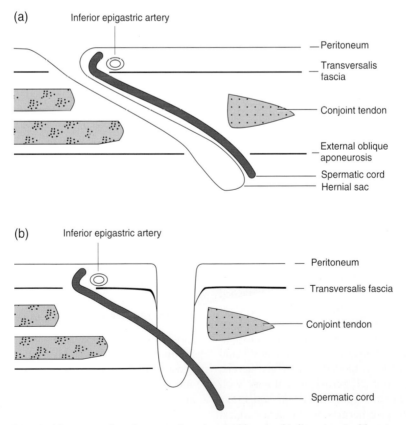

Fig. 43.4 Types of inguinal hernias (right side): (a) indirect inguinal hernia; (b) direct inguinal hernia.

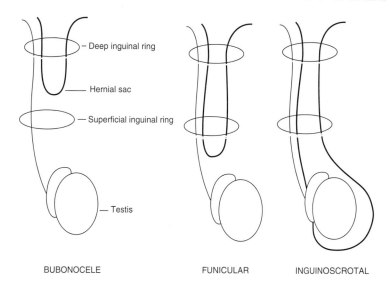

Fig. 43.5 Types of indirect inguinal hernias.

- Integrity of the posterior wall of the inguinal canal: weakness of the conjoint tendon reduces the strength of the posterior wall of the inguinal canal and reduces support behind the superficial inguinal ring.
- Oblique direction of the inguinal canal: if the deep and superficial inguinal rings enlarge, they may almost overlie each other and obliquity of the canal is lost.

Indirect inguinal hernia

The hernial sac of an IIH is a patent processus vaginalis, and the neck of the sac is situated at the deep inguinal ring, lateral to the inferior epigastric artery. The sac accompanies the spermatic cord along the inguinal canal towards the scrotum for a varying distance (see below). The sac lies in front of the cord and is enclosed by the coverings of the cord. Except in children and infants, the essential cause of an IIH is (i) failure of the processus vaginalis to become completely obliterated to form the ligamentum vaginale, which normally occurs within a few days after birth, and (ii) loss of integrity of the inguinal canal. Even though the sac of an IIH is congenital, herniation may not occur until later in life, when there is failure of the normal mechanisms that maintain the inguinal canal.

The incidence of IIH is approximately 800–1000 per million male population. IIH is approximately four times more common than DIH, occurs at any time during life, and has a male to female ratio of about 10 : 1.

Classification of indirect inguinal hernias

These hernias are classified according to the length of the hernial sac (Figure 43.5).
- Bubonocele: the sac is confined to the inguinal canal.
- Funicular: the sac extends along the length of the inguinal canal and through the superficial inguinal ring but does not extend to the scrotum or labium majora.
- Complete, scrotal or inguinoscrotal: the sac passes through the inguinal canal and superficial inguinal ring and extends into the scrotum or labium.

Direct inguinal hernia

A DIH protrudes directly through the posterior wall of the inguinal canal, medial to the inferior epigastric artery and deep inguinal ring. The essential fault with a DIH is weakness of the inguinal canal and is invariably associated with poor abdominal musculature. Herniation occurs at a site where the transversalis fascia is not supported by the conjoint tendon or the transversus aponeurosis, an area known as Hesselbach's triangle. The boundaries of Hesselbach's triangle are medially the lateral edge of the rectus sheath, superolaterally the inferior epigastric vessels, and inferiorly the inguinal ligament. Occasionally, the hernia sac straddles inferior epigastric vessels and is then known as a 'pantaloon hernia'.

DIH is rare in females and does not occur in children. It is more common on the right side after appendicectomy, suggesting that damage to the iliohypogastric and ilioinguinal nerves with subsequent weakness of the internal oblique and transversus abdominis muscles is an aetiological factor.

Clinical features of inguinal hernias

Inguinal hernias present with inguinal discomfort, with or without a lump. Discomfort is due to stretching of the tissues of the inguinal canal and occurs typically when IAP is increased. Pain may also be referred to the testis because of pressure on the spermatic cord and ilioinguinal nerve. Severe inguinal or abdominal pain suggests obstruction or strangulation. A lump is usually obvious to the patient, is often precipitated by increasing IAP, and may reduce completely with rest and lying down.

The patient initially is examined standing to demonstrate the lump and possible 'cough impulse', and then lying down to allow the hernia to be reduced. An IIH protrudes along the line of the inguinal canal for a variable distance towards the scrotum or labia; a DIH appears as a diffuse bulge at the medial end of the inguinal canal. The significance of a cough impulse, or sudden bulging of the inguinal region with coughing, must be interpreted carefully. A generalised weakness in the inguinal region will result in a diffuse bulge appearing with coughing, but this condition (known as Malgaigne's bulge) is not the same as a hernia, in which the cough impulse is discrete and confined to the area of herniation. Abdominal examination is performed to detect organomegaly, a mass or ascites.

Indirect or direct inguinal hernia?

An IIH is prevented from appearing by applying pressure over the deep inguinal ring, a DIH by pressure medial to the deep inguinal ring. The deep inguinal ring lies just above the midpoint of the inguinal ligament. The midpoint of the inguinal ligament lies halfway between the anterior superior iliac spine and the pubic tubercle; these are the attachments of the inguinal ligament to the pelvis. The midpoint of the inguinal ligament differs from the mid-inguinal point. The mid-inguinal point is halfway between the anterior superior iliac spine and the pubic symphysis. The femoral pulse can be palpated, below the inguinal ligament at the mid-inguinal point.

To distinguish an indirect from a direct inguinal hernia pressure is applied to the deep inguinal ring (midpoint of the inguinal ligament) and the patient is asked to cough; if the hernia is controlled, it is an IIH; if the hernia is not controlled, it is a DIH.

Sliding inguinal hernia

A sliding inguinal hernia is a variant in which part of a viscus (usually the colon) is adherent to the outside of the peritoneum forming the hernial sac beyond the hernial orifice. Thus, the viscus and the hernial sac, which may contain another abdominal viscus, lie within the inguinal canal (Figure 43.6). Sliding hernias are more common on the left side (where they contain part of the sigmoid colon) than on the right (where they contain part of the caecum). Sliding hernias occasionally contain part of the bladder or an ovary and ovarian tube. A sliding hernia may be indirect or direct. They are nearly always found in males. A sliding hernia should be suspected if the neck of the hernia is bulky, or if the hernial sac does not separate easily from the cord at operation.

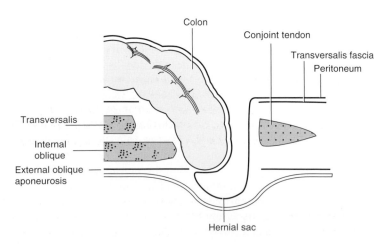

Fig. 43.6 Section through sliding inguinal hernia.

Inguinal hernias in infants and children

Inguinal hernias are always indirect in infants and children and are due to a patent processus vaginalis. The majority (90%) occur in males and more commonly on the right side, presumably due to the slightly later descent of the right testis. Approximately 10–20% are bilateral. If the contralateral side is also explored in a child undergoing unilateral inguinal hernia repair, a patent processus is found in approximately 50% of cases. Irreducibility is common and occurs in about 50% of hernias presenting within the first year of life. Strangulation appears to be rare. Testicular infarction can occur if a large irreducible hernia severely compresses the spermatic cord and is more common than infarction of the hernial contents.

Inguinal hernias in children should be repaired surgically. The hernial sac is very thin and because the superficial and deep inguinal rings are almost superimposed upon one another in children, the sac can be mobilised and ligated through the superficial inguinal ring. Herniotomy is all that is required.

Treatment of inguinal hernias

Inguinal hernias are treated surgically and the surgery can be performed open or laparoscopically. Open inguinal hernia surgery can be undertaken under general, regional or local infiltration anaesthesia. Open repair is performed through a skin-crease incision centred over the inguinal canal. The sac is dissected carefully from the cord, opened and the contents returned to the abdominal cavity. In an IIH, the sac is ligated at the deep inguinal ring and excised (herniotomy), whereas in a DIH the sac is formed from layers of the posterior wall of the inguinal canal and so is not excised. A procedure to strengthen the posterior wall of the inguinal canal is performed (herniorrhaphy or hernioplasty).

Herniorrhaphy

Herniorrhaphy refers to repair of the posterior wall of the inguinal canal behind the spermatic cord by one of several methods, together with repair of the external oblique aponeurosis in front of the cord. There are a variety of described techniques.

Hernioplasty

Hernioplasty refers to insertion of a prosthetic mesh (e.g. polypropylene) to cover and support the posterior wall of the inguinal canal. The mesh encircles the cord at the deep ring, covers the posterior wall behind the cord and is attached along the inguinal ligament from the pubic tubercle to lateral to the deep inguinal ring. Alternatively, the mesh can be inserted via an extraperitoneal approach and placed deep to the defect in the posterior wall.

Laparoscopic hernia repair

Laparoscopic repair is performed under general anaesthesia, using either a transperitoneal or extraperitoneal approach. The sac is dissected from the spermatic cord (or round ligament) and reduced. A mesh is inserted behind the posterior wall and deep ring to strengthen the area.

Management after inguinal hernia repair

Patients require analgesia for the first few days. They should avoid straining and lifting for 2 weeks after surgery, and slowly resume physical activity and work over the next 4 weeks. It takes about 6 weeks to fully recover.

Potential complications of inguinal hernia repair

In addition to the complications of any surgical procedure (haemorrhage, haematoma, wound and chest infection, deep vein thrombosis, pulmonary embolus, anaesthetic complications) there are a number of potential complications specific to inguinal hernia repair.

- Urinary retention: elderly male patients are particularly susceptible to retention of urine. Prostatic symptoms should be identified and treated before the hernia is repaired.
- Scrotal swelling and haematoma: oedema, swelling and bruising of the scrotum are common (especially with bilateral repairs) and resolve spontaneously. Scrotal support may bring symptomatic relief. Large haematomas require operative drainage.
- Wound infection: a deep wound infection which does not settle with antibiotics requires removal of the prosthetic mesh.
- Recurrent hernia: recurrence is related to surgical technique and expertise, experience of the operator, postoperative infection and haematoma, and failure to correct factors predisposing to hernia formation. Recurrence rates should be less than 2%. About 50% of recurrences appear within 5 years after the initial repair, and approximately 50% of recurrences are indirect hernias. A first recurrence is treated along the principles outlined in the previous section.

- Nerve injury: injury to the ilioinguinal nerve, which lies below the spermatic cord in the inguinal canal and passes out through the superficial inguinal ring, occurs in 10–20% of inguinal hernia repairs, resulting in paraesthesia or numbness below and medial to the wound over the pubic tubercle and proximal scrotum.
- Persisting wound pain: this is uncommon, and results from nerve entrapment or damage, neuroma formation, osteitis pubis if sutures have been inserted into the pubis, displacement of a mesh repair, or pressure on the spermatic cord. Pain may be a symptom of recurrent herniation. Local anaesthetic or phenol injections may help, and surgical exploration is indicated for severe or persistent pain.
- Testicular ischaemia and atrophy: interruption of the testicular arterial supply (testicular artery and indirectly from the cremasteric artery and the artery of the vas deferens) can occur during dissection of an indirect sac from the cord. Ischaemia produces testicular pain, tenderness and swelling. Testicular atrophy is observed in 1–5% of males.
- Hydrocele: a long-term complication probably resulting from the repair being too tight or scarring, with subsequent compression of lymphatics of the cord.
- Injury to the vas deferens: a rare complication that is most likely to occur when a recurrent hernia is repaired.
- Visceral injury: viscera in a sliding hernia are at risk for injury when the sac is being dissected away from them.

Femoral hernia

A femoral hernia occurs when the transversalis fascia which normally covers the femoral ring is disrupted, so that a peritoneal sac and hernial contents pass through the femoral ring into the femoral canal. The femoral canal is the most medial compartment of the femoral sheath and lies medial to the femoral vein. Femoral hernias are two to three times more common in females than males, and occur in the older age group, often after a period of weight loss. Femoral hernias are never congenital and are twice as common in parous as in nonparous females. Inguinal hernias are more common than femoral hernias in females (see Table 43.2). Approximately 60% of femoral hernias are on the right, 30% on the left and 10% bilateral. A femoral hernia is the commonest site for a Richter's

hernia. Aetiological factors in femoral hernia formation are:
- localised weakness at the femoral ring
- factors which increase IAP (see Box 43.1).

Presentation

A femoral hernia presents as either discomfort in the groin together with a lump, or acutely as intestinal obstruction with or without strangulation. A small hernia may be difficult to palpate, especially in the obese patient. The hernia is frequently irreducible and may not have a cough impulse.

On examination, the bulge of a femoral hernia appears in the region of the saphenous opening. The neck of the sac is always located below the line of the inguinal ligament, even though the fundus may appear to be above the ligament. This is because once within the femoral canal, the hernial sac is prevented from continuing inferiorly down the thigh with the femoral vessels because the femoral sheath (which encloses the femoral vessels and the femoral canal) becomes narrow and tapers to a point around the vessels. The hernia is therefore directed forwards through the fossa ovalis and is quite superficial at this point (Figure 43.7). It cannot continue down the thigh in a subcutaneous plane because the superficial fascia of the thigh is attached to the lower border of the fossa ovalis and is firmer than the superficial fascia above the level of the foramen ovalis. As the hernia enlarges, it turns upwards into the looser areolar tissue beneath the skin of the groin crease and may be confused with an inguinal hernia.

Thus, the direction taken by a femoral hernia is initially downwards through the femoral canal, then forwards through the fossa ovalis, and then upwards in the loose areolar tissue of the upper thigh. Therefore, in attempting to reduce the hernia, pressure is applied in the reverse order, i.e. initially downwards, backwards and then upwards.

Inguinal or femoral hernia?

Inguinal and femoral hernias are distinguished by their positions relative to the inguinal ligament and pubic tubercle. The inguinal ligament is identified by palpating the anterior superior iliac spine and the pubic tubercle; an imaginary line drawn between the two points is the line of the inguinal ligament. The neck of an inguinal hernia is above the inguinal ligament and pubic tubercle, and the hernia protrudes initially from above the ligament even though it may descend into the scrotum. The hernia passes medial to the pubic tubercle as it

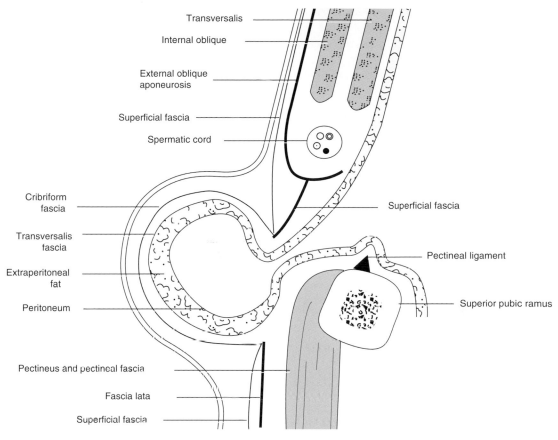

Fig. 43.7 Sagittal section of a femoral hernia.

descends from the superficial inguinal ring, into the scrotum or labia. The neck of a femoral hernia is below the inguinal ligament and lateral to the pubic tubercle, and the hernia protrudes initially from below the ligament.

Treatment

Surgical treatment of a femoral hernia should always be advised because of the risk of obstruction and strangulation. Surgery involves opening and emptying the sac and performing a herniorrhaphy to prevent recurrence. Herniorrhaphy aims to reduce the size of the femoral ring and is performed by inserting several sutures between the inguinal and pectineal ligaments, thereby effectively closing off the femoral canal. One of two operative approaches is used.
- A 'low' or subinguinal approach is used for small uncomplicated femoral hernias by making an incision over the hernia below the level of the inguinal ligament.
- The 'high' or supra-inguinal approach is recommended for large or complicated femoral hernias in an emergency situation. The extraperitoneal

space between the peritoneum and abdominal wall muscles is accessed through an abdominal incision. The sac is identified and opened to inspect the contents. The intestine is resected if necessary and the sac is excised. The femoral ring is repaired from this intra-abdominal approach.

Incisional hernia

An incisional hernia is a protrusion of the peritoneum (the sac) and underlying abdominal contents (hernial contents) into the subcutaneous plane through a defect at the site of an abdominal scar. The true incidence is difficult to ascertain but is on the order of 5% at 5 years and 10% at 10 years. There is a higher preponderance in males. Patients present a bulge at the site of a previous incision. Incisional hernias increase in size with time and frequently become irreducible.

The main predisposing factors for incisional hernia are poor surgical techniques, local wound complications, impaired wound healing and increased IAP (Box 43.2).

Box 43.2 Aetiological factors in incisional hernias

Poor surgical technique
- Angulated incision
- Parallel incisions
- Devitalised tissue in wound
- Tightly sutured wound
- Poor technique of abdominal wound closure
- Absorbable sutures of short duration

Local wound factors
- Infection
- Haematoma
- Foreign body
- Wound edges not in apposition

Impaired wound healing
- Malnutrition
- Corticosteroids, anti-proliferative and immunosuppressive drugs
- Uraemia
- Jaundice
- Diabetes
- Anaemia

Raised intra-abdominal pressure
See Box 43.1

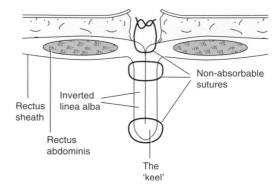

Fig. 43.8 Keel repair.

Treatment

Incisional hernias should be repaired because (i) they increase in size with time and become more difficult to repair as they become larger; (ii) they are at risk of becoming irreducible, obstructed and strangulated, especially if the neck is narrow; and (iii) patients request repair because of discomfort and unsightly appearance. Preoperative weight reduction in obese patients aims to facilitate the repair and to reduce postoperative respiratory problems and likelihood of recurrence. Diabetes and smoking contribute to higher rates of surgical failure, so patients need good preoperative diabetic control and should stop smoking.

Operation involves defining the sac and neck, returning the contents to the abdominal cavity, and repairing the hole in the abdominal wall. If the edges of the defect can be apposed without tension, the defect is closed directly with strong non-absorbable sutures; if not, the defect is reinforced with prosthetic mesh.

Mesh hernia repairs can be performed open or laparoscopically. Laparoscopic repairs are used for small (<5 cm diameter) defects and the mesh is placed intraperitoneally. For larger (>5 cm) defects an open mesh repair is favoured. The mesh can be placed over the abdominal closure in the subcutaneous space (on-lay repair). The mesh can be placed intraperitoneally and the musculo-aponeurotic layer is closed over the mesh (inlay technique). Alternatively, a sub-lay technique can be used. The mesh is placed over the closed posterior rectus sheath and peritoneum, with rectus muscles overlying the mesh and the anterior rectus sheath closed.

Epigastric hernia

An epigastric hernia is a protrusion of extraperitoneal fat, with or without a small sac of peritoneum, through a defect in the linea alba anywhere between the xiphisternum and the umbilicus. The defect is characteristically small, often about 1 cm in diameter, and seen as a transverse split in the linea alba. The hernia is usually easier to feel than to see, and is diagnosed by palpation of a small, often very tender, lump in the linea alba. Ultrasound may be helpful when a hernia is suspected but cannot be palpated. Epigastric hernias are usually irreducible and may be multiple.

Treatment

Surgery is undertaken to relieve symptoms. The hernia is marked preoperatively because it may be difficult to palpate when the patient is anaesthetised. If there are multiple hernias, the linea alba is exposed through a vertical incision, the extraperitoneal fat is excised and each defect is repaired. Small defects can be suture repaired by simple closure, 'keel' repair or 'Mayo' repair. A 'keel' repair is performed by inserting two or more layers of sutures into the linea alba and anterior rectus sheath, each successive layer covering the previous layer so that the repaired tissue resembles the keel of a boat (Figure 43.8). A 'Mayo' repair (Figure 43.9) is where the upper and lower edges of the defect are

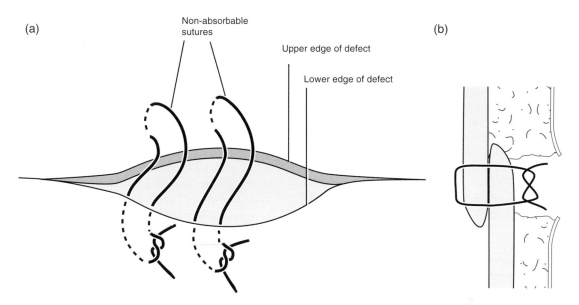

Fig. 43.9 Mayo repair. (a) Insertion of two sutures through upper and lower edges of hernial defect. (b) Sagittal section of linea alba after repair.

overlapped with interrupted sutures ('pants over vest' repair). Large defects are repaired with mesh.

Umbilical hernia in children

An umbilical hernia in a child is a congenital defect in which a peritoneal sac protrudes through a patent umbilical ring and is covered by normal skin. Approximately 5–10% of Caucasian infants have an umbilical hernia at birth. About one-third of hernias close within a month of birth, and they rarely persist beyond the age of 3–4 years. The hernia is noticeable whenever the child cries, coughs or vomits, and is a cause of concern for parents. Umbilical hernias in children rarely become irreducible or strangulate.

Umbilical hernia is a separate entity from exomphalos (omphalocele). Exomphalos is a rare congenital condition in which the midgut fails to return to the abdominal cavity during the first trimester, with subsequent failure of the abdominal wall to close at the umbilicus. At birth, the intestine protrudes into the base of the umbilical cord and is covered by a thin opaque sac of amnion, not normal skin.

Treatment

An expectant approach can be adopted as nearly all hernias close or greatly reduce in size. Repair is recommended for unusually large hernias or if the hernia is still present at school age. A short transverse subumbilical incision is made, the sac is excised, and the defect is closed by either edge-to-edge apposition or a Mayo repair (see Figure 43.9). The umbilical cicatrix is preserved. Recurrence is rare.

Para-umbilical hernia in adults

A para-umbilical hernia in an adult is an acquired condition and quite distinct from the umbilical hernia of childhood. A para-umbilical hernia protrudes through one side of the umbilical ring, while the umbilicus still retains its fibrous character within the linea alba, although it becomes effaced by the pressure of the hernial contents and has an eccentric 'half-moon' or crescentic furrow. Para-umbilical hernias initially contain extraperitoneal fat but, as the hernial orifice enlarges, omentum enters the sac. The contents typically adhere to the sac so that the hernia becomes loculated and irreducible. Para-umbilical hernias occasionally become very large and contain transverse colon and small intestine.

Treatment

Para-umbilical hernias are treated surgically because of the risk of obstruction, strangulation and, rarely, excoriation and ulceration of the skin overlying the hernia. The classic operative procedure is a Mayo repair (see Figure 43.9), but repairs with mesh are performed increasingly.

Hernias related to intestinal stomas

A hernia may occur through the abdominal wall at the site of an intestinal stoma (see Chapter 25). The surgically created defect through which the stoma is fashioned enlarges due to raised IAP and allows protrusion of the peritoneum (the hernial sac) through the defect to lie adjacent to the stoma (Figure 43.10).

Parastomal hernias eventually occur in about 10–30% of patients with colostomies and ileostomies. Correct surgical technique when fashioning intestinal stomas is of paramount importance in prevention. For example, stomas should be brought out through the aponeurotic part of the abdominal wall, not the muscular part, and they should not be sited in the main abdominal wound or the umbilicus.

Treatment

Surgery is required if the bulge of the hernia causes poor fitting of the stoma appliance and consequent leakage from beneath the appliance. Also, intestinal obstruction and strangulation may occur. Operation involves reducing the size of the stomal orifice by closing the abdominal wall tissues around the stoma, but this method has a high recurrence rate. Insertion of prosthetic mesh in an extraperitoneal or extraparietal plane to cover the defect in the abdominal wall generally provides a good repair but runs the risk of infection of the mesh. Relocation of the stoma and complete closure of the previous stoma site provides the best chance of cure.

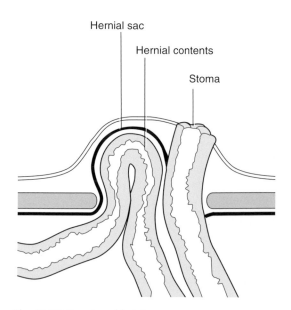

Fig. 43.10 Parastomal hernia.

Spigelian hernia

Spigelian hernias are rare. A Spigelian hernia occurs through a defect lateral to the rectus muscle through the semilunar line. The semilunar line marks the outer border of the rectus muscle. A Spigelian hernia protrudes through a defect lateral to the rectus muscle, through the Spigelian fascia. The hernia is limited laterally by the internal oblique muscle fibres and medially by the insertion of the external oblique aponeurosis to form the anterior rectus sheath.

Clinically, the diagnosis of a Spigelian hernia may be difficult. The patient, who typically is a middle-aged female, presents with diffuse aching pain in the area of the hernia, which is small and may not be palpable. Pain is often present during the day but may recede at night if the hernia reduces and may be made worse by raising the arm on the affected side. If a lump is not palpable, the diagnosis may be confirmed by ultrasound or CT scanning. The hernia usually contains omentum but may contain small or large bowel. A Richter's hernia may occur, and obstruction and strangulation are well-recognised complications.

Treatment

Spigelian hernias should be treated surgically because of the severity of symptoms and the risk of complications. An open or laparoscopic technique can be used.

Lumbar hernias

Lumbar hernias are rare. They occur typically in individuals with poor muscle tone, either spontaneously or following trauma, surgery, or paralysis of paravertebral muscles secondary to poliomyelitis. Differential diagnosis includes a lipoma, lumbar abscess or haematoma.

Lumbar hernias occur through two triangular sites of weakness in the lumbar region of the abdominal wall.

- Inferior lumbar triangle hernia (triangle of Petit): herniation occurs between the iliac crest inferiorly, the posterior edge of external oblique muscle anteriorly, and the anterior edge of latissimus dorsi posteriorly. The 'floor' of the triangle through which the hernia protrudes is formed by the internal oblique and transversus abdominis muscles.
- Superior lumbar triangle (triangle of Grynfeltt–Lesshaft): the hernia occurs between the lowermost edge of serratus posterior inferior muscle and the 12th rib superiorly, the anterior border of internal oblique muscle anteriorly, and the lateral edge

of erector spinae muscle medially. Grynfeltt's triangle lies superior to Petit's triangle, and the 'floor' is formed by the quadratus lumborum muscle. The hernia is covered by the latissimus dorsi.

Treatment

Treatment of lumbar hernias is difficult because of their anatomical boundaries, their size, the type of patient in whom they occur, and because they are bounded in part by muscle rather than tough aponeurotic tissue. Prosthetic mesh repair is required.

Obturator hernia

An obturator hernia is rare. It protrudes through the obturator canal or foramen, which is a normal anatomical structure between the obturator groove on the inferior aspect of the superior pubic ramus and superior border of the obturator membrane. The obturator canal carries the obturator nerve and vessels. When large, the hernial sac passes between the pectineus and adductor longus muscles and protrudes forwards to produce a diffuse bulge in the femoral triangle, where it can be mistaken for a femoral hernia. It is more common on the right side.

The hernia occurs most often in elderly females, particularly in those who have become debilitated and lost weight rapidly. Usually, the patient presents with intestinal obstruction of unknown cause. An abdominal and pelvic CT scan may make the diagnosis preoperatively. Otherwise, the hernia is diagnosed at operation. Patients may complain of diffuse pain in the groin together with pain in the medial side of the thigh and knee because of pressure on the obturator nerve. The hernia may be felt in the femoral triangle and also on vaginal examination. A Richter's hernia may occur with strangulation of the entrapped part of the intestinal wall.

Treatment

Laparotomy or laparoscopy is performed and the entrapped segment of bowel is released. The hernial defect is often found to be small. Care is taken not to damage the obturator nerve when either closing the defect or covering it with prosthetic mesh.

Sciatic hernias

Sciatic hernias are very rare and occur when a peritoneal sac enters the greater (gluteal hernia) or lesser sciatic foramina. Pain caused by pressure on the sciatic nerve or a palpable swelling and tenderness in the buttock suggests the diagnosis. Most commonly, sciatic hernias are discovered at laparotomy for intestinal obstruction. The sac is excised but attempts to close the defect run the risk of sciatic nerve damage.

Further reading

Cheek CM, Black NA, Devlin HB, Kingsnorth AN, Taylor RS, Watkin DFL. Groin hernia surgery: a systematic review. *Ann R Coll Surg Engl* 1998;80:S1–S80.

Fitzgibbons RJ, Greenburg AO (eds) *Nhyus and Condon's Hernia*. Philadelphia: Lippincott, Williams & Wilkins, 2001.

MCQs

Select the single correct answer to each question. The correct answers can be found in the Answers section at the end of the book.

1 The commonest type of hernia is:
   a inguinal
   b femoral
   c epigastric
   d incisional
   e umbilical

2 The most serious and urgent complication of a hernia is:
   a pressure on the spermatic cord
   b irreducibility
   c obstruction
   d strangulation
   e neuralgia

3 Indirect inguinal hernias:
   a can hardly ever be distinguished from direct inguinal hernias by clinical examination
   b rarely occur in children
   c can be treated by herniotomy, herniorraphy and hernioplasty
   d should not be treated laparoscopically
   e arise beneath the inguinal ligament

4 Femoral hernias:
   a may occasionally appear above the inguinal ligament in young children
   b should always be repaired surgically
   c can be treated with a surgical truss
   d are caused by a defect in the cribriform fascia
   e may compress the femoral artery

5 A strangulated hernia:
   a is easily reducible
   b can be observed and treated electively
   c requires urgent surgery
   d is more comfortable with a truss
   e has a strong cough impulse

Section 9
Skin and Soft Tissues

44 Tumours and cysts of the skin

Rodney T. Judson

University of Melbourne and Royal Melbourne Hospital, Melbourne, Victoria, Australia

Introduction

The skin has many functions, including the provision of a physical barrier between the body and the environment, and temperature regulation. The skin structure, of epithelium and appendages with the underlying dermis, forms a complex and interactive grouping of tissues and cells to serve these functions. It is not surprising that genetically determined processes and external factors can interact to produce lesions that by their superficial placement are both obvious and deserving of attention. The common lesions of the skin possibly requiring surgical therapy will be dealt with under the headings of cysts, benign tumours, malignant lesions and malignant tumours.

Cysts of the skin

These are common lesions whose only importance is their cosmetic effect and their propensity to become infected.

Epidermal or epidermoid cysts

Epidermal or epidermoid cysts are the most common cysts, and are frequently misnamed sebaceous cysts in the mistaken belief that they arise from sebaceous glands. True sebaceous cysts do occur but are rare. Epidermal cysts are inclusion cysts lined by fully differentiated epidermis. They are filled by laminated keratin, which forms the characteristic, white, unpleasant-smelling content. Clinically they are characterised by the presence of a small punctum or sinus on their surface They occur most commonly on the face, the scalp, the back and the scrotum and may be shelled out under local anaesthesia if uninfected or enucleated through small incisions to provide optimal cosmetic results. Infected cysts should be treated by incision and drainage, with later excision to avoid recurrence.

Milia are tiny multiple epidermal cysts that occur on the face, particularly around the eyes, and can be shelled out for cosmesis.

Dermoid cysts

Dermoid cysts are congenital inclusion cysts that occur at points of fusion, particularly in the face. Their structure differs from epidermal cysts in that they show multiple skin appendages rather than epidermis alone. They can be treated by excision but are less readily enucleated than epidermal cysts.

Post-traumatic dermoid cysts result from implantation of epidermis and appendages under the skin surface by penetrating injury and occur most commonly in the hands and fingers. Such cysts are often densely adherent to the underlying dermis but are readily excised.

Benign epidermal tumours

These are extremely common and arise from the epidermis itself, or more rarely from the skin appendages.

Seborrhoeic keratosis

Seborrhoeic keratoses are the most common of these lesions and occur on the trunk or limbs of the middle-aged or elderly. They develop initially as flat plaques with a waxy surface that progressively thickens, often with pigmentation due to haemosiderin deposition. Exuberant keratin and parakeratin production results from simple proliferation of keratinocytes for unknown cause, without any dermal involvement, so that the lesions are said to have a 'painted on' appearance. Because of their protruding nature the lesions are prone to trauma and subsequent low-grade infection. Keratoses can be removed or shaved under local anaesthesia if unsightly or irritated.

Textbook of Surgery, Fourth Edition. Edited by Julian A. Smith, Andrew H. Kaye, Christopher Christophi and Wendy A. Brown.
© 2020 John Wiley & Sons Ltd. Published 2020 by John Wiley & Sons Ltd.

Actinic keratosis

Actinic keratosis represents a progressive dysplastic change in the epidermis and the underlying dermis as the result of exposure to ultraviolet (UV) light. There is a build-up of keratin and parakeratin, with thickened elastic fibres (elastosis) in the dermis due to damaged fibroblasts. The lesions occur most commonly on sun-exposed areas, such as the ears in the male, the nose, the backs of the hands and forearms. They appear as rough crusty areas of thickening that may bleed when traumatised. Actinic keratoses are unquestionably premalignant, in contradistinction to seborrhoeic keratosis. They can be managed by the application of cytotoxic creams or by surgical excision if there is any suspicion that malignant change has already occurred.

Keratoacanthoma

Keratoacanthoma is a benign lesion that presents on the cheek, nose, ear or back of the hand in the elderly as a rapidly growing nodule which develops a characteristic central keratin plug. The lesions usually develop to several centimetres in diameter over the course of a few weeks and then regress spontaneously and rapidly. They can thus be treated expectantly.

Keratoacanthomas may occur in patients receiving immunosuppression, such as transplant recipients, and in these circumstances should be treated as squamous carcinoma because they may behave aggressively.

Malignant epithelial tumours

The most common tumours arise from the cells of the epidermis in the form of basal and squamous carcinomas and melanoma, which will be considered with pigmented lesions.

Basal cell carcinoma

Basal cell carcinoma (BCC) is the most common form of skin cancer and occurs almost exclusively on sun-exposed areas of the skin in the adult white population over the age of 40 years. They are rare in the oriental population and almost never occur in black-skinned races.

Between 75 and 80% of the lesions occur in the head and neck, usually above a line running from the corner of the mouth to the ear, with the remainder being situated on the limbs and a minority on the trunk. Although the cell of origin was presumed to be the basal cell in the epidermis, it is probable that the true progenitor is a potential epithelial cell in pylosebaceous tissue. Exposure to UVB is believed to be the precipitating factor, and there is no clear genetic basis for the disease apart from race, except in some rare conditions such as the naevoid BCC syndrome, where BCC occurs in childhood, often in non-sun-exposed areas and with associated odontogenic cysts of the mandible, medulloblastoma and tumours of the reproductive organs.

Clinical presentation

Basal cell carcinoma presents in a wide variety of forms, but the most common is as a waxy translucent nodule with a thin overlying epithelium and a fine network of vessels traversing the margins, probably the result of tumour-induced angiogenesis. Central regression may lead to depressions in the centre of the lesion, which may progress to ulceration to show the classical 'rodent ulcer' appearance. The tumours may be multifocal and as they grow tend to become infiltrative and may involve deeper tissues. They may thus become locally aggressive but only rarely metastasise.

Treatment

Optimal treatment for nodular BCC depends on size. Lesions less than 1 cm in diameter are rarely deeply invasive and can be treated by electro-desiccation with curettage, by cryosurgery or by excision with a narrow margin in terms of depth and width. Radiotherapy is an alternative form of therapy but not in areas close to cartilage. Lesions greater than 1 cm in size are best treated by excision with perioperative confirmation of clear margins of excision, which should not be less than 1 mm.

If treatment has been adequate, recurrence is rare, except in the case of sclerosing BCC, which may require multiple procedures to achieve control.

Squamous cell carcinoma

Squamous cell carcinoma (SCC) is the second most common tumour of the skin. The major aetiological factor is again exposure to UV light. Although such lesions are most commonly seen in the elderly, they are now becoming increasingly frequent in young adults because of excessive sun exposure in childhood. As expected from its aetiology, the lesions are most common in white populations and are seen most frequently on the face and ears, lip, the back of hands and forearms.

Clinical presentation

Clinical presentation is initially as an area of crusting that is clinically indistinguishable from solar keratosis but which on excision shows the cellular atypia that provides the diagnosis of carcinoma *in situ* before the breaching of the basement membrane at the dermoepidermal junction to form frank invasive carcinoma. If the lesions are untreated at this stage, they will progress to form a nodule or plaque that is irregular in shape and may ulcerate with a pink rolled edge. Unlike BCC, SCC can metastasise, usually to the regional lymph nodes but also systemically, although this is unusual unless the lesions are large or neglected. It should be noted that immunosuppression is associated with a much higher incidence of SCC, as for example in renal transplant recipients in whom the normal 4 : 1 ratio of BCC to SCC is reversed; BCCs are also more common in such patients than in the normal age- and sex-matched population.

Treatment

Treatment of SCC is primarily surgical with excision to a margin of at least 0.5 cm in depth and peripherally, as determined on clinical grounds, although this margin may be reduced in the head and neck to avoid unnecessary cosmetic problems. If lesser margins are used, frozen section should be utilised to ensure that complete excision of the lesion has occurred. Tumour thickness is closely related to outcome. Local recurrence is unusual with lesions less than 4 mm in thickness and metastasis is more common in lesions which are greater than 10 mm in thickness (Table 44.1). Adjuvant radiotherapy is only used when the margins of excision are compromised by vital structures. Radiotherapy as a primary treatment is almost as effective as surgery but should be reserved for those patients not fit for surgery. As nodal involvement with cutaneous SCC is unusual, prophylactic lymph node dissection is not used and therapeutic

Table 44.1 Excision margins related to tumour thickness.

Thickness of melanoma	Stage (TNM)	Excision margin
In situ	pTis	5 mm
<1.5 mm	pT1, pT2	1 cm
1.5–4 mm	pT3	1–2 cm
>4 mm	pT4	2–3 cm

dissection is only indicated when there are enlarged glands that prove on biopsy to demonstrate involvement with tumour. Prognosis is good, with at least 95% disease-free survival at 5 years. Local recurrence is rare following pathologically confirmed complete surgical excision.

Pigmented lesions

Pigmented tumours of the skin are common. Their major importance is the propensity of some lesions to progress to the formation of melanoma, or the initial clinical differentiation from primary melanoma. A number of lesions that may become pigmented, such as seborrhoeic keratoses or BCC, have been dealt with previously.

Naevus

The term *naevus* should refer by definition to any congenital lesion of the skin, but by convention is used to describe any congenital or acquired neoplasm of melanocytes.

Acquired naevus

Acquired or naevocellular naevi are common. An Australian survey demonstrated 15 such lesions per person in an adult white Caucasian population. They are most common on sun-exposed areas of the body. They are formed by melanocytes that have been transferred from their usual dendritic single-cell position among the basal layers of keratinocytes to form aggregates along the dermoepithelial junction. This aggregation of cells forms a junctional naevus. The cells of such naevi show little individual change, and mitotic figures are not numerous.

The clinical appearance of each form of naevus is thus important, although it must be understood that clinical interpretation of any pigmented skin lesion is not always accurate and any lesion where there is uncertainty about its nature must be subjected to excisional biopsy. The junctional naevus is impalpable, pale to dark brown in colour and is usually small, rarely being more than 1 cm in diameter. They may appear in childhood but usually become obvious around puberty, growing slowly until the cessation of skeletal growth in late adolescence. In contrast, compound naevi are palpable, because of the size of the collection of melanocytes in the papillary dermis. These naevi are usually darker in colour than junctional naevi. The transitional phase between junctional and compound naevus means that some lesions show the characteristics of both.

Dysplastic naevus (atypical moles)

Dysplastic naevi (BK moles) occur as large (>5 mm in diameter) flat macules or slightly raised plaques that are present in large numbers all over the body surface but with a particular concentration on the trunk. These naevi, in contrast to those already described, are frequent in non-sun-exposed areas. They commonly have an irregular contour and variable colour, particularly being darker in the centre than on the periphery. Histologically, there is replacement of the normal basal cell layer of the epidermis by naevus cells at the dermoepithelial junction with elongation of rete ridges. In the majority of cases there is a strong family history of such naevi and sometimes an additional family history of melanoma. Where there is an established family history of melanoma in association with dysplastic naevi, the trait is inherited in an autosomal dominant fashion. Dysplastic naevi may be a pleiotropic manifestation of the 1p36 familial melanoma gene, designated *CMM1*.

The management of such patients requires excisional biopsy of a typical lesion to establish the diagnosis, with genetic studies where appropriate and regular review with photographs and measurement of lesions for comparison, allowing excision of suspicious lesions at an early stage. Where there is no family history of melanoma, there is a much lesser chance of development of melanoma, and review can be less intense.

Juvenile naevus

Juvenile naevus (Spitz naevus) is most common in children and adolescents but may also occur in adults. It presents as a pink nodule that rapidly increases in size and on excision shows frequent mitoses and cellular pleomorphism which may raise questions of malignancy. Melanoma is comparatively rare in children and it is probable that some cases reported in the past have actually been Spitz naevi, which appear to have no malignant potential. However, this is not to say that melanoma does not occur in children. Indeed, when it does occur it may be aggressive in its behaviour and have a poor prognosis.

Melanoma

Aetiology and pathology

Melanomas are composed of malignant cells arising from melanocytes in the skin but can also arise in oral and anogenital mucosa, and in the eye.

Cutaneous melanomas, like naevocellular naevi, are a disorder of white-skinned Caucasian populations, with the highest incidence being in white populations living close to the equator who are exposed to UV light during both work and recreation. There has been a rapidly increasing incidence in such populations, even in susceptible populations in northern Europe with a much lower regular exposure to sunlight. It is probable that this is a real increase in incidence rather than a process of earlier detection, although public education programs now lead to much earlier presentation of the disease. The role of UV light is well established, with melanoma being most common on sun-exposed skin such as that of the upper back in males and females and also on the lower leg in females.

Melanoma can be classified into four types: lentigo maligna, superficial spreading, nodular, and acral lentiginous. As noted previously, a melanoma gene has been mapped to chromosome 1p36, and a second, designated *CMM2*, to chromosome 9p21, with the cell cycle regulator *CDKN2A* as the candidate gene. Mutations in this gene are the most common cause of inherited melanoma. The risk of melanoma in *CDKN2A* mutation carriers is approximately 14% by age 50, 24% by age 70 and 28% by age 80 years.

Lentigo maligna

Lentigo maligna occurs in elderly patients, usually more than 70 years of age, and is more common in men than in women. It appears as an extensive melanotic lesion (Hutchinson's melanotic freckle) on the cheek or temple. It is characteristically dark brown in colour and develops over many years as a superficial impalpable lesion unless malignant change occurs. Malignant change is manifested by the development of palpable darker nodules with an irregular edge, and this change is often multicentric. Hutchinson's freckle itself requires no specific treatment apart from regular observation, but lesions demonstrating suspicious changes should be removed by excisional biopsy. If malignant on biopsy, the entire lesion should be widely excised. Prognosis is good, with at least 95% disease-free survival at 10 years. There is a tendency for lateral and superficial spread of tumours long before vertical invasion occurs.

Superficial spreading melanoma

Superficial spreading melanoma is the most common form of melanoma and can occur in any site and at any age, although it is most common in middle age and commonly arises from a pre-existing naevus as already discussed. Characteristically, it is slightly raised above the skin surface, is variegated in colour (often with a dark brown or even black component) and has an irregular edge. Over a variable period, the lesion remains within the epidermis and then involves the reticular dermis. It is rare for metastasis to occur at this phase of radial growth. If untreated, an invasive vertical growth phase supervenes, with progressive involvement of the deeper dermis and underlying tissues and the development of metastatic potential. It is now possible to use a variety of melanoma antigens to discriminate between benign melanotic lesions, *in situ* melanoma, the radial and vertical growth phases of invasive melanoma, and finally metastatic melanoma. These tests give clear indications of differences in cell behaviour at these various phases.

The treatment for superficial spreading melanoma is excisional biopsy with a margin that varies with the size of the primary lesion and subsequent assessment of depth of invasion. This is determined by the use of Clark's levels of invasion, which define six levels in terms of the anatomy of the epidermis and dermis, or by the thickness of the lesion, as described by Breslow. Although Clark's levels have some correlation with prognosis, it is clear that simple measurement of the thickness of the lesion gives an even better correlation. For those with a thickness of less than 0.75 mm, 95% 10-year survival can be expected. This contrasts with only 25% survival at 10 years if the thickness is greater than 4 mm. There has been much controversy about the margins of excision in the past. It had been felt that radical excision with at least a 5-cm margin was necessary for all melanomas, but it is clear that with superficial spreading melanoma a limited margin is quite adequate.

There is also controversy about the role of elective lymph node dissection (ELND). On present evidence, as nodal metastasis is rare in lesions less than 1 mm thick, ELND should not be performed in such cases. As patients with invasive lesions more than 4 mm thick are unlikely to survive in any event, the operation is superfluous.

Of particular interest has been the development of lymphatic mapping following intradermal injection of radiolabelled colloids around the primary site, with removal of 'sentinel nodes' and histological and histochemical examination with subsequent full node dissection if positive. This procedure was examined in a large multicentre international trial and found not to provide any survival advantage and thus is not routinely recommended.

Nodular melanoma

Nodular melanoma presents as its name suggests with a protruding lesion usually arising from a pre-existing naevus, the nodular form being one component of vertical invasion. The nodule may be dark or may be amelanotic. As it is really a particular form of invasive melanoma, it is treated on its merits in terms of thickness by wide local excision with consideration of therapeutic lymph node dissection and adjuvant therapy.

Acral lentiginous melanoma

Acral lentiginous melanoma occurs in all races in non-pigmented areas, such as the palms of the hands, the soles of the feet, the subungual area and on mucosal surfaces. They are often pink in colour with little in the way of pigmentation, and there is often delay in diagnosis because of this non-specific appearance. Treatment is as for superficial spreading melanoma, depending on the thickness of the lesion. Late presentation often means that there is a significant invasive element and wide excision with or without adjuvant therapy may be necessary.

Adjuvant therapy

Chemotherapy

The benefits of combining surgery with adjuvant chemotherapy are now clear in relation to some cancers. This is undertaken in the belief that metastasis will often have occurred before patients present for primary surgery, although this may not be clinically apparent, and that systemic therapy is most likely to be effective in such patients when the bulk of tumour has been removed by surgery and the residual tumour burden is low.

Limb perfusion

For melanoma of poor prognosis confined to a limb, an additional form of treatment aimed at controlling presumed in-transit metastasis is perfusion of the isolated limb at high temperatures through an oxygenated circuit that contains phenylalanine mustard, which is selectively taken up by melanoma cells (at least in theory). The role of isolated limb perfusion as an adjuvant to surgical treatment in primary treatment remains unclear and is generally not recommended especially in the light of recent advances in immunotherapy.

Radiation therapy

Radiation therapy has no role as an adjuvant to surgery for localised disease that is treatable by wide excision, but is of value in the treatment of recurrent or inoperable disease with effective local control, particularly of nodal metastases.

Systemic therapy

Immunotherapy with anti-CTLA4 (cytotoxic T-lymphocyte-associated protein 4) has become a standard treatment for metastatic melanoma and BRAF (serine/threonine protein kinase B-raf) inhibitors have demonstrated a rapid but sometimes short-lived effect in patients with oncogene-addicted BRAF-mutant metastatic melanoma. The most appropriate sequencing of therapeutic agents remains under investigation as does the role of these agents as neoadjuvant therapy for high-risk locally advanced melanoma.

Further reading

Jakub JW, Racz JM, Hieken TJ *et al*. Neoadjuvant systemic therapy for regionally advanced melanoma. *J Surg Oncol* 2018;117:1164–9.

Menzies AM, Long GV. Systemic treatment for BRAF-mutant melanoma: where do we go next? *Lancet Oncol* 2014;15:e371–e381.

Singh B, Shah JP. Skin cancers of the head and neck. In: Shah JP, Patel SG (eds) *Cancer of the Head and Neck*. Hamilton, Ontario: BC Decker, 2001, chapter 4.

MCQs

Select the single correct answer to each question. The correct answers can be found in the Answers section at the end of the book.

1 A 70-year-old man presents with a 1-cm painless nodule on the side of his nose. This has been present for 3 weeks. The centre of the lesion appears to contain a plug of hard skin. What is the most likely diagnosis?
   a squamous cell carcinoma
   b basal cell carcinoma
   c keratoacanthoma
   d Merkel cell carcinoma
   e seborrhoiec keratosis

2 A 45-year-old motor mechanic presents with a nodule on the tip of his finger. This has been present for 12 months and it bothers him now when he presses on that finger. He seems to remember injuring that finger at work several years earlier. On examination there is a 0.5-cm nodule and the overlying skin is intact. What is the most likely diagnosis?
   a dermoid cyst
   b epidermoid cyst
   c pyogenic granuloma
   d dermatofibroma
   e cylindroma

3 The parents of a 4-week-old boy are concerned about a lump above the infant's right eye. It has been present since birth and has not changed in size. The skin over the 1-cm lump is intact and the lump appears to be attached to the underlying tissues. What is the most likely diagnosis?
   a dermoid cyst
   b epidermoid cyst
   c cystic hygroma
   d branchial cyst
   e osteoma

4 A 75-year-old man has what appears to be a 1-cm basal cell carcinoma on the side of his nose immediately below his left eye. What would be the most appropriate treatment?
   a radiotherapy
   b application of 5-fluorouracil cream
   c injection of vinblastine
   d excision and split-skin graft
   e excision and full-thickness graft

5 A 17-year-old girl presents with a painless swelling on the anterior aspect of her right leg. This has been present for about 6 months and does not bother her much, except that it itches occasionally. The lump is pink and firm, and the overlying skin is intact. What is the most likely diagnosis?
   a basal cell carcinoma
   b epidermoid cyst
   c Bowen's disease
   d dermatofibroma
   e malignant melanoma

45 Soft tissue tumours

Peter F. Choong

University of Melbourne, St. Vincent's Hospital and Peter MacCallum Cancer Centre, Melbourne, Victoria, Australia

Introduction

Primary soft tissue tumours include benign and malignant tumours. Malignancies of skin such as basal cell carcinomas, squamous cell carcinomas and melanomas are dealt with in Chapter 44. The most common soft tissue tumours are benign. Sometimes differentiating these from malignant tumours (sarcoma) can be very difficult because sarcomas are rare and experience in both identification and treating this entity may be lacking.

The approach to managing soft tissue tumours is focused on differentiating benign from malignant forms. To this end, a good history and examination coupled with appropriate investigations and biopsy are essential to avoid the complications of inadvertent excision of sarcoma. Important characteristics on history include the temporal nature of tumour occurrence and the presence of symptoms (pain and compression). The tumour's physical characteristics should be described in terms of size, site, shape, consistency, border, underlying structures, and overlying structures. Cystic structures may be transilluminated and vascular sturctures may be pulsatile.

Investigations include ultrasound, anatomic and functional imaging. Anatomic imaging includes computed tomography (CT) and magnetic resonance imaging (MRI). The latter is the most accurate means of characterising the anatomy and nature of soft tissue tumours because it provides unparalleled soft tissue contrast. Ultrasound, although very easy to obtain, is prone to misdiagnosis and is best reserved solely for determining whether the lesion is solid or cystic. Differentiating the malignant potential based on ultrasound is fraught.

Most benign tumours may be excised alone and rarely require adjuvant therapy. Sarcomas, in contrast, require expert centre-based multidisciplinary care.

Benign soft tissue tumours

Lipoma

The commonest benign tumour is the lipoma (Figure 45.1). Originating from the mesenchyme, fatty tissue is one of the ubiquitous supportive tissues in the body that separate anatomical parts. In this regard, lipomas may arise from almost any part of the body. Typically, lipomas have a long history (years) and may be characterised by slow growth. Occasionally, there may be a history of fast growth (months). Often this is less a case of exponential growth but more of a large lipoma emerging (herniating) from between muscle fibres, septae or anatomical compartments.

Lipomas are slow-growing, thus allowing the adjacent fascial tissue to expand and adapt around it. Rather than being fixed and constraining, the membranous capsule around a lipoma adapts and is the reason why lipomas are often soft and pliable. Lipomas are often solitary but may be multiple. Dercum's disease is a syndrome of multiple painful lipomata.

Atypical lipomas are a variant of lipomas where there is a mild cellular atypia. These are thought to have malignant potential leading to the formation of well-differentiated lipoma-like liposarcoma.

CT often shows a well-encapsulated lesion with a predominance of fatty attenuation. What should raise suspicion is the presence of obvious fibrous striations running through the substance of the tumour. Histology is the key to making the diagnosis, with the presence of cells with size differences and some level of atypia. Lipoblasts tip the diagnosis towards sarcoma. More recent investigations include molecular profiling, which has identified *MDM2* gene amplification as a hallmark of sarcomatous change.

Lipomas may be excised if large or cosmetically unacceptable. Sometimes, lipomas may recur and intramuscular varieties have a greater likelihood for this.

Textbook of Surgery, Fourth Edition. Edited by Julian A. Smith, Andrew H. Kaye, Christopher Christophi and Wendy A. Brown.
© 2020 John Wiley & Sons Ltd. Published 2020 by John Wiley & Sons Ltd.

(a)   (b)

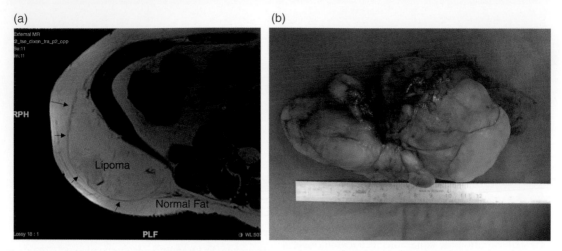

Fig. 45.1 (a) Lipoma of the flank: MRI showing typically encapsulated lesion (arrows) with signal attenuation identical to surrounding normal fat. (b) Surgical specimen is encapsulated, greasy and yellow in colour.

Nerve sheath tumour

Nerve sheath tumours comprise schwannomas and neurofibromas. Schwannomas are peripheral nerve sheath tumours that arise from the myelin-producing supporting cells (Schwann cells) that surround the nerves and their fibrils. They usually occur as solitary lesions, lying along the line of skin or motor nerves. They may vary in size from small pea-sized tumours to much larger tumours that can occupy whole anatomic compartments. These tumours are associated with hypersensitivity when touched or knocked. Neurofibromas are small benign tumours that also arise from peripheral nerves. In almost all cases (90%), these are sporadic. However, the remainder may be associated with an abnormality of the neurofibromatosis (*NF1*) gene. Neurofibromatosis is an autosomal dominant inherited abnormality characterised by a constellation of cutaneous, visceral and musculoskeletal abnormalities as well as pain syndromes and occasionally cognitive deficits.

The key investigation here is MRI, which classically demonstrates a round encapsulated lesion with a 'rat's tail' appearance of the nerve entering and leaving the mass (Figure 45.2).

Nerve sheath tumours can usually be left alone unless they are symptomatic (exquisitely tender). If they arise from important sensory or motor nerves, careful intraneural dissection may be required to preserve the continuity of the affected nerve.

Haemangioma

Haemangiomas are a variety of vascular malformation and are common (Figure 45.3). They may occur in any tissue and may be superficial or deep.

Haemangiomas comprise tortuous channels of blood vessels often embedded in lipomatous tissue. They may be predominantly arterial or, more commonly, low-flow venous types. When deep, haemangiomas may be first noticed as a lump that increases and decreases in size. Other times, the lump may be heralded by acute pain and swelling caused by thrombosis and pain.

Haemangiomas of the skin are often referred to as birthmarks. They may be very localised and small like the strawberry naevus seen on the foreheads of young babies that often involute with age, or the wide permanent areas often referred to as port wine stains. When on the face, these may follow a dermatomal pattern.

Haemangiomas may be associated with a number of well-described syndromes, including Sturge–Weber syndrome, Klippel–Trenaunay syndrome, Bean syndrome and Proteus syndrome.

Deep-seated haemangiomas which cause a mass can be excised if well circumscribed. If the haemangioma is more extensive without clear boundaries, repeated embolisation may help to reduce its size. Surgery for this variety is more challenging.

Angiomyoma

Angiomyomas are small painful tumours often found near joints. They are mostly in a subcutaneous position and the knee and ankle are common sites. They arise from the tunica media of blood vessels and present as discrete firm nodules or lumps. They are exquisitely tender when touched and can mimic neuromas. They are often well circumscribed. Angiomyomas are easily excised and rarely recur.

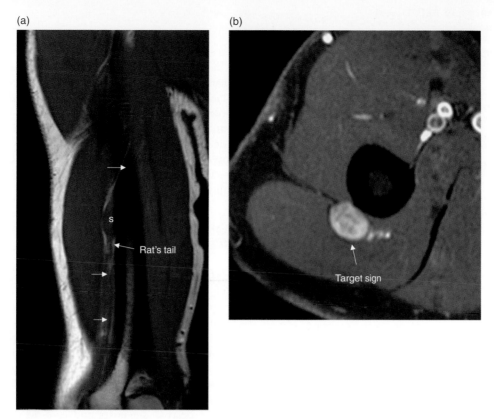

Fig. 45.2 (a) MRI of schwannoma (S) of the upper arm demonstrating ovoid lesion in the line of the radial nerve (arrows) which give the characteristic 'rat's tail' appearance. (b) Axial MRI showing characteristic concentric light–dark–light rings within schwannoma giving rise to the 'target' sign.

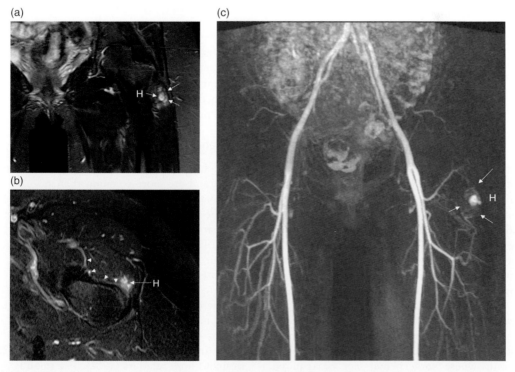

Fig. 45.3 (a) MRI showing haemangioma (H) in proximal vastus lateralis (arrows). Note the large cavernous spaces within the haemangioma. (b) MRI showing vascular supply to the haemangioma (arrowheads). (c) MRI angiogram demonstrating vascular tree with tributary (arrows) to haemangioma.

Myxoma

An intramuscular myxoma is a mucin-producing tumour that is found deep within muscle. Although it is poorly encapsulated and merges with the surrounding musculature, its defining characteristic is its mobility within muscle and it is sometimes likened to the 'breast mouse' (fibroadenoma). Generally paucicellular, this entity produces abundant myxoid tissue and can grow to large sizes. This can sometimes be difficult to differentiate from a low-grade myxoid sarcoma.

Excision of a myxoma, once confirmed from biopsy, is not associated with any recurrence, despite the surgery often leaving residual tumour behind because of its embedment within muscle.

Desmoid

Desmoid tumours arise from the fibroblast lineage and are characterised by a craggy hard mass. The condition is also known as fibromatosis. They are usually solitary but may be multiple. As they arise from the mesenchyme, they may occur in any location. They commonly occur in women between 20 and 40 years of age and are found on the nape and flank. They may also occur in the limbs.

They are often slow-growing, although their growth pattern may be irregular and unpredictable. A sudden acceleration during or after pregnancy and their predominance in women suggest a correlation with hormonal regulation. Although benign, desmoid tumours may grow in critical localities compromising vital structures such as organs, vessels and nerves. At worse, desmoid tumours may also prove fatal because of impingement on these vital structures.

Desmoid tumours may also be syndromic, such as in Gardner's syndrome, a variant of familial adenomatous polyposis (FAP). FAP is an autosomal dominant inherited condition characterised by multiple colonic polyps with a predisposition to colonic carcinoma. In Gardner's syndrome, there is also the presence of multiple extracolonic abnormalities including osteomas, fibromas, thyroid malignancies, epidermoid cysts and desmoid tumours.

The treatment of desmoid tumours may be challenging. The presence of peripheral microscopic extensions make recurrence of the tumour highly likely if resected with close margins. Adjuvant radiotherapy has been shown to reduce the likelihood of recurrence if combined with resection, although radiotherapy alone may result in size reduction to the point where surgery may not be required. Conventional chemotherapy is not normally used because of the poor response, but other agents such as hormonal/antihormonal drugs and other novel agents have been tried with some success. Predicting which tumour is likely to respond is difficult. Occasionally, desmoid may behave in an idiosyncratic fashion and disappear after needle biopsy alone. This has led to one option which is to merely observe desmoid until such time as it becomes a problem, then a choice of surgery or surgery plus adjuvants may be exercised.

Primary malignant soft tissue tumours (sarcomas)

Soft tissue sarcoma (STS) is of mesenchymal origin and may arise in any tissue layer of the body. Despite being rare, over 70 subtypes exist, attesting to the complexity of diagnosis and confusion that may sometimes arise in identifying the nature of a soft tissue lump. Fewer than 1% of all soft tissue tumours and only 0.1% of all cancers are sarcomas, meaning that the lack of familiarity of pathologists and clinicians with this entity often leads to incorrect or delayed diagnoses and care. Modern sarcoma management is best conducted in expert centres where multidisciplinary care may be provided by clinicians with a specialist interest in sarcoma treatment, and in this setting patients with sarcoma are afforded the best outcomes for local and systemic control of disease. Surgery is the mainstay of sarcoma management and is often combined with radiotherapy in a neoadjuvant or adjuvant setting. Chemotherapy is sometimes used in combination with surgery, although this is not regarded as conventional and depends on institutional preferences.

Incidence

Soft tissue sarcomas arise in 2–4 per 100 000 population and are more common than primary bone sarcomas. There is a male predominance (1.4 : 1) and the median age of occurrence is approximately 60 years. STS have a bimodal presentation with peaks in the fifth and eighth decades. Specific tumour types are associated with each of these peaks. For example, synovial sarcoma and myxoid liposarcoma arise in younger patients whereas undifferentiated pleomorphic sarcoma is mainly found in middle-aged and older adults.

STSs occur most commonly in the limbs, with lower limb tumours being twice as common (28%) as upper limb tumours (12%). The thigh is by far the most common site for STS. Over 50% of STSs occur deep to the deep fascia and may grow to substantial sizes if they arise in the thigh and pelvic cavity. The median size of an STS is approximately 8 cm.

Behaviour

Soft tissue sarcomas grow in a centrifugal manner and displace adjacent tissue. More aggressive lesions may show an 'invasive' character rather than a 'pushing' character. STSs may be mistaken for lipomas, which are by far the most common soft tissue lumps. While lipomas may grow to enormous sizes, they are often soft and pliable which reflects their slow rate of growth and adaptation of the surrounding tissue to their slow growth. STSs, on the other hand, are often firm or hard, which reflect their rapid growth within the confines of a tissue boundary or the tumour's pseudocapsule. The pseudocapsule is a boundary of compressed normal tissue or inflammatory adventitia that forms due to the growth of the tumour and the stimulation of an inflammatory response at the periphery of the tumour by tumour cytokines. STSs are known to have satellite lesions within the inflammatory zone at the periphery of the tumour. This is an important characteristic of a STS that mandates appropriate surgical margins and adjuvant treatment.

STSs recur locally or systemically. The reason for local recurrence is the existence of residual tumour after resection or local metastasis in the setting of a very aggressive tumour. Control of local recurrence is achieved through adequate surgical margins in the first instance.

STSs may also metastasise and these occur most commonly to the lungs. Pulmonary metastases account for 50% of all metastases and may be unilateral or bilateral. Often pulmonary metastases are solitary or low in numbers and are amenable to resection (pulmonary metastasectomy). Metastases occur via the haematogenous route but may also occur via lymphatic spread in rare cases. Examples of tumours that may metastasise to the lymph nodes include synovial sarcoma, alveolar soft part sarcoma and epithelioid cell sarcoma.

Classification

The World Health Organization Classification of Tumours of Soft Tissue and Bone is an attempt at developing a common nomenclature to describe this rare tumour (Table 45.1)and is based on the most differentiated cell type within the array of malignant cells. Its adoption allows more meaningful comparisons of tumour types and treatment regimens. The most significant change to the classification since the 2000s has been to drop the entity 'malignant fibrous histiocytoma' and its variants, which was previously the most frequent diagnosis made. This term was used to describe a grab-bag of tumours that could not otherwise be classified into distinct histological types according to the most differentiated cell type observed. Today, an STS that cannot be classified according to histology is referred to as undifferentiated pleomorphic sarcoma (UPS) and this is often a diagnosis of exclusion. Newer modalities of pathological interrogation, including molecular, chromosomal and immunohistochemical techniques, have aided in refining the diagnostic process and accuracy.

Tumour grade

The grade of a tumour relates to its histological appearance, which also correlates with its clinical behaviour. A variety of grading systems exist. Increasing cellular pleomorphism, hyperchromatism, spontaneous tumour necrosis, intratumoral vascular invasion, mitotic activity and lack of cellular differentiation are hallmarks of higher-grade tumours. Higher-grade tumours are associated with a higher risk of local and systemic recurrence of disease. A four-grade (I–IV) histological system to grade tumours is commonly used. Grades I and II may also be referred to as low grade, while grades III and IV may be referred to as high grade.

Diagnosis

Diagnosis relies on a high index of clinical suspicion, and the judicious use of appropriate investigations (anatomical, functional) that culminate in biopsy.

History

Soft tissue sarcomas undergo a regular and rapid doubling rate. Therefore, patients often report the presence of a lump that appeared spontaneously and which seemed to remain a certain size before rapidly increasing its dimensions over a period of months. The rapid increase is due to tumour cells reaching the exponential phase of growth. The lump is often painless and because of this there is often a delay in presentation. It is surprising, however, the number of patients who present with enormous tumours. Synovial sarcoma is one that has contrasting behaviour to other STSs. It is often detected at a younger age, smaller size and a hallmark of presentation is pain.

Table 45.1 Primary soft tissue tumours.

Tissue type	Subtype	
Adipose	Benign	Lipoma
	Malignant	Well-differentiated lipoma-like liposarcoma
		Myxoid liposarcoma
		Round cell liposarcoma
		Pleomorphic liposarcoma
Fibrous	Benign	Desmoid (fibromatosis)
		Nodular fasciitis
	Malignant	Fibrosarcoma
		Myxofibrosarcoma
Cartilage	Benign	Enchondroma
		Osteochondroma
	Malignant	Central chondrosarcoma
		Dedifferentiated chondrosarcoma
		Clear-cell chondrosarcoma
		Mesenchymal chondrosarcoma
Bone	Benign	Osteoma
	Malignant	Conventional osteosarcoma
		Parosteal osteosarcoma
		Periosteal osteosarcoma
		Low-grade central osteosarcoma
Skeletal muscle	Benign	Myoma
	Malignant	Alveolar rhabdomyosarcoma
		Embryonal rhabdomyosarcoma
Smooth muscle	Benign	Leiomyoma
	Malignant	Leiomyosarcoma
Vascular	Benign	Haemangioma
	Malignant	Haemangioendothelioma
		Haemangiopericytoma
		Angiosarcoma
Nerve sheath	Benign	Neurofibroma
		Schwannoma
	Malignant	Malignant peripheral nerve sheath tumour
		Neuroepithelioma
		Malignant granular cell tumour
Synovial	Benign	Pigmented vilonodular synovitis (giant cell tumour of tendon sheath)
	Malignant	Synovial sarcoma
Unclassified	Malignant	Undifferentiated pleomorphic sarcoma

All lumps greater than 5 cm (golf ball size) or deep to the deep fascia should be considered a sarcoma until proven otherwise.

Investigations

All lumps suspected of being a sarcoma must undergo appropriate anatomical and functional imaging prior to biopsy. The reason for biopsy following imaging is that imaging modalities such as MRI may be difficult to interpret in the setting of a biopsy-induced imaging artefact (e.g. inflammation, haematoma, altered anatomy). To avoid unnecessary or inadequate imaging, all lumps suspected of being a sarcoma should be referred to a tumour centre specialising in sarcoma management for definitive investigation and treatment.

Plain radiography

Plain radiography is seldom indicated as an initial investigation for STS. However, this modality may be useful for differentiating a soft tissue mass from a bony protruberance such as an osteochondroma. Plain radiography may also detect ossification within a soft tissue mass and this may be characteristic of myositis ossificans, heterotopic ossification, phleboliths within a haemangioma or a synovial sarcoma.

Magnetic resonance imaging

MRI provides unsurpassed soft tissue contrast and is essential for evaluating soft tissue tumours (Figure 45.4). MRI scans can be used to accurately characterise the site, size, shape, consistency, and relation of the mass to adjacent structures. Fine detail provided by MRI may also allow evaluation of invasion of the tumour into adjacent bone and soft tissue structures. Peritumoral oedema is an important finding which reflects the possibility of tumour extension. Spontaneous tumour necrosis may also be suggested by a heterogeneous MRI signal reflecting a high-grade tumour.

The most viable tumour tissue is present in the more solid areas and at the periphery of the tumour. These areas should be targeted for biopsy. Centrally necrotic or haemorrhagic areas should be avoided in order to prevent a false-negative diagnosis. These features are readily identifiable on MRI, which can be used to plan the approach to biopsy. Because MRI is so sensitive to any soft tissue perturbation, it is essential that these scans are performed prior to biopsy to avoid confounding signals generated by biopsy or surgical artefact that may make interpretation difficult leading to under- or over-diagnosis.

The entire tumour-bearing compartment should be scanned to ensure that any satellite lesions are detected so that these can be included as part of the resected specimen. Moreover, MRI scans are extremely useful for delineating adjacent neurovascular structures and the involvement of specific muscular compartments. Such anatomical information assists in determining tumour resectability and the anticipated quality of surgical margins.

Computed tomography

CT scans are ubiquitous and are easily obtained where MRI is either not available or contraindicated such as in patients with pacemakers, vascular stents or embedded metal shrapnel. These scans are particularly good for detecting fine calcifications and this modality may be useful when evaluating the nature of periosteal reactions, bone destruction or soft tissue calcification (Figure 45.5).

CT scans of the lungs are essential for assessing the systemic spread of disease because the lungs are the commonest site for metastases.

Percutaneous CT-guided core needle biopsy is now the standard for obtaining tissue for diagnosis. This modality allows accurate placement of the biopsy needle, planning of the biopsy tract, and a scan to be obtained of the needle in position to confirm adequacy and appropriateness of the biopsy.

Functional scans

Functional scans are used to evaluate the metabolic activity of a tumour. Highly metabolic lesions are more likely to be malignant; in the context of a confirmed STS, a highly metabolic tumour is likely to be a higher-grade lesion. Functional scans are invaluable for identifying the most metabolically active location within a tumour and this location may then be co-registered with a CT scan and used to

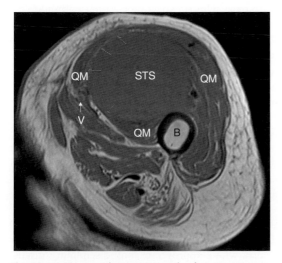

Fig. 45.4 MRI provides unsurpassed soft tissue contrast. Fatty tissue (blue arrows) around soft tissue sarcoma (STS) within the quadriceps musculature (QM) provides different signal characteristics from the tumour and is invaluable for determining the boundary of the tumour. MRI clearly demonstrates important neighbouring structures such as the femoral vessels (V) and the uninvolved cortex and intramedually canal of bone (B).

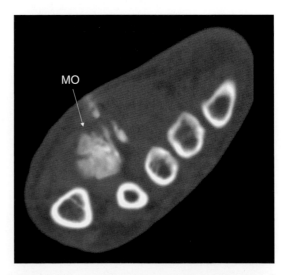

Fig. 45.5 CT scan of foot demonstrating calcification of myositis ossificans (MO) on plantar aspect.

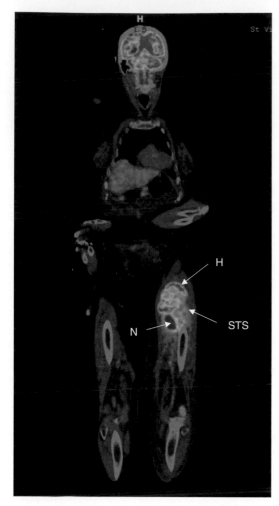

Fig. 45.6 PET scan of a soft tissue sarcoma (STS) within the quadriceps muscle. Note high metabolic activity (H) in tracer-avid region of tumour, and low tracer avidity in area of central tumour necrosis (N). This helps to demonstrate both response to treatment and also areas that should be targeted or avoided during image-guided biopsy.

up thallium when activated. Such tissues that take up ^{201}Tl on a thallium scan stand out as a 'hotspot'. Glucose is also used as an energy source by highly metabolically active tumours. This characteristic is exploited in PET scans where radioactively labelled glucose is used as the nuclear tracer.

Both types of scan may be used effectively for tumours of the limbs. However, PET is more useful for intra-abdominal and pelvic STSs as the high amount of visceral uptake of ^{201}Tl can sometimes obscure any tracer-avid tumour.

Biopsy

Biopsy is essential for the appropriate treatment of STS. No soft tissue tumour should be excised without an accurate diagnosis and biopsy is the most effective way of obtaining this. Biopsy should be performed at the completion of all other anatomical and functional investigations. This is because biopsy may confound the findings of anatomical and functional scans if done before imaging, because of the post-biopsy imaging artefact. In addition, imaging provides an ideal resource for targeting the optimal site for biopsy in order to obtain the most representative and highest-grade component of a tumour.

Biopsy may be performed in a number of ways, namely fine-needle aspiration biopsy, percutaneous core needle biopsy, open biopsy and excisional biopsy. Fine-needle biopsy requires a highly skilled cytologist who is expert in sarcoma pathology for interpretation of cellular findings and these individuals may not be readily available in all institutions. For optimal care, open biopsy should be undertaken at a tumour centre where experts in sarcoma surgery are available to plan the biopsy entry site in relation to the definitive procedure. This is because the biopsy tract will need to be excised en bloc with the tumour mass to ensure local control of disease. The placement of the biopsy site is critical for appropriate surgical management because errors in biopsy placement or procedure may compromise subsequent surgery or reconstruction. At worst, an error in biopsy may lead to amputation of the affected limb. Excisional biopsy should never be done except in a tumour centre where appropriate multidisciplinary discussion can occur prior to the procedure and all the relevant imaging modalities scrutinised. Image-guided core needle biopsy is now a standard method for obtaining biopsy material (Figure 45.7). Image guidance allows accurate targeting of representative tissue and the procedure is less invasive or harmful than open biopsy, where the complications of haemorrhage and infection are a finite risk that

target the biopsy. Functional scans may also be used to evaluate the tumour's response to neoadjuvant treatment such as radiotherapy or chemotherapy. Functional scans may be used to differentiate recurrent tumour from postoperative granulation. If a patient is referred after inadvertent resection of an STS, functional scans may be useful for identifying gross residual tumour.

Two types of functional scan in use include the thallium scan and positron emission tomography (PET) (Figure 45.6). Thallium-201 (^{201}Tl) is a radioactive chemical analogue of potassium and its uptake by metabolically active tissue relies on the sodium potassium pump. Cardiac muscle, bowel and active muscle are examples of tissue that take

(a) (b)

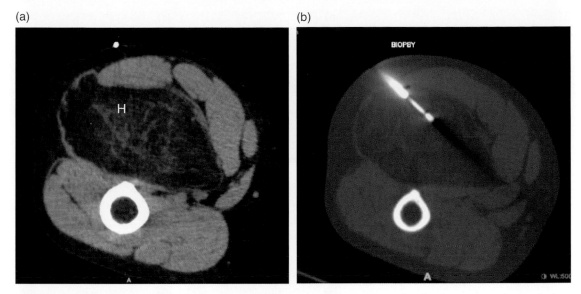

Fig. 45.7 (a) Heterogeneous area (H) within lipomatous tumour raising suspicions that this 'lipoma' may be atypical. (b) Image-guided biopsy can target suspicious areas.

may affect subsequent treatment. Image-guided core needle biopsy requires skill and experience in this field, and the modality is best sought from a centre specialising in sarcoma care.

Staging of tumours

Staging of tumours is the process whereby extensive data are collected on tumours. Preoperative local staging includes all the imaging modalities described to better understand the local extent of the tumour. Systemic staging includes a CT scan of the chest and functional scans in order to assess the occurrence of metastatic spread. Preoperative staging studies also include the biopsy.

Restaging studies after neoadjuvant treatment and prior to surgery include these same tests but without the need for a second biopsy. The purpose of the restaging studies is to evaluate the response of the tumour to neoadjuvant treatment, whether metastases are visible after the treatment or whether there has been any change in lesions suspected of being metastases. The features of response may include a change in size, shape, number, consistency, presence of intratumoral haemorrhage or cystic change, and the appearance of a true capsule around the tumour. Functional scans are valuable for assessing the metabolic response to neoadjuvant treatment and is a measure of tumour 'kill'.

Treatment

The mainstay of treatment is surgical resection. This is usually combined with radiotherapy.

Chemotherapy is sometimes provided as an institutional preference.

Surgery

The most important goal of surgical care is to achieve adequate surgical margins. Doing so ensures the lowest risk of local recurrence of disease. Surgical margins are planned preoperatively with the use of the staging studies. MRI provides unsurpassed soft tissue contrast and is critical for planning surgical margins. Surgery should be performed with oncological goals and not with the view to reducing reconstruction (aesthetic goals).

Surgical margins may be classified as intralesional, marginal, wide or radical margins (Figure 45.8). Intralesional margins are seen when the excision passes through the tumour capsule. Marginal margins are seen when the excision passes through the inflammatory zone around the tumour. This zone contains satellite lesions or extensions of the tumour which may be responsible for the high rate of local recurrence should a resection pass through this zone. Wide margins include a cuff of normal tissue around the tumour itself. This can be achieved when there is a named anatomical layer of normal tissue around the tumour in the radial direction and there is 2–5 cm of normal tissue in the longitudinal axis of the tumour. Radical margins are achieved when the entire tumour-bearing compartment is excised.

Intralesional or marginal margins are inadequate surgical margins. Occasionally, marginal margins are required to preserve vital structures such as

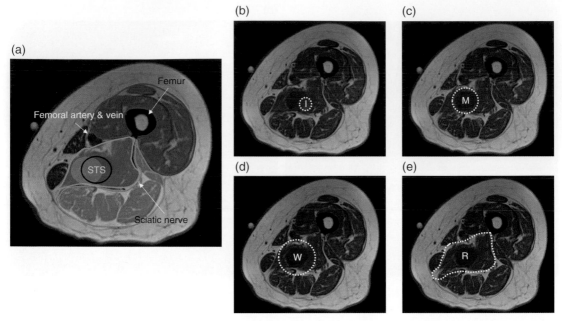

Fig. 45.8 (a) MRI of soft tissue sarcoma (STS) within adductor magnus muscle. Note adductor compartment (green), hamstring compartment (orange) and quadriceps compartment (blue). (b) Intralesional margin (dotted line) passes through the capsule of the tumour. (c) Marginal margin (dotted line) passes through the inflammatory pseudocapsule of the tumour. (d) Wide margin (dotted line) passes outside the inflammatory zone through a cuff of normal tissue. (e) Radical margin (dotted line) includes the entire tumour-bearing compartment, which in this case is the adductor compartment.

nerves, vessels and viscera. In this scenario, radiotherapy is often used to upgrade the quality of the margin and when combined with marginal margins is equal to wide margins alone. Intralesional margins should never be knowingly employed.

Resection of an STS usually leaves a large dead space or exposed soft tissue defect. In both cases, soft tissue reconstructions are required to diminish dead space and provide skin cover or to provide a functional reconstruction. If following resection a limb is not expected to be functional or if the defect cannot be closed, then amputation should be considered.

Inadequate surgery should be avoided where possible. Inadvertent resection with positive margins is associated with a higher risk of death from disease, inferior survival and local recurrence. Surgery for STS should be performed at a tumour centre specialising in sarcoma care.

Radiotherapy

The combination of radiotherapy and surgery provides better local control of disease than either surgery or radiotherapy alone. Radiotherapy is able to upgrade the quality of the surgical margins and this

is particularly important where the margin has to be close because of an attempt to preserve vital neurovascular structures or viscera.

Radiotherapy is usually given to a total dose of 50.4 cGy and delivered over 5–6 weeks. During this time, the patient may develop skin reactions in the field of radiotherapy and this may be characterised by erythema, desquamation or blistering. Surgery is usually performed 4–5 weeks after completion of radiotherapy to allow the soft tissue reaction to settle.

Chemotherapy

There is debate as to the role of chemotherapy in the management of primary STS. It is not conventionally used, but some institutions do prescribe chemotherapy and cite a local control advantage. Some suggest the use of chemotherapy in the setting of a high-risk tumour (large and high grade).

Chemotherapy does have a role in metastatic disease. In a palliative setting, chemotherapy may control growth for a period of time and may be able to provide some relief for patients with symptomatic disease.

There is growing interest in next-generation sequencing for identifying genetic aberrations that may be linked with mechanisms for tumour progression. Identifying these aberrations may pave the way for novel therapy in appropriate candidates.

Further reading

Trieu J, Sinnathamby M, Di Bella C *et al*. Biopsy and the diagnostic evaluation of musculoskeletal tumours: critical but often missed in the 21st century. *ANZ J Surg* 2016;86:133–8.

Vodanovich DA, Choong PF. Soft-tissue sarcomas. *Indian J Orthop* 2018;52:35–44.

MCQs

Select the single correct answer to each question. The correct answers can be found in the Answers section at the end of the book.

1 Soft tissue sarcomas are commonest in:
   a abdomen and retroperitoneum
   b head and neck
   c lower limb
   d upper limb
   e thorax

2 The commonest site of metastasis for soft tissue sarcomas is:
   a regional lymph nodes
   b liver
   c bone
   d lungs
   e brain

3 Which of the following is an indication for removal of a lipoma?
   a a 3-cm lipoma in the tibialis anterior
   b a 3-cm lipoma in the subcutaneous fat of the anterior abdominal wall
   c a 3-cm lipoma in the subcutaneous fat of the buttock
   d a lipoma of many years standing which has not changed in size
   e a lipoma on CT scanning of heterogeneous density

4 Desmoid tumours:
   a are commoner in women as they age
   b occur in the root of the mesentery in association with FAP syndrome
   c cause death by metastasis
   d tend not to recur locally
   e metastasise to regional lymph nodes

5 Soft tissue sarcomas:
   a are often greater than 5 cm
   b often engage the deep fascia
   c should be treated at a sarcoma centre
   d need to be investigated and biopsied at a sarcoma centre
   e all the above

46 Infection of the extremities

Mark W. Ashton¹ and David M.A. Francis²

¹ University of Melbourne and Royal Melbourne Hospital, Melbourne, Victoria, Australia
² Department of Urology, Royal Children's Hospital, Melbourne, Victoria, Australia and Department
of Surgery, Tribhuvan University Teaching Hospital, Kathmandu, Nepal

Introduction

Infections of the extremities may be broadly grouped into those arising from fungal and those arising from bacterial organisms. Bacteria may secondarily infect fungal disease. Whilst most patients will have no underlying medical problems, particular care needs to be taken in treating patients with a compromised immune system, especially those with diabetes, immunosuppression and alcoholism.

Fungal infections of the extremities

Fungal infections are probably the most common of the infections involving the extremities, particularly the lower limb. Almost everyone has either experienced personally or knows someone who has had a fungal infection. Fungi thrive in warm, moist, dark environments, and are broadly divided into two groups, yeasts and moulds. Yeasts are unicellular and round or oval in shape whereas moulds are multicellular and filamentous or threadlike in shape. Both yeasts and moulds can infect humans.

The most common types of fungi causing disease in humans are called dermatophytes. These are aerobic fungi that require keratin for growth and hence they invade and infect the skin, hair and nails. In general, these infections are superficial and the fungi do not cause invasive disease except in immunocompromised patients. Dermatophytes are usually spread by direct contact from other people, animals or soil. However, they can also be spread via non-living objects that are capable of transferring infection. These objects are called *fomites* and common examples are skin cells, hair, clothing, bedding and mattresses.

The clinical disease varies by the type of organism, the site of infection and the host response.

Tinea pedis

This is probably the most common fungal infection in the extremities and may be caused by either a mould or a yeast. The moist occluded areas of footwear, particularly in the presence of sweat, provide an ideal environment for fungi. These fungi also thrive in the warm humid atmosphere of public showers, saunas, spas and steam rooms, and consequently transmission between individuals can occur readily in these environments.

Tinea pedis appears in three ways.

- In the *interdigital* skin, where it appears as white macerated soggy skin that may or may not be accompanied by an odour.
- As *patches* of recurrent vesicular eruptions that are itchy and red, commonly on the instep of the foot.
- On the soles of the foot, where it appears as dry and scaly skin that is frequently itchy; there may be cracking, fissuring and thickening of the skin.

The treatment of tinea pedis initially involves changing the environment in which the fungi are growing. These measures are aimed at reducing the amount of available moisture, and include proper drying of the feet after bathing, open footwear, and using natural fibres such as cotton or wool to reduce sweating. Patients are advised to avoid contact with high-risk areas by the use of sandals.

Conservative treatment may be combined with antifungal agents. These may be administered either topically or systemically. Topical treatment with tolnaftate or miconazole creams, for example, is best used in superficial infection, as these agents are unable to penetrate thick keratin layers such as those found on the heel. These topical treatments usually need to be applied daily for a minimum of 6 weeks. Recurrence of tinea pedis is often due to patients discontinuing the treatment once the symptoms disappear.

Textbook of Surgery, Fourth Edition. Edited by Julian A. Smith, Andrew H. Kaye, Christopher Christophi and Wendy A. Brown.
© 2020 John Wiley & Sons Ltd. Published 2020 by John Wiley & Sons Ltd.

In severe or chronic cases, oral treatment with griseofulvin may be considered. The newer generation of oral treatments have shorter treatment times and higher cure rates with fewer side effects.

Onychomycosis

This is a fungal infection of the nail. In general, it is much more difficult to treat than tinea pedis. It is broadly grouped into four distinctive types.
- *Distal* or lateral side of the nail: this is the most common.
- *Proximal*: this is often chronic.
- *Superficial*: the nail plate becomes white. It usually develops from distal to proximal.
- *Total*: the whole nail is affected and may result from any of the above.

In all these categories the nail takes on a characteristic appearance. The nail becomes white and thickened, there may be white or yellow vertical striations, and the nail plate may lift off the underlying nail bed.

The treatment of fungal infection of the nail depends on number of nails involved, the clinical type and the severity of infection. In general, distal and superficial disease can be treated with a topical agent whereas systemic treatment is always required in proximal infection. Topical treatments are usually unable to cure proximal nail infection because of inadequate nail penetration. In general, monotherapy tends to be less effective than combination therapy, and daily application for a long period of time is usually required, sometimes up to a year.

In severe or chronic cases, oral or systemic treatment may be considered. As with the treatment of tinea pedis, the newer generation of oral treatments have replaced the older treatments. These agents have shorter treatment times and higher cure rates with fewer side effects. In severe cases oral treatments may be combined with nail removal and topical agents.

Despite these newer agents, the rate of recurrence in proximal disease remains high, and therefore alternative treatments such as photodynamic therapy may represent future treatment options.

Ringworm

Ringworm is a fungal infection of the skin. Typically, it results in a red, itchy, scaly circular rash. It may be associated with hair loss and multiple areas of skin can be affected simultaneously. About 40 different types of fungi can cause ringworm. Treatment is the same as for tinea pedis and involves keeping the area clean and dry, reducing moisture and the use of topical antifungal creams.

Bacterial infection of the extremities

Bacterial infection of the extremity may arise following injury to the arm or leg or may arise as a manifestation of a systemic infection. Bacterial infection may rapidly progress and can lead to significant loss of tissue, the amputation of the limb, or death. Patients particularly at risk are those with a compromised immune system, such as those with diabetes, alcoholism or HIV infection, and therefore any history obtained from a patient must specifically question the individual's immune status. In almost every case, bacterial infection of the extremities will respond to rest and elevation of the affected limb, and indeed this is the mainstay of the treatment of bacterial infection of the extremities.

Bacterial infection of the extremities covers a diverse range of disease, extending from the minor to the rapidly progressing infection that is life-threatening. The most common infections involve organisms that are usually seen on the skin surface of otherwise healthy individuals. The most common of these are *Staphylococcus aureus* and group A *Streptococcus*. *Streptococcus* species are particularly important as they produce an enzyme called streptokinase that breaks down the body's defence systems and allows rapid spread of *Streptococcus* (and other bacteria) significantly beyond the original site of contamination.

Usually these organisms are sensitive to simple antibiotics. However, in environments where there is a high usage of penicillin antibiotics, a resistant form of *Staphylococcus aureus* (the most common of which is meticillin-resistant *Staphylococcus aureus* or MRSA) is able to proliferate, and hence normal penicillins and β-lactam antibiotics are not effective, and more sophisticated antibiotics may be required. The environments in which these MRSA bacteria are found include, but are not limited to, hospitals, nursing homes, emergency departments and doctors' surgeries. Therefore, in treating bacterial infection acquired in these environments the practitioner should consider MRSA infection, particularly if the wound is not responding to traditional antibiotic therapy.

Simple contained bacterial infections of the hand and foot

Felon

A felon is an abscess of the pulp space of the digit or the toe (Figure 46.1). It usually occurs after trauma to the pulp in which bacteria are introduced beneath the skin surface. Treatment involves drainage of the

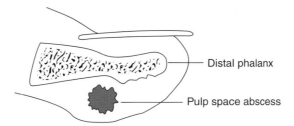

Fig. 46.1 Longitudinal section of the finger tip with a pulp space abscess. Source: courtesy of Mr David M.A. Francis.

abscess, removal of any retained foreign body (such as a splinter of wood), copious lavage, elevation and splinting of the digit to limit movement, and antibiotics.

Paronychia

Paronychia, sometimes called a whitlow, is an abscess of the nail fold and nail bed (Figure 46.2). The infection is usually due to *Staphylococcus aureus* or *Staphylococcus epidermidis* and most commonly follows minor injury to the nail fold. Pus forms around the nail fold and may extend under the nail to involve the nail bed or proximally to involve the subcutaneous tissue between the nail fold and distal interphalangeal joint. In rare circumstances, the infection may extend into the joint, causing a septic arthritis.

Treatment consists of elevation and splinting of the finger or hand, antibiotics and, if pus is present, surgical drainage.

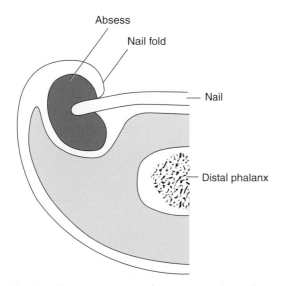

Fig. 46.2 Transverse section of acute paronychia with subungual extension. Source: courtesy of Mr David M.A. Francis.

Synovial sheath infection

In certain circumstances, infection may extend into the synovial sheath surrounding the flexor tendons. This is more common in the hand and usually involves a penetrating injury. When this occurs a classic combination of signs appears, called Kanavel's four cardinal signs of flexor sheath infection:
- sausage-shaped fusiform swelling of the digit
- stiffness of the finger in a semi-flexed position
- tenderness of the sheath extending proximally into the palm
- pain when the finger is passively extended.

This diagnosis is important because if the infection is left untreated the tendon may rupture, or the inflammation may lead to adhesions forming between the tendon and its sheath, leading to limitation of movement and compromised hand function.

Treatment involves surgical washout or lavage of the tendon sheath, usually on multiple occasions, elevation and splinting of the hand, antibiotics and, once the infection is treated, aggressive hand therapy to prevent adhesion formation and maintenance of hand function.

Infection of the metacarpophalangeal joint

This infection is common after bare-fisted fights and results from a clenched fist striking the teeth and mouth. The mechanism of injury is a tooth lacerating the skin and extensor tendon overlying the joint and entering the joint capsule of the metacarpophalangeal joint (MCPJ). This is a surgical emergency as the infection and septic arthritis may destroy the joint cartilage, resulting in permanent damage to the joint itself. Because the patient invariably presents with their hand in a flat or open position, the communication between the laceration and the joint is usually not immediately apparent, and the diagnosis may be missed. It is only when the patient is asked to remake a clenched fist and flex the MCPJ to 90° that the direct continuation of the laceration into the joint cavity becomes clear. On examination, the soft tissue around the joint is

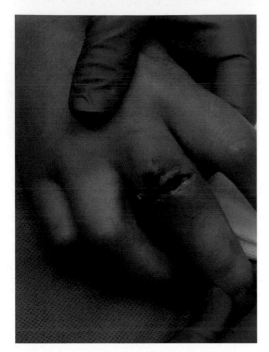

Fig. 46.3 This laceration overlying the proximal interphalangeal joint needs to be explored to ensure the laceration does not communicate with the joint. This is best done by asking the patient to make a fist to reproduce the joint position at the time of injury.

usually swollen and movement of the MCPJ is painful. A history of recently being involved in a fight is helpful but is not always given. Treatment is similar to that of flexor tendon sheath infection and involves multiple surgical washouts of the joint, elevation and splinting of the hand, and antibiotic therapy. An injury overlying an interphalangeal joint is shown in Figure 46.3 and the organisms most commonly isolated in bite wounds to the hands are listed in Box 46.1.

Ingrown toenail (onychocryptosis)

This is a painful condition that occurs when the sharp corner or the edge of the toenail cuts into the skin at the distal end or side of the toe. Whilst pain and inflammation are common, occasionally the condition can progress to infection and then abscess formation. The disorder is particularly common in adolescents and young adults. Whilst any toenail can become involved, it is most common in the great toe. It is thought that tight shoes and high heels are risk factors as they force the toes to be compressed. Particular care should be taken in treating people with diabetes and those who are immunosuppressed.

> **Box 46.1 Organisms most commonly isolated in bite wounds to the hands**
>
> **Human bites: these are the most dangerous**
> - *Staphylococcus*
> - *Streptobacillus*
> - *Eikenella corrodens*
> - Anaerobes
>
> **Dog bites**
> - *Pasteurella multocida*
> - *Streptobacillus*
> - *Staphylococcus*
> - Anaerobes
>
> **Cat bites**
> - *Pasteurella multocida*

In its early stages, the offending segment of the nail can be cut back or the sharp edge of the nail plate lifted with a splint so that the underlying soft tissue of the nail bed is protected. In more advanced cases, the entire nail may need to be surgically removed. Treatment of an associated abscess involves removing the nail and draining the underlying infection. For recurrent or chronic ingrown toenails, a lateral matricectomy is performed in which the germinal matrix from which the nail grows is surgically removed.

Disseminated bacterial infections of the extremities (Box 46.2)

Impetigo

Impetigo is a highly contagious common superficial skin infection caused by *Staphylococcus aureus* or *Streptococcus pyogenes* (group A *Streptococcus*). It typically appears as yellow crusts on the face, arms or legs, but may also develop into superficial blisters. It is spread by direct contact and hence is common in schools, day care facilities, nursing homes and areas in which crowding occurs. Left alone the infection usually clears in 2–3 weeks, but the infection can be treated with topical or systemic antibiotics. Patients should keep the sores clean and dry and should avoid spreading the fluid of the sores onto unaffected skin or other non-affected people.

Cellulitis

Cellulitis is a bacterial infection of the skin and is one of the most common infections of the extremities. Typically, the skin progressively becomes red, swollen and painful. It takes on a shiny glossy appearance and may begin to weep, particularly in

Box 46.2 How to treat bacterial infection of the extremities

- Rest and elevation of the limb (critically important)
- Debridement of non-viable tissue and cleansing of the wound
- Antibiotic therapy targeted to the organism
- Frequent review to ensure the treatment is effective and the infection is subsiding

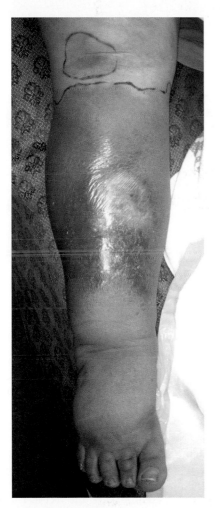

Fig. 46.4 Significant cellulitis of the lower leg. The skin is red, shiny and oedematous.

the lower leg (Figure 46.4). Most infections are caused by bacteria that are normally present on the individual's skin surface, and of these the most common organisms are *Staphylococcus aureus* and *Streptococcus* species.

Whilst it usually only affects the superficial tissues of the leg, sometimes the infection may extend to involve the deeper tissues of fat and fascia, particularly in individuals whose immune system is compromised such as diabetics and alcoholics. There may or may not be a history of trauma to the leg or hand, and diabetics or people with venous hypertension in the lower legs may notice that cellulitis seems to appear for no obvious reason. Patients at risk are those with immune compromise, diabetes, eczema, tinea and other fungal infections, and venous insufficiency.

Cellulitis can spread proximally, particularly in the presence of group A *Streptococcus*, and it may enter the lymphatics where it induces inflammation characterised by linear red streaks extending up the arm or leg to the cubital fossa, axilla or groin lymph nodes (lymphangitis) (Figure 46.5). In severe cases cellulitis is associated with systemic signs such as fever, fatigue, sweating, aches, chills and shaking. The immediate treatment is to rest and immobilise the affected limb, preferably with a splint made from plaster of Paris or fibreglass, so that the splint closely contours the limb and is therefore more comfortable and patient compliance is better. It is important that the hand is placed in a neutral position, or *position of function* (Figure 46.6) to avoid contracture of the ligaments and short muscles of the hand. In the lower limb, it is important to place the ankle at 90° to avoid contracture of the Achilles tendon and muscle flexors of the ankle joint (Figure 46.7). The limb should be elevated and the patient confined to bed.

The most common organisms are sensitive to the penicillins and cephalosporins. This antibiotic therapy should be commenced immediately, either through intravenous or oral administration. Usually, once the exact organism is subsequently identified, the antibiotic therapy is modified depending on the sensitivities obtained from microbiology. Importantly, the treatment of lower leg cellulitis should also include antithrombolytic therapy such as enoxaparin sodium or heparin to minimise the risk of subsequent deep venous thrombosis in the setting of extended bed rest.

Once the cellulitis is controlled, the underlying cause should be identified and treated. This may involve referral to an endocrinologist to treat and/or better control the patient's diabetes, a dermatologist to treat the fungal infection or eczema, or a vascular surgeon to treat the venous insufficiency. Occasionally, in severe cellulitis there may be loss of skin and the patient will need referral to a plastic surgeon for skin grafting.

Hidradenitis suppurativa

This is an infection of the apocrine sweat glands and is most common in the axillae, groin, external genitalia and perianal areas. The apocrine sweat

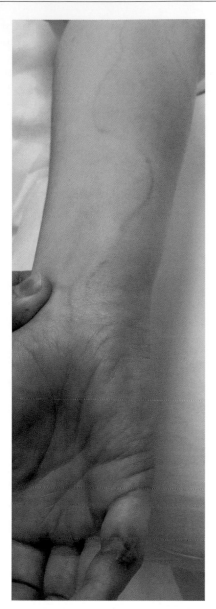

Fig. 46.5 The infection in the little finger has spread and has resulted in lymphangitis along the ulnar border of the forearm.

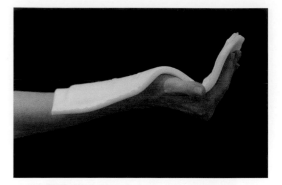

Fig. 46.6 The ideal splinting position for the hand. Note that the wrist is extended and the metacarpophalangeal joints are at 90°.

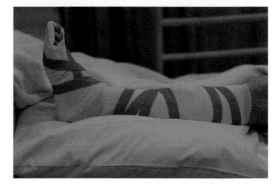

Fig. 46.7 The ideal splinting position for the foot and lower leg.

glands produce a thick secretion and easily become blocked, particularly at adolescence. The secretions subsequently become infected with staphylococci, Gram-negative and anaerobic organisms leading to abscesses, cellulitis and sinuses. The infections are often recurrent, leading to significant scarring. Unfortunately, antibiotics alone are often unable to control recurrent infection and surgery may be required to excise the infected and scarred tissue. In severe cases the entire area may need to be removed and replaced with either a skin graft or skin flap (see Chapter 47).

Bairnsdale ulcer (also known as Buruli ulcer)

This unusual infection caused by *Mycobacterium ulcerans* tends to occur in the cooler months, particularly in maritime or coastal environments. It was first described in Bairnsdale in eastern Victoria, Australia in the 1930s, but has been described in coastal areas from far northern Queensland to Adelaide. Interestingly, it is quite variable as to who contracts the disease and it is not clear how it is spread. There is some evidence to suggest the mosquito may be the vector. The infection's hallmark is a non-healing shallow ulcer, usually on the extremities, that slowly enlarges over weeks to months and is not responsive to antibiotics. It is usually single, and often starts as a small red lump. Treatment involves good wound care and dressings. Heat therapy in which the ulcer is treated with a heat lamp has been shown to be beneficial

Necrotising fasciitis

This is a rapidly progressive and dangerous bacterial infection that can affect any part of the body, but most commonly the extremities. It often has an insidious onset and may result from the most trivial damage to the skin. It is followed by rapid progression of infection that occurs below the skin surface, and hence the extent of the infection may be far greater than is initially clinically apparent. It often involves the deep fascia and may lead to muscle necrosis. The rapid spread is due to the presence of β-haemolytic *Streptococcus*, usually in association with other organisms particularly mixed anaerobes. It is most commonly seen in patients who are immunocompromised such as diabetics, alcoholics and patients with HIV. The diagnosis is notoriously difficult in the early stages, as the skin and soft tissues appear relatively normal. The key to an early diagnosis is the presence of severe pain out of keeping with the skin appearance, and the presence of associated signs such as tachycardia, fever, sweats and occasionally episodic hypotension. Interestingly, the majority of infections are caused by organisms that normally reside on the individual's skin. Most infections manifest more than one type of bacteria, the most common organisms being group A *Streptococcus*, *Staphylococcus aureus* and MRSA, *Klebsiella*, *Clostridium*, *Escherichia coli* and *Aeromonas hydrophila*.

Treatment involves aggressive early surgical debridement and lavage, often on multiple occasions. Frequently, large areas of skin and soft tissue are removed and hence most patients require some form of skin grafting or flap repair. Amputation of either part or all of the limb is not uncommon. Untreated, the infection rapidly leads to death.

Gas gangrene

This is a life-threatening, rapidly progressive bacterial infection classically associated with *Clostridium perfringens* (Boxes 46.3 and 46.4). Clostridia are anaerobic, spore-forming, Gram-positive bacilli found in soil, manure and decaying plants and animals. They produce potent exotoxins such as haemolysin, collagenase, hyaluronidase and other proteolytic enzymes that break down tissue and facilitate the spread of bacteria. In a similar manner to necrotising fasciitis, the infection spreads along deep muscle and fascial tissue planes and the overlying skin may appear relatively normal and apparently uninvolved. Gas gangrene derives its name from the presence of small bubbles of gas within the integument, which give the soft tissue a 'crackling' sound when the skin is pressed. Mortality is high (25–40%).

Treatment involves resuscitation from the shock that frequently accompanies this infection, high-dose

---

> **Box 46.3 What is gangrene?**
>
> Gangrene is the death of tissue due to either:
> - lack of blood flow, or
> - serious bacterial infection.
>
> The difference between these two causes can often be determined by whether the gangrene is 'wet' or 'dry'.
> - Wet indicates a bacterial cause: there is usually swelling and blistering. It often has a rapid onset.
> - Dry indicates lack of blood flow (ischaemia): there is usually minimal swelling and no blistering. The onset is slow. Note that ischaemic gangrene can become infected.

> **Box 46.4 Flesh-eating bacteria**
>
> Flesh-eating bacteria is a misnomer: the bacteria do not eat the tissue but rather destroy tissue by releasing toxins.

---

intravenous antibiotics and urgent surgical exploration and debridement of dead muscle and soft tissue with copious lavage of the wounds. The debridement and lavage is repeated on a daily basis until all the infected and necrotic tissue is removed. This is usually associated with an improvement in the patient's systemic condition and can serve as a monitor that the surgical debridement is adequate. Because soft tissue loss is frequently extensive, a skin graft is often required. Most patients are critically ill and will need support in an intensive care unit to treat their renal failure, severe shock and multiple organ failure.

Meningococcal septicaemia

Meningococcal septicaemia is the systemic disease caused by *Neisseria meningitidis*. It is a life-threatening, rapidly progressive bacterial infection and systemic disease that in addition to causing systemic shock and multiple organ failure also leads to multiple areas of skin, muscle and bone necrosis in the extremities. The loss of tissue in the extremities may be severe and frequently involves a segment or whole compartments of tissue. These segments of tissue loss are usually multiple and distributed over the entire body. Amputation of limbs is common, and death inevitable without aggressive early treatment.

In the early stages of infection, patients complain of severe lethargy and tiredness. There may not be any skin manifestations. Indications of septicaemia and progressive severe infection include the development of a blotchy and then purpuric rash, and high fever. Patients rapidly become shocked. This infection is a life-threatening emergency. Patients should be given high doses of penicillin or cephalosporin immediately, by whatever means available, and urgently transferred to hospital. It is important not to wait until a rash appears before commencing treatment if a diagnosis is suspected.

Neisseria meningitidis is endemic, with up to 20% of the population carrying the bacteria at any one time without ever becoming ill. It normally resides in the nose and throat and is transmitted between individuals via mucus and saliva. The mechanism by which a bacterium that may harmlessly reside in one individual but which becomes life-threatening when transferred to another is not well understood. The meningococcal disease accompanying septicaemia is most common in young children and adolescents. It is thought this is because the transfer of saliva and mucus is more common in these age groups through mouthing of objects and kissing. There are five main strains of the organism and vaccines protecting against them are available.

Further reading

Australian Government National Health and Medical Research Council. Therapeutic Guidelines, Antibiotic Version 15 (2014). Available at http://www.tg.org.au/index.php?sectionid=41

Neligan PC (ed.) *Plastic Surgery*, 4th edn. Elsevier, 2017.

Royal Australasian College of Surgeons. Infection Control in Surgery. Prevention of healthcare associated infection in surgery. Ref. No. FES-PST-009 Available at https://www.surgeons.org/media/297157/2015-05-20_pos_fes-pst-009_prevention_of_healthcare_associated_infection_in_surgery.pdf

Weinzweig, J (ed.) *Plastic Surgery Secrets Plus*, 2nd edn. Philadelphia: Mosby Elsevier, 2010.

Williams JD, Taylor EW (eds) *Infections in Surgical Practice*. London: Hodder Arnold Publication, 2003.

MCQs

Select the single correct answer to each question. The correct answers can be found in the Answers section at the end of the book.

1 Which of the following measures is the mainstay for treatment of cellulitis?
   a bed rest and elevation of the affected limb
   b antibiotics
   c frequent changing of the dressings
   d ensuring the patient is not a diabetic or is immunosuppressed
   e minimising any causative factors such as recurrent trauma

2 Fungal infection:
   a is not usually transferred by direct contact
   b is not able to be transferred by a non-living object
   c is uncommon in warm moist environments
   d of the proximal nail is best treated with topical antifungal creams
   e usually requires a combination of conservative measures and antifungal medication for a prolonged period

3 Which of the following statements about hand infection is correct?
   a following a fist fight, MCPJ joint involvement and infection is easy to diagnose
   b paronychia is not linked with septic arthritis
   c the mainstay of treatment of bacterial hand infection is rest, elevation and splinting in a neutral position
   d flexor tendon sheaths can become infected, but the signs are not characteristic and are highly variable
   e patients should be encouraged to return to work and use their hand as much as possible so that it does not stiffen up

4 Meningococcal septicaemia is:
   a not associated with a purple rash
   b usually seen in elderly patients, while healthy young adolescents are safe
   c is not life-threatening and is slowly progressive
   d is caused by a bacterium that harmlessly resides in the nasopharynx of up to 20% of the population
   e not an indication to urgently administer penicillin or cephalosporin antibiotics, and it is best to wait until the patient gets to hospital and let the emergency doctors do microbiological cultures first

5 Which of the following features are shared by necrotising fasciitis and gas gangrene?
   a both are very easy to detect in their early stages
   b both are relatively harmless
   c skin overlying the infection is usually red, shiny and weeping
   d surprisingly, the patient is otherwise quite well
   e an early diagnosis is made by the dichotomy of a gravely ill patient, with fever, shock and fatigue, in the presence of relatively normal-looking soft tissue

47 Principles of plastic surgery

Mark W. Ashton

University of Melbourne and Royal Melbourne Hospital, Melbourne, Victoria, Australia

Introduction

Despite its name, plastic surgery has nothing to do with plastic. Both the surgical specialty, and the malleable compound that we all know, derive their name from the Greek word *plastikos* and the Latin word *plasticus*. Both words refer to the capacity to 'mold' or 'transform'. The application of these terms to the now ubiquitous 'plastic' material makes sense. The relevance to plastic surgery requires a little more explanation.

Plastic surgery, as a specialty, developed in the First World War. This war, unlike others before it, was characterised by trench warfare using high-powered but relatively low-velocity guns, heavy artillery that released huge amounts of shrapnel on detonation, and a developing air war using the new aeroplanes made of highly flammable wood, canvas, lacquers and paint. These planes had no parachutes.

Surviving casualties of this war fell roughly into two broad groups: those suffering grossly disfiguring compound wounds to the face and limbs and those with severe full-thickness burns. In the unlikely event these soldiers and airmen could be saved, they returned home with horrific disfiguring injuries. They were outcast, stared at and excluded. Re-assimilation into mainstream society was uncommon and suicide rates were high.

In an effort to help these young men a series of special units initially comprising ear nose and throat surgeons, oral and maxillofacial surgeons, neurosurgeons and general surgeons were developed to reconstruct and restore these men's horrific injuries. The task was enormous. Whilst well-known historical methods of transferring tissue around the body were utilised as much as possible, these proved somewhat limited in being able to provide adequate reconstruction. The sheer complexity and severity of injury required these new units to be ingenious, in an unheralded way, by inventing and developing new techniques of tissue transfer. (In recognition of the uncertainty of outcome, and the adventurous nature of the surgery, one of these units in the Second World War became affectionately known as the Guinea Pig Club.) Many operations were multi-staged and it was not uncommon for a patient to undergo 10, or even 20, individual operations (Figure 47.1). Unsure of what to call themselves, these new surgeons coined the term 'plastic surgery' as they were molding and transforming tissue. One could also say they were molding and transforming the soldiers themselves, giving them, for the first time, a real chance to re-integrate back into society.

At its most basic core, plastic surgery involves the transfer of tissue from one part of the body to the other. It may be very close (local) or far away (distant). The tissue that is transferred may remain attached to the body, in which case it is called a flap, or it may be completely detached and therefore must gain access to a new blood supply at the recipient site into which it is inset. These tissue transfers are called grafts.

A special situation exists in which the tissue to be transferred is isolated on its specific blood supply. The artery and vein supplying the tissue is identified and tagged. At the recipient site, a separate artery and vein of the same calibre are also identified and tagged. Using a microscope and fine micro-surgical instruments and sutures, the artery and veins are divided and the tissue transferred to the new site, completely free of its original blood supply. The vessels are then re-anastomosed and the blood supply re-established. These flaps are called 'free flaps' and were first described in Melbourne, Australia. The advantages of these flaps are that the tissue can be transferred over great distances in a single operation and that the surgeon is able to customise, or choose, what components are in the

Textbook of Surgery, Fourth Edition. Edited by Julian A. Smith, Andrew H. Kaye, Christopher Christophi and Wendy A. Brown.
© 2020 John Wiley & Sons Ltd. Published 2020 by John Wiley & Sons Ltd.

(a)   (b)

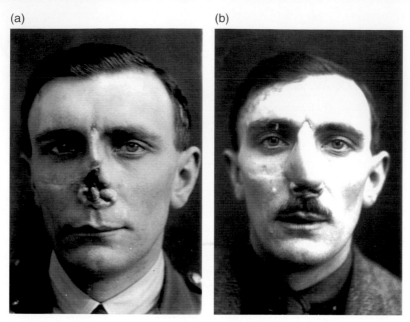

Fig. 47.1 (a) Captain J.G.H. Budd was admitted to hospital in May 1919 missing most of his nose. (b) His appearance in December 1919 after six operations at Sidcup. Source: gilliesarchives.org.uk. Reproduced with permission of Royal College of Surgeons London.

flap – skin only, muscle only, nerve, bone or a combination, all these permutations are possible.

Integral to every successful plastic surgical procedure is a comprehensive understanding of blood supply. Much of the disappointment in the early plastic surgical procedures resulted from tissue being transferred that did not have a reliable circulation. Despite all the hard work and long hours of surgery, the surgeon and patient would subsequently watch on in despair as the tissue that was transferred went purple, and then black, as it died.

Many of the advances in plastic surgery have therefore come from a new understanding of the blood supply of tissue, and in particular the volume, type and extent of tissue that may be safely transferred on a single artery and vein. Through a thorough knowledge of soft tissue blood supply, plastic surgeons are now able to safely transfer large volumes of complex tissue predictably and reliably. As an example, patients suffering from head and neck cancer can now have their jaw, tongue and mouth removed and then replaced using the fibula bone and skin and soft tissue of the leg on the peroneal artery and vein in a single operation. Patients having a mastectomy for breast cancer can have the breast reconstructed using skin and fat tissue from the lower abdomen transferred on the deep inferior epigastric vessels. And patients suffering severe mutilating gunshot wounds to the face can have a face transplant using donor soft tissue transferred on the facial artery and vein.

Plastic surgeons talk of two important concepts – 'like with like' and a 'reconstructive ladder' – in repairing defects. In essence, these two principles refer to matching the donor tissue as closely as possible to the defect, and using the most simple and straightforward technique that will achieve the reconstructive outcome. As the term ladder implies, the initial techniques to be considered are the most straightforward, graduating in complexity to microsurgical free tissue, which is considered the most complex. With increasing complexity comes an increase in demands on staff, infrastructure and the patient, but the capacity to individualise the reconstruction is unparalleled.

These techniques are discussed in the following sections.

Direct closure

This is the most simple of the techniques of wound closure, but has a number of pitfalls for the unwary. The technique involves directly suturing or opposing the wound edges together. This may be done at the time of injury, which is called primary closure, or some days or weeks later, when it is called secondary or delayed closure. This latter technique is incredibly useful in contaminated or infected wounds, or in wounds in which the viability of the wound edges is in question. If ever in doubt, a surgeon is well advised to delay closure. Delaying closure for up to 72 hours does not affect wound healing or the final scar. In contrast, prematurely closing a wound by direct suture may result in infection, abscess formation, wound breakdown and further tissue loss.

The principles of direct wound closure are to excise the wound edges back to clean, healthy, non-infected tissue. The wound edges are then opposed using sutures that may pass vertically through the skin surface as a series of interrupted sutures, or horizontally just below the surface of the skin in the dermis, either in an interrupted or continuous fashion. It is important to eliminate dead space and hence additional sutures may be employed to oppose fat, fascia or muscle in the depths of the wound. An important principle is that the wound is closed without tension.

A clean dressing should be applied to absorb any fluid and draw it away from the wound edges. The wound should then be splinted and the patient rested. Depending on the degree of contamination, additional antibiotics may be prescribed for a week following wound closure. Tetanus prophylaxis is mandatory.

If the wound edges are unable to be opposed without excessive tension, then the surgeon should move up the 'reconstructive ladder', and there are now two quite different techniques that may be used to achieve closure of the wound. Again, wound closure may be primary (at the time of injury) or secondary.

Skin grafts

Split-thickness skin grafts

The first technique involves the harvesting of a thin layer of skin, called a split-thickness skin graft, from somewhere else in the body. It is called 'split thickness' because the thickness is such that only the top layers of the epidermis and dermis are included in the tissue harvested, and deeper structures in the dermis such as the sweat glands and hair follicles are left behind. This is important because these structures are lined with epithelial cells, and it is the epithelial cells within these structures that proliferate to re-epithelialise the donor wound and re-establish the epithelial lining, thereby healing the donor site.

Split-thickness skin grafts have the advantage of allowing for very large areas of skin to be harvested, and because the epithelial cells regrow over the donor site, the skin graft harvesting may be repeated many times. Not surprisingly, this is the method of choice for closing large full-thickness burn wounds.

The disadvantage of a split-thickness skin graft is that the harvested skin does not contain all the elements of normal skin, and in particular the lack of deep dermal structures means that it is quite fragile and does not tolerate friction or shearing forces. These grafts are intimately dependent on the vascularity and quality of the tissue bed onto which they are laid, and hence should not be used to cover infected wounds, bare bone or tendon, or tissue in which the vascularity is poor such as irradiated tissue. Split-thickness skin grafts also contract as they heal and therefore should not be used on the face, as this contraction will lead to distortion of mobile structures such as the eyelid, mouth or lip.

Full-thickness skin grafts

If the skin is harvested deeper, below the lowest part of the dermis, all layers of the skin are included in the graft. This is called a full-thickness skin graft. There is no possibility of regeneration of the donor site as all the sweat glands and hair follicles containing the epithelial cells are also included in the graft. The donor site must therefore be closed by direct suture. The advantage of full-thickness skin grafts is that they are more durable and resistant to shear forces. Because all the components of the skin are included, these grafts are able to maintain normal skin colour and are less like to fade or go pale. Full-thickness skin grafts are therefore the graft of choice for facial defects, particularly the eyelid and nose. Because the donor site must be sutured directly, there is a limit to the possible sites available for harvesting. In general, skin that is closest to the wound will provide the best colour match and hence the skin behind the ear or the neck is used for the face, and the inguinal groin crease used for other parts of the body.

Other grafts

In much the same way that skin may be harvested as a graft to replace skin that is missing following an injury or surgery, other tissues may also be transferred as a graft. The most common of these is nerve tissue and tendons, but bone and cartilage can also be transferred. Combinations of tissue can also be grafted and these are called composite grafts. The limiting factors are the volume of the graft and the tissue bed into which the graft is inset. As the graft does not have its own blood supply it is initially dependent on oxygen and nutrients diffusing into the cells composing the graft from the recipient bed. Over time, blood vessels grow into the graft and re-vascularise it; however, this ingrowth of blood vessels takes somewhere between 3 days and a week. The graft cells are therefore entirely dependent on oxygen diffusion until revascularisation occurs, and subsequently there is a limit as to the volume or dimensions of tissue that can be safely and reliably transferred.

Flaps

Flaps are the second alternative for closing a wound when the wound edges will not meet to close the defect. Flaps differ from grafts in that they carry with them their own blood supply. Because flaps are not reliant on the initial diffusion of nutrients and oxygen from the recipient bed for their survival, they are less dependent on the vascularity and characteristics of the recipient bed and may therefore be used to close a greater variety of wounds. Flaps may be broadly categorised into those that are close, or local, and those that are distant. As with grafts, flaps may be composed of skin, fat, muscle, nerve or bone. Because they have their own blood supply, much greater volumes of tissue can be safely transferred, and hence it is not uncommon for a composite flap comprising all types of different tissue to be included in a single transfer. The key principle here is an understanding of which tissues derive their blood supply from the identified source vessel supplying the flap and then ensuring that this blood supply is included in the transfer.

Several surgical techniques have been described for transferring flaps, and this has allowed a further classification. The principle in planning a flap is an assessment of skin laxity and working out which tissue can be safely harvested for transfer without significant distortion of the remaining body contour. This tissue is then selected as the flap. The most simple is a rotation flap (Figure 47.2) but others, such as transposition, V–Y (Figure 47.3) and Z-plasty (Figure 47.4), are regularly used. More complicated flaps have been extensively used, such as the tubed pedicle, in which the flap is attached to an intermediate site for a period of 3 weeks before being further transferred to the final destination, and cross leg or arm flaps, in which tissue from one leg or arm is transferred to the other. With increased understanding of the blood supply to tissue, there has been a refinement in flap transfer. It is now possible to preoperatively determine what tissue is required, what artery and vein supply that tissue, and then harvest that desired tissue on its specific blood supply. If the targeted donor tissue is adjacent to the surgical defect, it may be transferred directly. If the defect is at a distance from the donor site, the artery and vein are divided and re-anastomosed to vessels at the defect site with the aid of a microscope.

As with grafts, flaps may be composed of skin only, muscle only, nerve, bone, cartilage or tendon. It is usual for the flap to contain more than one type of tissue. These flaps are called composite flaps. As with all plastic surgery, the best aesthetic result is achieved when the transferred tissue matches as closely as possible the tissue that was lost at the time of injury or surgical resection.

Cosmetic surgery

It quickly became apparent that the plastic surgical techniques used to repair injury could also be used to repair congenital defects such as cleft lip and palate, and also to reverse the signs of ageing or to change someone's appearance. Cosmetic surgery may therefore be defined as:

> Any invasive procedure where the primary intention is to achieve what the patient perceives to be a more desirable appearance and where the procedure involves changes to bodily features that have a normal appearance on presentation to the doctor.

It is understood that 'normal appearance' is a subjective notion, and what appears normal to the surgeon may not in fact appear normal to the patient. In contrast, surgery performed with the goal of achieving a normal appearance, where bodily

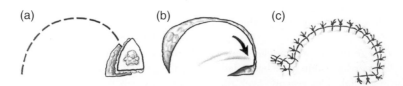

Fig. 47.2 Rotation flap. (a) Design of flap. Lesion/defect triangulated and flap designed as semicircular arc from apex of defect. (b) Flap incised, elevated and rotated into defect. (c) Flap sutured into position with secondary defect closed directly.

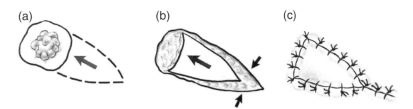

Fig. 47.3 A V–Y advancement flap.

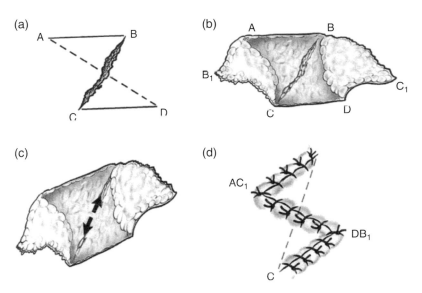

Fig. 47.4 A Z-plasty flap.

features have an abnormal appearance on presentation due to congenital defects, developmental abnormalities, trauma, infections, tumours or disease, does not fall under the definition of cosmetic surgery. This is best described as reconstruction of the whole.

An important principle is that there is a continuum between reconstruction and cosmetic surgery, and that at its very core reconstruction aims to make the patient at least the same, if not more attractive than they would otherwise be. Any practitioner operating within reconstructive surgery must have a clear understanding of what is 'normal', but must also possess an appreciation of the nuance of beauty and attractiveness. In this respect, one may argue that an arbitrary distinction between reconstructive and cosmetic surgery is somewhat simplistic, as the two are intimately intertwined and surgical techniques shared extensively across the two aspects of plastic surgery. It is often said that the hallmark of a master reconstructive surgeon is a beautiful cosmetic result. This is clearly apparent in the field of breast reconstruction after mastectomy, but could equally be applied to facial reconstruction after cancer or hand reconstruction after trauma.

The principle is to achieve an outcome that is normal in appearance and where possible aesthetically pleasing or even beautiful.

The most common cosmetic operations are breast reduction, breast enlargement, abdominoplasty and facial plastic procedures such as facelifting, eyelid reduction and rhinoplasty. These operations all use the same plastic surgical techniques of flap repair, and are also critically dependent on a robust and reliable blood supply. Advances in our understanding of tissue perfusion and vascular anatomy has revolutionised all aspects of plastic surgery, and cosmetic surgery has benefited from this increased understanding. As an example, breast reduction surgery can now be performed reliably and predictably, and even very large breasts causing back and neck pain can be safely made smaller without the need for nipple grafting. An advanced understanding of nipple and areolar blood and nerve supply means that the nipple is now transferred on a neurovascular pedicle that remains attached to the underlying breast tissue. It has the advantage that nipple sensation is preserved, and that patients are able to breastfeed after surgery.

In face-lifting surgery, an increased understanding of the blood supply of the face and what tissues can be safely moved has resulted in facial tissue being tightened at a deeper, relatively avascular surgical plane below the superficial muscles of facial expression. This results in less bruising and swelling, and the ability to place tension on deeper structures, and not on wound edges, means that the very tight appearance that plagued traditional techniques is avoided. These are just two examples, but the principle underlying these operations, and plastic surgery in general, remains the same: the tissue that is to be transferred must have a robust blood supply, and the morbidity associated with harvesting that tissue must be minimised.

Finally, is not possible to eliminate risk, and all surgery, even so-called non-surgical cosmetic surgery, can go wrong. This is critically important in elective cosmetic procedures that are not medically required. Any decision to proceed to surgery must be based on a sound understanding of the risks involved in surgery and the other forms of treatment that may be available. The surgeon at all times needs to ensure that full informed consent of the outcome of surgery, and the risks involved, is clearly and carefully explained.

Further reading

Neligan PC (ed.) *Plastic Surgery*, 4th edn. Elsevier, 2017.
Weinzweig, J (ed.) *Plastic Surgery Secrets Plus*, 2nd edn. Philadelphia: Mosby Elsevier, 2010.

MCQs

Select the single correct answer to each question. The correct answers can be found in the Answers section at the end of the book.

1 Which of the following statements is correct?
   a plastic surgery developed in the 1970s as a response to breast augmentation
   b advances in plastic surgery have come from a reappraisal and increased understanding of blood supply to tissue
   c it is not possible to breastfeed after a breast reduction
   d 'non-surgical' cosmetic procedures are entirely safe and carry no risk
   e grafts differ from flaps in that they carry with them their own blood supply

2 Closing a wound at the time of injury with a split-thickness skin graft:
   a is best described as direct closure
   b is best described as secondary closure
   c is best described as primary wound closure
   d can be safely and reliably performed in the presence of contamination

3 A composite graft or flap may contain:
   a skin
   b fat
   c bone
   d muscle
   e all of the above

4 Which of the following describes how split-thickness skin grafts differ from full-thickness skin grafts?
   a hair follicles and sweat glands are harvested with the graft
   b can only be harvested from the donor site once
   c are best used in areas of friction and shear, such as the sole of the foot
   d do not contract and are therefore the graft of choice for eyelid reconstruction
   e none of the above

Section 10
Trauma

48 Principles of trauma management

Scott K. D'Amours[1], Stephen A. Deane[2] and Valerie B. Malka[1]

[1] University of New South Wales and Department of Trauma Services, Liverpool Hospital, Sydney, New South Wales, Australia
[2] Macquarie University, Sydney, and University of Newcastle, Newcastle, New South Wales, Australia

General principles

Good trauma management recognises the importance of a number of key issues (Box 48.1).

Trauma as a disease

Injury is a major economic burden to societies such as Australia. Recent estimates suggest a massive total economic burden on Australia's economy annually of A$27 billion (an increase from the 1990 estimate of A$13 billion), including both direct and indirect costs. Injury is the most frequent cause of death in Australians less than 45 years of age, and is a major cause of death in all age groups. Most importantly, it accounts for more years of productive life lost than cancer and heart disease combined. The major impact of injury deaths and disability is borne by the young adult segment of the population and disproportionately by males. Although road traffic-related injuries account for only 30% of injury admissions to major trauma services, importantly this group accounts for 75% of those with serious multi-trauma and about 75% of those who die in hospital from injury.

Many of the advances in trauma care in recent years have been derived from experience with injuries suffered in war or with penetrating injuries resulting from interpersonal violence, particularly in the USA. However, the proportion of patients admitted to hospitals in Australia with injuries resulting from gunshot wounds or stabbings is low, varying between 2 and 7%. Even within this population, stabbings predominate.

It needs to be recognised that for every patient who dies from injury, 10 more are admitted to hospital with serious injury and two will suffer significant long-term disability.

Trauma system planning

When examining deaths due to injury, there has been a fairly consistent finding worldwide that where systems of trauma care have not been specifically organised, 15–30% of the deaths can be deemed to have been potentially preventable. In addition, approximately two-thirds of deaths in the absence of serious head injury have been deemed to be potentially preventable. Much has been done to improve this situation with respect to education, standardised care and reorganisation, but more progress is still needed.

Considerable attention has been given internationally in recent years to the appropriate design of regional systems of trauma care that enable patients with potentially serious injuries to access a process that minimises the time from injury to definitive care. The aim is to 'get the right patient to the right hospital in the right time'. The essential components of such a plan are outlined here.

Pre-hospital triage

Triage is the process of grouping injury victims according to risk of death or other adverse outcome. Pre-hospital care providers are trained to carry this out using a criteria-based system usually employing four simple groups of factors.
- *Physiology*: the vital signs, such as pulse over 120/min, systolic blood pressure less than

Box 48.1 General principles of good trauma management

- The importance of injury as a public health issue including surveillance, prevention, economic impact and functional outcomes.
- The importance of the injury mechanism in predicting actual injuries.
- The differing implications of blunt and penetrating injury.
- The importance of triage and a team-based approach.
- The importance to the triage process of:
  o injury mechanism
  o physiological status
  o evident injuries.
- The differing risk exposures and injury patterns in children, young adults and the elderly.
- The patterns of associated injuries that are commonly observed.
- The commonly documented deficiencies in acute injury management.
- The importance of an integrated trauma treatment service in a hospital.
- The value of clinical practice guidelines for the assessment and management of acute injury.
- The importance of regional systems of trauma care that link injury prevention activities, pre-hospital care, acute care hospitals with differing roles, rehabilitation services and the overall return to premorbid functioning.

90 mmHg, Glasgow Coma Scale (GCS) score less than 15, point-of-care testing (e.g. blood gases).
- *Anatomy*: the immediately evident injuries such as fractured long bones, pelvic fractures, spinal cord injury, flail chest, positive FAST (focused assessment using sonography for trauma).
- *Mechanism of injury*: for example fall of more than 2 m, injury to two or more body regions, vehicle crash with ejection, penetrating injury, significant burns.
- *Patient factors*: extremes of age, use of anticoagulants, pregnancy.

Pre-hospital treatment and transport decisions

On the basis of the triage process, certain predetermined decisions are made that attempt to direct the transport of patients to the most appropriate hospital. Pre-hospital care providers are trained to recognise and treat life-threatening problems in the field, including airway interventions, chest decompressions, application of splints and pelvic binders and administration of blood products. The most appropriate hospital is not necessarily the nearest

hospital: the pre-hospital triage process should identify patients who need to bypass the nearest hospital for one that has the resourcing and expertise to care for all types of serious injuries.

Categorisation of hospitals

The role of a hospital within a regional system of trauma care is designated by the appropriate health authority. A major trauma service (level 1) has the facilities and internal organisation to support its role as the most appropriate primary destination for patients with potentially serious injuries. Some patients can be appropriately triaged to level 2 and 3 centres in the urban environment if the above criteria are not met. In semi-rural, rural and remote environments, strategically located regional trauma services (levels 2–4) are required. These smaller trauma services must have strong links with a major trauma service. Even in remote environments trauma care education, trauma service planning, and strong links with the rest of the regional network need to be continuously promoted.

Hospital trauma response and trauma teams

Initial assessment of trauma patients requires an organised trauma response that aims to minimise the time from injury to definitive care (Box 48.2). Such trauma responses or teams have a predetermined multidisciplinary membership, a triage device to trigger mobilisation, predetermined roles for members, and standardised approaches to the performance of primary survey, resuscitation,

Box 48.2 Goals of trauma assessment and resuscitation

General goals
The sequence of goals in the initial assessment of an individual trauma patient is as follows.
1 Save life: this requires knowledge of the causes of death
2 Prevent major disability: this requires knowledge of the causes of disability
3 Diagnose and appropriately manage all injuries
4 Avoid unnecessary investigations or interventions

Achieve by:
1 Minimise the time from injury to definitive care
2 Do not allow obvious injuries to distract from diagnosing other, less obvious injuries
3 Follow the principles of ABCDE
4 Always have a clear management plan
5 Assess response to intervention by re-evaluation of the patient

secondary survey and investigations. Most importantly the presence of a senior surgeon has been shown to facilitate timely decision-making, investigations and both operative and non-operative management resulting in better patient outcomes.

Disaster management

Certain natural and human disasters, as well as terror-related incidents, can result in multiple casualties that may overwhelm otherwise well-resourced hospitals. The increasing incidence of these events requires pre-planned disaster responses, training of personnel and simulation exercises to ensure that the principles of acceptable injury management are applied. The principles of disaster management are designed to achieve the best outcomes for the greatest possible number of casualties using standardised approaches.

Blunt and penetrating mechanisms of injury

The patterns and severity of injury differ dramatically between blunt and penetrating injury. The severity of injuries relates to the amount of energy transferred in the injury process and the amount of the body across which the energy is transferred. Serious injury from blunt trauma is typified by victims of traffic-related injury or by falls from a significant height. In these situations, large amounts of energy are often transferred across broad and multiple regions of the body without breaching the walls of the body cavities. Accordingly, certain injury patterns can only be broadly anticipated and occult injuries are not uncommon.

Penetrating injuries are divided into those that result from gunshot wounds and those from stabbings. A further small group are patients who suffer impalement. It is important to recognise that interpersonal violence can combine mechanisms (gunshot wounds, stabbings and blunt injury from a fist or a boot). Possible injuries from stab wounds can often be fairly confidently predicted as energy transmission and tissue disruption is limited to the penetrating tract. However, gunshot wounds can pose additional difficulties because the missile path may not be predictable and energy transmission and tissue disruption can cause gross destruction of surrounding soft tissues through cavitation and other aspects of ballistics and the physical features of the missile such as velocity, size, mass and impact surface. Because of the uncertainties posed by these features and the potentially serious nature of possible injuries, a lower threshold usually exists for comprehensive investigation and surgical exploration in the presence of gunshot wounds than with stab wounds.

Deaths

Deaths from injury can be broadly divided into four groups that link the cause of death to the time from injury to death: death at the scene; death within 'minutes'; death within 'hours'; and death over 'days' (some examples are given in Box 48.3). Many patients in the fourth group are recognised as 'late septic complications' or 'multiple organ failure'. However, the foundations for these late complications are often laid in the first hour or two following injury; they relate to the extent and duration of physiological disturbance. It is therefore clear that they can also relate to the promptness and completeness of early assessment and resuscitation measures. Prevention of death can be linked broadly to the principles in Box 48.4.

Disability

Disability principally relates to:
- cognition
- locomotion
- manipulation skills
- chronic pain.

While definitive care of the actual injuries plays a major role in preventing these categories of disability, it must be recognised that ensuring adequate oxygen delivery to brain and to muscle groups also plays a major role, especially in the first hour or two after injury. As with death, prevention of disability is linked to specific measures (Box 48.5).

Initial assessment

Efficient initial assessment of a trauma patient derives from the broad principles outlined previously in Box 48.1, a clear understanding of the patterns of death and disability (Boxes 48.3, 48.4 and 48.5) and recognition of the following factors.
- Trauma patient assessment is different from that of the usual patient. The traditional approach of taking a full history, doing a full physical examination, determining a provisional diagnosis and a list of differential diagnoses, and deriving a logical plan for investigation and treatment needs to be laid aside in order to first ensure a patient's survival and then to ensure the smallest possible risk of major complications (see later).
- Minimise the time from injury to definitive care, with special attention to recognition and management of haemorrhage.

Box 48.3 Causes of death from injury

Deaths at scene/incompatible with life
- Brainstem transection
- High spinal cord transection
- Decapitation
- Major thoracic vascular injury with free intrapleural bleeding
- Major tracheobronchial disruption
- Liver avulsion
- Cardiac rupture

Death within minutes
- Hypoxia: airway obstruction, tension pneumothorax, open pneumothorax, massive flail chest
- Major bleeding: external (amputation), thoracic (haemothorax), abdominal (spleen, liver, mesentery, major vessels), pelvic fracture
- Pericardial tamponade (cardiac rupture)
- Rapid tentorial herniation: rapid rise in intracranial pressure (ICP)

Death within hours
- Hypoxia: severe pulmonary contusion, tracheobronchial rupture, diaphragm rupture
- Sepsis: perforated hollow viscus (e.g. thoracic oesophagus, abdominal viscera)
- Bleeding: external (face, massive wounds); thoracic aortic rupture; lungs, chest wall (haemothorax); liver, spleen, retroperitoneum; pelvis fracture; long-bone fractures
- Coagulopathy
- Brain: increasing ICP (haematoma, swelling)

Death over days
- Brain: high ICP from brain swelling, no cerebral perfusion
- Respiratory failure: pneumonia, severe pulmonary contusions, fat emboli, type 2 respiratory failure in elderly (i.e. hypoxaemia in setting of hypercapnia)
- Renal failure: crush injury, acute on chronic, contrast nephropathy
- Gastrointestinal failure, especially liver, gut mucosal barrier
- Sepsis: pulmonary, abdominal, wound
- Ischaemia: muscle groups, liver, gut
- Myocardial infarction
- Pulmonary embolus

Box 48.4 Prevention of death

General measures
- Optimise oxygenation (A, B)
- Optimise perfusion acutely (C)
- Meticulous continuing fluid management
- Thrombosis prophylaxis
- Adequate nutrition by appropriate route

Local measures
- Arrest or minimise bleeding (C)
- Correct raised ICP (D)
- Control 'leaks' (tracheobronchial, oesophageal, abdominal hollow viscera, pancreas, urinary)
- Decompress or revascularise ischaemic tissue promptly
- Debride dead tissue aggressively
- Debride and clean contaminated wounds

Box 48.5 Prevention of disability

General measures
- Optimise oxygenation (A, B)
- Optimise perfusion (C)
- Protect spine (A and following measures)
- Correct raised ICP (D)

Local measures
- Reduce dislocations as soon as possible
- Realign fractures as soon as possible
- Correct local ischaemia early
- Diagnose and decompress compartment syndromes early
- Prevent secondary damage to nerves (iatrogenic injury, ischaemia, compression, e.g. dislocations)
- Debride ischaemic tissue early
- Debride contaminated wounds early
- Find the 'minor injuries' to ligaments, joints and small bones (tertiary survey)

- Any single measurement of physiology (e.g. pulse, respiratory rate, GCS and blood pressure) is of limited value. Overall trends and specific tests (blood gases, viscoelastic testing) are more informative.
- Life-threatening injuries may be occult, multiple life-threatening injuries may coexist in different body regions, and the injuries that appear most dramatic may not be those that pose the greatest risk.

- The concept of the 'golden hour' is important, a 1–2 hour period during which all opportunities need to be taken to discover injuries that may cause death within minutes and then to discover injuries that may cause death within hours.
- Pre-planned protocols or evidence-based guidelines help to prevent errors in care.

Figure 48.1 outlines a well-accepted approach to the first 24 hours of injury management. The term 'initial assessment' applies particularly to the elements of primary survey, resuscitation, secondary survey, monitoring/reassessment and specific investigations. The term 'definitive care' relates to specific treatment (operative or non-operative) aimed at establishing the optimal conditions for the healing of specific injuries.

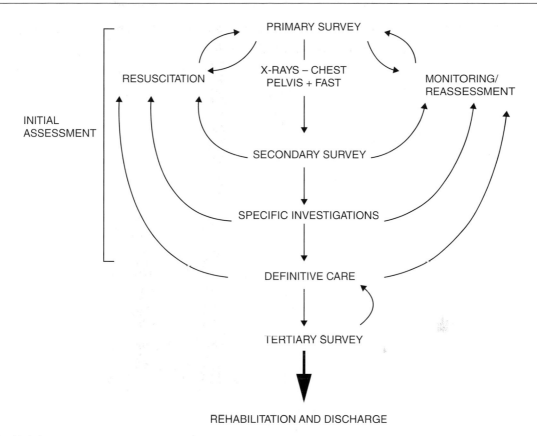

Fig. 48.1 Acute trauma management procedure.

Primary survey and resuscitation

The strategy for primary survey and resuscitation is outlined in Figure 48.2. The ABCDE sequence prioritises the importance of specific injuries and assists clinical performance. Primary survey is the process used to assist the recognition of acutely life-threatening injuries and should proceed concurrently with resuscitation. As the primary survey assessment scheme is followed, intervention should be taken immediately to correct the problems that are identified with each step. Note the emphasis given to using simple measures to protect the cervical spine when attending to the adequacy of the airway. External bleeding must be controlled; direct pressure is usually effective.

In a hospital with a major trauma service and an effective trauma-team response there will be enough team members to perform some parts of the primary survey concurrently, together with the necessary resuscitative interventions. However, when resources are limited the framework illustrated in Figure 48.2 assumes even greater importance.

Table 48.1 provides further detail regarding primary survey and resuscitation. Effective primary survey requires awareness of a limited number of life-threatening entities, rapid and simple systems of physiological assessment, and awareness of a menu of interventions that can be applied to correct the identified problem. Some aspects of care during the primary survey need special emphasis.

Imaging

The only appropriate imaging at the time of the primary survey should be directed towards proving or excluding a source for haemorrhage leading to haemodynamic instability. These include a chest X-ray, a pelvic X-ray and a FAST examination. Lateral C-spine X-rays (previously routine) are not required in initial patient assessment given the primacy of haemorrhage identification and control. In major trauma patients, spinal injuries are presumed until excluded by further assessment and CT scanning (with or without MRI). It is important to minimise movement of the cervical and thoracolumbar spine until after the completion of the primary survey or later if other injuries or unstable physiology take priority.

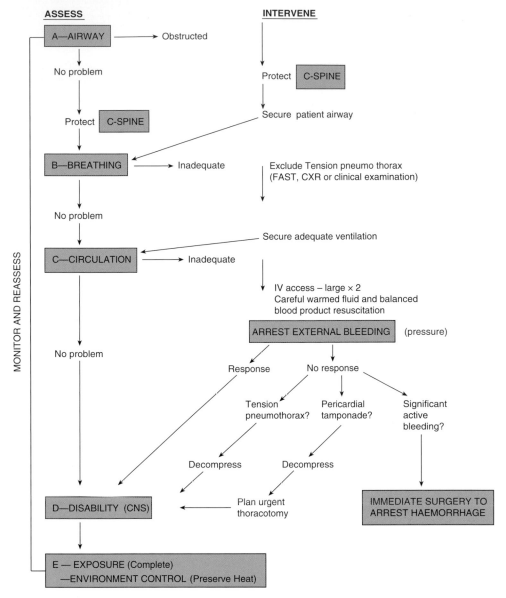

Fig. 48.2 Outline of strategy for primary survey and resuscitation.

Table 48.1 Primary survey and resuscitation.

	Problem	Assess	Intervene
Airway	Direct trauma: disruption/oedema Obstruction: Foreign bodies Blood and vomitus Soft tissue oedema Deteriorating consciousness	Cyanosis Tachypnoea Voice Stridor Confusion 'Respiratory distress' Air movement	Gloved finger, light, suction Laryngoscope, forceps Oxygen Chin lift/jaw thrust Oropharyngeal airway Nasopharyngeal airway Orotracheal tube Supraglottic airway Video-assisted laryngobronchoscopy Surgical airway: Cricothyroidotomy Urgent tracheostomy

Table 48.1 (Continued)

	Problem	Assess	Intervene

C-spine	Unstable fracture	Assume if:
		  Unconscious
		  Head injury
		  Face injury
			Protect C-spine/limit mobility
			  Collar
			  Sandbags

Breathing	Tension pneumothorax Massive haemothorax Open pneumothorax Massive flail Reduction in level of consciousness/poor effort High spinal cord injury	Cyanosis Tachypnoea Confusion 'Respiratory distress' Shallow respiration Poor expansion Asymmetric expansion Hyperinflation Hyperresonance Breath sounds Tracheal shift Diaphragmatic breathing	Oxygen Ventilation Needle or finger thoracostomy Tube thoracostomy Tracheal intubation Cover open wound: three-sided dressing

Circulation	Bleeding:
	  External (scene, bed, floor)
	  Chest (X-ray)
	  Abdomen (FAST or DPA/DPL)
	  Pelvis (X-ray)
	  Femurs (clinical examination)
	  Combination
	
	Heart:
	  Tension pneumothorax
	  Pericardial tamponade
	  Contusion
	  Infarction
		Pale, clammy, cool
		Peripheral cyanosis
		Confusion
		Tachycardia
		Low pulse volume
		Slow capillary refill
		Neck veins
		Heart sounds (muffled)
			Haemorrhage control (direct pressure or surgery)
			Oxygen
			Intravenous access (large-bore ×2)
			Warmed crystalloid/blood products (packed red blood cells, fresh frozen plasma or plasma concentrate, platelets, cryoprecipitate)
			Blood warming
			Gastric tube
			Surgery
			Urinary catheter
			Needle/finger tube thoracostomy
			Resuscitative thoracotomy
			Cross-clamp aorta/REBOA

Disability (CNS)	Secondary brain injury
	Intracranial haematoma
	Brain:
	  Compression
	  Contusion
	  Laceration
	  Swelling
		Alert
		Voice response
		Pain response
		Unresponsive
		Lateralising signs
		Pupils
			A, B, C
			C-spine protection
			Limited hyperventilation (aim Pa_{CO_2} low end of normal)
			Osmotic agents:
			Hypertonic saline
			Mannitol

Exposure	Concealed injuries	Prepare for secondary survey	Remove all clothes
Environment control	Hypothermia		Warm fluids External warming devices (bear hugger, warmed blankets) Ambient room temperature

DPA/DPL, diagnostic peritoneal aspiration or lavage; FAST, focused assessment using sonography for trauma; REBOA, resuscitative endovascular balloon occlusion of the aorta.

Shock

A primary goal in minimising death and disability is to ensure adequate oxygen supply to peripheral tissues. The most urgent threat to achieving this is interruption of oxygen supply (airway). The next most urgent threat is interference with alveolar oxygen exchange (breathing). The third most important threat is failure of peripheral delivery of oxygen (via the circulation). The adverse effects of shock occur at the microcirculation level, and early recognition of shock depends on clinical observations of:

- the microcirculation of the skin (pale, cold, clammy)
- the brain (level of consciousness: confusion, agitation, anxiety, etc.)
- the kidneys (timed urinary output via urinary catheter).

The acid–base status of the patient, as manifested in the results of arterial blood gases, gives an indication of the magnitude of the microcirculatory failure and is an invaluable tool for assessing shock and the response to resuscitation in a critically injured patient.

Cardiac arrest

From time to time, injured patients present in actual or impending cardiac arrest. It is generally agreed that attempted resuscitation of patients who have no vital signs at the scene of injury will not restore life except in some circumstances where hypothermia is extreme.

When patients who have arrived with recordable vital signs deteriorate rapidly so that cardiac arrest is imminent, there is no time even to carry out a rapid systematic primary survey. Management is simplified by rapidly instituting the maximum response to potential problems with airway and breathing and circulation. This involves endotracheal intubation and controlled ventilation with 100% oxygen, insertion of bilateral intercostal catheters and insertion of at least two large-bore intravenous cannulas to facilitate infusion of warmed blood. External bleeding must be rapidly controlled by direct pressure.

Although victims of blunt trauma who arrive at hospital without vital signs are unlikely to be salvaged by the most aggressive resuscitation, patients with sub-diaphragmatic haemorrhage and circulatory collapse may be salvageable with limitation of systemic circulation (resuscitative endovascular balloon occlusion of the aorta, thoracic aortic cross-clamping via left anterolateral thoracotomy), volume resuscitation and immediate definitive surgical intervention.

In the setting of penetrating injury leading to cardiac arrest, there is greater opportunity for patient salvage. These patients require immediate resuscitative thoracotomy with or without pericardotomy and/or aortic cross-clamping in the emergency department to restore central perfusion (heart and brain). Patients will then need definitive surgical management in the operating room.

Gastric tube

Insertion of a gastric tube can be a life-saving manoeuvre if it is used to decompress a full stomach and avoid aspiration of gastric contents. A gastric tube should be inserted, usually towards the end of the primary survey, in all trauma patients with major abdominal injury, major chest injury, spinal injury, brain injury, major burns and shock. Gastric distension is particularly common in injured children. In most situations the gastric tube can be placed through the nasal route; however, in patients with a high likelihood of basal skull or cribriform plate fractures it should *only* be placed by the oral route.

Urinary catheter

There is no great urgency to insert a urinary catheter but it is helpful if used in patients with potentially serious injury and is inserted at the end of the primary survey. The observation of gross haematuria or documentation of microscopic haematuria may have important diagnostic implications. However, once the bladder is empty, monitoring of the hourly urine output is an important part of assessing the response to intravenous fluid resuscitation. In nearly all patients a urinary catheter can be placed by an experienced operator. If it cannot be gently advanced, it is advisable to seek urologist support or suprapubic catheter placement needs to be considered.

Secondary survey

The emphasis in secondary survey is on identifying anatomical injuries and providing clinical information that will determine the need for plain X-rays and other special investigations. It is a careful and methodical physical examination from head to toe. It requires close inspection, careful palpation and appropriate auscultation. Common omissions resulting in delayed identification of injury include examination of the entire scalp, careful inspection of the back (always needing a log-roll), inspection of the perineum and inspection of the axillae.

Table 48.2 outlines a useful sequence for the execution of the secondary survey. It also indicates the common general abnormalities that may be observed and highlights some simple procedures that assist with pain relief, reduce the risk of infection and lead into the definitive-care phase of early trauma management.

Monitoring

Injuries may be multiple and occult and therefore repeated examination and close monitoring are essential, particularly in the first 24 hours following

Table 48.2 Secondary survey: look! listen! feel!

Head-to-toe

Glasgow Coma Scale	**Assess for the following**
Scalp	Tenderness
Ears (including tympanic membranes)	Lacerations (including entry, exit wounds)
Eyes (including pupils, acuity, fundoscopic exam)	Swelling (including haematoma)
Facial bones	Structural deformity (i.e. bones)
Mouth (including teeth)	Discoloration (e.g. bruising)
Neck (C-spine, soft tissues, trachea)	Crepitus (including subcutaneous)
Clavicles	Ischaemia (i.e. limbs)
Chest:	Functional impairment:
Chest wall	Visceral (lungs, heart,
Chest movement	bowel)
Lungs	Musculoskeletal
Heart	neurological
Abdomen	**Proceed with the following**
Pelvis	Take photos of wounds
Hips	Sterile pad on wounds
Thighs	Pressure on bleeding sites
Knees	Splint fractures: traction where indicated
Legs	Application of pelvic binding device if indicated
Ankles	Pain relief
Feet	Tetanus prophylaxis
Upper arms	Antibiotics if indicated
Elbows	
Forearms	
Wrists	
Hands	
Fingers	
Back and flanks (log-roll)	
Perineum, genitalia	
Rectal examination	
Urinalysis	

injury. Injuries may also progress to become life- or limb-threatening, and recognition of these possible patterns of progression are essential. Table 48.3 identifies some common injury progression patterns to be wary of.

The monitoring strategy varies with the known injuries, comorbidity and age factors, other anticipated injuries and the potential consequences or complications of the known injuries or their management.

Monitoring of oxygenation (airway and breathing) may include skin colour, level of consciousness, respiratory rate and depth, physical examination of the respiratory system, chest X-rays, pulse oximetry, capnography, arterial blood gases and ventilation pressures.

Monitoring of the circulation may include pulse rate, blood pressure, skin colour and temperature, level of consciousness, urinary output, assessment of volume status and cardiac function, serial haemoglobin, arterial blood gases, drain outputs (e.g. chest tube), as well as repeated physical examination of the abdomen and wound dressings.

Monitoring of the central nervous system relies heavily on physical examination and serial CT scans. When CT scans reveal significant injury, an intracranial pressure monitoring device may be required. Serial documentation of the GCS score is imperative in patients who are not sedated and paralysed.

Early detection and treatment of sepsis are important. Temperature regulation and avoidance of extremes are important in limiting adverse consequences such as coagulopathy with hypothermia or secondary brain injury with hyperthermia.

Definitive care

Definitive care is the phase of early trauma management when particular injuries receive their specific treatment. Much of this takes place in the operating theatre, and in situations of multiple major injuries a number of surgical subspecialty teams may be involved. Figure 48.1 emphasises the need for resuscitation to be continuing, and for monitoring and reassessment of a patient's responses to resuscitation to be conducted, throughout this and all other phases of care. Any deterioration in a patient's physiological status should lead to urgent reassessment of the primary survey priorities and immediate intervention when acutely life-threatening events are identified.

Definitive care continues through any necessary stay in the intensive care unit (ICU) and through early convalescence on the hospital ward. As our systems of trauma care improve, the interface between acute care and rehabilitation should become progressively more invisible.

Tertiary survey

The tertiary survey is a repeat clinical examination along the lines of the primary and secondary surveys. It is performed with the aim of identifying injuries that have been missed during initial assessment. It is best performed after the early phase of definitive care and is most likely to be done if viewed

Table 48.3 Common injuries and potentially dangerous sequelae.

Finding	Beware
Fractured mandible: patent airway when patient sitting upright	Acutely obstructs if the patient lies down
Small pneumothorax: patient not compromised	Enlarges to become life-threatening complete pneumothorax or develops tension
Small pulmonary contusions: patient well	Progression of oedema or haemorrhage resulting in major alterations to pulmonary compliance and oxygen exchange
Small intracranial haematoma: GCS >13	Enlarges leading to GCS drop, increased intracranial pressure
Contained arterial vascular disruptions: haemodynamics normal	Free rupture and massive haemorrhage
Arterial intimal injuries: no distal organ/tissue compromise	Thrombotic or embolic events, e.g. stroke, gut or limb ischaemia, renal infarction
Crushed or reperfused extremity muscles	Compartment syndrome, rhabdomyolysis, renal failure

as the first routine clinical task on the morning after admission of the patient to hospital. In addition to clinical examination, all X-rays and CT scans should be reviewed (along with final consultant radiologist reports) and new X-rays or other tests organised as indicated from the physical examination.

Injuries that may not have been identified during primary survey often have great functional importance and impact the return of the patient to normal occupational, family and social functions. They usually pose little threat to life but often would lead to locomotor or manipulative disability if undetected and untreated. Examples include cervical spine injury without neurological deficit, fractures of small bones in the hands and feet, ligamentous injuries to the knee or ankle, dislocated acromioclavicular joint and peripheral nerve injuries. Review of previous X-rays will sometimes result in a new diagnosis of pneumothorax, widened mediastinum, pelvic fracture or rib fractures that require specific management. Visceral injury (solid organ or hollow viscus) may not be appreciated on clinical examination or even on CT imaging, and must be considered especially in patients who then develop subtle signs (e.g. mild tachycardia, change in abdominal examination). In addition, mild traumatic brain injury may have no initial signs other than amnesia. These patients should be formally assessed using a test such as the post-traumatic amnesia test, which is administered in the hours to days following injury.

Outcomes

Prevention of deaths and disability

In accordance with these strategies, deaths that are avoidable can usually be prevented. Diagnosis of any problems must be early. Surgery must be prompt. Application and extension of the principles outlined for prevention of death will also succeed in minimising disability.

Trauma registries and performance improvement

It is critical that any mature or maturing trauma system has a functional trauma registry that incorporates information on injuries sustained and specific criteria of initial assessment and management that can also be used as markers indicating adequate or inadequate care. Additionally, it is important that details of complications and information on outcomes and lengths of stay are included. It is only with this information that objective comparisons can be made and assessments of adequacy of care undertaken.

Performance improvement refers specifically to a process whereby care is objectively assessed and strategies are implemented to either better the process of care or result in better patient outcomes. This approach requires objective collection of information, a robust system of review or audit, strategies to ameliorate demonstrated deficiencies, and repeated collection of data to assess efficacy of changes. It is only with repeated cycles of assessment and change that better overall results and outcomes can be achieved.

Further reading

Boffard KD (ed.) *Manual of Definitive Surgical Trauma Care incorporating Definitive Anaesthetic Trauma Care*, 5th edn. Boca Raton, FL: CRC Press, 2019.

Gabbe BJ, Simpson PM, Sutherland AM *et al.* Improved functional outcomes for major trauma patients in a regionalized, inclusive trauma system. *Ann Surg* 2012; 255:1009–15.

Mattox KL, Moore EE, Feliciano DV (eds) *Trauma*, 7th edn. New York: McGraw-Hill, 2013.

MCQs

Select the single correct answer to each question. The correct answers can be found in the Answers section at the end of the book.

1 Which of the following critical determinants of patient outcome following injury is *incorrect*?
   a time from injury to definitive care
   b presence of a well-organised regional system of trauma care
   c protocols and guidelines when clinical experience is limited
   d early mobilisation of teams led by doctors to most scenes of injury
   e thrombosis prophylaxis

2 Which of the following does *not* result in hypovolaemic shock?
   a pulmonary laceration
   b extradural haemorrhage
   c pelvic fracture
   d femur fracture
   e laceration to scalp

3 A restrained 32-year-old male involved in a head-on motor vehicle collision presents with chest pain and the following vital signs on arrival in the emergency department: heart rate, 120/min; blood pressure, 86/50 mmHg; GCS score, 10; and oxygen saturation, 92%. Which of the following takes first priority?
   a urgent CT scan of the head to rule out an extradural haemorrhage with midline shift
   b rapid resuscitation with two large-bore intravenous cannulas and warmed fluids
   c ECG and an echocardiogram to eliminate cardiac contusion as the cause of his hypotension
   d obtaining an urgent cross-match
   e elimination of tension pneumothorax as a cause of his symptoms/signs

4 Which of the following is *not* considered an immediate threat to life?
   a fracture of T6 with a complete spinal cord transection
   b splenic injury with ongoing bleeding
   c open pneumothorax
   d rapidly rising intracranial pressure
   e aspiration

49 Burns

Ioana Tichil and Heather Cleland

Victorian Adult Burns Service, Alfred Health, Melbourne, Victoria, Australia

Introduction

Burns are common. From sunburn to scald injuries to major flame burns, anyone can be affected due to the accidental and often unpredictable nature of the injuries. Most are minor and will heal on their own with little or no medical intervention. However, severe burns are a life-changing event, with potentially devastating consequences for physical, emotional, psychosocial and economic function. Therefore, burn treatments have been an area of interest and research in medicine from ancient times, and have principally involved the use of various topical applications applied in the hope of aiding spontaneous healing. More recently, the acute surgical management of even massive burns, made possible by improvements in critical and supportive care, has resulted in significantly better prognoses for burn-injured patients.

Epidemiology and aetiology of burns

Incidence, cause, pattern, gender and age groups affected by burns vary greatly between low- and middle-income countries and high-income countries. In Australia and New Zealand, it is estimated that every year 1% of the population suffers a burn that requires medical attention. Of these, 10% will require hospitalisation and of these 10% will have life-threatening injuries. Thus, severe burns are relatively uncommon in Australia and New Zealand, where adults and children alike are most likely to be injured at home in the kitchen or in the bathroom. For adults, workplace injuries and burns sustained during recreational activities are also frequent. Scalds are the third most common cause of injury in the general population and the most frequent form of injury amongst the paediatric population. For adults requiring admission to burn units, flame is the commonest cause of injury. However, scalds are the commonest cause of burns in the elderly, and have a high mortality rate. Chemical and electrical injuries are much less common than thermal injuries (for more information see Burns Registry of Australia and New Zealand, www.branz.org).

Skin anatomy and physiology

Skin is the largest human organ, comprising 16% of total body weight. Its main role is to protect the body from the environment and to facilitate interaction via sensory input, to insulate and thermoregulate, and to aid in immune defence and vitamin D production.

Skin is composed of two layers, the epidermis and the dermis, which rest on the panniculus adiposus (known as the hypodermis) and sometimes considered to be the third layer of the skin (Figure 49.1). The epidermis is a stratified squamous epithelium containing keratinocytes in progressive stages of differentiation, designated from deep to superficial layers as stratum basale, stratum spinosum, stratum granulosum, stratum lucidum and stratum corneum. Among the keratinocytes are melanocytes, antigen-processing Langerhans cells and pressure-sensing Merkel cells. Dermis contains collagen, elastic fibres, blood vessels, sensory structures, appendages and fibroblasts. It is composed of two layers: a superficial layer, the papillary dermis, and a deep layer, the reticular dermis. The papillary dermis contains vascular plexuses, free nerve endings and Meissner's corpuscles and the reticular dermis contains hair follicles, sebaceous glands, sweat glands, hair follicles, Pacinian corpuscles and Ruffini's endings.

The capacity of a burn to heal without the need for surgical intervention is largely determined by the depth of burn: the epithelial elements of the dermis are destroyed by deep burns and therefore cannot heal by proliferation of epithelial stem cells remaining in the wound bed.

Textbook of Surgery, Fourth Edition. Edited by Julian A. Smith, Andrew H. Kaye, Christopher Christophi and Wendy A. Brown.
© 2020 John Wiley & Sons Ltd. Published 2020 by John Wiley & Sons Ltd.

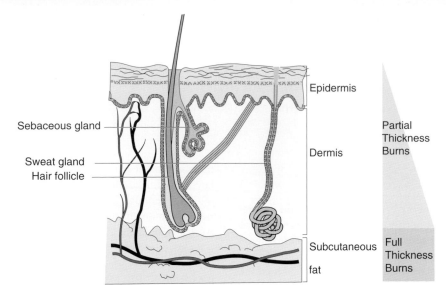

Fig. 49.1 Burn depth in relation to skin structure.

Classification of burns

Burns are classified by extent (percent body surface area involved and depth) and by cause. It is important to accurately assess a burn injury, as extent determines treatment (transfer, resuscitation, surgical management) and prognosis.

Assessment of extent of burn

Size of burn is expressed as a percentage of total body surface area (TBSA) and is best assessed with the assistance of diagrams. For adults, the 'rule of nines' is used (Figure 49.2). Each arm is approximately 9% TBSA, the head 9% TBSA, each leg 18% TBSA, and the front and back of the torso 18% TBSA each. The palmar surface of the hand (including fingers) is approximately 1% TBSA. For children, who depending on age have a relatively larger head and smaller legs relative to torso, use the Lund and Browder chart (Figure 49.3) or equivalent. These are guidelines only and are less accurate in the morbidly obese. Superficial burns should not be included in extent estimates.

Assessment of burn depth

Depth of burn is classified according to anatomy (Table 49.1). Superficial burns involve the epidermis only. They clinically manifest as painful erythema and late blistering ('peeling' or dry scaling). They heal spontaneously within a few days and do not require specialised care. Severe sunburn is a typical superficial burn.

Superficial dermal (partial-thickness) burns

Superficial dermal (partial-thickness) burns extend to involve the papillary dermis. They are very painful because of the exposed nerve endings. Capillary return is brisk as dermal vasculature is intact. Serous blisters are characteristic. The skin covering the blister is dead and is separated from the base by inflammatory oedema fluid (Figure 49.4). When the blister ruptures the underlying papillary dermis is exposed, which presents as pink, moist and shiny. These burns heal spontaneously by epithelialisation within 14 days.

Deep dermal (partial-thickness) burns

Deep dermal (partial-thickness) burns extend into the reticular dermis, i.e. the epidermis, papillary dermis and reticular dermis are affected. Blisters may be present on examination but have typically burst and sloughed very early (Figure 49.5). Exposed dermis is pale, or red due to red cell extravasation, and capillary refill is very slow. Some nerve endings may be intact so the burn can be sensate but are generally less painful than more superficial burns. They tend to be dry. These burns have the potential to heal through a combination of granulation, wound contraction and epithelialisation from deep dermal appendages and the wound edges with conservative management, but typically take 3 weeks or more to heal and are at high risk of hypertrophic scarring if allowed to do so.

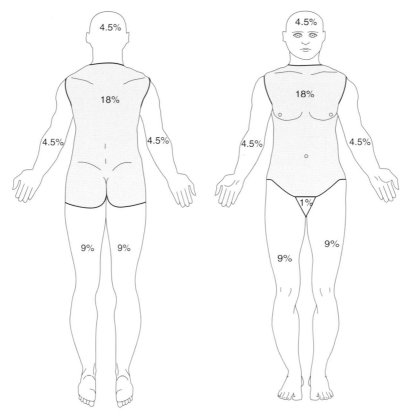

Fig. 49.2 'Rule of nines' for estimating extent of burns in adults.

Mid-dermal (partial-thickness) burns

Mid-dermal partial-thickness burns are burns that present as neither superficial nor deep partial thickness. It is not possible to predict soon after injury whether these will go on to heal within 3 weeks, and generally this will become evident only after 5–7 days, as the burn wound evolves.

Full-thickness burns

Full-thickness burns extend to the hypodermis. All layers of the skin are affected, no dermal structures are preserved and underlying hypodermic fat may be implicated. There is no blistering; the wounds are dry with a charred leathery appearance, known as eschar, and underlying thrombosed blood vessels. These wounds do not heal with conservative management.

Burn mechanism

Most burns are due to thermal injury and are the result of flame, hot liquids (i.e. scalds), contact with hot objects, or radiant heat. Chemical and electrical injuries are uncommon.

Electrical injuries

Electrical injuries are classified into high and low voltage. Sources of low-voltage current (<1000 V) include domestic power supplies (240 V Australia and New Zealand), motor vehicle batteries (12 V) and industrial switchboards (415 V). They can result in significant usually localised tissue damage, and less commonly other effects such as cardiac arrhythmias. High voltage is defined as greater than 1000 V and is related to electrical distribution systems, including high-tension power lines (11 000–33 000 V), power stations and substations.

Tissue damage is, in simple terms, the result of heat generated by resistance to current transfer. However, the precise mechanism of tissue damage may be multifactorial, especially in high-voltage injuries: electrical field changes can damage cell membranes (a cause of rhabdomyolysis).

In high-voltage injuries, in addition to damage due to current flow, arcing over a distance may produce a flash type of burn without direct contact with the current source. Arcs may also ignite clothing and result in flame burns. In high-voltage injury, current may be conducted according to a composite resistance across all tissues: limbs (especially at

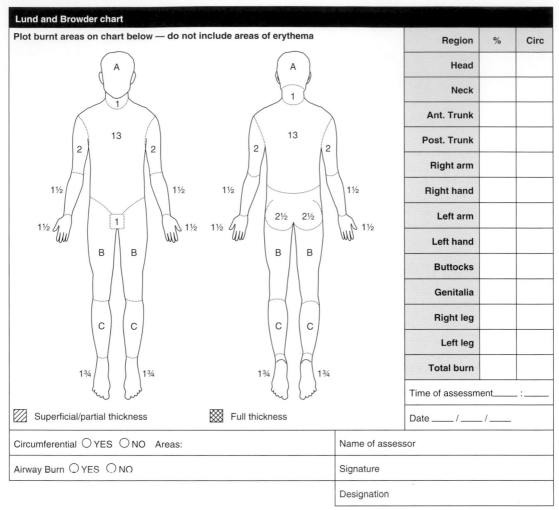

Lund and Browder chart

Plot burnt areas on chart below — do not include areas of erythema

Region	%	Circ
Head		
Neck		
Ant. Trunk		
Post. Trunk		
Right arm		
Right hand		
Left arm		
Left hand		
Buttocks		
Genitalia		
Right leg		
Left leg		
Total burn		

Time of assessment_____ : _____

Date ____ / ____ / ____

☒ Superficial/partial thickness   ☒ Full thickness

Circumferential ○ YES ○ NO   Areas:

Airway Burn ○ YES ○ NO

Name of assessor

Signature

Designation

Age (years)	0	1	5	10	15	Adult	
A – ½ of head	9 ½	8 ½	6 ½	5 ½	4 ½	3 ½	Relative percentage of areas affected by growth
B – ½ of one thigh	2 ¾	3 ¼	4	4 ¼	4 ½	4 ¾	
C – ½ of one leg	2 ½	2 ½	2 ¾	3	3 ¼	3	

Fig. 49.3 Lund and Browder chart for estimating extent of burns in children. Source: Shutterstock.

Table 49.1 Assessment of burn depth.

	Superficial partial thickness dermal burn	Deep partial thickness dermal burn	Full-thickness burn
Colour	Pink	Pale/red	White/red
Blisters	Late	Early	Epidermis destroyed
Circulation	Present	Sluggish	Absent
Sensation	Hypersensitive: painful	Decreased	Anaesthetic
Healing	<2–3 weeks	>3 weeks	No

joints, where there is localised increased resistance) will be more damaged than the torso. High-voltage injuries tend to cause extensive deep tissue damage and are associated with high amputation and mortality rates.

Chemical burns

Most chemical burns occur as a result of the mishandling of household cleaners and other chemicals. Because of occupational health and

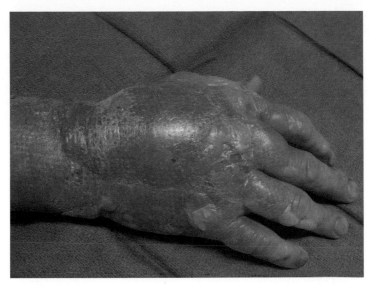

Fig. 49.4 Superficial partial-thickness burn at 24 hours with intact blister. Note hyperaemic underlying dermis.

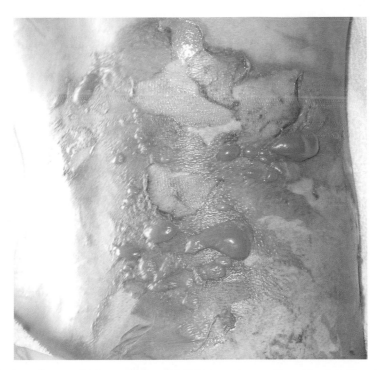

Fig. 49.5 Mixed depth predominantly deep partial- and full-thickness burns. Note necrotic epidermis which has largely sloughed.

safety standards in Australia and New Zealand, industrial exposures are rare. However, when they occur they can be life-threatening due to the high concentrations of toxic chemicals used in these settings.

The severity of a chemical burn depends on the agent's concentration, quantity, manner and duration of exposure, penetration and mechanism of action. There is a wide variety of chemicals that can damage tissues in many ways. Two broad categories are acids and alkalis. As a general rule, acids such as sulphuric, hydrochloric and hydrofluoric produce injury by coagulation necrosis and precipitation of proteins, while alkaline substances such as potassium hydroxide, sodium hypochlorite (bleach) or cement lead to liquefying necrosis that allows further penetration into the tissues resulting in deeper, more severe and more extensive burns. In addition to direct tissue damage, chemical compounds injure by various mechanisms including exothermic reaction and tissue dehydration. In some cases, additional systemic manifestations may be associated with exposure (which can occur by inhalation as well as direct contact with skin), including metabolic acidosis and alkalosis, hypocalcaemia, and liver or kidney damage.

First aid is aimed at removing the offending agent, removing affected clothing, and application of copious water irrigation for a minimum of 30 minutes. Irrigation should be prolonged if pain persists. The use of specific neutralising agents is generally not indicated for most agents, although hydrofluoric acid exposure should be managed with calcium gluconate applied topically or injected subcutaneously or intra-arterially. Diphoterine® is a neutralising solution effective against a wide range of chemicals (but not hydrofluoric acid), in addition to acids and alkalis, and is used for first aid in industrial settings, although is not generally available in hospital emergency departments. Cutaneous chemical burns are often deep and require surgical management.

Inhalation injury

Inhalation of the toxic products of combustion may occur in association with burn injury, and is likely if burns are sustained in enclosed spaces. Damage can be due to thermally or chemically induced injury to the upper and lower respiratory tract and may be classified into three groups.

- Most fire-related deaths result not from cutaneous burns but from inhalation of toxic combustion products. Carbon monoxide and other toxic gases produce hypoxia that can result in altered conscious state and death.
- Heat and chemical damage to the upper airway produces swelling and respiratory obstruction over a period of hours after injury.
- Inhalation of irritant chemicals such as hydrogen chloride, nitrogen oxide and aldehydes cause acute pulmonary oedema and chemical pneumonitis and may progress to adult respiratory distress syndrome, with secondary infection.

Bronchoscopy is a useful diagnostic and therapeutic tool, but chest X-ray has been shown to be an insensitive diagnostic investigation for inhalation injury. Treatment starts with administration of 100% oxygen. Where upper airway injury is suspected, early intubation is indicated to protect the airway, especially if the patient is to be transported.

Emergency management of burn patients

The principles of initial management of a patient with a severe burn consist of immediate first aid, followed by primary and secondary survey, with institution of simultaneous resuscitation. Burns are obvious but should not distract from the possibility of coexistent other trauma, especially in patients who have been involved in motor vehicle accidents or have suffered a high-voltage electrical or blast injury.

First aid at the scene

First aid should always be aimed at stopping the burning process and cooling the burn with running water, ideally for 20 minutes within the first 3 hours from injury, while avoiding hypothermia. Ice or iced water should never be used, as the subsequent vasoconstriction will deepen burns and increase the risk of hypothermia. The patient should not be allowed to become hypothermic during irrigation. Children especially are susceptible to the development of hypothermia, and irrigation should be discontinued if this occurs. It is important to remember to cool the burn and warm the patient.

Patients with major burns have suffered significant trauma, and in addition to assessment of the burn wound should undergo a routine primary and secondary survey in order to identify all injuries. Features of particular relevance with respect to burn-injured patients are discussed in the following sections.

Primary survey

A: Airway maintenance and cervical spine control

Patients with upper airway swelling due to inhalation injury may present with a hoarse voice or (a late sign) stridor, which is an emergency and an indication for intubation.

B: Breathing, ventilation and oxygen supplementation

Circumferential full-thickness chest and abdomen burns may impede ventilation and are an indication for escharotomy. Be aware of the possibility of carbon monoxide poisoning where 'cherry-red' appearance can mask tissue hypoxaemia.

C: Circulation with haemorrhage control

Circumferential full-thickness limb burns can, especially with fluid resuscitation, produce constriction of limbs and distal ischaemia. This is an indication for escharotomy.

Patients with extensive burns rapidly become hypovolaemic due to fluid losses. Insert two large-bore intravenous lines preferably through unburnt tissue, take bloods and start fluid resuscitation.

D: Disability and neurological status

Altered consciousness may be due to inhalation injury.

E: Exposure with environmental control

Remove clothing and jewellery, log roll to assess the posterior surface, keep patient warm and estimate the percentage of burn area in relation to total body surface area.

Resuscitation

Before proceeding to the secondary survey certain therapeutic steps must be taken. In adults with burns of more than 15–20% TBSA, early fluid resuscitation should be started in order to reduce the risk of irreversible organ damage due to hypoperfusion. Delayed or inadequate replacement of intravascular volume in the setting of major burns results in suboptimal tissue perfusion associated with end-organ failure and death. Multiple resuscitation formulas are available but are a *guide only* to resuscitation, and should be titrated based on clinical parameters.

A commonly used effective formula is the Parkland Formula, which uses intravenous warmed crystalloids (Hartmann's solution) as follows:

$$3 - 4\,mL \times weight(kg) \times \%TBSA\ burn$$

Half is administered in the first 8 hours after injury and the remainder in the subsequent 16 hours. The efficacy of fluid resuscitation is monitored primarily by urine output: a rate of 0.5 mL/kg per hour should be the aim in adults. A urinary catheter should be inserted for monitoring.

Fluid management in paediatric burns

Fluid management in children with burns is both similar to and different from that of adults with burns. Intravenous fluid resuscitation is reserved for children whose total body surface burned exceeds the definition for a major burn, and volumes and rates are commenced in accordance with the modified Parkland Formula. Once fluid resuscitation is commenced, optimal urine output and vital signs are the primary determinants for the ongoing rate of intravenous fluid resuscitation. Therefore, urinary catherisation is strongly recommended for all children receiving fluid resuscitation, as this provides the most accurate measure of urine output and its response to changes in fluid rates.

The preferred choice of fluid resuscitation is no different from that of adults (i.e. crystalloid) and both Hartmann's solution and normal saline (0.9% NaCl) are in common use. Colloid has no current routine place in fluid resuscitation for paediatric burns, albeit the crystalloid versus colloid debate continues in the paediatric literature as it does in the adult burns literature. The differences in burn fluid management with respect to children versus adults include the following.

- *Definition of major burn*: resuscitation fluids are commenced for children with burns in excess of 10% TBSA.
- *Optimal urinary output*: 1 mL/kg per hour.
- *Cerebral oedema risk*: children receiving excessive resuscitation fluids are at increased risk of cerebral oedema, especially in the setting of hyponatraemia. This risk can be mitigated by careful monitoring of fluid rates and keeping the child 'head up' in the first 24 hours.
- *Maintenance fluids*: these are given *in addition* to any resuscitation fluids. Fasting children require maintenance fluids to meet their physiological requirements. They are particularly susceptible to hypoglycaemia due to limited hepatic glycogen stores. Therefore, the maintenance fluid must contain glucose (or dextrose), and the child's blood glucose should be checked regularly during initial stabilisation and transport.

As with resuscitation fluid choices, the ideal maintenance fluid for the injured child remains an area of controversy. There is consensus that hypotonic fluids, such as 0.18% NaCl with 4% dextrose, should not be used as they expose children to risks of severe iatrogenic hyponatraemia. Recent evidence supports increased use of isotonic maintenance fluids such as normal saline or PlasmaLyte to avoid hyponatraemia.

Maintenance rates are calculated according to a standard and internationally recognised paediatric formula. This formula, commonly referred to as the '4:2:1 rule', can be summarised as follows:

4 mL/h for the first 10 kg of body weight +

2 mL/h for each kg of body weight over 10 kg and less than 20 kg body weight +

1 mL/h for each kg of body weight over 20 kg of body weight

Secondary survey

This consists of two components: history and head-to-toe examination.

History

Salient points of the history can be summarised by the mnemonic AMPLE.

A   Allergies
M   Medications
P   Past medical illness
L   Last meal
E   Events and circumstances related to injury

Of particular importance in the history is to ascertain when the injury occurred, and what treatment, including fluid resuscitation, has been administered since. The mechanism and place of occurrence are also relevant in helping to assess the likely severity of the burn and likelihood of inhalation injury.

Examination

- *Head and neck*: check for corneal burns using fluorescein staining. Look for indications of possible inhalation injury, such as burns or blistering of the nose and mouth, singeing of nasal hairs, soot in the mouth or pharynx, and blisters or oedema of the tongue. Carefully check for signs of cervical spine injury.
- *Chest*: examine the whole chest, assessing the burn and noting whether it is compromising respiration.
- *Abdomen*: assess if abdominal burns are restricting respiration, especially in children who are predominantly diaphragmatic breathers.
- *Perineum*: check for perineal burns and other injuries.
- *Limbs*: assess the burns to determine if they are full-thickness and circumferential. Such burns may cause constriction as swelling occurs and impair venous return from the limb, leading to further swelling and eventual cessation of arterial inflow, producing tissue ischaemia and necrosis.

Ensure adequate analgesia, as burns are often very painful injuries. Make sure the patient does not become hypothermic. Ascertain adequate tetanus prophylaxis.

In order to minimise swelling, affected limbs and the head and neck region should be elevated. Patients with deep circumferential burns that impair circulation and ventilation may require escharotomy prior to transfer. Escharotomy is an emergency damage control procedure that entails incision of circumferential deep burns down to subcutaneous fat along the mid-axial lines of limbs, and incision of chest and abdominal burns in order to relieve constriction caused by unyielding eschar over swelling deeper tissues.

Indications for transfer to a burns unit

Small superficial burns can be managed in an outpatient setting with appropriate dressings and follow-up. Patients with deep burns that will not heal within 3 weeks are likely to require surgical treatment and should be referred for operative management. Indications for referral and transfer to a burns unit include:

- more than 10% TBSA burn (adults) and more than 5% TBSA burn (children)
- electrical burn
- chemical burn
- associated inhalation injury
- circumferential deep burns
- special areas (perineum/hand/face)
- poor-risk patient (comorbidities/pregnancy)
- non-accidental injury (suspected child or elder abuse)
- associated trauma.

Burn wound care

For patients with significant injuries who require transfer to a burns unit, simple temporary dressings for transfer are recommended, such as plastic cling film wrap, hydrogel or paraffin gauze dressings. Superficial dermal and some mid-dermal burns that are expected to heal by epithelisation within 2–3 weeks with minimal scarring should be managed conservatively with dressings (Figure 49.6).

A burn wound should be cleaned and loose devitalised tissue removed. The ideal burn dressing will promote moist wound healing, protect against infection and assist in pain management. Non-stick dressings that can be kept intact for several days are particularly useful when treating burns in a paediatric population, where the aim is to minimise distress brought about by changes of dressings and to avoid infection.

It should be noted that burn wounds evolve over time and require dressings with different characteristics as they progress to healing. Early after injury, burns produce significant amounts of exudate, and dressings should be absorptive. The necessity for this capacity decreases after the first few days. Even relatively minor burns are not 'set and forget'

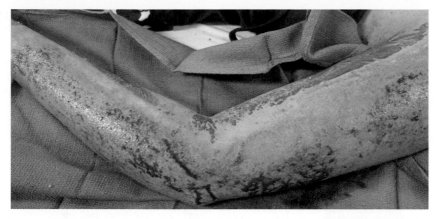

Fig. 49.6 Healing superficial burn 10 days after injury. Note that more superficial periphery of injury has healed, and the islands of regenerating epithelial cells which will proliferate to resurface the rest of the wound.

injuries and require regular review to ensure they are progressing to healing. Silver-impregnated dressings are widely available in a variety of forms, but evidence for their value in superficial non-contaminated injuries is lacking. Principles for informing choice of definitive dressing and alternative types of dressing can be found at www.vicburns.org.au.

Deep dermal and full-thickness burns do not heal spontaneously: their natural progression is to granulate, contract and epithelialise from the edges. This may take several weeks or months, during which time wounds are susceptible to infection. Subsequent scarring is very often hypertrophic and contracted and may lead to distorted local anatomy and significant functional impairment. This is why treatment of deep burns is primarily surgical and aimed at early excisional debridement and wound closure using autologous skin grafting.

Systemic effects of burn injury

Cutaneous burns larger than 20% in adults and 10% in children can have an impact on the entire body. A systemic inflammatory response syndrome (SIRS) consequent on a massive surge of inflammatory mediators is characteristic of extensive burns. The most notable early effect of this is 'burns shock', characterised by hypovolaemia secondary to fluid losses and oedema formation, and is a result of generalised increased capillary membrane permeability. Decreased cardiac contractility also contributes to burns shock. Prior to the recognition of this phenomenon and the consequent need for active fluid resuscitation in the early twentieth century, many people with severe burns died from shock secondary to fluid losses.

Major burns affect multiple organ systems. They elicit a hypermetabolic response characterised by tachycardia and hyperthermia leading to protein breakdown and muscle wasting. Adequate nutritional support is required for all burns exceeding 20% TBSA. Immune system compromise due to inhibition of the humoral and cellular pathways contributes to susceptibility to infection, which is the leading cause of mortality in these patients. Gut barrier function may be affected and result in bacterial translocation, which may be ameliorated by early enteral feeding. Patients with extensive burns are also at increased risk of gastric ulceration. Acute respiratory distress syndrome (ARDS) can manifest in the absence of inhalation injury as part of the body's SIRS response to injury.

Various systemic effects can persist for months and even years after all wounds have healed and range from central disposition of fat to decreased muscle growth and bone mineralisation. In children this can lead to a permanent reduction in growth.

Management of the major burn wound

Early excisional debridement of burn eschar, preferably within 24 hours of injury, may result in benefits such as decreased SIRS response, decreased blood loss, decreased length of stay, and decreased risk of invasive wound infections, particularly in massive burns. Tangential excision, whereby successive thin layers of tissue are removed until healthy well-perfused tissue forms the wound bed, is preferred to en bloc fascial debridement (Figure 49.7). Several methods are used to minimise blood loss during surgery, such us tourniquets, infiltration of tumescent adrenaline solutions, use of topical diluted adrenaline, diathermy and various fibrin-based tissue glues.

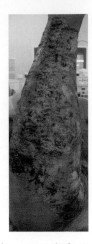

Fig. 49.7 Excised burn wound of mixed full and partial thickness depth showing preservation of deep dermis in areas of deep partial thickness depth and hypodermis (fat) in areas of full-thickness burn excision.

It is rarely a good idea to excise an extensive burn wound and close the wound with autologous split-skin graft at the same sitting, especially in the setting of acute excision, when the patient is still undergoing resuscitation. After the burn is excised, the wound should be closed with a skin substitute until such time as the patient is stable, when wound closure can be performed in a semi-elective, and frequently staged, manner. This is especially the case when donor sites are insufficient for total wound coverage.

There are different surgical algorithms for managing such wounds (Figure 49.8). It is essential to have a consistent and structured approach to wound closure in patients with major burns, as survival ultimately depends on timely wound healing.

Donor skin can be harvested as a split-thickness graft with the use of an electrical dermatome from most sites of the body; thighs are preferred, but in

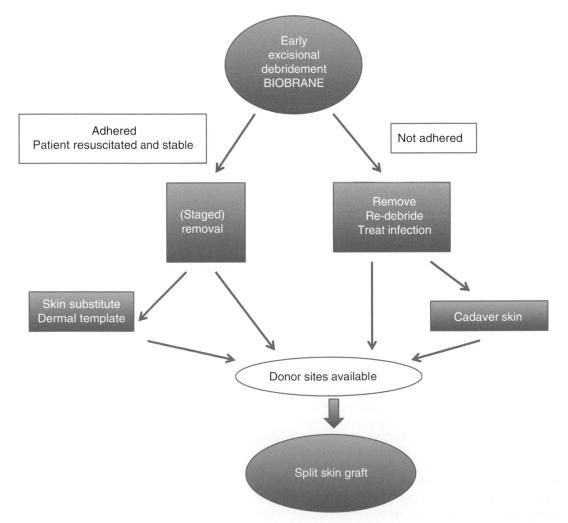

Fig. 49.8 Surgical algorithm for large burn wound management.

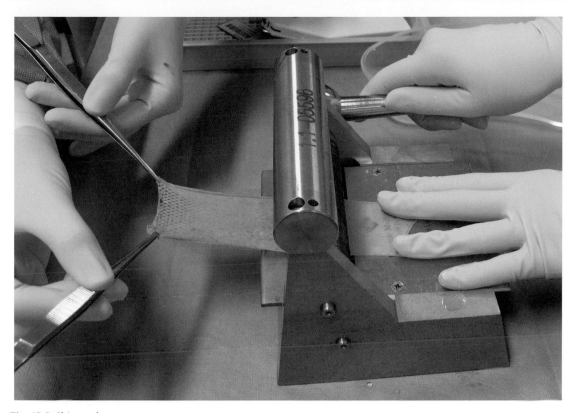

Fig. 49.9 Skin mesher.

case of major burns any unburned skin can potentially be used. Donor sites heal by epithelialisation from epithelial stem cells in dermal appendages and may be reharvested when healed; depending on patient factors and thickness of grafts, this may be as soon as 7–10 days. Skin grafts can be used as sheets when repairing functional or aesthetic areas such as hands, face, neck and upper chest and they can also be meshed to allow for expansion and coverage of larger areas (Figure 49.9). This technique is useful in large burns where donor sites are limited. Widely meshed skin grafts rely on epithelial migration to fill the gaps in the mesh, which will take longer to heal and result in suboptimal aesthetic outcomes. In the case of large burns with very limited donor sites, specialised centres may employ an alternative to skin grafting by using tissue engineering techniques to produce cultured epithelial autografts (CEA). Otherwise, temporising measures to close the wound prior to skin grafting, in the form of various epithelial or dermal substitutes or cadaver allografts, can be life-saving procedures because of their ability to close excised burn wounds (thereby decreasing the risk of wound infection) until donor sites heal and become available for reharvesting.

Several skin substitutes are currently commercially available in Australia. Their main advantage in acute burns is due to their ability to temporarily close extensive wounds while patients are stabilised and donor sites for skin grafts become available. For example, Biobrane™ is an epidermal substitute consisting of a nylon woven mesh coated with pig collagen and sealed with a thin silicone membrane. This adheres to open wounds and produces physiological wound closure, until removed and replaced with an autologous skin graft. Other products are designed to act as dermal templates and are generally also bilayered constructs. The deeper layer is composed of animal collagen and supports ingrowth and vascularisation from the wound bed. When this has occurred, the superficial sealing layer is removed and the vascularised deeper layer now composing the wound bed is skin grafted.

Teamwork in burn care

Specialised burn care is a complex undertaking, delivered in burn units by a multidisciplinary team of healthcare professionals. Burns surgeons work closely with nursing staff, emergency physicians, anaesthetists, pain specialists, infectious disease physicians, intensivists, physiotherapists and occupational therapists, speech pathologists, dietitians, psychologists and social workers to deliver care to this complex patient group.

Conclusion

Knowledge of burn pathophysiology, and in particular the systemic effects of burn injury, is a relatively recent achievement, and most major developments in burn care have been made in the last 60 years. Improvements in resuscitation, infection control, nutritional support, treatment of inhalation injuries, wound management with early debridement and coverage of wounds, and a multidisciplinary approach to treatment have significantly lowered, and continue to lower, the mortality rate for patients with severe burns, and improve scarring outcomes and quality of life for survivors. The future holds great promise for further improvements through scientific developments in the areas of skin tissue engineering and wound healing, and that improved understanding of the pathophysiology of contractures and hypertrophic scar formation produces better treatments.

Acknowledgement

The authors are grateful to Warwick Teague, Paediatric Surgeon and Director, Trauma Service, Royal Children's Hospital, Melbourne for his advice on paediatric burn resuscitation.

Further reading

Burns Registry of Australia and New Zealand, www. branz.org
Herndon, D. *Total Burn Care*, 5th edn. Elsevier, 2018.
Klasen HJ. *History of Burns. Rotterdam: Erasmus*, 2004.
Victorian Adult Burns Service, www.vicburns.org.au

MCQs

Select the single correct answer to each question. The correct answers can be found in the Answers section at the end of the book.

1 A 49-year-old male, weighing 70 kg, suffers a scald burn from freshly boiled water while handling a pot in the kitchen. The distribution of the burns mostly affects the anterior limbs and truck as shown in the figure below. All of it is blistered and the epidermis is peeling off. What is the approximate affected TBSA?

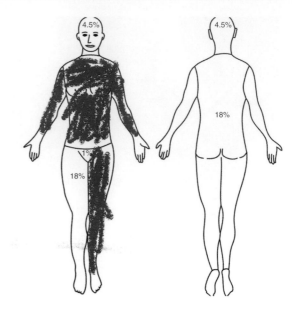

a 60%
b 54%
c 40%
d 25%
e 36%

2 With regard to the patient in question 1, what would adequate first aid consist of?
a wrap the affected area with a cold, wet towel/ flannel
b cool using ice or ice water, wrap in cling film and transport to hospital
c cover with silver-based dressings and see GP for follow-up
d cool running water for 20 minutes within the first 3 hours
e aloe vera cream

3 With regard to the patient in question 1, what is the correct amount of resuscitation fluid that he requires within the first 8 hours?
a 5000 mL
b 4500 mL
c 4000 mL
d 5500 mL
e 10 000 mL

4 Surgical management may include:
a formal scrub in theatre
b early excision of burns
c use of dermal substitutes
d temporised skin grafting
e all of the above

Section 11
Orthopaedic Surgery

50 Fractures and dislocations

Peter F. Choong

University of Melbourne and St. Vincent's Hospital, Melbourne, Victoria, Australia

Fractures

Definitions

A fracture is a loss in the normal continuity of bone following the application of a direct or indirect force to that bone. A fracture may involve a part or the entire circumference of the cortex.

Classification of fractures

Closed

A closed fracture is one that is not associated with a breach in the overlying skin or mucous membrane.

Open

An open fracture is one where there is direct communication between the fracture and the externa through a breach in the overlying skin or mucous membrane. Open fractures are at significant risk for infection.

Types of fractures

- Transverse
- Oblique
- Spiral
- Comminuted (more than two fragments)
- Displaced
- Angulated
- Impacted
- Rotated
- Distracted
- Greenstick: this occurs when only one cortex of the bone is seen to be fractured on the X-ray, and there is usually minimal deformity. This most commonly occurs in the paediatric age group

- Intra-articular: fractures that extend to the articular surface of a joint
- Special fractures:
  - Pathological fracture: fracture through an abnormal bone
  - Stress fracture: fracture through repeated minor trauma to a normal bone (Figure 50.1)

Clinical presentation

All fractures are painful. There is normally a history of trauma except in pathological fractures where minimal trauma or no trauma is the rule. Fractures are tender, swollen, occasionally deformed, mobile at the fracture site, and associated with loss of limb function.

Investigations

Radiography

All suspected fractures should be X-rayed in two planes (anteroposterior, lateral) (Figure 50.2).

Bone scans

Suspected fractures that are not obvious on plain radiographs may be identified by bone scan, which show increased isotope uptake corresponding to the site of the fracture. This may be less apparent in the geriatric group where an osteoblastic response may be less prominent. In the elderly, a delay of 1 week before bone scanning is usually required to show a positive scan. Bone scans are useful for detecting femoral neck and pelvic fractures in the elderly and carpal injuries in younger patients.

Computed tomography

Computed tomography (CT) is excellent for delineating cortical and trabecular bone. The plane of

Textbook of Surgery, Fourth Edition. Edited by Julian A. Smith, Andrew H. Kaye, Christopher Christophi and Wendy A. Brown.
© 2020 John Wiley & Sons Ltd. Published 2020 by John Wiley & Sons Ltd.

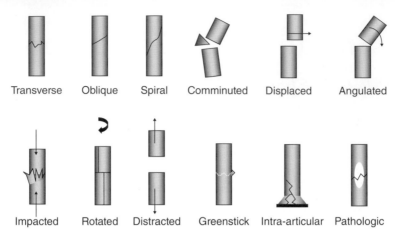

Transverse Oblique Spiral Comminuted Displaced Angulated

Impacted Rotated Distracted Greenstick Intra-articular Pathologic

Fig. 50.1 Types of fractures.

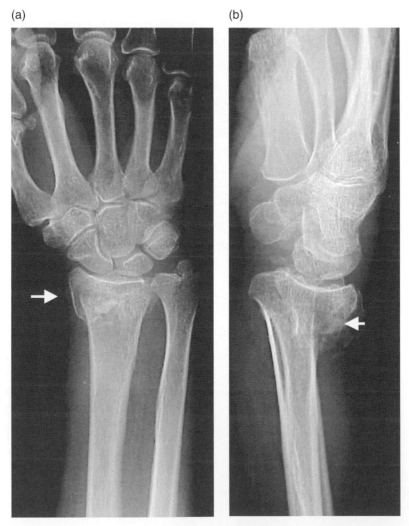

(a) (b)

Fig. 50.2 Colles fracture. (a) Anteroposterior X-ray of comminuted distal radial metaphyseal fracture. Note shortening and slight radial angulation of the fracture. An important sign that denotes a fracture are overlapping cortices (arrow). (b) Lateral X-ray of comminuted distal radial fracture. Dorsal displacement, dorsal tilt and shortening is typical of a Colles fracture.

the CT should be perpendicular or oblique to the fracture line to detect the fracture. CT is good for demonstrating periosteal new bone formation and may be valuable for diagnosing subtle stress fractures such as minimally displaced femoral neck fractures, pelvic ring fractures and rib fractures.

Magnetic resonance imaging

Limited magnetic resonance imaging (MRI) in the coronal or surgical plane is excellent for demonstrating fractures which are suspected but not readily apparent on plain X-rays. T1-weighted MRI is able to detect the fracture immediately after injury and T2-weighted images can differentiate soft tissue inflammation from intraosseous oedema. MRI scans are excellent for early detection of undisplaced scaphoid and femoral neck fractures.

Treatment

Closed fractures

The principles of management of a closed fracture include:
• correction of the deformity (reduction)

• immobilisation of the fracture
• protection until the fracture has consolidated
• rehabilitation of the muscles and joints of the affected limb.

Closed reduction

Under appropriate anaesthesia (local, regional, general) the fracture fragments should be manipulated and reduced into normal alignment. In reducing the fracture, combinations of distraction, increasing and then reducing the deformity of the fracture, and holding the reduction with three-point fixation are employed. This technique of reduction is also used with open fractures (Figure 50.3).

Open reduction

Open reduction is indicated when closed manipulation of bone fragments has failed to reduce the fracture into a satisfactory position, if reduction is impossible or if reduction is lost after initial closed reduction. Open reduction may be indicated to stabilise fractures securely to allow safe and effective management of the patient with multiple other bone or soft tissue injuries, or if movement of the adjacent joint is paramount.

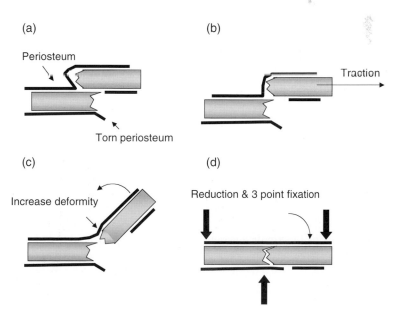

Fig. 50.3 Principles of the technique of fracture reduction. (a) Most fractures are displaced, impacted and shortened. It is common that the periosteum on one side of the fracture is intact, while that on the other side is torn. (b) The first step in reducing a fracture is disimpaction, where traction is applied along the axis of the bone to draw the fracture ends apart. In young patients, this may be difficult because of the very thick and resilient periosteum. (c) The next step is to increase the deformity so that the opposing ends of the fracture may be approximated. (d) The final step of reduction once the fracture ends are opposed is to correct the deformity and to apply three-point fixation to hold the fracture reduction (arrows). The arrows point to areas where pressure must be applied while shaping the plaster-of-Paris cast.

Open fractures

Open fractures are at risk of developing infections (acute and chronic osteomyelitis). The principles of management include the following.

- Cleaning of contaminated tissue. This is usually accomplished by irrigation with copious amounts of sterile irrigation solution. In heavily contaminated wounds, pulsatile irrigation devices are used to agitate the wound to assist in dislodging and diluting foreign debris. The use of soaps or iodinated solutions has been shown to reduce the bacterial load in contaminated wounds.
- Debridement of traumatised wound edges and tissue. This step is important for removing necrotic or ischaemic tissue, which may become foci for infection if colonised by infective organisms. Careful surgical handling of the tissue is mandatory to prevent extension of tissue injury.
- Stabilisation of fractures. Stability of the fracture is important for protecting the surrounding soft tissue from further injury, which may occur if the sharp fracture ends were allowed to move. The method of stabilisation is important and will depend on the extent of the soft tissue injury (see later section).
- Closure of exposed bone by adequate soft tissue cover. On completion of wound debridement, the soft tissue defect may be closed either by direct suture or tissue grafts. Tissue grafts may be in the form of split-skin grafts or tissue flaps. The decision regarding closure will depend on the degree of contamination and size of the defect.
- Temporary wound closure using vacuum-assisted dressings helps to minimise serous collections within the wound defect, stimulate granulation tissue, maintain a closing tension on the wound to reduce skin edge retraction, and prepares the wound for subsequent primary or graft closure (Figure 50.4).

Classification of open fractures

Open fractures are classified according to the severity of the injury and the modality of injury.

- Type 1: puncture of overlying of skin or mucous membrane by a bony spike from within.
- Type 2: laceration less than 1 cm overlying the fracture.
- Type 3: laceration greater than 1 cm overlying a fracture.
- Type 3A: raising of a soft tissue flap around the fracture.
- Type 3B: absolute skin loss around a fracture.
- Type 3C: deep and highly contaminated wound such as after a farm injury, gunshot injury and fractures associated with neurovascular injury.

(a)

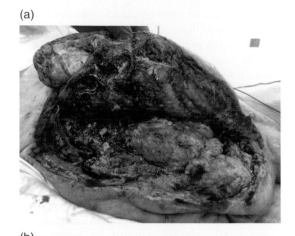

(b)

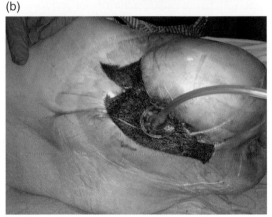

Fig. 50.4 (a) Large pelvic wound after amputation requiring multiple debridements prior to definitive closure. (b) Vacuum-assisted dressing facilitates drainage of serous collections, enhances local vascularity and granulation, and assists wound closure by drawing in wound edges to reduce the size of the actual skin defect through suction.

Surgical considerations of open fractures

- Type 1 and 2 open fractures that can be thoroughly debrided and cleansed with copious amounts of fluid (6 L) may be able to be fixed with internal fixation devices. Such injuries are also treated with prophylactic perioperative antibiotics for 48 hours, such as cefazolin 2 g i.v. 8-hourly.
- Type 3 open fractures are usually fixed with external fixation devices after thorough debridement, cleansing and fracture reduction. Frequently, soft tissue reconstruction is required to provide closure of the wound. Administer cefazolin 2 g i.v. 8-hourly.
- Type 3C injuries are associated with a poor prognosis and amputation may be required in up to 60% of cases. A course of antibiotics is usually prescribed and the selection of antibiotic will

depend on the type of contamination introduced into the wound, for example vancomycin 1 g i.v. 12-hourly (adjusted to pre-administration levels) and ceftriaxone 1 g i.v. 12-hourly.

Fracture immobilisation

Splintage

Minor fractures such as those affecting the phalanges of the fingers may be treated using small metal or plastic splints.

Plaster of Paris cast

Plaster of Paris cast immobilisation is a conventional method of immobilising the fracture following closed reduction. This may be either a completely encircling moulded cast or an incompletely encircling cast (plaster slab).

Traction

Some fractures, particularly those involving the lower limb, may be treated temporarily or definitively by the application of traction along the line of the limb. Traction encourages normal alignment of the fracture and the increased tension of the surrounding soft tissue helps to provide internal splintage of the fracture.

External fixation

External fixation is the application of transfixing pins and bars to create a construct that lies external to the limb and acts to hold the fracture following either open or closed reduction. This method of immobilisation is selected if unstable fractures cannot be held using traditional non-operative techniques. External fixation is also indicated when an open and contaminated fracture is at risk of infection and therefore must be held immobilised by a system which does not introduce into the wound any foreign material such as metal plates and screws.

Internal fixation

Internal fixation is indicated when closed reduction has failed, when further displacement is anticipated, when closed non-operative immobilisation constitutes a risk to the patient, or when internal fixation allows earlier mobilisation, rehabilitation and earlier return to normal function. Internal fixation includes the use of transfixing wires, inter-fragmentary screws, metal plates and intramedullary rods.

Outcome

Fracture union

Fractures treated with closed reduction are said to have united when no mobility occurs at the fracture site. Early union is normally associated with some tenderness on stressing of the fracture, whilst complete union and consolidation is said to be evident when there is no tenderness of the fracture site and stressing does not reproduce symptoms of pain. Radiographic assessment of union is made by observing the development of fracture callus and the gradual disappearance of the fracture line.

Rigid internal fixation with internal fixation devices may reduce the amount of callus formation and because of the rigidity of the fracture immobilisation may make clinical assessment of union difficult. When fractures have been openly reduced and internally fixed, the union is assessed using radiography to demonstrate the disappearance of the fracture line.

Fracture protection

All healing fractures must be protected against re-fracture by gradually permitting stresses along the fractured bone that is commensurate with the strength of that healing bone. In the lower limb, this may be undertaken as a combination of graduated weight bearing of the fractured limb and the use of external supports such as crutches, splints and braces after 6–8 weeks of non-weight bearing. In the upper limb, weighted activity may commence after 4–6 weeks.

Complications

Haemorrhage

Bleeding may occur from laceration of adjacent soft tissue, vascular structures or through fracture ends. Significant amounts of bleeding may occur into soft tissue depending on the bone fracture, for example closed femoral fractures may lose up to 2 L of blood into the thigh, and pelvic fractures up to 4 L into the pelvic cavity.

Infection

Infection is a risk for all open injuries. Adequate prophylactic measures must be taken to prevent infection in the setting of an open fracture or when internal fixation is employed.

Intra-articular extension

Some fractures extend from bone into the joint. Displacement of articular fragments must be treated by anatomical reduction to reduce the risk of post-traumatic arthritis.

Vascular compromise

Excessive bleeding or swelling into the soft tissue may induce a compartment syndrome where excessive pressures within the tissue compartment prevent adequate blood flow to that compartment. Unless this is treated expediently necrosis of soft tissue and subsequent scarring may cause loss of limb function or loss of the limb itself. The signs of a compartment syndrome are dominated by pain that is not responsive to analgesia. Increasing pain following limb surgery mandates an examination to exclude a compartment syndrome. Other signs of limb ischaemia include pallor, paraesthesia, paralysis, poikilothermia and pulselessness.

Late complications

Delayed union

Delayed union occurs when a fracture has not united in a period of time that is at least 25% longer than the expected average time for fracture union at that site. The causes of delayed union include inadequate immobilisation, infection, avascular necrosis of bone, and soft tissue interposition between fracture ends. Delayed union is assessed radiographically.

Non-union

Non-union is said to have occurred when no evidence of union is seen on sequential X-rays over a 6-month period. Non-union is associated clinically with movement or pain at the fracture site. If there is copious callus formation but without bridging of the fracture, a state of hypertrophic non-union is said to exist and requires rigid internal fixation for cure. If there is no evidence of callus formation, then a state of hypotrophic non-union is said to exist and bone grafting and internal fixation is required for treatment.

Malunion

Malunion occurs when the fracture unites with a loss of anatomical alignment. Malunion by shortening may be acceptable but angulation and rotation of the bone following union may not be acceptable and may interfere with normal function.

Rehabilitation

On removal of a plaster cast, the joints adjacent to a fractured limb require rehabilitation to prevent or treat stiffness. This involves passive and active range of motion exercises and proprioception exercises to improve the sense of balance in the recovering joint. In addition, it is important to return the strength and endurance of the muscles in the injured limb by a regime of exercises.

Limbs treated with internal fixation may undergo earlier mobilisation because the fracture is usually more stable than those treated by plaster immobilisation.

Dislocations

Definition

Dislocation is a complete loss of contact between the articular surfaces of the bones forming a joint. Subluxation is displacement of the joint with loss of normal congruity but the articular surfaces remain in partial contact with each other (Figure 50.5).

Clinical presentation

Subluxations and dislocations normally follow direct or indirect trauma. These conditions may also occur voluntarily in patients with ligamentous laxity. Dislocations may also follow an epileptic seizure or electrocution, and the classic injury is a posterior shoulder dislocation. Patients complain of pain, deformity and loss of function. Examination demonstrates loss of normal contour of the joint, marked restriction of movement and pain on attempted passive motion of the joint.

Investigations

Radiography

Plain radiographs are sufficient to demonstrate dislocations and subluxations. Radiography in two planes (anteroposterior and lateral) are essential for confirming the diagnosis. Occasionally, associated fractures may be seen and care should be taken not to displace these fractures in an attempt to reduce the dislocation.

It is wise to obtain plain radiographs of all suspected dislocations to avoid the complication of attempting closed reduction of a fracture or

(a)   (b)

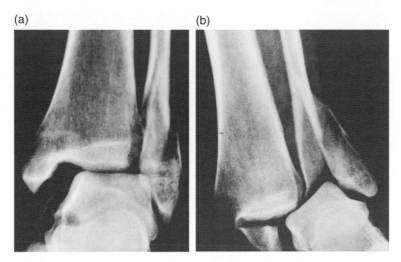

Fig. 50.5 (a) Fracture subluxation of the ankle. (b) Fracture dislocation of the ankle.

unwittingly converting an undisplaced crack into a complete and displaced fracture.

Treatment

The principles of treatment are to reduce the dislocation, immobilise the joint and to rehabilitate the joint.

Closed reduction of the joint under adequate anaesthesia and analgesia is undertaken with the combination of traction, rotation and angulation. At all times forceful manipulation of the joint should be avoided in order to prevent fracture of adjacent bones or neurovascular trauma.

Open reduction is undertaken when closed reduction has failed. This may occur because of the interposition of tissue or the entrapment of the dislocated bone by capsular or ligamentous attachments. Open reduction may also be undertaken if the dislocation is associated with a complex fracture or neurovascular injury that requires exploration and repair.

Chronic dislocations, i.e. joints that have been dislocated for more than 1 week, are usually treated by open reduction because soft tissue scarring and fibrosis within the joint would normally prevent normal reduction.

Immobilisation

Immobilisation of the joint may be performed using a sling or splints. The purpose of immobilisation is to rest the joint to allow capsular and ligamentous healing.

Physiotherapy

Movement of the joint following reduction may be encouraged after an adequate period of time where healing of the soft tissues has occurred. Supervised movement by a physiotherapist is normally encouraged to prevent re-dislocation. The purpose of physiotherapy is to strengthen the periarticular musculature to provide joint stability and also to improve the range of motion that is normally restricted because of capsular scarring. Strengthening exercises of the joint are only encouraged after full range of motion has been achieved.

Complications

- Neurovascular injury
- Joint stiffness
- Recurrent dislocation
- Fracture

Further reading

Strudwick K, McPhee M, Bell A, Martin-Khan M, Russell T. Review article: Best practice management of of neck pain in the emergency department (part 6 of the musculoskeletal injuries rapid review series). *Emerg Med Australas* 2018;30:754–72.

Strudwick K, McPhee M, Bell A, Martin-Khan M, Russell T. Review article: Best practice management of closed hand and wrist injuries in the emergency department (part 5 of the musculoskeletal injuries rapid review series). *Emerg Med Australas* 2018;30:610–40.

Strudwick K, McPhee M, Bell A, Martin-Khan M, Russell T. Review article: Best practice management of common shoulder injuries and conditions in the emergency department (part 4 of the musculoskeletal injuries rapid review series). *Emerg Med Australas* 2018;30:456–85.

Strudwick K, McPhee M, Bell A, Martin-Khan M, Russell T. Review article: Best practice management of common knee injuries in the emergency department (part 3 of the musculoskeletal injuries rapid review series). *Emerg Med Australas* 2018;30:327–52.

Strudwick K, McPhee M, Bell A, Martin-Khan M, Russell T. Review article: Best practice management of common ankle and foot injuries in the emergency department (part 2 of the musculoskeletal injuries rapid review series). *Emerg Med Australas* 2018;30:152–80.

Strudwick K, McPhee M, Bell A, Martin-Khan M, Russell T. Review article: Best practice management of low back pain in the emergency department (part 1 of the musculoskeletal injuries rapid review series). *Emerg Med Australas* 2018;30:18–35.

MCQs

Select the single correct answer to each question. The correct answers can be found in the Answers section at the end of the book.

1 Radiological evidence of an acute fracture includes:
  a loss of continuity in cortical bone
  b osteoporosis
  c sclerosis of bone
  d reduced adjacent soft tissue markings
  e gas in the surrounding muscle

2 In assessing the severity of an acute fracture, one must always:
  a examine for subcutaneous emphysema
  b examine for evidence of gangrene
  c examine the status of the neurovascular system of the fractured part
  d examine for a temperature and arrhythmia
  e examine for evidence of a fat embolism

3 The cardinal feature of a compartment syndrome is:
  a pain
  b hyperthermia
  c rubor
  d punctate ecchymosis
  e limb hyperactivity

4 When a plaster cast is applied for a fractured wrist, care must be taken to instruct the patient on symptoms of:
  a pulmonary embolism
  b fat embolism
  c air embolism
  d compartment syndrome
  e Choong–Baker syndrome

5 Dislocation may be missed in which of the following circumstances?
  a posterior dislocation of the hip
  b posterior dislocation of the shoulder
  c posterior dislocation of the elbow
  d posterior dislocation of the sternoclavicular joint
  e posterior dislocation of the knee

51 Diseases of bone and joints

Peter F. Choong

University of Melbourne and St. Vincent's Hospital, Melbourne, Victoria, Australia

Infections

Acute osteomyelitis

Acute osteomyelitis is an acute bacterial infection of bone. It occurs more commonly in paediatric and geriatric patients, and in those who are immunocompromised. Infection may also follow trauma that is associated with major contamination of bone or joints.

Organism

The commonest organism involved is *Staphylococcus aureus*. Other organisms include *Streptococcus pneumoniae*, *Streptococcus* spp., *Haemophilus influenzae*, Gram-negative organisms and mycobacteria.

Aetiology

Bacteria pass from a distant source (e.g. dental infections, open sores, urinary tract infections) via the bloodstream to the metaphysis of bone (haematogenous spread). Manipulation of infected areas (e.g. tooth extractions, urethral catheterisation) may cause a bacteraemia that can lead to osteomyelitis. Here the entrapped organisms multiply to create an acute inflammatory, then suppurative lesion in metaphyseal bone. Spread of infection from the intramedullary canal through to the cortex may cause a subperiosteal abscess. Involvement of the adjacent joint may cause a suppurative arthritis while spread of the infection across the growth plate in the paediatric age group may cause growth abnormalities (Figure 51.1).

Elevation of the periosteum by the abscess together with intraosseous pressure caused by the metaphyseal abscess may result in a vascular infarction of the involved bone. The necrotic bone is referred to as a *sequestrum*. In time, the elevated periosteum generates new bone that surrounds the sequestrum. The new tube of bone that is formed is referred to as an *involucrum*. A communication from the intramedullary abscess through the skin to form a sinus is referred to as a *cloaca*, which may discharge pus and necrotic debris. The presence of a sequestrum, involucrum and cloaca is referred to as chronic osteomyelitis.

Clinical presentation

There is often a history of minor trauma to the affected part. Trauma may give rise to a haematoma which then forms a locus of decreased resistance to infection (locus minoris resistentia). Several days later the patient presents with a painful and swollen limb where pressure over the infected area elicits marked tenderness. Children may be reluctant to use the affected limb. With progression of infection the patient becomes constitutionally unwell (fever, rigors, sweat, nausea, vomiting, anorexia). Fluctuance denotes the development of a subperiosteal abscess.

Investigations

Blood tests

Full blood examination reveals elevated white cell count, left shift, increased band forms, and elevated erythrocyte sedimentation rate (ESR) and C-reactive protein (CRP).

Blood cultures

Blood should be taken for aerobic and anaerobic cultures on diagnosis (two sets of cultures 1 hour apart) and at times of high fevers (>38.5°C). Blood cultures should be obtained prior to the commencement of antibiotic therapy.

Textbook of Surgery, Fourth Edition. Edited by Julian A. Smith, Andrew H. Kaye, Christopher Christophi and Wendy A. Brown.
© 2020 John Wiley & Sons Ltd. Published 2020 by John Wiley & Sons Ltd.

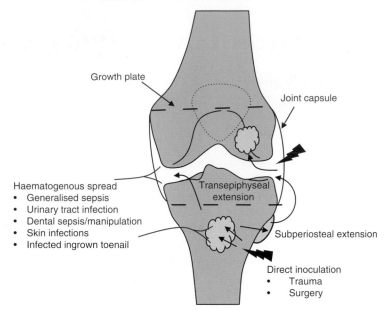

Fig. 51.1 Mechanisms of entry of infective organisms into bone and joints.

In the figure:
- Growth plate
- Joint capsule
- Haematogenous spread
  - Generalised sepsis
  - Urinary tract infection
  - Dental sepsis/manipulation
  - Skin infections
  - Infected ingrown toenail
- Transepiphyseal extension
- Subperiosteal extension
- Direct inoculation
  - Trauma
  - Surgery

Radiography

Radiographs early in disease commonly demonstrate soft tissue swelling or an associated joint effusion but no bone changes. After 10–14 days, radiographic changes include periosteal new bone formation, which signifies elevation or inflammation of the periosteum by oedema or infective material and regional osteopenia.

Bone scans

Infections induce a marked inflammatory response with hyperaemia of bone and increased bone turnover. Nuclear bone scans, using technetium-99 methylene diphosphonate (^{99m}Tc-MDP) or gallium-67, demonstrate increased tracer uptake at the affected site (hot scan). Indium white cell scans demonstrate acute white cell collections (abscess).

Magnetic resonance imaging

MRI is a very sensitive test for inflammation and bony oedema. Marked marrow and soft tissue changes on TI- and T2-weighted films can be expected. The sensitivity of MRI sometimes confounds the interpretation of marked bone and soft tissue oedema, where bone oedema arising as a sympathetic response to overlying cellulitis may be interpreted as osteomyelitis.

Differential diagnosis

Important differential diagnoses for a painful swollen bone include:
- primary bone tumour, e.g. osteosarcoma, Ewing's sarcoma
- secondary bone tumour, e.g. breast, lung, prostate
- haematological malignancy, e.g. lymphoma, myeloma
- fracture, e.g. stress fracture.

Treatment

Antibiotic therapy

Intravenous antibiotics are initiated after blood cultures have been taken (flucloxacillin 2 g i.v. 4-hourly and cefazalin 2 g i.v. 8-hourly) and continued until the organism(s) has been identified and antibiotic sensitivities known. There is usually a rapid response to the initiation of antibiotics with an improvement in constitutional symptoms and signs.

Immobilisation

The affected limb should be immobilised and elevated to reduce oedema and pain.

Analgesia

Combination of oral and intramuscular analgesia may be required.

Surgery

Surgery is indicated if:
- there is evidence of a subperiosteal or soft tissue abscess
- the patient's condition deteriorates despite adequate antibiotics therapy, and there is radiological evidence of an intramedullary collection.

Outcome

Modern antibiotic therapy is associated with good and often complete resolution of infection. Occasionally a remnant nidus of infection will cause repeated flare-ups for which repeated courses of antibiotic therapy will be necessary. If a sequestrum develops and is colonised, a state of chronic osteomyelitis may develop.

Acute septic arthritis

This is an acute bacterial infection of a joint. It is commonly monoarticular but may occasionally affect several joints concurrently.

Organism

The commonest organism involved is *Staphylococcus aureus*. Other organisms include *Haemophilus* and *Neisseria* species.

Aetiology

Septic arthritis may arise from haematogenous spread, direct inoculation, transepiphyseal spread of osteomyelitis or direct spread from a subperiosteal collection of pus (see Figure 51.1).

Clinical presentation

The patient is often febrile and toxic. Any movement of the joint causes extreme pain. In the elderly, symptoms may be less dramatic than in younger patients and the diagnosis may be missed. The elderly are also prone to multifocal infections, with several joints being affected at the same time. The joint is swollen, tender and warm. The joint need not be erythematous. An antecedent history of trauma to the limb may exist, or acute septic arthritis may follow as a complication of a local skin or bone infection. Examination of the cardiac valves is necessary to ensure that these are not the source of infections (bacterial endocarditis) or a consequence of septic arthritis.

Investigations

Blood tests
Full blood examination shows elevated white cell count, left shift, increased band forms, and elevated ESR and CRP.

Blood cultures
Blood should be taken for aerobic and anaerobic cultures on diagnosis (two sets of cultures 1 hour apart) and at times of high fevers (38.5°C). Blood cultures should be obtained prior to the commencement of antibiotic therapy.

Radiography
Radiographs early in disease commonly demonstrate soft tissue swelling or an associated joint effusion with elevation of the extra-articular fat pad. There are usually no bone changes.

Bone scans
Infections induce a marked inflammatory response with hyperaemia of bone and increased bone turnover. Nuclear bone scans (e.g. ^{99m}Tc-MDP, gallium-67) demonstrate increased tracer uptake at the affected site (hot scan). Indium white cell scans demonstrate acute white cell collection (abscess).

Ultrasound
Joints that are difficult to palpate (e.g. shoulder, hip) may be examined with ultrasound scans.

Joint aspiration
An experienced doctor should perform a joint aspiration under sterile conditions with a large-bore needle and the fluid should be submitted for microbiological examination, culture and antibiotic sensitivities. Ultrasound or CT guidance can be valuable.

Differential diagnoses

Important differential diagnoses for an acutely swollen and painful joint include:
- gout
- haemarthrosis, e.g. post-traumatic, haemophilic, coagulopathic
- trauma, e.g. osteochondral injury or fracture, intra-articular ligament injury
- inflammatory arthritis
- degenerative arthritis.

Treatment

Surgery
Arthrotomy, irrigation and drainage of the joint.

Antibiotic therapy
Antibiotics are instituted following blood cultures and culture of joint fluid (flucloxacillin 2 g i.v. 4-hourly and ampicillin 1 g i.v. 6-hourly) until an organism is identified and sensitivities known.

Immobilisation
The limb should be immobilised in a splint and elevated until symptoms resolve.

Physiotherapy

Gradual physiotherapy should be prescribed after symptoms resolve to regain joint motion.

Outcome

Early and adequate treatment is important to prevent cartilage destruction (chondrolysis) that may lead to stiffness and arthritis.

Chronic infective arthritis

Chronic infective arthritis is uncommon and is usually seen following *Mycobacterium tuberculosis* infections.

Pathology

Joint infection usually follows seeding from a distant site such as the lung or kidneys. In addition, chronic tuberculosis osteomyelitis may also extend from the metaphysis or epiphysis into the articular cavity.

Clinical presentation

Pain in the joint is variable and may be extreme or slight. Typically, this is most severe at night when the patient relaxes and joint movement during sleep causes severe attacks of pain (night cries). Constitutionally, the patient is unwell with fever, lassitude and loss of weight.

Affected joints are swollen with a doughy synovial thickening, effusion and gross muscle wasting. There is restriction and pain with movement, but this is not as severe as in acute suppurative arthritis. There may be joint sinuses and marked stiffness (fibrous or bony ankylosis).

Investigations

Blood tests

Full blood examination demonstrates an elevated lymphocyte count, elevated ESR and anaemia of chronic infection.

Mantoux test

Mantoux test is positive; however, in overwhelming disease there may be no reaction.

Joint aspiration and culture

Joint aspiration and culture may demonstrate acid-fast bacilli. More recent tests using polymerase chain reaction (PCR) techniques can demonstrate the characteristic DNA pattern of mycobacteria.

Treatment

- Arthrotomy, irrigation and drainage of the joint if the infection is in its acute phase.
- Immobilisation of the limb until the disease is quiescent.
- Commence anti-tuberculous medication following joint and tissue culture.
- Commence physiotherapy after the disease has become quiescent.

Outcome

Anti-tuberculous therapy is usually successful in controlling or eradicating the infection. However, complications include:

- stiffness from intra-articular fibrosis
- deformity from destruction of the growth plate
- degenerative arthritis from cartilage destruction
- osteomyelitis from local spread
- haematogenous dissemination.

Arthritides

Degenerative arthritis

Degenerative arthritis is one of the commonest conditions in orthopaedics and a major cause of life years lost through disability. The commonest joints involved include the hip, knee, shoulder and lumbar spine. Other joints less commonly involved include the carpometacarpal joint, elbow and ankle. Degenerative arthritis is a progressive condition that is initiated by an acute or chronic repetitive insult.

Causes

- Idiopathic
- Trauma
- Infection
- Inflammation
- Metabolic, e.g. gout, pseudogout
- Avascular necrosis, e.g. steroid induced, osteochondritis dissecans

Clinical presentation

Pain

Pain typically occurs with movement or with weight bearing (mechanical pain). This may radiate to involve the whole limb if it is advanced. Referred pain is common, for example knee pain in severe hip arthritis.

Stiffness

Patients note a restricted range of motion, develop a limp and are unable to function normally, such as to run, climb stairs or twist their leg to put their shoes on.

Deformity

With progressive loss of motion and the development of contractures the patient loses symmetry of the joints. This results in an abnormal gait or posture (Figure 51.2).

Investigations

Radiography

The four main radiological features of arthritis include loss of joint space, subchondral sclerosis, osteophyte formation and cyst formation (Figure 51.3).

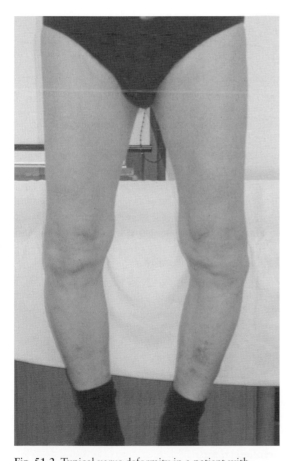

Fig. 51.2 Typical varus deformity in a patient with osteoarthritis of the knees where that part of the limb distal to the joint is deviated towards the midline. This contrasts with the knees of a patient with rheumatoid arthritis where that part of the limb distal to the joint is deviated away from the midline (valgus).

Treatment

Non-operative

This usually consists of pain relief with oral analgesics and anti-inflammatory medication. The use of a walking aid such as a walking stick for lower limb arthritis and splints for upper limb arthritis may also be helpful. Physiotherapy to maintain range of motion and to prevent further loss is valuable. A mobile arthritic joint is better than a stiff arthritic joint.

Operative

- Prosthetic joint replacement: this is usually recommended in the advanced stages of arthritis when the severity of symptoms of functional loss has reduced the quality of life to an intolerable state. The commonest sites of arthritis requiring joint replacement are the hip, knee, shoulder and elbows. It is a very successful procedure, with the survival of joint replacements approaching 95% at 15 years from initial surgery.
- Osteotomy: this is the division of bone and may be used to correct the deformity of arthritis and realign the limb biomechanically to allow passage of forces through less-affected parts of the joints, thus reducing the pressure across the arthritic part of the joint. Osteotomy has an important role in managing knee arthritis and may provide the patient with many years of pain relief before joint replacement, which in many cases is inevitable. Osteotomy is also used with good success for the management of hallux valgus.
- Arthrodesis: this is the surgical fusion of a joint, which is usually undertaken in the smaller joints of the feet or hands or in very young patients. Fusion results in permanent loss of motion but a successful fusion can also result in complete pain relief because the arthritic joint is no longer mobile.

Outcome

Arthritis is a progressive disease characterised by remissions and relapses. Non-operative treatment may slow the rapidity of symptoms. Whilst X-rays demonstrate the extent of arthritis, symptoms may not always correlate with the severity of radiological features.

Inflammatory arthritis

This is a spectrum of seropositive and seronegative arthritides characterised by acute and subacute chronic and relapsing joint inflammation. Joint

(a) (b)

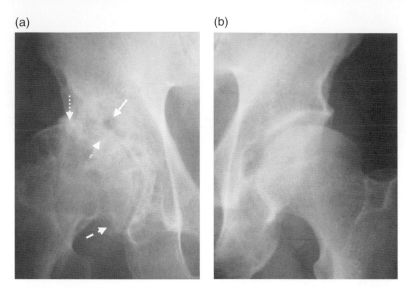

Fig. 51.3 The radiological features of (a) osteoarthritis include joint space narrowing (dotted arrow), subchondral cyst formation (solid arrow), osteophyte formation (dashed arrow) and subchondral sclerosis (double body arrow). Compare this with (b) a normal joint.

involvement is part of a clinical picture that may manifest in multiple large and small joints at the same time or be limited to only one or a few joints. Inflammatory arthritis may also affect bones, tendons and other organs.

Pathology

The cause of inflammatory joint disease is thought to be an autoimmune process beginning with a synovitis that causes articular cartilage destruction, disruption of the joint capsule and a proliferative synovitis.

Types

- Rheumatoid arthritis (seropositive)
- Psoriatic arthritis (seropositive and seronegative varieties)
- Ankylosing spondylitis (seronegative)
- Reiter's disease (seronegative)
- Inflammatory bowel disease (seronegative)
- Behçet's disease (seronegative)

Presentation

Typically, patients complain of stiffness, pain and joint swelling. Characteristic exacerbations and remissions are noted, and constitutional symptoms may be present, with acute joint involvement.

Patients with rheumatoid arthritis may present with bilateral symmetric involvement of the small joints of hand, wrist and feet, and triggering of tendons. Eventually involvement of the hips, knees, shoulders and ankles are noted. Valgus deformities of the knee or a 'windswept' appearance with varus deformity of one knee and valgus of the other are typical. Ulnar deviation and swan-neck and boutonniere deformities of the fingers are characteristic.

Patients with seronegative arthritis usually present with monoarticular arthritis involving the large joints such as the knee and hip, although small joint involvement of the hand with nail changes are also seen in psoriatic arthritis. These patients also present with low back pain. Progressive vertebral stiffness, kyphosis and sacroiliitis are typical of advancing ankylosing spondylitis. Visceral involvement of the heart, lungs, liver, spleen, bowel and eyes may occur.

Investigations

Blood tests
Full blood examination reveals elevated white cell count and elevated ESR.

Serological tests
- Rheumatoid factor
- Anti-nuclear antibody
- Anti-double-stranded DNA antibody
- HLA-B27

Radiography
- Seropositive disease: radiographs demonstrate soft tissue swelling, osteopenia, joint erosions or narrowing, and symmetric bilateral joint deformity of the hands and feet.
- Seronegative disease: monoarticular involvement, sacroiliitis, syndesmophytes, bamboo spine, enthesopathy, and ossification of the capsular margins.

Bone scans
Generalised uptake around joint. Increased uptake in arterial phase demonstrating active synovitis. Bone scans are useful for identifying stress fractures from associated or steroid-induced osteoporosis.

Treatment

- Rest and immobilisation of affected joints.
- Analgesia, anti-inflammatory medication and corticosteroids.
- Disease-modifying medication such as methotrexate, penicillamine and gold.
- Splints or braces to prevent or correct deformities.
- Surgery to correct deformities or joint destruction (osteotomy, arthrodesis, joint replacement).
- Synovectomy is the removal of inflamed synovium. This is usually indicated in early disease and may be performed by open surgery, arthroscopy, or radiotherapy with intra-arterial instillation of a radioisotope.

Metabolic conditions of bones

Rickets

Rickets is an uncommon condition of the immature skeleton characterised by poor mineralisation of osteoid. It is caused by a dietary lack of calcium and vitamin D or a lack of exposure to sunlight. It is usually seen in malnourished patients such as those in developing countries. Rickets may also be seen in malabsorption syndromes.

Presentation

Joint tenderness, swelling and deformity. Bones typically involved include the tibia (genu varum) and ribs (rickety rosary).

X-rays

Gradual deformation of long bones is seen. In addition, there is expansion and loss of cortical definition of the metaphyseal region of bone. The costochondral junctions may be expanded (rickety rosary).

Treatment

- Correction of malabsorption syndromes
- Supplementation of vitamin D and calcium.
- Surgical correction of long-standing bone deformity

Osteomalacia

This is a condition of the adult skeleton characterised by inadequate bone mineralisation. The main causes of this include vitamin D deficiency, vitamin D resistance (renal failure), impaired vitamin D synthesis (liver failure, renal failure) and other metabolic disturbances.

Presentation

Patients present with pathological fractures or radiological evidence of bone loss (Looser's zones), and muscle aches and pains. There is no growth abnormality because osteomalacia is a condition of the mature skeleton.

Investigations

Blood tests
- Elevated serum alkaline phosphatase
- Reduced serum calcium
- Reduced serum vitamin D

Radiography
- Looser's zones in areas of stress, e.g. pubic rami, femoral neck
- General osteopenia

Bone biopsy
Bone biopsy shows deficient mineralisation with widened unossified seams of osteoid.

Treatment

- Correction of metabolic irregularity
- Supplement calcium and vitamin D
- Fixation of fractures if appropriate

Hormonal conditions of bones

Hyperthyroidism (see Chapter 37)

A reduction of thyroid hormone produces growth abnormalities in infant and paediatric patients.

There is stunted growth, a delay in walking and cretinism. The late appearance of secondary ossification centres suggests hypothyroidism. Early treatment with thyroid hormone supplementation is important to prevent mental retardation.

Hyperparathyroidism (see Chapter 38)

Hyperparathyroidism is due to increased secretion of parathyroid hormone. This may be caused by hypersecretion by a parathyroid adenoma or a secondary response to chronic renal failure. Increasing the secretion of parathyroid hormone raises serum calcium through bone resorption. Bone resorption results in a bone-softening condition wherein pathological fractures are frequent.

Clinical picture

Nausea, vomiting, weight loss, abdominal pain, bone pain and muscular weakness.

Investigations

Radiography

There is a generalised reduction in bone density. Late in the disease bone resorption manifests as bone cysts. Mottling of the skull and subperiosteal erosions of the phalanges are commonly seen. Other manifestations of hypercalcaemia such as renal calculi or heterotopic calcification are seen.

Blood tests
- Elevated serum calcium
- Decreased serum phosphate
- Elevated urinary phosphate
- Elevated parathyroid hormone

Treatment
- Correction of metabolic irregularity
- Surgical removal of adenoma or partial removal of the parathyroid glands

Congenital/developmental conditions

Osteogenesis imperfecta

Osteogenesis imperfecta is an extremely rare condition characterised by bone fragility.

Pathology

This is an inherited condition, and results from an abnormality in the metabolism of type 1 collagen.

The fragility leads to bone deformity and/or fractures and soft tissue abnormalities.

Classification

Type	Inheritance	Clinical features
I	Autosomal dominant	Childhood fractures, hearing loss, blue sclera ± opalescent teeth, commonest
II	Autosomal recessive	Lethal, multiple fractures, flattened vertebrae, blue sclera, very rare
III	Autosomal recessive	Birth fractures and progressive deformity; short stature, ± opalescent teeth; white sclera, spinal deformity and costovertebral anomalies
IV	Autosomal dominant	Skeletal fragility, no hearing loss, moderate growth failure, white sclera, may have opalescent teeth

Presentation

Patients with the severe form of osteogenesis imperfecta die at or soon after birth with multiple fractures. Patients who survive at birth may present as an abnormality of development with a typical globular-shaped head, frontal bossing, stunted growth, kyphoscoliosis and hypermobility of joints. There is commonly a history of multiple fractures following minimal trauma. If presentation occurs during adolescence, normal skeletal development is seen and fracture incidence declines with increasing maturity. Fracture healing is normal but remodelling is abnormal, giving rise to bone deformities. Many survivors have blue sclera, which is due to the abnormally thin and translucent sclera highlighting the dark choroid behind it.

Radiography

Radiographs show multiple healing or old fractures, bone deformities, ribbon-shaped ribs and Wormian bones in the skull and a trefoil pelvis.

Pathology

The condition is characterised by marked cortical thinning and attenuation of trabeculae. There may be persistence of hypercellular woven bone.

Treatment

Patients require protection from injury particularly when young. Treatment is aimed at correcting limb deformities by multiple osteotomies and a transfixing pin or rod. Fracture healing is excellent.

Dyschondroplasia

Also known as Ollier's disease, or multiple enchondromata, dyschondroplasia is characterised by the development during youth of multiple asymmetric intraosseous cartilage masses.

Pathology

There is an abnormality of metaphyseal bone organisation. Although metaphyseal growth ceases after puberty, enchondromata may continue to grow.

Clinical presentation

Patients present with metaphyseal swelling that may be particularly severe in the fingers. This may affect joint function and the length of the bone. Limb length discrepancies are not unusual.

Investigations

Radiography
Radiographs show areas of lucency with central calcific stippling and endosteal scalloping. Shortening, angulation and expansion of bone can be seen.

Bone scans
Increased ^{99m}Tc-MDP uptake in the lesions implies ongoing growth and remodelling of surrounding bone. Activity in the lesions itself can be demonstrated by avidity for thallium or pentavalent dimercaptosuccinic acid (DMSA).

Treatment

Troublesome lesions may be excised or curetted. The prognosis is good. Rarely, transformation to low-grade chondrosarcoma may occur. This should be suspected in lesions that show a recent increase in size and pain, and radiographs that demonstrate lysis, expansion/remodelling of bone, endosteal erosion and cortical breach. Wide resection is recommended.

Outcome

A normal life expectancy is usual.

Hereditary diaphyseal aclasis

Also known as multiple cartilaginous exostoses, hereditary diaphyseal aclasis is a skeletal condition that usually presents in childhood and affects the growing ends of long bones. Occasionally, ribs, vertebrae and the pelvis may also be involved.

Pathology

There is an aberration in physeal regulation with the development of cortical exostoses at the growing end of bones with a cartilage cap of varying thickness. This is an autosomal dominant condition in which abnormalities of chromosomes 18, 11 and 19 have been identified.

Clinical presentation

Patients present with problems of:
- impingement
- deformity
- limb length discrepancy
- malignant transformation to chondrosarcoma.

Investigations

Radiography
Exostoses are sessile or pedunculated. Trabecular bone of the diaphysis is confluent with that of the exostosis and the cortex of the osteochondroma is continuous with that of the bone from which it arises.

Bone scans
Increased ^{99m}Tc-MDP uptake in the lesions implies ongoing growth and remodelling of surrounding bone. Activity in the lesions itself can be demonstrated by avidity for thallium or DMSA.

Computed tomography
CT scans are excellent for demonstrating cortical erosion, endosteal scalloping and the large cartilage cap.

Magnetic resonance imaging
MRI is excellent for demonstrating the soft tissue component, intramedullary changes and the thickness of the cartilage cap (if >1 cm, suspect malignancy).

Treatment

Simple excision of the lesion at its base should suffice. Occasionally, correction of angular deformities is required. Malignant transformation is uncommon but when it occurs transformation to a low-grade chondrosarcoma is noted. Like the sarcomatous transformation noted in dyschondroplasia, removal of the tumour requires wide resection.

Outcome

A normal life expectancy is usual.

Achondroplasia

This is an autosomal dominant condition characterised by abnormalities in limb length in the presence of a normal-sized trunk and an enlarged head. It is the most common skeletal dysplasia.

Pathology

It is a hereditary defect of cartilage modelling, caused by a mutation in the gene for fibroblast growth factor receptor protein. Normal chondral calcification does not occur. Periosteal bone formation is normal. This causes thickening of bone but not lengthening of bone. Membranous bones are not affected.

Clinical presentation

The classic achondroplastic dwarf has short limbs, a normal trunk, a large head with frontal bossing and a flattened root of the nose. Patients develop the typical bow-legged appearance and an increase in lumbar lordosis. Lumbar canal stenosis is common because of short pedicles and the increased lordosis.

Radiography

Radiographs show short tubular bones with wide metaphyses.

Treatment

Corrective osteotomies may be required for abnormality in joint alignment, and limb-lengthening surgery may be useful for increasing height and reach. Limb bowing may lead to degenerative knee arthritis where osteotomy or joint replacement may be required. Canal stenosis may be severe enough to cause significant nerve root impingement symptoms that may require surgical decompression.

Outcome

A normal life expectancy is usual.

Bone conditions of unknown origin

Paget's disease

Paget's disease is a condition of adults in middle age and onwards. It is a deforming condition characterised by disorganised bone formation and bone resorption. Two stages exist, an acute hyperaemic and bone-softening phase and a chronic brittle phase.

Pathology

It is thought to be of viral origin, as viral inclusion bodies have been noted within osteoclasts from affected bones.

Presentation

Patients may complain of a painless deformity of a long bone such as the femur and tibia. Alternately, patients may also complain of pain, which is usually dull and constant and not related to activity. Pain may be due to Paget's disease, stress fractures or malignant change. Common bones to be involved include the skull, pelvis, femur, tibia and single vertebrae. Patients may also develop symptoms of nerve compression, pathological/stress fractures, and high-output failure from the regional hyperaemia which may act like an arteriovenous shunt.

Investigations

Blood tests
Elevated serum alkaline phosphatase.

Urinary tests
Elevated urinary calcium and hydroxyproline excretion.

Bone biopsy
Biopsy demonstrates abundant disorganised woven bone with abnormal cement lines and abnormal-shaped lamelli, so-called crazy pavement.

Radiography
Radiographs show coarse trabeculae, thickened cortices, flame-shaped lysis, stress fractures, bone deformity, enlarged bone and malignant change.

Bone scans
Bone scans show markedly increased uptake of radioactive tracer in active Paget's disease.

Treatment

- Pain relief: oral analgesia, non-steroidal anti-inflammatory drugs
- Anti-osteoclastic drugs: bisphosphonate, calcitonin
- Surgery: joint replacement, correction of deformity

Outcome

Paget's may become burnt out with established deformities and hard, brittle and pain-free bone. Fractures through this bone are not uncommon because of their brittle nature. Abnormality in bone architecture may predispose to arthritis. Sometimes, differentiation between the pain of Paget's disease and arthritis may be difficult. Rarely malignant transformation may occur, which carries a very poor prognosis.

Osteoporosis

Osteoporosis is an absolute loss of bone mass with an increase in fracture risk.

Pathology

There is normal mineralisation of osteoid, but the absolute amount of bone is decreased. Osteoporosis may be associated with calcium deficiency, secondary hyperparathyroidism, excess alcohol intake, immobilisation, steroid use and malignancy.

Clinical presentation

Osteoporosis has an insidious onset characterised by a gradual loss of height with increasing age, the development of kyphoscoliosis and a predisposition to fracture after minor trauma or falls. Specific areas prone to fracture include vertebrae, the pelvis and radius. Stress fractures of the tibia and pelvis are common.

Investigations

Blood tests
Primary osteoporosis has a normal blood profile. If associated with other causes, blood derangements may be typical of those other conditions.

Radiography
Lumbar vertebrae are bioconcave with herniation of the disc into and through the endplate of the vertebrae (fish-shaped). There may be osteoporotic wedge fractures of the vertebrae. Stress fractures may be seen in the pubic rami, sacrum, medial tibia and sometimes the distal tibia. The shafts of bone may look washed out with a pencilled-in cortex.

Bone mineral density scans
Bone mineral density scans show low mineralised bone content. Results are compared to age- and sex-matched control data to determine the risk of fracture.

Bone biopsy
Bone biopsy may be required if the diagnosis and cause for apparent bone loss is unclear. Tetracycline labelling protocol is required to determine the rate and amount of bone formation within a given time.

Treatment

- Correction of metabolic deficiencies
- Correction of the underlying medical condition
- Reduction of bone resorption (bisphosphonates)
- Oestrogen supplementation
- Vitamin D supplementation

Fibrous dysplasia

This is a deforming condition of bone that may begin in young adulthood. It is characterised by abnormal development of cysts and fibrotic areas within bone associated with gradual deformation. When associated with McCune–Albright syndrome, fibrous dysplasia is associated with precocious puberty, hormonal dysfunction and pituitary abnormalities.

Presentation

The patient may complain of pain or the condition may be an incidental finding on X-ray.

Investigations

Radiography
Radiographs demonstrate thickened bone, with lytic areas containing matrix with a typical ground-glass appearance. Bone deformities include 'shepherd's crook' abnormality of the proximal femur, thickened cortices and expanded diaphysis.

Biopsy
Biopsy demonstrates normal trabeculae of bone broken up into tiny islands of bone by fibrous stroma and bland cells giving a 'Chinese character' type appearance.

Outcome

There may be gradual deformity in a weight-bearing bone. Pathological fractures may also occur. Malignant change occurs rarely.

Conditions of joints

Charcot's disease

Charcot's disease is the consequence of conditions that result in denervation or loss of proprioceptive sense, predisposing to bone and joint destruction (neuropathic joint).

Pathology

Repeated trauma leads to fracture, poor healing and joint derangement. Predisposing causes include diabetes, alcoholism, syringomyelia, syphilis and trauma.

Presentation

Patients present with painless, deformed and swollen joints. The ankle and knee are the most commonly affected joints. Syringomyclia should be suspected with Charcot's disease of the shoulder. Patients may also present with the complications of deformed joints (e.g. chronic non-healing ulcers overlying bone prominences).

Radiography

Typical radiographic signs include dense bone, destruction of joint, para-articular bone debris, and deformity.

Treatment

Bracing
Deranged joints may be stabilised with external braces or splints. The purpose of this is to prevent further deformity rather than to correct it, which is usually permanent.

Surgery
Surgery to correct the deformity or to arthrodese the joint is usually met by failure. Amputation is considered if the joint becomes useless and is an impediment to limb function or is complicated by persistent infection.

Gout

Gout is an abnormality of purine metabolism characterised by excess production of uric acid or a reduction in the excretion of uric acid. Deposition of urate crystals and the subsequent inflammatory response elicits painful joint symptoms and other visceral complications. Pseudogout is a replica of gout, but the crystals are rhomboid and positively birefringent and the major abnormality is that of high levels of calcium pyrophosphate in the joint.

Clinical features

Patients present with acutely painful swollen and tender joints. If severe, there may be constitutional symptoms. Joint symptoms can be mistaken for septic arthritis. Typically, the metatarsophalangeal joint of the big toe is affected. In chronic gout, deposits of urate crystals in the soft tissue (tophi) are common and these can be seen on the ear and on the phalangeal joints of the fingers and toes. Other associated conditions include cardiac disease, hypertension and renal failure.

Investigations

Radiography
Radiographs may show peri-articular erosions, joint deformities and soft tissue calcifications.

Blood tests
Elevated serum uric acid. This may be normal in 30% of patients. The white cell count is elevated, in addition to elevated ESR and CRP.

Joint aspiration
Joint aspirations should be performed under sterile conditions and fluid submitted for biochemical and microbiological examination including culture. Typically, negatively birefringent needle-shaped crystals are noted.

Treatment

- Rest immobilisation and elevation of joint
- Oral and intramuscular analgesia
- Anti-inflammatory medication
- Colchicine
- Allopurinol
- Dietary control

Outcome

Patients with gout often have recurring attacks. Uncontrolled gout may lead to joint destruction and renal tubular failure.

Pigmented villonodular synovitis

This is a rare condition characterised by localised nodular or papillary overgrowth and inflammation of the synovium. This may cause bone erosions, subchondral cysts and large soft tissue masses. There is controversy as to whether this is an inflammatory or true neoplastic process.

Clinical presentation

Patients may present with a range of symptoms including recurrent joint swelling and pain, soft tissue masses and osteoarthritis.

Investigations

Radiography
Radiographs show generalised joint narrowing if the diffuse form of the disease is present. Typically, subchondral cyst are large and situated at a distance from the joint.

Magnetic resonance imaging
MRI demonstrates an articular soft tissue haemosiderin-laden carpet of synovium, or a well-circumscribed mass. Synovitis is well demonstrated by this scan.

Treatment

- Synovectomy
- Radiation synovectomy with intra-articular isotopes
- Joint replacement

Synovial chondromatosis

This is a metaplastic condition of the synovium resulting in the formation of numerous intra-articular cartilaginous loose bodies.

Clinical presentation

These may cause painful catching or locking or osteoarthritis of the joint.

Investigation

Radiography
Radiographs demonstrate intra-articular loose bodies if they are calcified. If the loose bodies remain cartilaginous, they may not be detectable on radiographs.

Magnetic resonance imaging
MRI demonstrates cartilage very well and is excellent for detecting intra-articular loose bodies.

Treatment

- Synovectomy
- Removal of loose body
- Joint replacement in severe disease with associated articular degeneration

Osteochondritis dissecans

Osteochondritis dissecans is a condition of adolescence and young adulthood that is characterised by local avascular necrosis of epiphyseal bone causing fracture and/or separation of an osteoarticular fragment.

Clinical presentation

The commonest joints involved are the knee, elbow and ankle. It presents initially with pain on weight bearing activity. Repeated joint effusions or clicking or locking of the joint may be noted.

Investigations

Radiography
Early in the condition this may be normal. Late in the condition a defect of bone may be seen and a loose fragment may be noted. Typical areas include the lateral side of the medial femoral condyle, superomedial corner of the dome of the talus, the head of the second metatarsal and the capitellar surface.

Bone scans
Bone scans may show increased focal activity.

Computed tomography
CT scans are excellent for demonstrating a subchondral fracture.

Magnetic resonance imaging
MRI is excellent for demonstrating lesions that are not visible on radiography or CT scans. MRI can detect oedema and inflammation surrounding the area of necrosis.

Treatment

- Acute pain may be treated by rest, partial weight bearing and use of crutches.

- Arthroscopy and drilling of the fragment may assist and encourage a new blood supply and thus healing of the fragment.
- Open reduction internal fixation is indicated if the osteochondral fragment is large.
- *Ex vivo* autogenous chondrocyte culture and reimplantation is a new and exciting technique for treating this condition.

Outcome

Lesions that remain attached usually proceed to heal. Detached lesions may heal after internal fixation, but if too small may simply be discarded. The residual defect does not heal normally and may predispose to osteoarthritis if it is large and on the weight-bearing surface of bone.

Orthopaedic malignancies

Malignant primary tumours of bone

Sarcomas are primary malignancies of bone and soft tissue. The cells of origin arise from mesenchymal and neuroectodermal tissue. Two peak incidences exist (<20 years and >55 years). Males are more commonly affected. The commonest site for bone sarcomas is the lower limb, particularly around the knee.

Clinical presentation

Sarcomas present with a mass. Bone sarcomas are painful; characteristically, the pain is constant, unremitting, nocturnal and responds poorly to oral analgesia. It is important to note that bone pain that is unremitting and not responsive to simple analgesia should raise suspicions of a tumour.

The most frequent bone sarcomas are osteosarcoma, Ewing's sarcoma and chondrosarcoma.

Investigation

All investigations must be completed prior to biopsy because biopsy can produce imaging artefacts that may confound the final histological definition. Inappropriate biopsy site or procedure may jeopardise limb-sparing surgery.

Radiography

All suspected bone tumours should be radiographed. Typical patterns are recognised for most tumours.

Computed tomography

CT scans provide excellent imaging of cortical and trabecular destruction. Pulmonary scans are mandatory for determining systemic spread.

Magnetic resonance imaging

MRI provides excellent multiplanar imaging with unsurpassed soft tissue contrast. MRI is important for determining the site, size, shape, consistency and vascularity of a tumour, and the relationship of adjacent structures. This modality is extremely important for assessing surgical margins.

Nuclear scans

^{99m}Tc-MDP bone scans are excellent for demonstrating multicentric bone involvement. Such scans are also important for determining response to treatment. More recently, functional nuclear scans (e.g. thallium, positron emission tomography) allow an assessment of tumour activity (Figure 51.4).

Biopsy

Biopsy is important for confirming the diagnosis and for determining histological subtype. Biopsy may be performed percutaneously with fine- or wide-bore needles, or through a formal incision. More invasive methods carry a higher risk of complications and contamination of tissue planes. Each year 30% of limbs are lost through inappropriate biopsy site and technique. In principle, biopsies should be performed at a tumour centre by a musculoskeletal specialist in tumour surgery.

Treatment

Chemotherapy

All osteosarcomas and Ewing's sarcomas are treated with protocols of preoperative chemotherapy unless the patient's renal or cardiac function prohibits the use of chemotherapy. Chondrosarcoma is resistant to chemotherapy.

Radiotherapy

Radiotherapy is usually indicated for soft tissue sarcomas and is also combined with chemotherapy in certain cases of Ewing's sarcoma. This may be provided preoperatively or postoperatively. The benefit of preoperative radiotherapy is the smaller target of irradiation. Postoperative radiotherapy requires targeting of the entire operative field. The complications of preoperative versus postoperative radiotherapy are comparable.

Surgery

Surgical margins may be classified as intralesional (tumour capsule is transgressed), marginal

(a)　　　　　　　(b)　　　　　　　(c)　　　　　　　(d)

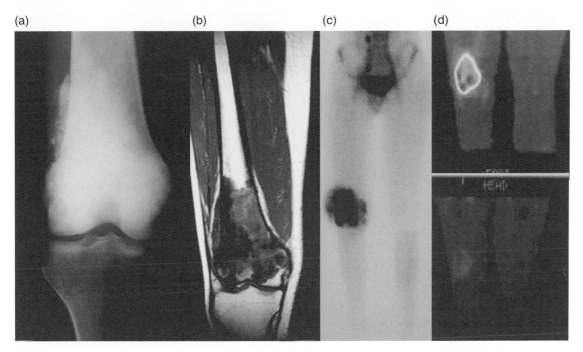

Fig. 51.4 (a) Radiograph of a distal femoral osteosarcoma showing typical areas of mixed lytic and blastic changes within the tumour. Note the periosteal new bone formation (arrow). (b) MRI clearly shows the intraosseous and extraosseous extension of the tumour. (c) Bone scanning shows the activity of new bone formation stimulated by the tumour. The changes before and after chemotherapy on bone scanning may indicate response to treatment. (d) Functional metabolic imaging (thallium or positron emission tomography) shows the metabolic activity of the tumour itself before chemotherapy (upper panel) and after chemotherapy (lower panel), where a good response is noted by the marked reduction in nuclear tracer activity.

(pericapsular inflammatory zone is transgressed), wide (surrounding cuff of normal tissue) and radical (entire tumour-bearing compartment is excised). All sarcomas should be excised with at least wide margins. Intralesional and marginal margins are regarded as inadequate and are associated with the highest local recurrence rates.

Outcome

The 5-year metastasis-free survival for osteosarcoma is 75%, for Ewing's sarcoma 50% and for chondrosarcoma 80%. All patients should follow a regular program of surveillance with clinical examination, pulmonary CT scans and imaging of the operated area.

Secondary malignancies

Metastatic carcinomas are the commonest malignant tumours of bone. Carcinomas that commonly metastasise to bone include breast, prostate, lung, kidney and thyroid. The majority are osteolytic although prostate is unique because 95% of bone lesions are osteoblastic.

Clinical presentation

Patients present with pain, pathological fracture or loss of limb function, or as an incidental finding on other imaging. Solitary metastases are uncommon. Up to 30% of bone metastases are the initial presenting feature of carcinoma.

Investigations

Radiography
Radiographs of the affected limb are vital for determining the extent of disease and the likelihood of fracture.

Bone scans
Bone scans are important for determining multicentricity of bone disease. All hotspots should be radiographed.

Magnetic resonance imaging
MRI may be important for assessing the quality and extent of bone involvement if reconstruction is being considered.

Computed tomography

CT is helpful for determining cortical destruction. CT scans of the chest, abdomen and pelvis are important for identifying the site of the primary tumour.

Blood tests

Routine blood tests may indicate the extent of marrow involvement. Elevation of specific markers such as prostate-specific antigen (prostate), carcinoembryonic antigen (gastrointestinal), alpha-fetoprotein (gastrointestinal) and ESR (myeloma) may assist diagnosis.

Treatment

- Radiotherapy is very useful for controlling pain, lysis or growth of the tumour.
- Chemotherapy has an important role in specific carcinomas.
- Surgery is indicated for the prevention of impending pathological fracture, or the treatment of fracture. In almost all cases, pain is a major reason for surgical intervention.

Outcome

In general, the surgical treatment of metastatic disease of bone is palliative. On occasion, resection of solitary renal or thyroid disease may affect cure.

Further reading

Allen KD, Choong PF, Davis AM *et al*. Osteoarthritis: models for appropriate care across the disease continuum. *Best Pract Res Clin Rheumatol* 2016;30:503–35.

Clark JC, Dass CR, Choong PF. Current and future treatments of bone metastases. *Expert Opin Emerg Drugs* 2008;13:609–27.

Hatzenbuehler J, Pulling TJ. Diagnosis and management of osteomyelitis. *Am Fam Physician* 2011;84:1027–33.

Kalunian KC. Current advances in therapies for osteoarthritis. *Curr Opin Rheumatol* 2016;28:246–50.

Ta HT, Dass CR, Choong PF, Dunstan DE. Osteosarcoma treatment: state of the art. *Cancer Metastasis Rev* 2009;28:247–63.

Trieu J, Sinnathamby M, Di Bella C *et al*. Biopsy and the diagnostic evaluation of musculoskeletal tumours: critical but often missed in the 21st century. *ANZ J Surg* 2016;86:133–8.

MCQs

Select the single correct answer to each question. The correct answers can be found in the Answers section at the end of the book.

1 Degenerative arthritis is a common condition characterised by:
   a joint pain, stiffness, contracture and deformity
   b recurrent haemarthroses, joint swelling and a Charcot joint
   c high temperature, exquisite joint pain and constitutional symptoms
   d flitting arthralgia, skin rash and sore throat
   e single joint swelling, conjunctivitis and urethritis

2 Which of the following radiological features of degenerative arthritis is correct?
   a syndesmophytes, bamboo spine
   b joint narrowing, subchondral sclerosis, osteophyte formation, cyst formation
   c joint debris, density, derangement and destruction
   d osteoporosis, valgus knee, marked joint synovitis
   e soft tissue swelling, fracture, fluid–fluid levels and gas in soft tissue

3 Crystal arthropathy may be seen in which of the following conditions?
   a hyperuricaemia
   b chondrodysplasia
   c haemochromatosis
   d Osgood–Schlatter disease
   e osteochondritis dissecans

4 Septic arthritis is associated with which of the following features?
   a exquisite pain with attempted joint motion
   b minimal constitutional symptoms
   c low incidence in children
   d low incidence in the elderly
   e never associated with trauma

5 Septic arthritis should be managed urgently with:
   a amputation
   b arthrodesis
   c arthrocentesis
   d arthrocutaneous fistula
   e arthroplasty

Section 12
Neurosurgery

52 Head injuries

Andrew H. Kaye

Department of Surgery, University of Melbourne and Royal Melbourne Hospital, Melbourne, Victoria, Australia

Introduction

Trauma is the leading cause of death in youth and early middle age, and death is often associated with major head trauma. Head injury contributes significantly to the outcome in more than half of trauma-related deaths. There are approximately 2.5 deaths from head injury per 10 000 population in Australia each year and road traffic accidents are responsible for about 65% of all fatal head injuries.

Head injury may vary from mild concussion to severe brain injury resulting in death. Management of patients requires careful identification of the pathological processes that have occurred.

Pathophysiology of head injury

Most head injuries result from blunt trauma, as distinct from a penetrating wound of the skull and brain caused by missiles or sharp objects. The pathological processes involved in a head injury include:
- direct trauma
- cerebral contusion
- intracerebral shearing
- cerebral swelling (oedema)
- intracranial haemorrhage
- hydrocephalus.

In addition, it is likely that following the initial injury there is a 'secondary injury' leading to further tissue damage, involving a complex series of destructive biochemical events. These include the possible release of excitotoxic neurotransmitters such as glutamate, and lipid peroxidation initiated by free oxygen radicals originating from the injured tissue, which leads to a cascade of oxidative damage.

Direct trauma

In penetrating injuries the direct trauma to the brain produces most of the damage, but in blunt injuries the energy from the impact has a widespread effect on the brain.

Cerebral contusion

Cerebral contusion may occur locally, under the position of the impact, but often occurs at a distance from the area of impact as a result of a contracoup injury. As the brain is mobile within the cranial cavity, sudden acceleration/deceleration will result in the opposite 'poles' of the brain being forced against the cranial vault. A sudden blow to the back of the head will cause the temporal and frontal lobes to slide across the skull base, causing contusion to the undersurface of the brain and to the temporal and frontal poles of the brain as they are jammed against the sphenoid ridge and frontal bones, respectively.

Intracerebral shearing

Intracerebral shearing forces result from the differential brain movement following blunt trauma, causing petechial haemorrhages, and tearing of axons and myelin sheaths.

Cerebral swelling

Cerebral swelling occurs either focally around an intracerebral haematoma or diffusely throughout the brain. The process involves a disturbance of vasomotor tone causing vasodilatation and cerebral oedema.

Intracranial haemorrhage

Intracranial haemorrhage following trauma may be intracerebral, subdural or extradural. Intracranial haematoma or cerebral swelling may cause cerebral herniation. The medial surface of the hemisphere may be pushed under the falx (subfalcine), the uncus and parahippocampal gyrus of the temporal lobe herniate through the tentorium causing pressure on

Textbook of Surgery, Fourth Edition. Edited by Julian A. Smith, Andrew H. Kaye, Christopher Christophi and Wendy A. Brown.
© 2020 John Wiley & Sons Ltd. Published 2020 by John Wiley & Sons Ltd.

the third nerve and midbrain (Figure 52.1), or there may be caudal displacement of the brainstem and/or cerebellum herniating into the foramen magnum.

Hydrocephalus

Hydrocephalus occurs occasionally early after a head injury and may be due to obstruction of the fourth ventricle by blood or swelling in the posterior fossa, or a result of a traumatic subarachnoid haemorrhage causing a communicating hydrocephalus. This is also an uncommon but important cause of delayed neurological deterioration.

Concussion

Concussion usually involves an instantaneous loss of consciousness as a result of trauma. The term *concussion* is not strictly defined in respect to the severity of the injury. However, a minimum criterion is that the patient will have had a period of amnesia. The retrograde amnesia of most cerebral concussion is usually short term, lasting less than 1 day. The initial retrograde amnesia may extend over a much longer period but gradually diminishes. A more reliable assessment of the severity of the head injury is the post-traumatic amnesia. The concussion is regarded as being severe if the amnesia following the head injury lasts more than 1 day.

The exact definition of concussion remains a contentious issue. The American National Football League established a Committee on Mild Traumatic Brain Injury (MTBI) that has established a much broader definition for concussion as follows: alteration of awareness or consciousness including being 'dazed', 'stunned' and with features of a 'post-concussion syndrome' that include headache, vertigo, light-headedness, loss of balance, blurred vision, drowsiness and lethargy. This definition is particularly relevant in the sports injury context where it informs the timing of commencing physical activity and returning to the sporting activity. Most sporting codes now have strict guidelines regarding the return to activity after a concussion. In addition, there is increasing concern regarding the likelihood of the cumulative effects of multiple concussions resulting in delayed permanent serious neurological consequences such as cognitive decline and possibly other neuropsychiatric disorders.

Associated injuries

Cranial nerves

The cranial nerves may be injured as a result of direct trauma by the skull fracture, cerebral swelling, brain herniation or the movement of the brain. The olfactory nerves are most commonly affected.

Eighth nerve damage is often associated with a fracture of the petrous temporal bone and deafness may be

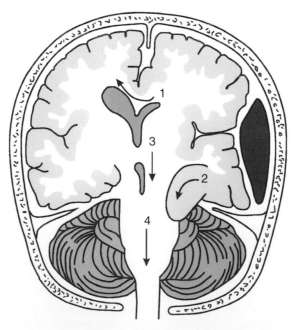

Fig. 52.1 Brain herniation: 1, subfalcine; 2, herniation of the uncus and hippocampal gyrus of the temporal lobe into the tentorial notch, causing pressure on the third nerve and midbrain; 3, brainstem caudally; 4, cerebellar tonsils through foramen magnum. Source: adapted from Kaye AH. *Essential Neurosurgery*, 3rd edn. Oxford: Blackwell Publishing, 2005. Reproduced with permission of John Wiley & Sons.

conductive, due to a haemotympanum, or sensorineural, as a result of injury to the inner ear or nerve itself.

Facial paralysis is usually associated with a fracture through the petrous temporal bone. It may be either immediate, as a result of direct compression of the nerve, or delayed, due to bleeding and/or swelling around the nerve.

The sixth cranial nerve has a long subarachnoid course and is easily damaged by torsion or herniation of the brain.

The third cranial nerve may also be damaged by direct trauma or by brain herniation, with the herniated uncus of the temporal lobe either impinging on the midbrain or directly stretching the nerve.

Skull fractures

Trauma may result in skull fractures that are classified as simple (a linear fracture of the skull vault), depressed (when bone fragments are depressed beneath the vault; Figure 52.2) or compound (when there is a communication with the external environment, usually from a laceration over the fracture). A fracture of the base of the skull may have a direct connection outside the vault, via the air sinuses.

Scalp lacerations

The extent of the scalp laceration does not necessarily indicate the degree of trauma to the underlying brain.

Traumatic intracranial haematomas

Intracranial haematoma formation following head injury is the major cause of fatal injuries in which death may potentially have been avoidable. Delay in the evacuation of the haematoma may also increase morbidity in survivors.

The general classification of traumatic intracranial haematoma depends on the relationship of the haematoma to the dura and brain. They are classified as extradural, subdural or intracerebral.

Extradural haematoma

Extradural haematomas are more likely to occur in the younger age group because the dura is able to strip more readily off the underlying bone. Although an extradural haematoma may occur in the presence of a severe head injury and coexist with a severe primary brain injury, its important feature is that it may occur when the injury to the underlying brain is either trivial or negligible.

The most common sites of extradural haematoma are the temporal region followed by the frontal area. Posterior fossa and parasagittal extradural haematomas are relatively uncommon. In most cases the haemorrhage is from a torn middle meningeal artery or its branches, but haematomas may also develop from haemorrhage from extradural veins or the venous sinuses. A fracture overlies the haematoma in nearly all (95%) adults and most (75%) children.

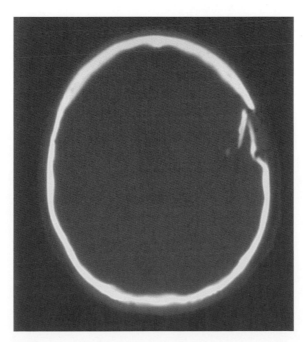

Fig. 52.2 Depressed skull fracture.

Clinical presentation

Frequently, extradural haematoma occurs following a head injury that has resulted in only a transient loss of consciousness, and in approximately 25% of cases there has been no initial loss of consciousness. In these patients the most important symptoms are:

- headache
- deteriorating conscious state
- focal neurological signs (dilating pupil, hemiparesis)
- change in vital signs (hypertension, bradycardia).

Headache is the main initial symptom in patients who have either not lost consciousness or who have regained consciousness. The headache is often followed by vomiting.

A deteriorating conscious state is the most important neurological sign, particularly when it develops after a 'lucid' interval. It is essential that the drowsiness that occurs in a patient following a head injury is not misinterpreted as just the patient wishing to sleep.

Focal neurological signs will depend on the position of the haematoma. In general, a temporal haematoma will produce a progressive contralateral spastic hemiparesis and an ipsilateral dilated pupil. Further progression will result in bilateral spastic limbs in a decerebrate posture and dilated pupils related to uncal herniation. Occasionally, the hemiparesis may initially be ipsilateral due to compression of the contralateral crus cerebri of the tentorial edge, but only rarely is the opposite pupil involved first.

A change in vital signs shows the classical Cushing response to increased intracranial pressure (ICP), i.e. bradycardia accompanied by an increase in blood pressure. Disturbances in respiration will develop into a Cheyne–Stokes pattern of breathing.

Radiological investigations

A computed tomography (CT) scan will show the typical hyperdense biconvex haematoma with compression of the underlying brain and distortion of the lateral ventricle (Figure 52.3).

Treatment

The treatment of extradural haematoma is urgent craniotomy with evacuation of the clot.

As soon as an extradural haematoma is suspected clinically, the patient should have an urgent CT scan. In some cases the rate of neurological deterioration may be so rapid that there is not sufficient time for a CT scan and the patient should be transferred immediately to the operating theatre. Infusion of mannitol (25% solution, 1 g/kg) or frusemide (20 mg i.v.) may temporarily reduce the ICP during transfer to the operating theatre. If unconscious, the patient should be intubated and hyperventilated during the transfer. It is essential that there should be no delay in evacuating the haematoma. An extradural haematoma is a surgical

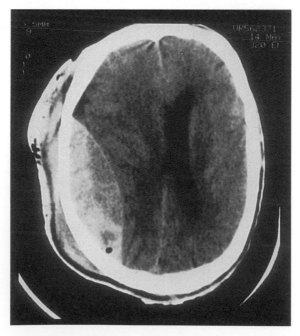

Fig. 52.3 Extradural haematoma with typical biconvex configuration.

emergency because the haematoma will result in death if not removed promptly.

Subdural haematoma

Subdural haematomas have been classified depending on the time at which they become clinically evident following injury: acute (<3 days), subacute (4–21 days) and chronic (>21 days). However, a CT scan enables a further and clinically more relevant classification depending on the density of the haematoma relative to the adjacent brain. An acute subdural haematoma is hyperdense (white) and a chronic subdural haematoma is hypodense. Between the end of the first week and the third week the subdural haematoma will be isodense with the adjacent brain.

Acute subdural haematoma

Acute subdural haematoma frequently results from severe trauma to the head and commonly arises from cortical lacerations.

An acute subdural haematoma usually presents in the context of a patient with a severe head injury whose neurological state is either failing to improve or deteriorating. The features of a deteriorating neurological state (decrease in conscious state and/ or increase in lateralising signs) should raise the possibility of a subdural haematoma.

A CT scan will show the characteristic hyperdense haematoma, which is concave towards the brain with compression of the underlying brain and distortion of the lateral ventricles (Figure 52.4). More than 80% of patients with acute subdural haematomas have a fracture of either the cranial vault or base of skull.

Chronic subdural haematoma

Chronic subdural haematoma may follow some time after a significant and often severe head injury, but in approximately one-third of patients there is no definite history of preceding head trauma. The aetiology of the subdural haematoma in this non-traumatic group is probably related to rupture of a fragile bridging vein in a relatively atrophic 'mobile' brain. A relatively trivial injury may result in movement of the brain, like a walnut inside its shell, with tearing of the bridging vein. The majority of patients in this group are more than 50 years of age.

If the patient is being treated in hospital for a head injury, the presence of a chronic subdural haematoma should be considered if the neurological state deteriorates. Alternatively, a patient may present without the history of a significant head injury in one of three characteristic ways.

• Raised ICP with or without significant localising signs such as a hemiparesis or dysphasia. Headache, vomiting and drowsiness, even in the

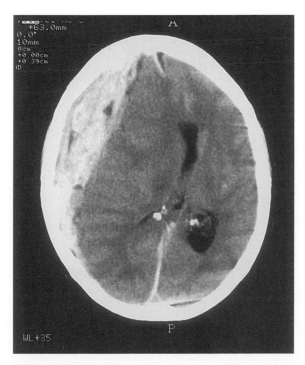

Fig. 52.4 Acute subdural haematoma with compression of ventricles.

absence of focal neurological signs, indicate the possible differential diagnosis of a cerebral neoplasm or chronic subdural haematoma.
- Fluctuating drowsiness.
- Progressive dementia.

Chronic subdural haematoma will be diagnosed on CT scan as a hypodense extracerebral collection causing compression of the underlying brain (Figure 52.5). In 25% of cases the haematoma is bilateral. The chronic subdural haematoma can usually be drained through burr holes, but a small craniotomy is sometimes necessary, especially if there is evidence of subdural membranes indicating the presence of multiple loculated chronic subdural haematomas.

Intracerebral haematoma

Intracerebral haematomas occur as a result of a penetrating injury (e.g. missile injury), a depressed skull fracture or following a severe head injury. They are frequently associated with a subdural haematoma.

An intracerebral haematoma should be suspected in any patient with a severe head injury or a patient whose neurological state is deteriorating. A CT scan will show the size and position of the haematomas.

A large intracerebral haematoma usually needs to be evacuated. Small intracerebral haematomas are not removed but should be monitored because the haematoma may expand and require evacuation.

Initial management

The key aspects in the management of patients following head injury are:
- clinical assessment of the neurological and other injuries
- determination of the pathological process involved
- recognition that a change in the neurological signs indicates a progression or change in the pathological processes.

Immediate treatment at the site of the accident is critical to the outcome and involves rapid restoration of an adequate airway and ventilation, circulatory resuscitation, first-aid treatment of other injuries, and the urgent transfer of the patient to hospital. It is essential to avoid hypoxia and hypotension because both will cause further brain injury.

Clinical assessment

In the management of head injury, it is essential to know the type of accident that caused the head inujury and whether the neurological condition is deteriorating. An assessment of the patient's initial neurological condition can be obtained from bystanders at the site of the accident or from the ambulance officers.

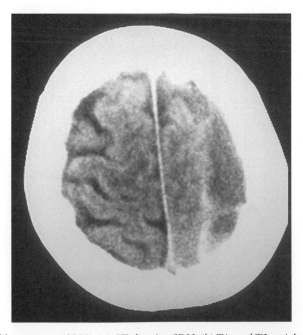

Fig. 52.5 Chronic subdural haematoma (SDH): (a) CT showing SDH; (b) T1- and T2-weighted MRI showing bilateral SDH; (c) MRI FLAIR showing bilateral SDH.

Neurological examination

Neurological examination will help to determine the type and position of the pathological process and provide a baseline for comparison with subsequent examinations. Although a full neurological examination should be undertaken, special emphasis should be given to:

- the conscious state
- pupillary size and reaction
- focal neurological signs in the limbs.

An assessment should be made of the retrograde amnesia and post-traumatic amnesia, if possible.

There is a continuum of altered consciousness from the patient being alert and responding appropriately to verbal command to those who are deeply unconscious. Drowsiness is the first sign of a depressed conscious state. As the level of consciousness deteriorates, the patient will become confused. The use of the words 'coma', 'semi-coma' or 'stuporose' should be avoided because they convey different meanings to different observers. The assessment is more accurate and reproducible if the Glasgow Coma Scale (GCS) is used (Table 52.1). This scale gives a numerical value to the three most important parameters of the level of consciousness: eye opening, best verbal response and best motor response. The exact response can be shown on a chart or the level of consciousness can be given as a numerical score (the sum of the three parameters of the GCS). A score of 8 or less indicates a severe brain injury. However, it is essential to realise that following a head injury the neurological state can deteriorate rapidly and there must be no complacency even in patients with a GCS score of 14 or 15.

In fact in older patients (>60 years) a GCS score of 12 indicates a serious injury, with the possibility of poor outcome.

Careful evaluation of the pupil size and response to light is essential at the initial clinical assessment and during further observation. Raised ICP causing temporal lobe herniation will cause compression of the third nerve, resulting in pupillary dilatation that nearly always occurs initially on the side of the raised pressure. The pupil will initially remain reactive to light but will subsequently fail to respond to light in any way. As the ICP increases, this same process commences on the opposite side.

Neurological examination of the limbs will assess tone, power and sensation. A hemiparesis will result from an injury of the corticospinal tract at any point from the motor cortex to the spinal cord. Following a severe brain injury the limbs may adopt an abnormal 'posturing' attitude. The decerebrate posture consists of the upper limbs adducted and internally rotated against the trunk, extended at the elbow and flexed at the wrist and fingers, with the lower limbs adducted, extended at the hip and knee with the feet plantar flexed. Less frequently the upper limbs may be flexed, probably due to an injury predominantly involving the cerebral white matter and basal ganglia, corresponding to a posture of decortication.

Particular attention must be given to the patient's ventilation, blood pressure and pulse. At all times it is essential to ensure the patient's ventilation is adequate. Respiratory problems may result either as a direct manifestation of the severity of the head injury or due to an associated chest injury.

Table 52.1 Glasgow Coma Scale.

Parameter	Response	Numerical value
Eye opening	Spontaneous	4
	To speech	3
	To pain	2
	None	1
Best verbal response	Oriented	5
	Confused	4
	Inappropriate	3
	Incomprehensible sounds	2
	None	1
Best motor response to painful stimulus	Obeys commands	6
	Localises to pain	5
	Flexion to pain (withdrawal)	4
	Flexion (abnormal)	3
	Extension to pain	2
	None	1
Total		3–15

Pyrexia frequently occurs following a head injury. A raised temperature lasting more than 2 days is usually due to traumatic subarachnoid haemorrhage or may occur in patients with a severe brainstem injury.

General examination

Careful assessment must be made of any other injuries. Chest, skeletal, cardiovascular or intra-abdominal injury must be diagnosed and the appropriate management instituted. Hypotension or hypoxia may severely aggravate the brain injury.

Radiological assessment

Radiological assessment following the clinical evaluation will be essential unless the injury has been minor. A CT scan will show the macroscopic intracranial injury and should be performed if:

- the patient is drowsy or has a more seriously depressed conscious state
- the patient has a continuing headache
- there are focal neurological signs
- there is neurological deterioration
- there is cerebrospinal fluid (CSF) rhinorrhoea
- there are associated injuries that will entail prolonged ventilation so that ongoing neurological assessment will be difficult.

The indications for a skull X-ray have diminished since the introduction of CT, especially as the bony vault can be assessed by the CT scan using the bone 'windows'.

It is important to note that radiological assessment of the cervical spine is essential in all patients who have sustained a significant head injury, particularly if there are associated facial injuries. Radiological assessment of the full spine is necessary in all patients who are unconscious and should be considered in all patients who have focal spinal pain or tenderness depending on the mechanism of injury.

Further management

Following the clinical and radiological assessments, subsequent management will depend on the severity of the injury and the intracranial pathology.

Minor head injury

Any patient who has suffered a head injury must be observed for at least 4 hours. The minimum criteria for obligatory admission to hospital are given in Box 52.1. Further management of these patients will be by careful observation, and neurological

> **Box 52.1 Minimum criteria for obligatory admission to hospital after head injury**
>
> - Loss of consciousness (post-traumatic amnesia) for more than 10 minutes
> - Persistent drowsiness
> - Focal neurological deficits
> - Skull fracture
> - Persisting headache, nausea or vomiting after 4 hours' observation
> - Lack of adequate care at the patient's home

observations should be recorded on a chart displaying the GCS scores.

Should the patient's neurological state deteriorate, an immediate CT scan is essential to re-evaluate the intracranial pathology. Further treatment will depend on the outcome of the scan.

Severe head injury

The management of a patient following a severe head injury depends on the patient's neurological state and the intracranial pathology resulting from the trauma. In general, the following applies.

The patient has a clinical assessment and CT scan as described previously. If the CT scan shows an intracranial haematoma causing shift of the underlying brain structures, then this is evacuated immediately.

Following the operation, or if there is no surgical lesion, the patient should be carefully observed and the neurological observations recorded on a chart with the GCS scores. Measures to decrease brain swelling should be implemented, including management of the airway to ensure adequate oxygenation and ventilation (hypercapnia will cause cerebral vasodilatation and so exacerbate brain swelling), elevation of the head of the bed to 20°, and maintenance of fluid and electrolyte balance. Normal fluid maintenance with an intake of 3000 mL per 24 hours is optimum for the average adult. Blood loss from other injuries should be replaced with colloid or blood, not with crystalloid solutions. Pyrexia may be due to hypothalamic damage or traumatic subarachnoid haemorrhage, but infection as a cause of the fever must be excluded. The temperature must be controlled because hyperthermia can elevate ICP, will increase brain and body metabolism, and predisposes to seizure activity. Adequate nutrition must be maintained as well as routine care of the unconscious patient, including bowel and bladder care, and pressure care.

More aggressive methods to control ICP are advisable if the patient's neurological state continues to deteriorate and the CT scan shows evidence of cerebral swelling without an intracranial haematoma, there is posturing (decerebrate) response to stimuli, or the GCS score is less than 8.

An ICP monitor will also be useful in patients requiring prolonged sedation and ventilation as a result of other injuries. Measurement of ICP will provide another useful monitoring parameter, and any sustained rise in the pressure will be an indication for careful reassessment and, if necessary, CT scan.

The techniques used to control ICP include controlled ventilation maintaining $Paco_2$ at 33–38 mmHg, CSF drainage from a ventricular catheter, and diuretic therapy using intermittent administration of mannitol or frusemide. Mild hypothermia, achieved by cooling the patient to 34°C, is possibly of benefit. Other techniques such as administration of barbiturates (to reduce cerebral metabolism and ICP) and hyperbaric oxygen have been advocated in the past but have not been shown to have any proven benefit. Steroid medication is of no proven benefit in head injury.

The role of a large decompressive craniectomy, involving removal of a large component of the skull, in severe brain injury remains controversial. Whilst some studies have shown possible benefit, a large prospective study (the DECRA study reported in the *New England Journal of Medicine* in 2011) showed no advantage and even possible detrimental outcome. At present most neurosurgeons would advise its use only in carefully selected patients in whom the ICP continues to rise despite using the measures described here.

Management of associated conditions

Scalp injury

A large scalp laceration may result in considerable blood loss. When the patient arrives in the emergency department, 'spurting' arteries should be controlled with haemostatic clips prior to a sterile bandage being applied to the head. After initial assessment and stabilisation the wound should be closed without delay. The hair should be shaved widely around the wound, which should be meticulously cleaned and debrided. The closure should be performed in two layers if possible, with careful apposition of the galea prior to closing the skin.

If the scalp wound has resulted in loss of soft tissue, the wound may need to be extended to provide an extra 'flap' of healthy tissue so that the skin edges can be approximated without tension.

Skull fractures

Simple fracture

There is no specific management for a simple skull fracture without an overlying skin injury, although it is an indication that the trauma was not trivial and it should provide a warning that a haematoma may develop beneath the fracture.

Compound fracture

A skull fracture may be compound because of an overlying scalp laceration or if it involves an air sinus. The scalp wound should be debrided and closed. A short course of prophylactic antibiotics should be administered to reduce the risk of infection.

Depressed skull fracture

If the depressed skull fracture is compound, prophylactic antibiotics and tetanus prophylaxis should be administered. Surgery, usually requiring a general anaesthetic, should be performed as soon as possible.

Cerebrospinal fluid rhinorrhoea

A fracture involving the base of the anterior cranial fossa may cause tearing of the dura, resulting in a fistula into the air sinuses. This type of fistulous connection should also be suspected if the patient suffers an episode of meningitis or if the radiological investigations show a fracture in the appropriate site. An intracranial aerocele is proof of a fistulous connection. CSF rhinorrhoea may also occur as a result of a fistula through the tegmen tympani into the cavity of the middle ear and leakage via the eustachian tube.

Surgery should be performed if CSF leakage persists, if there is an intracranial aerocele or if there has been an episode of meningitis in a patient with a fracture of the anterior cranial fossa.

Rehabilitation

Some form of rehabilitation is essential following any significant head injury. If the injury has been relatively minor, then the rehabilitation necessary may involve only advice and reassurance to the patient and family. Following a severe head injury, rehabilitation will also usually involve a team of paramedical personnel, including physiotherapists, occupational therapists, speech therapists and social workers.

Further reading

American Academy of Neurology. Practice parameter. The management of concussion in sports. *Neurology* 1997;48:581–5.

American Congress of Rehabilitation Medicine. Definition of mild traumatic brain injury. *J Head Trauma Rehabil* 1993;8:86–7.

Collins M, Grindal S. Relationship between concussion and neuropsychological performance in college football players. *JAMA* 1999;282:964–70.

Hsiang JNK, Yeung T, Yu ALM, Poon WS. High-risk mild head injury. *J Neurosurg* 1997;87:234–8.

Kaye AH. *Essential Neurosurgery*, 3rd edn. Oxford: Blackwell Publishing, 2005.

Sahuquillo J, Poca M-A, Arridas M, Garnacho A, Rubio E. Interhemispheric supratentorial intracranial pressure gradients in head-injured patients: are they clinically important? *J Neurosurg* 1999;90:16–26.

Zhao W, Alonso OF, Loor JY, Busto R, Ginsberg MD. Influence of early posttraumatic hypothermia therapy on local cerebral blood flow and glucose metabolism after fluid-percussion brain injury. *J Neurosurg* 1999;90:L510– L519.

MCQs

Select the single correct answer to each question. The correct answers can be found in the Answers section at the end of the book.

1 In the treatment of head injury, which of the following is correct?
   a steroids are regularly used
   b patients with a GCS score less than 8 are usually intubated and ventilated
   c antibiotics are routinely used
   d pyrexia is nearly always due to severe infection
   e severe fluid restriction is necessary

2 Which of the following is the best investigation for patients with severe head injury?
   a CT scan
   b skull X-ray
   c EEG
   d ultrasound
   e MRI

3 Traumatic intracerebral haematomas following blunt trauma:
   a can usually be diagnosed by skull X-ray
   b are usually associated with severe brain injury
   c always need to be drained
   d should be treated with fluid restriction
   e are always associated with a skull fracture

4 An acute subdural haematoma:
   a shows a characteristic hyperdense extracerebral mass
   b is often associated with only a minor head injury
   c virtually never needs surgical excision
   d can always be managed with diuretic therapy
   e usually causes an ipsilateral hemiparesis

53 Intracranial tumours, infection and aneurysms

Andrew H. Kaye

Department of Surgery, University of Melbourne and Royal Melbourne Hospital, Melbourne, Victoria, Australia

Introduction

This chapter provides a brief overview of three important neurosurgical conditions: intracranial tumours, cerebral aneurysms and intracranial infection. A brief description of each of these pathologies will be given and the principles of treatment discussed.

BRAIN TUMOURS

Brain tumours are responsible for approximately 2% of all cancer deaths. However, central nervous system (CNS) tumours comprise the most common group of solid tumours in young patients, accounting for 20% of all paediatric neoplasms.

The general brain tumour classification is related to cell of origin and is shown in Box 53.1. Table 53.1 shows the approximate distribution of the more common brain tumours, some of which are described in this chapter.

Aetiology

Epidemiological studies have not indicated any particular factor, either chemical or traumatic, that causes brain tumours in humans. Generally, there is no inherited genetic predisposition to brain tumours, but many specific chromosome abnormalities involving chromosomes 10, 13, 17 and 22 have been noted in a wide range of CNS tumours. There is considerable conjecture regarding the role of trauma, electromagnetic radiation and organic solvents in the development of brain tumours, but as yet no convincing evidence has been forthcoming.

Molecular biology techniques have enabled the identification of a variety of alterations in the genome of the tumour cell, including those of brain tumours. These include alterations in the genes (such as the receptor tyrosine kinases) that control the numerous complex cell signalling pathways that regulate cell proliferation, survival and migration. It is also clear that numerous epigenetic mechanisms, such as methylation and microRNA, play a vital role in gene expression. Tumour suppressor genes are normally present in the genome and act as a 'brake' on cell transformation. Mutations in the *TP53* tumour suppressor gene are the most common gene abnormality found in tumours to date and have been shown to occur in both astrocytomas and meningiomas.

Cerebral glioma

Gliomas comprise the majority of cerebral tumours and arise from neuroglial cells. There are four distinct types of glial cells: astrocytes, oligodendroglia, ependymal cells and neuroglial precursors. Each of these gives rise to tumours with different biological and anatomical characteristics.

Astrocytoma

The most common gliomas arise from the astrocytes, which comprise the majority of intraparenchymal cells of the brain. The tumours arising from the astrocytes range from the relatively benign to the highly malignant. The term *malignant* for brain tumours differs from its usage for systemic tumours, in that intrinsic brain tumours very rarely metastasise (except for medulloblastoma and ependymoma) and instead refers to the aggressive biological characteristics and poor prognosis.

There are many classifications of brain tumours in general and gliomas in particular. The World Health Organization (WHO) classification of

Textbook of Surgery, Fourth Edition. Edited by Julian A. Smith, Andrew H. Kaye, Christopher Christophi and Wendy A. Brown.
© 2020 John Wiley & Sons Ltd. Published 2020 by John Wiley & Sons Ltd.

Box 53.1 General classifications of brain tumours

Neuroepithelial tumours
  Gliomas
    Astrocytoma (including glioblastoma)
    Oligodendrocytoma
    Ependymoma
    Choroid plexus tumour
  Pineal tumours
  Neuronal tumours
    Ganglioglioma
    Gangliocytoma
    Neuroblastoma
  Medulloblastoma
Nerve sheath tumour
  Acoustic neuroma
Meningeal tumours
  Meningioma
Pituitary tumours
Germ cell tumours
  Germinoma
  Teratoma
Lymphomas
Tumour-like malformations
  Craniopharyngioma
  Epidermoid tumour
  Dermoid tumour
  Colloid cyst
Metastatic tumours
Local extensions from regional tumours
(e.g. glomus jugulare, carcinoma of ethmoid)

Source: Kaye AH. *Essential Neurosurgery*, 3rd edn. Oxford: Blackwell Publishing, 2005. Reproduced with permission of John Wiley & Sons.

Table 53.1 Incidence (%) of common cerebral tumours.

Neuroepithelial	52
Astrocytoma (all grades including glioblastoma)	44
Ependymoma	3
Oligodendroglioma	2
Medulloblastoma	3
Metastatic	15
Meningioma	15
Pituitary	8
Acoustic neuroma	8

Source: Kaye AH. *Essential Neurosurgery*, 3rd edn. Oxford: Blackwell Publishing, 2005. Reproduced with permission of John Wiley & Sons.

cerebral gliomas recognises four grades. Grade I is assigned to the pilocytic astrocytoma, an uncommon tumour that is very slow-growing and biologically distinct from the diffuse astrocytomas, which are classified as astrocytoma (WHO grade II), anaplastic astrocytoma (WHO grade III) and glioblastoma multiforme (WHO grade IV) and which comprise over 50% of the astrocytoma tumours. The most recent 2016 revision of the WHO classification includes the use of both histological appearance and molecular features, such as isocitrate dehydrogenase (IDH) mutation and 1p/19q status to classify glioma.

Pathology

The hallmark of the pathology of cerebral gliomas is invasion of tumour cells into the adjacent normal brain. Although in certain areas the margin of the tumour may seem to be macroscopically well defined from the brain, there are always microscopic nests of tumour cells extending well into the brain. The histological appearance of the tumour varies with the tumour grade, with increasing cellular atypia, mitoses, endothelial and adventitial cell proliferation and necrosis with increasing grade of the tumour.

Clinical presentation

The presenting features of all intracranial tumours can be classified under:
- raised intracranial pressure (ICP)
- focal neurological signs
- epilepsy.

The duration of symptoms and the evolution of the clinical presentation will depend on the grade of the tumour (i.e. rate of growth). A patient presenting with a low-grade astrocytoma (grade I or II) may have a history of seizures extending over many years antedating the development of progressive neurological signs and raised ICP. Patients with the more common higher-grade tumour present with a shorter history, and glioblastoma multiforme is characterised by a short illness of weeks or a few months.

Raised ICP is due to the tumour mass, surrounding cerebral oedema and hydrocephalus due to blockage of cerebrospinal fluid (CSF) pathways. The main clinical features of raised ICP are headaches, nausea and vomiting, drowsiness and papilloedema.
- *Headache* associated with increased ICP is usually worse on waking in the morning and is relieved by vomiting. ICP increases during sleep, probably as a result of vascular dilatation due to carbon dioxide retention.
- *Nausea and vomiting* are usually worse in the morning.

- *Drowsiness* is the most important clinical feature of raised ICP. It is the portent of rapid neurological deterioration.
- *Papilloedema* is the definitive sign of raised ICP. The early features of increased pressure on the optic nerve head are those of dilatation or failure of normal pulsations of retinal veins. As the ICP rises, the nerve head becomes more swollen and the disc margins become blurred on fundoscopic examination. Flame-shaped haemorrhages develop, particularly around the disc margins and along the vessels.
- *Sixth nerve palsy* causing diplopia may result in raised ICP owing to stretching of the sixth cranial nerve by cordal displacement of the brainstem. This is a so-called false localising sign.
- *Focal neurological signs* are common in patients presenting with cerebral gliomas, and the nature of the deficit will depend on the position of the tumour.

Patients presenting with tumours involving the frontal lobes may sometimes have pseudo-psychiatric problems, with personality change and mood disorders. Limb paresis results from interference of the pyramidal tracts, either at a cortical or subcortical level, and field defects are associated with tumours of the temporal, occipital or parietal lobes. Dysphasia, either expressive or receptive, is a particularly distressing symptom in patients involving the relevant areas of dominant hemisphere.

Investigations

Computed tomography (CT) and magnetic resonance imaging (MRI) of the brain are the essential radiological investigations and an accurate diagnosis can be made in nearly all tumours on MRI.

Low-grade gliomas show decreased density on CT and T1-weighted MRI, with minimal surrounding oedema and usually no enhancement with contrast (Figure 53.1). Calcification may be present. High-grade gliomas are usually large and enhance vividly following intravenous injection of contrast material and have extensive surrounding oedema (Figure 53.2).

MRI, particularly when used with gadolinium contrast enhancement, improves the visualisation of cerebral gliomas. Gadolinium enhancement is more likely to occur in high-grade tumours. The use of MRI spectroscopy to measure biochemical changes in the tumour and surrounding brain as well as blood flow and blood volume helps to further define the exact diagnosis.

Management

Following the presumptive diagnosis of a glioma, the management involves surgery and radiation and chemotherapy.

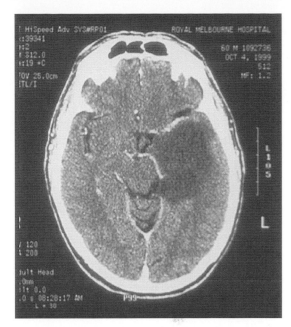

Fig. 53.1 Low-grade glioma with decreased density on T1-weighted MRI.

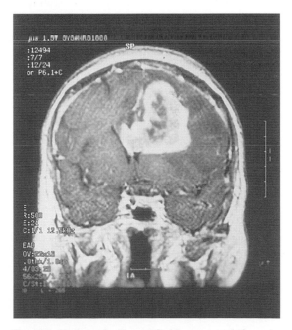

Fig. 53.2 High-grade glioma (glioblastoma multiforme) showing vivid enhancement after intravenous injection of contrast material.

Surgery

The aim of surgery is to:
- make a definitive diagnosis
- reduce the tumour mass to relieve the symptoms of raised ICP
- reduce the tumour mass as a precursor to adjuvant treatments.

There is still some debate regarding the oncological benefit of tumour resection in the treatment of glioma as complete resection of high-grade (and most low-grade) gliomas is not possible and the high-grade glioma will inevitably recur despite what is considered by the surgeon as a 'complete' resection. Nevertheless, it is advisable to resect as much tumour as possible provided that the patient is not inflicted with a neurological deficit.

RADIOTHERAPY AND CHEMOTHERAPY
Postoperative combined radiation therapy and temozolomide chemotherapy (known as the Stupp protocol) is often used as an adjunct to surgery in the treatment of high-grade gliomas, especially in patients under 70 years of age.

The adjuvant treatment for low-grade astrocytoma is more controversial as these tumours are less responsive to adjuvant therapies. However, studies have shown possible survival benefit with radiation and chemotherapy, although the long-term complications, especially cognitive decline associated with radiation effects on the normal brain, remain a concern and has tempered the use of these treatments routinely. However, radiation and possibly chemotherapy are usually advised for the larger tumours in patients over 40 years of age as these patients have a poorer prognosis.

Oligodendroglioma is more responsive to chemotherapy than other types of glioma and adjuvant treatment may be considered either following the initial resection or when there is evidence of tumour recurrence or progression on MRI.

Prognosis

At present there is no satisfactory treatment for cerebral glioma. In a large prospective study of the treatment of high-grade glioma (glioblastoma multiforme), the median survival following surgery and the Stupp protocol of combined radiation and temozolomide chemotherapy was 14.6 weeks, with a 2-year survival of 26% and 5-year survival of 10%. However, most series report significantly less promising survival results.

Oligodendroglioma

Oligodendrogliomas are much less common than the astrocytoma group, being responsible for approximately 5% of all gliomas. Oligodendrogliomas have the same spectrum of histological appearance as astrocytomas but, as distinct from the astrocytoma series, are more likely to be slow-growing. Calcium deposits are found in 90% of these tumours (Figure 53.3). The 2016 WHO classification includes

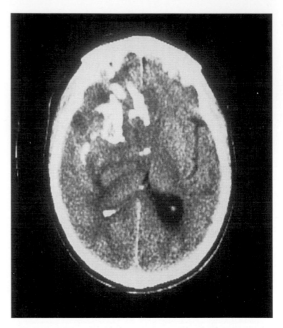

Fig. 53.3 Oligodendroglioma that is highly calcified.

the requirement for these tumours to have an IDH mutation and 1p/19q deletion for the diagnosis.

The clinical presentation is essentially the same as for the astrocyte group, but as these tumours are more likely to be slow-growing, epilepsy is more common.

The principles of treatment are the same as for the astrocytoma group. Surgery is necessary to make a definitive diagnosis and debulking the tumour will relieve the features of raised ICP as well as reducing the tumour burden for adjuvant therapies. Radiotherapy is probably helpful in reducing the rate of growth of any remnant tumour. Chemotherapy has been shown to be more beneficial in helping to control those tumours with an oligodendroglial component, especially those tumours with proven loss of heterozygosity on chromosome 1p or 19q.

Metastatic tumours

Metastatic tumours are responsible for 15% of brain tumours in clinical series, but up to 30% of brain tumours reported by pathologists. Approximately 30% of deaths are due to cancer and 20% of these will have intracranial metastatic deposits at postmortem. The metastatic tumours most commonly originate from:

- carcinoma of the lung
- carcinoma of the breast
- metastatic melanoma
- carcinoma of the kidney
- gastrointestinal carcinoma.

In 15% of cases a primary origin is never found. Most metastatic tumours are multiple and one-third are solitary. In about half of the solitary tumours, systemic spread is not apparent. The incidence of tumours in the cerebrum relative to the cerebellum is 8 : 1. Metastatic tumours are often surrounded by intense cerebral oedema.

Clinical presentation

The interval between diagnosis of the primary cancer and cerebral metastasis varies considerably. In general, secondary tumours from carcinoma of the lung present relatively soon after the initial diagnosis, with a median interval of 5 months. Although cerebral metastases may present within a few months of the initial diagnosis of malignant melanoma or carcinoma of the breast, some patients may live many years before an intracranial tumour appears.

The presenting clinical features for cerebral metastasis are similar to those described for other tumours, namely raised ICP, focal neurological signs and epilepsy.

Radiological investigations

CT or MRI will diagnose metastatic tumour and show whether or not the deposits are solitary or multiple. Most metastatic tumours are isodense on unenhanced scan and they enhance vividly after intravenous contrast material. MRI following gadolinium contrast may demonstrate small metastatic tumours often not visible on a CT scan (Figure 53.4).

Treatment

Steroid medication will control cerebral oedema and should be commenced immediately if there is raised ICP.

Surgery to remove the metastasis is indicated if:

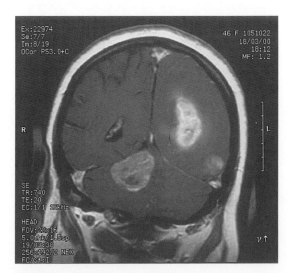

Fig. 53.4 Multiple metastatic tumours.

- there is a solitary metastasis in a surgically accessible position
- there is no systemic spread.

Excision of multiple metastases may occasionally be indicated if the tumours are causing symptoms, and are in a surgically accessible position and especially if the tumour is known to be resistant to radiation therapy.

Removal of a metastasis is preferable if the primary site of origin has been, or will be, controlled. Excision of a single or even multiple metastases will provide excellent symptomatic relief and consequently may be indicated even if the primary site cannot be treated satisfactorily.

Radiotherapy, together with steroid medication to control cerebral oedema, is often used to treat patients with multiple cerebral metastases and may be advisable following excision of a single metastasis. Stereotactic radiosurgery, which uses a highly focused beam of radiation, can be used to treat single and multiple cerebral metastases if the tumour is less than 3 cm in diameter, especially if the tumour is known to be radiation sensitive.

Prognosis

The survival for patients who have undergone surgical excision of a metastatic deposit depends on control of the primary tumour and the effectiveness of oncological therapies.

Paediatric brain tumours

Intracranial tumours are the most common form of solid tumours in childhood, with 60% of tumours occurring below the tentorium cerebelli. The most common supratentorial tumours are astrocytomas, followed by anaplastic astrocytomas and glioblastoma multiforme.

Posterior fossa paediatric tumours

Of paediatric brain tumours, 60% occur in the posterior fossa. The relative incidence of tumours is:
- cerebellar astrocytoma, 30%
- medulloblastoma (infratentorial primary neuroectodermal tumour), 30%
- ependymoma, 20%
- brainstem glioma, 10%
- miscellaneous (choroid plexus papilloma, haemangioblastoma, epidermoid, dermoid, chordoma), 10%.

Clinical presentation

The presenting clinical features of posterior fossa neoplasms in children are related to raised ICP and focal neurological signs.

RAISED INTRACRANIAL PRESSURE

Raised ICP is the most common presenting feature. It is due to hydrocephalus caused by obstruction of the fourth ventricle and is manifest by headaches, vomiting, diplopia and papilloedema. The raised ICP may result in a strasbismus causing diplopia due to stretching of one or both of the sixth (abducens) cranial nerves (a false localising sign).

FOCAL NEUROLOGICAL SIGNS

Focal neurological signs are due to the tumour invading or compressing the cerebellum, brainstem and cranial nerves. Truncal and gait ataxia result particularly from midline cerebellar involvement. Horizontal gaze paretic nystagmus often occurs in tumours around the fourth ventricle. Vertical nystagmus is indicative of brainstem involvement. Disturbance of bulbar function, such as difficulty in swallowing, with nasal regurgitation of fluid, dysarthria and impaired palatal or pharyngeal reflexes, result from brainstem involvement. Compression or tumour invasion of the pyramidal tracts may result in hemiparesis or sensory disturbance.

Investigations

CT and MRI will confirm the position of the tumour and whether there is hydrocephalus (Figure 53.5).

Management

The treatment of posterior fossa tumours involves surgery, radiotherapy and chemotherapy.

A CSF shunt may need to be performed to control raised ICP due to hydrocephalus. The CSF diversion can be achieved with either an external drain or ventriculoperitoneal shunt. The shunt will provide immediate and controlled relief of intracranial hypertension and the subsequent posterior fossa operation can be performed as a planned elective procedure. A criticism of preoperative ventriculoperitoneal shunt is that it may promote the metastatic spread of these tumours.

In general, the treatment of medulloblastoma and ependymoma involves surgery to excise the tumour, followed by radiation therapy, which may be to the whole neuraxis as the tumour may spread throughout the CNS, followed by chemotherapy.

The survival of patients with medulloblastoma depends on the genetic subtype of the tumour, the spread of the tumour at the time of diagnosis, the extent of resection and the age of the patients. Overall 5-year survival is 70–80%, for children with high-risk disease 50–60%, and for infants 30–50%. The prognosis for ependymoma depends on similar factors and overall 5-year survival is 70–75%.

(a)

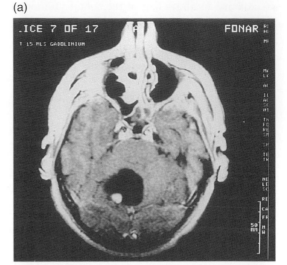

(b)

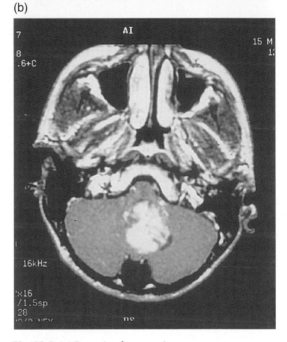

Fig. 53.5 (a) Posterior fossa cystic astrocytoma with small tumour nodule and large cyst. (b) Enhancing midline posterior fossa tumour (medulloblastoma).

Many cerebellar astrocytomas have a small single nodule surrounded by a large cyst. These tumours can often be cured by excision of the nodule alone, and adjuvant therapy is not necessary. In contrast, the treatment of brainstem glioma usually involves only a biopsy of the tumour to confirm the diagnosis, possibly followed by radiotherapy and/or chemotherapy. These tumours usually cause death within 24 months of diagnosis, although some patients with low-grade tumours will live longer.

Benign brain tumours

The most common benign brain tumours are:
- meningioma
- acoustic neuroma
- haemangioblastoma
- dermoid and epidermoid tumours
- colloid cysts
- pituitary tumours
- craniopharyngioma.

Meningiomas

Meningiomas are the most common of the benign brain tumours and constitute about 15% of all intracranial tumours, comprising about one-third the number of gliomas. However, the true incidence of meningioma is much higher, as many are small asymptomatic meningiomas that are only diagnosed on CT or MRI undertaken for investigation of headache or other neurological symptoms. Although they may occur at any age, they reach their peak incidence in middle age and are very uncommon in children.

Unlike gliomas, where the classification system is based on the histological appearance of the tumours, meningiomas are usually classified according to the position of origin rather than histology. The reason for this is that, in general, the biological activity of the tumour, presenting features, treatment and prognosis all relate more to the site of the tumour than the histology (Table 53.2).

Whilst there are numerous histological subtypes of meningioma, approximately 10–15% are regarded as showing 'atypical' features, which indicate a much higher risk of recurrence. Only 2% are regarded as being malignant.

Clinical presentation
Meningiomas present with features of raised ICP, focal neurological signs and epilepsy. The position

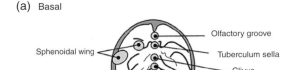

(a) Basal

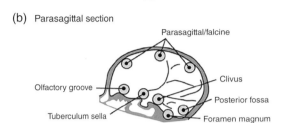

(b) Parasagittal section

Fig. 53.6 Classical positions of meningiomas.

of the tumour (Figure 53.6) will determine the features of the clinical presentation. The tumours often grow slowly and there is frequently a long history, often of many years, of symptoms prior to diagnosis.

- *Parasagittal tumours* often arise in the middle third of the vault, and the patient may present with focal epilepsy and paresis, usually affecting the opposite leg and foot, as the motor cortex on the medial aspect of the posterior frontal lobe is affected. Urinary incontinence is occasionally a symptom for a large frontal tumour, especially if it is bilateral.
- *Convexity tumours* often grow around the position of the coronal suture. Patients present with raised ICP, and more posterior tumours will cause focal neurological symptoms and epilepsy.
- *Inner sphenoidal wing meningioma* will cause compression of the adjacent optic nerve and patients may present with a history of uniocular visual failure.
- *Olfactory groove meningioma* will cause anosmia, initially unilateral and later bilateral. The presenting features may include symptoms of raised ICP. Large frontal tumours, especially those arising in the midline and causing compression of both frontal lobes such as tumours arising from the olfactory groove, may present with cognitive decline.
- *Suprasellar tumours* arise from the tuberculum sellae and will cause visual failure with a bitemporal hemianopia.
- *Posterior fossa tumours* may arise from the cerebellar convexity or from the cerebellopontine angle or clivus. Tumours arising in the cerebellopontine angle or extending into the basal cisterns

Table 53.2 Position (%) of intracranial meningioma.

Parasagittal and falx	25
Convexity	20
Sphenoidal wing	20
Olfactory groove	12
Suprasellar	12
Posterior fossa	9
Ventricle	1.5
Optic sheath	0.5

Source: Kaye AH. *Essential Neurosurgery*, 3rd edn. Oxford: Blackwell Publishing, 2005. Reproduced with permission of John Wiley & Sons.

around the brainstem (such as petro-clival meningiomas) may initially present with cranial nerve abnormalities, such as hearing loss or facial sensory disturbance before the development of ataxia or hemiparesis related to brainstem compression.

Radiological investigations

CT and MRI show tumours that enhance vividly following intravenous contrast (Figure 53.7). Hyperostosis of the cranial vault may occur at the site of attachment of the tumour, and these bony changes may often be seen on plain skull X-ray or better on the bone windows of the CT scan.

Treatment

The treatment of clinically significant meningiomas is surgical excision, if possible including obliteration of the dural attachment. Although this objective is often possible, there are some situations where complete excision is not possible because of the position of the tumour. Surgery may be preceded by embolisation of the main vascular supply of the tumour.

Incomplete resection carries the possibility of tumour recurrence, especially in those tumours that show 'atypical' histological features. In these tumours postoperative radiation therapy may be recommended to reduce the risk of recurrence.

Small asymptomatic meningiomas may be managed conservatively and followed with regular MRI.

Acoustic neuroma

Acoustic schwannomas arise from the eighth cranial nerve and account for 8% of intracranial tumours. The tumours are schwannomas, with their origin from the vestibular component of the eighth cranial nerve in or near the internal auditory meatus.

Clinical presentation

The clinical presentation of an acoustic schwannoma will depend on the size of the tumour at the time of diagnosis. The earliest symptoms are associated with eighth nerve involvement. Tinnitus and unilateral partial or complete sensory neural hearing loss are the earliest features. With extension into the cerebellopontine angle, the tumour will compress the trigeminal nerve, resulting in facial numbness, and the cerebellum, causing ataxia. Compression of the pyramidal tracts due to a large tumour causing brainstem compression will cause a

(a)

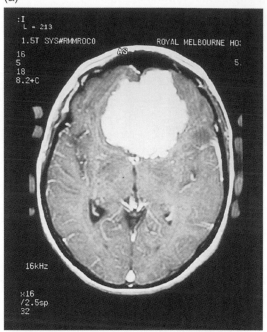

(b)

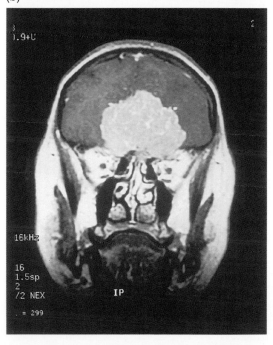

Fig. 53.7 (a) Axial and (b) coronal MRI showing meningioma with vivid contrast enhancement arising from floor of anterior carnial fossa (olfactory groove) and growing into superior frontal lobes.

contralateral hemiparesis, and a large tumour will also cause obstructive hydrocephalus. Smaller tumours can cause a communicating hydrocephalus due to raised protein in the CSF.

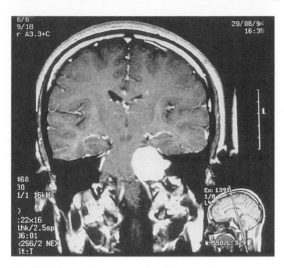

Fig. 53.8 Acoustic neuroma showing extension to tumour into internal auditory canal.

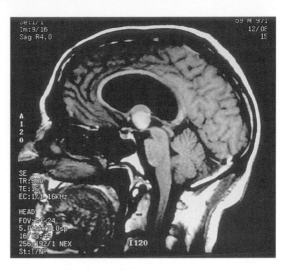

Fig. 53.9 Colloid cyst of third ventricle.

Radiological investigations

MRI will show an enhancing tumour usually in the internal auditory canal and with extension into the cerebellopontine angle. The internal auditory meatus and canal will be widened, indicating the tumour has arisen from the eighth cranial nerve (Figure 53.8). This is often best appreciated on CT scan that shows bone structures better than the MRI.

Treatment

The treatment of a large acoustic neuroma is surgical. Stereotactic radiosurgery has been advocated by some for smaller tumours (<2 cm diameter), with tumour control rates being in excess of 90%. However, the risks of surgery are higher in those patients in whom radiation fails to control the tumour and there remains a concern regarding the possible carcinogenic effects of radiation in the long term, especially in younger patients. Intracanalicular or small tumours in the elderly may be just observed and treatment advised only if there is evidence of tumour growth.

Colloid cyst of third ventricle

A colloid cyst of the third ventricle is situated in the anterior part of the ventricle and applied to the roof just behind the foramen of Munro. As the cyst grows it causes bilateral obstruction to the foramen of Munro resulting in raised ICP from hydrocephalus.

Radiological investigations include MRI and CT, which show a round tumour in the anterior third ventricle that usually enhances following intravenous contrast (Figure 53.9). The treatment is surgical excision.

Pituitary tumours

Pituitary tumours account for 8–10% of all intracranial tumours.

Pathology

Historically, three main types of pituitary tumours were defined by their cytoplasmic staining characteristics: chromophobic, acidophilic and basophilic. The development of immunoperoxidase techniques and electron microscopy have provided a more refined classification of pituitary adenomas based on the specific hormone produced. This classification is shown in Table 53.3. The tumours can be further classified by size, with microadenomas (<1 cm diameter) and macroadenomas (>1 cm diameter) being confined to the sella or with extrasellar extension (Figure 53.10).

Clinical presentation

The presenting clinical features of pituitary tumours are due to the size of the tumour and endocrine disturbance. Headache occurs principally in patients with acromegaly and is uncommon in other types of pituitary tumours.

VISUAL FAILURE

Suprasellar extension of the pituitary tumour causes compression of the optic chiasm resulting in bitemporal hemianopia. Optic atrophy will be evident in patients with long-standing compression of the chiasm. Extension of the tumour into the cavernous sinus may cause compression of the third, fourth or sixth cranial nerves.

ENDOCRINE DISTURBANCE

Endocrine disturbance is due to either hypopituitarism or excess secretion of a particular pituitary hormone.

Table 53.3 Classification of pituitary adenomas.

Hormone secreted	Percentage of tumours
Prolactin	40
Growth hormone	20
Null cell and endocrine inactive tumours	20
ACTH	15
Prolactin and growth hormone	5
FSH/LH	1–2
TSH	1
Acidophil stem cell (no hormone)	1–2

FSH, follicle-stimulating hormone; LH, luteinising hormone; TSH, thyroid-stimulating hormone.
Source: Kaye AH. *Essential Neurosurgery*, 3rd edn. Oxford: Blackwell Publishing, 2005. Reproduced with permission of John Wiley & Sons.

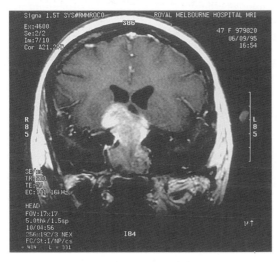

Fig. 53.10 Large pituitary tumour with marked suprasellar extension causing compression of the optic chiasma.

Hypopituitarism

Hypopituitarism results from failure of the hormone secreted by the adenohypophysis. The endocrine secretions are not equally depressed, but there is selective failure and the order of susceptibility is as follows: growth hormone, gonadotrophin, corticotrophin, thyroid-stimulating hormone. Hypopituitarism initially results in vague symptoms including lack of energy and tiredness, sexual impairment, undue fatiguability, muscle weakness and anorexia, and when prolonged or severe will cause low blood pressure. Clinical hypothyroidism is manifest by physical and mental sluggishness and a preference for warmth. When the hypopituitarism is severe episodic confusion occurs and the patient will become drowsy.

Pituitary apoplexy

Pituitary apoplexy results from sudden spontaneous haemorrhage into the pituitary tumour. It is characterised by sudden severe headache followed by transient and more prolonged loss of consciousness, with features of neck stiffness or vomiting and photophobia. Extension into the suprasellar cistern may cause visual failure and diplopia, but extension laterally into the cavernous sinus may cause compression of the nerves controlling ocular motility (third, fourth and sixth cranial nerves).

Prolactinoma

Prolactin-secreting tumours may be a microadenoma or a macroadenoma. Patients with microadenomas are usually women who present with infertility associated with amenorrhoea and galactorrhoea. These tumours can usually be treated with dopamine agonists such as bromocriptine or cabergoline, which have a direct inhibitory effect on the lactotroph cells via stimulation of dopamine D_2 receptors. Very large macroadenomas may occur in males who present with features of hypopituitarism and visual failure due to suprasellar extension.

Acromegaly

Acromegaly is caused by growth hormone-secreting pituitary adenomas. Growth hormone (GH) is a 191-amino acid single-chain polypeptide whose secretion is under the control of GH releasing and inhibiting factors transported via the hypothalamic–pituitary portal system. The anabolic effects of GH are mostly mediated through the production of insulin-like growth factor (IGF)-1 in the liver. The clinical features of acromegaly are numerous and include bone and soft tissue changes, as evidenced by an enlarged supraciliary ridge, enlarged frontal sinuses and increased mandibular size, which causes the chin to project (prognathism), and severe arthritis (especially in weight-bearing joints) and arthralgias. The hands and feet enlarge, and the skin becomes coarse and greasy and sweats profusely. The voice becomes hoarse and gruff. Systemic problems include hypertension, cardiac hypertrophy and diabetes. The clinical diagnosis must be confirmed by laboratory investigations that include measurement of both GH and IGF-1.

Cushing's disease

Cushing's disease is due to adrenocorticotropic hormone (ACTH)-producing pituitary adenomas. Over

80% of the tumours are microadenomas and there is a marked female predominance. The onset is often insidious and the disease may affect children or adults. Severe obesity occurs, the skin is tense and painful, and purple striae appear around the trunk. Fat is deposited, particularly on the face (moon-face), neck, cervicodorsal junction (buffalo hump) and trunk. The skin becomes purple due to vasodilatation and stasis. Spontaneous bruising is common. The skin is greasy, acne is common and facial hair excessive. Osteoporosis predisposes to spontaneous fractures and there is wasting of the muscles. Glucose tolerance is impaired and hypertension occurs. Laboratory investigations are vital to confirm the diagnosis and to differentiate Cushing's disease due to a pituitary ACTH-producing tumour from either an adrenal tumour or ectopic source of ACTH production such as small cell carcinoma of the lung.

Treatment

The treatment of patients with pituitary tumours depends on whether the patient has presented with features of endocrine disturbance or with problems related to compression of adjacent neural structures.

Surgical excision will be used as the primary method of treatment for the following.

- Large tumours (other than prolactin tumours) with extrasellar extension and especially if causing compression of adjacent neural structures, particularly the visual pathways.
- Growth hormone-secreting tumours causing acromegaly.
- ACTH-secreting tumours causing Cushing's disease.
- The occasional treatment of a prolactin-secreting adenoma when medical treatment using a dopamine agonist is not tolerated or is ineffective in reducing the size of the tumour.

Most tumours can be excised via the trans-sphenoidal approach to the pituitary fossa.

The treatment of patients with persistent acromegaly or Cushing's disease following surgery now involves pharmacological therapies, all of which have variable effectiveness. Dopamine agonists and somatostatin analogues (e.g. octreotide and lanreotide) are used in acromegaly. The most effective agents for Cushing's disease are those that inhibit adrenal steroidogenesis, such as ketoconazole, and those that inhibit cortisol synthesis, such as metyrapone. Radiotherapy may be indicated if the endocrine abnormality persists after trial of pharmacological agents and if there is tumour recurrence in non-secreting tumours.

Pineal region tumours

Tumours arising in the pineal region are relatively uncommon, accounting for 0.5% of all brain tumours, although they are much more common in China and Japan where their incidence is 5%. Most occur in the age group 10–30 years. The two major groups of tumours are germ cell tumours and pineal cell tumours. Germinomas are the commonest pineal region tumour, and teratoma the next most common germ cell tumour. These most frequently occur in children and adolescents. Pineocytoma and pineoblastoma more commonly occur in young adults.

Patients with pineal region tumours present with the following.

- Raised ICP due to obstructive hydrocephalus.
- Focal neurological signs: compression of the superior quadrigeminal plate causes limitation of upgaze, convergence paresis with impaired reaction of the pupils to light, and accommodation (Parinaud's syndrome).
- Endocrine disturbances are uncommon but include precocious puberty (nearly always in males) and diabetes insipidus.

The diagnosis is made by MRI and shows an enhancing tumour in the pineal region (Figure 53.11) and the likely associated hydrocephalus. The tumour markers alpha-fetoprotein and β-human chorionic gonadotrophin are specific for malignant germ cell elements. If present, biopsy may not be necessary and the tumour can be managed with radiation and chemotherapy.

If hydrocephalus is present, this is best treated by an endoscopic third ventriculostomy, at which time a biopsy of the tumour can also be obtained. Germinomas are very radiosensitive and may be treated with radiation, but the other tumours with negative tumour markers will require resection.

SUBARACHNOID HAEMORRHAGE AND CEREBRAL ANEURYSM

The sudden onset of a severe headache in a patient should be regarded as subarachnoid haemorrhage until proven otherwise. The most common cause of subarachnoid haemorrhage in adults is rupture of a berry aneurysm. Subarachnoid haemorrhage in children is much less common than in the adult population, and the most common paediatric cause is rupture of an arteriovenous malformation. Cerebral aneurysm as a cause of subarachnoid haemorrhage becomes more frequent than arteriovenous malformation in patients over the age of 20 years.

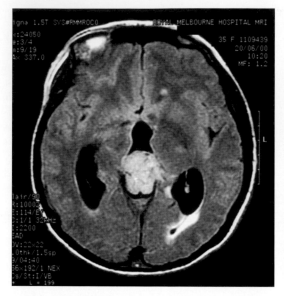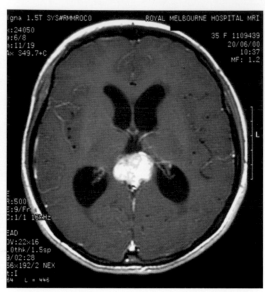

Fig. 53.11 T1-weighted MRI with enhancement showing pineal tumour.

Subarachnoid haemorrhage

Clinical presentation

HEADACHE

The sudden onset of a severe headache of a type not previously experienced by the patient is the hallmark of subarachnoid haemorrhage. A relatively small leak from an aneurysm may result in a minor headache, sometimes referred to as a 'sentinel headache', and this may be the warning episode of a subsequent major haemorrhage from the aneurysm.

DIMINISHED CONSCIOUS STATE

Most patients have some deterioration of their conscious state following subarachnoid haemorrhage. This varies from only slight change, when the haemorrhage has been minor, to apoplectic death resulting from massive haemorrhage.

MENINGISMUS

Blood in the subarachnoid CSF will cause the features of meningismus (headache, neck stiffness, photophobia and fever or vomiting).

FOCAL NEUROLOGICAL SIGNS

Focal neurological signs may occur in subarachnoid haemorrhage due to concomitant intracerebral haemorrhage, the local pressure effects of the aneurysm itself (such as a third cranial nerve palsy resulting from pressure from a posterior communicating artery aneurysm) or cerebral vasospasm that follows subarachnoid haemorrhage.

Clinical assessment

The major differential diagnosis of subarachnoid haemorrhage is meningitis, although a minor haemorrhage is often misdiagnosed as migraine. Confirmation of the clinical diagnosis of subarachnoid haemorrhage should be undertaken as soon as possible by CT scanning (Figure 53.12). If there is any doubt that subarachnoid blood is present on the CT scan, as may occur following more minor haemorrhages, a lumbar puncture is essential. The presence of xanthochromia (yellow staining) in the CSF will confirm subarachnoid haemorrhage. This can be assessed visually, by examining the supernatant following centrifugation of the CSF sample, or by spectrophotometry.

Cerebral angiography (Figure 53.13) will confirm the cause of the subarachnoid haemorrhage and will determine the subsequent treatment.

Cerebral aneurysm

Cerebral aneurysms are the most common cause of subarachnoid haemorrhage in the adult population. The great majority of aneurysms arise at branch points of two vessels and are situated mainly on the circle of Willis, about 85% on the anterior half of the circle and 15% in the posterior circulation (Box 53.2). Aneurysms occur in more than one position in approximately 15% of cases.

Management

Management of patients following rupture of a cerebral aneurysm is determined by three factors:
- severity of the initial haemorrhage
- rebleeding of the aneurysm
- cerebral vasospasm.

About 30% of all patients suffering a subarachnoid haemorrhage from a ruptured aneurysm either undergo apoplectic death or are deeply comatose as

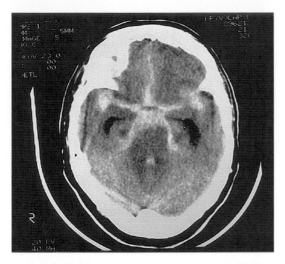

Fig. 53.12 Diffuse blood in the basal cisterns confirming the diagnosis of subarachnoid haemorrhage.

(a)

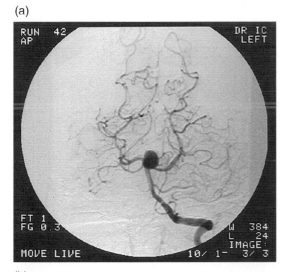

(b)

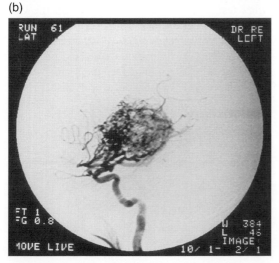

Fig. 53.13 (a) Cerebral aneurysm on angiogram.
(b) Arteriovenous malformation.

Box 53.2 Position of cerebral aneurysm

Anterior circle of Willis
Anterior communicating artery
Middle cerebral artery: bifurcation or trifurcation
Internal carotid artery
   Posterior communicating artery
   Terminal bifurcation
   Anterior choroidal artery
   Ophthalmic artery
   Intracavernous
   Pericallosal artery

Posterior circulation (15%)
Terminal basilar artery: most common
Vertebrobasilar junction
Posterior inferior cerebellar artery
Anterior inferior cerebellar artery
Superior anterior cerebellar artery
Superior inferior cerebellar artery
Posterior cerebral artery

Source: Kaye AH. *Essential Neurosurgery*, 3rd edn. Oxford: Blackwell Publishing, 2005. Reproduced with permission of John Wiley & Sons.

---

a result of the initial haemorrhage. Rebleeding occurs in about 50% of patients within 6 weeks and in 25% of patients within 2 weeks of the initial haemorrhage. The only certain way to prevent the aneurysm rebleeding is to occlude it from the circulation. Cerebral vasospasm usually does not commence until 72 hours after the initial haemorrhage. It occurs in 50% of patients following subarachnoid haemorrhage and in 25% it results in serious neurological complications. Clinical vasospasm is treated using hypertension and volume expansion, and consequently the treatment is most effective if the aneurysm has been occluded.

Surgery or endovascular occlusion
Although in the past surgery has often been delayed for fear that it might exacerbate cerebral vasospasm, the current treatment of cerebral aneurysm is immediate obliteration of the aneurysm by either surgery or an endovascular technique. Active intervention is usually not performed on patients who are comatose or have features of decerebrate posturing unless the CT scan shows a large intracerebral haematoma resulting from the ruptured aneurysm that needs to be evacuated, or hydrocephalus as a cause of the poor neurological state. Evacuation of intracerebral haematoma or drainage of the hydrocephalus should be performed urgently, and the aneurysm occluded.

The surgical procedure involves a craniotomy with occlusion of the neck of the aneurysm, usually with a titanium clip. Endovascular techniques, using detachable coils, have been shown to have an increasing role in the treatment of cerebral aneurysms, particularly for posterior fossa (basilar tip) aneurysms. Most centres treating aneurysms utilise endovascular coiling in over 60% of cases.

INTRACRANIAL INFECTION

Although infections involving the nervous system may present in many ways and involve a large variety of pathogens, the most common infections involving the neurosurgeon are acute bacterial meningitis and cerebral abscess.

Meningitis

Bacterial meningitis is a serious life-threatening infection that requires urgent treatment with the appropriate antibiotic. Most of the common organisms that cause bacterial meningitis are related to the patient's age and to the presence and nature of any underlying predisposing disease. Table 53.4 shows the common organisms causing bacterial meningitis related to age.

The bacteria reach the meninges and CSF by three main routes:
- haematogenous spread from extracranial foci of infection
- retrograde spread via infected thrombi within emissary veins from infections adjacent to the CNS such as sinusitis, otitis or mastoiditis
- direct spread into the subarachnoid space such as from osteomyelitis of the skull and infected paranasal sinuses.

Table 53.4 Common organisms causing primary bacterial meningitis related to age.

Age	Organism
Neonate (0–4 weeks)	Group B streptococcus, *Escherichia coli*
4–12 weeks	Group B streptococcus, *Streptococcus pneumoniae*, *Salmonella*, *Haemophilus influenzae*, *Listeria monocytogenes*
3 months to 5 years	*Haemophilus influenzae*, *Streptococcus pneumoniae*, *Neisseria meningitidis*
Over 5 years and adults	*Streptococcus pneumoniae*, *Neisseria meningitidis*

Source: Kaye AH. *Essential Neurosurgery*, 3rd edn. Oxford: Blackwell Publishing, 2005. Reproduced with permission of John Wiley & Sons.

Clinical presentation

Bacterial meningitis is usually an acute illness with rapid progression of the clinical signs. The major presenting features are high fever and meningismus, including headache, neck stiffness, photophobia and vomiting. Although patients are usually alert at the commencement of the illness, they will frequently become drowsy and confused.

In infants, neonates, the elderly and the immunocompromised, the presentation of bacterial meningitis may be different. Neck stiffness and fever are often absent and the presentation includes listlessness and irritability in the young and confusion or obtundation in the elderly. A careful search must be made for a skin rash. Meningococcal infection frequently manifests a coexisting petechial rash, which occurs less frequently in other bacterial or viral infections.

In some patients the original source of the infection, for example sinusitis, bacterial endocarditis, otitis media or mastoiditis, may be evident and many patients have evidence of pharyngitis – bacterial meningitis sometimes follows another respiratory tract infection.

The diagnosis is made by CSF examination obtained by lumbar puncture, which should be performed immediately once the diagnosis is suspected. If the patient is drowsy, has other signs of raised ICP or if there are focal neurological signs, an urgent CT scan must be performed prior to lumbar puncture to exclude an intracranial space-occupying lesion.

The CSF features in a lumbar puncture are:
- raised cell count, predominantly a polymorphonuclear leucocytosis
- protein level greater than 0.8 g/L
- glucose level less than 2 mmol/L
- positive Gram stain in more than 70%.

Other tests that should be performed on the CSF include examination for *Cryptococcus neoformans* and for *Mycobacterium tuberculosis*. Other investigations should include blood cultures and radiological investigations to detect the source of the infection (chest X-ray, CT scan or skull X-ray for sinusitis).

The differential diagnoses include:
- other types of meningitis (viral, fungal, carcinomatosis)
- subdural empyema (patients are drowsy, with focal neurological signs, and usually have seizures)
- subarachnoid haemorrhage
- viral encephalitis.

Treatment

High-dose intravenous antibiotic therapy should be commenced immediately, and the selection of the antibiotic depends on the initial expectation of the most likely organism involved, taking into account the age of the patient, source of infection, CSF microbiology studies and the antibiotic that has best penetration to CSF.

There are many antibiotic regimens, but if bacterial meningitis is suspected empirical antibiotic therapy must commence immediately as follows.

- Neonates (under 3 months): cefotaxime or ceftriaxone plus benzylpenicillin or amoxicillin/ampicillin.
- 3 months to 15 years: cefotaxime or ceftriaxone.
- 15 years to adults: cefotaxime/ceftriaxone plus benzylpenicillin or amoxicillin.
- Add vancomycin if Gram-positive streptococci are seen in the CSF or if *Streptococcus pneumoniae* is suspected clinically (e.g. by the presence of sinusitis or otitis) to cover the possibility of intermediate and/or resistant *S. pneumoniae*.

When the organism has been identified, the most appropriate antibiotic should be used, depending on sensitivities and the ability of the antibiotic to penetrate the CSF.

The usual specific antimicrobial therapy following identification of the organism is as follows.

- *Streptococcus pneumoniae* or *Neisseria meningitidis*: benzylpenicillin (child: 60 mg/kg up to 1.8–2.4 g i.v. 4-hourly). If the organism is not sensitive to penicillin or the patient is allergic to penicillin, use cefotaxime (child: 15 mg/kg 6-hourly or ceftriaxone 100 mg/kg daily). If a meningococcal rash is present or there are signs of septicaemia, systemic antibiotic treatment must be instituted immediately before diagnostic tests. About half the patients with meningococcal meningitis have petechiae or purpura. Subclinical or clinical disseminated intravascular coagulation often accompanies meningococcaemia and may progress to haemorrhage, infarction of the adrenal glands, renal cortical necrosis, pulmonary vascular thrombosis, shock and death. The antibiotic therapy must be accompanied by intensive medical supportive therapy. If *S. pneumoniae* is resistant to both penicillin and third-generation cephalosporins (cefotaxime and ceftriaxone), then vancomycin is recommended.
- *Haemophilus influenzae*: amoxicillin/ampicillin if organism is susceptible. If the patient is allergic or organism resistant, use cefotaxime or ceftriaxone.
- *Listeria*: benzylpenicillin or amoxicillin/ampicillin or trimethoprim and sulfamethoxazole.
- Hospital-acquired meningitis: vancomycin plus ceftazidime or vancomycin plus meropenem.

The decision regarding the most appropriate antibiotic must be made in conjunction with an infectious disease consultant.

In addition, intravenous dexamethasone may be indicated but this must be discussed with an infectious disease specialist and/or neurosurgeon before commencement. Current evidence favours early treatment with dexamethasone in *Haemophilus* meningitis in childhood and in adults with pneumococcal meningitis and should be given before the first dose of antibiotics. However, antibiotic treatment *must not be delayed* if dexamethasone is unavailable.

Complications of bacterial meningitis

Complications are more likely to occur if treatment is not commenced immediately. The major complications are:

- cerebral oedema
- seizures
- communicating hydrocephalus, which may occur early in the disease or as a late manifestation
- subdural effusion, particularly in children, with most resolving spontaneously but some requiring drainage.

Rarer complications include:

- subdural empyema, which usually requires drainage
- brain abscess.

Brain abscess

Cerebral abscess may result from:

- haematogenous spread from a known septic site or occult focus
- direct spread from an infected paranasal or mastoid sinus
- trauma causing a penetrating wound.

Metastatic brain abscesses arising from haematogenous dissemination of infection are frequently multiple and develop at the junction of white and grey matter. Most common sites of infection include skin pustules, chronic pulmonary infection (bronchiectasis), diverticulitis, osteomyelitis and bacterial endocarditis. The site of origin of haematogenous spread is unknown in approximately 25% of patients.

Direct spread from paranasal sinuses, mastoid air cells or the middle ear are the most common pathogenic mechanisms in many series. Infection from the paranasal sinuses spread either into the frontal or temporal lobe and the abscesses are usually single and located superficially. Frontal sinusitis may cause an abscess in the frontal lobe. Middle ear infection may spread into the temporal lobe and uncommonly the cerebellum.

Table 53.5 Cerebral abscess: pathogenesis and principal organisms.

History	Site of infection	Predominant organism
Sinusitis: frontal	Frontal lobe	Aerobic streptococci *Streptococcus milleri* *Haemophilus* species
Mastoiditis, otitis	Temporal lobe	Mixed flora Aerobic and anaerobic streptococci Enterobacteria *Bacteroides fragilis* *Haemophilus* species
Haematogenous, cryptogenic	Brain	Aerobic streptococci Anaerobic streptococci Enterobacteria
Trauma	Brain	*Staphylococcus aureus*

Source: Kaye AH. *Essential Neurosurgery*, 3rd edn. Oxford: Blackwell Publishing, 2005. Reproduced with permission of John Wiley & Sons.

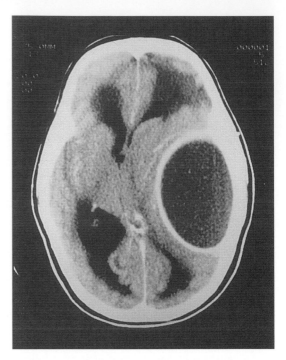

Fig. 53.14 Cerebral abscess: a ring-enhancing mass. Source: Kaye AH. *Essential Neurosurgery*, 3rd edn. Oxford: Blackwell Publishing, 2005. Reproduced with permission of John Wiley & Sons.

Bacteriology

Table 53.5 details the pathogenesis and principal organisms in cerebral abscess. Streptococci are isolated from approximately 80% of brain abscesses. The most common single species is the α-haemolytic carboxyphilic *Streptococcus milleri*, whose major habitat is the alimentary tract including the mouth and dental plaque. Otogenic abscesses usually yield mixed flora, including *Bacteroides*, various streptococci and members of the Enterobacteriaceae. *Staphylococcus aureus* is often the pathogen in abscesses resulting from trauma.

Presenting features

- An intracranial mass (raised ICP, focal neurological signs, epilepsy)
- Systemic toxicity (fever and malaise in 60% of cases)
- Clinical features of the underlying source of infection (sinusitis, bacterial endocarditis, diverticulitis)

Diagnosis

CT and MRI (Figure 53.14) show a ring enhancing mass often surrounded by considerable oedema.

Management

The principles of treatment are:
- identify the bacterial organism
- institute antibiotic therapy
- drain or excise the abscess.

A specimen of pus is essential for accurate identification of the organism. Antibiotic therapy should be commenced as soon as the pus has been obtained. The initial choice of antibiotic, before culture results are available, will depend on the probable cause of the brain abscess and the Gram stain. The therapy will be refined once the organism is known. Anticonvulsant medication should be commenced as there is an incidence of seizures of 30–50%.

The abscess may need to be treated by either single or repeat aspiration. Surgical excision of the abscess may be necessary if there is persistent reaccumulation of the pus, or if a fibrous capsule develops that fails to collapse despite repeat aspirations. A cerebellar abscess requires excision.

Further reading

Colli BC, Carlotti CG, Machado HR, Assirati JA. Intracranial bacterial infections. *Neurosurg Q* 1999;9: 258–84.

Dorsch NWC, King MT. A review of cerebral vasospasm in aneurysmal subarachnoid haemorrhage. *J Clin Neurosci* 1994;1:19–26.

International Subarachnoid Aneurysm Trial (ISAT) Collaborative Group. International Subarachnoid Aneurysm Trial (ISAT) of neurosurgical clipping vs endovascular coiling in 2143 patients with ruptured intracranial aneurysms: a randomised trial. *Lancet* 2002;360:1267–73.

Kaye AH. *Essential Neurosurgery*, 3rd edn. Oxford: Blackwell Publishing, 2005.

Kaye AH, Black PMcL. *Operative Neurosurgery*. Edinburgh: Churchill Livingstone, 1999.

Kaye AH, Laws ER. *Brain Tumors*, 2nd edn. Edinburgh: Churchill Livingstone, 2001.

Stephanov S. Surgical treatment of brain abscess. *Neurosurgery* 1988;22:724–30.

Stupp R, Mason WP, van den Bent MJ *et al.* Radiotherapy plus concomitant and adjuvant temozolomide for glioblastoma multiforme. *N Engl J Med* 2005;352:987–96.

Weir B. Unruptured intracranial aneurysms: a review. *J Neurosurg* 2002;96:3–42.

MCQs

Select the single correct answer to each question. The correct answers can be found in the Answers section at the end of the book.

1 Which of the following statements is correct?
   a meningioma is the most common malignant adult brain tumour
   b brain tumours are rare in children
   c high-grade cerebral gliomas are invariably fatal
   d metastatic cancer in the brain is uncommon
   e oligodendroglioma is the most common type of glioma

2 Which of the following statements about cerebral gliomas in adults is correct?
   a do not infiltrate through the brain
   b are best managed with chemotherapy
   c rarely cause raised intracranial pressure
   d are best visualised by MRI
   e most frequently occur in the cerebellum

3 Which of the following statements about brain tumours in children is correct?
   a most commonly occur in the posterior fossa
   b can be cured with surgery
   c never metastasise
   d invariably have an excellent prognosis
   e most frequently present with epilepsy

4 Which of the following statements about cerebral aneurysms is correct?
   a usually occur on the peripheral intracranial vessels
   b can be definitively diagnosed by a CT scan
   c are the most common cause of subarachnoid haemorrhage in adults
   d are virtually always multiple
   e usually present with focal seizures

5 Which of the following statements about subarachnoid haemorrhage is correct?
   a is most commonly due to ruptured arteriovenous malformation in adults
   b usually presents as an epileptic seizure as the initial symptom
   c must be evacuated as an emergency
   d is characterised by the onset of a sudden severe headache
   e is frequently due to haemorrhage from a tumour

6 Which of the following statements about pituitary tumours is correct?
   a the tumour is always confined to the sella
   b adults frequently present with growth retardation
   c prolactin-secreting tumours are best treated with surgery
   d ACTH-secreting tumours cause Cushing's disease
   e posterior pituitary function is almost always absent in patients presenting with large tumours

54 Nerve injuries, peripheral nerve entrapments and spinal cord compression

Andrew H. Kaye

Department of Surgery, University of Melbourne and Royal Melbourne Hospital, Melbourne, Victoria, Australia

Introduction

Peripheral nerves may be trapped, compressed or injured at any position along their course, although there are certain regions where they are especially vulnerable. Injury to the nerve occurs when the nerve is either relatively superficial and exposed, or lying adjacent to bone so that the jagged fractured ends of the bone may directly injure the nerve. Nerve entrapments occur particularly where the peripheral nerve passes through a tunnel formed by ligaments, bone and/or muscle.

Acute nerve injuries

Peripheral nerve anatomy

The axon projects from the cell body and is surrounded by a basement membrane and myelin sheath. The axon is covered by the endoneurium, the innermost layer of connective tissue, and a number of axons are grouped together in a bundle called a fascicle, which is invested by a further connective tissue sheath called the perineurium. The peripheral nerve consists of a group of fascicles covered by the outermost layer of connective tissue, the epineurium.

Classification of nerve injuries

There is no single classification system that can describe all the many variations of nerve injury. Most systems attempt to correlate the degree of injury with symptoms, pathology and prognosis. Seddon in 1943 introduced a classification of nerve injuries which forms the basis for more refined classifications. It is based on three main types of nerve fibre injury and whether there is continuity of the nerve (Table 54.1).

Neurotmesis

Neurotmesis is the most severe injury. The nerve is completely divided and complete distal Wallerian degeneration occurs. There is complete loss of motor, sensory and autonomic function.

Although the term *neurotmesis* implies a cutting of the nerve, the term is also used when the epineurium of the nerve is still in continuity but the axons have been destroyed and replaced by scar tissue to such a degree that spontaneous regeneration is impossible. If the nerve has been completely divided, axonal regeneration causes a neuroma to form in the proximal stump.

Axonotmesis

Axonotmesis is characterised by complete interruption of the axons and their myelin sheaths, but with preservation of the epineurium and perineurium. Spontaneous regeneration will occur, with the intact endoneurial sheaths guiding the regenerating fibres to their distal connections. Axonotmesis is initially clinically indistinguishable from neurotmesis because there is complete and immediate loss of motor, sensory and autonomic function distal to the lesion with a similar picture on electromyogram (EMG). Regeneration occurs at a rate of 1–2 mm per day so that the time of recovery will depend on the distance between a lesion and the end organ, as well as on the age of the patient. The major types of injuries causing axonotmesis include compression, traction, missile and ischaemia.

Textbook of Surgery, Fourth Edition. Edited by Julian A. Smith, Andrew H. Kaye, Christopher Christophi and Wendy A. Brown.
© 2020 John Wiley & Sons Ltd. Published 2020 by John Wiley & Sons Ltd.

Table 54.1 Classification of nerve injuries.

	Neurotmesis	Axonotmesis	Neurapraxia
Pathological			
Anatomical continuity	May be lost	Preserved	Preserved
Essential damage	Complete disorganisation, Schwann sheaths preserved	Nerve fibres interrupted	Selective demyelination of larger fibres, no degeneration of axons
Clinical			
Motor paralysis	Complete	Complete	Complete
Muscle atrophy	Progressive	Progressive	Very little
Sensory paralysis	Complete	Complete	Usually much sparing
Autonomic paralysis	Complete	Complete	Usually much sparing
Electrical phenomena			
Reaction of degeneration	Present	Present	Absent
Nerve conduction distal to the lesion	Absent	Absent	Preserved
Motor-unit action potentials	Absent	Absent	Absent
Fibrillation	Present	Present	Occasionally detectable
Recovery			
Surgical repair	Essential	Not necessary	Not necessary
Rate of recovery	1–2 mm/day after repair	1–2 mm/day	Rapid, days or weeks
March of recovery	According to order of innervation	According to order of innervation	No order
Quality	Always imperfect	Perfect	Perfect

Source: adapted from Seddon H. *Surgical Disorders of the Peripheral Nerves*, 3rd edn. Oxford: Blackwell Publishing, 2005. Reproduced with permission of John Wiley & Sons.

Neurapraxia

Neurapraxia is the most mild form of injury and is likened to a transient 'concussion' of the nerve, where there is a temporary loss of function that is reversible within hours to months of the injury (with an average of 6–8 weeks). If there is initially a complete loss of function, neurapraxia cannot be distinguished from the more serious type of injury but will be recognised in retrospect when recovery of function has occurred sooner than would be possible following Wallerian degeneration.

Causes of peripheral nerve injury

The type of trauma will determine the nature of the injury to the nerve (Box 54.1).

Management of nerve injuries

The basis of management depends on a precise assessment of the damage that has been done to the nerve (Box 54.2). The types of injuries vary considerably, from an isolated single nerve lesion to a complex nerve injury in a patient with multiple trauma.

Brachial plexus injury

The mechanisms of injury are the same as for any peripheral nerve (see Box 54.1).

Birth injuries

Birth injuries include Erb's palsy due to damage to the upper trunk of the brachial plexus, Klumpke's paralysis due to damage to the lower trunk of the brachial plexus (C8 and T1; resulting from the arm being held up while traction is applied to the body during a breech delivery), and paralysis of the whole arm as a result of severe birth trauma.

Adolescents and adults

In adolescents and adults the most common cause is severe traction on the brachial plexus, resulting most frequently from a motorbike or motor vehicle accident. The trauma may result in damage to any part of the plexus but severe traction may result in

---

Box 54.1 Types of trauma and the nature of nerve injury

- Lacerations cause neurotmesis, with complete or partial division of the nerve.
- Missile injuries may cause the spectrum of nerve injury from complete disruption of the nerve to a mild neurapraxia.
- Traction and stretch trauma may result in either complete disruption of the nerve or, if minor, a neurapraxia. This type of mechanism is responsible particularly for brachial plexus injuries following motorbike accidents, radial or peroneal nerve injuries. It is a common mechanism of nerve injuries associated with skeletal fractures.
- Fractures or fracture dislocation may cause nerve injuries when the adjacent nerve is either compressed by the displaced bone fragments or, less commonly, severed by the jagged edge of the bone.
- Compression ischaemia may produce a neurapraxia in mild cases or, if prolonged and severe, axonotmesis or neurotmesis. It is the cause of the pressure palsies following improper application of a tourniquet or the 'Saturday night palsy', in which the radial nerve has been compressed against the humerus.
- Injection injury results from either direct trauma by the needle or the toxic effect of the agent injected. As would be expected, the sciatic and radial nerves are the most commonly affected.
- Electrical and burn injuries are uncommon causes of serious peripheral nerve damage.

Box 54.2 General guidelines for management of nerve injuries

- Determination of the exact nerve involved by (i) the clinical deficit and (ii) the position of the injury.
- Assessment of the type of nerve damaged by the mechanism of injury.
- If a neurapraxia or axonotmesis is suspected on clinical grounds, there is no specific surgical treatment for the nerve but physiotherapy should commence as soon as possible to prevent stiffness of the joints and contractures.
- Immediate or early exploration of the nerve should be undertaken in the following circumstances:
- When it is highly probable that the type of injury (e.g. laceration) has caused the nerve to be severed.
- If the nerve injury has been caused by a displaced fracture that needs reduction by open surgery, it is appropriate to explore the nerve at that time.
- Delayed exploration of the nerve will be indicated if the clinical and EMG findings indicate failure of regeneration of the nerve beyond the time expected, i.e. the injury has resulted in a neurotmesis rather than an axonotmesis or neurapraxia.

tearing of the arachnoid and dura with nerve root avulsion from the spinal cord.

Management

The management involves determination of the exact neurological injury, particularly the part of the brachial plexus involved (Figure 54.1). The presence of Horner's syndrome is evidence there has been avulsion of the nerve roots from the spinal cord.

Magnetic resonance imaging (MRI) may show the pseudomeningocele characteristic of nerve root avulsion. Electrical studies provide useful baseline data for future comparison. It is reasonable to obtain these studies 8 weeks after the injury.

There is debate concerning the indications for surgical intervention for closed brachial plexus injuries in adults. In general there is limited benefit from early exploration of the plexus in closed injuries, although some surgeons do advocate exploration approximately 4 months after the injury if clinical and electrical evidence shows the lesion to

be complete. If the injury is improving there is no indication for surgery and management includes intensive physiotherapy and mobilisation of the joints. There is no place for surgical repair of the injured nerve itself if there is evidence of nerve root avulsion from the cord, but nerve and tendon transfer procedures may considerably improve the functional outcome.

Peripheral nerve entrapment

Entrapment neuropathies occur particularly when nerves pass near joints. Less common forms of entrapment neuropathies may lie at a distance from a joint. Box 54.3 lists the common and less frequent entrapment neuropathies.

Carpal tunnel syndrome

This is by far the most common nerve entrapment and women are affected four times more frequently than men.

Anatomy

The carpal tunnel is a fibro-osseous tunnel on the palmar surface of the wrist (Figure 54.2). The dorsal and lateral walls consist of the carpal bones,

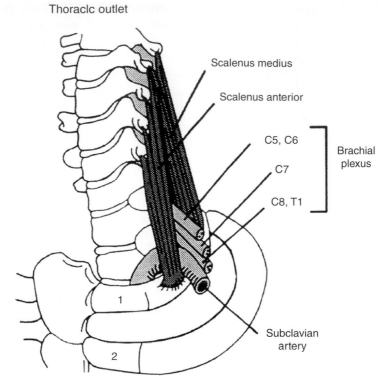

Thoracic outlet

Scalenus medius

Scalenus anterior

C5, C6

C7

Brachial plexus

C8, T1

Subclavian artery

Fig. 54.1 The brachial plexus passing through the cervicobrachial junction. Source: Kaye AH. *Essential Neurosurgery*, 3rd edn. Oxford: Blackwell Publishing, 2005. Reproduced with permission of John Wiley & Sons.

Box 54.3 Entrapment neuropathies (the more common ones are shown in bold)

Median nerve
- **Carpal tunnel syndrome**
- Supracondylar entrapment
- Cubital fossa entrapment
- Anterior interosseus nerve entrapment

Ulnar nerve
- **Tardy ulnar palsy**
- Deep branch of ulnar nerve

Radial nerve (posterior interosseus nerve)
Suprascapular nerve
Meralgia paresthetica (lateral femoral cutaneous nerve of thigh)
Sciatic nerve
Tarsal tunnel syndrome
Thoracic outlet syndrome

---

which form a crescentic trough. A tunnel is made by the fibrous flexor retinaculum, which is attached to the pisiform and hook of the hamate medially and the tuberosity of the scaphoid and crest of the trapezium laterally. The contents of the tunnel are the median nerve and flexor tendons of the flexor digitorum superficialis, flexor digitorum profundus and flexor pollicis longus.

Aetiology

The initial symptoms occur in women during pregnancy and in both sexes when they are performing unusual strenuous work with their hands, although the features of carpal tunnel syndrome may present at any stage throughout the adult years. A number of systemic conditions are associated with, and may predispose to, carpal tunnel syndrome:
- pregnancy and lactation
- contraceptive pill
- rheumatoid arthritis
- myxoedema
- acromegaly.

Any local condition around the wrist joint that decreases the size of the carpal tunnel will also predispose to carpal tunnel syndrome. These include a ganglion, tenosynovitis, unreduced fractures or dislocations of the wrist or carpal bones, and any local arthritis.

Clinical features

The principal clinical features of carpal tunnel syndrome are pain, numbness and tingling.

The pain, which may be described as burning or aching, is frequently felt throughout the whole hand and not just in the lateral three digits. There is

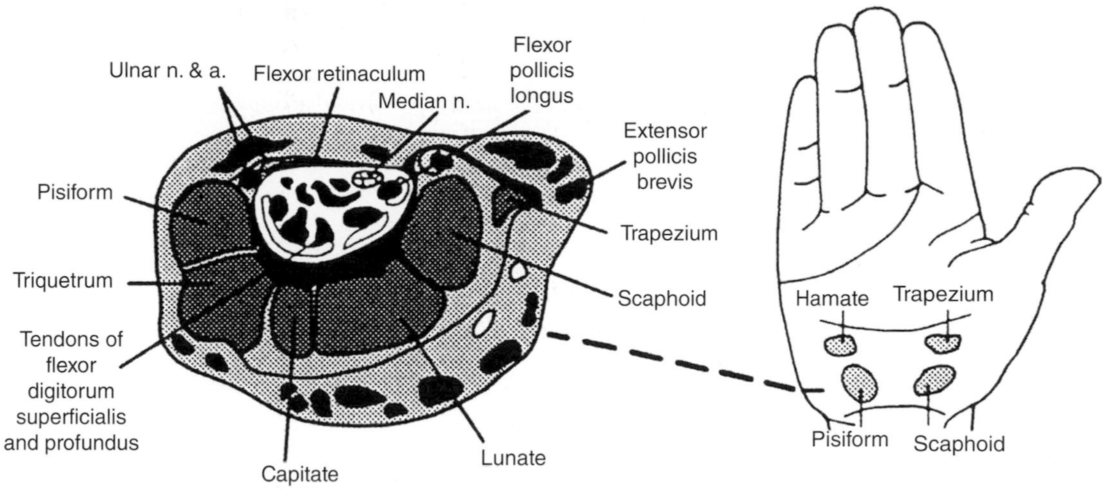

Fig. 54.2 The carpal tunnel just distal to the wrist. Source: Kaye AH. *Essential Neurosurgery*, 3rd edn. Oxford: Blackwell Publishing, 2005. Reproduced with permission of John Wiley & Sons.

often a diffuse radiation of the pain up the forearm to the elbow and occasionally into the upper arm. The symptoms are particularly worse at night, and on awakening the patient has to shake the hand to obtain any relief.

Numbness and tingling principally occur in the lateral three and a half fingers, in the distribution of the median nerve, although the patient frequently complains of more diffuse sensory loss throughout the fingers. This symptom is also worse at night and with activity involving the hands. The patient frequently complains that the hand feels 'clumsy', but with no specific weakness.

There are often only minimal signs of median nerve entrapment at the wrist. The Tinel sign (tingling in the median nerve-innervated thumb, index and middle finger) may be elicited by tapping over the median nerve but its absence has little diagnostic value.

If the compression has been prolonged there may be signs of median nerve dysfunction, including wasting of the thenar muscle, weakness of muscles innervated by the distal median nerve, especially abductor pollicis brevis, and diminished sensation over the distribution of the median nerve in the hand. The clinical diagnosis can be confirmed by EMG.

Treatment

Surgery involving division of the flexor retinaculum is a simple and effective method of relieving the compression and curing the symptoms. However, conservative treatment involving the use of a wrist splint and non-steroidal anti-inflammatory agents is appropriate if the symptoms are mild or intermittent or if there is a reversible underlying precipitating condition, such as pregnancy or oral contraceptive pill.

Ulnar nerve entrapment at the elbow

Anatomy

The ulnar nerve runs behind the medial epicondyle of the humerus and enters the forearm through a fibro-osseous tunnel formed by the aponeurotic attachment of the two heads of flexor carpi ulnaris, which span from the medial epicondyle of the humerus to the olecranon process of the ulnar forming the cubital tunnel (Figure 54.3). During flexion of the elbow the ligament tightens and the volume of the cubital tunnel decreases, putting increasing pressure on the underlying nerve. Compression can also be due to injuries in the region producing deformity of the elbow, although the features of ulnar nerve entrapment do not usually appear for some years. This delay in the appearance of symptoms led to the term 'tardy ulnar palsy'.

Aetiology

In most cases there is no particular predisposing cause. In a minority there are underlying factors that predispose to nerve entrapment, including lengthy periods of bed rest from coma or major illness, and poor positioning of the upper limbs during long operations causing prolonged pressure on the nerve. Other causes include arthritis of the elbow, ganglion cysts of the elbow joint and direct trauma.

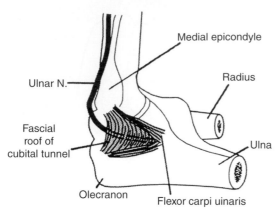

Fig. 54.3 The ulnar nerve passing behind the medial epicondyle of the humerus and through the cubital tunnel. Source: Kaye AH. *Essential Neurosurgery*, 3rd edn. Oxford: Blackwell Publishing, 2005. Reproduced with permission of John Wiley & Sons.

Clinical features

The clinical features include paraesthesia and numbness in the ring and little finger of the hand and the adjacent medial border of the hand, wasting of the hypothenar eminence and interossei muscles, and weakness.

In advanced cases, entrapment of the ulnar nerve will lead to weakness of the muscles of the hypothenar eminence, the interossei, the medial two lumbricals, adductor pollicis, flexor digitorum profundus (ring and little finger) and flexor carpi ulnaris. Paralysis of the small muscles of the hand causes 'claw hand', this posture being produced by the unopposed action of their antagonists. As the interossei cause flexion of the fingers at the metacarpophalangeal joints and extension at the interphalangeal joints, when these muscles are paralysed the opposite posture is maintained by the long flexors and extensors causing flexion at the interphalangeal joints and hyperextension at the metacarpophalangeal joints. This is most pronounced in the ring and little fingers as the two radial lumbricals, which are innervated by the median nerve, compensate to some degree for the impaired action of the interossei on the index and middle fingers. Froment's sign is demonstrated by asking the patient to grasp a piece of cardboard between the index finger and thumb against resistance. There will be flexion of the interphalangeal joint of the thumb because the median innervated flexor pollicis longus is used rather than the weakened adductor pollicis.

Treatment

Conservative treatment may be tried if the clinical features are minor and not progressive. The patient should avoid putting pressure on the nerve at the elbow during reading, sitting or lying and should cease heavy work with the arms.

Surgery involves decompression of the nerve and is indicated if there are progressive symptoms or signs and if there is any wasting or weakness.

Meralgia paresthetica

Meralgia paresthetica results from entrapment of the lateral cutaneous nerve of the thigh beneath the inguinal ligament, just medial to the anterior superior iliac spine. At this position the nerve passes between two roots of attachment of the inguinal ligament to the iliac bone and there is a sharp angulation of the nerve as it passes from the iliac fossa into the thigh.

Prolonged standing or walking and an obese pendulous anterior abdominal wall accentuates the downward pull on the inguinal ligament and may predispose to entrapment of the nerve. The syndrome is most frequently seen in middle-aged men who are overweight and in young army recruits during strenuous training.

The principal symptom is a painful dysaesthesia in the anterolateral aspect of the thigh, with the patient often describing the sensation as 'burning', 'pins and needles' or 'prickling'. The only neurological sign is diminished sensation over the anterolateral aspect of the thigh in the distribution of the lateral cutaneous nerve.

The symptoms may be only minor and the patient may be satisfied with reassurance. The unpleasant features may resolve with conservative treatment, including weight reduction in an obese patient. Surgery may be necessary if the symptoms are debilitating and the procedure involves decompression of the nerve; if that fails, occasionally division of the nerve may be necessary.

Spinal cord compression

Compression of the spinal cord is a common neurosurgical problem and requires early diagnosis and urgent treatment if the disastrous consequences of disabling paralysis and sphincter disturbance are to be avoided. Although there are a large range of possible causes of spinal cord compression in clinical practice, the majority are due to the following.

- Extradural
  - Trauma
  - Metastatic tumour
  - Extradural abscess

- Intradural, extramedullary
  - Meningioma
  - Schwannoma
- Intramedullary
  - Glioma (astrocytoma and ependymoma)
- Syrinx

Presenting features

The two major presenting features that are the hallmark of spinal cord compression are pain and neurological deficit. There is considerable variation in the manner in which these two major features present, and depend on the pathological basis, the site of the compression and the speed of the compression.

Pain

Pain is a typical early feature of spinal cord compression and is especially common in extradural compression due to metastatic cancer. Pain often precedes any neurological disturbance, sometimes by many months. The pain is due to involvement of local pain-sensitive structures, such as the bone of the vertebral column. Involvement of a spinal nerve root will cause pain radiating in the affected region. Thoracic cord compression with involvement of the thoracic nerve root will often be associated with pain radiating around the chest wall. This 'girdle' pain is an important feature associated with a lesion which may cause spinal cord compression. In addition, there is also a 'central' pain due to spinal cord compression, which is described as an unpleasant diffuse dull ache with a 'burning' quality.

Flexion or extension of the neck may cause 'electric shock' or tingling sensations radiating down the body to the extremities. This is called Lhermitte's sign, and is typically associated with cervical cord involvement. It is an ominous sign of impending spinal cord compression.

Neurological deficit

The neurological features of spinal cord compression consist of progressive weakness, sensory disturbance and sphincter disturbance.

Motor impairment

The motor impairment will be manifest as a paralysis, and the level of the weakness will depend on the position of the cord compression. Thoracic cord compression will result in a progressive paraparesis of the lower limbs and if the cervical cord is involved the upper limbs will also be affected. Compression of the corticospinal pathways will result in upper motor neurone weakness with little or no wasting, increased tone, increased deep tendon reflexes and positive Babinski response. As the cord becomes more severely compressed a complete paraplegia will result. The compressing mass will also cause weakness of the nerve root segment at the involved level. In the cervical region this will result in a lower motor neurone weakness of the involved nerve roots in the upper limbs. In the lumbar region involvement of the conus medullaris may produce a mixture of lower motor neurone and upper motor neurone signs in the lower limbs. Cauda equina compression produces a lower motor neurone pattern of weakness.

Sensory disturbance

A sensory level is the hallmark of spinal cord compression. In the thoracic region the sensory level will be to all modalities of sensation over the body or trunk, although there may be some sparing of some modalities in the early stages of compression. A useful guide is to remember that the T4 dermatome lies at the level of the nipple, T7 at the xiphisternum and T10 at the umbilicus.

Sphincter involvement

Sphincter disturbance often follows compression of the spinal cord, with the first symptom being difficulty in initiating micturition, which is followed by urinary retention, often relatively painless. Constipation and faecal incontinence will subsequently occur. The clinical signs include an enlarged palpable bladder, diminished perianal sensation and decreased anal tone.

In summary the clinical features of spinal cord compression are:
- pain, local and radicular
- progressive weakness of the limbs
- sensory disturbance, often with a sensory level
- sphincter disturbance.

Management

Spinal cord compression is a *neurosurgical emergency*. Investigation and treatment must be undertaken as a matter of urgency once the diagnosis is suspected.

The radiological studies undertaken to confirm the diagnosis of spinal cord compression include:
- plain spinal X-ray
- MRI (Figures 54.4 and 54.5)
- CT scan to show detail of bone involvement.

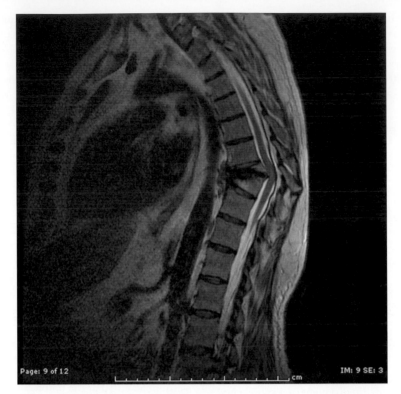

Fig. 54.4 MRI of thoracic fracture causing spinal cord compression.

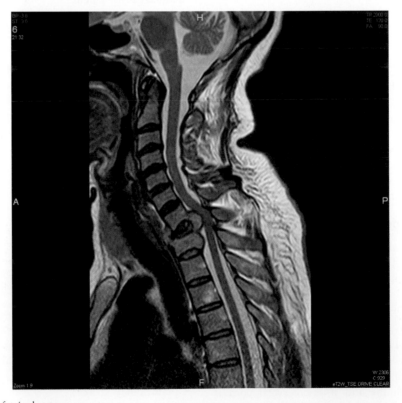

Fig. 54.5 MRI of spinal metastases.

MRI is of considerable value in diagnosing the cause and position of spinal cord compression and is by far the best investigation, as it will clearly show the pathological changes in the vertebral body, spinal canal, spinal cord and paravertebral region, thereby aiding with planning the treatment. Plain X-ray and CT scan will help show the focal bony destruction.

Treatment

The standard treatment for spinal cord compression is urgent surgery, except in some cases of compression due to malignant tumour known to be radiosensitive, in which treatment with high-dose glucocorticosteroids and radiotherapy may be indicated.

Common causes of spinal cord compression

Malignant spinal cord compression

By far the most common cause of spinal cord compression, this results from extradural compression by malignant tumours. The most common tumours involved are:

- carcinoma of the lung
- carcinoma of the breast
- carcinoma of the prostate
- carcinoma of the kidney
- lymphoma
- myeloma.

Surgical management for malignant spinal cord compression utilises either:

- decompressive laminectomy (posterior approach)
- vertebrectomy and fusion (anterior approach).

Urgent radiotherapy, combined with high-dose glucocorticosteroids, may be effective in controlling the tumour causing spinal cord compression and is sometimes advisable if the patient has a known primary tumour that is radiosensitive and if there is a partial incomplete neurological lesion that is only slowly progressive.

Schwannoma (neurofibroma)

Schwannomas are the most common of the intrathecal tumours and may occur at any position. They arise invariably from the posterior nerve roots and grow slowly to compress the adjacent neural structures. Occasionally, the tumour extends through

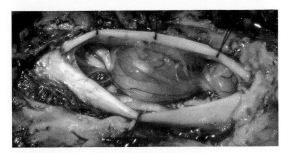

Fig. 54.6 Spinal schwannoma at operation causing spinal cord compression.

the intervertebral foramen to form a 'dumb-bell' tumour, which may rarely present as a mass in the thorax, neck or posterior abdominal wall.

The presenting features are those of a slow-growing tumour causing cord compression. There is frequently some degree of Brown–Séquard syndrome due to the lateral position of the tumour (see section Incomplete lesions; Figure 54.6). The treatment is surgical excision.

Spinal meningioma

Spinal meningiomas are intradural and most frequently occur in the thoracic region (Figure 54.7). They occur particularly in middle-aged or elderly patients and there is a marked female predominance. The tumour grows extremely slowly and there is usually a long history of ill-defined back pain, often nocturnal, and a slowly progressive paralysis prior to diagnosis.

Intramedullary tumours

Ependymoma (Figure 54.8) and astrocytoma of the spinal cord are uncommon, with the presenting features depending on the level of cord involvement. Ependymomas not infrequently arise in the filum terminale and will cause features of cauda equina compression. There is often a history of low back and leg pain, progressive weakness in the legs (often with radicular features), sensory loss over the saddle area and eventually sphincter disturbance.

It is usually possible to resect ependymomas, but surgical resection of astrocytomas is not possible as they spread diffusely through the spinal cord.

Intervertebral disc prolapse

Intervertebral disc herniation is a common cause of nerve root compression, but if the disc prolapses directly posteriorly (centrally) it will cause

(a)

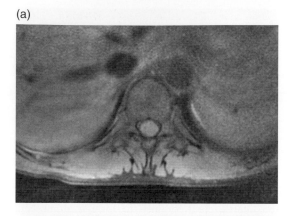

(b)

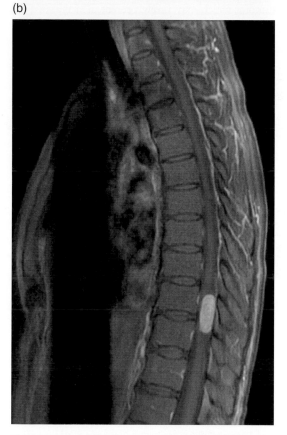

Fig. 54.7 T1-weighted contrast-enhanced MRI of thoracic meningioma: (a) axial; (b) sagittal.

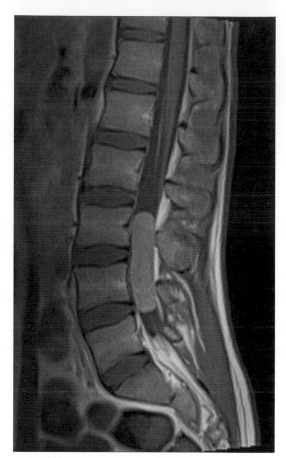

Fig. 54.8 T1-weighted post-contrast sagittal MRI of lumbar ependymoma.

compression of the spinal cord in the cervical or thoracic region and of the cauda equina in the lumbar region. Urgent surgery is essential to relieve the compression.

Spinal abscess

Spinal abscess may be secondary to an infection in the intervertebral disc or vertebral body (osteomyelitis of the vertebra) or an infection in the epidural space, usually from an infective source elsewhere in the body. It requires urgent treatment. The spinal cord compression is due to both inflammatory swelling and pus, and presenting features include severe local spinal pain with rapidly progressive neurological features of spinal cord compression. There are frequently constitutional features of infection such as high fever, sweating and tachycardia. MRI is the preferred investigation and treatment consists of urgent surgery with appropriate antibiotic medication.

Cervical myelopathy

Cervical myelopathy results from cervical cord compression due to a narrow cervical vertebral canal. The constriction of the canal enclosing the cervical cord is due to a combination of congenital narrowing, and cervical spondylosis involving hypertrophy of the facet joints and osteophyte formation, hypertrophy of the ligamenta flava and bulging of the cervical disc. The myelopathy results from both direct pressure on the spinal cord and ischaemia of the cord due to compression and obstruction of the small vessels within the cord or to compression of the feeding radicular arteries within the intervertebral foramen.

There is frequently a history of slowly progressive disability, although it is not unusual for the neurological disability to deteriorate rapidly, particularly following what might be even a minor or trivial injury involving sudden movement of the neck.

Muscular weakness, manifest by clumsiness involving the hands and fingers, impairment in fine-skilled movements and dragging or shuffling of the feet, is the most common initial symptom. *Sensory symptoms* are frequent, and occur as diffuse numbness and paraesthesia in the hands and fingers.

MRI will confirm the severity of the cord compression and show the exact pathological basis for the compression. An additional benefit of MRI is that it may show myelomalacia (high signal within the cord) indicating the severity of the compression and a poorer prognosis following surgery.

Surgery is indicated for clinically progressive or moderate or severe myelopathy. The operation may involve either a posterior decompressive laminectomy or, if the compression is predominantly anterior to the cord, an anterior approach with excision of the compressive lesion involving the intervertebral disc and/or vertebral osteophytes followed by fusion is preferred.

Spinal injuries

Trauma to the spinal column occurs at an incidence of approximately 2–5 per 100 000 population. Adolescents and young adults are the most commonly affected, with most serious spinal cord injuries being a consequence of road traffic accidents and water sports (especially diving into shallow water), skiing and horse riding accidents.

Mechanism of injury

Although severe disruption of the vertebral column usually causes serious neurological damage, it is not always possible to correlate the degree of bone damage with spinal cord injury. Minor vertebral column disruption does not usually cause neurological deficit, but occasionally may be associated with severe neurological injury. The mechanism of the injury will determine the type of vertebral injury and neurological damage.

Trauma may damage the spinal cord by direct compression by bone, ligament or disc,

haematoma, interruption of the vascular supply and/or traction.

Cervical spine

Flexion and flexion–rotation injuries are the most common type of injury to the cervical spine, with the C5/6 level being the most common site. There is often extensive posterior ligamentous damage and these injuries are usually unstable. Compression injuries also most frequently occur at the C5/6 level. The wedge fracture injuries are often stable because the posterior bony elements and longitudinal ligaments are often intact. However, those with a significant retropulsed fragment are likely to have disruption of the associated ligaments and are considered unstable. When combined with a rotation force in flexion, a 'tear drop' fracture may occur, with separation of a small anterior–inferior fragment from the vertebral body, and these should also be considered unstable.

Hyperextension injuries are most common in the older age group and in patients with degenerative spinal canal stenosis. The bone injury is often not demonstrated and the major damage is to the anterior longitudinal ligament secondary to hyperextension.

Thoracolumbar spine

Flexion–rotation injuries most commonly occur at the T12/L1 level and result in anterior dislocation of T12 on the L1 vertebral body. Compression injuries are common with the vertebral body being decreased in height. These injuries are usually stable and neurological damage is uncommon. Open injuries may result from stab or gunshot wounds that result in damage to the spinal cord.

Neurological impairment

There is a state of diminished excitability of the spinal cord immediately after a severe spinal cord injury, which is referred to as 'spinal shock'. There is an areflexic flaccid paralysis. The duration of spinal shock varies, with minimal reflex activity appearing within a period of 3–4 days or being delayed up to some weeks.

Complete lesions

The most severe consequence of spinal trauma is a complete transverse myelopathy in which all neurological function is absent below the level of the lesion, causing either a paraplegia or quadriplegia (depending on the level), impairment of autonomic function including bowel or bladder function, and sensory loss.

Incomplete lesions

There are numerous variations of neurological deficit manifest in incomplete lesions but with some specific syndromes.

- *Anterior cervical cord syndrome*: this is due to compression of the anterior aspect of the cord resulting in damage to the corticospinal and spinothalamic tracts, with motor paralysis below the level of the lesion and loss of pain, temperature and touch sensation but relative preservation of light touch, proprioception and position sense, which are carried by the posterior columns.
- *Central cord syndrome*: this is due to hyperextension of the cervical spine with damage located centrally causing the most severe injury to the more centrally located cervical tracts, which supply the upper limbs. There is disproportionate weakness in the upper limbs compared with the extremities. Sensory loss is usually minimal.
- *Brown–Séquard syndrome*: from hemisection of the cord resulting in ipsilateral paralysis below the level of the lesion with loss of pain, temperature and touch on the opposite side.

Management of spinal injuries

As little can be done to repair the damage caused by the initial injury, major efforts are directed towards prevention of further spinal cord injury and complications resulting from the neurological damage. The general principles of management are:

- prevention of further injury to the spinal cord
- reduction and stabilisation of bony injuries
- prevention of complications resulting from spinal cord injury
- rehabilitation.

The initial first-aid management of patients with injuries to the spinal column and spinal cord require the utmost caution in turning and lifting the patient. The spine must be handled with great care to avoid inflicting additional damage. Sufficient help should be available before moving the patient in order to provide horizontal stability and longitudinal traction. Spinal flexion must be avoided. A temporary collar should be applied if the injury is to the cervical spine. Hypotension and hypoventilation immediately follow an acute traumatic spinal cord injury and this may not only be life-threatening but may also increase the extent of neurological impairment. Respiratory insufficiency may require oxygen therapy and ventilatory assistance. Loss of sympathetic tone may result in peripheral vasodilatation with vascular pooling and hypotension. Treatment will include the use of intravascular volume expanders, α-adrenergic stimulators and intravenous atropine.

Careful attention should be paid to body temperature as the spinal patient is poikilothermic and will assume the temperature of the environment. A nasogastric tube should be passed to avoid problems associated with vomiting due to gastric stasis and paralytic ileus and a urinary catheter is necessary. Prophylaxis for deep vein thrombosis and subsequent pulmonary embolus should be commenced as soon as possible.

Radiological investigations will include plain X-ray, CT and MRI.

High-dose dexamethasone is usually administered as soon as possible for patients with spinal cord compression but there is no conclusive proof of its effectiveness.

Spinal reduction and stabilisation

Skeletal traction for restoration and/or maintenance of normal alignment of the spinal column is an effective treatment, with a variety of cervical traction devices available. The traction must be commenced under X-ray or fluoroscopic control and great care should be taken to avoid distraction at the fracture site, as traction on the underlying cord will worsen the neurological injury. Reduction of facet dislocations may involve either manipulation under fluoroscopic control with the patient under general anaesthesia or may require open surgery. This management must only be undertaken in specialised neurosurgical or spinal injury departments. In patients where the fracture/dislocation is considered unstable a spinal fusion is usually performed, utilising either an anterior or posterior approach. In cervical injuries this may be augmented using halo immobilisation.

In the past most injuries of the thoracolumbar spine were managed conservatively by postural reduction in bed, but now unstable injuries are managed with surgical fixation.

There has been considerable controversy over surgical intervention with spinal cord injuries. The damage to the spinal cord occurs principally at the time of the injury and there has been no evidence to show improved neurological function from acute operative decompression of the spine. The following are the general indications for surgical intervention.

- Progression of neurological deficit is an absolute indication.
- Patients with a partial neurological injury who fail to improve, with radiological evidence of persisting compression of the spinal cord.
- An open injury from a gunshot or stab wound.
- Stabilisation of the spine if there is significant instability or if it has not been possible to reduce locked facets by closed reduction.

Further management

Following reduction and immobilisation of fractures, the principles of continuing care involve avoidance of potential complications in patients who are paraplegic or quadriplegic and early rehabilitation, which commences as soon as the injury has stabilised.

Further reading

Kaye AH. *Essential Neurosurgery*, 3rd edn. Oxford: Blackwell Publishing, 2005.

Kline DG, Judice DJ. Operative management of selected brachial plexus lesions. *J Neurosurg* 1983;58:631–49.

Pang D, Wessel HB. Thoracic outlet syndrome. *Neurosurgery* 1988;22:105–21.

MCQs

Select the single correct answer to each question. The correct answers can be found in the Answers section at the end of the book.

1 Which of the following statements about carpal tunnel syndrome is correct?
   a most frequently occurs in men
   b is due to compression of the ulnar nerve at the wrist
   c usually causes severe weakness in the hand
   d is especially associated with pregnancy and lactation
   e causes decreased sensation on the dorsum of the hand

2 Which of the following statements about spinal cord compression is correct?
   a the most common cause is an intramedullary spinal cord tumour
   b management of compression by a malignant metastatic tumour is best undertaken utilising chemotherapy
   c the usual treatment for spinal cord compression due to malignant tumours is urgent surgery or radiotherapy
   d spinal pain is a late feature of spinal cord compression
   e metastatic tumours are rarely a cause of spinal cord compression

3 Which of the following statements about nerve injuries is correct?
   a a neurapraxia almost never recovers
   b neurotmesis is a mild form of injury, likely to be transient
   c Erb's palsy is due to damage of the upper trunk of the brachial plexus
   d Horner's syndrome in association with a brachial plexus injury is indicative of an excellent prognosis
   e injury to the radial nerve in the upper arm causes weakness of finger flexion

4 Which of the following statements about peripheral nerve entrapments is correct?
   a the ulnar nerve is frequently trapped at the elbow in front of the medial epicondyle
   b carpal tunnel syndrome is due to entrapment of the radial nerve at the wrist
   c meralgia paresthetica is due to entrapment of the lateral cutaneous nerve of the thigh
   d the principal symptom of meralgia paresthetica is weakness of the leg
   e the early features of ulnar nerve entrapment at the elbow is numbness involving the thumb and index finger

Section 13
Vascular Surgery

55 Disorders of the arterial system

Raffi Qasabian and Gurfateh Singh Sandhu

Royal Prince Alfred Hospital, Sydney, New South Wales, Australia

Introduction

Diseases of the arterial tree such as atherosclerosis affect all arterial beds and so a patient who presents with an ischaemic limb is also susceptible to stroke and myocardial infarction.

Epidemiology

Patients with peripheral arterial disease usually die from coexistent coronary or cerebrovascular disease. Heart, stroke and vascular disease combined caused 29% of all deaths in Australia in 2017, more than any other disease group. The prevalence of diabetes has doubled over the last 20 years and now affects 8% of the adult population.

Atherosclerosis

In 90% of adults with peripheral arterial disease, the cause is atherosclerosis. The other 10% comprise less common causes, including peripheral thromboembolism, aneurysmal disease, trauma, fibromuscular disease and rare inflammatory conditions.

The pathogenesis of atherosclerosis is complex and can begin in the second decade of life, with implications for the timing of preventive measures. It may take many years for atherosclerotic plaques to enlarge sufficiently to narrow an artery. Peripheral vascular disease may therefore remain asymptomatic for many years.

The earliest detectable pathological feature of atherosclerosis is the fatty streak, which later evolves into the fibrous plaque. More complex lesions occur with intra-plaque haemorrhage, calcification or disruption of the overlying fibrous cap.

Once the diameter of an artery starts to reduce, collateral circulation develops to compensate. The clinical outcome of arterial occlusion depends on the adequacy of the arterial collateral. If there is little collateral present (as would occur in acute occlusion), then ischaemia can be severe. With well-developed collaterals, arterial occlusion may even be asymptomatic.

Aneurysms

> If you see an aneurysm in one place, look and feel for it in another.
>
> *R. Qasabian, vascular surgeon*

An *aneurysm* is a greater than 50% dilatation of an artery's diameter compared with the expected diameter of that artery. A true aneurysm is one in which the dilated segment involves all three layers of the vessel wall. They may be morphologically distinguished as either saccular or fusiform.

A false aneurysm or *pseudoaneurysm* is when there is a collection of blood outside the vessel lumen but remaining in continuity with the circulation. It is not actually an aneurysm at all, but rather a defect in the artery wall, with the surrounding tissues preventing exsanguination. They are most commonly due to vessel trauma, especially iatrogenic, but can also be due to anastomotic disruption, infection of a vessel, or contained rupture of a pre-existing true aneurysm.

The clinical consequences of aneurysm formation are as follows.

- *Rupture*: the most feared complication, most likely to occur in the thoracic and abdominal aorta and iliac vessels, and in visceral aneurysms.
- *Thrombosis*: popliteal aneurysms form laminated thrombus that can embolise and cause distal ischaemia. Thrombus accumulation within aneurysms can also lead to complete occlusion.
- *Local compression*: any aneurysm can cause local mass effect, impinging on veins and causing venous hypertension or deep vein thrombosis, compression of nerves causing pain, sensory and motor loss, and occasionally erosion of adjacent bone.

Textbook of Surgery, Fourth Edition. Edited by Julian A. Smith, Andrew H. Kaye, Christopher Christophi and Wendy A. Brown.
© 2020 John Wiley & Sons Ltd. Published 2020 by John Wiley & Sons Ltd.

A patient with an abdominal aortic aneurysm is likely to have other aneurysms involving the iliac arteries in 40% and popliteal arteries in 15%. Popliteal artery aneurysms are the most common peripheral aneurysms and account for 80% of all peripheral aneurysms; 50% of these are bilateral. Conversely, aortic aneurysms are present in about 40% of patients with bilateral popliteal aneurysms.

Epidemiology

The prevalence of abdominal aortic aneurysm increases with age, from 5% in men aged 65–69 years to 11% in men aged 80–83 years and is higher in Caucasian males who smoke and have hypertension. The mortality from a ruptured abdominal aortic aneurysm is over 75%, with most patients dying before they can reach hospital. Even with surgery there is a 50% mortality rate. Every effort must therefore be made to identify and treat abdominal aortic aneurysm before rupture occurs.

Once an aneurysm reaches a diameter greater than 5 cm, the risk of rupture increases exponentially with further expansion: at a diameter of 5–6 cm the annual risk of rupture is 5%, at 6–7 cm 15%, and at over 7 cm approaches 40% (Table 55.1).

Aetiology

The aetiology of abdominal aortic aneurysms is multifactorial, with matrix metalloproteinases in the media of the vessel, localised haemodynamic stress and genetic predisposition all contributing. There is a 15% familial association in first-order siblings and an association with genetic disorders such as Marfan or Ehlers–Danlos syndromes.

Clinical presentation

Most abdominal aortic aneurysms are asymptomatic unless rupture is impending, in which case the presentation can be dramatic, with hypotension and abdominal pain radiating through to the back and syncope or presyncope. More usually, an abdominal aortic aneurysm is an unexpected finding, either on astute routine physical examination or on incidental ultrasound or CT scanning.

Evaluation and treatment

Evaluation of a patient with a suspected aortic aneurysm must begin with a thorough history to ensure they are not symptomatic and to ascertain risk factors and comorbidities, followed by a clinical examination in which the abdomen and lower and upper limb pulses are palpated. Whilst a plain film X-ray may delineate the calcium lining of an aneurysm, ultrasound is the initial imaging modality of choice for confirming a suspected abdominal aortic or popliteal aneurysm. Ultrasound is also the mainstay of surveillance of known aneurysms that are not in the chest.

Contrast-enhanced CT angiography (CTA) offers detailed information with regard to the anatomy of the aneurysmal segment and the access vessels, and is routinely performed prior to surgical repair of an aortic aneurysm. It is also important in the detection of aneurysmal disease in the thorax, which is difficult to demonstrate on ultrasound due to the presence of the ribs.

Asymptomatic aortic aneurysms should be treated when the rupture risk is higher than the accepted surgical mortality of 5%, which occurs at a diameter of 5–5.5 cm. Aneurysms can be treated by open surgery or endovascular means and the type of operation depends on anatomical considerations such as access and complexity, on patient age, medical comorbidities, and the preference and skills of the surgeon and the equipment available.

Table 55.1 Demonstration of the exponential increase in rupture risk with increasing diameter of abdominal aortic aneurysm (AAA).

AAA diameter (cm)	Risk of rupture per year (%)	Surveillance and surgery
<3	Negligible	Ultrasound surveillance
3–3.9	0.4	
4–4.9	1.1	
5–5.9	3.3	Consider repair: open or endovascular
6–6.9	9.4	
7–7.9	24	

Source: Cronenwett JL, Johnston KW (eds). *Rutherford's Vascular Surgery*, 8th edn. Philadelphia: Elsevier Saunders, 2014. Reproduced with permission of Elsevier.

Endoluminal repair of aneurysms (see also Chapter 58)

The endovascular method of treating an abdominal aortic aneurysm involves the radiologically guided insertion of an aortic stent-graft (a covered stent) through the common femoral artery via a catheter, avoiding the morbid open abdominal incision and the physiological stress of clamping arteries and thereby interrupting blood flow.

Not all patients are suitable for treatment by the endoluminal method. In order to anchor the aortic endograft, sufficient normal aorta (>2.5 cm) is needed below the renal arteries to securely fix the device in place. Secure fixation may be impossible if this segment of aorta is too dilated. The femoral and iliac vessels may be occluded, narrow, calcified and/or tortuous, preventing access with the stent-graft. Some of these anatomical limitations may be overcome with further technical advances in endograft design and delivery systems such as bespoke fenestrated and branched stent-grafts custom-made for individual patients. The same concept can be extended to treat other peripheral aneurysms, for example in the thoracic aorta or popliteal artery.

Open surgical repair of aneurysms

The open method of treating an abdominal aortic aneurysm has been used for more than 50 years, and late graft failure and rupture is rare. Conventional repair of an abdominal aortic aneurysm involves a laparotomy, clamping of the aorta and sewing in a prosthetic arterial graft to replace the aneurysmal aorta. This can be done in a straight or bifurcated configuration.

In other settings, the aneurysm can be ligated and circulation maintained by a bypass procedure. This is the commonest form of treatment for popliteal aneurysms.

Complications

Randomised trials have confirmed a short-term advantage with endovascular repair, with a lower perioperative mortality of 1.2% compared with 4.6% for open repair. General complications, particularly cardiorespiratory, are more common with open repair, but there is a higher incidence of local vascular or implant-related complications after endovascular repair.

It is not yet known if the immediate advantage of endovascular repair will be sustained in the longer term because of late problems that can develop. For this reason, ongoing surveillance of the aneurysm

Table 55.2 Types of endoleak.

Type	Description
Ia	Periprosthetic at proximal attachment
Ib	Periprosthetic at distal attachment
II	Back-bleeding lumbars or inferior mesenteric artery
III	Graft component separation
IV	Graft damage or porosity
V	Aneurysm sac enlarging in absence of demonstrable endoleak

Source: White GH, May J, Waugh RC, Chaufour X, Yu W. Type III and type IV endoleak: toward a complete definition of blood flow in the sac after endoluminal AAA repair. *J Endovasc Surg* 1998;5:305–9. Reproduced with permission of SAGE Publications.

repaired endovascularly is crucial. Device failure may occur due to migration, occlusion (usually of an iliac limb) or endoleak (flow of blood into, and pressurisation of, the aneurysm sac; Table 55.2).

Serious complications of both open and endovascular aneurysm repair include renal dysfunction, paraplegia, ischaemic colitis and prosthetic graft infection. Aorto-enteric fistulas are very rare but occur more commonly following open repair.

Ruptured aneurysms or more extensive aneurysms involving the thoracoabdominal aorta have been generally regarded as not suitable for treatment by the endoluminal method, although more and more centres are embracing endovascular approaches as a treatment option for these complex pathologies.

Chronic limb ischaemia

Chronic limb ischaemia is the commonest clinical problem occurring in patients with peripheral vascular disease (Box 55.1).

Clinical presentation

Claudication

Patients may present with intermittent claudication, a characteristic muscle pain induced by exercise, relieved by rest and recurring on walking the same distance again. Similar pain occurs less commonly on a neurogenic basis from spinal cord or nerve root compression but can be distinguished from arterial claudication by physical examination and exercise testing. Referred pain from arthritic joints can also mimic intermittent claudication.

Box 55.1 Patterns of disease affecting the lower limb

Superficial femoral artery (approximately 60%)
The most common site for atherosclerotic occlusion or stenosis is at the lower end of the superficial femoral artery (adductor hiatus) where it passes through the hiatus in the adductor magnus muscle into the popliteal fossa.

Aorto-iliac disease (approximately 30%)
Common patterns include disease of the lower aorta involving the common iliac arteries and disease of the external iliac artery extending into the common femoral and profunda femoris arteries. Severe aorto-iliac disease can result in Leriche syndrome involving buttock and thigh claudication with impotence and the absence of femoral pulses.

Combined disease (approximately 10%)
These patients have significant disease of both systems. Other recognised patterns include disease of the common femoral or profunda femoris artery and disease of the tibial arteries associated with diabetes.

The risk of limb loss is low, with a less than 1% chance of amputation in 5 years. A mortality of 30% at 5 years can be expected from associated medical comorbidities, with coronary events the usual cause of death. The outlook is considerably worse in claudicants with diabetes who continue to smoke.

Critical limb ischaemia

A patient is said to have critical limb ischaemia when they have rest pain for more than 2 weeks or tissue loss (ulceration or gangrene) secondary to objectively proven arterial occlusive disease. Rest pain is described as a burning sensation felt in the toes, made worse by elevation of the leg and relieved by placing the foot in a dependent position, thus allowing gravity to improve the delivery of blood flow to the peripheral tissues.

Without restoration of adequate blood supply in a patient with critical limb ischaemia, the chance of amputation is about 30% within 3 months. A mortality rate of 10% per year can be expected, with the higher mortality reflecting the more severe, generalised disease in such patients.

Clinical evaluation

Evaluation of a patient's pulses can reveal valuable information about the level of an arterial occlusion or thrombosis, and the size and characteristics of the artery itself. The aorta and femoral pulses should be palpated in every routine physical examination. The femoral pulse is generally easy to feel and therefore a good site to check cardiac rate and rhythm. The degree of arterial calcification can be estimated by the rigidity of the pulse. Palpation of the popliteal artery is more difficult. Whenever the popliteal pulse is prominent and easy to feel, a popliteal aneurysm should be suspected. The dorsalis pedis and posterior tibial pulses must also be palpated.

Investigations

As atherosclerosis is a generalised disease, investigations should be carried out to assess risk factors and the involvement of other arterial beds, thinking particularly of the coronary and carotid arteries.

Measurement of ankle pressure

The ankle–brachial index (ABI) can be derived by dividing the highest ankle systolic pressure by the arm systolic blood pressure. This measurement adds a degree of objectivity to the detection and grading of any arterial occlusive disease present. The ABI has the following characteristics.
- Normal range: 0.95–1.2
- Intermittent claudication: 0.9–0.4
- Rest pain: 0.4–0.15
- Gangrene: less than 0.15

Patients with diabetes or chronic renal failure may have highly calcified incompressible arteries, especially in the lower limbs, resulting in falsely elevated ABI determination.

Duplex ultrasound imaging

Ultrasound can also be used to image blood vessels, with the anatomical display of the artery using B-mode (or brightness-mode) imaging combined with spectral waveform analysis using the Doppler equation to calculate blood velocity. This is the simplest and most cost-effective way to confirm the diagnosis and anatomical location of suspected peripheral arterial disease but the acquisition of a good-quality study is highly operator dependent.

Angiography

Angiography is regarded as the diagnostic gold standard. Angiography can be CT, MRI or catheter-based. The complication rate is low, and is related to arterial injury or adverse reaction to the contrast agent used. Ultrasound has replaced angiography for many applications because these risks are avoided. Catheter-based angiography has the added advantage of being therapeutic as well as diagnostic and is now more selectively used on an 'intention-to-treat' basis after duplex imaging.

Management (Figure 55.1)

Atherosclerosis is the underlying cause of most peripheral vascular disease. All patients should be advised to modify their risk factors for atherosclerosis, and therefore all patients with peripheral vascular disease should be encouraged to cease smoking. They should be taking an antiplatelet agent such as aspirin and a cholesterol-lowering and plaque-stabilising agent such as a statin. Their blood pressure should be well controlled with antihypertensive agents and any diabetes tightly controlled.

The type and timing of operative intervention for chronic limb ischaemia is dependent naturally on the degree of ischaemia, its effect on the patient and the complexity of the culprit lesions.

Claudication

Historically speaking, patients suffering from claudication have been offered elective operative intervention only when it is short distance and is significantly affecting quality of life or ability to work. With the advent of percutaneous procedures, which carry a lower risk than open surgery, there has been a paradigm shift towards offering claudicants these reasonably safe procedures to improve their quality of life.

Critical limb ischaemia

Patients with critical limb ischaemia (tissue loss, rest pain) are treated more urgently and aggressively for limb salvage. This may include open surgery (endarterectomy, bypass) or percutaneous balloon angioplasty with or without stenting, or a combination.

In general terms, the more extensive the disease and the more distal the disease within the arteries, the more difficult the treatment and the poorer the outcome.

Endovascular procedures (see also Chapter 58)

Arterial stenoses or occlusion may be dilated or stented by minimally invasive catheter technology.

Depending on the procedure and patient, this may be done under a local anaesthetic. Balloon angioplasty enlarges the lumen by a controlled dissection. The risk of serious complications is about 2%. In the iliac arteries an initial success rate of about 90% is well maintained over a period of 5 years. In the superficial femoral artery the results are less satisfactory. Metallic stents may be deployed to maintain the lumen after angioplasty, improving durability of arterial dilatation but adding to the cost of intervention. Many of the local complications of balloon angioplasty can be controlled by stent placement. The use of paclitaxel-coated balloon angioplasty is used in recurrent disease to minimise the risk of scarring and luminal narrowing. Furthermore, technologies such as directional atherectomy, which aim to remove the culprit plaque, are also in early stages of use. The benefit of using drug-eluting stents in the lower limb is still not known and is the subject of randomised controlled trials.

Operative management

Arteries may be cleared by endarterectomy, i.e. surgically removing atherosclerotic plaque from the intima and part of the media of the artery wall. Longer occlusions may be bypassed surgically, by anastomosing a conduit to carry blood around an occluded arterial segment, even down to the tibial arteries in the foot. A prosthetic graft may be needed if autogenous vein, the preferred graft material, is unavailable.

Femoropopliteal bypass has an operative mortality of 1–2% and a 5-year patency of 50–70%, with the best results achieved when autogenous vein can be used as graft material. Aortofemoral bypass has an operative mortality of 2–5% and a 5-year patency of 80%.

Open operations are being performed with decreasing frequency because of the comparable results and lower morbidity of endovascular methods. A patient may initially receive percutaneous treatment, with open options reserved for failure of percutaneous treatment or for young patients who have a longer life expectancy or for those anatomically not suitable for percutaneous approaches.

Surveillance

Whether the patient has been treated by endovascular means or bypass surgery, regular surveillance is required to detect and correct late structural

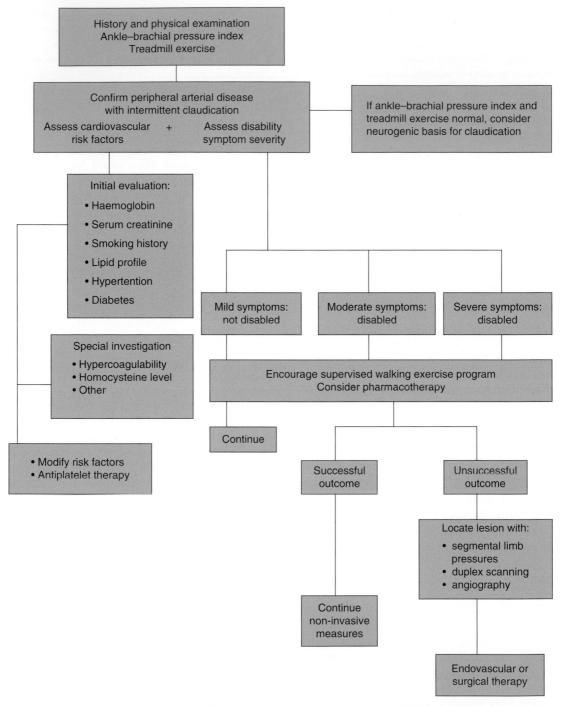

Fig. 55.1 Suggested management algorithm for intermittent claudication. Source: modified from Dormandy JA, Rutherford RB. Management of peripheral arterial disease (PAD). *J Vasc Surg* 2000;31:S1–S296. Reproduced with permission of Elsevier.

problems. Re-stenosis is usually due to neointimal hyperplasia (scarring), which occurs most frequently in the first 18 months after intervention and can be detected by ABI measurement and ultrasound scanning.

The diabetic foot: sepsis, arterial inflow and risk factors

Patients with long-standing diabetes mellitus are predisposed to foot complications on the basis of arterial occlusive disease, neuropathy and infection.

Coexistent arterial disease, with calcification of the tibial arteries, is most likely in diabetics who smoke.

Diabetic neuropathy may affect motor, sensory and autonomic nerves. Sensory neuropathy results in loss of pain sensation. Motor neuropathy results in paralysis and atrophy of the small muscles of the foot. This produces clawing of the toes and disturbance of the foot architecture, with neuropathic ulceration forming under the metatarsal heads, the maximum area of load bearing. Autonomic neuropathy results in dry skin (due to sweat gland dysfunction) and subsequent cracking of the skin, allowing a portal for infection. It also plays an important role in bone resorption associated with Charcot foot deformities.

The key to managing the diabetic foot is to control sepsis, optimise arterial inflow, 'offload' the neuropathic foot and manage risk factors.

Sepsis

Control infection with antibiotics or debridement of infected tissue:

- if patient is haemodynamically stable and not persistently febrile, antibiotics are usually enough to control sepsis
- if unstable, patient should have emergency debridement/amputation for source control.

Arterial inflow

If there is significant tissue loss and suspected arterial occlusive disease, then improve the arterial flow in the foot ideally prior to amputation or debridement.

Offloading

Podiatrists play an important role in ensuring the diabetic foot is adequately offloaded with suitable footwear to aid in the healing of pressure ulcers and to minimise their risk of recurrence.

Risk factors

There should be medium- to long-term control of blood glucose levels to limit microvascular disease and continuation of antiplatelet drugs and statins.

Clinical presentation

The foot lesion may be the presenting feature of maturity-onset non-insulin-dependent diabetes mellitus. The patient may present with a 'punched-out' ulcer or an area of localised gangrene, or acutely with a major infection in the foot.

Assessment is directed at determining the extent of local tissue damage and the adequacy of the blood supply. Plain X-ray of the foot may reveal any underlying orthopaedic abnormality such as bony changes associated with Charcot foot, metatarsophalangeal dislocation or evidence of osteomyelitis.

Management

Prevention is a major goal by careful control of the diabetes, and foot care to removing callus that can precede ulceration. Surgery plays an important role, requiring interdisciplinary cooperation. Vascular surgeons are involved in improving lower extremity blood supply and orthopaedic surgeons in correcting local bone or soft tissue complications of diabetes to improve foot architecture and function and aid with offloading of the foot. The outlook is worst for patients with diabetic foot ulceration due to peripheral arterial disease who continue to smoke.

Acute limb ischaemia

Acute arterial ischaemia can be caused by trauma (see section Vascular trauma) or non-traumatic conditions, notably arterial embolism or thrombosis of a pre-existing diseased arterial segment. Unless blood flow is restored within hours, irreversible tissue damage will occur, leading to possible amputation. The acuity of onset means that collaterals have not had time to develop to compensate for the ischaemia.

Pathophysiology

The common causes of non-traumatic acute limb ischaemia are embolus, thrombosis or graft occlusion following prior surgery. The most common site of origin of an embolus is the heart, due to atrial fibrillation or after myocardial infarction. Arterial thrombosis can be precipitated by pre-existing arterial disease, resulting in sudden occlusion at the site of an atheromatous arterial stenosis.

Evaluation

Features such as rapid onset of ischaemia, presence of atrial fibrillation or recent myocardial infarction, or absence of a history of claudication are more common in patients with embolus. The ABI will indicate the severity of the ischaemia. In almost all cases, angiography (either CTA or catheter-based angiography) is necessary to define the site and extent of obstruction. In these patients, the ischaemic lower limb is characterised by:

- pain
- pulselessness
- pallor
- perishingly cold
- paraesthesia
- paralysis.

Treatment

The survival of the limb is threatened if there is loss of sensation and muscle tenderness or weakness. The aim is to restore arterial inflow by thrombolytic therapy to dissolve the occluding thrombus (which is successful in 30% of cases), open thrombectomy or embolectomy, or bypass. The mortality remains on the order of 10% and the rate of amputation about 20%.

Upper extremity

Upper extremity ischaemia occurs far less commonly than lower extremity ischaemia and is usually due to non-atherosclerotic causes. Embolus, from atrial fibrillation or in the context of hypercoagulable states (e.g. malignancy, thrombophilias, polycythaemia), can lodge in the axillary or subclavian arteries. These require urgent thrombectomy.

Thoracic outlet syndrome

The subclavian artery and vein and T1 nerve root pass over the first rib to enter the arm. These structures can be compressed in the presence of cervical ribs or with the hypertrophic musculature that follows hard work or in athletes.

The clinical presentation will vary, depending on whether the artery, vein or nerve is predominantly compressed. In selected patients, removal of the first rib, usually by a transaxillary approach, will relieve arterial, venous or neural compression.

Vasospastic disorders

Raynaud's syndrome describes the changes which result from intermittent vasospasm of the arterioles in the hands or feet that occurs after exposure to cold. There is a classic sequence of colour change, from pallor to cyanosis to redness as the arterioles first spasm then slowly recover. This can be secondary to an underlying connective tissue disorder such as scleroderma or rheumatoid arthritis.

Management is directed towards treating the underlying condition but with severe digital ischaemia causing tissue loss, vasodilator therapy or occasionally endoscopic surgical sympathectomy is indicated to dilate the digital arteries and improve cutaneous circulation.

Vascular trauma

Vascular injury may be blunt or penetrating. Most arterial injury in Australia is due to blunt trauma sustained in motor vehicle accidents, but there is an increasing incidence of penetrating trauma related to urban violence.

Patterns of arterial injury

Arterial transection

This will present with haemorrhage and evidence of distal ischaemia. The severity of the ischaemia depends on the collateral circulation. With complete transection, arterial spasm and contraction occurs so that bleeding may spontaneously stop as the distal end of the artery thromboses. With partial transection, arterial contraction cannot occur so bleeding can be profuse while the distal pulses remain present.

Arteriovenous fistula

If a penetrating injury involves the adjacent artery and vein, a fistula between the two may develop, with shunting of blood from artery to vein. External bleeding may therefore be minimal.

Closed injury/intimal dissection

This type of injury is most commonly encountered with blunt injury and is dangerous because there may be no external haemorrhage and therefore the possibility of arterial injury overlooked. The artery wall usually remains intact but may weaken, producing a false aneurysm classically seen with traumatic dissection of the thoracic aorta.

Certain orthopaedic injuries, such as supracondylar fracture of the humerus or dislocation of the knee, are associated with concomitant arterial injury.

Clinical presentation

Vascular injury should be suspected when there is pulsatile bleeding, signs of distal ischaemia, an expanding haematoma, or a thrill or bruit overlying a site of suspected arterial injury.

Diagnosis

Regular clinical review with a high index of suspicion is essential in detecting arterial injury. Prompt assessment in an operating theatre, ideally equipped for intraoperative angiography, is required for arterial injury associated with ongoing haemorrhage or acute ischaemia. Less obvious arterial injury will usually be detected with measurement of the ABI, duplex scanning and diagnostic angiography. Arterial spasm should not be assumed as an explanation for limb ischaemia after injury unless intimal disruption has been excluded by angiography, ultrasound or surgical exploration.

Treatment

Arterial inflow must be restored within 4–6 hours of acute injury to prevent permanent muscle damage and limb loss.

The technique of arterial repair depends on the pathology of the injury. In some cases of lacerated wounds direct repair can be performed. If a segment of artery has been damaged, an interposition graft may be necessary to bridge the defect. Covered stents are also used in selected cases.

Reperfusion syndrome can occur when blood supply is restored to muscle damaged by ischaemia, so that the breakdown products from ischaemic muscle necrosis are washed into the general circulation. Systemic features of reperfusion syndrome include hyperkalaemia and myoglobinuria that can cause sudden death, adult respiratory distress syndrome and cardiac or renal failure.

If muscle swelling is anticipated following restoration of blood flow, a fasciotomy will relieve high intra-compartmental pressure.

Further reading

Adam DJ, Beard JD, Cleveland T. Bypass versus angioplasty in severe ischaemia of the leg (BASIL): multicentre, randomised controlled trial. *Lancet* 2005;366:1925–34.

Australian Bureau of Statistics. Australia's leading causes of death, 2017. Australian Bureau of Statistics 3303.0 Causes of Death, *Australia*, 2017.

Greenhalgh RM, Brown LC, Powell JT. Endovascular versus open repair of abdominal aortic aneurysm. *N Engl J Med* 2010;362:1863–71.

Hirsch AT, Haskal ZJ, Hertzer NR *et al.* ACC/AHA 2005 practice guidelines for the management of patients with peripheral arterial disease (lower extremity, renal, mesenteric, and abdominal aortic): executive summary. *Circulation* 2006;113:e463–e654.

Mohiuddin SM, Mooss AN, Hunter CB. Intensive smoking cessation intervention reduces mortality in high-risk smokers with cardiovascular disease. *Chest* 2007; 131:446–52.

Norgren L, Hiatt WR, Dormandy JA *et al.* Inter-society consensus for the management of peripheral arterial disease (TASC II). *Eur J Vasc Endovasc Surg* 2007; 33(Suppl 1):S1–S75.

Perler BA, Sidawy AN (eds) *Rutherford's Vascular Surgery and Endovascular Therapy*, 9th edn. Philadelphia: Elsevier, 2018.

MCQs

Select the single correct answer to each question. The correct answers can be found in the Answers section at the end of the book.

1 Which of the following statements about a pulsatile mass in the abdomen is correct?
  a it must be an aortic aneurysm
  b an ultrasound would be the best initial investigation
  c no imaging is needed if the mass is not tender
  d immediate surgery is indicated
  e immediate angiography is indicated

2 Which of the following suggest that acute arterial ischaemia is due to embolus in a 70-year-old woman?
  a she is in atrial fibrillation
  b her symptoms developed slowly over a month
  c she has had long-standing intermittent claudication
  d she smokes
  e she is an insulin-dependent diabetic

3 Which of the following statements about arterial trauma is correct?
  a all arterial injury is associated with pulsatile bleeding
  b the commonest cause in Australia is penetrating injury
  c the distal pulses will be absent
  d there is no relationship to major joint dislocations
  e bleeding is more likely with partial than with complete arterial transection

4 Which of the following statements about diabetic foot complications is correct?
  a the neuropathy is only sensory
  b there is no relation to ongoing smoking
  c the metatarsophalangeal joints do not dislocate
  d the prognosis is worse with arterial disease and ongoing smoking
  e there is no place for surgical management

56 Extracranial vascular disease

Raffi Qasabian and Gurfateh Singh Sandhu

Royal Prince Alfred Hospital, Sydney, New South Wales, Australia

Introduction

The four major arteries that supply the brain are the vertebral arteries, which originate from the subclavian arteries to form the basilar artery and supply the posterior cerebral circulation, and the internal carotid arteries, which arise from the carotid bifurcation in the neck and lead onto the middle cerebral arteries, the most important branches in the anterior cerebral circulation. The circle of Willis provides potential communication between the anterior and posterior cerebral circulations but may be inadequate to fully compensate for an occluded internal carotid artery in about 20% of individuals. Disease in these vessels may be due to atheromatous and non-atheromatous causes and may be asymptomatic or symptomatic, presenting as strokes or transient ischaemic attacks (TIAs).

The term 'stroke' refers to an acute loss of focal cerebral function with symptoms that last more than 24 hours. Neurological symptoms or signs that last less than 24 hours are called TIAs. Stroke is the third most common cause of death worldwide and is the principal cause of neurological deficit. About 40 000 Australians have a stroke each year, one-third of which are fatal while another third are left with significant neurological deficit. Predominantly middle-aged males are affected but the incidence of stroke increases exponentially with age, with 50% of all strokes occurring in patients over 75 years of age. The risk factors for stroke are listed in Box 56.1.

> ### Box 56.1 Risk factors for stroke
>
> Hypertension
> Tobacco smoking
> Heavy alcohol consumption
> Hypercholesterolaemia
> Obesity
> Diabetes
> Sedentary lifestyle

Pathogenesis (Box 56.2)

Haemorrhagic stroke can be readily differentiated from ischaemic stroke by computed tomography (CT) or magnetic resonance imaging (MRI) and will not be considered further.

Atherosclerosis affecting the extracranial circulation most commonly occurs at the carotid bifurcation, particularly at the origin of the internal carotid artery, where there is a region of turbulent flow as the common carotid artery divides into the high-resistance external carotid artery and low-resistance internal carotid artery.

There are two main theories of how disease at the carotid bifurcation may cause TIAs and stroke.
- *Embolic theory*: embolisation of atherosclerotic material or thrombus can arise from the carotid bifurcation. This is more likely to occur with complicated atherosclerotic plaques forming a tight (>70%) stenosis.
- *Haemodynamic theory*: blood flow to the brain may be reduced by a tight stenosis or occlusion of the carotid arteries. The effect of such lesions will depend on the extent of the intracranial collateral circulation. This is the mechanism of stroke after profound hypotension from any cause.

> ### Box 56.2 Pathogenesis of stroke
>
> **Ischaemia (85%)**
> - Atherosclerosis of large arteries and atherothromboembolism (65%): internal carotid artery origin is the most common site of atherosclerosis
> - Cardiac embolism (15%): atrial fibrillation, myocardial infarction
> - Small vessel occlusions: usually related to hypertension causing lacunar infarcts (5%)
>
> **Haemorrhage (15%)**
> - Intracerebral haemorrhage (intraparenchymal) (11%)
> - Subarachnoid haemorrhage (4%)

These theories are not mutually exclusive, as the likelihood of embolisation from carotid plaque and occlusion of the internal carotid artery increases with the degree of stenosis.

Clinical presentation

Cerebrovascular disease may be asymptomatic, found incidentally on clinical examination and imaging, or symptomatic (TIAs, stroke). The neurological symptoms will depend on whether the culprit lesion is within the internal carotid arteries (anterior circulation) or vertebral arteries (posterior circulation) or is due to global hypoperfusion.

Asymptomatic

This is often detected by the presence of a bruit, which may lead to duplex ultrasound investigation. The presence or loudness of a bruit has no correlation with the degree of arterial stenosis. Only 20% of bruits are associated with carotid disease, the remainder being caused by valvular and coronary artery disease.

Symptomatic

TIAs and stroke caused by carotid disease classically cause:
- ipsilateral retinal ischaemia manifesting as amaurosis fugax (fleeting blindness described as 'a curtain coming down over the eye')
- focal contralateral upper, with or without lower, limb sensory and/or motor loss
- dysphasia with speech disturbance, which is common particularly when the dominant hemisphere is affected (usually the left hemisphere in a right-handed individual).

Symptomatic vertebrobasilar disease

When the vertebrobasilar system is involved, the symptoms are less specific but may affect both sides of the body, with bilateral visual disturbance. Symptoms such as ataxia, imbalance, unsteadiness and vertigo can also be caused by middle ear disorders or bradycardia causing the patient to collapse (Stokes–Adams attacks).

Subclavian steal

Another mechanism of haemodynamic cerebral hypoperfusion occurs on basis of 'subclavian steal'.

If the left subclavian artery or more rarely the innominate artery is stenosed or occluded, then the vertebral artery becomes an important collateral pathway to sustain blood flow to the arm. When the arm is exercised, vertebral arterial flow reverses resulting in cerebral hypoperfusion. This is usually asymptomatic unless there is coexistent internal carotid stenosis.

Non-atheromatous carotid disease

Carotid aneurysm
A rare condition. Patients most commonly present with pulsatile mass, dissection or embolisation.

Carotid dissection
This is associated with head or neck pain and cranial nerve palsy, and presents as traumatic, iatrogenic or spontaneous. Anticoagulation and antihypertensives are the mainstay of treatment.

Carotid body tumour
Carotid body tumours are rare and originate from the preganglionic chemoreceptor cells of the carotid body. They are highly vascular and therefore should not be biopsied. They present as a mass in the neck and often mimic other neck lumps; 5% are locally malignant, 5% systemically malignant and 5% bilateral. Surgical excision is the treatment of choice.

Carotid arteritis
Giant cell arteritis is a systemic granulomatous inflammatory condition affecting the medium and large arteries in elderly patients. It mostly affects the aortic arch and the extracranial carotid arteries.

Takayasu's arteritis is a non-specific arteritis of unknown aetiology that can manifest as arterial occlusions, stenoses or aneurysms. There is a female preponderance and it can affect the entire aorta and its branches. Cerebrovascular involvement in the form of carotid or brachiocephalic disease is common. Arteritides are usually treated with steroids and other immune-modulating medications.

Fibromuscular dysplasia
Fibromuscular dysplasia (FMD) is a non-atherosclerotic, non-inflammatory vascular disease that primarily involves long unbranched segments of medium-sized and small arteries and is characterised by segmental irregularity of small and medium-sized muscular arteries, most commonly renal and carotid (although mesenteric, subclavian and iliac arteries can be involved). This can give a characteristic 'string of pearls' appearance on angiography.

There are several types, although medial fibroplasia accounts for 70–95%. Females are more commonly affected than males, typically aged 30–50 years old.

The aetiology is unknown but theories include the following.
- Humoral: hormones, pregnancy
- Mechanical stresses: ptosis of right kidney, increased severity with right-sided disease
- Blood vessel wall ischaemia
- Genetic:
  - High incidence in some families and in Caucasians
  - Autosomal dominant inheritance pattern
  - HLA-DRw6 association with FMD
- Smoking
- Vasculitis
- Infective: rubella

In general terms, FMD responds very well to balloon angioplasty alone, but the indications for treatment in the carotid arteries is not well defined, and is usually limited to those with symptomatic or progressive disease.

Investigations

With the advent of CT and carotid duplex scanning it has become easier to define those patients who are likely to have hemispheric neurological symptoms on the potentially correctible basis of thromboembolic phenomena arising from the carotid bifurcation.

General medical evaluation includes blood pressure measurement to detect hypertension and electrocardiography to assess any cardiac rhythm disturbance like atrial fibrillation or evidence of coexistent coronary artery disease. Haematological disorders such as polycythaemia, leukaemia or coagulopathies can cause stroke and should be sought. Similarly, renal function and lipid and glucose levels are measured to exclude renal failure, hyperlipidaemia and diabetes, respectively.

CT or MRI will identify intracranial blood if a haemorrhagic stroke has occurred and will demonstrate cerebral infarction or space-occupying lesions such as a brain tumour. Although sophisticated three-dimensional reconstruction of the extracranial vasculature can be done with both MRI and CT, these are usually not the first-line investigations to assess the carotid arteries.

Duplex ultrasound is used in most centres as the initial diagnostic test to evaluate the carotid arteries and as the definitive investigation by many vascular surgeons in planning carotid endarterectomy. Duplex ultrasound is operator dependent but can

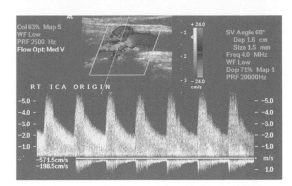

Fig. 56.1 Carotid duplex scan showing turbulent flow at the origin of the internal carotid artery with a peak systolic velocity of 571.5 cm/s and an end-diastolic velocity of 198.5 cm/s indicating more than 80% stenosis of the artery.

show the morphology of the carotid bifurcation and accurately identify the degree of stenosis present (Figure 56.1).

Carotid angiography, considered the diagnostic gold standard, is now used very selectively and particularly if the ultrasound findings are uncertain or if the major aortic arch branches need to be imaged in planning carotid stenting (Figure 56.2).

Treatment

Best medical management (Box 56.3) is indicated for all patients and comprises a single/dual antiplatelet, statin, antihypertensive and cessation of smoking.

Symptomatic carotid disease

Symptomatic carotid stenosis requires prompt treatment, with the most benefit obtained for stenoses of greater than 70% and when surgery is performed within 2 weeks of symptom onset. This is based on the North American Symptomatic Carotid Endarterectomy Trial (NASCET) which showed that the risk of stroke in symptomatic patients with greater than 70% stenosis of the relevant internal carotid artery could be reduced at 2 years from 26% to 9% with carotid endarterectomy, provided that the surgery is done with an acceptably low morbidity and mortality. A recent audit of carotid surgery in New South Wales confirmed that in an Australian setting, carotid endarterectomy is being performed with less than 2–3% combined stroke/death rate, in keeping with NASCET recommendations. Box 56.4 is a summary of the findings of the NASCET and another randomised controlled trial the European Carotid Surgery Trial (ECST) that guide surgical practice.

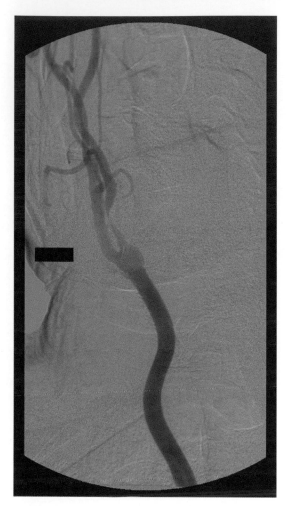

Fig. 56.2 Carotid angiogram showing more than 80% stenosis at the origin of the internal carotid artery.

Asymptomatic carotid disease

In the Australian setting, surgery is generally only offered for severe (>80%) asymptomatic carotid stenosis. Best medical management with antiplatelet drugs and statins is the treatment of choice for stenoses of less than 70% or in patients who have a very high surgical risk or limited life expectancy (<5 years). The Asymptomatic Carotid Atherosclerosis Study (ACAS) suggested a modest benefit of carotid endarterectomy versus best medical therapy in patients with carotid stenosis of greater than 70%. The number needed to treat to prevent a stroke at 5 years was 20, which is significantly higher than that for high-grade symptomatic stenosis. Surgery reduced the absolute risk by 6% and relative risk by 60% at 5 years. Although there was therapeutic benefit at 1 year, the benefit was greater at 5 years. The benefit appeared greater for men than women. This in turn accounts for the considerable variability in treatment of asymptomatic carotid stenosis, with the majority of Australian surgeons offering surgery for stenoses of greater than 80%, some selectively for stenoses of greater than 60%, and some only best medical management for all degrees of asymptomatic stenosis.

Carotid endarterectomy

The aim of this surgery is to remove the culprit atherosclerotic plaque and thus reduce the risk of thromboembolisation to the brain. The patient may receive general or local anaesthetic depending on suitability and surgical preference. The skin incision may be transverse or longitudinal anterior to the border of the sternocleidomastoid. Traversing through the platysma and deep fascia, the surgeon identifies

Fig. 56.3 After the carotid arteries are clamped, the plaque (a) is removed (b) and the arteriotomy closed either primarily or with a patch (c).

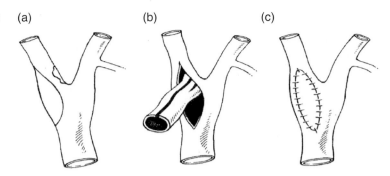

(a) (b) (c)

and preserves the marginal mandibular branch of the facial nerve. The common facial vein is a useful marker of the site of the carotid bifurcation which is carefully exposed, taking extreme care not to over-handle the diseased carotid. One careless flick or retraction prior to distal clamping could cause the culprit plaque to thromboembolise and the patient to have a significant stroke. The hypoglossal and vagus nerves are also identified and preserved. Heparin 5000 units is administered and the carotid arteries clamped so that the artery can be opened to endar-terectomise the atherosclerotic plaque (Figure 56.3). There is a plane between the diseased portion of the carotid artery and the outer media so that a smooth surface can be restored to the artery.

Transcranial Doppler and/or sensory and motor evoked potentials may be used to monitor for changes in middle cerebral artery velocities or brain function, respectively, after internal carotid artery clamping; if significant changes are found, the sur-geon may use a shunt to maintain cerebral perfu-sion whilst clamping. This is particularly important if the patient has significant contralateral carotid disease or posterior circulation disease. Most units in Australia are selective shunters. After the surgeon is confident that all atherosclerotic material has been removed, the lumen of the artery is flushed with heparinised saline and the artery closed. Many surgeons close the artery with a patch made of vein, Dacron or polyurethane to ensure a widely patent lumen and to reduce the incidence of carotid re-ste-nosis due to neointimal hyperplasia after surgery. A drain is placed in the wound and the platysma and skin are closed.

Carotid stenting

Carotid artery stenting (CAS) is a more recent tech-nical advance and remains a controversial aspect of carotid therapy. There has been continuing improve-ment in the reported results of balloon dilatation and stenting for atherosclerotic carotid arterial dis-ease. The proposed benefit of CAS is that an anaesthetic can be avoided as can the neck incision and risk of cranial nerve injury.

Patients who have symptomatic carotid stenosis but with contraindications to surgery may be suit-able for CAS. CAS is preferable when carotid lesions are anatomically unfavourable in cases of re-stenosis, high cervical or intrathoracic lesions or post radiation. The American Stroke association also recommends CAS over carotid endarterectomy in patients at increased risk of surgery.

There have been concerns about a higher risk of periprocedural cerebral embolisation and stroke and late recurrent stenosis. The risk of periprocedural stroke has been reduced with cerebral protection devices, designed to catch embolic material before it can pass into the brain.

Controlled clinical trials should resolve the rela-tive merits of carotid stenting and endarterectomy. Until that time, carotid endarterectomy is the estab-lished intervention for high-risk patients with high-grade symptomatic internal carotid stenosis.

Angioplasty and stenting is usually indicated for treating subclavian artery stenosis or occlusion causing subclavian steal. Carotid angioplasty has for some time been the therapy of choice for symp-tomatic FMD, a relatively rare condition occurring in fewer than 3% of patients with symptomatic carotid arterial disease. Stenting is rarely needed in this setting.

Perioperative management

Close monitoring is essential after any form of cer-ebrovascular intervention to observe for neurological deficit, guide blood pressure control and decrease the risk of adverse cardiovascular events. Patients are usually kept on their regular antiplatelet ther-apy soon after surgery to decrease the risk of thrombosis at the endarterectomy site.

Re-stenosis is more common after stenting. Postoperative surveillance using ultrasound is com-monly done to monitor the operated or stented carotid artery.

Procedural complications

There is a 2–3% risk of ipsilateral stroke after carotid endarterectomy (higher after CAS) related to embolisation from the carotid during the manipulation of intervention or to the interruption of cerebral blood flow. Labile blood pressure is common and hypertension is related to the risk of postoperative intracerebral haemorrhage. Coexistent coronary artery disease is an important cause of postoperative myocardial infarction and death.

Carotid endarterectomy can be complicated postoperatively by the following.

- Cranial nerve injuries: can include the hypoglossal and recurrent laryngeal nerves. Sensory loss in the distribution of the greater auricular nerve and the transverse cervical nerve of the cervical plexus is commonly observed.
- Neck haematoma: if severe can obstruct respiration, requiring prompt return to the operating theatre.

Future developments

There is an increased focus on preventing stroke by risk factor modification and by identification of subgroups at high risk of stroke who will benefit from prophylactic intervention. Furthermore, the concept of plaque morphology as an alternative to degree of stenosis in predicting stroke risk and indication for surgery is an evolving area that may change future practice.

Further reading

Ahn SH, Prince EA, Dubel GJ. Carotid artery stenting: review of technique and update of recent literature. *Semin Intervent Radiol* 2013;30:282–7.

Cronewett JL, Johnston KW (eds) *Rutherford's Vascular Surgery*, 8th edn. Philadelphia: Elsevier Saunders, 2014.

Ferguson GG, Eliasziw M, Barr HW *et al.* The North American Symptomatic Carotid Endarterectomy Trial: surgical results in 1415 patients. *Stroke* 1999;30: 1751–8.

Halliday A, Mansfield A, Marro J *et al.* Prevention of disabling and fatal strokes by successful carotid endarterectomy in patients without recent neurological symptoms: randomised controlled trial. *Lancet* 2004;363: 1491–502.

Mughal MM, Khan MK, DeMarco JK, Majid A, Shamoun F, Abela GS. Symptomatic and asymptomatic carotid artery plaque. *Expert Rev Cardiovasc Ther* 2011;9: 1315–30.

Robicsek F, Roush TS, Cook JW, Reames MK. From Hippocrates to Palmaz-Schatz, the history of carotid surgery. *Eur J Vasc Endovasc Surg* 2004;27:389–97.

Walker MD, Marler JR, Goldstein M. Endarterectomy for asymptomatic carotid artery stenosis. *JAMA* 1995; 273:1421–8.

MCQs

Select the single correct answer to each question. The correct answers can be found in the Answers section at the end of the book.

1 Which of the following statements about the anatomy of extracranial arterial disease is *incorrect*?
a the left subclavian artery arises directly from the aortic arch
b the vertebral artery is a branch of the subclavian artery
c the vertebral arteries form the basilar artery
d there is no communication between the anterior and posterior cerebral circulations
e there is a low-resistance flow pattern in the internal carotid artery

2 An 80-year-old woman presents with transient right hemiparesis lasting 15 minutes and resolving completely. She is otherwise healthy and independent. Her carotid duplex scan shows >80% stenosis of her left internal carotid artery. Despite aspirin therapy, she has a further episode. Which of the following statements is true?
a she is best managed on warfarin therapy
b left carotid endarterectomy is indicated
c carotid stenting is a preferred option to surgery
d she is facing a cumulative 5% stroke risk within the next 3 years
e lowering her blood cholesterol level will reduce her immediate risk of stroke

3 Which of the following statements about the pathology of extracranial arterial disease is correct?
a atherosclerosis is the commonest cause of internal carotid stenosis
b recurrent stenosis occurs in more than 50% of patients after carotid endarterectomy
c carotid body tumours arise from the vertebral arteries
d fibromuscular disease is commonest in young men
e Takayasu's disease is commonly known as 'pulsing disease'

4 Which of the following statements about carotid endarterectomy is correct?
a it is associated with a high (>5%) risk of perioperative stroke
b closure with a patch decreases the risk of recurrent stenosis

c there is a plane between the atheromatous plaque and the intima

d it is the procedure of choice for fibromuscular disease

e it precludes the use of a carotid stent for recurrent stenosis

5 A 65-year-old man presents with angina, and a left neck bruit is heard. Which of the following statements is correct?

a the first priority is investigation of the bruit

b the bruit may be arising from the aortic valve

c a carotid angiogram in indicated

d there is no relationship between angina and a carotid bruit

e the left internal carotid artery must be occluded

57 Venous and lymphatic diseases of the limbs

Hani Saeed[1] and Michael J. Grigg[2]

[1,2] Eastern Health, Melbourne, Victoria, Australia
[2] Monash University, Melbourne, Victoria, Australia

Varicose veins

Varicose veins are a common condition, occurring in 20% of adults. The characteristics of varicose veins are that they are

- visible
- dilated
- elongated
- tortuous.

Varicose veins result from incompetent valves in the venous system.

Anatomy of the venous system

The veins of the lower limb can be classified into three groups: superficial, deep and perforating.

Superficial veins

The superficial veins are collected in two major systems. These are the tributaries and main trunks of the long and short saphenous veins.

The long saphenous system begins on the dorsum of the foot and runs anterior to the medial malleolus, along the medial aspect of the calf and thigh and ends at the saphenofemoral junction, where it joins the common femoral vein. This junction is 2–3 cm below and lateral to the pubic tubercle. A major tributary, the posterior arch vein, joins the long saphenous vein just below the knee. This drains blood from much of the medial side of the calf and communicates with the deep venous plexus of the calf by way of several perforating veins, so named because they 'perforate' the deep fascia. In the thigh, there are large medial and lateral tributaries and thigh perforating veins. A number of tributaries join the long saphenous vein close to its termination. These are important in the surgery for saphenofemoral incompetence since failure to deal with these will result in recurrence of the varicose veins.

The short saphenous system begins behind the lateral malleolus of the ankle and runs along the lateral and then the posterior aspect of the calf to penetrate the deep fascia in the upper calf. It terminates in the popliteal fossa by joining the popliteal vein in the vicinity of the knee crease. The exact level of the junction is variable and may be either a few centimetres above or below the knee crease.

Deep veins

The deep veins run as venae comitantes of the major arteries in the foot and calf, where they receive tributaries from the muscles of the calf, including the venous sinusoids in the calf muscles. The venous sinusoids within the calf muscles are important as part of the venous pump mechanism. They are a frequent site of origin for venous thrombosis. The deep system also receives the perforating veins from the superficial system. At about the level of the knee joint a single popliteal vein is formed in most cases. This runs proximally in company with the main artery to become the femoral vein and then the external iliac vein as it passes beneath the inguinal ligament.

Perforating veins

The perforating veins join the superficial and deep systems. They contain valves which direct blood flow from the superficial to the deep system. Perforating veins are variable in number and position, but usual sites are the medial side of the lower third of the calf between the posterior arch vein and the posterior tibial veins and at about the junction of the middle and lower thirds of the thigh between the long saphenous vein and the femoral vein. Other perforating veins join the anterior tibial veins, the

Textbook of Surgery, Fourth Edition. Edited by Julian A. Smith, Andrew H. Kaye, Christopher Christophi and Wendy A. Brown.
© 2020 John Wiley & Sons Ltd. Published 2020 by John Wiley & Sons Ltd.

peroneal veins and the superficial veins. The inconstancy of these veins makes precise localisation difficult and is an important reason for the development of recurrent varicose veins following treatment.

Physiology

The superficial veins collect blood from the superficial tissues. During the relaxation phase of the calf muscle cycle, the pressure in the superficial veins is greater than the pressure in the deep veins and thus blood flows from superficial to deep. Each contraction of the calf muscles results in high pressure (approximately 250 mmHg) being generated in the calf compartments. This empties the veins in the muscles and transmits a pulse of blood proximally.

Retrograde flow, or reflux, due to gravity is prevented by valves. If the valves in the veins directing venous return proximally or the perforating veins are incompetent the venous return from the leg is less efficient. This results in higher pressures in the superficial system and progressive dilatation occurs, causing more valves to become incompetent. This is accompanied by elongation of the superficial veins, which results in tortuosity. The high pressure in the superficial veins, particularly in the most gravitationally dependent part of the leg around the ankle, may be sufficient to impair the nutrition of the subcutaneous tissue and dermis and contribute to ulcer formation.

Varicose veins are a disorder of the superficial and perforating veins. In most cases the disorder is inborn, although the mode of inheritance is uncertain. Varicose veins often first appear in young adults. Females are affected more commonly and the veins are more prominent during pregnancy due to the combined effects of the muscle-relaxing effects of hormonal (especially progesterone) changes and the pressure effects of the pregnant uterus, which also acts as an arteriovenous fistula in the pelvis. Partial regression occurs following delivery but there is progression of the varicosities with succeeding pregnancies. Tributaries of the internal iliac vein and even the ovarian vein may be involved, producing posterior thigh and vulval varices (pelvic venous insufficiency).

Clinical presentation

Patients with varicose veins most commonly present for cosmetic reasons. Some patients present with tiny veins – telangiectasia or venous flares. Others present with large veins that may have been present for 10–20 years or longer.

Symptoms

Symptoms result from fluid congestion of gravitationally dependent superficial tissues due to inadequate venous return and increased venous pressure. Patients may complain of tiredness and aching of the lower legs at the end of the day. This is relieved by rest and elevation of the legs. They may develop mild ankle swelling, particularly in warmer weather but significant lower limb oedema is not a characteristic of varicose veins. Leg pain is a common complaint and the presence of varicose veins may be coincidental.

Complications

Thrombophlebitis

Thrombosis in a segment of varicose vein is common. The patient presents with signs of inflammation spreading from a hard lump, which is the thrombosed vein. The redness, pain and heat falsely suggest the presence of infection. The condition usually resolves over a period of days provided the thrombosis does not extend into the deep venous system, when pulmonary embolus becomes a risk. Hence thrombus extending from the long saphenous vein into the common femoral vein can be very dangerous. The thrombus often extends 15 cm or more proximal to the clinical signs of inflammation, and a duplex scan will readily demonstrate the true level of the clot. Urgent treatment, usually by way of full anticoagulation, needs to be considered for thrombophlebitis extending above the level of the knee joint. If there is a contraindication to anticoagulation, urgent saphenofemoral ligation can be undertaken.

Haemorrhage

The subcutaneous varices of the lower calf and around the ankle may rupture through the skin causing profuse bleeding. This bleeding will continue unabated whilst the limb remains dependent, even to the point of exsanguination. The patient should lie down immediately and elevate the limb. Pressure should be applied directly over the bleeding point. This pressure can be reinforced by a firm bandage. A tourniquet should not be used as a rise in venous pressure can be produced and may actually worsen the bleeding.

Ulceration

Prior to the advent of duplex scanning, which enables non-invasive evaluation of the venous system, it was mistakenly believed that superficial varicose veins rarely caused venous ulceration. It is now realised that severe long-standing varicose veins are a common cause of leg ulcers. Before the development of frank ulceration, secondary venous tissue changes occur, including pigmentation due to haemosiderin deposition, lipodermatosclerosis and atrophie blanche.

Other complications

Rare presentations occur in children and are associated with major congenital abnormalities of the venous system, often associated with arteriovenous malformations.

Examination

The purpose of the examination is to determine (i) the distribution of the varicose veins, (ii) if there are secondary venous tissue changes, and (iii) if lower limb pulses are present (this is particularly important if compressive stockings are to recommended).

The patterns of disease are:
• long saphenous incompetence
• short saphenous incompetence
• incompetence of thigh or calf communicating veins
• combinations of the above.

The patient is initially examined standing, which makes the veins more obvious. The size and distribution of varicose veins are examined. If the veins are predominantly medial and if they involve the thigh, it is likely that the long saphenous vein is involved. If they are posterior and lateral in the calf, it is likely that the short saphenous vein is involved. It should be remembered that there are many communications between the two systems so that, for example, incompetence in the long saphenous system may fill varices on the posterior and lateral aspects of the calf. An incompetent vein will transmit a cough impulse.

The examiner should also be aware of findings which signify that the patient does not have a 'straightforward' varicose vein problem, such as in the following circumstances.
• Varices of the medial aspect of the upper thigh may indicate pelvic venous insufficiency.
• The presence of significant leg oedema is unlikely to be due to varicose veins alone.
• Prominent superficial veins extending above the level of the inguinal ligament in the suprapubic area suggest that these veins are dilated

collaterals which have formed in response to deep venous obstruction.
• Ulcers sited proximal to the mid-calf level are unlikely to have a venous aetiology and are more likely to be neoplastic.

With the availability of ultrasound examination, eponymously named tourniquet tests are now of historical interest only.

Investigations

Duplex ultrasound

Duplex ultrasound incorporates both B-mode ultrasound (image) and Doppler ultrasound (blood flow). It is used to identify sites of valvular incompetence and to determine the presence of deep venous incompetence and the presence of venous thrombosis.

Venography

Venography is an obsolete investigation for these patients and should be avoided because of the poor risk-to-benefit ratio.

Treatment

There are few serious sequelae of untreated varicose veins (see earlier section Complications) so treatment is not essential, except in those patients with pre-ulcerative secondary venous tissue changes in the lower calf or with complications (see section Symptoms).

Elastic stockings

Elastic stockings will not cure varicose veins but will provide relief from symptoms of swelling and tiredness in the legs and prevent complications. They are particularly helpful for the pregnant patient with varices. A range of stockings are available: low-, medium- and high-grade compression and below- and above-knee lengths. For patients with varicose veins, a below knee-stocking of moderate compression (grade 2, 20–30 mmHg pressure) will suffice. If there is doubt that the veins are the cause of the symptoms in a particular patient, relief of symptoms while wearing stockings supports the diagnosis of varicose veins and, conversely, failure of stockings to relieve symptoms suggests that other causes should be sought. Graduated compression stockings should be prescribed with caution for patients in whom pedal pulses are not palpable.

Injection–compression therapy

Injection therapy should not be considered while there are major uncontrolled sites of deep to superficial incompetence. When these sites have been controlled, injections may be used to control small veins that may remain. An important part of injection therapy is compression, which keeps together the surfaces irritated by the sclerosant. This facilitates fibrous organisation and inhibits recanalisation of the vein. Recently, techniques have been introduced for injecting very small cutaneous veins. These often cause cosmetic disability because they are prominent blue or red lines in the skin that are hard to disguise.

Operation

Operation is an appropriate method of control for major sites of incompetence. The aims of operation are to obliterate the major sites of deep to superficial incompetence and to remove the larger varicose veins. The presence of varicose veins predisposes to the development of postoperative deep vein thrombosis so appropriate prophylaxis should be undertaken.

Saphenofemoral ligation

Saphenofemoral ligation is the procedure performed most commonly. The saphenofemoral junction is exposed through a skin crease incision about 3 cm long placed below and lateral to the pubic tubercle and 1 cm above the groin crease. The long saphenous vein and its tributaries are dissected. All tributaries are ligated and divided. Once the junction between the long saphenous and femoral veins has been clearly identified, the long saphenous vein is divided and ligated flush with the femoral vein. The femoral vein is explored for 1 cm proximal and distal to the junction to ensure that there are no more tributaries entering the vein. Any that are found are ligated and divided.

Saphenopopliteal ligation

Saphenopopliteal ligation is carried out in a manner analogous to saphenofemoral ligation. The dissection may be difficult because of the fat in the popliteal fossa and is greatly facilitated by precise knowledge from duplex ultrasound scanning of the exact level of the saphenopopliteal junction. Care is necessary to avoid inadvertent injury to the sural nerve which runs with the short saphenous vein.

Stripping

Stripping of the long saphenous vein from the groin to the knee removes a large dilated vein which, if left, may be the site of thrombophlebitis or recurrence. A varicose long saphenous vein is not useful for later coronary or leg artery bypass. Stripping the long saphenous vein between the ankle and the knee should not be performed since it is unnecessary and may result in troublesome neuritis of the saphenous nerve.

Multiple extractions

Most of the obvious varicosities are removed through multiple small incisions. The veins are then grasped either by small artery forceps or specially designed hooks. As much as possible of the dilated vein is removed. The next incision is made 2–4 cm away and the process repeated until all the major varices have been removed.

Ligation of incompetent perforating veins

This usually involves an incision over the perforating vein as it passes through the deep fascia. Preoperative duplex scan provides accurate localisation. The vein is ligated and divided beneath the deep fascia. Ligation of perforating veins is usually reserved for patients undergoing operation for recurrent veins or those who have significant secondary venous tissue changes or ulceration. It is not a cosmetic procedure.

Postoperative care

The leg is firmly bandaged to promote haemostasis from the extraction sites. Early and continued mobility is encouraged to reduce the risk of deep vein thrombosis. Patients having bilateral operations or operation for major recurrences usually stay in hospital overnight. The outer bandages are removed 24–48 hours after operation and elastic stockings are applied. These are worn for about 2 weeks while there is a tendency for the leg to swell.

Prognosis and results of surgery

The result of surgery that has been carefully planned and carried out should be good. With well-performed surgery the recurrence rate is 15–20% at 5 years. Injection therapy may be used to obliterate telangiectatic vessels that it is not possible to remove surgically.

Complications

Deep venous thrombosis is uncommon if prophylaxis is employed. Wound infections can occur in relation to skin crease incisions but respond well to antibiotics as no prostheses are implanted. Recurrence is perhaps the most important issue for patients and this can occur for four reasons: (i) there was unrecognised pre-existing valvular incompetence at a site other than where operation was performed; (ii) operation was not adequate where a major tributary has been missed; (iii) remote (from operative site) valvular incompetence has developed subsequent to operation; and (iv) neovascularisation has occurred (the development of multiple tiny channels between the deep and superficial systems through scar tissue at the site of ligation).

Other techniques of venous ablation

Radiofrequency ablation

The radiofrequency catheter delivers radiofrequency energy to achieve heat-induced venous spasm and collagen shrinkage. Under ultrasound guidance, a sheath is introduced into the vein at an appropriate point near the knee crease using a Seldinger technique. The radiofrequency applicator is passed through the sheath and into the great saphenous vein under ultrasound control. The tip is usually positioned approximately 2 cm below the saphenofemoral junction. The radiofrequency ablation catheter is then withdrawn at a controlled rate and treatment stopped once the catheter has entered the sheath.

Endovenous laser therapy

Endovenous laser therapy releases thermal energy both to the blood and to the venous wall, causing localised tissue damage. Tumescence fluid (0.9% saline with local anaesthetic) is injected into the saphenous compartment to reduce risk of skin burn. A laser sheath is inserted in a similar way to radiofrequency ablation and a laser fibre is inserted into the sheath. A laser generator is used to provide laser energy as the catheter is pulled back at a controlled rate.

Both these techniques can be performed under local anaesthesia and on an outpatient basis.

Lymphoedema

Lymphoedema is the consequence of abnormal amounts of fluid and protein in the interstitial spaces of the skin and subcutaneous tissues, particularly with respect to the limbs. The high protein content of the fluid distinguishes this type of swelling, or brawny oedema, from that seen occurring as a result of the filtration oedema of heart and kidney failure, venous obstruction and hypoproteinaemia (pitting oedema).

Incidence

This is an unusual cause of limb swelling. There are two principal types:
- a congenital abnormality of the lymphatic channels (primary lymphoedema)
- secondary lymphatic obstruction resulting from infection, trauma (including surgery and radiotherapy), secondary metastatic tumours and, occasionally, primary tumours such as lymphoma.

Physiology

The brain and the spinal cord are the only body tissues that do not have significant lymphatic vessels. For all other structures, lymphatic vessels function to collect lymph – tissue fluid including protein that leaks from the capillary bed – and convey this to the regional lymph nodes, to the major lymphatic trunks and ultimately into the thoracic duct, which terminates by joining the junction of the subclavian and internal jugular vein in the left side of the neck.

The lymphatic capillaries are thin-walled endothelial tubes, the endothelium being supported on collagen with occasional smooth muscle cells. The onward progression of the lymph in these channels is maintained by the presence of valves and the compression applied by neighbouring structures, such as the contraction of muscles and the varying pressures and movements of the gut in the abdominal cavity. The onward flow is also enhanced by the changes in intrathoracic pressure generated by respiration. The composition of the lymph will vary with the drainage site; for example, in the intestine it will contain chylomicrons. In all cases there is a high concentration of albumin. The lymph flow in the thoracic duct varies from 1 to 4 L per day and the proportions of its final composition will depend on the relative flow from the various sites of the body and the food intake at the time.

Pathogenesis and pathology

The pathogenesis of lymphoedema is invariably a consequence of inadequate lymphatic flow, either because the lymph vessels are congenitally abnormal or deficient or because of obstruction to the vessels or the draining lymph nodes. Less frequently, temporary lymphoedema can occur in a limb on account of muscle inactivity, as occurs with prolonged sitting, but resolves swiftly with muscle activity.

Primary lymphoedema

Primary or idiopathic lymphoedema refers to swelling due to intrinsic abnormalities of the lymphatic vessels. This can be a familial abnormality and is often bilateral and symmetrical. The lymphatic vessels are aplastic in 15% and hypoplastic in 65% of patients, being fewer and smaller in calibre than is normal. They may be varicose, dilated and incompetent in 20% due to fibrosis in the draining lymph nodes. In this group with an intrinsic abnormality present at birth, lymph may reflux into the skin, leak through the skin (especially between the toes), into the peritoneum as chyloperitoneum, into the thorax as chylothorax and into the urine as chyluria.

Acquired lymphoedema

Acquired lymphoedema often affects only one limb, except when the obstructing lesion is due to an infective agent such as the filarial nematode *Wuchereria bancrofti*. This is a mosquito-borne parasite of tropical regions. The other infective agents that cause secondary lymphoedema are lymphogranuloma inguinale, tuberculosis and recurrent non-specific infection.

Tumour-induced secondary lymphoedema is most commonly associated with metastatic tumour of the breast, causing upper limb lymphoedema, and pelvic tumours of the cervix, ovary and uterus in the female and of the prostate in males, giving rise to lower limb lymphoedema.

Iatrogenic or trauma-induced lymphoedema occurs most frequently as a result of block dissections of either the axilla or groin, or in association with radiation of the same region.

The pathological complications of lymphoedema include recurrent infection such as cellulitis and chronic thickening of the skin with hyperkeratosis. In the very long term, lymphangiosarcoma may develop (see Chapter 45).

Clinical presentation

Primary lymphoedema

Primary or idiopathic lymphoedema can manifest clinically at various ages. Congenital lymphoedema is apparent at, or within a few weeks of, birth, often in association with some other congenital abnormality.

Lymphoedema praecox refers to lymphoedema not present at birth but which appears before the age of 35 years. It usually affects adolescent women.

Lymphoedema tarda becomes evident after the age of 35 years. This group of patients, usually females, may have unilateral or bilateral limb swelling which can affect the upper or lower limbs. There may be a temporal relationship with a minor injury or surgery on the limb that precedes the onset of the swelling. Initially the swelling is soft and pitting but with time the tissues become more indurated and fibrous. This change is hastened and accentuated by attacks of cellulitis.

Lymphoedema tends to affect the foot and the toes. In the later stages, the skin becomes thickened and hyperkeratotic with wart-like excrescences. In the severe and chronic stage, the limb has a tree trunk-like appearance and can be distinguished from venous oedema by the absence of prominent pigmentation and the chronic venous ulceration commonly seen in severe venous insufficiency oedema.

Secondary lymphoedema

The swelling of secondary lymphoedema develops more rapidly, often in an older age group and may be associated with dragging discomfort. This form of lymphoedema is frequently secondary to an obstructing lesion; thus there may be changes at the site of obstruction such as scarring, swelling and local erythema. As with primary lymphoedema, these patients are prone to episodes of cellulitis and lymphangitis.

Investigation

It is important to distinguish lymphoedema involving the lower limbs from venous oedema (deep venous incompetence or obstruction). The clinical presentation, history and examination will usually suggest either of these conditions but each can be readily excluded by the use of duplex scanning of the lower limb venous system. If the scan does not demonstrate venous obstruction or deep venous valvular incompetence, the swelling is more likely to be lymphatic in origin. It is important to ensure that the iliac venous system has been sonographically interrogated before a venous cause is excluded.

Oedema associated with generalised problems, such as hypoproteinaemia, nephrotic syndrome or cardiac failure, will be excluded on clinical examination, biochemical tests (e.g. liver function tests, serum protein levels, urea, creatinine and electrolytes) and examination of the urine for protein.

Specific investigations for lymphoedema are not usually employed as they rarely impact on management, but include lymphoscintigraphy. Radioactive labelled colloids can be injected into the interdigital spaces and should appear within 30 minutes in the regional nodes if the lymphatic vessels are normal. Reduced uptake implies hypoplastic or obliterated lymphatic vessels. In obstructive secondary lymphoedema, the radionuclide uptake in the regional nodes is often normal. It may be slow in the more proximal nodes, indicating an obstruction at that level.

Computed tomography of the regional node area will allow an assessment of nodal enlargement if these are obstructive; in primary lymphoedema the number and size of nodes may be diminished. Lymphangiography is now seldom used because it may accentuate the obliterative process of primary lymphoedema and give rise to infection or an inflammatory process that may relate to the contrast medium used. It provides information about the type and site of lymphatic obstruction and valvular incompetence in the lymph vessels in particular cases.

Hence the diagnosis of lymphoedema, particularly primary lymphoedema, tends to be a diagnosis of exclusion. The major aim when investigating a patient with lymphoedema is to determine whether or not underlying pathology exists. The extent and severity of lymphoedema should be determined and recorded as baseline information to gauge subsequent treatment. The minimum is precise measurements of limb circumference with reference to defined bony points, for example 2 cm above the medial malleolus.

Treatment

The treatment of lymphoedema is essentially conservative. Conservative treatment aims to preserve the quality of the skin, prevent lymphangitis and reduce limb size. Skin quality can be maintained by careful avoidance of trauma and regularly applying a water-based skin lotion. Non-skin-drying soaps should be used to minimise the loss of oil from the skin.

Patients with lymphoedema are predisposed to cellulitis and spreading lymphangitis. The problem is that infection will further damage the lymphatic system. Patients should be warned to avoid trauma and to seek early and aggressive management of skin sepsis. Streptococci are the most common organisms causing cellulitis. Early treatment with systemically administered penicillin is indicated if any form of skin sepsis develops. The most common portal of entry is via associated interdigital fungal infection with tinea pedis. If a patient has recurrent attacks of cellulitis, long-term prophylaxis with pencillin 250 mg twice daily is appropriate. For those allergic to penicillin, erythromycin may be given as treatment for acute infections. Any interdigital fungal infection should be treated regularly with an antifungal powder; if there is an established infection, oral griseofulvin can be taken. If the infection fails to respond to standard treatment, alternative antibiotics can be considered.

Limb swelling is best managed with graded compression stockings. The patient should sleep with the foot of the bed elevated on the equivalent of two house bricks and graded compression stockings fitted before the patient gets out of bed. The stockings may range from 30 to 50 mmHg in their compression depending on the tolerance of the patient. For those with whole limb swelling, the pantyhose or thigh stocking should be used. Similar stockings can be used for those with arm oedema.

Intermittent pneumatic compression may help to reduce limb swelling. The pneumatic compression is applied as a multi-cell unit arranged concentrically. The multi-cell unit inflates successively from peripheral to proximal and thus has a 'milking' action that drives fluid from the periphery to the centre. The use of compression stockings and the intermittent use of external pneumatic compression devices will achieve very satisfactory limb size control in the majority of patients.

Surgical treatment is rarely performed, being reserved for the few patients who cannot have their swelling controlled by compression, have repeated bouts of sepsis or in whom skin changes and the persisting swelling might suggest there is a risk of a neoplasm. Surgery may either involve excision of subcutaneous tissue (Charles operation) or attempts at lymphatic bypass, the latter being still experimental.

Prognosis and results of treatment

The majority of patients can control their leg swelling with compression stockings during the day and nocturnal elevation. The ability to achieve this goal is largely dependent on the determination and compliance of the patient. This can be facilitated by putting the patient in touch with the local lymphoedema society (see Further reading).

Further reading

Australasian Lymphology Association, www.lymphoedema.org.au

Davies D, Rogers M. Morphology of lymphatic malformations: a pictorial review. *Australas J Dermatol* 2000;41:1–5.

Fitridge RA, Thompson MM (eds) *The Mechanisms of Vascular Disease: A Reference Book for Vascular Specialists.* Adelaide: University of Adelaide Press, 2011:497–510.

Gloviczki P. Principles of surgical treatment of chronic lymphoedema. *Int Angiol* 1999;18:42–6.

Merchant RF, Pichot O. Long-term outcomes of endovenous radiofrequency obliteration of saphenous reflux as a treatment for superficial venous insufficiency. *J Vasc Surg* 2005;42:502–9.

Moore WS (ed.) *Vascular and Endovascular Surgery: A Comprehensive Review*, 8th edn. Philadelphia: Elsevier Saunders, 2013, chapter 51.

Rabe E, Schliephake D, Otto J, Breu FX, Pannier F. Sclerotherapy of telangiectases and reticular veins: a double-blind, randomized, comparative clinical trial of polidocanol, sodium tetradecyl sulphate and isotonic saline (EASI study). *Phlebology* 2010;25:124–31.

Sidawy AN, Perler BA (eds) *Rutherford's Vascular Surgery and Endovascular Therapy*, 9th edn. Philadelphia: Elsevier, 2018.

Szuba A, Rockson SG. Lymphoedema: classification, diagnosis and therapy. *Vasc Med* 1998;3:145–56.

MCQs

Select the single correct answer to each question. The correct answers can be found in the Answers section at the end of the book.

1 Which of the following statements about varicose veins is *incorrect*?
   a varicose veins are dilated, tortuous and visible when the patient is standing
   b valvular incompetence is an integral component of the pathogenesis of varicose veins
   c the principal superficial venous systems of the lower limbs are the long and the short saphenous systems
   d the principal route of venous drainage from the lower limb is via the superficial venous system
   e the principal driver of venous drainage from the legs in the erect position is the calf pump

2 Which of the following statements about patients with varicose veins is *incorrect*?
   a they experience calf pain after walking 200 m that is relieved by resting for 5 minutes
   b present with a superficial ulcer on the ankle
   c experience aching discomfort in the calf after prolonged standing
   d present with superficial thrombophlebitis
   e show spontaneous bleeding from a varix

3 Which of the following statements is correct?
   a venography is an accurate method for investigating varicose veins
   b duplex scanning has little to add to the preoperative investigation of varicose veins
   c the most frequent cause of recurrent varicose veins is neovascularisation
   d due to frequent and serious late complications, all patients with varicose veins should be advised to have surgery
   e patients with varicose veins and who have haemosiderin deposits and liposclerosis at the ankle should be treated

4 Which of the following statements about the management of patients with varicose veins is *incorrect*?
   a below-knee elastic stockings may be definitive treatment in the patient in whom surgery is contraindicated because of comorbidities
   b injection with a sclerosing agent followed by elastic compression for 4–6 weeks can be beneficial
   c using a below-knee elastic stocking may help decide if calf symptoms are due to varices
   d surgical trials have demonstrated that it is not necessary to remove the long saphenous vein in the thigh
   e incompetent perforating veins should be subfascially ligated if there are secondary skin changes

5 Primary lymphoedema:
   a should be differentiated from oedema due to varicose veins with a duplex scan
   b should be investigated with lymphoscintigraphy before deciding on treatment
   c is due to an underlying malignancy
   d is cured by diuretic therapy
   e the response to therapy can be monitored by serial measurement of limb circumference

58 Endovascular therapies

Timothy Buckenham

Monash University and Department of Imaging, Monash Health, Melbourne, Victoria, Australia

Introduction

The management of vascular disease has made a steady movement toward minimally invasive therapies over the last 20 years. These minimally invasive techniques when applied to arteries are called endovascular or endoluminal, meaning the therapy is delivered through the lumen of the artery. This change in practice has been driven by the rapid development of new technologies and the increasing sophistication of multiplanar imaging, facilitating accurate planning and deployment of endoluminal devices. Most endovascular procedures require the use of ionising radiation (X-rays) and contrast media (ionic or gaseous) and therefore have risks as well as benefits for the patient, but overall endovascular procedures are attractive for their low morbidity and mortality and rapid recovery of the patient. High-resolution imaging, particularly modalities not utilising ionising radiation such as ultrasound and magnetic resonance imaging (MRI), has improved the efficacy of endovascular repair by allowing the detection of treatment failure or facilitating intervention to prevent treatment failure. This is particularly important in endovascular repair of arteries as secondary intervention is much more common than in traditional open surgery and durability is often dependent on these secondary interventions

Equipment requirements for endovascular therapy

Angiography suite

Imaging

The majority of endovascular interventions are carried out in an angiography suite (also known as a catheter laboratory) or an operating theatre equipped with a high-quality angiographic imaging system (hybrid theatre) (Figure 58.1). The angiographic equipment has a number of features that facilitate endovascular procedures, including a C-arm that may be floor or ceiling mounted and allows the X-ray tube and the detector to rotate around the patient to facilitate multiplanar imaging. The table is made of carbon to ensure radiolucency and it floats, meaning the operator can easily raise or lower the table or move it side to side or end to end by depressing a table-side control. Essential to the procedure is the ability to subtract out background so that only the detailed image provided by the contrast media is visible; this is called *digital subtraction angiography*. Another important feature is the ability to superimpose live fluoroscopic imaging on a stored image (called a 'road map') and, on some equipment, to superimpose CT or MRI images to help complex interventions. Radiation protection for both the patient and the operator is important. Therefore, equipment characteristics include virtual collimation, lead shields and a low-dose mode, and operators wear lead gowns, lead glasses and increasingly commonly lead helmets.

Ultrasound

Ultrasound located within the angiographic suite allows rapid and safe access to a range of arteries, usually the femoral although other commonly used access sites include the brachial, radial and pedal arteries. With the common use of closure devices to facilitate haemostasis, ultrasound has an important role in selecting the optimal access site. Many endovascular procedures require large-access catheters up to 24F and ultrasound can help assess the optimal point of puncture. Ultrasound can also be used to assess the intraoperative outcome of an endovascular procedure in superficial arteries and conduits

Textbook of Surgery, Fourth Edition. Edited by Julian A. Smith, Andrew H. Kaye, Christopher Christophi and Wendy A. Brown.
© 2020 John Wiley & Sons Ltd. Published 2020 by John Wiley & Sons Ltd.

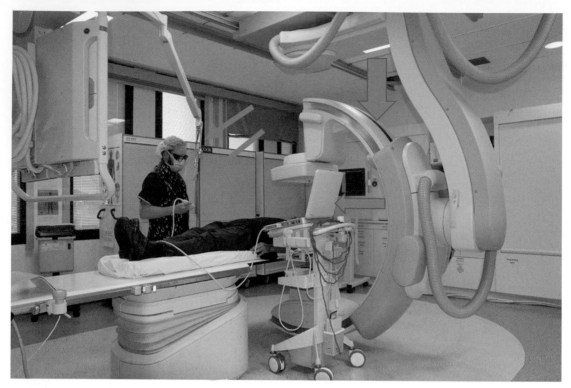

Fig. 58.1 Angiography suite: note the ceiling-mounted C-arm configuration (vertical arrow) with ultrasound machine to assist with vessel access (horizontal arrow). The operator is wearing a lead apron and lead glasses and is standing behind a lead window to maximise radiation protection (double arrow).

Endoluminal devices

It is beyond the scope of this chapter to detail the huge range of devices available for endovascular procedures but they can be divided into a number of groups.

Devices used for arterial occlusion

Arteries may be occluded with a range of materials called embolic agents. These are delivered through the lumen of an arterial catheter into the target arterial lumen. Embolic agents maybe solid, particulate or liquid. A common example of a solid embolic agent is a metallic coil made of stainless steel or tungsten. These coils are linear when loaded into the lumen of the delivery catheter but on entering the arterial lumen assume a predetermined coil shape that occludes the target artery. An example of a liquid embolic agent is cyanoacrylate, which is not radiopaque but when mixed with contrast media can be seen and injected into target arteries with great accuracy, where it sets as a glue cast that occludes the vessel. Particulate embolic material usually takes the form of polyvinylalcohol

microspherules with a wide range of diameters, the diameter being matched to the diameter of the target arteries.

Devices for reopening diseased arteries

Angioplasty balloons are the most important tool for revascularising stenotic and occluded arteries. They are delivered into the body over a guidewire and inflated when traversing the diseased segment. Angioplasty balloons come in a wide range of diameters and lengths that the operator matches to the arterial segment being treated. The balloons are inflated to a predetermined pressure using an inflation manometer. Some balloons have a drug coating mixed with an excipient that allows controlled transfer of the drug (usually paclitaxel) to the wall of the artery to reduce re-stenosis by inhibiting smooth muscle proliferation.

Arterial stents (Figure 58.2) are designed to act as a scaffold that hold the treated arteries open and are used to improve patency or manage an injury to the artery such as a dissection or a rupture; some of these stents are drug-eluting. Stents come in two basic designs.

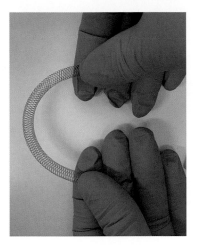

Fig. 58.2 A flexible self-expanding stent.

- Self-expanding stents: these are often made of Nitinol and have a thermal memory, re-forming to a particular size when released by the delivery catheter and warmed by the blood. These stents tend to be more flexible that balloon-expandable stents.
- Balloon-expandable stents: these are commonly made of stainless steel and are deployed by inflating an angioplasty balloon on which the stent is loaded. Once the stent achieves the diameter determined by the delivery balloon, the balloon is removed and the stent remains in position expanding the arterial lumen. Balloon-expandable stents are usually shorter and more rigid than self-expanding stents and are used mainly above the inguinal ligament where the need for flexibility is less significant.

Endografts or covered stents have a covering made of PTFE or Dacron and may be mounted on a balloon-expandable or self-expanding stent platform. These stents are primarily used to exclude aneurysms but are used for revascularisation particularly in the suprainguinal circulation, but they require much larger delivery catheters and therefore much larger percutaneous access site punctures.

Devices for excluding aneurysms

There are many endoluminal devices that are designed to exclude aneurysms, particularly abdominal and thoracic aortic aneurysms. They all have a fabric covering (usually PTFE or woven polyester) attached to a metal endoskeleton or exoskeleton and are deployed through a sheath (Figure 58.3). Most consist of multiple components: a body with a long and a short limb. After infrarenal deployment of the graft body, the short limb is extended with an endograft into the contralateral common iliac artery. The longer graft limb, ipsilateral to the side the body

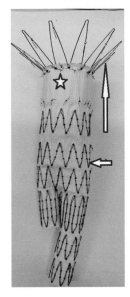

Fig. 58.3 Bifurcated endograft for exclusion of an abdominal aortic aneurysm. Note the uncovered suprarenal fixating tines (vertical arrow) and the V-shaped metallic exoskeleton (horizontal arrow). The proximal covered segment of the aortic graft provides the infrarenal sealing zone (star).

has been deployed from, is then extended with an endograft into the common iliac artery giving an aorto bi iliac configuration (Figure 58.3). Some of these grafts have tines or similar that cross the renal arteries and fix in the suprarenal aorta, while others are deployed entirely inferior to the renal arteries. Most require ballooning to ensure graft apposition, with the sealing zones below the renal arteries and in the common iliac arteries and at the junctions of the components.

Endovascular procedures: the basics

Seldinger technique

This technique underpins all percutaneous arterial access and was described by the Swedish radiologist Sven Seldinger in 1953 (Figure 58.4). Its modern iteration involves introduction of a soft guidewire into the arterial lumen through the barrel of a hollow bevelled needle. The needle tip is placed in the lumen of the access artery percutaneously, usually under ultrasound guidance. Once the guidewire is successfully deployed in the arterial lumen, a suitably sized access sheath can be advanced over the guidewire into the access artery. After passing the sheath, the guidewire is withdrawn. Other devices such as catheters, balloons and stents can then be introduced through the access sheath.

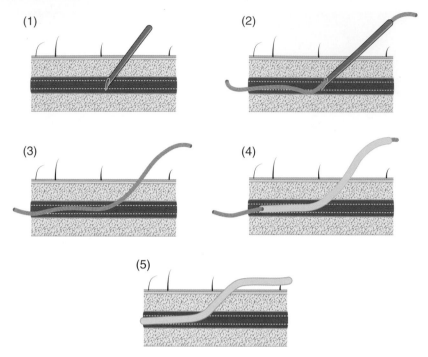

Fig. 58.4 Seldinger technique. (1) The artery is punctured with a hollow needle; (2) a flexible guidewire is introduced through the needle; (3) the needle is withdrawn, leaving the guidewire in the artery; (4) the arterial catheter is introduced over the guidewire; (5) the guidewire is removed and the catheter remains in the vessel.

Selective arterial catheterisation

Pre-shaped catheters, with names such as Cobra and Sidewinder, allow access to all major arteries in the body, and are used in conjunction with guide-wires of varying stiffness and lubricity. In small arteries (<4 mm), microcatheters may be used. These are placed inside the lumen of the shaped catheter and pass over a very fine guidewire lying centrally in the lumen.

Arteriography

Opacification of the lumen of the access artery, of an arterial segment for revascularisation or exclusion or of target arteries for embolisation requires the injection of contrast media through a catheter and the rapid acquisition of digitally subtracted images. Pre-shaped or selective cathe-ters have a single end hole, but if larger volumes of contrast are required in order to opacify the aorta a multi-holed pigtail catheter is used. Contrast media can be positive or negative. Iodinated contrast is positive as it attenuates the X-ray beam, but is associated with allergy and renal dysfunction. Carbon dioxide is a negative contrast and displaces blood and reduces attenu-ation of the X-ray beam. Carbon dioxide is non-allergenic and non-nephrotoxic but may be uncomfortable for the patient.

Access artery closure

On completion of an endovascular procedure, access site haemostasis needs to be achieved. If a small access sheath such as 5F or 6F has been used, manual compression for 10 minutes is usually ade-quate and safe. If larger access sheaths have been used, for example over 20F in thoracic endovascular aneurysm repair (TEVAR) and endovascular aneu-rysm repair (EVAR), multiple suture closure devices may be used. These devices deploy an endoluminal needle that is deflected by a cup and recaptured by the device, allowing the suture to be tightened and closing the access site. There are multiple other per-cutaneous closure devices that use alternative tech-nologies, such as collagen plugs and Nitinol clips.

Endovascular management of arterial aneurysm disease

Aortic aneurysmal disease

Indications

The indications for EVAR of abdominal aortic aneu-rysm are similar to those for open surgery, i.e. diam-eter of 55 mm, rapid expansion on serial imaging, or are symptomatic. CT scanning will determine the diameter and suitability for EVAR. These parameters include adequate infrarenal aortic neck (undiseased non-dilated parallel segment of aorta), adequate-sized iliac arteries for access and common iliac arteries that are suitable for distal sealing.

The indications for TEVAR of thoracic aortic aneurysms are again similar to those for surgery, i.e. diameter of 60 mm, rapid expansion on serial imaging, or symptomatic.

Procedure and outcomes

Aortic aneurysmal disease is characterised by structural dysfunction of the aortic wall, with gradual expansion that can progress to rupture. This commonly occurs in the abdominal aorta and less frequently in the thoracic aorta. The aim of aortic aneurysm repair is to prevent aneurysm rupture and aneurysm-related death by excluding the aneurysm from the aortic circulation. There are two options for the treatment of aneurysms: traditional open surgery and endovascular repair. Open surgical repair has higher risks of morbidity and mortality compared with the minimally invasive often percutaneous EVAR. EVAR has a 30-day mortality of around 2% compared with 4% for open surgical repair, but interestingly all-cause mortality is equal at 5 years and the periprocedural survival advantage is not sustained. Patients undergoing EVAR have a significant re-intervention rate of around 30% within 5 years, mainly to correct endoleaks, and the very long term durability is still uncertain. Despite advancing technology not all aortic aneurysms can be repaired with EVAR. In abdominal aneurysms, this is usually related to an unfavourable sealing zone in the infrarenal abdominal aorta, which can be overcome with more complex EVAR procedures that involve apertures or fenestrations to maintain visceral artery patency, the sealing zone in these cases being the suprarenal aorta. In TEVAR, similar limitations apply. In thoracic aortic aneurysm disease most endoluminal repair is performed distal to the left subclavian artery but the proximal landing zone (the segment of aorta just distal to the left subclavian artery) may be inadequate, requiring more proximal aortic landing with graft fenestrations for the carotid and subclavian arteries. Similar re-intervention rates to EVAR are seen in TEVAR but a greater proportion of these secondary interventions are with open surgery rather than minimally invasive techniques which are predominant in EVAR.

Limitations and complications

The Achilles heel of both EVAR and TEVAR is the high incidence of endoleaks (Figure 58.5). An endoleak is when systemically pressurised arterial blood enters the aneurysm sac external to the endograft. This may occur around the sealing zones (type 1) or more commonly via retrograde flow from lumbar or visceral branch arteries such as the inferior mesenteric artery (type 2). Other sources of endoleak are from the junctional zones (type 3) or through the fabric (type 4). Sac expansion secondary to a type 2 endoleak or the presence of a type 1 or 3 leak merits treatment to prevent aortic rupture. Other complications are access site and access artery trauma and kidney injury from contrast media.

Current status of EVAR and TEVAR

Endoluminal repair is currently the preferred treatment modality for thoracic aortic aneurysms distal to the left subclavian artery and infrarenal abdominal aortic aneurysms because of low morbidity and mortality and inpatient stay of 24–48 hours. Similar endoluminal techniques are also applied in the treatment of other aortic pathology such as acute type B dissection, aortic trauma, mycotic aneurysms, fistulas and penetrating atheromatous ulcers.

Endovascular management of peripheral vascular disease

Chronic limb ischaemia

Lower limb arterial disease may result in ischaemia which develops over time and may present as non-limb-threatening claudication or as chronic critical limb ischaemia (CCLI), which results in rest pain and tissue loss. The classification usually used for determining the severity of chronic limb ischaemia is the Rutherford system (Table 58.1). Thus Rutherford grade I patients (claudicants) may be managed conservatively and have a low lifetime risk of amputation. Patients with grades II and II CCLI require revascularisation using endovascular or open surgical procedures. Given that atherosclerosis is a systemic disease, patients with CCLI are likely to have coexistent coronary and carotid disease, making minimally invasive techniques attractive due to their low morbidity and mortality.

Which arterial lesions are amenable to endovascular therapy?

The Trans-Atlantic Inter-Society Consensus Document on Management of Peripheral Arterial Disease (TASC II) has divided the lower limb arterial

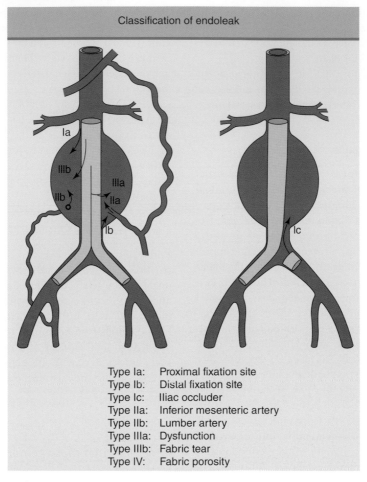

Classification of endoleak

Type Ia: Proximal fixation site
Type Ib: Distal fixation site
Type Ic: Iliac occluder
Type IIa: Inferior mesenteric artery
Type IIb: Lumber artery
Type IIIa: Dysfunction
Type IIIb: Fabric tear
Type IV: Fabric porosity

Fig. 58.5 Endoleak classification.

Table 58.1 Rutherford classification for chronic limb ischaemia.

Grade	Category	Clinical description	Objective criteria
0	0	Asymptomatic: no haemodynamically significant occlusive disease	Normal treadmill or reactive hyperaemia test
	1	Mild claudication	Completes treadmill exercise; AP after exercise >50 mmHg but at least 20 mmHg lower than resting value
I	2	Moderate claudication	Between categories 1 and 3
	3	Severe claudication	Cannot complete standard treadmill exercise, and AP after exercise <50 mmHg
II	4	Ischaemic rest pain	Resting AP <40 mmHg, flat or barely pulsatile ankle or metatarsal PVR; TP <30 mmHg
III	5	Minor tissue loss: non-healing ulcer, focal gangrene with diffuse pedal ischaemia	Resting AP <60 mmHg, ankle or metatarsal PVR flat or barely pulsatile; TP <40 mmHg
	6	Major tissue loss: extending above TM level, functional foot no longer salvageable	Same as category 5

AP, ankle pressure; PVR, pulse volume recording; TM, transmetatarsal; TP, toe pressure.

tree into components with recommendations as to the appropriateness of endovascular treatment. In summary, most iliac disease is amenable to percutaneous repair, including complex occlusive disease involving the aorta and iliac arteries. New technology has allowed safer and more effective treatment of complex suprainguinal disease. An example of this is covered endovascular repair of the aortic bifurcation (CERAB), where two covered iliac stents are introduced into an aortic stent creating an endovascular version of an aorto bi-iliac graft (Figure 58.6).

Lesions below the inguinal ligament in patients with CCLI are treated with an angioplasty first if the lesion is judged amenable to angioplasty and stenting. With long-segment occlusions and very distal disease, surgical bypass with autologous venous conduits have an important role

Acute limb ischaemia

Acute limb ischaemia (ALI) usually results from *in situ* thrombosis of an atheromatous artery with acute clot or occlusion from an embolus that may originate in the heart or a more local source such as a popliteal artery aneurysm. ALI has a separate classification to CCLI (Table 58.2). Rutherford grade IIa and IIb patients may benefit from catheter-directed therapy in the acute phase, primarily aspiration thromboembolectomy or catheter-directed thrombolysis. Both these techniques require a catheter to traverse the acutely occluded arterial segment and the clot is removed through the lumen of the catheter

(a)   (b)

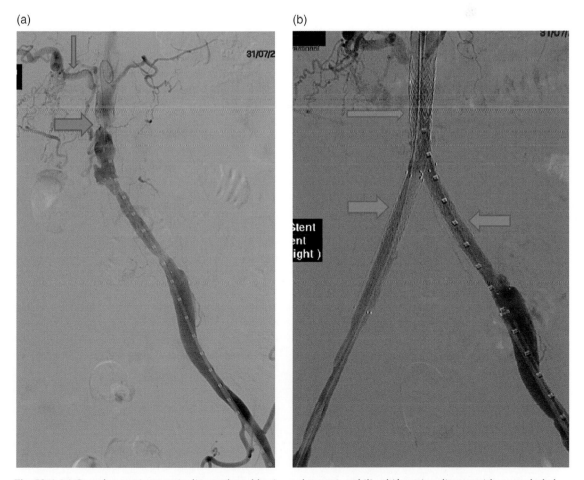

Fig. 58.6 (a) Complex aortic stenotic disease (broad horizontal arrow) and iliac bifurcation disease with an occluded right common iliac artery (not seen). Note the extensive collateral circulation (vertical arrow). (b) Arteriogram after percutaneous revascularisation using an aortic stent and bilateral iliac stents (arrows), the CERAB technique, in a patient with intermittent claudication.

Table 58.2 Rutherford classification for acute limb ischaemia.

		Findings		Doppler signal	
Category	Description/prognosis	Sensory loss	Muscle weakness	Arterial	Venous
I Viable	Not immediately threatened	None	None	Audible	Audible
II Threatened					
a Marginally	Salvageable if promptly treated	Minimal (toes) or none	None	Inaudible	Audible
b Immediately	Salvageable with immediate revascularisation	More than toes, associated rest pain	Mild, moderate	Inaudible	Audible
III Irreversible	Major tissue loss or permanent nerve damage inevitable	Profound, anaesthetic	Profound, paralysis	Inaudible	Inaudible

manually or by mechanical suction or it is laced with a lytic agent such as urokinase (which is infused across the occluded segment though a catheter with multiple small side holes). The therapeutic management of ALI often needs careful thought as time frames to achieve revascularisation are crucial and the ischaemic limb may require other interventions such as fasciotomy. Given these constraints, endovascular techniques play a secondary role to surgical embolectomy, thrombectomy and bypass.

Endovascular treatment of haemorrhage

Endovascular techniques have an important role in the management of acute haemorrhage, particularly bleeding from the colon usually presenting as haematochezia or in the management of traumatic injury complicated by bleeding. Multidetector CT is capable of identifying the source of bleeding in many cases, allowing rapid and focused closure of the bleeding point with embolisation. The principle of embolisation requires the operator to isolate the bleeding segment by embolising both proximal and distal to the site of bleeding ('closing the front and back doors'). As previously discussed, delivery of embolic material such as coils or glue causes rapid artery closure. In non-traumatic haemorrhage it is important to recognise that embolisation is not treating the underlying lesion and further investigation is important. In the colon this may be diverticular disease or a neoplasm and colonography or colonoscopy is required. In some cases lesions that are associated with a high risk of bleeding are prophylactically embolised, for example pancreatic pseudoaneurysms and psuedoaneurysmis associated with tumours such as angiomyolipomas

(Figure 58.7). Not all bleeding arteries are treated with embolisation and if end-organ ischaemia is a potential problem, the bleeding site may be excluded with a covered stent.

Other applications of endovascular therapy

Endovascular therapy is widely used in the venous circulation to treat conditions such as May–Thurner syndrome (compression of the left common iliac vein by the right common iliac artery), acute lower limb deep venous thrombosis and Paget–Schroetter disease (effort thrombosis of the subclavian and axillary veins). Other applications include the endovascular management of failing dialysis fistulas and central venous obstruction from all causes. Chemoembolisation has an important role in the treatment of tumours, particularly in the liver, and the management of stroke and subarachnoid haemorrhage has been revolutionised by endovascular techniques that can remove intracerebral clot and treat leaking cerebral aneurysms.

Conclusion

Endovascular management of vascular disease is an attractive minimally invasive treatment option that is rapidly increasing in scope as technology provides more devices and the miniaturisation and improvement of current devices. However, the best approach for each patient is a knowledgeable discussion of medical, surgical and endovascular options.

(a) (b) (c)

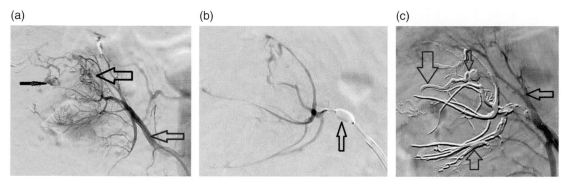

Fig. 58.7 Catheter arteriogram of a highly vascular renal carcinoma of the right kidney (a) shows a selective catheterisation (red arrow) and arteriography of the right renal artery demonstrating abnormal tumour circulation in a renal carcinoma (black arrows), (b) shows a balloon occluding catheter placed proximal to the tumour prior to embolization (open arrow), (c) shows an arteriogram after the injection of liquid embolic agent (red arrow) into the tumour circulation. Untreated arteries are indicated by black arrow.

Further reading

Conte SM, Vale PR. Peripheral vascular disease. *Heart Lung Circ* 2018;27:427–32.

England A, McWilliams R. Endovascular aortic aneurysm repair (EVAR). *Ulster Med J* 2013;82:3–10.

Robertson L, Paraskevas KI, Stewart M. Angioplasty and stenting for peripheral arterial disease of the lower limbs: an overview of Cochrane Reviews. *Cochrane Database Syst Rev* 2017;(2):CD 012542.

MCQs

Select the single correct answer to each question. The correct answers can be found in the Answers section at the end of the book.

1 Which of the following statements about elective endovascular repair (EVAR) of an abdominal aortic aneurysm is correct?
a only infrarenal aortic aneurysms can be repaired
b preoperative imaging with ultrasound is sufficient
c 30-day operative mortality is lower with EVAR than open surgical repair
d type 2 endoleaks are the least common type of endoleak after EVAR
e requires open surgical access to the femoral arteries

2 Which of the following is *not* a relative contraindication to percutaneous balloon angioplasty in a 70-year-old woman with short-distance bilateral intermittent claudication?
a the femoral artery lesion is a 90% stenosis over a length of 1 cm
b the ipsilateral common femoral artery is severely diseased with calcified plaque
c obesity
d prior ipsilateral groin surgery
e a >10 cm heavily calcified femoral arterial occlusion

3 Which of the following statements about percutaneous arterial embolisation is *incorrect*?
a solid organ arterial injury associated with bleeding demonstrated on a CT angiogram may be suitable
b a common indication is haematochezia
c complete arterial transection of the femoral or popliteal arteries is an indication
d embolic agents maybe solid, liquid or particulate
e embolisation of lumbar arteries may be required to treat a type 2 endoleak

4 Which of the following statements about thoracic aortic endovascular repair (TEVAR) is *incorrect*?
a coarctation is an indication
b acute complicated type B dissection is an indication
c an extra anatomical graft from the carotid to subclavian artery may be required to allow coverage of the origin of the left subclavian artery
d complications include spinal cord ischaemia
e aneurysmal disease of the descending thoracic aorta is unsuitable for TEVAR

Section 14
Urology

59 Benign urological conditions

Anthony J. Costello[1], Daniel M. Costello[2] and Fairleigh Reeves[1]

[1] University of Melbourne, Melbourne, Victoria, Australia
[2] St. Vincent's Hospital, Melbourne, Victoria, Australia

Anatomy of the urinary tract

Kidneys

The kidneys lie in the retroperitoneum at the level of T12 to L3 with the right slightly lower than left due to the bulk of the liver. The renal hilum faces medially and contains the renal vein, renal artery and ureter, in that order from anterior to posterior. Blood supply is from the aorta via single renal arteries, although up to 30% of people have accessory arteries. The renal vein, single on both sides, drains to the inferior vena cava. The left renal vein crosses anterior to the aorta.

Ureters

The ureters are approximately 25 cm long and travel behind the peritoneum into the pelvis before swinging forward and medially at the level of the ischial spine to enter the bladder. The ureter narrows at the pelviureteric junction, at its crossing of the pelvic brim and at its oblique entrance into the bladder wall (vesicoureteric junction). The ureteric blood supply is derived from multiple vessels as it descends from abdomen to pelvis.

Bladder

The bladder lies within the pelvis, with a distended volume of 400–500 mL. The ureteric orifices and bladder neck form the triangular area known as the trigone at the bladder base. Bladder arterial supply derives from branches of the internal iliac artery with named superior and inferior vesical arteries. Venous drainage is by the internal iliac veins. Lymphatics run with the blood vessels.

Prostate

The prostate is a fibromuscular gland (plum-sized in the male after 50 years, walnut-sized in the postpubertal male) that lies beneath the bladder and above the urogenital diaphragm. The prostatic urethra traverses the prostate and receives the prostatic and ejaculatory ducts, the latter being formed by the seminal vesicles and vas deferens. The prostate anatomically is described by surfaces, lobes and zones. Its base abuts the bladder neck, and apex opens into the membranous urethra which is surrounded by the horseshoe-shaped striated muscle of the external urethral sphincter. Its inferolateral surfaces are cradled by levator ani and its posterior surface lies in front of the rectum and is palpable on digital rectal examination. The prostate has left and right lobes and a median lobe at the bladder neck. Zonal anatomy comprises a peripheral zone, where prostate cancer usually begins, a transition zone (the site of benign prostatic hyperplasia, which can obstruct urinary outflow), and a 'central zone' surrounding the urethra. There is also an anterior fibromuscular zone that can be difficult to target with traditional transrectal ultrasound biopsy technique. Blood supply is predominantly from the inferior vesical artery with variable additional supply. Venous drainage is through the vesico-prostatic plexus to the internal iliac veins. Lymph drainage is to internal and external iliac, obturator, presacral and para-aortic nodes.

Stones

Aetiology

Calcium-based stones account for the vast majority of all renal calculi (80–85%). These are usually due to elevated urinary calcium, uric acid or oxalate or decreased urinary citrate (an inhibitor of stone formation). Conditions which lead to hypercalcaemia such as hyperparathyroidism may be causative. However, in many patients an underlying metabolic defect cannot be identified.

Infection stones (struvite stones) account for 1–5% of all stones. These stones can grow rapidly and commonly present as a staghorn calculus. They contain magnesium, ammonium and phosphate. Urea-splitting organisms (such as *Proteus*, *Pseudomonas* and *Klebsiella*) produce urease, which catalyses the conversion of urea into ammonia and carbon dioxide, resulting in alkalinisation of the urine and providing an environment conducive to this type of stone formation.

Less than 5% of all stones are uric acid based. Risk factors for uric acid stones include diabetes, gout, myeloproliferative disease, rapid weight loss, chemotherapy treatment, haemolytic anaemia and chronic diarrhoea. These stones are characteristically radiolucent on X-ray and can be dissolved with urinary alkalinisation to a pH above 6.5.

Cysteine stones are uncommon (only 1–2% of all stones). They occur due to a genetic metabolic defect leading to increased urinary cysteine. These patients begin forming stones at a young age and have a high recurrence rate, and therefore need close observation and medical management for the prevention of stones.

Aetiology of renal calculi is often multifactorial. Dehydration certainly increases the risk of urolithiasis, with a higher incidence of stones being seen in hot dry climates. Individual patients may also have underlying structural (any condition that leads to urine stasis) or metabolic (as highlighted above) disorders that increase their risk of stone formation.

Clinical presentation

Non-obstructing intrarenal calculi rarely cause any symptoms and are often detected incidentally on imaging done for other reasons. In contrast, renal colic, perhaps more accurately considered ureteric colic, results in severe pain that has a sudden onset and a typical 'loin to groin' distribution. An acute abdomen must be excluded. Those with renal colic characteristically shift in bed constantly struggling to get comfortable, in stark contrast to the patient with peritonitis who will be lying very still. Clinical examination in renal colic tends to be rather unremarkable. Patients may have renal angle tenderness but have a soft abdomen with no signs of peritonism. A urinalysis often demonstrates haematuria, but this is not diagnostic as it may be absent and can also be seen in other conditions.

If someone presents with renal colic, coexisting urinary infection must also be excluded as the presence of an infected obstructed kidney is a surgical emergency and mandates urgent drainage of the infected system.

Investigation

The majority (90%) of all renal calculi are radiopaque and can therefore be visualised on plain X-ray (Figure 59.1). For initial diagnosis, however, CT of the kidneys, ureters and bladder (non-contrast; Figure 59.1b) is the imaging modality of choice as not only will it identify calculi, but also provides helpful information with regard to their anatomical location as well as any associated hydronephrosis indicating obstruction. CT intravenous pyelography (contrast study including delayed phase) can be used to delineate the urinary system to differentiate phleboliths or other external calcification from ureteric calculi. If CT is contraindicated (pregnancy), ultrasound may reveal hydronephrosis and can sometimes demonstrate renal calculi, although ultrasound has a low sensitivity for detecting ureteric calculi.

Patients with renal calculi should have initial metabolic screening with serum urea, creatinine and electrolytes including calcium, magnesium, phosphate and uric acid. Urine should also be sent for microscopy and culture and pH evaluation.

More formal metabolic testing is indicated in patients with recurrent calculi or other risk factors, and a 24-hour urine collection (particularly for recurrent stone formers) should be evaluated for pH, volume, calcium, oxalate, citrate and uric acid; this may reveal an underlying metabolic abnormality that can be targeted to prevent future episodes.

Management

Many ureteric calculi can be managed conservatively. The smaller the stone and the more distal, the more likely it will pass spontaneously. Approximately 70% of stones less than 5 mm in size will pass. Acute renal colic pain is best managed by non-steroidal anti-inflammatory drugs rather than opioids. Medical expulsion therapy with alpha-blockers such as tamsulosin is often prescribed to improve rate of spontaneous stone passage, although the evidence regarding efficacy is unclear. In patients who elect for conservative management, follow-up imaging to ensure stone

(a)

(b)

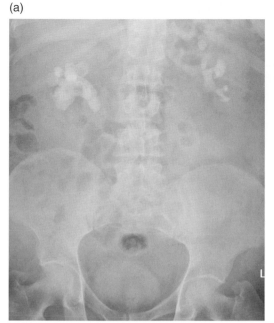 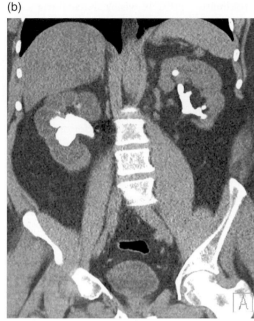

Fig. 59.1 X-ray of kidneys, ureters and bladder (a) and non-contrast abdominal CT (b) showing bilateral staghorn calculi.

passage is important as symptoms may resolve despite persistence of an obstructing calculus due to autoregulation of renal blood flow. Patients who fail conservative management after 4–6 weeks warrant surgical intervention to prevent renal impairment. Indications for intervention include infection, obstruction in a solitary kidney, bilateral obstruction and uncontrolled pain.

In the setting of an infected obstructed kidney, resuscitation, antibiotics and urgent drainage of the collecting system should be undertaken. Decompression can be achieved either by cystoscopic insertion of a ureteric stent or radiological insertion of a nephrostomy tube. Once the sepsis has been adequately treated, definitive stone treatment is undertaken on an elective basis.

Non-obstructing intrarenal stones do not always require treatment depending on size and associated symptoms. The risk of a symptomatic episode for small non-obstructing renal calculi is 10–25% per year. However, all staghorn calculi should be treated as they may lead to progressive renal damage and infection if left. Indications for treating smaller intrarenal stones include infection, symptoms (pain/haematuria), patient preference, stones larger than 5 mm, high-risk stone formers and social circumstances that would make seeking future medical attention difficult should an emergency arise.

Definitive stone treatment depends on the size, location and composition (if known) of the stone.

Large intrarenal calculi (including staghorns) are best managed with percutaneous nephrolithotomy. Smaller ureteric or renal calculi may be managed with ureteroscopy/pyeloscopy and stone fragmentation (usually with laser) or extraction, or extracorporeal shockwave lithotripsy (ESWL). As highlighted earlier, some stones may be amenable to dissolution therapy.

All stone formers should be given general dietary advice to increase oral fluid intake, decrease sodium and meat intake, and have a moderate calcium intake (as risk of stone formation can increase with calcium intake that is either too low or too high). If a metabolic defect is isolated, treatment should be targeted at correction of this.

Haematuria

Differential diagnosis

Haematuria may originate anywhere along the urinary tract. Differential diagnoses of haematuria include benign (trauma, infection, calculi, iatrogenic, intrinsic renal disease, benign prostatic hypertrophy, inflammation, stricture) and malignant causes.

Haematuria may be macroscopic (visible) or microscopic (evident on testing but not visible). The distinction is important as the risk of malignancy is significantly higher if the haematuria is visible (approximately 20% in visible haematuria compared to 5% for microscopic haematuria). Associated symptoms and timing of macroscopic haematuria can assist in determining the source of haematuria. For example, initial haematuria is suggestive of anterior urethral pathology compared with terminal haematuria from the posterior urethra, whereas blood throughout the urinary stream suggests the pathology is coming from the bladder or higher.

Investigation

Radiological investigation for haematuria is best done using CT intravenous pyelography. This has the best sensitivity and specificity for identifying upper tract causes for haematuria, but generally radiological imaging provides inadequate evaluation of the bladder. Therefore, a cystoscopy is also required to complete investigation of the lower urinary tract. Urine cytology may also be performed.

Management

Management of haematuria should be directed at underlying pathology. Acutely, any coagulopathy should be corrected, and anticoagulants should be withheld. If the patient has a stable haemoglobin and is voiding well, haematuria may be investigated as an outpatient. If there is evidence of urinary retention due to clot, then a urinary catheter is required for bladder washout. In some cases, if this fails to resolve the haematuria, a patient may need emergency endoscopic evaluation to evacuate remaining clots in the bladder and coagulate active bleeding or resect tumour if present.

Lower urinary tract symptoms

Benign prostatic hyperplasia

Presentation

Benign prostatic hyperplasia (BPH) is commonly seen in older men, affecting more than 80% of men in their eighties. As men age, there is a normal increase in the amount of prostatic stroma and smooth muscle tone, which may ultimately result in bladder outlet obstruction (BOO). In contrast to prostate cancer, which tends to occur in the peripheral zone of the prostate (and therefore rarely presents with local symptoms), BPH occurs in the periurethral transition zone and therefore readily affects voiding. BPH can result in a range of symptoms including weak and/or intermittent stream, hesitancy, terminal dribbling and nocturia. Patients

may also have poor bladder emptying. In the long term, the bladder may become overworked, manifesting either with urgency and frequency from detrusor overactivity, or with inadequate contractions leading to retention or overflow incontinence.

Investigation

When assessing patients with lower urinary tract symptoms it is important to establish if their symptoms are prostatic in origin or if there may be other underlying pathology or contributing factors. A thorough history should be taken and examination, including of the prostate per rectum, and urinalysis performed in all. A bladder diary is a valuable tool to gain insights into patients voiding patterns and likely aetiology.

A urinary tract ultrasound is not essential for investigation of all cases of lower urinary tract symptoms but can be helpful in triaging patients, by identifying complications of BPH (e.g. presence of hydronephrosis or bladder calculi). Also, although prostate size does not correlate with patient symptoms, this information can be useful in guiding appropriate BPH treatment selection.

A poor voiding flow rate supports a diagnosis of BOO. However, in complex cases where it is unclear if poor flow is due to obstruction or detrusor failure, formal urodynamic testing will confirm high detrusor pressure in the setting of BOO.

For men with a life expectancy of 10 years of more, testing for prostate-specific antigen (PSA) should be considered because a diagnosis of prostate cancer may change treatment choices.

Management

The decision to treat BPH largely comes down to the degree of inconvenience the patient experiences. If a man is not bothered by his lower urinary tract symptoms, it is reasonable to defer treatment in most cases as not all patients with BPH will have progression of their symptoms. For most men with BPH, medical management will be first line. Alpha-blockers and 5α-reductase inhibitors are the mainstay of pharmacological management, either alone or in combination.

Alpha-blockers act by relaxing the smooth muscle of the bladder neck and prostate, with symptom improvement noted within a few days of initiation of treatment. They are generally well tolerated with relatively few side effects (retrograde ejaculation, dizziness and postural hypotension). Hypotension is now seen less frequently, as selective alpha-blockers (such as tamsulosin) target only the

α_{1A} receptor subtype (localised to the bladder, prostate, vas deferens and seminal vesicles), sparing the α_{1B} receptors (located in blood vessels) which caused troublesome hypotension with previous generation non-selective drugs.

The 5α-reductase inhibitors (e.g. finasteride or dutasteride) block the conversion of testosterone to dihydrotestosterone, which results in reduction of prostate volume over time. This ultimately leads to improvement of urinary flow as well as reduction in risk of urinary retention and need for surgery. However, due to the mechanism of action noticeable symptom improvement is generally only achieved after 6–9 months of treatment. Logically, considering their effect relates to reduction of prostate volume, these drugs tend to work best in larger glands (>40 mL). When prescribing 5α-reductase inhibitors, patients need to be counselled about the possible side effects, which include erectile dysfunction, decreased libido, decreased ejaculate volume and gynaecomastia as these can cause significant distress. It is also import to note that 5α-reductase treatment is associated with a decrease un PSA of approximately 50% after treatment for 9–12 months. This must be kept in mind when considering a patient's PSA results. Because of their difference in mechanism of action and onset of symptom relief, alpha-blockers and 5α-reductase inhibitors can be effectively combined if required.

An absolute indication for surgical relief of obstruction is the presence of hydronephrosis and renal impairment due to high-pressure retention (obstructive uropathy). Other indications for surgical intervention include voiding symptoms refractory to medical therapy, recurrent urinary retention, infections, gross haematuria or bladder calculi.

Transurethral resection of the prostate (TURP) is considered the gold standard for surgical management of BPH. It involves endoscopic resection of the prostate using a cutting diathermy loop to shave away chips of prostate to leave a wide-open prostatic fossa. Potential complications include bleeding, infection, retrograde ejaculation, stricture, and transurethral resection syndrome (collection of symptoms/signs including hyponatraemia, hypervolaemia, hypertension, nausea, vomiting, visual disturbance and altered conscious state due to excess absorption of hypotonic irrigation fluid).

Although TURP still remains a mainstay in many urology practices, other surgical options also exist. In small prostates where there is simply a tight bladder neck, the bladder neck may be incised endoscopically without formally resecting any tissue. Very large prostates may be more safely and effectively treated with an open *simple* prostatectomy to enucleate the adenomatous tissue, leaving behind the prostatic capsule. The threshold to elect for open surgery will vary from surgeon to surgeon, although a prostate volume of in excess of 100–150 cm^3 would be considered too large for TURP by many. As technology and surgical expertise advance, lasers are being used to tackle glands that were previously considered too large for endoscopic intervention. Lasers can be used to either vaporise BPH tissue (GreenLight photoselective vaporisation of the prostate, usually utilised in small to moderate-sized glands) or enucleate the prostate (holmium laser enucleation of the prostate, which achieves a similar outcome to open prostatectomy in large glands with reduced blood loss). One of the drawbacks of laser therapies is a higher rate of irritative voiding symptoms postoperatively.

Urethral stricture

A stricture is an abnormal narrowing, and in the urethra this obstructs the usual passage of urine, leading to a weak flow. Some patients may also describe spraying or a double urinary stream as well as frequency, dysuria or haematuria.

Acquired urethral strictures are common in men and are usually due to previous infection (historically most commonly gonococcal urethritis) or trauma, such as catheterisation, surgical instrumentation or external trauma such as a straddle injury or pelvic fracture. A retrograde urethrogram (Figure 59.2) is important in evaluating these

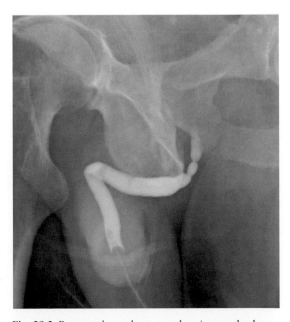

Fig. 59.2 Retrograde urethrogram showing urethral stricture.

patients as it will demonstrate the extent and location of any stricture and can help guide management.

Urethral dilatation or urethrotomy (endoscopic incision of stricture) will usually relieve any symptoms, but in many cases the stricture will recur. Urethroplasty involves formal repair of the stricture and has a higher chance of long-term success. For short strictures, excision of the stricture with end-to-end anastomosis may be used, but longer strictures require grafting of the affected area (usually with buccal mucosa). Alternatively, patients can keep the urethral lumen patent with intermittent self-catheterisation.

Nocturia

Nocturia is defined as waking once or more at night to void. Although it is commonly related to BPH in men, there are many other causes that must be considered. These causes can be grouped into three broad categories: (i) polyuria (voided volume >2800 mL per 24 hours); (ii) nocturnal polyuria (amount voided overnight is more than one-third the daily total volume, which may be due to behavioural issues or underlying medical disease); and (iii) bladder capacity problems (including BOO, overactive bladder, neurogenic bladder). Management needs to be directed at the underlying cause.

Urinary tract infections

Urinary tract infection (UTI) is a common condition that a variety of clinicians will manage in their practice. The urologist's role is to manage complicated cases and recurrent infection. UTIs most commonly present with symptoms of infection of the bladder (cystitis), but may also involve other parts of the urinary tract including epididymis, testis (see section Epididymitis) and prostate (see section Prostatitis) in men, and kidney in both sexes.

Often empirical treatment will be commenced based on a clinical diagnosis made in the presence of symptoms of UTI and pyuria, but definitive diagnosis requires urine culture. Specimen for culture should be a clean catch and midstream. In an era of increasing antibiotic resistance, culture results can be valuable in directing therapy.

Recurrent UTI

Recurrent infection may be due to incomplete treatment of a UTI (unresolved) or a truly recurrent UTI where there is an intervening negative culture and re-infection occurs either as a result of bacterial persistence within the urinary tract or from new infection.

Upper tract infection

Upper tract infection most often occurs in the setting of ascending Gram-negative infection but may also arise from haematogenous spread (often Gram positive). A spectrum of disease can be seen: progression of pyelonephritis can lead to renal or perinephric abscess. If a patient with presumed pyelonephritis fails to respond to appropriate antibiotics, an abscess should be excluded. Upper tract infection can also occur in the setting of stone disease (see section Stones).

Prostatitis

The prostate can be a source of infection and inflammation. Four different categories of prostatitis are recognised: (i) acute bacterial prostatitis, (ii) chronic bacterial prostatitis, (iii) chronic pelvic pain and (iv) asymptomatic inflammatory prostatitis.

Acute bacterial prostatitis is most commonly due to *Escherichia coli* infection. Patients present with systemic signs of infection (such as fever) along with pain and lower urinary tract symptoms. A total of 4–6 weeks of antibiotics are required. Failure to respond to antibiotics should prompt pelvic CT to exclude a prostatic abscess. In the setting of urinary retention, a catheter (possibly a suprapubic catheter) is required to allow bladder drainage.

Chronic bacterial prostatitis describes lower-grade recurrent symptomatic infections, which tend to affect older men. This may require prolonged antibiotic therapy, and after initial treatment may even need low-dose suppressive therapy to prevent recurrent infection. In these men it is also sensible to consider TURP to remove infected tissue and prevent recurrence.

Chronic pelvic pain is a very important entity that is gaining increasing recognition. It is a complex and debilitating condition that is associated with pain and urinary, bowel, psychological and sexual symptoms. Treatment requires a multidisciplinary approach, with the team often comprising a urologist, specialised pelvic floor physiotherapist, psychologist and pain specialist.

Asymptomatic bacteriuria

Asymptomatic bacteriuria is commonly seen in clinical practice. Predisposing conditions include catheter use (permanent or intermittent), bowel incorporated into the urinary system (e.g. ileal conduit, bladder augmentation), diabetes and institutionalised elderly patients. Treatment of asymptomatic bacteriuria can lead to emergence of resistant bacteria, so is not recommended in most situations. An exception is in pregnancy. Pregnant women should be screened and treated, as asymptomatic bacteriuria confers at least a 20- to 30-fold risk of progression to pyelonephritis in pregnancy, which is associated with preterm labour and low birthweight.

Penis

Anatomy (Figure 59.3)

The penis facilitates urination and the process of erection and ejaculation for sexual intercourse. It has a root, body and glans and comprises three cylinders of erectile tissue, the two corpora cavernosa dorsally and the corpus spongiosum ventrally. The penile urethra travels within the corpus spongiosum, which expands distally to form the glans penis. The corpora are filled with sinusoidal tissue that becomes engorged with blood during erection. The penis is invested with penile skin which is

continued from the skin of the anterior abdominal wall, and folds back on itself at its distal end over the glans, forming the foreskin (prepuce). Arterial supply is from branches of the internal pudendal artery. Venous drainage is through a complex of veins, culminating in superficial dorsal and deep dorsal veins, to the vesico-prostatic plexus. The deep dorsal vein carries the majority of the penile venous return. Control of this vein by ligation is an essential step in radical (cancer) prostatectomy. The lymph drainage of the penile skin, the corporal tissue and glans penis is to the superficial and deep inguinal nodes. The penis is richly supplied by pudendal nerves via the dorsal nerves, which follow the course of the dorsal arteries, and are especially prevalent in the sensitive glans. The cavernous nerves ramify in the erectile tissue, providing sympathetic and parasympathetic supply to the erectile tissue. Neural control of erections is parasympathetic causing vasodilation, while sympathetic and somatic nerves stimulate contraction and ejaculation. The neurovascular bundle runs alongside the prostate in a groove above the rectum. It contains

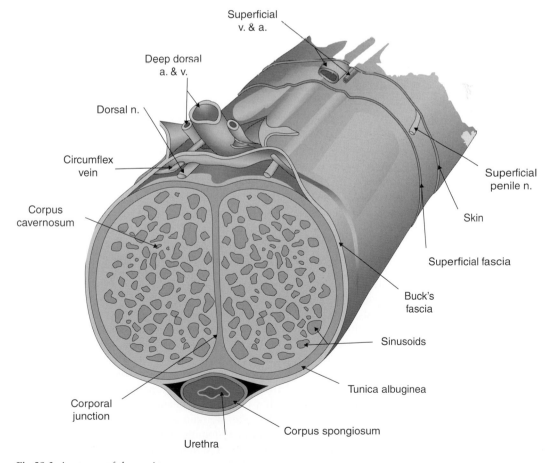

Fig.59.3 Anatomy of the penis.

sympathetic nerves from the hypogastric plexus (T12–L1) and parasympathetics (S2–S4).

Penile conditions

Phimosis

Phimosis describes a tight foreskin that cannot be retracted fully behind the glans. This can lead to overgrowth of smegma bacillus under the foreskin due to inability to cleanse the area and may be associated with voiding dysfunction with urine ballooning behind the tight foreskin.

Phimosis is physiological in the paediatric population, but beyond puberty the foreskin is retractile in almost all men. In adults, phimosis may be due to a pathological scarring process called lichen sclerosis (previously known as balanitis xerotica obliterans).

Circumcision effectively treats phimosis.

Paraphimosis

Paraphimosis describes an inability to replace the retracted foreskin over the glans. It is often associated with significant oedema and pain and may result in tissue necrosis if not corrected. One of the common causes in hospital is failure to replace the foreskin after inserting a urinary catheter.

Compression and manual reduction is successful in most cases. If this fails then a dorsal slit to release the constricting band is needed. Many patients will require an elective circumcision to prevent recurrence.

Priapism

Priapism is defined as a persistent erection (lasting greater than 4 hours) unrelated to, or lasting beyond, sexual stimulation. There are two distinct types of priapism.

The most common is ischaemic priapism, also known as low flow or venous occlusive. This is a urological emergency as the penis is engorged with deoxygenated blood, which can lead to penile necrosis and long-term erectile dysfunction if not treated. Emergency drainage of the blood from the corpora cavernosa is required. Risk factors for ischaemic priapism include injectable medications for the treatment of erectile dysfunction and sickle cell disease or other hypercoagulable states as well as certain medications.

The less common, non-ischaemic priapism (also known as arterial, high flow or non-occlusive) accounts for less than 5% of all priapism. These cases are due to unregulated arterial blood flow and are often due to trauma. The diagnosis can be confirmed with cavernosal blood gas and treatment is not an emergency as the penile tissue continues to receive oxygenated blood.

Peyronie's disease

Abnormal penile curvature is commonly due to Peyronie's disease, in which plaques of fibrotic tissue develop in the tunica albuginea of the corpora cavernosa that limits expansion, resulting in curvature in the opposite direction during erection. The cause is unknown but may relate to trauma. Peyronie's disease is linked to Dupuytren's contracture of the hands and Ledderhose disease of the feet.

Peyronie's disease has an initial acute phase which is often associated with pain. This usually settles after 6–18 months as the condition stabilises and the chronic phase begins. Once stable, surgical correction can be undertaken if the curvature is interfering with intercourse.

Scrotum and testes (see also Chapter 79)

Anatomy

Scrotum

The scrotum is a bag-like structure which hangs below the penis and contains the male reproductive units, the testes, and associated structures. The scrotum is divided into spaces by a fibromuscular septum in the form of the median raphe and is covered by hair-bearing skin, thrown up into multiple rugae. Under the skin lies the dartos muscle layer. Arterial supply is from the external pudendal arteries anteriorly and the perineal arteries posteriorly. The venous drainage of the scrotum is via external pudendal veins to the great saphenous vein. Scrotal skin receives multiple sources of innervation, including the ilioinguinal nerve anteriorly and branches of the pudendal nerve posteriorly.

Testes

The adult testes are paired ovoid-shaped reproductive glands of approximately 30 mL in volume. They produce sperm and the hormone testosterone. The testes descend *in utero* just before birth from an intra-abdominal position. They take coverings from the abdominal wall layers as they pass through the inguinal canal. In some cases, they fail to descend before birth. The undescended (cryptorchid) testis is more prone to malignancy. The external oblique muscle continues as the external spermatic fascia, and the internal oblique muscle continues as the cremasteric muscle. The internal spermatic fascia is a continuation of the transversalis fascia and the tunica vaginalis is a continuation of the peritoneal layer. These layers constitute the spermatic cord, which also contains the vas deferens, testicular artery and vein, nerves and lymphatics and adipose tissue. The testes themselves are surrounded by tunica vaginalis, which has two layers, a visceral and a parietal layer. This is a potential space that can normally contain 2–3 mL of fluid. This space can be the origin of a fluid sac called a hydrocele. The tiny appendix testis is attached to the superior surface of the tunica vaginalis. Deep to the tunica vaginalis lies the extremely tough tunica albuginea, the dense fibrous capsule of the testes. The seminiferous tubules leading from the lobules of the testes coalesce and enter the rete testis, which passes into the epididymis. This combines to become a single vas deferens, travelling upward in the spermatic cord.

The testis draws its own blood supply with it from the abdomen, and thus the testicular artery which travels in the spermatic cord originates from the aorta. Further arterial supply to the testis comes from the artery to the vas, and a large area of anastomosis occurs at the epididymis between these arteries and the cremasteric artery, allowing for a rich supply to the testis.

The testis is drained by many veins that anastomose extensively forming the pampiniform plexus. These veins join forming two to three branches in the inguinal canal and ultimately a single gonadal (testicular) vein, which drains into the inferior vena cava on the right and the renal vein on the left (related to varicocele formation).

The delineation of scrotal lymph drainage from that of the testes is of vital importance in the surgical treatment of testis cancer. The skin of the scrotum is drained by the superficial inguinal lymph nodes of the ipsilateral side. The testis drains via the spermatic cord to the para-aortic nodes on the same side. This implies that scrotal integrity should not be breached when performing an orchidectomy for testis cancer, as this will ensure that two areas of lymphatic drainage are now involved.

The testes are supplied by sympathetic nerves from the renal and aortic plexuses, as well as by contributions from the pelvic plexuses accompanying the vas deferens. The testes have a rich sensory innervation, and thus even minor trauma can be followed by severe pain in the testes, which is often felt as a more generalised abdominal pain due to the sensory fibre mediation by T10 dorsal root ganglions.

Scrotal pain and masses

Testicular torsion

Torsion is a surgical emergency. It involves rotation of the testis and spermatic cord that compromises the blood supply to the testis, leading to ischaemia and ultimately necrosis if not corrected urgently. It tends to occur in males 12–18 years of age or newborns but may occur at any age. Risk factors for torsion include undescended testis and 'bell clapper' deformity where the tunica vaginalis inserts high on the spermatic cord, allowing the testis to rotate freely.

Patients present with sudden-onset, severe, unilateral testicular pain and swelling. On examination the testis is extremely tender and often high-riding due to cremasteric spasm.

Clinical suspicion of torsion mandates urgent surgical exploration. Although Doppler ultrasonography may show lack of testicular blood flow, theatre should not be delayed for imaging as the time this takes may result in death of the testicle. In addition, there is a risk of a false negative result. The best chance for testicular survival is if the torsion is corrected within 6 hours of symptom onset. After the testis has been untwisted, both testes are fixed to the scrotum to prevent recurrence.

Torsion of testicular appendices is an important differential diagnosis in acute scrotal pain.

Hydrocele

A hydrocele is a collection of fluid within the tunica vaginalis. It often obscures palpation of the underlying testis and is readily transilluminable. Although it is usually painless, it can become quite large. If bothersome, it can be treated. While aspiration may provide relief, fluid frequently reaccumulates. Therefore, surgical hydrocelectomy is preferable.

Hydroceles may represent primary pathology or occur in response to another process (such as tumour, trauma or infection). Ultrasound (Figure 59.4) is essential to exclude underlying pathology prior to treatment.

Spermatocele/epididymal cyst

These fluid collections usually occur in relation to the head of the epididymis. They often present as a painless palpable lump or are noted incidentally on

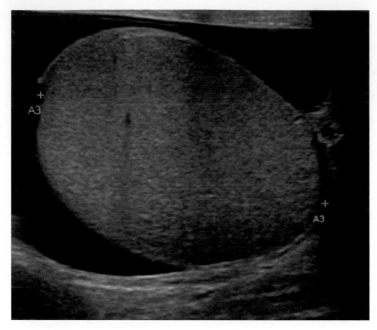

Fig. 59.4 Testicular ultrasound showing hydrocele.

imaging for another reason. Many patients are asymptomatic and generally require no treatment. If they are large and uncomfortable, they may be excised surgically.

Varicocele

A varicocele is a group of dilated veins of the pampiniform plexus. They occur more commonly on the left and usually develop slowly over time. Although often asymptomatic, a varicocele may cause a dull ache that increases with standing and worsens over the course of the day. Discomfort is typically relieved with lying down. In some, but not all, cases it may be associated with impaired fertility or atrophy of the affected testicle.

Scrotal examination classically reveals a 'bag of worms' that is more readily appreciated when examining the patient standing and with Valsalva manoeuvre.

If symptomatic or associated with infertility, it may be treated with surgical ligation or radiological embolisation of the gonadal vein.

Epididymitis

Epididymitis or epididymo-orchitis can also present with significant scrotal pain and enlargement. In contrast to torsion, symptoms usually have a gradual onset. There may also be other associated lower urinary tract symptoms of infection such as dysuria or frequency. Urinalysis will often be suggestive of infection and urine should be sent for microscopy and

culture. Scrotal ultrasound typically demonstrates an enlarged epididymis with increased blood flow.

In men younger than 35 years old, epididymitis is usually due to a sexually transmitted infection, whereas in older men or young children it is most often due to a urinary pathogen (such as *E. coli*). Treatment involves bed rest, scrotal support, analgesia and empirical antibiotics directed at the most likely causative organism until culture results are available to direct therapy.

Further reading

American Urological Association Guidelines, http://www.auanet.org/guidelines

European Association of Urology Non-Oncology Guidelines, https://uroweb.org/individual-guidelines/non-oncology-guidelines/

Wieder JA. *Pocket Guide to Urology*, 5th edn. J. Wieder Medical, 2014.

MCQs

Select the single correct answer to each question. The correct answers can be found in the Answers section at the end of the book.

1 A 14-year-old boy presents to the emergency department with 2 hours of left testicular pain. Which of the following statements is *incorrect*?

   a history of undescended testis is associated with a higher risk of torsion

b pain may be due to appendix testis torsion

c an ultrasound should be done to check testicular blood flow as the pain may be due to testicular torsion

d the best chance for testicular survival is if torsion is corrected within 6 hours of symptom onset

e the patient should be taken to theatre immediately if there is a clinical suspicion of torsion

2 Which of the following statements about haematuria is correct?

a blood throughout the urinary stream suggests that bleeding is coming from the urethra

b if it resolves it does not need further investigation

c the risk of malignancy is the same if haematuria is detected on microscopy or is visible (macroscopic)

d if the CT intravenous pyelogram is normal, a cystoscopy does not need to be performed

e it always needs investigation as it may be due to malignancy

3 A 54-year-old woman presents to the emergency department with acute flank pain. You suspect she has renal colic from a ureteric stone. What is the correct response?

a X-ray of the kidneys, ureters and bladder is the investigation of choice

b patients with renal stones should be encouraged to decrease calcium intake to prevent future stone episodes as most stones contain calcium

c non-steroidal anti-inflammatory drugs are more effective than opioids for controlling renal colic pain

d if her urinalysis shows no haematuria, it is unlikely that she has a stone

e if there are signs of infection, the stone can be managed conservatively if the patient is given antibiotics

4 A 75-year-old man describes poor urinary flow and nocturia. Which of the following statements about his condition is correct?

a obstructive symptoms in this age group are most often due to stricture

b nocturnal polyuria may be the cause of his nocturia (defined as the production of more than one-quarter of 24-hour urine output between midnight and 8 a.m.)

c even if he is not bothered by his symptoms he should have treatment

d BPH occurs in the periurethral transition zone of the prostate

e a bladder diary is only necessary if the patient is a poor historian

5 Which of the following statements about UTIs is *incorrect*?

a urinary stasis is a risk factor for infection

b asymptomatic bacteriuria should always be treated to avoid development of clinical infection

c definitive diagnosis requires urine culture

d presence of sepsis in the setting of an obstructing ureteric calculus is a surgical emergency

e empirical antibiotics for epididymo-orchitis in a sexually active 30-year-old man should treat sexually transmitted infections

60 Genitourinary oncology

Homayoun Zargar and Anthony J. Costello

University of Melbourne and Department of Urology, Royal Melbourne Hospital, Melbourne, Victoria, Australia

Prostate cancer

Prostate cancer (PC) is the most commonly diagnosed cancer and the second most common cause of cancer death in men in Australia. In Australia, the lifetime prevalence of PC is one in six. Most men with PC die of other causes and only 3% of men with PC will die of their disease.

Aetiology and pathology

The prevalence of PC increases with age and development of PC before age of 40 is rare. Men with a family history of PC in a first-degree relative have a higher risk of developing PC. This risk further increases if more than one first-degree relative has had PC. History of breast or ovarian cancer in a first-degree relative also increases the lifetime risk of developing PC in the same manner. Mutations in the tumour suppressor genes *BRCA1* and *BRCA2*, involved with DNA repair mechanisms, have been identified in men with a strong family history of PC. The lifetime prevalence of PC is higher in African-American men.

Adenocarcinoma is the most common type of PC and the majority cancers arise from the peripheral zone of the prostate. PC is a heterogeneous disease and often multifocal on diagnosis. PC generally progresses slowly but this also is influenced by the stage and grade of the cancer.

Clinical presentation

The majority of PC patients are asymptomatic on diagnosis. PC can also be diagnosed incidentally in prostatic tissue resected in men undergoing transurethral resection of the prostate (TURP) for benign prostatic enlargement (10% of TURP procedures) or in the prostate of patients treated with cystoprostatectomy for bladder cancer (40–60% of bladder specimens).

In cases of locally advanced disease, patients can present with difficulty urinating, urinary retention or haematuria. Metastatic disease can present with bony pain, pathological fractures or spinal cord compression due to metastatic deposits in the thoracic/lumbar spine.

Investigations

Prostate-specific antigen

Prostate-specific antigen (PSA) is a serine protease produced by the prostate. It is a physiologically important enzyme for the process of semen liquefaction. Raised PSA levels are observed in 90% of men with PC, although elevated PSA levels are not specific to PC. Any process affecting the prostate, including benign enlargement, prostatitis, urinary tract infection and urological instrumentation, can cause a rise in PSA levels.

PSA as a screening tool for detection of PC has become a controversial topic in recent years. Screening leads to earlier cancer detection and improvement in survival in men with clinically significant PC but at the same time can lead to over-diagnosis, psychological stress and over-treatment of men with non-significant PC.

Patient with minimum 10 years' life expectancy should be counselled about the risks, benefits and limitations of PC screening prior to PSA testing. PSA screening should accompany digital rectal examination. PSA screening should start from the age of 40 and the screening interval should be guided by the initial PSA level. If initial PSA is less than 1 ng/mL, the next assessment can be made at age 45. PSA screening should be performed annually after the age of 50.

Textbook of Surgery, Fourth Edition. Edited by Julian A. Smith, Andrew H. Kaye, Christopher Christophi and Wendy A. Brown.
© 2020 John Wiley & Sons Ltd. Published 2020 by John Wiley & Sons Ltd.

Prostate imaging

Transrectal ultrasound imaging of the prostate allows assessment of the size and shape of the prostate but cannot accurately identify PC. Multiparametric magnetic resonance imaging (MRI) uses various sequences and can identify PC in 80–90% of the cases. This can aid in targeting the abnormal areas during prostate biopsy. Prostate biopsy and histological assessment of the samples is the only method for the identification of PC. Prostate biopsy can be performed via the transrectal or transperineal route.

Staging

PC spreads locally to periprostatic tissues, via lymphatics to pelvic and retroperitoneal lymph nodes and via vascular spread to bones and viscera. TNM staging is outlined in Table 60.1.

Grading

The Gleason grading system is based on the architectural pattern of the prostate glands under low-magnification light microscopy. The two most abundant tumour patterns are graded from 1 to 5. The Gleason score is reported as the most common grade plus the second most common grade, followed by the sum (e.g. 3 + 4 = 7). Higher-grade tumours are associated with higher risks of recurrence, metastasis and death from PC. The newer International Society of Urological Pathology (ISUP) grading system aims at simplifying PC grading and reporting. The relationship between Gleason score and ISUP grading system is as follows.

- ISUP Group 1, equivalent to Gleason score ≤6 (3 + 3 and below)
- ISUP Group 2, equivalent to Gleason score 3 + 4 = 7
- ISUP Group 3, equivalent to Gleason score 4 + 3 = 7
- ISUP Group 4, equivalent to Gleason score 8 (4 + 4, 3 + 5 or 5 + 3)
- ISUP Group 5, equivalent to Gleason scores 9 and 10

Risk groups

Based on pre-biopsy PSA, clinical T stage (cT stage) and grading of the tumour, patients can be stratified into low-, intermediate- and high-risk groups (D'Amico risk groups; Table 60.2). The risk groups have prognostic implications and guide in tailoring treatment for PC patients.

Table 60.1 The 2010 TNM (tumour, node, metastasis) staging of prostate cancer.

T Primary tumour	
Tx	Primary tumour cannot be assessed
T0	No evidence of primary tumour
T1	Clinically tumour not palpable or visible by imaging
T1a	Tumour incidental histological finding in 5% or less of tissue resected
T1b	Tumour incidental histological finding in more than 5% of tissue resected
T1c	Tumour identified by needle biopsy, e.g. due to elevated prostate-specific antigen (PSA) level
T2	Tumour confined within the prostate
T2a	Tumour involves half of one lobe or less
T2b	Tumour involves more than half of one lobe, but not both lobes
T2c	Tumour involves both lobes
T3	Tumour extends through the prostatic capsule
T3a	Extracapsular extension (unilateral or bilateral) including microscopic bladder neck involvement
T3b	Tumour invades seminal vesicle(s)
T4	Tumour is fixed or invades adjacent structures other than seminal vesicles: external sphincter, rectum, levator muscles, and/or pelvic walls
N Regional lymph nodes	
Nx	Regional lymph nodes cannot be assessed
N0	No regional lymph node metastasis
N1	Regional lymph node metastasis
M Distant metastasis	
Mx	Distant metastasis cannot be assessed
M0	No distant metastasis
M1	Distant metastasis
M1a	Non-regional lymph node(s)
M1b	Bone(s)
M1c	Other site(s)

Table 60.2 Risk groups for prostate cancer.

D'Amico risk group	Criteria
Low	PSA <10 and Gleason score ≤6 and cT1 or cT2a
Intermediate	PSA 10–20 or Gleason score 7 or cT1 or cT2b or cT2c
High	PSA >20 or Gleason score >7 or cT3

Treatment

Treatment for patient with PC is influenced by many factors, including patient factors (age, comorbidities, personal preferences, presence of urinary symptoms), disease factors (stage and grade of PC) as well as access to healthcare (e.g. proximity to a hospital or radiation centre). For patients with localised PC, treatment options include active surveillance, watchful waiting, surgery or radiation.

Active surveillance versus watchful waiting

Low-risk PC typically progresses slowly and has a low potential for metastasis. Treatment of PC regardless of modality utilised is associated with some degree of decline in quality of life with regard to urinary control and sexual function. The concept of active surveillance is to closely monitor the men with low-grade (and typically small-volume) PC and as long as the disease remains stable (established by regular examination, PSA test, MRI and regular interval biopsies) definitive treatment can be avoided. If during the course of surveillance the disease progresses (changes in stage or grade), the patient still remains a good candidate for definitive therapy.

Watchful waiting follows a similar pattern but is considered in patients with comorbidities who are not candidates for definitive therapies. The patients are followed up, but only treated symptomatically. If the patients develop systemic disease, then they are offered hormonal therapy (not curative) in order to minimise the complications of PC. The majority of men on watchful waiting do not require any treatment in their lifetime and die with but not due to their PC.

Surgery (radical prostatectomy)

Radical prostatectomy is the surgical removal of the *entire* prostate and seminal vesicles. Depending on the risk of spread to the lymph nodes, it can be accompanied by pelvic lymph node dissection. The surgery can be performed via an open, laparoscopic or robotic-assisted approach. If performed by an expert surgeon there is no difference in the outcomes of surgery performed by different modalities. Robotic-assisted surgery allows this complex surgery to be performed in a minimally invasive fashion, with reduction in pain, blood loss, transfusion rate, hospital stay and postoperative complications.

Surgery provides over 90% 10-year disease-free survival in patients with organ-confined disease (this may vary depending on the grade of PC). Urinary control is initially compromised after radical prostatectomy but over time this function recovers for most men. Certain technical manoeuvres during surgery have been associated with earlier continence recovery. Pelvic floor muscle exercises implemented by a specialist pelvic physiotherapist have been shown to improve continence rate in men undergoing radical prostatectomy. The continence continues to improve for the first year post surgery. The rate of persistent urinary incontinence after surgery is around 7–15%.

Depending on the risk, surgery can be modified to include sparing of neurovascular bundles responsible for male erectile function. With high-risk disease, where the risk of extraprostatic spread is high, wide local excision of neurovascular bundles are performed and this leads to erectile dysfunction.

Both urinary incontinence and erectile dysfunction occurring after radical prostatectomy can be addressed by future surgeries with successful outcomes.

Radiotherapy

The other curative treatment option for PC is radiotherapy. Radiation can be delivered via external beam radiotherapy (typically, daily treatment over period of 6 weeks) or in selected patients radioactive seeds can be planted within the prostate gland (brachytherapy). A combination of the two treatments can also be delivered. The rate of erectile dysfunction and incontinence after radiotherapy is similar to surgery but these often occur later. Depending on PC risk, radiotherapy needs to be accompanied by up to 2 years of androgen deprivation therapy. Some of the side effects of radiotherapy, such as bladder and bowel toxicity (bowel/bladder frequency that can be accompanied by recurrent bleeding) or urethral stricture, are rare but are often difficult to treat and can be permanent.

Ablative therapies

This approach should not be considered as a mainstream treatment and remains experimental. Ablative energy (cryotherapy, high-intensity focal ultrasound, laser or irreversible electroporation) is applied to part or all of the prostate gland with the aim of killing cancer cells without damaging the neurovascular bundles or urinary continence mechanism. Whole-gland treatment has a similar side-effect profile to radiation, and focal ablation has a significant rate of disease recurrence as PC is often multifocal and ablating only part of the prostate does not treat cancer elsewhere in the gland.

Systemic therapy

Androgen deprivation therapy (ADT) has long been used to suppress PC in patients with locally advanced or metastatic disease. ADT does not improve survival but minimises complications associated with metastatic disease such as bony fractures or spinal cord compression. ADT achieves chemical castration and as PC cells rely on testosterone to grow, ADT suppresses their growth initially. Both surgical (bilateral orchiectomy) and medical castration can achieve this goal. Medical castration can be achieved by the means of luteinising hormone-releasing hormone analogues, gonadotropin-releasing hormone antagonists, antiandrogens or in combination.

ADT causes andropause, which leads to hot flushes, adverse lipid profile, diabetes, cardiovascular disease, weight gain, loss of muscle mass, gynaecomastia, anaemia, osteoporosis, depression and decline in cognition. Men on ADT should be well counselled about these side effects. Close monitoring of cardiovascular risk factors and addressing them, physical activity, weight-bearing exercises, calcium and vitamin D supplements, and psychological counselling can counteract some of the adverse effects of ADT.

Some men with PC will develop castrate-resistant prostate cancer after a period of ADT. These men can be treated with chemotherapy and/or novel antiandrogen agents such as abiraterone acetate or enzalutamide. Such agents are increasing used at earlier stages of the systemic disease with or without ADT with very encouraging results.

Urothelial cancer

The epithelial lining of the urinary tract, from renal collecting tubes to urinary meatus, is termed urothelium. Urothelial cancer (UC), previously known as transitional cell cancer, can arise from urothelium anywhere within the urinary tract. UC of the bladder is the most common followed by UC in the renal pelvis and the ureters, also termed upper tract urothelial cancer (UTUC). UC is the most common form of bladder cancer. Other, less common types of bladder cancer include squamous cell carcinoma (SCC) and adenocarcinoma.

Aetiology and pathology

Cigarette smoking is the most common cause for bladder cancer. Occupational exposure to aniline dyes and petroleum products has also been associated with an increased rate of bladder cancer, seen in those working in the textile, dye, leather and petroleum industries. Other known risk factors include iatrogenic exposure (radiation, cyclophosphamide, and phenacetin – no longer used) and chronic inflammatory conditions including *Schistosoma haematobium* infection (bladder SCC). Bladder cancer is more common in men than women.

Clinical presentation

The most common presentation is painless haematuria. Haematuria can be gross (visible) or microscopic. Haematuria is a serious symptom and should never be dismissed and always requires full investigation.

Some patients can present with frequency and urgency or a history of recurrent bladder infections. Patients with UTUC can present with symptoms similar to renal colic (clot colic) or with symptoms due to ureteric obstruction.

Investigations

In patients presenting with haematuria or those suspected to have bladder cancer, after history and risk assessment urological evaluation of the bladder with cystoscopy is essential. For the assessment of the upper tracts, CT intravenous pyelography is the gold standard. It visualises the urothelial linings of the kidneys and ureters. It will not detect small bladder lesions. Ultrasound can visualise the kidneys but cannot assess the ureters adequately. For patients with contrast allergy or renal impairment, magnetic resonance urography is an alternative. Urine cytology has poor sensitivity for low-grade tumours but is often positive in patients with high-grade cancers and should be considered as part of the work-up. The 2010 TNM staging system for bladder cancer is shown in Table 60.3.

Treatment

Treatment of UC is governed by the grade, stage and location of the tumour.

Upper tract urothelial cancer

The gold standard treatment for UTUC is nephro-ureterectomy, which involves removal of the entire

Table 60.3 The 2010 TNM (tumour, node, metastasis) staging of bladder cancer.

T Primary tumour

Tx	Primary tumour cannot be assessed
T0	No evidence of primary tumour
Ta	Non-invasive papillary tumour
Tis	Carcinoma *in situ* (CIS): always high grade
T1	Tumour invades lamina propria (subepithelial connective tissue)
T2	Tumour invades muscularis propria (bladder muscle)
T3	Tumour invades perivesical tissue
T3a	Microscopically
T3b	Macroscopically
T4	Tumour invades prostate, seminal vesicles, uterus, vagina or pelvic/abdominal wall

N Regional lymph nodes

Nx	Lymph node metastasis cannot be assessed
N0	No distant metastasis
N1	Single regional lymph node metastasis
N2	Multiple regional lymph node metastasis
N3	Lymph node metastasis to common iliac and beyond

M Distant metastasis

M0	No distant metastasis
M1	Distant metastasis

kidney and ipsilateral ureter and a cuff of the bladder around the concerned ureter. This can be achieved via an open, laparoscopic or robotic approach. In a select few cases when the tumour is small and low grade, ablation of the tumour with laser can be attempted but such patients require intense follow-up and are likely to require retreatment as UC is often a recurrent problem. Patients with UTUC also require periodic cystoscopy for the assessment of the bladder as this is a common site of recurrence.

Bladder cancer

Nearly two-thirds of bladder cancers on presentation are limited to the superficial layer of the bladder, not involving the muscularis propria of the bladder. These tumours are termed 'non-muscle invasive bladder cancer' and are generally resected by transurethral resection of bladder tumour (TURBT). During this procedure, an instrument mounted on a cystoscope is passed via the urethral meatus into the bladder and the bladder tumour is resected or ablated using an energy source (electricity or laser). The resected specimen is removed and assessed for grade and stage. The staging of bladder cancer is outlined in Table 60.3. The grade of the tumour (low grade vs. high grade) is also assessed. High-grade tumours are more likely to recur or progress (to higher stages). Instillation of chemotherapeutic agents (mitomycin C as well as others) in the bladder after TURBT has been associated with reduction in the rate of tumour recurrence.

For those patients with high risk of disease recurrence or progression (CIS, T1 or high-grade Ta disease), intravesical instillation of bacillus Calmette–Guérin (BCG) can reduce the risk of disease recurrence and progression. BCG treatment is not without risks and can cause local symptoms such as frequency and urgency and rarely can lead to systemic mycobacterial infection.

When the disease is muscle invasive, TURBT is no longer a curative option. The treatment of choice in such instances is radical cystectomy. This is often preceded by a course of systemic chemotherapy (neoadjuvant chemotherapy) with cisplatin-based agents and this approach has shown to improve patient survival. Radical cystectomy includes removal of prostate in men and removal of uterus and upper vagina in women. After radical cystectomy the urinary stream needs to be diverted. The diversion can be incontinent (ileal conduit) or continent (catheterisable urinary reservoir, neobladder).

Bladder-sparing therapy, employing a combination of TURBT and chemoradiotherapy in patients whom due to comorbidities cannot undergo surgery, is an alternative. The risk of disease recurrence after this approach remains high.

Metastatic bladder cancer has a very poor prognosis. Palliative chemotherapy and recently immunotherapy can reduce the symptoms and modestly improve patient survival.

Renal cell carcinoma

With the global increase in the use of cross-sectional imaging, the majority of renal masses are identified incidentally. The term 'small renal mass' (SRM) applies to renal lesions of less than 4 cm. Around 20–30% of SRMs are benign but the available imaging techniques cannot differentiate between benign and malignant lesions. Renal biopsy is increasingly used to help further identify these lesions. The biopsy can differentiate benign from malignant tumours in the majority of cases but is not always 100% accurate and is highly dependent on the quality of the biopsy specimen taken. For example, it can be difficult to differentiate an oncocytoma (benign) from a chromophobe-type renal cell carcinoma (malignant). The treatment options for a SRM include surveillance, extirpative therapy (partial or radical nephrectomy) or ablation (using various energy sources including cryotherapy, radiofrequency ablation or microwave).

A renal mass can be solid or cystic. Cystic lesions are classified according to the Bosniak classification (I–IV) that stratifies the lesions based on their radiological appearance and risk of malignancy. Solid lesions can be benign (angiomyolipoma, oncocytoma) or malignant (renal cell cancer, Wilms' tumour or metastatic disease).

Aetiology and pathology

Renal cell carcinoma (RCC) is the most common type of primary renal cancer. The risk of RCC is higher in patients with a history of smoking, obesity and hypertension. Patients with certain genetic predispositions and hereditary syndromes are at increased risk for developing RCC. These include von Hippel–Lindau syndrome (clear cell RCC), Birt–Hogg–Dubé syndrome (clear cell, chromophobe and oncocytoma) and tuberous sclerosis (RCC and angiomyolipoma). RCC is often clear cell type but can also be papillary, chromophobe or unclassified variety. These subtypes are based on histological assessment and have prognostic implications.

Clinical presentation

The triad of abdominal pain, haematuria and flank mass is the tell-tale sign of late RCC presentation and is seldom seen these days. Increasingly RCCs are diagnosed incidentally (see description of SRM). In men, development of left-sided varicocele due to obstruction of the gonadal vein can be seen with RCCs. Around 20–30% of patients with RCC develop paraneoplastic syndromes due to circulating cytokines and hormones produced by the tumour cells. Paraneoplastic syndromes include toxic effects such as fever, cachexia, anaemia, deranged liver function test (Stauffer's syndrome) and high erythrocyte sedimentation rate; and endocrine effects such as polycythaemia (erythropoietin production), hypertension (renin production) and hypercalcaemia (parathyroid hormone-like substances).

Investigations

An abdominal CT scan with and without contrast is the investigation of choice for the assessment of renal masses. The presence of post-contrast enhancement (surrogate for tumour vascularity) is often seen with RCCs. The presence of fat within the lesion points toward angiomyolipoma (benign tumour).

Staging

The local staging for RCCs is outlined in Table 60.4. Chest imaging (X-ray or CT) is mandatory at the time of diagnosis. Further imaging such as bone scan or CT of the head is recommended when there are symptoms suspicious for metastatic disease.

Treatment

Surveillance

SRMs can be treated in many ways. For a small lesion (<3 cm) even when malignant the tendency for spread beyond the kidney remains low. The risk of malignancy for an SRM is 70–80% and the risk of spread over a period of 3 years is around 1%. Given this, in a patient with coexisting comorbidities surveillance of an SRM with or without biopsy offers a safe strategy, as such patients often live the rest of their lives without any need for further therapy.

Ablation techniques

Ablation therapies using various energy sources delivered laparoscopically or percutaneously are

Table 60.4 The 2010 TNM (tumour, node, metastasis) staging of renal cancer.

T Primary tumour	
Tx	Primary tumour cannot be assessed
T0	No evidence of primary tumour
T1	Tumour 7 cm or less confined to the kidney
T1a	Tumour 4 cm or less confined to the kidney
T1b	Tumour 4–7 cm confined to the kidney
T2	Tumour >7 cm confined to the kidney
T2a	Tumour >7 cm but ≤10 cm confined to the kidney
T2b	Tumour >10 cm confined to the kidney
T3	Tumour extends to major veins or perinephric fat but confined to Gerota's fascia
T3a	Tumour extends to renal vein or perinephric fat
T3b	Tumour extends to the vena cava below the diaphragm
T3c	Tumour extends to the vena cava above the diaphragm or the wall of the vena cava
T4	Tumour invades beyond Gerota's fascia (including extension into the ipsilateral adrenal gland)
N Regional lymph nodes	
Nx	Lymph node metastasis cannot be assessed
N0	No distant metastasis
N1	Regional lymph node metastasis
M Distant metastasis	
M0	No distant metastasis
M1	Distant metastasis

minimally invasive and offer 80–90% success rate depending on tumour location and energy source used. In cases of recurrences (10–15%), further ablation can be attempted. These therapies have minimal impact on renal function and are ideal for patients where surgery is not suitable.

Surgery

Surgery is the gold standard for the treatment of renal malignancies. For certain tumours, depending on size, location, kidney function and presence of the contralateral kidney, surgical removal of the tumour with sparing of the rest of the kidney (partial nephrectomy or nephron-sparing surgery) is recommended. The remaining nephrons within the operated kidney can continue to perform their function and the risk of renal impairment is mitigated. Partial nephrectomy can be done in an open fashion or laparoscopically. Robotic platforms allow this complex surgery to be performed in a minimally invasive fashion and with minimal complications. For larger tumours, radical nephrectomy is recommended (open or laparoscopic). The prognosis of the patient is determined by the stage of the disease as well as histological characteristic of the tumour. Larger tumours carry a worse prognosis. Up to 25% of patients with kidney tumours have metastatic disease or develop it within the first year of diagnosis.

After surgical removal of the kidney, in addition to oncological follow-up renal function needs to be closely monitored. Such patients need to see their GPs a few times per year and any modifiable factors contributing to renal impairment (hypertension, diabetes, smoking) should to be identified and mitigated.

Testicular cancer

The majority of testicular tumours are germ cell tumours (90–95%) with stromal tumours such as Leydig cell and Sertoli cell tumours being the minority. Germ cell tumours are divided into seminoma or non-seminoma. Non-seminoma tumours can have embryonal, yolk sac, choriocarcinoma or teratoma elements.

Aetiology and pathology

Undescended testis or cryptorchidism is a risk factor for the development of testicular cancer. Other conditions, such as HIV infection, chromosomal abnormalities, infertility and family and personal history of testicular cancer, also increase the risk of testicular cancer.

Clinical presentation

A palpable painless lump is the most common presentation but up to 10% of patients present with pain. Metastatic disease can present with back pain or abdominal pain in cases with extensive bulky retroperitoneal disease.

Investigations

Clinical examination should include careful inspection of both testes including assessment of size. Assessment of the lymph nodes, breasts (gynaecomastia is seen in some cases), abdomen (retroperitoneal mass) and neurological system is essential.

Scrotal ultrasound can identify and characterise testicular lesions. Tumour markers, such as alphafetoprotein, human chorionic gonadotropin and lactate dehydrogenase, are part of staging. Once the diagnosis is confirmed, CT of chest and abdomen is required for complete staging.

Treatment

Radical orchiectomy removes the primary tumour and provides local staging information. The surgery is performed via the inguinal approach (rather than scrotal) in order to keep the lymphatic drainage of the testes unaltered. Testes lymphatics drain into the retroperitoneum, but in patients with scrotal surgery this drainage path can be altered and hence lymphatic spread can occur in an unpredictable fashion. Depending on the staging and characteristics of the tumour (size, lymphovascular invasion), surveillance or chemotherapy might be required. The retroperitoneum is the most common site of testicular metastasis. In cases where a retroperitoneal mass after chemotherapy persists, retroperitoneal lymph node dissection is performed to remove all the residual testicular tumours.

Penile cancer

Penile cancer is a rare cancer and SCC accounts for more than 95% of the cases.

Aetiology and pathology

Human papillomavirus (HPV), smoking, poor hygiene (particularly if uncircumcised) and chronic inflammation are associated with SCC of the penis.

Clinical presentation

An ulcerative painless penile lesion is a common presentation. The lesion can become fungating and can be associated with inguinal lymphadenopathy. If phimosis is present the lesion might not be visible.

Investigations

Biopsy of the lesion, ideally excisional biopsy, can confirm the diagnosis. MRI can provide further details about the depth of the lesion. Inguinal lymph nodes are the most common sites of metastasis and should be imaged and/or biopsied depending on the clinical situation. Chest imaging as well as cross-sectional abdominal/pelvic imaging in patients with nodal disease are mandatory.

Treatment

Excision of the lesion with a surgical margin is the goal of treatment. For low-grade small tumours, depending on the location, penile-sparing surgery can be offered. For larger high-grade lesions, partial or total penectomy plus inguinal lymph node dissection is recommended.

Further reading

European Association of Urology Guidelines, https://uroweb.org/guidelines/

McAninch JW, Lue TF (eds) *Smith and Tanagho's General Urology*, 18th edn. New York: McGraw-Hill, 2013.

Wein AJ, Kavoussi LR, Partin AW, Peters CA (eds) *Campbell-Walsh Urology*, 11th edn. Philadelphia: Elsevier, 2016.

Wieder JA. *Pocket Guide to Urology*, 5th edn, 2014. Available at http://www.pocketguidetourology.com/

MCQs

Select the single correct answer to each question. The correct answers can be found in the Answers section at the end of the book.

1 Which of the following statements about prostate cancer is correct?
   a prostate cancer is always visible on transrectal ultrasound imaging
   b prostate cancer is always associated with elevated PSA
   c some patients with prostate cancer have a normal serum PSA reading
   d MRI detects more than 95% of prostate cancers

2 Which one of the following findings leads to the diagnosis of high-risk prostate cancer?
   a PSA >15
   b Gleason score of 4 + 3 on biopsy
   c palpable nodule on digital rectal examination
   d ISUP grade 4 prostate cancer

3 Which of the following statements about bladder cancer is correct?
   a the majority of bladder cancers at diagnosis do not involve the muscle layer
   b haematuria is the most common mode of presentation of bladder cancer
   c haematuria always requires investigation
   d all of the above

4 Which of the following is a risk factor for the development of bladder cancer?
   a smoking
   b occupational exposure
   c radiation
   d all of the above

5 Which one of the following is *not* a serum marker for testicular cancer?
   a β-human chorionic gonadotropin
   b alpha-fetoprotein
   c alkaline phosphatase
   d lactate dehydrogenase

Section 15
Cardiothoracic Surgery

61 Principles and practice of cardiac surgery

James Tatoulis[1] and Julian A. Smith[2]

[1] University of Melbourne and Royal Melbourne Hospital, Melbourne, Victoria, Australia
[2] Department of Surgery, Monash University and Department of Cardiothoracic Surgery, Monash Health, Melbourne, Victoria, Australia

Introduction

Cardiac surgery is a modern surgical specialty. The development of the heart–lung machine in 1953 provided total circulatory support and oxygenation while intracardiac procedures were performed on the empty, and preferably still (asystolic), heart. Other milestones were the successful introduction of cardiac valve replacement in 1960, and coronary artery bypass graft (CABG) surgery in 1968.

In addition, complex and lethal conditions such as acute dissection of the thoracic aorta, cardiac wall and valve rupture after myocardial infarction, and infective endocarditis can be dealt with and mechanical cardiac assist devices and transplantation for the failing heart have become routine techniques.

Cardiopulmonary bypass: heart–lung machine

Cardiopulmonary bypass (CPB) revolutionised cardiac surgery, allowing precise intracardiac repair while vital organ perfusion, oxygenation and function were maintained. The essential components of the CPB circuit are described in Box 61.1.

The duration of CPB for most operations is between 1 and 2 hours. Complex operations may require 3–4 hours of CPB and occasionally several days or weeks (see section Circulatory support). Major shortcomings are blood cell destruction (roller pump) leading to haemoglobinuria and thrombocytopenia, coagulation factor consumption and systemic inflammatory response (due to contact with silastic tubing), as well as neurological, pulmonary, renal and hepatic dysfunction. All these problems are time-related, becoming noticeable after 2 hours of CPB.

Hypothermia (30–34°C) is used to help protect vital organ function against brief periods of possible hypotension. Haemodilution (haematocrit 21–25%) is used to help reduce blood product use, reduce red cell loss during surgery, and improve small vessel blood flow in hypothermic conditions. For complex surgery of thoracic aortic arch aneurysm, CPB is used to cool the patient to 18°C (profound hypothermia), blood is drained into the CPB reservoir, and the circulation arrested for up to 60 minutes, allowing excellent and rapid asanguineous access to major vessels, yet maintaining cerebral and renal protection. At the completion of the vascular procedure the patient is rewarmed to 37°C over 30–40 minutes.

Deep hypothermic circulatory arrest techniques are also used to facilitate surgery on or within the inferior vena cava, especially in venous extensions of renal neoplasms into the renal vein and inferior vena cava, where precise safe clearance of these endovascular extensions is required.

CPB is not always necessary. CABG can be performed without using the heart–lung machine and indeed is the preferred technique for some surgeons either routinely or when the aorta is 'hostile', when any manipulation of the aorta may result in an embolic stroke, and in 'closed' cardiac surgery (see later section).

Myocardial protection

In some conditions it is possible to perform an excellent cardiac operation using CPB but with the heart normally perfused and beating, for example closure of an atrial septal defect (ASD). However, precise coronary artery anastomoses and complex

---

Box 61.1 Cardiopulmonary bypass circuit

Venous cannula(s)	Drains blood from right atrium or both venae cavae
Suckers	Return shed blood from operative field to the reservoir
Reservoir	Drainage sump for venous and shed blood to be collected, and then oxygenated
Oxygenator	Venous blood oxygenated across a membrane
Heat exchanger	Cools and rewarms blood (and thereby the patient)
Roller or centripetal pump	Performs function of left ventricle, flow rates of 4–6 L/min
Arterial cannula	Returns oxygenated blood to the distal ascending thoracic aorta or other major artery

Box 61.2 Cardiac surgery without CPB

PDA closure
Coarctation of aorta repair
Mitral valvotomy (for mitral stenosis)
Pericardiectomy
Coronary bypass (selected cases)

valvular procedures are best performed in a still flaccid heart.

Ideally, this state is achieved by clamping the distal ascending thoracic aorta and infusing 'cardioplegia solution' (oxygenated blood with additional potassium, magnesium, lidocaine and amino acid substrates) at 10–20°C in order to arrest the heart, reduce its metabolic requirements and provide appropriate substrates, thus protecting the heart while being operated upon and being deprived of its normal coronary blood flow. There are many formulas of cardioplegic solutions, and methods of administration, although the principles remain the same.

Cardioplegia is also frequently administered retrogradely via the coronary sinus (the main venous drainage of the myocardium) using specially designed cannulas, in addition to antegrade administration. This technique is particularly useful for protecting the myocardium downstream from very stenotic or occluded coronary arteries or when the heart is positioned such that it is difficult or inefficient to easily administer further antegrade cardioplegia (aortic valve incompetence).

The usual cardiac arrest times are 45–90 minutes, although up to 180 minutes is possible with preservation of cardiac function. Sinus rhythm is usually restored within 1–2 minutes of re-establishing coronary blood flow.

Closed cardiac surgery

Many procedures do not require CPB. The early operations were performed with the heart beating. Such operations are possible where they are remote from the heart, such as closure of patent ductus arteriosus (PDA), or where disruption of cardiac function is transient and can be well tolerated (mitral valvotomy).

With the evolution and refinement of imaging and technology, many 'closed' and some 'open' (CPB-requiring) operations have been replaced by endovascular or percutaneous transcatheter techniques, for example dilatation of aortic coarctation, PDA closure, atrial and ventricular septal defects and, more recently, aortic, pulmonary and mitral valve replacements and mitral valve repair (see later).

Operations commonly performed without CPB are listed in Box 61.2. The vast majority (>90%) of cardiac operations worldwide are performed using CPB.

Coronary artery surgery

Coronary atherosclerosis is a major disease process in western countries and is rapidly increasing in incidence in developing countries. Coronary angiography (by retrograde cannulation of the coronary ostia via the femoral or radial artery under local anaesthetic) was introduced in 1962. Coronary bypass surgery became established in 1968 and coronary angioplasty in 1978.

Pathology

Atherosclerotic stenotic lesions develop proximally at the origins of main coronary branches or at major branching points. The coronary vessels are usually free of disease distally. A stenosis of more than 50% diameter loss is considered significant. Atheromatous plaques may disrupt, occlude or suffer from intraplaque haemorrhage, causing acute spasm, occlusion or thrombosis. Gradual progressive chronic stenosis causes angina. Acute spasm results in ischaemic chest pain at rest, and thrombotic occlusion results in acute myocardial infarction.

Risk factors for coronary artery disease include family history, male gender, diabetes, hypertension, smoking, hypercholesterolaemia and obesity.

Symptoms

Angina pectoris on exertion is the most common symptom. Ischaemic chest pain occurring spontaneously at rest (unstable angina) also occurs and is associated with spasm in the vicinity of the stenotic plaque and/or transient coronary artery occlusion. Myocardial infarction occurs with prolonged or permanent coronary occlusion resulting in severe chest pain lasting several hours. Diabetic patients may not experience chest pain because of neuropathy.

Between 10 and 15% of patients, especially women, may experience atypical symptoms such as back pain and epigastric, throat or jaw discomfort. Myocardial infarction must not be confused with the symptoms of acute aortic dissection, which presents as sudden and dramatic severe interscapular pain, as opposed to the progressive crescendo of myocardial infarction.

Investigations

- Chest X-ray may indicate cardiomegaly or left ventricular aneurysm as a result of prior myocardial infarction.
- Electrocardiogram (ECG) may show ST-segment elevation or depression with acute chest pain, or 'Q' waves due to old myocardial infarction.
- Stress test (treadmill or bicycle with ECG monitoring), where positive, will result in chest pain, ST-segment depression and a fall in blood pressure.
- Thallium, sestamibi and positron emission tomography (PET) scans may indicate areas of hypoperfusion, ischaemia, viability and reversibility of left ventricular function.
- Computed tomography (CT) is useful for screening, especially in young patients presenting with chest pain. If negative, this excludes coronary artery disease (99% specificity). Conversely, a high calcium score indicates a high chance of coronary artery disease. Currently, coronary angiography is then required as the definitive investigation to outline the number, location and severity of the stenotic lesions, and the size and quality of the vessels beyond.
- Intravascular (coronary) ultrasound details the extent, severity and nature of coronary artery plaques, especially useful when evaluation on coronary angiography is uncertain.
- Fractional flow reserve (FFR) is measured by an intracoronary pressure wire at the time of angiography and provides a physiological assessment of the degree of ischaemia distal to the stenotic lesion. A pressure drop of more than 20% across the stenotic lesion (FFR <0.80) is considered significant and allows an objective evidence-based and targeted strategy towards revascularisation, which in turn results in better short- and long-term outcomes.

The SYNTAX score, developed for a randomised trial of coronary stenting versus CABG, allows scoring of the 'severity and complexity' of coronary lesions and choice of appropriate revascularisation strategy: angioplasty and stenting for discrete short lesions in one or two arteries; CABG for complex or bifurcation lesions in multiple coronary branches.

Medical management

Low-dose aspirin, nitrates (sublingual, spray or topical), beta-blockers (metoprolol, atenolol), calcium antagonists (nifedipine, amlodipine) and cholesterol-lowering agents (statins) are used.

Indications for intervention

- Uncontrolled symptoms: where symptoms persist despite appropriate medical therapy or where medication cannot be tolerated.
- Prognosis: patients with severe stenoses in the left main coronary artery, proximally in a large left anterior descending artery, or when all the main coronary arteries (left anterior descending, circumflex and right coronary artery) have severe stenoses, revascularisation has been clearly shown to provide major long-term prognostic benefit.

Percutaneous coronary intervention: coronary angioplasty and stenting

Discrete stenotic plaques in one or two arteries may be treated by percutaneous transluminal coronary angioplasty (PTCA) to dilate the plaque to its normal lumen size (2–2.5 mm), with the plaque held open by placement of a stent. Advances include drug-eluting stents, which inhibit proliferation of neointima and have reduced in-stent re-stenosis rates to 1–5% at 1 year.

Coronary artery bypass graft surgery

Multiple severe coronary artery stenoses associated with chronic uncontrolled angina, or unstable angina, are best treated surgically. CABG comprises 60% of all adult cardiac operations. There are many variations of surgical techniques but the general principles are as follows.

Sternotomy is performed. The left internal thoracic artery (LITA) is harvested and is usually anastomosed

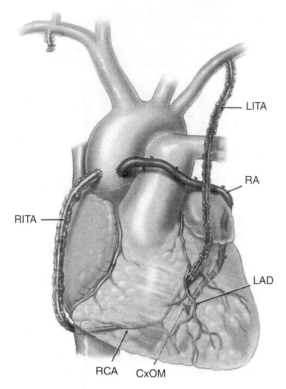

Fig. 61.1 Typical coronary artery revascularisation of the anterior, lateral and inferior walls of the heart. LITA, RITA, left and right internal thoracic artery; RA, radial artery; LAD, left anterior descending artery; RCA, right coronary artery; CˣOM, circumflex (obtuse) marginal artery.

to the left anterior descending artery (LAD), which is considered to be the most important artery. In younger patients (<70 years), the right internal thoracic artery (RITA) is harvested and anastomosed to the second most important affected coronary vessel. Other coronary vessels are grafted using either the radial artery (Figure 61.1) or saphenous vein.

CPB is used, and the heart is arrested and protected with cardioplegia while performing the distal anastomoses. The proximal graft anastomoses may be performed to the ascending thoracic aorta while the heart is arrested or using a specially designed clamp. Alternatively, the proximal inflow may be from the subclavian artery or via the construction of pedicled grafts off the internal thoracic artery (ITA). A typical operation takes 3–4 hours, including cardiac arrest for 30–60 minutes and bypass times of 60–90 minutes, depending on the number of bypasses performed (average of three to four). The pericardium is usually loosely closed to protect the right ventricle in future re-sternotomy, drain tubes placed behind the sternum and into the pleural cavities if they have been entered, and the sternum re-wired so that it is extremely stable.

The patient spends 24–48 hours in the intensive care unit, where blood pressure, right atrial pressure, pulmonary artery pressure, left atrial pressure, and cardiac and urine outputs are measured and interventions performed as appropriate.

The patient is mobilised on the first or second postoperative day, and aspirin, a statin, and beta-blocker and calcium antagonists are recommenced. Most patients are discharged from hospital 5–7 days postoperatively. Recovery is rapid, with most returning to 'office work' in 4–6 weeks and to full activity within 3 months.

Results of CABG surgery

The operative mortality is 1% (although higher in re-operations or where left ventricular function is poor). The main morbidity relates to perioperative stroke (1%), myocardial infarction (1%), sternal and mediastinal infections (1%) and haemorrhage (2%) (see section Complications of cardiac surgery). Graft patency is best for the left ITA and worst for the saphenous vein (Table 61.1).

Long-term freedom from recurrent angina pectoris is 85% at 5 years and 70% at 10 years (recurrence rate of approximately 3% per annum). Long-term survival is excellent: 90–95% at 5 years and 80–85% at 10 years. Survival is significantly influenced by age at surgery (current mean age 68 years), presence of diabetes, degree of left ventricular dysfunction, and control of risk factors after surgery. The presence of one or more ITA grafts enhances survival and long-term freedom from angina. A patent LITA to the LAD appears to be the most important prognostic component of myocardial revascularisation (Figure 61.2). Multiple large longitudinal studies (beyond 10 years) have shown that the use of multiple arterial grafts (including radial artery grafts) is associated with identical perioperative results but with superior long-term survival and fewer cardiac events and re-operations compared with when the majority of bypass grafts are with saphenous vein.

Table 61.1 Coronary bypass graft patency.

Conduit	5 years	10 years	20 years
Left internal thoracic artery	96%	95%	90%
Right internal thoracic artery	93%	90%	80–90%
Radial artery	90%	85–90%	80–90%
Saphenous vein	75%	50%	25–30%

(a)   (b)   (c)

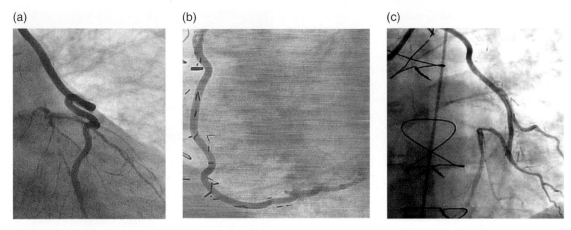

Fig. 61.2 Postoperative angiography of (a) the left internal thoracic artery sequentially to the diagonal and left anterior descending coronary arteries; (b) an aortocoronary radial artery to the posterior descending coronary artery; and (c) a radial artery placed sequentially to the first and second circumflex marginal arteries.

In general, for every 100 patients undergoing CABG, 10 more 'multi-arterial' patients will be alive at 10 years (80% vs. 70%).

Coronary surgery confers prognostic benefits (over medical management and percutaneous coronary intervention) to patients with stenosis of the left main coronary artery, those with high-grade proximal LAD stenoses, those with triple vessel coronary disease (LAD, right and circumflex coronary arteries), where there is left ventricular dysfunction, and in diabetics. These groups account for approximately 85% of patients undergoing coronary surgery.

Surgery for complications of myocardial infarction

Complications of coronary artery disease, especially myocardial infarction, may require treatment in conjunction with CABG surgery. Myocardial infarction involving the left ventricular wall, including papillary muscles of the mitral valve, in combination with left ventricular dilatation may result in severe ischaemic mitral regurgitation. This would need correction by mitral valve repair or replacement (operative mortality approximately 10%). Left ventricular aneurysms, particularly in relation to occlusion of the LAD, may require excision and repair (operative mortality 3%).

Extensive infarction may result in left ventricular free wall rupture into the pericardium (tamponade) or rupture of the interventricular septum (acute cardiogenic shock). These complications, treated conservatively, are almost universally fatal. Surgical repair using appropriate techniques (patches and biological glues) is essential, although operative mortality is high (25%), relating predominantly to the extensive myocardial damage and to the precarious preoperative state of the patients.

Off-pump coronary surgery

Devices and techniques have been developed that allow excellent stabilisation of the coronary arteries, making it possible to perform precise coronary anastomoses, especially to the LAD and diagonal arteries (anterolateral aspects of the heart), while the heart is beating and maintaining circulation. Similarly, the circumflex and right coronary arteries may be grafted.

Potential advantages are avoidance of CPB and manipulation of the aorta (by cannulas and clamps), which may be an important factor in older patients or where the aorta is atheromatous or calcified, thereby reducing the possibility of bleeding or stroke. There are also potential economic gains through avoidance of CPB, with savings on consumables and personnel and potential to reduce intensive care and hospital stays, although this has not been proved thus far.

However, there are also potential disadvantages, with greater operative technical difficulty, possible coronary artery damage, and episodes of hypotension with excessive displacement and manipulation of the heart. The role of off-pump coronary artery bypass is still being debated. Randomised controlled trials have not shown perioperative differences, nor differences in cognitive function. However, there appears to be reduced graft patency, earlier return of angina, a greater need for re-intervention and compromised long-term survival. Conversely, it may be associated with better short-term results in high-risk patients with poor left ventricular function and 'hostile' atheromatous aortas.

New concepts in CABG surgery

Endoscopic harvesting techniques for saphenous vein and radial arteries minimise incisions, discomfort and infection. 'Hybrid' procedures are those where the LAD is bypassed with the LITA via a small left thoracotomy and other stenoses are addressed by stents, either at the same time in a 'hybrid' operating room (with angiographic and CT facilities) or as sequential procedures (LITA–LAD first). These may be used in older higher-risk patients to minimise surgical trauma and facilitate recovery.

The application of robotic techniques in CABG surgery is still in its infancy.

Cardiac valve surgery

The initial valve operations were performed on the beating heart (closed mitral valvotomy). The first successful aortic and mitral valve replacements were performed in 1960. Valve pathology is still a significant factor in clinical cardiac disease. A high incidence of rheumatic valve disease persists in developing countries (India, China, Indonesia, South America) and also in Australia's Northern Territory. In western countries the most common valve problems are due to degenerative processes and ageing, which have increased in incidence, while rheumatic pathology has declined.

Pathology

The two most common valve pathologies in western countries are calcific aortic stenosis and degenerative myxomatous mitral regurgitation. Aortic stenosis results from dystrophic calcification of a bicuspid aortic valve (including calcification as part of the degenerative ageing process) and is more commonly seen in older patients (a result of improved living standards and longevity). There is progressive narrowing of the aortic valve orifice with resultant left ventricular hypertrophy and left ventricular failure in advanced cases. Aortic valve distortion may also result in aortic regurgitation with additional deleterious effects (Figure 61.3).

Myxomatous degeneration predominantly affects the mitral valve (collagen and elastin abnormalities, and increased mucopolysaccharide deposition). It results in annulus dilatation, chordae tendineae elongation, leaflet redundancy and prolapse and, in extreme cases, chordal rupture and mitral leaflet flail, resulting in massive mitral regurgitation. Sequelae are left ventricular and left atrial dilatation, left heart failure, atrial fibrillation (AF) and

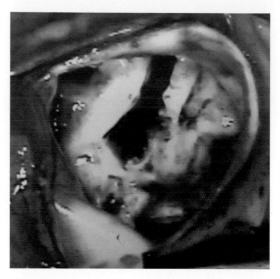

Fig. 61.3 Severe calcific aortic stenosis with associated aortic valve insufficiency secondary to the rigidity and distortion of the aortic valve leaflets.

pulmonary hypertension. Myxomatous degeneration affecting the aortic valve results in progressive aortic regurgitation.

The chronic effects of rheumatic fever are cardiac valve leaflet thickening and retraction. In the aortic valve this results in a combined lesion of aortic stenosis and regurgitation. In the mitral valve, stenosis is the predominant effect of leaflet thickening, fusion at commissures and shortening of chordae tendineae. Regurgitation occurs with severe leaflet fibrosis, retraction and failure of leaflet coaptation.

Symptoms

The key symptom is dyspnoea, although this occurs late in the course of valve disease as each of the valve pathologies is generally well tolerated because of left ventricular reserve and the initial compliance of the left atrium. Dyspnoea requires immediate investigation and aggressive intervention because it indicates exhaustion of the cardiac compensatory mechanism and a poor prognosis and rapid demise for the patient if left untreated.

Angina and syncope may be additional symptoms in aortic stenosis due to pressure loss across an extremely stenotic aortic valve and resultant poor coronary and cerebral perfusion.

Cerebral emboli or endocarditis may occur if the valve lesions are complicated by valvular or left atrial thrombus, infections or vegetations.

Investigations

Chest X-ray may show cardiomegaly, calcification in the aortic or mitral valves, and pulmonary

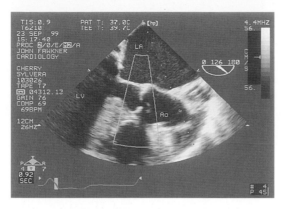

Fig. 61.4 Transoesophageal echocardiogram to evaluate the aortic valve (centre of image). LA, left atrium posteriorly; LV, left ventricle; Ao, ascending thoracic aorta. Dots represent 1-cm markings.

congestion. ECG may show left ventricular hypertrophy, a wide bifid P wave in severe mitral stenosis, or AF.

Echocardiography is the key investigation in valvular heart disease. Accurate measurements can be made of the cardiac chambers, pulmonary artery pressure and the valvular orifices. Calcification, degree of stenosis or regurgitation, leaflet excursion, flow, valve area, gradient and annular size can be precisely measured and compared with prior or future measurements. Transthoracic echocardiography is an excellent screening tool. Transoesophageal echocardiography (TOE) gives greater anatomical detail of valves and their pathologies and is particularly useful in planning for and predicting surgical outcomes and in the intraoperative setting (Figure 61.4).

Coronary angiography is performed in patients older than 40 years to screen for coexistent coronary artery disease, with 30% of patients undergoing cardiac valve surgery requiring concomitant CABG surgery.

Medical management

Where patients are asymptomatic, and echocardiography shows normal function and cardiac chamber size and normal pulmonary artery pressures, conservative management is indicated. Peripheral vasodilating medications such as calcium antagonists (nifedipine, amlodipine) or angiotensin-converting enzyme (ACE) inhibitors (perindopril, ramipril, etc.) are useful in aortic regurgitation and mitral regurgitation for reducing the afterload for left ventricular ejection. Diuretics (frusemide) are required for pulmonary congestion. Warfarin anticoagulation and digoxin may be required if there is AF.

Aortic valve surgery

A mean gradient of more than 40 mmHg in aortic stenosis or a left ventricular end-diastolic diameter of more than 60 mm in aortic regurgitation are indications for surgery. The mean age for aortic valve replacement (AVR) is 69 years. Sternotomy and CPB are required. The aorta is opened transversely 2–3 cm above the aortic valve. Occasionally the valve can be repaired. The valve is excised, all calcium removed from the annulus and an aortic valve prosthesis is placed using non-absorbable sutures. The aortotomy is then closed, and air is evacuated from the heart prior to re-establishment of circulation through the heart. Carbon dioxide in the operative field (heavier and more soluble than oxygen and nitrogen) is used to minimise potential air embolism. The ascending aorta is usually occluded for 60 minutes, CPB time is 80 minutes and total operative time approximately 3 hours.

Where the predominant pathology is aortic valve regurgitation, and the leaflets are nearly normal, it is possible to repair such valves by plicating prolapsed leaflets or enhancing leaflet coaptation by tailoring the aortic annulus and the aortic root (David, Yacoub, Lansaac procedures), which preserves the natural leaflets and avoids long-term warfarin. These procedures are complex but are appropriate for young patients with aortic valve incompetence.

Mitral valve surgery

Rheumatic mitral stenosis may be treated by percutaneous balloon valvuloplasty. The procedure is carried out by catheterisation of the femoral vein, passing superiorly into the right atrium, across the interatrial septum into the left atrium and eventually dilatation of the mitral valve.

Alternatively, and now rarely used, closed mitral valvotomy via a left thoracotomy and trans-left atrial or trans-left ventricular dilatation of the mitral valve is performed. These procedures are performed under TOE guidance and are best when the valve leaflets are pliable and there is no valve calcification nor thrombus in the left atrium.

Valve leaflet thickening, calcification, fused chordae and left atrial thrombus are all indications for open operation (via sternotomy and CPB), which may include commissurotomy to free the fused commissures between the anterior and posterior mitral leaflets, debridement of calcification, and fenestration or resection of portions of thickened chordae. A severely distorted valve, especially if additionally regurgitant, will require replacement.

Myxomatous degenerative mitral valve regurgitation is due to elongated and ruptured chordae, leading to prolapse and flail of the mitral valve leaflets, usually in combination with mitral annular dilatation. If the gross changes are localised to a specific part of the valve (e.g. central scallop of the posterior leaflet), mitral valve repair is possible. If the changes are widespread with multiple areas of prolapse, flail and lack of leaflet coaptation, repair is more complex and challenging and then valve replacement may be indicated, especially in older patients (tissue valve).

Mitral valve repair is performed via a sternotomy, CPB and direct left atriotomy. Many techniques are used and include quadrangular resection of the flail or prolapsed segment, annulus and leaflet repair, and placement of an annuloplasty ring to reinforce the annulus repair and correct annular dilatation and valve geometry. Leaflet prolapse can also be corrected by replacing elongated or ruptured chordae (Gore-Tex neochordae). Retention of the native mitral valve avoids the need for warfarin anticoagulation in the long term (if the patient is in sinus rhythm) and maintains the geometry and function of the left ventricle.

Mitral valve replacement is performed if the valvular pathology is too extensive. However, as much of the subvalvular mechanism (including leaflet tissue, chordae and papillary muscles) is retained to maintain left ventricular geometry and function, hence resulting in a low operative mortality and improved long-term left ventricular function and patient survival. Low profile mechanical valves are used in patients aged less than 70 years (see following section). Warfarin anticoagulation is always required when a mechanical valve prosthesis has been placed.

Many patients with mitral valve pathology have AF. This is addressed by closure of the left atrial appendage (where thrombi and potential emboli may occur) and incorporating by a Maze procedure to isolate the pulmonary veins where AF originates, disrupt macro re-entry circuits and create an antegrade pathway for atrial conduction to the atrioventricular node. This is usually performed with a set of 'cryolesions' and adds approximately 20–30 minutes to the procedure. It has a 50–80% success rate in converting AF to sinus rhythm in the longer term and is more likely to be successful if the atrium is not too dilated, and the AF has been more recent (<5 years).

Extensive or recurrent myocardial infarction may lead to left ventricular and mitral annular dilatation, and failure of the mitral leaflets to meet and coapt results in mitral regurgitation. Although not primarily a leaflet problem, severe mitral valve regurgitation that leads to pulmonary hypotension, heart failure and dyspnoea may be addressed by a restrictive mitral rigid annuloplasty ring to enforce the leaflet coaptation, or via mitral valve replacement (as the left ventricular muscle pathology cannot be addressed).

Cardiac valve prosthesis

There are two categories of valve prosthesis available for implantation: mechanical and tissue (Figure 61.5).

Mechanical valves are made of pyrolytic carbon with a Dacron sewing cuff, are low profile and inert, and commonly have two semicircular leaflets (St Jude, ATS/ Medtronic). Mechanical valves always require warfarin anticoagulation maintaining

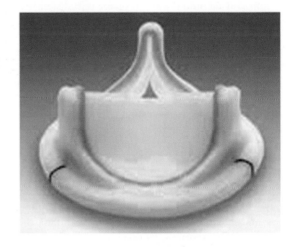

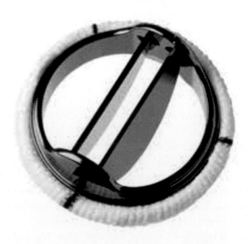

Fig. 61.5 Prosthetic cardiac valves: (*top*) pericardial xenograft tissue valve; (*bottom*) bileaflet mechanical (pyrolytic carbon) mechanical valve.

Table 61.2 Cardiac valve prosthesis.

Valve type	Advantages	Disadvantages
Mechanical	Durable	Warfarin anticoagulation Higher bleeding and thromboembolic rates
Tissue	No anticoagulation Better haemodynamics (stentless valves)	15-year durability (Ca^{2+}, dehiscence), re-operation

international normalised ratio (INR) values between 2.5 and 3.5.

Tissue valves (bioprostheses) are derived from humans (human cadaver aortic valve allograft), pulmonary valve autografts (discussed later) or xenografts (specially treated porcine or bovine valves). Additionally, tissue valves may be mounted on a stent for ease of implantation, or may be stentless to enhance haemodynamics, allowing a larger valve into any anatomical situation. The advantages and disadvantages of each type of valve are indicated in Table 61.2.

In the mitral position, mechanical valves are used in patients younger than 70 years or if the patient is to be on long-term warfarin (AF). Xenograft tissue valves may be used in older patients, which allow lesser degrees of warfarin anticoagulation. However, xenografts fail rapidly in young patients (<60 years).

In the aortic position, there are a number of choices determined by age and patient lifestyle. In patients older than 70 years, a xenograft tissue valve is generally used. Only low-dose aspirin is required long term if the patient is in sinus rhythm.

In patients younger than 70, generally a mechanical valve together with warfarin anticoagulation is used. A human cadaver allograft is used if warfarin is to be avoided (e.g. patient lives in a remote area, patient participates in contact sports) or when there is endocarditis affecting the aortic valve annulus. However, allografts are relatively difficult to procure and are in short supply.

Some younger patients (15–50 years) have a pulmonary autograft (Ross) procedure in which the diseased aortic valve is replaced with the patient's own pulmonary valve, which in turn is replaced with a human cadaver pulmonary valve allograft. This is an extensive procedure, but well tolerated in young patients. Anticoagulation is avoided. However, long-term results beyond 15 years are not established. Women of childbearing age requiring mitral replacement have tissue valves to avoid

warfarin, which can be teratogenic, but recognising that further surgery will be required.

Unfortunately, all tissue valves are subject to wear and tear and gradual degeneration. Inevitably, if any type of bioprosthesis is used in patients younger than 60, there is a very high probability that re-operation will be required, although this is uncommon within 10 years.

Recent developments in cardiac valve surgery

Small incisions

Short (5 cm) upper sternal and right parasternal incisions have been used for aortic valve surgery, and right submammary and short lower sternal incisions for mitral, atrial septum and tricuspid valve surgery. These approaches are facilitated by video telescope assistance, especially designed long-shafted instruments and peripheral (femoral vessel) cannulation for CPB. Left submammary incisions may be used for isolated coronary bypass to the LAD.

Advantages include cosmesis, less bleeding and fewer wound infections. Disadvantages include a substantial learning curve, longer CPB times, less certain myocardial protection, potential retrograde emboli where there is aortic atheroma, and limb vascular problems as femoral vessel cannulation has been complicated by aortic dissection, leg ischaemia and venous thrombosis. Limited exposure may compromise safety and lengthen the duration of the procedure. Overall the results in experienced centres are similar to those by established techniques.

Sutureless rapid deployment aortic tissue valves

These can be efficiently implanted once the diseased valve has been excised. Advantages include shorter operative times, especially when multiple cardiac procedures are required. Such valves predominantly depend on expansion of the stents or scaffolds they are mounted upon. Disadvantages include higher degrees of heart block and occasional paravalvular leaks. Implantation techniques are particularly suited to aortic valve replacement via small incision access.

Other developments

- Robotic techniques are also used for mitral and atrial septum surgery. The results are similar but there is a substantial learning curve and greater expense which have limited their application.

- Percutaneous transcatheter aortic valve implantation and mitral procedures are now also widely practised.
- Tissue aortic valves on nitinol stents can be crimped onto a catheter and implanted into the aortic valve position via the femoral artery, axillary artery or ascending thoracic aorta, or antegradely by the left ventricular apex. Once in position the old diseased (stenotic) aortic valve leaflets are pushed laterally into the capacious sinuses of Valsalva, and the new aortic valve is aligned and expanded into position.
- Mitral valve clips (MitraClip) or mitral valve prostheses can be introduced percutaneously via the femoral vein across the interatrial septum and used to enhance coaptation between the two mitral leaflets (MitraClip) or replace the mitral valve.

These techniques are highly reproducible and have been very successful in older, inoperable or high-risk patients, with procedural mortalities of less than 5%, rapid recovery and promising early results out to 5 years.

Postoperative management

Perioperative prophylactic antibiotics are given to protect against endocarditis (prior to anaesthesia, and for 48 hours postoperatively) and meticulous care taken to avoid any sepsis. Warfarin anticoagulation (if appropriate) is commenced 24 hours postoperatively, and a therapeutic INR of 2.5–3.5 achieved by day 7. Warfarin is continued indefinitely (except in mitral repair or where aortic tissue valves have been used). Diuretics and ACE inhibitors are usually required for several weeks or months. General postoperative management and progress is similar to that of patients undergoing coronary artery surgery.

Other valve conditions

Severe infective endocarditis affecting either the aortic or mitral valve is usually caused by *Staphylococcus aureus* and results in fever, aortic and/or mitral regurgitation, and eventual renal and hepatic dysfunction. It is best managed aggressively with appropriate antibiotic loading and early surgery to eradicate the infection and either replace or repair (uncommon but sometimes possible) the affected valve.

Tricuspid valve surgery is uncommon. Tricuspid regurgitation may be the end product of chronic aortic or mitral valve disease, left heart failure and pulmonary hypertension. The mechanism is that of right ventricular and tricuspid valve annular dilatation and loss of central leaflet coaptation. The leaflets and chordae are otherwise normal.

Tricuspid valve annuloplasty to correct tricuspid annulus size and shape to normal is performed at the time of aortic or mitral surgery. Organic tricuspid valve stenosis or regurgitation due to rheumatic disease is rare and is managed following the principles of mitral valve surgery.

Results

Operative mortality varies from 1% (AVR, mitral valve repair) to 3% (mitral valve replacement). Operative mortality for combined CABG and valve surgery is 3–5%, and for re-operation is 5–8%. Long-term results are excellent. Survival following mitral valve repair or AVR is 90% at 5 years, and 80% at 10 years. Survival following mitral valve replacement is a little less than this due to late referral and excision of the subvalvar apparatus in the previous era.

Morbidity of valve replacement surgery

Unfortunately, each valve prosthesis has a group of long-term problems associated with its use:
- anticoagulant-related haemorrhage, which may be extremely serious (cerebral, gastrointestinal)
- thromboembolism from small thrombi that form around the annulus or within the prosthetic valve
- endocarditis from an infection on the valve prosthesis
- perivalvular leaks, or structural deterioration of tissue valve which, when severe enough, would require re-operation.

Each of these complications occurs with an annual incidence of approximately 0.5–1.0%, and hence the potential for a patient to be totally free from any one of these complications over the course of 10 years is only of the order of 70%.

Congenital cardiac surgery

Cardiac anomalies occur in 8 per 1000 live births. The range of anomalies is extensive. Only the common ones are discussed here. Congenital cardiac abnormalities are best corrected as early as possible after birth (preferably in the first 3 months). Some, such as a large persistent PDA, which creates a huge shunt from the aorta to the pulmonary artery, or severe coarctation of the aorta, which places a large afterload on the left ventricle, need urgent correction at birth.

Patent ductus arteriosus

PDA allows blood flow from the pulmonary artery trunk to the aorta when the lungs and pulmonary circulation are not functioning *in utero*. The PDA usually closes at birth. A persistent small PDA is vulnerable to endocarditis. A persistent large PDA allows shunting of blood from the aorta back into the pulmonary circulation, overloading it as well as the right heart, eventually leading to pulmonary hypertension and right heart failure. Closure of the PDA is essential and this can be achieved either by percutaneous catheter closure or by direct suture ligation or division and oversewing via a small left thoracotomy.

Coarctation of the aorta

The most common site is just distal to the left subclavian artery, with the lumen of the aorta often narrowed to 1–2 mm. Left untreated, upper body hypertension, left ventricular hypertrophy and left ventricular failure develop. Correction is by either percutaneous retrograde (from the femoral artery) catheter balloon dilatation or surgical resection and repair via a small left thoracotomy.

Atrial septal defect

Atrial septal defect is the most common congenital cardiac defect and occurs as a result of developmental failure of the interatrial septum and can be high (sinus venosus), mid (ostium secundum) or low (ostium primum) defects. A significant ASD is more than 1 cm in diameter and if left uncorrected results in a persistent left atrium to right atrium shunt, eventually leading to right heart overload, right atrial and ventricular enlargement, AF and pulmonary hypertension. Life expectancy may be reduced by 10–30 years (depending on the size of the ASD and shunt).

Echocardiography gives excellent depiction of the anatomical location, size of the ASD and flow through it, as well as the size of the cardiac chambers and pressure in the right ventricle and pulmonary artery.

ASD closure is indicated if pulmonary circulatory flow is more than 1.5 times the systemic circulatory flow. Surgical repair is readily performed (using CPB) by either direct suture or a patch of autologous pericardium, and has an extremely low mortality (1 in 400). Percutaneous ASD closure via the femoral vein with a catheter-mounted baffle-type device is applicable where the ASD is well circumscribed with a defined circumferential rim.

Ventricular septal defect

Ventricular septal defect (VSD) occur when ventricular septal development is incomplete and may

be single or multiple and placed either just below the tricuspid valve and the origin of the great vessels, or more inferiorly in the body of the muscular septum. Most commonly, VSDs occur in isolation but may also be present as part of a more complex cardiac anomaly (e.g. tetralogy of Fallot). Small VSDs, particularly in the central muscle septum, may close spontaneously with cardiac growth. Larger VSDs associated with pulmonary-to-systemic flow ratios of more than 1.5 : 1 are repaired to avoid endocarditis, and also the sequelae of pulmonary and right heart overload (see preceding section). Surgical closure is by using CPB, and by direct suture or patch. Percutaneous closure is also possible. The main specific complication is heart block as the conducting bundle passes near the inferior rim of the VSD, and care is taken not to damage the conducting bundle with sutures at VSD closure.

Other congenital abnormalities

Other congenital abnormalities that may be surgically corrected with excellent long-term results include pulmonary valve stenosis, tetralogy of Fallot, transposition of the great vessels and endocardial cushion defects (atrioventricular canal). However, there are numerous rarer, more complex conditions (e.g. hypoplastic left heart syndrome, single ventricle, tricuspid atresia) where surgery is also possible, but often multiple procedures are required, with suboptimal results. (The reader is directed to texts of paediatric cardiology and cardiac surgery.)

Surgery of the thoracic aorta

Aneurysms of the thoracic aorta, especially the transverse arch, are challenging. The most common pathologies are atheromatous or myxomatous degeneration of the aortic wall media, leading to aneurysmal dilatation and eventual rupture or dissection. Marfan's syndrome (autosomal dominant inheritance) is one entity that is part of the spectrum of myxomatous degeneration of connective tissues. Hypertension and atherosclerosis are now better controlled in the population and are less common contributing factors to thoracic aneurysms. Dilatation of the thoracic aorta to a diameter of more than 5 cm is associated with a marked increase in the possibility of rupture or dissection and so elective repair/replacement is advised (Figure 61.6).

The patients are usually asymptomatic. The aneurysm is often noted on routine chest X-ray. Rupture or dissection is associated with dramatic, sudden, severe chest and interscapular pain, possibly collapse,

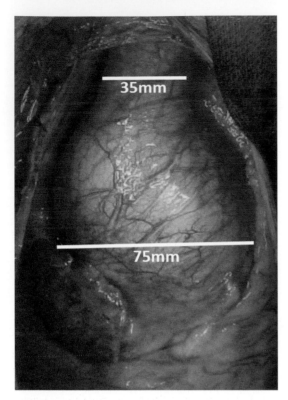

Fig. 61.6 Large aneurysm of the ascending thoracic aorta that preferentially affects the aortic root and the proximal ascending thoracic aorta.

hypotension (due to blood loss into the mediastinum, pleural cavity or pericardium) and unequal pulses (due to dissection around the origins of the large artery). The ECG is usually normal.

CT and TOE are the most important diagnostic tests and should be performed urgently. They will show the size and location of the aneurysm, any dissection flaps, the site of the aortic wall tear, extent of dissection, and the function of the aortic valve, which may partly dehisce from the outer aortic wall and become regurgitant.

Elective repair is indicated when the aneurysm is more than 5 cm in diameter. This will involve replacement of the aneurysm with a Dacron tube graft, but may also require AVR, re-implantation of the coronary artery ostia or even replacement of the transverse arch with re-implantation of the great vessels. Results of elective surgery are excellent, with operative mortality generally less than 3%.

If rupture or dissection has occurred, emergency surgery is indicated. Over 50% of patients die before reaching hospital. The systolic blood pressure should be kept at approximately 90 mmHg en route to surgery (nitroprusside, glyceryl trinitrate, beta-blockers). Similar operative techniques are used, preserving the aortic valve if possible. Biological

glues are used to bind and stiffen the fragile myxomatous layers of the aorta at the site of anastomoses and repair. This complex surgery is usually facilitated by use of deep hypothermia (18°C) and total circulatory arrest (see section Cardiopulmonary bypass: heart–lung machine). Major morbidity may result from these urgent difficult operations and includes postoperative haemorrhage, stroke and renal dysfunction. The operative mortality is between 10 and 30%, depending on the preoperative clinical state, organ or limb malperfusion prior to surgery and age.

Vigilant long-term follow-up with control of hypertension, and serial CT scans or echocardiograms, are required because other parts of the aorta (descending thoracic or abdominal) may dilate over time.

Pacemaker and dysrhythmia surgery

Degenerative fibrosis associated with age can affect the cardiac conduction mechanism to produce heart block. The heart rate may fall to 30 beats/min (ventricular escape rhythm) and result in dizziness or syncope. This is a common clinical problem in older patients. Occasionally, heart block may result from trauma to the conducting bundle at cardiac surgery or from some antiarrhythmic medications (verapamil, sotolol).

Treatment is relatively simple and achieved by implantation of a pacing lead into the right ventricle via the cephalic or subclavian vein below the clavicle and implantation of a lithium-powered, low-profile pacemaker generator, all performed under local anaesthesia. The pacing rate is adjusted to 70–80 beats/min as required by telemetry. An atrial lead can also be inserted to allow sequential atrial–ventricular pacing, which is more efficient. The pacemaker may be programmed to allow spontaneous increase of pacing rates according to patient activity.

Programmed sequential biventricular pacing may be beneficial in patients with left ventricular dilatation, severe dysfunction and cardiac failure.

Rapid atrial arrhythmias (AF, atrial flutter, junctional tachycardia) that remain uncontrolled on medication (digoxin, sotolol, amiodarone) and which are significantly symptomatic can be treated either surgically or, more commonly, by percutaneous catheter radiofrequency ablation.

Life-threatening rapid ventricular arrhythmias (ventricular tachycardia, ventricular fibrillation), which may occur in cardiomyopathies, chronic ischaemia and hypertrophic obstructive cardiomyopathy for example, may also be treated by implantable cardioverter defibrillators with minimal operative mortality and morbidity, and excellent long-term results.

Circulatory support

Circulatory support may be required to allow time for cardiac recovery after a temporary but reversible insult, or permanently.

Afterload-reducing agents

Nitroprusside and glyceryl trinitrate infusions allow rapid peripheral, arterial and venous dilatation, and reduction of cardiac preload and afterload. Calcium antagonists (nifedipine, amlodipine) and ACE inhibitors (perindopril, ramipril) are oral medications that also cause peripheral vasodilatation and reduce cardiac afterload, allowing myocardial (left ventricular) contraction and ejection of stroke volume against a lower systemic vascular resistance.

Inotropic agents

Inotropic agents are usually given as infusions for short-term use (hours or days). They include dopamine, dobutamine, adrenaline, isoprenaline, milrinone, levosimendan and calcium. All have varying properties and effects, but the underlying mechanism is an enhanced inotropic effect on the myocardium. Milrinone is a potent vasodilator (and inotrope), particularly useful in pulmonary hypotension. Additionally, intravenous or oral prostacyclin (iloprost), bosentan, glyceryl trinitrate, sildenafil and inhaled nitric oxide are effective in severe pulmonary hypertension or where the right ventricle is failing.

Intra-aortic balloon pump

Intra-aortic balloon pump (IABP) is indicated when hypotension and poor cardiac output persist despite appropriate inotropic support. A catheter with a 30 or 40 mL balloon is introduced into the descending thoracic aorta, usually percutaneously by the femoral artery. The balloon inflates (helium) and deflates in sequence with the ECG. It inflates in diastole, suddenly increasing diastolic pressure, mean blood pressure and organ perfusion, especially coronary blood flow and myocardial perfusion. The balloon rapidly deflates just prior to cardiac systole, dramatically reducing the afterload on the left ventricle. The usual duration of IABP support is between 1 and 5 days but use up to 21 days has been reported.

Potential problems include leg ischaemia, systemic infection and mechanical blood cell destruction leading to anaemia and thrombocytopenia.

Ventricular assist devices

Ventricular assist devices provide additional (and superior) mechanical support when inotropes and IABP are insufficient. Typically, cannulas are placed on the inlet side (left atrium or apex of the left ventricle) and into the outlet side (aorta) with a mechanical device in between, effectively performing the work of the left ventricle. (A similar circuit can be constructed for the right side of the heart.) Numerous devices are available (Thoratec, Novacor, Heartmate, Abio-Med) with varying characteristics relating to size, implantability, portability, ease of use and expense. Ventricular assist devices may be *in situ* from 3 to more than 300 days.

Ventricular assist devices may allow myocardial recovery over weeks or months or be used to optimise the patient's clinical state as a bridge to transplantation. Total artificial hearts can also be implanted as a bridge to transplantation or potentially (in the USA) as 'destination therapy'. The devices are compromised by thromboembolism (or bleeding), infection and mechanical failures. However, they do allow a reasonable quality of ambulant life in the interim. The 'drives' are external, about the size of a large handbag, and allow excellent patient mobility.

Extracorporeal membrane oxygenation

Where temporary (days to weeks) but major support of either (or both) the circulation and oxygenation is required (where oxygenation cannot be maintained with mechanical ventilation, 100% oxygen and maximum positive end-expiratory pressure), extracorporeal membrane oxygenation (ECMO) can be used. ECMO is identical to regular CPB but with special cannulas and circuit modifications for long-term use. The management is extremely demanding as the patient requires anticoagulation and constant supervision.

Respiratory indications include pneumonia, influenza and asthma, where the cause is potentially reversible, and in the meantime the patient cannot be kept alive via mechanical ventilation with 100% oxygen.

Cardiac indications include support after cardiac operations, after massive myocardial infarctions and drug overdoses (e.g. tricyclic antidepressants), and for acute cardiomyopathies in conditions where heart function is deemed recoverable and the patient is relatively young (<70 years). ECMO use is now expanding into witnessed cardiac arrests with ongoing cardiopulmonary resuscitation, providing it can be instituted within 60 minutes.

Cardiac transplantation

The first human cardiac transplant was performed in 1967 by Dr Christiaan Barnard in South Africa. This was preceded by extensive laboratory work by Dr Norman Shumway and colleagues at Stanford University, USA. The initial results were suboptimal because of difficulties with rejection and fulminating infections.

Ciclosporin, which was introduced in 1980, dramatically reduced the severity of the rejection and infection episodes to manageable levels, promoting renewed interest. Other advances included superior donor heart preservation, better tissue typing, myocardial biopsy surveillance and more efficient anti-rejection regimens.

Indications for cardiac transplantation include permanent severe heart damage and failure from myocarditis, cardiomyopathy and multiple myocardial infarctions. Donor hearts are usually procured following brain death from motor vehicle or cerebral trauma. Recipients are usually less than 65 years of age with no other significant coexisting medical or psychological problems.

The surgery is straightforward: reconnection of the atria, pulmonary artery trunk and ascending thoracic aorta after removal of the failing heart. The challenges are in logistics, personnel and postoperative management.

The results of cardiac transplantation are very good, with an operative mortality of 2–3%, 1-year survival of 90% and 5-year survival of 80%. Approximately 100 cardiac transplants are performed in Australia each year and almost 3000 are performed annually worldwide; however, numbers are limited by donor shortages. In response to this, much development is centred on implantable artificial hearts.

Complications of cardiac surgery

Operative mortality

Most cardiac operations have an operative mortality of approximately 1% (including the first 30 days post operation). Mortality rates are increased in re-operations (5%), multiple procedures (5%) and with increasing age (>80 years,

5–10%), age being a marker for multiple associated comorbidities.

Stroke

The incidence of major neurological events in the perioperative period is 1–2%. Causes include primary cerebrovascular disease in older patients, atheroembolism from the ascending thoracic aorta, hypoperfusion during CPB, and air or particulate embolism during valve surgery. Fortunately, there is usually a significant recovery. Subtle neuropsychological dysfunction can also occur, with abnormalities lasting up to 6 months.

Sternal and mediastinal infection

Sternal and mediastinal infection is a devastating complication, with an incidence of 1–2%. Risk factors include diabetes, obesity, bilateral ITA grafting, prolonged preoperative hospitalisation and multiple instrumentations/procedures. Prophylactic antibiotics are used in all cardiac surgery. Protection against mediastinitis is afforded by closure of the thymus and pericardium behind the sternum. Bacteria commonly involved include *Staphylococcus aureus* (including meticillin-resistant *S. aureus*).

Clinical features include fever, increased sternal discomfort, redness and movement of a previously stable sternum. Early diagnosis is essential, as established mediastinitis has a mortality of 30%.

Treatment depends on the extent of pathology, from intravenous antibiotics, to local debridement and sternal rewiring, to extensive debridement and use of omental and myocutaneous flaps.

Postoperative haemorrhage

Postoperative haemorrhage occurs with an incidence of 2–5%. Specific causes include bleeding from suture lines, branches of grafts and the ITA bed. However, in the majority no specific bleeding point is found but re-operation is useful to remove retained blood and clots from the pericardium, mediastinum and pleural cavities, and establish haemostasis in the oozing areas. Aspirin and other more potent antiplatelet drugs (clopidogrel, ticagrelor) or newer anticoagulants (dabigatran, rivaroxaban) within 5 days of cardiac surgery may be contributing factors.

Numerous other complications may also develop, including AF, pulmonary atelectasis, pneumonia, pleural and pericardial effusions, pneumothorax and fluid retention. These are all readily treatable and reversible.

Box 61.3 Percutaneous cardiac procedures

Balloon angioplasty and coronary stents
Closure of ASD, VSD, PDA, paravalvular leaks
Balloon valvotomy for mitral, aortic and pulmonary valve stenosis
Balloon dilatation of coarctation
Mitral valve repair (MitraClip)
Valve implantation: aortic, mitral, pulmonary
Thoracic aorta stent grafts
Radiofrequency ablation for atrial fibrillation
Left atrial appendage closure
Septal muscle ablation for hypertrophic cardiomyopathy

The future of cardiac surgery

Over the past 10 years there has been much interest in less (minimally) invasive surgery, reducing trauma, improving cosmesis and, where possible, avoiding the potentially deleterious effects of CPB. Earlier return to work and activity, especially for younger patients is usual. These techniques are based on smaller incisions, peripheral cannulation for CPB or off-pump surgery. These have been discussed within the relevant topic areas.

Advances in imaging with CT, echocardiography and MRI with three-dimensional reconstruction, and ingenious developments in technology and instrumentation have enabled an ever-increasing number of potentially definitive cardiac treatments and procedures to be accomplished by percutaneous catheter-based platforms under local anaesthesia. This list will continue to expand (Box 61.3).

The number of cardiac operations performed worldwide per annum continues to increase. Interventional cardiology techniques such as angioplasty have changed the spectrum of 'open' cardiac surgery to more complex and redo operations, and the mean age of patients is older.

Robotics for cardiac surgery is being developed and promises to assist minimally invasive techniques, while substantial endeavour continues in improving prosthetic cardiac valve and artificial heart technology.

Further reading

Buxton BF, Frazier OH, Westaby S (eds) *Ischaemic Heart Disease: Surgical Management*. Mosby International, 1999.

Cohn LM, Adams DH (eds) *Cardiac Surgery in the Adult*, 5th edn. New York: McGraw-Hill Education, 2018.

Fuster V, Harrington RA, Narula J, Eapen ZJ (eds) *Hurst's The Heart, 14th edn*. New York: McGraw-Hill Education, 2017.

Sellke FW, del Nido PJ, Swanson SJ (eds) *Sabiston and Spencer's Surgery of the Chest*, 9th edn. Philadelphia: Elsevier, 2017.

MCQs

Select the single correct answer to each question. The correct answers can be found in the Answers section at the end of the book.

1 The coronary artery bypass conduit with the highest patency after 5 and 10 years is:
   a left internal thoracic artery
   b right internal thoracic artery
   c left radial artery
   d right radial artery
   e left or right long saphenous vein

2 Which of the following statements about the results of coronary artery bypass grafting is correct?
   a an operative mortality of over 10% is common
   b patients with poor left ventricular function have a higher operative mortality
   c older patients have less postoperative morbidity
   d diabetes has no influence on postoperative morbidity
   e the use of an internal mammary artery improves survival but does not provide long-term freedom from angina

3 Which of the following statements about cardiac valve prostheses is correct?
   a mechanical valves require no long-term anticoagulation
   b tissue valves are highly durable
   c mechanical valves have lower bleeding and thromboembolic rates
   d tissue valves are generally preferred in the mitral position
   e structural failure is extremely rare in mechanical valves

4 The complications of cardiac valve replacement surgery include:
   a anticoagulant (warfarin)-related haemorrhage
   b cerebral thromboembolism
   c prosthetic valve endocarditis
   d structural deterioration of tissue valves after 10–15 years
   e all of the above

62 Common topics in thoracic surgery

Julian A. Smith

Department of Surgery, Monash University and Department of Cardiothoracic Surgery, Monash Health, Melbourne, Victoria, Australia

Introduction

Thoracic surgical topics discussed in this chapter are related to disorders of the chest wall, pleural space, lungs and mediastinum. Other conditions frequently managed by general thoracic surgeons include diseases of the oesophagus and chest trauma. Both of these topics are presented in Chapters 14, 15 and 48.

Presentation of thoracic disorders

Symptoms

Common thoracic symptoms include cough, chest pain, shortness of breath (on exertion or at rest), excessive or abnormal sputum production, haemoptysis, wheeze or stridor. Many conditions (especially neoplasms) are asymptomatic and are first detected on chest X-ray.

Examination findings

On examination, the patient may appear quite normal or severely short of breath (e.g. from a spontaneous pneumothorax). Clues to intrathoracic problems may be found in the other parts of the body, such as clubbing of the fingernails, peripheral cyanosis and lymphadenopathy. The jugular venous pressure may be elevated (e.g. from neoplastic superior vena caval obstruction or tension pneumothorax) and the trachea may be deviated from the midline. Signs found in the chest in some common thoracic conditions are shown in Table 62.1. Again, in some conditions, the findings on examining the chest can be completely normal.

Non-invasive diagnostic investigations

Chest X-ray

All patients with a suspected thoracic problem should have an erect posteroanterior and lateral chest X-ray. This will help define the location and extent of the problem.

Pulmonary function testing and arterial blood gases

Pulmonary function tests (PFTs) help to define the degree of respiratory impairment on presentation, the amount of functional reserve, and hence the ability of the patient to tolerate lung surgery and, at follow-up, the response to therapy. There are two major types of PFT:
- those that assess the movement of air in and out of the lungs (e.g. forced expiratory volume in 1 second, forced vital capacity, peak flow, total lung capacity, residual volume)
- those that measure the ability to transfer gas across the alveolar–capillary membrane (e.g. tests of carbon monoxide diffusing capacity).

When considering surgical therapy for a given patient, it may be evident that the patient has insufficient ventilatory capacity to withstand a chest wall incision or a major pulmonary resection, and alternative therapies will need to be offered.

Arterial blood gas analysis is an important investigation in patients with acute and chronic thoracic conditions. Parameters measured include Pao_2, $Paco_2$, pH, bicarbonate level and arterial oxygen saturation.

Computed tomography

High-resolution images of the chest wall, pleural space, lungs and mediastinum are provided in

---

Table 62.1 Physical signs in thoracic disease.

	Chest wall movement	Mediastinum and trachea	Tactile/vocal fremitus	Percussion note	Breath sounds
Large pleural effusion	Reduced on affected side	Shift to opposite side	Absent	Stony dull	Absent. May be bronchial above fluid level
Large pneumothorax	Reduced on affected side	Shift to opposite side	Decreased	Increased	Decreased
Massive lung collapse	Reduced on affected side	Shift to affected side	Absent	Dull	Decreased
Pneumonic consolidation	Reduced on affected side	Central	Increased	Dull	Bronchial
Advanced emphysema	Reduced on both sides ('barrel chest')	Central	Decreased	Increased	Decreased

cross-section. Tissue density is quantified and a fairly accurate map of pathological lesions throughout the chest is obtained. Serial computed tomography (CT) is helpful in following up suspicious lesions. Percutaneous needle biopsy of pulmonary or pleural lesions is frequently performed under CT guidance. The upper abdomen should also be scanned in patients with known or suspected pulmonary malignancy to assess the liver and adrenal glands, which are common sites for secondary deposits. Magnetic resonance imaging (MRI) is also used in centres where it is available.

Positron emission tomography

Positron emission tomography (PET), performed in isolation or in combination with CT (PET/CT), is a nuclear medicine imaging modality that uses fluorodeoxyglucose as a tracer to assess the metabolic activity of lung lesions and possible metastases in lymph nodes or elsewhere.

Invasive and operative investigations

Bronchoscopy

Diagnostic bronchoscopy, using a flexible or rigid instrument, provides direct visualisation of airway lesions for biopsy. Lesions of the lung parenchyma or lymph nodes in the subcarinal space may be biopsied using a transbronchial technique. Most commonly, diagnostic bronchoscopy is performed by respiratory physicians using the flexible bronchoscope and a combination of topical anaesthesia and intravenous sedation. More difficult and potentially complicated situations are handled by thoracic surgeons in the operating room. Occasionally,

therapeutic rigid bronchoscopy is required to control massive haemoptysis, remove aspirated foreign bodies, or clear retained inspissated sputum leading to postoperative lung or lobar collapse.

Endobronchial ultrasound-guided biopsy

Endobronchial ultrasound images are obtained by passing an endoscope fitted with an ultrasound processor into the patient's airway. Biopsy specimens from mediastinal masses, lung lesions or nearby lymph nodes may be obtained by passing a needle through the wall of the airway under ultrasound guidance. This has proven to be a valuable method for staging the mediastinum in patients with lung cancer and has avoided the need for the more invasive procedure mediastinoscopy (see next section) in many instances.

Mediastinoscopy

The mediastinoscope is a lighted cylindrical instrument used to biopsy paratracheal and subcarinal lymph nodes, most commonly in the work-up to stage a patient with known or suspected lung cancer. This investigation usually precedes any major pulmonary resection for lung cancer. It is also used in the investigation of mediastinal masses. The instrument is introduced via a transverse suprasternal incision and passed caudally in a plane deep to the pretracheal fascia. The mediastinoscope passes close to the superior vena cava (to its right), the innominate artery and arch of aorta (in front) and the recurrent laryngeal nerves (to the left and right posterolaterally). Care should be taken to avoid biopsying vascular structures such as the superior vena cava, azygos vein and pulmonary artery. Access is obtained to the upper middle and posterior mediastinum except for the subaortic area below the aortic arch, which is best approached via an anterior mediastinotomy.

Anterior mediastinotomy

Anterior mediastinotomy is a left parasternal intercostal incision employed to access tissue from the anterior mediastinum (e.g. thymic lesions). A short horizontal or vertical incision may be made either in the second or third intercostal space or by resecting a costal cartilage. A left anterior mediastinotomy allows excellent access to the subaortic lymph nodes, the primary site of spread for tumours in the left upper lobe.

Pleural aspiration and biopsy

When a pleural effusion is present (Figure 62.1), pleural fluid may be aspirated (thoracocentesis) using a needle and syringe. Cytological, microbiological and biochemical analyses may provide a clue as to the cause of the pleural effusion. Pleural biopsy can be performed at the same time using an Abram's needle.

Percutaneous biopsy

Many chest wall, pleural, pulmonary or mediastinal masses can be biopsied under CT control. This allows a tissue diagnosis to be made prior to any surgical intervention. It must be noted that a negative biopsy result does not exclude malignancy.

Video-assisted thoracoscopic surgery

Thoracoscopy, the thoracic equivalent of laparoscopy, uses cameras, telescopes and television monitors to inspect the pleural space, lung and mediastinum. Biopsy material may be taken from lesions in all these areas. The most common application is for lung and pleural biopsy. Three ports made by 2-cm incisions in the chest wall are used in the hemithorax, one for the telescope with the camera and light source and two for the instruments. Some therapeutic procedures, especially the management of recurrent spontaneous pneumothorax, recurrent pleural effusions and thoracodorsal sympathectomy, are routinely carried out using video-assisted thoracoscopy (VATS) techniques. More recently, minor and major resections of lung tissue such as a lobectomy have been performed in this way. VATS techniques have resulted in patients experiencing less postoperative pain, having a shorter in-hospital stay and returning to a normal life and/or work sooner.

Thoracotomy

Rarely, a diagnostic thoracotomy is required when less invasive procedures are inappropriate or have failed to provide a diagnosis. Access is obtained to the mediastinal lymph node groups, the great vessels, oesophagus, lung and pericardium for tissue sampling. Frozen section analysis usually provides an immediate diagnosis and this result will determine what further intraoperative measures, if any, are required.

Basic thoracic surgical techniques

Pleural aspiration

Pleural aspiration may be used in diagnosis, as the primary treatment of a pleural collection or as a preliminary measure prior to the insertion of a chest tube for the drainage of a pleural effusion. The presence of fluid should be confirmed on physical examination and chest X-ray (see Figure 62.1) prior to commencement. With the patient in a comfortable position sitting up, the chest is widely prepared and the puncture site chosen. Local anaesthetic is infiltrated liberally down to the pleura. The aspiration needle is inserted at the upper edge of the rib and up to 1 L can safely be removed at a given sitting. Upon completion, the needle is removed and a small dressing applied. A chest X-ray is then performed to exclude a pneumothorax.

Chest tube insertion and management

Common indications for chest tube insertion include spontaneous pneumothorax, tension pneumothorax, a large pleural effusion or empyema and post-traumatic haemothorax. Chest tubes are placed routinely at the completion of intrathoracic

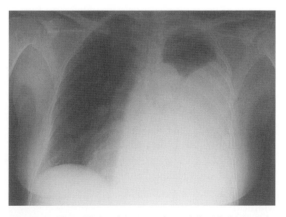

Fig. 62.1 Chest X-ray showing a large left-sided pleural effusion.

operations. In all situations, it is mandatory that an experienced operator insert the tube, because a badly performed placement is extremely dangerous.

The usual site for insertion is the fourth or fifth intercostal space in the mid-axillary line, but for the drainage of specific air, fluid or blood collections, the appropriate location on the chest wall should be chosen. The patient should be in a comfortable and relaxed position, and adequate local analgesia is essential. Following antiseptic skin preparation and infiltration of local anaesthetic into the skin, muscle layers and pleura, a skin incision is made over the middle of the chosen intercostal space. The incision is deepened using blunt dissection (with artery forceps) down to and through the pleural layer. Final dissection into the pleural space is made with a finger, and the point of entry can be widened by opening the artery forceps widely in two directions at 90° to each other. If a tension pneumothorax is present, this manoeuvre will result in a rush of air and immediate relief for the patient. The chest drain is inserted through the chest wall and firmly retained in position with strong non-absorbable sutures. The drain tube is then connected to an underwater drainage system. In almost all situations the drain should be connected to wall suction, usually high flow and low pressure (e.g. 20 cmH$_2$O). A chest X-ray must always be performed following chest tube insertion to confirm tube position and to exclude a large pneumothorax.

A chest drain should be removed only when all air leak and fluid drainage has ceased. The lung should be fully expanded on chest X-ray. A chest tube must never be 'clamped' prior to removal. The patient is asked to breathe in maximally while the tube is briskly removed and an occlusive dressing placed over the wound.

Tracheostomy

Tracheostomy is the making of a surgical opening in the trachea. Recent modifications have included percutaneous tracheostomy and minitracheostomy.

Indications

The common indications for tracheostomy are listed in Box 62.1. The benefits of a tracheostomy are that it overcomes respiratory tract obstruction, allows control of secretions, reduces respiratory dead space and allows mechanical ventilation other than via an endotracheal tube.

Method

An elective surgical tracheostomy is performed in the operating room usually under general

---

Box 62.1 Indications for tracheostomy

- Respiratory tract obstruction
- Tracheobronchial toilet/retained secretions
- Prolonged mechanical ventilation
- Elimination of respiratory dead space
- Radical laryngeal surgery

---

anaesthesia. Alternative settings include the intensive care unit (percutaneous tracheostomy) or the bedside (minitracheostomy). Via a midline lower cervical incision, a stoma is created at the level of the second and third tracheal rings through which a cuffed tracheostomy tube is placed. The lower airway is suctioned with a fine catheter and, after the tube is secured in position and the cuff inflated, ventilation can commence.

Complications

The complications of tracheostomy are listed in Box 62.2.

Thoracotomy

Posterolateral thoracotomy

Posterolateral thoracotomy is the standard approach for major pulmonary resections. The incision is located below the inferior angle of the scapula, the latissimus dorsi is divided and the pleural space is entered along the superior surface of the fifth or sixth rib.

Lateral thoracotomy

Lateral thoracotomy is used when only limited access is required, such as in the operative treatment of recurrent pneumothorax. The incision is made between the anterior and posterior axillary lines.

Box 62.2 Complications of tracheostomy

Operative
- Haemorrhage
- Pneumothorax
- Tube malposition

Postoperative
- Tube obstruction or dislodgement
- Haemorrhage
- Tracheal stenosis
- Dysphagia
- Tracheo-oesophageal fistula
- Tracheo-innominate fistula

Anterior thoracotomy

Anterior thoracotomy is commonly used for open lung biopsy. An incision is made beneath the male nipple or female breast. There is a low incidence of post-thoracotomy neuralgia using this approach.

Median sternotomy

Median sternotomy or 'sternal split' gives excellent access to the anterior mediastinum, pericardium, heart and great vessels. Anterior mediastinal tumours (e.g. thymomas) and apices of each lung (in lung volume reduction operations) can be removed via this approach.

Common thoracic disorders

Chest wall

A classification of common chest wall conditions is given in Box 62.3. Chest injuries are presented in Chapter 48. Soft tissue tumours and primary bone tumours will not be discussed further (see Chapters 45 and 51).

Pectus excavatum

In pectus excavatum or 'funnel chest', there is a variable amount of depression of the sternum, lower costal cartilages and ribs. Frequently asymmetric, the deformity may displace the heart into the left chest. Heart and respiratory function are seldom impaired. Surgery, when indicated, is entirely cosmetic to correct the deformity.

Pectus carinatum

In pectus carinatum or 'pigeon chest', the opposite deformity exists, where the sternum protrudes forward like the keel of a boat. Again, surgical correction is possible if the deformity is cosmetically unacceptable.

Secondary chest wall tumours

Involvement of the ribs and sternum by secondary tumours far exceeds that by primary bone tumours. Direct extension to the chest wall may occur in breast or lung carcinomas. Chest wall mestatases are often multiple and commonly originate in the lung, prostate, kidney, thyroid, stomach, uterus or colon. Tumours with multiple chest wall secondary deposits usually have a very poor prognosis.

Chest wall infections

De novo infections of the chest wall are extremely rare, and currently infection is most associated with a recent sternotomy or thoracotomy wound. Risk factors for postoperative wound infection include diabetes and morbid obesity. Abscesses can occur within the soft tissue planes and very rarely an empyema thoracis can 'point' through the chest wall (empyema necessitans).

Pleural effusion

The pleural space is a potential cavity that normally contains negligible amounts of fluid due to equilibrium between its production and absorption. The accumulation of fluid within this space may be a manifestation of local or systemic disease.

Classification and aetiology

There are two types of pleural effusion: a transudate or exudate. The common causes of each are given in Box 62.4.

Pathophysiology

A transudate (specific gravity <1.016 and protein content <3 g/dL) results from the altered production or absorption of pleural fluid. There is elevated systemic or pulmonary capillary pressures, lowered

---

> **Box 62.3 Classification of chest wall conditions**
>
> - Congenital anomalies: pectus excavatum, pectus carinatum
> - Chest injuries
> - Soft tissue tumours: lipomas, neurofibromas, fibrosarcomas, liposarcomas
> - Primary bone tumours: chondromas, fibrous dysplasia, osteosarcomas, Ewing's tumour, myeloma
> - Secondary chest wall tumours
> - Chest wall infections
> - Thoracic outlet syndrome

> **Box 62.4 Causes of pleural effusion**
>
> **Transudates**
> - Congestive heart failure
> - Cirrhosis
> - Nephrotic syndrome
> - Hypoalbuminaemia
>
> **Exudate**
> - Infective (post-pneumonic)
> - Malignancy
> - Chylothorax

plasma oncotic pressure or lowered intrapleural pressure. There is no disorder of the pleural surfaces. An exudate (specific gravity >1.016 and protein content >3 g/dL) is found in the presence of diseased pleural surfaces or lymphatics where there is increased capillary permeability or lymphatic obstruction.

Surgical pathology

Pneumonia of any cause may be complicated by the formation of a pleural effusion. Should pus form within the pleural space, the collection is known as an empyema thoracis. Currently, the most common cause of a post-pneumonic pleural effusion and empyema is bacterial infection.

Malignant pleural effusions can result from secondary pleural deposits, extension of the primary (lung) tumour to the pleural surface or lymphatic obstruction. Metastatic lung or breast carcinoma is the most common cause of malignant pleural effusions, but other common primary sites include the ovary, colon and kidney. There are frequently associated pulmonary metastases, but in some instances the intrathoracic metastatic lesion may be confined to the pleural space. The effusions are often blood-stained (serosanguineous), with positive cytology in up to 70% and a positive pleural biopsy in 80% of malignant effusions.

Chylothorax refers to the accumulation of chyle within the pleural space due to disruption of the thoracic duct. Very rarely a congenital anomaly of the thoracic duct and seldom from tumour involvement, chylothorax is usually the result of surgical trauma to the duct somewhere along its course.

Clinical features

Common symptoms of a pleural effusion include pleuritic chest pain, shortness of breath, cough and haemoptysis (malignant effusion). The physical signs of a large pleural effusion are shown in Table 62.1.

Investigations

Investigations are listed in Box 62.5. Chest X-ray (see Figure 62.1) will determine the extent of the effusion and may demonstrate underlying lung disease. CT will also reveal significant intrathoracic disease. Diagnostic pleural aspiration will reveal the type of effusion based on appearance and cytological, microbiological and biochemical analyses. Pleural biopsy should be performed utilising VATS if the diagnostic pleural aspiration is unsuccessful

> **Box 62.5 Investigations of pleural effusion**
>
> - Chest X-ray
> - CT scan of chest
> - Diagnostic pleural aspiration
> - Pleural biopsy (needle, video-assisted thoracoscopy or thoracotomy)
> - Bronchoscopy

or non-diagnostic. Should the effusion prove to be the result of a malignant process, it is important to adequately stage the disease prior to the commencement of therapy.

Management

Therapy should be directed to any underlying cause such as pneumonia (antibiotics), congestive heart failure (diuretics) or malignancy (chemotherapy or radiotherapy).

The prognosis in patients with a malignant pleural effusion is poor; an average survival of 6 months follows diagnosis. Treatment of the effusion is therefore, at best, palliative. Closed chest tube drainage will provide short-term symptomatic relief, but the effusion usually re-accumulates on tube removal. An attempt should be made to obliterate the pleural space (pleurodesis) to prevent the effusion re-accumulating. This may be achieved by introducing a sclerosing agent (e.g. talc) into the pleural space via a chest tube or at operation (VATS or thoracotomy) following drainage of the effusion.

Chylothorax usually responds to non-operative therapy: chest tube drainage of the collection and measures to reduce chyle flow (no-fat diet, parenteral nutrition). Should the effusion persist or re-accumulate, operative intervention (thoracic duct ligation and/or pleurodesis) is indicated.

Empyema is managed in its early stages with dependent chest tube drainage. The pleural space may be irrigated with antiseptic solution. In chronic cases, a thick fibrous wall or cortex forms around the pus-filled pleural space. Treatment options include prolonged closed-chest tube drainage, open chest tube drainage after resection of a segment of rib and open surgical decortication to remove the entire abscess wall. This releases the restricted chest wall and diaphragm and allows the lung to re-expand.

Pneumothorax

Pneumothorax refers to the presence of air within the pleural space. The air usually originates from the lung itself, but it may come from outside (after penetrating trauma) or from the oesophagus (after endoscopic perforation). The common types of pneumothorax are listed in Box 62.6. Traumatic pneumothorax is discussed in the chapter on chest injuries (see Chapter 48).

Primary spontaneous pneumothorax

Primary spontaneous pneumothorax is the most common type of pneumothorax and usually results from the rupture of a tiny bleb or bulla at the lung apex. Occurring in tall, thin, young adults of either sex, it presents with acute chest pain and shortness of breath. Physical findings are given in Table 62.1. Chest X-ray reveals an absence of peripheral lung markings and often a poorly defined line marking the border between lung and air (Figure 62.2). The lung may be completely collapsed at the hilum.

If the pneumothorax is small, it may need no therapy other than observation and a repeat chest X-ray to confirm lung re-expansion or it may be aspirated with a needle. If the pneumothorax is large or under tension (discussed later) or if there is an associated pleural effusion, a formal chest tube should be inserted. As air is evacuated from the pleural space, the lung expands and presses against the chest wall, thereby sealing the site of the air leak. Once the tube stops bubbling it can be removed.

Secondary spontaneous pneumothorax

Secondary spontaneous pneumothorax occurs in the presence of significant underlying lung or pleural disorders, such as primary or secondary malignancy, chronic airway disease (especially bullous emphysema) and pulmonary infections (bronchiectasis and lung abscess). The clinical features reflect the underlying disorder, and the presentation and initial management of the pneumothorax is as discussed in the preceding section.

Tension pneumothorax

A tension pneumothorax is present when the site of air leak in the lung acts as a one-way valve such that air enters the pleural space during inspiration and coughing but its escape is prevented during expiration, thus raising the pressure within the pleural space. Such pressure or tension compresses the lung and shifts the mediastinum towards the other side. This compresses the normal lung and may also kink and distort the superior vena cava. The diagnosis should be suspected when signs of a large pneumothorax are associated with mediastinal shift and an elevated jugular venous pressure. This constitutes a medical emergency. A large-bore needle should be inserted to the affected side and if the diagnosis is correct will be met by the hiss of escaping air and relief of the immediate problem. A formal chest tube should then be inserted.

Recurrent spontaneous pneumothorax

Approximately 30% of primary spontaneous pneumothoraces will recur and after a second episode this figure rises to 70%. If the same side has been affected twice or more, and especially if tension has occurred, a definitive procedure should be considered. Approaches via VATS or a limited thoracotomy include stapling of apical bullae to prevent further air leakage, and pleurodesis (either abrasive or chemical) or pleurectomy, which allows the visceral pleura to adhere to the parietal pleura or the bare chest wall.

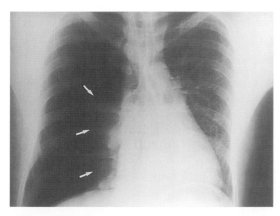

Fig. 62.2 Chest X-ray showing a large right-sided spontaneous pneumothorax. Arrows show the collapsed lung edge.

Carcinoma of the lung

Carcinoma of the lung is the most common cause of cancer deaths in males and the second most common cause of cancer deaths after breast cancer in females. Usually occurring in patients older than 50, the overall incidence in both sexes continues to rise.

Aetiology

Cigarette smoking is the single most common predisposing factor. Environmental or occupational exposure to asbestos, arsenic, nickel, chromium and hydrocarbons also play a role. The highest geographical incidence is in parts of Scotland, suggesting a possible genetic influence.

Surgical pathology

The pathological types of lung carcinoma are listed in Box 62.7.

Squamous cell carcinoma accounts for about 35% of all lung carcinomas. Most often centrally located, these tumours arise from metaplasia of the normal bronchial mucosa. Varying degrees of differentiation are seen depending on the presence of keratin, epithelial pearls, prickle cells, basal pallisading, cell size and mitotic activity.

Adenocarcinoma represents about 45% of lung carcinomas. More often found in women and located peripherally in the lung, the histopathology reveals acinar or papillary glandular elements. The tumour may form in long-standing scars (e.g. post-tuberculosis) and spreads via the bloodstream. Alveolar cell carcinoma is a highly differentiated form of adenocarcinoma. Tall columnar epithelial cells proliferate and spread along the alveolar walls. The tumour may be solitary, multinodular or diffuse (pneumonic). It may be indistinguishable from metastatic adenocarcinoma to the lung.

Large cell carcinoma comprises another 15% of malignant lung tumours. Peripherally located, there is abundant cell cytoplasm with a cellular pattern that is predominantly anaplastic.

Adenosquamous carcinoma is the most common of the mixed non-small-cell types of lung carcinoma.

Tending to be peripheral in location, their behaviour is based on the most prominent cell type.

Small-cell carcinomas make up about 10% of malignant lung tumours. Mostly centrally located, they are the most malignant and carry the worst prognosis. The cells are small, round or oval in appearance ('oat cell'). Ectopic formation of adrenocorticotropic hormone (ACTH) or antidiuretic hormone (ADH) may occur. Lymphatic and pleural invasion is common. Extrathoracic involvement at presentation is seen in 70% of tumours.

Clinical features

Approximately 10–20% of lung cancers are asymptomatic and present as a chance finding on routine chest X-ray. Symptoms may be thoracic or extrathoracic.

Thoracic symptoms include cough, haemoptysis, shortness of breath, chest pain (pleuritic or retrosternal), hoarseness of voice (involvement of recurrent laryngeal nerve), arm pain and weakness (Pancoast's syndrome; apical tumour involving brachial plexus).

Extrathoracic symptoms include those of metastases (e.g. bone, central nervous system, liver, adrenals) and those of non-metastatic paraneoplastic syndromes. These include the production of ectopic ACTH, ADH and parathyroid hormone. Wrist and ankle pain due to hypertrophic osteoarthropathy and a variety of myopathies are also found.

Physical findings include hypertrophic pulmonary osteoarthropathy, fingernail clubbing, supraclavicular and cervical lymphadenopathy, signs of brachial plexus involvement, Horner's syndrome (ptosis, miosis, anhidrosis, enophthalmos from involvement of the cervical sympathetic ganglia), elevated jugular venous pressure and facial oedema (superior vena caval obstruction). In the chest there may be signs of a pleural effusion or lung collapse (see Table 62.1).

Investigations

Investigations are listed in Box 62.8 and will provide a tissue diagnosis and aid in determining the extent of intrathoracic disease. Figure 62.3 shows typical findings on chest X-ray and CT scan. If metastatic disease is suspected in sites such as bone or the brain, additional scans of these areas should be included so as to accurately stage the disease and avoid unnecessary surgical intervention. PET scanning is important in the evaluation of regional lymph nodes and also distant metastases. The radioactive tracer fluorodeoxyglucose detects differences

---

Box 62.7 Pathological types of lung carcinoma

Non-small-cell lung cancer
- Squamous cell carcinoma
- Adenocarcinoma
- Large-cell carcinoma
- Mixed (adenosquamous)

Small-cell carcinoma

Box 62.8 Investigations for lung carcinoma

- Chest X-ray
- Sputum cytology
- CT scan of chest and upper abdomen
- PET scan
- Needle biopsy under CT control
- Bronchoscopy and biopsy
- Mediastinoscopy or anterior mediastinotomy
- Video-assisted thoracoscopic biopsy

(a)

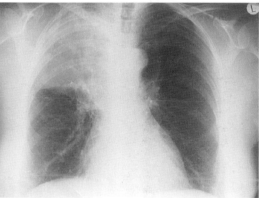

(b)

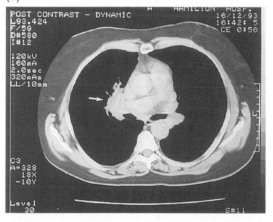

Fig. 62.3 (a) Chest X-ray showing a right hilar lung cancer with collapse and consolidation of the right upper lobe. (b) CT scan showing the right hilar lung cancer.

in metabolism between normal and malignant tissue. Metastatic disease has been found in up to 15% of lung cancers thought to have resectable disease. The number of these investigations required by a given patient is determined by the ease with which a tissue diagnosis and accurate staging is reached.

Staging of lung cancer

Staging of non-small-cell lung cancer is clinical and based on descriptors for the size and location of the primary tumour (T), the spread to lymph nodes within the thorax (N) and to the presence or absence of distant metastases (M). TNM subsets are grouped together into stages 0 through IV and these stages provide information about prognosis, allow a comparison of outcomes from different clinical series and also guide therapy.

Differential diagnosis

Carcinoma of the bronchus presenting as a solitary pulmonary nodule ('coin lesion') in the lung periphery should be differentiated from:
- secondary tumours
- benign lung tumours (bronchial adenoma)
- non-specific granuloma
- tuberculous granuloma.

Management

Unfortunately, two-thirds of patients are incurable at presentation owing to spread evidenced by one or more of the following:
- distant metastases
- a malignant pleural effusion
- involved cervical lymph nodes
- superior vena caval obstruction
- recurrent laryngeal nerve palsy.

If the patient has an otherwise resectable tumour and adequate respiratory reserve, surgical resection offers the only hope of long-term survival.

Surgical treatment consists of a thoracotomy with removal of the entire lung or lobe along with regional lymph nodes and contiguous structures. Where possible, lobectomy is the procedure of choice. Pneumonectomy is used if the tumour involves the main bronchus, extends across a fissure or is located such that wide excision is required. Survival following 'curative' resection is approximately 30% at 5 years and 15% at 10 years. The best results are found in squamous cell carcinoma followed by large-cell carcinoma and adenocarcinoma. There are very few survivors of small-cell carcinoma beyond 2 years.

Radiotherapy may be 'curative' in patients with early-stage disease unfit for surgical resection. However, the usual role for radiotherapy is in the palliation of pain from bone secondaries, superior vena caval obstruction or haemoptysis. Combinations of radiotherapy and platinum-based chemotherapy provide the best palliation for patients with good performance status and non-resectable disease.

Multi-agent chemotherapy is indicated for small-cell carcinoma. There is a small survival benefit from palliative combination chemotherapy in non-small-cell lung cancer. Trials are currently under-way to determine whether there is a role for induction chemotherapy in patients with locally advanced non-small-cell lung cancer. Responders, if down-staged, can be offered surgical resection with a view to long-term survival. This management strategy remains controversial and should currently only be offered in the context of a properly con-ducted randomised clinical trial.

Solitary pulmonary nodule

A solitary pulmonary nodule is a single well-defined opacity up to 3 cm in diameter seen radiologically. Frequently asymptomatic and found on chest X-ray screening (Figure 62.4), there are numerous possi-ble causes (Box 62.9) but malignant lesions must be excluded. Those less than 1 cm in diameter carry a low chance of being malignant and can be observed. Where possible, increases in size should be deter-mined by sequential imaging and such occurrence mandates non-surgical biopsy or surgical resection. However, stable lesions over a 2-year period may also be observed. Investigative modalities (Figure 62.4) are similar to those used for patients

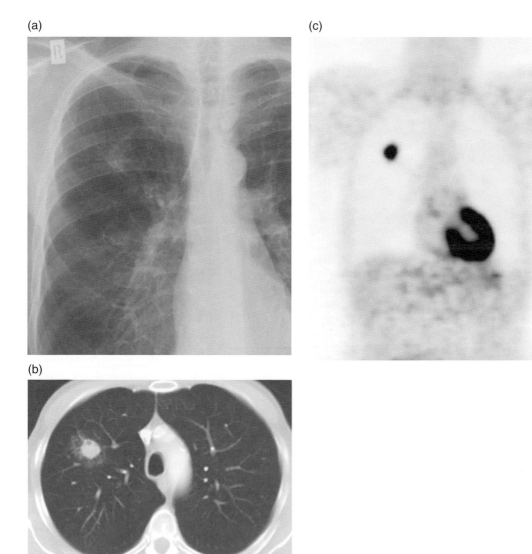

(a)

(b)

(c)

Fig. 62.4 (a) Chest X-ray, (b) CT scan and (c) PET scan appearance of a solitary pulmonary nodule.

Box 62.9 Causes of a solitary pulmonary nodule

Benign
- Infectious granuloma (tuberculosis, atypical mycobacteria, histoplasmosis, coccidioidomycosis)
- Hamartoma
- Arteriovenous malformation

Malignant
- Lung carcinoma
- Solitary metastasis (from breast, colon, kidney)
- Malignant carcinoid tumour
- Extranodal lymphoma

Box 62.10 Classification of primary mediastinal tumours

Anterosuperior masses
- Germ cell tumours
- Thymoma
- Lymphadenopathy
- Retrosternal thyroid
- Aneurysm of the aortic arch

Middle mediastinal masses
- Lymphadenopathy
- Mediastinal cysts
- Aneurysm of ascending aorta

Posterior mediastinal masses
- Neurogenic tumours (benign and malignant)
- Peripheral intercostal nerves: neurofibroma, neurilemmoma
- Sympathetic ganglia: ganglioneuroma, neuroblastoma
- Paraganglia: phaeochromocytoma, paraganglioma
- Oesophageal: duplication, tumours, diverticulae
- Hiatus hernia
- Bronchogenic cyst

---

with suspected lung carcinoma. A negative needle biopsy does not exclude a malignant cause and so a surgical biopsy/excision may be required regardless of the needle biopsy finding.

Mediastinal tumours

The mediastinum is a midline space between the pleural cavities. It is divided into the superior, anterior, middle and posterior compartments. Mediastinal tumours may be primary or secondary in origin. Secondary neoplasms most often result from lymphatic spread to mediastinal lymph nodes. Common primary sites are lung, oesophagus, larynx, thyroid and stomach. A classification of primary mediastinal tumours is given in Box 62.10.

Clinical presentation

Approximately half are asymptomatic and have no abnormal findings on examination. They are discovered by chance on a plain chest X-ray. Lesions in the young and those with symptoms are more likely to be malignant.

Thoracic symptoms result from compression of adjacent structures and include pain (back or chest), shortness of breath, cough or dysphagia. Systemic symptoms may be fever, malaise, weight loss and night sweats. Local findings include cervical lymphadenopathy, facial and/or arm swelling and tracheal shift. General findings may include testicular masses, hepatosplenomegaly and muscle weakness.

Surgical pathology

Neurogenic tumours are the most common mediastinal tumours and are found almost exclusively in the posterior mediastinum. About 10% are malignant and this feature is more frequent in children. All nerve types may be affected (Box 62.10).

Germ cell tumours are the most common anterior mediastinal tumours and are more common in the young. Types include teratoma, seminoma and non-seminomatous. Tumour markers may be elevated in non-seminomatous types and can be used to monitor the response to therapy.

Mediastinal lymphoma is usually associated with widespread disease and is seldom the only site (5%). The majority (90%) are either lymphoblastic (Hodgkin's) or diffuse large cell (non-Hodgkin's) in type.

Thymoma is more common in adults than children. About 30% of patients have myasthenia gravis and about 15% of patients with myasthenia gravis develop thymoma. The differentiation between benign (encapsulated) and malignant (invasive) thymoma can be difficult.

Investigations

Investigations are summarised in Box 62.11. In some instances, the combination of clinical features and findings on imaging allow a precise diagnosis. A patient with myasthenia gravis and an anterior mediastinal mass will most likely have a thymoma. The site of the lesion will determine the type of biopsy required.

Box 62.11 Investigation of mediastinal tumours

Imaging
- Chest X-ray
- CT scan with contrast
- MRI (neurogenic or vascular)
- Angiography (vascular)
- Barium swallow (posterior mediastinum)
- Radionuclide (thyroid or parathyroid; gallium for lymphoma)

Biochemistry
- Lactate dehydrogenase (elevated in lymphomas, seminomas)
- β-Human chorionic gonadotrophin (may be elevated in seminomas)
- Alpha-fetoprotein (non-seminomatous germ cell tumours)

Tissue diagnosis
- Fine-needle aspiration biopsy
- Mediastinoscopy
- Video-assisted thoracoscopy
- Thoracotomy

Box 62.12 Management of common mediastinal tumours

- Asymptomatic cysts
  - Pericardial: aspirate
  - Bronchogenic: observe
- Symptomatic cysts: surgical resection
- Neurogenic tumours
  - Benign, asymptomatic: may observe
  - Symptomatic: surgical resection
  - Malignant: surgical resection
- Thymoma
  - Benign: surgical resection
  - Malignant: surgical resection and chemotherapy
- Lymphoma: chemotherapy, radiotherapy (rarely surgical resection)
- Germ cell tumours: chemotherapy, radiotherapy, surgical resection

Management

Options in management include simple observation and follow-up, aspiration, surgical resection, radiotherapy, chemotherapy and combinations of surgical resection, radiotherapy and chemotherapy. A summary of the approach to management of the common primary mediastinal tumours is given in Box 62.12.

Further reading

Kaiser LR, Jamieson GG, Thompson SK (eds) *Operative Thoracic Surgery, 6th edn*. Boca Raton, FL: CRC Press, 2018.
LoCicero J, Feins R, Colson YL, Rocco G (eds) *Shields' General Thoracic Surgery, 8th edn, Vols 1 and 2*. Philadelphia: Wolters Kluwer, 2019.

MCQs

Select the single correct answer to each question. The correct answers can be found in the Answers section at the end of the book.

1 Which of the following clinical signs is *not* present in a patient with a tension pneumothorax?
   a tachypnoea
   b hypotension
   c elevated jugular venous pressure
   d tracheal deviation towards the side of the pneumothorax
   e hyperresonant percussion note on the side of the pneumothorax

2 Immediate insertion of a chest tube may be life-saving in which of the following conditions?
   a carcinoma of the lung
   b pulmonary embolism
   c tension pneumothorax
   d pleural effusion
   e lung abscess

3 Which of the following pathological types of carcinoma of the lung has the worst prognosis?
   a small-cell carcinoma
   b large-cell carcinoma
   c adenocarcinoma
   d squamous cell carcinoma
   e adenosquamous cell carcinoma

4 The greatest chance of long-term survival in a patient with a localised carcinoma of the lung is provided by:
   a chemotherapy
   b radiotherapy
   c combined chemotherapy and radiotherapy
   d surgical excision
   e immunotherapy

Section 16
Problem Solving

Section 16
Problem Solving

63 Chronic constipation

Kurvi Patwala[1] and Peter De Cruz[2]

[1] Austin Health, Melbourne, Victoria, Australia
[2] Inflammatory Bowel Disease Service, Austin Health, and University of Melbourne, Melbourne, Victoria, Australia

Introduction

Constipation is a common presenting symptom. The Rome IV consensus approach to the diagnosis of functional constipation requires the following.

1 Must include two or more of the following:
   a Straining during more than 25% of defecations
   b Lumpy or hard stools for more than 25% of defecations
   c Sensation of incomplete evacuation for more than 25% of defecations
   d Manual manoeuvres to facilitate more than 25% of defecations (e.g. digital evacuation, support of the pelvic floor)
   e Fewer than three spontaneous bowel motions per week
2 Loose stools are rarely present without the use of laxatives
3 Insufficient criteria for irritable bowel syndrome.

A more practical approach defines constipation as a syndrome related to bowel symptoms such as difficult or infrequent passage of stool, hardness of stool or a feeling of incomplete evacuation that may occur secondary to an underlying disorder or in isolation. Although constipation is a symptom and not a disease, it affects 6–30% of the population and, if associated with abdominal pain, results in poorer overall health and function. Management involves diagnosing the underlying cause and tailoring therapy towards improving quality of life (Figure 63.1).

Physiology

A solid meal passes from the mouth to the caecum in 4 hours and residue from this meal reaches the rectosigmoid junction by 24 hours. When luminal contents of the small intestine empty into the large intestine, distension of the colon activates the myenteric plexus leading to three patterns of motility:

- Retrograde peristalsis, which occurs mainly in the right colon
- Segmentation, which results in minimal transit over the colon and occurs mainly in the left colon
- Mass movement, which results in propelling contents over long distances but occurs only a few times daily.

Motility is likely controlled by a pacemaker in the transverse colon, which also acts as the main region of storage. Colonic motility is under enteric nervous and endocrine control. It can be significantly affected by physical activity, dietary fibre and emotional states.

Colonic motility causes the bowel contents to be retained and mixed to facilitate absorption. It takes 3–4 days for the meal residue to finally be evacuated in the stools. The frequency of bowel movements in most normal humans ranges from three per week to three per day and about 70% of stool consistency is water. Consequently, inadequate water intake may result in harder stools that are difficult to evacuate.

The rectum is usually empty until faeces arrives periodically from the colon. Distension of the rectal or pelvic muscle walls causes an urge to defecate. Initially, this can be suppressed by voluntary contraction of the anal sphincters and pelvic floor muscles. Further arrival of faeces will eventually make defecation unavoidable. At defecation, expulsion is aided by raised intra-abdominal pressure and colonic contraction. The pelvic floor muscles and the anal sphincters relax so the faeces can be discharged through the anus. Subsequently, the pelvic floor muscles and the anal sphincters resume their tone in order to maintain bowel continence.

Textbook of Surgery, Fourth Edition. Edited by Julian A. Smith, Andrew H. Kaye, Christopher Christophi and Wendy A. Brown.
© 2020 John Wiley & Sons Ltd. Published 2020 by John Wiley & Sons Ltd.

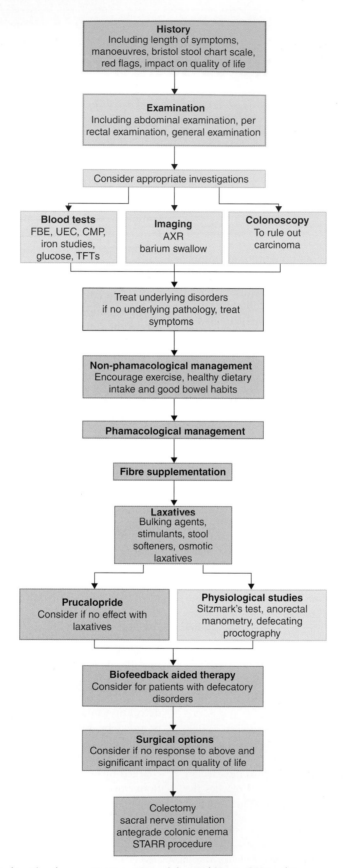

Fig. 63.1 Management algorithm for constipation. AXR, abdominal X-ray; CMP, calcium, magnesium, phosphate; FBE, full blood examination; TFTs, thyroid function tests; UEC, urea, electrolytes and creatinine.

Risk factors

Box 63.1 outlines the common risk factors associated with the development of constipation. Prevalence rates of constipation are higher in women, ethnic populations and elderly populations living in residential aged care facilities. Furthermore, elderly patients are more likely to be prescribed therapy for comorbidities that contribute to constipation. Common medications with constipation as an adverse effect are listed in Box 63.2.

Aetiology

A systematic approach incorporating history, examination and investigations is required to delineate underlying aetiology and ongoing management of constipation. A classification of the more common causes of constipation is given in Box 63.3.

Evaluation

History

Clinical assessment must begin with a detailed history that elicits the patient's symptoms of constipation. In particular, questions must be asked about the timing of onset, manoeuvres used to defecate and stool consistency based on a rating scale such as the Bristol Stool Scale. Self-reported stool frequency is a subjective measure and is often underestimated. Consequently, utilising a bowel diary may be of value. Furthermore, red flags such as sudden change in bowel habits, per rectal blood loss, weight loss or a family history of colon cancer must be addressed and investigated appropriately to rule out a sinister cause. The patient should be questioned about associated symptoms such as abdominal bloating, non-gastrointestinal symptoms (fatigue,

malaise) and impact on quality of life determined by use of laxatives, complications and interference with their sense of well-being. Lastly, it is important to elicit a thorough past medical history focusing on conditions associated with constipation, as outlined in Box 63.3.

Examination

Abdominal examination may be unremarkable or reveal distension secondary to a colon full of faeces. A perianal and rectal examination must be performed assessing for faecal soiling on perianal skin, haemorrhoids, anal fissure, rectocele, puborectalis tenderness and stool in the rectal vault. It is also important to assess anal resting tone and tone on straining.

Although the physical examination will concentrate on the abdomen and anorectum, careful systemic examination is also important to exclude systemic causes of constipation.

Investigations

Simple blood test investigations such as full blood count, renal function studies, electrolyte levels, iron studies, glucose and thyroid function tests should be considered to assess for complications or underlying causes of constipation. Evidence of anaemia, particularly microcytic iron deficiency anaemia, should prompt further investigation to rule out a malignancy. Deranged electrolytes or endocrinological abnormalities may suggest an underlying aetiology for constipation. A colonoscopy or double-contrast barium enema is often needed to exclude dangerous organic pathology such as a neoplasm. In chronic constipation, a barium enema may be preferable because the colon can be dilated and tortuous, especially with megacolon making colonoscopic intubation difficult.

Physiological testing

Physiological testing is based on colonic physiology and is performed in patients with chronic constipation that is refractory to fibre supplementation or laxative use. It can also be utilised when clinical suspicion of disordered defecation is high.

Slow transit constipation

This refers to colonic motor dysfunction, which may be due to a marked reduction in interstitial cells of Cajal and colonic intrinsic cells. Slow transit constipation can be determined using a Sitzmark test, which involves ingestion of a capsule

---

Box 63.1 Risk factors associated with the development of constipation

- Female
- Low socioeconomic status
- Lower parental education rates
- Less physical activity
- Living in a residential aged care facility
- Medications (see Box 63.2)
- Depression
- Physical and sexual abuse
- Stressful life events

Box 63.2 Medications associated with constipation

5-HT$_3$ antagonists: ondansetron
Analgesics
    Opioids: morphine
    NSAIDs: ibuprofen
Anticholinergic agents
    Tricyclic antidepressants: amitriptyline >
        nortriptyline
    Antiparkinsonian therapy: benztropine
    Antipsychotics: chlorpromazine
    Antispasmodics: dicyclomine
Antihistamines: diphenhydramine
Anticonvulsants: carbamazepine
Antihypertensives
    Calcium channel blockers: verapamil, nifedipine
    Diuretics: frusemide
    Centrally acting: clonidine
    Antiarrhythmics: amiodarone
    β_2 antagonists: atenolol
Bile acid sequestrants: colestyramine, colestipol
Cation-containing agents
    Aluminium
    Calcium
    Bismuth
    Iron supplements
    Lithium
Chemotherapy agents
    Vinca alkaloids: vincristine
    Alkylating agents: cyclophosphamide
Endocrine: pamidronate, alendronic acid
Other antidepressants: monoamine oxidase inhibitors
Other antipsychotics: clozapine, haloperidol, risperidone
Other antiparkinsonian drugs: dopamine agonists
Other antispasmodics: mebeverine, peppermint oil
Sympathomimetics: adrenaline, terbutaline
Miscellaneous: barium sulphate, oral contraceptive pill, polystyrene resins

Box 63.3 Aetiology of constipation

Dietary
Poor fibre intake
Poor fluid intake

Physiological
Slow transit constipation
Intestinal pseudo-obstruction (Ogilvie's syndrome)

Mechanical obstruction
Colon cancer
External compression from malignant lesion
Strictures
    Diverticular
    Post-ischaemic
Post-surgical abnormalities
Megacolon
Perianal: rectocele, anal fissure

Neuromuscular disease
Cerebral: cerebrovascular accidents, Parkinsonism, tumours
Spinal: cauda equina tumour, multiple sclerosis, paraplegia
Peripheral: Hirschsprung's disease, autonomic neuropathy, Chagas' disease
Myopathies: amyloidosis, scleroderma

Functional
Irritable bowel syndrome
Immobility: degenerative joint disease
Pregnancy
Psychiatric and psychological causes: depression, confusion, cognitive impairment

Endocrine and electrolyte disturbance
Diabetes mellitus
Hypothyroidism
Hyperparathyroidism
Hypercalcaemia
Hypokalaemia
Hypomagnesaemia

Other
Uraemia
Scleroderma
Heavy metal poisoning

containing 20–50 radiopaque markers followed by either serial abdominal X-rays until all markers are defecated or a single abdominal X-ray on day 5. The presence of more than 20% retained markers at day 5 is consistent with delayed transit constipation. Intraluminal assessments with manometry and barostat can be used, although these are imperfect surrogate markers for normal and abnormal colonic motor function. Colonic transit testing is not recommended in early assessment as it does not exclude the presence of defecatory disorders and further anorectal testing is often required.

Defecatory disorders

These are defined by impaired rectal evacuation with normal or delayed colonic transit. This may be caused by inadequate propulsive rectal forces or increased resistance to evacuation secondary to anismus (high resting anal pressure) or dyssynergia (incomplete relaxation or paradoxical contraction of the pelvic floor or external anal sphincters). Defecating proctography can be performed by

Table 63.1 Laxatives used in the management of constipation.

Class	Mechanism of action	Examples
Bulking agents	Absorption of water in colon to increase faecal bulk	Ispaghula husk Methylcellulose Sterculia
Stimulant laxatives	Increase intestinal motility through stimulation of colonic nerve endings	Bisacodyl Senna Sodium picosulphate
Stool softeners	Soften stool by assisting water to mix with faeces and lubricate stool to allow easier passage	Docusate Liquid paraffin
Osmotic laxatives	Increase colonic water absorption through osmosis and have local irritant effects to increase motility	Lactulose Fleet phosphosoda Magnesium sulphate

filling the rectum with radiological contrast and allowing the patient to attempt defecation on a radiolucent toilet seat. The progress of the contrast is assessed by fluoroscopy. Another option is the rectal balloon expulsion test, which monitors the patient's ability to evacuate a water-filled balloon. Requiring up to 5 minutes is considered normal.

Anorectal manometry assesses the integrity of the intrinsic innervation of the rectum and anus by inflating a rectal balloon and assessing for a transient drop in anal pressures. A clinically absent rectosphincteric reflex is suggestive of Hirschsprung's disease.

While these tests are useful in the diagnosis of defecatory disorders, they are often difficult to interpret given the difficulty patients face in performing these tests in a clinical and public environment. Therefore, an environment as private as possible is advised.

Management

The management of constipation is directed towards the underlying aetiology. If the primary pathology is not amenable to treatment or no pathology is identified, management is symptomatic. Non-pharmacological approaches suggest improving dietary practices and encouraging exercise. There is limited evidence for probiotic use or increasing fluid intake unless the patient is markedly dehydrated. Other simple behavioural practices such as developing a regular bowel routine and responding to the urge for defecation should be encouraged.

Over-the-counter therapy including fibre supplements and laxatives, enemas or suppositories form the bulk of outpatient constipation management. Soluble dietary fibre supplements, up to 30 g/day,

are significantly effective in reducing symptomatic constipation. However, patients should be counselled on their delayed effect, taking several weeks to reduce symptoms. A number of laxative options exist with varying pharmacological properties. Examples of each laxative option with the corresponding mechanism of action are described in Table 63.1. No evidence is currently available that indicates which laxative or laxative regimen is superior.

Treatment with prucalopride, a 5-HT$_4$ agonist, is appropriate for use in patients with chronic constipation unresponsive to laxatives and works by increasing colonic transit time. It can result in clinically significant improvements in the number of spontaneous bowel movements and reduction in severity of symptoms. There is a rapid onset of action and improvement is maintained for at least 12 weeks.

For patients with defecatory disorders, biofeedback-aided pelvic floor retraining plays a role. Using visual and auditory feedback recorded by manometry or electromyographic sensors, patients can learn to relax pelvic floor muscles and increase abdominal pressure during defecation. Biofeedback therapy is safe and evidence suggests that 55–82% of patients maintain symptom improvement. However, the expertise to perform this is not yet widely available.

Surgical intervention plays a role when non-surgical measures fail and symptoms significantly impact the patient's quality of life. For patients with documented slow transit constipation not responding to conservative therapy, a colectomy and ileorectal anastomosis can be performed. Although this treats primary symptoms, it is unlikely to improve abdominal pain and bloating. Other options for slow transit constipation or constipation refractory to laxative use include sacral nerve stimulation and antegrade colonic enemas, which have limited exposure in adults. Response to sacral nerve stimulation is variable and many patients have significant loss of efficacy after some time. Alterations in the pulse width or frequency of stimulation appear to have no significant effect on the improvement of symptoms in patients with constipation. For patients with defecatory disorders secondary to rectal intussusception or rectocele, a stapled transanal rectal resection (STARR) procedure can be considered. The STARR procedure involves stapling excess rectal mucosa with the aim of alleviating symptoms. However, long-term outcomes of patients are questionable and rates of complications, such as pelvic sepsis, fistula formation and bowel perforation, are relatively high.

Irritable bowel syndrome

Irritable bowel syndrome classically presents with abdominal discomfort that is relieved by defecation or is associated with a change in stool frequency or appearance in the absence of organic pathology. It can be divided into diarrhoea-predominant or constipation-predominant subtypes. Management is directed towards symptomatic relief of pain and bowel frequency, with counselling to avoid stress or precipitating factors, dietary advice and pharmacotherapy. More severely affected patients may require formal psychological management. The majority of patients will be satisfied with reassurance that dangerous diseases like colorectal cancer have been excluded.

Other causes

Specific conditions like rectal intussusception, sigmoidocele, Hirchsprung's disease (especially short-segment disease in adults) and Chagas' disease are relatively rare and discussed further in standard textbooks on colorectal surgery.

Further reading

Bharucha AE, Pemberton JH, Locke GR. American Gastroenterological Association technical review on constipation. *Gastroenterology* 2013;144:218–38.
Lehur PA, Stuto A, Fantoli M *et al*. ODS II Study Group. Outcomes of stapled transanal rectal resection vs. biofeedback for the treatment of outlet obstruction associated with rectal intussusception and rectocele: a multicentre, randomised, controlled trial. *Dis Colon Rectum* 2008;51:1611–18.

Saha L. Irritable bowel syndrome: pathogenesis, diagnosis, treatment and evidence-based medicine. *World J Gastroenterol* 2014;20:6759–73.

MCQs

Select the single correct answer to each question. The correct answers can be found in the Answers section at the end of the book.

1 A 22-year-old female has had constipation for 4 weeks since starting medical school. She occasionally has mild cramping abdominal pain. She has no other symptoms and no family history of colorectal cancer. Which of the following is the most appropriate management?
   a encouraging oral dietary fibre and fluids
   b colonoscopy and anorectal physiology tests
   c anorectal biofeedback therapy
   d right hemicolectomy
   e teaching self-digital extraction of faeces from rectum

2 An 88-year-old male with multiple comorbidities including Parkinson's disease, hypothyroidism and depression represents with a several-year history of ongoing constipation. A colonoscopy performed a year ago was normal with no evidence of obstruction, malignancy or stricturing. Which of the following is the most likely cause?
   a psychological
   b colon cancer
   c medication adverse effects
   d immobility
   e poor fibre and fluid intake

3 A 51-year-old male presents with a 1-year history of worsening constipation, abdominal cramps and weight loss. Blood test investigations reveal a microcytic iron deficiency anaemia. There is no family history of colon cancer. The most appropriate next step is:
   a anorectal physiology tests
   b colonoscopy
   c barium swallow
   d use a combination of laxatives and enemas
   e right hemicolectomy

4 A 43-year-old mother of two children complains of difficulty in initiating rectal evacuation. She feels there is a lump in the perineum which requires vaginal reduction prior to effective evacuation. Which of the following is the most appropriate management?
   a transit marker studies

b defecating proctogram
c anorectal biofeedback
d teach good hygienic practices
e use rectal enemas to assist bowel movements

5 After a previous hysterectomy, a 55-year-old mother of three children complains of constipation. Defecating proctogram showed a lack of relaxation of the puborectalis paradoxus at defecation. Which of the following is the most appropriate management?
a regular use of St. Mark's anal dilator prior to defecation
b mandatory use of squatting posture at defecation
c transit marker studies
d avoid laxatives but teach rectal washout instead
e anorectal biofeedback therapy

64 Faecal incontinence

Andrew Bui

University of Melbourne and Austin Health, Melbourne, Victoria, Australia

Introduction

Faecal incontinence is defined as an involuntary loss of liquid or solid stools. This symptom may be further divided into passive and urge incontinence. *Passive incontinence* means that the patient is not aware of the passage of stools and is mainly due to impaired internal anal sphincter or anorectal sensory dysfunction. *Urge incontinence* refers to the situation where the patient is aware of the signal to pass stools but is unable to prevent it from happening. It is due to dysfunction of contraction or neurological control of the external anal sphincters. Patients often present with mixed symptoms of passive and urge incontinence. Another term in use is *anal incontinence*, which refers to the loss of stools and flatus.

The estimated prevalence of faecal incontinence from various studies is 2–18%, with a higher prevalence of up to 25% among the older population and people in institutional care. The large variation in the prevalence reported is attributed to the different definitions of faecal incontinence used in various studies, sample size and population sampled. Additionally, there is under-reporting as most people find it embarrassing and distressing to discuss even with healthcare providers. A recent systematic review of the literature highlighted the difficulties and the inaccuracy of the prevalence studies of faecal incontinence and provided an estimated prevalence rate of 1 in 8 community adults.

Faecal incontinence is a distressing and socially isolating condition that leads to poor quality of life. It is also costly to the wider community: in Australia in 2010, the estimated cost per person was A$14 023, with an overall cost to the community of approximately A$66.7 billion, according to a study by Deloitte Access Economic.

Pathophysiology

The maintenance of normal faecal continence depends on complex interactions between various factors: an intact anorectal structure consisting of internal anal sphincter (IAS), external anal sphincter (EAS) and puborectalis, rectal reservoir and compliance, anorectal angle, stool consistency, intact sensory and motor neural pathways, and normal mental function (Figure 64.1).

The sphincter muscle complex, which controls the exit of stools, is composed of the puborectalis and internal and external sphincter muscles. The IAS is smooth muscle under involuntary control and mainly accounts for the resting anal tone. The puborectalis and EAS are striated muscle controlled by the pudendal nerve via the S2–S4 nerve roots.

The arrival of stool or gas in the rectum leads to distension and relaxation of the IAS and sampling of the contents by the richly innervated anal canal mucosa, which sends signals to the central nervous system (CNS) via the spinal cord for interpretation of whether evacuation is acceptable. If it is socially acceptable, the EAS is voluntarily relaxed for evacuation of rectal contents. If it is not, then the EAS is commanded to contract to close the anal canal and defer defecation.

Loss of continence therefore results from interruption of this complex coordination between neural and motor pathways, from impairment of the anorectum and sphincter complex, and from change in stool consistency.

Textbook of Surgery, Fourth Edition. Edited by Julian A. Smith, Andrew H. Kaye, Christopher Christophi and Wendy A. Brown.
© 2020 John Wiley & Sons Ltd. Published 2020 by John Wiley & Sons Ltd.

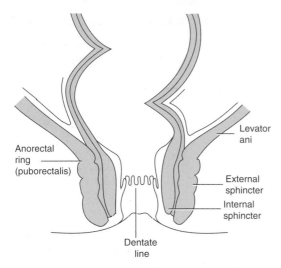

Fig. 64.1 Anal canal and rectum.

Labels in figure:
Levator ani
Anorectal ring (puborectalis)
External sphincter
Internal sphincter
Dentate line

> **Box 64.1 Causes of faecal incontinence**
>
> **Incontinence with abnormal sphincters and rectum**
> - Sphincter defect: obstetric, previous anorectal surgery, perineal trauma
> - Neuropathic sphincters: lower motor neurone lesions (e.g. stretch pudendal neuropathy, diabetes, demyelination), upper motor neurone lesions (e.g. stroke, cerebral tumours, demyelination)
> - Rectal prolapse and internal rectal mucosal intussusception
> - Loss of rectal capacity or compliance from rectal surgery, irradiation or IBD
> - Anorectal/pelvic cancer
> - Congenital anorectal abnormalities
>
> **Incontinence with normal sphincters and rectum**
> - Faecal impaction
> - Severe diarrhoea
> - Dementia or mental retardation

Causes of faecal incontinence

Faecal incontinence is due to impairment of the various factors involved in maintaining normal continence. They may be classified into the following broad categories.

- Impaired anal sphincter: injuries during childbirth account for the majority in female patients; impalement injuries from falls or motor vehicle accidents.
- Reduced rectal reservoir and sensation: proctitis from inflammatory bowel disease (IBD), radiation, resection of rectal cancer (low and ultra-low anterior resection).
- Change in stool consistency and frequency: infective diarrhoea or IBD.
- Impaired nerve function, pudendal neuropathy from stretch or chronic straining, diabetes.
- Spinal cord injuries.
- Impaired mental function.

The most common cause of faecal incontinence in females is obstetric injury, resulting from tearing of the perineum and anal sphincter muscle, stretching of the pudendal nerve and subsequent neuropathy. Sphincter damage may be detected clinically in 10–13% of all vaginal deliveries and occult injury may be detected by endoanal ultrasound in up to 80% of forceps deliveries. Other causes are shown in Box 64.1.

Diagnostic approach

History

Careful and sensitive history taking is key to dealing with patients with this embarrassing condition. Direct and tactful questioning will also be necessary to define the patient's symptoms and expectations. It is important to differentiate true faecal incontinence as defined previously from pseudo-incontinence due to overflow of liquid stools around faecal impaction in the rectum. Specific questions are outlined here.

- Enquire about onset of symptoms, precipitating events, urge or passive incontinence, stool consistency, frequency of incontinence, severity and impact on daily living and quality of life.
- Ask about risk factors such as obstetric history, with regard to baby size, prolonged labour, forceps delivery and perineal tear.
- Other risks include anorectal surgery such as haemorrhoidectomy, anal dilatation or sphincterotomy for fissure, and fistulotomy.
- Ask about other surgery such as spinal surgery affecting pelvic nerves, cholecystectomy or other upper gastrointestinal tract surgery causing diarrhea, colorectal surgery causing low anterior resection syndrome.
- Additional routine questions should enquire about medications and other medical illnesses such as thyroid disease, diabetes or multiple sclerosis.

Continence scoring systems

These are used to quantify the severity of faecal incontinence objectively for the purpose of monitoring progress and for research. The commonly used incontinence score systems include the Wexner incontinence score, Vaizey scale and Faecal Incontinence Quality of Life Scale. The Wexner incontinence score is probably the most widely

Table 64.1 Wexner score.

Type of incontinence	Frequency				
	Never	Rarely	Sometimes	Usually	Always
Solid	0	1	2	3	4
Liquid	0	1	2	3	4
Gas	0	1	2	3	4
Wears pad	0	1	2	3	4
Lifestyle alteration	0	1	2	3	4

Never, 0; rarely, <1/month; sometimes, <1/week, ≥1/month; usually, <1/day, ≥1/week; always, ≥1/day.
Totals: 0, perfect; 20, complete incontinence.

used and takes into account the frequency of incontinence to solid, liquid and gas, the use of pads and effects on lifestyle (Table 64.1).

Examination

Patients are usually examined in the left lateral position. It is also important to examine the patient in a comfortable and private setting to allay any anxiety. The perineum is inspected for faecal soiling, perianal scars, gaping deformity of the anal margin, skin tags or prolapsed rectal mucosa or haemorrhoids on straining. Descent of the perineum of more than 4 cm on straining indicates significant weakness of the pelvic floor. Digital examination is performed to assess the integrity of the anal sphincter, resting tone and voluntary contraction and any abnormal masses.

Sigmoidoscopy is performed to inspect the anal canal and rectal mucosa for internal prolapse, proctitis, tubulovillous adenoma or tumour.

Further investigations

Further investigations may be indicated, and these include colonoscopy to rule out malignancy, colitis or rectal tubulovillous adenoma. Specialised investigation of faecal incontinence includes endoanal ultrasound, anorectal manometry, pudendal nerve latency time and defecating proctogram

Endoanal ultrasound

Endoanal ultrasound uses a rigid ultrasound probe with a 360° rotating transducer that scans the anal canal to produce a circular picture of the puborectalis and IAS and EAS (Figure 64.2). It is highly

(a)

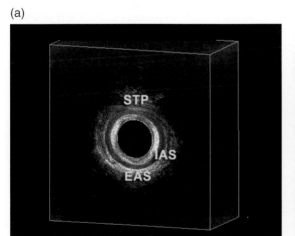

(b)

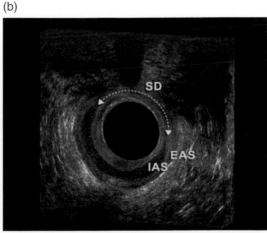

Fig. 64.2 Endoanal ultrasound: (a) mid-anal canal; (b) external and internal sphincter defects. EAS, external anal sphincter; IAS, internal anal sphincter; SD, sphincter defect; STP, superficial transverse perinei. Source: *Clinical Uses of Pelvic Ultrasound* by Dr. Marianne Starch, BK Medical Publication BG 0460-A/ March 2010.

sensitive for detecting structural defects in the IAS and EAS. The three-dimensional modality improves the accuracy and provides further structural detail of sphincter anatomy. It is the preferred modality for investigation of anal sphincters.

MRI is an alternative imaging technique, but is less accurate in detecting defects of the sphincter muscles compared with endoanal ultrasound. Furthermore, MRI is costly and less readily available.

Manometry

This provides an objective measure of the pressure within the anal canal. It involves the use of a balloon-tipped catheter with pressure sensors inserted into the anal canal to measure resting pressure and squeeze pressure. Low resting pressure reflects underlying IAS defect and low squeeze pressure poor EAS contraction.

Rectal compliance or capacity is measured by the response to inflation of the balloon at the tip of the catheter. The balloon is progressively inflated to various volumes and the patient is asked to indicate the sensation detected, as first sensation, urge sensation and maximal tolerated volume.

The rectoanal inhibitory reflex is measured by inflating the balloon rapidly and deflating it to see if there is relaxation of the IAS in response to balloon distension. Positive response is normal and indicates reflex.

Pudendal nerve latency time

The pudendal nerve latency time (PNLT) refers to the time between stimulation of the pudendal nerve and contraction of the EAS. This is measured by the St. Mark's electrode attached to the gloved index finger and connected to a special nerve stimulator and recorder. Delay in PNLT indicates pudendal nerve neuropathy but it does not appear to correlate fully with severity of incontinence. Measurement of PNLT is operator dependent and has not been shown to correlate with severity of incontinence.

Defecating proctogram

This is a fluoroscopic study of the defecation process after patients have been given an enema of diluted barium. It provides information on the anorectal angle, presence of enterocele, rectocele or internal rectal intussusception and the extent of full-thickness rectal prolapse. The concept of internal rectal intussusception is new and has been proposed by some colorectal surgeons to cause faecal incontinence, particularly in the group of patients with idiopathic incontinence.

Treatment

Treatment of faecal incontinence is challenging and needs to be individualised according to the underlying functional and structural defects, symptom severity and effects on quality of life, as well as the patient's wishes. The ideal management approach to this complex condition is with a multidisciplinary team of specialists comprising colorectal surgeons, urogynaecologists, continence nurses, physiotherapists and dietitians. Conservative measures and surgical therapies are not mutually exclusive and in fact they are often used to complement each other to improve patient outcome.

Conservative therapy

The first-line treatment measures are usually conservative and can be summarised as follows.
- Diarrhoea can be treated with antidiarrhoeal medications such as loperamide, while codeine phosphate helps to reduce stool frequency. Cholestyramine may be useful in patients who developed diarrhoea following cholecystectomy.
- Addition of bulking agents such as psyllium or bran to the diet will improve consistency of liquid stools. Often, formed solid stools are easier to be held back by a weakened sphincter.
- Pre-emptive measures to empty the rectum using glycerine suppository or enema before venturing out of the house will reduce the risk of faecal leakage and provide some confidence to individuals.
- Biofeedback therapy uses visual, auditory or verbal feedback techniques to assist patients in the training of the pelvic floor and sphincter muscles to improve their strength, sensation and coordination. It requires patients to be motivated and to have the ability to understand and follow instructions. Additional supportive counselling and practical advice regarding diet and skin care help to improve the success of this treatment. Non-randomised studies have reported 64–89% improvement in incontinence episodes.
- Anal plugs are disposable absorbent devices which may be useful in patients with minor incontinence or neurological impairment, such as spinal injuries.

Surgery

The indications for surgery are failed conservative therapy and when symptoms are sufficiently severe to warrant it. The principle of surgery is, first do no harm. Although faecal incontinence is a debilitating condition, it is not life-threatening and therefore the risks and benefits of surgery must be carefully considered for each individual patient. The operation can be broadly divided into the following groups: sphincter repair, sphincter augmentation, sphincter replacement, neuromodulation and stoma formation.

Anterior anal sphincter repair

This operation is used to repair the defect in the EAS, which is usually situated in the anterior portion of the sphincter complex. The EAS defect usually results from childbirth injury caused by tearing of the anterior portion of the external sphincter muscle. The torn ends of the EAS are dissected from the surrounding tissue and sutured in an overlapping manner using absorbable suture such as 0 PDS. Successful restoration of continence can be achieved in 60–80% of cases, but there is a tendency for deterioration over a 5-year period of time.

Post-anal repair (Park's operation) involves plication of the posterior aspect of the EAS to restore the acute anorectal angle. It is no longer a recommended treatment option for faecal incontinence.

Sphincter augmentation by injectables

This is the procedure where bulking agents are injected into the defect in the anal sphincter complex, usually in the IAS, to restore the normal contour of the anal canal. Various biological or synthetic materials have been trialled with varying success. These materials include autologous fat, glutaraldehyde cross-linked collagen, Teflon, PTFE, PTQ, NASHA (dextranomer in stabilised hyaluronic acid), and new agents such as Solesta and Sphin-Keeper™. The injection into the sphincter defect can be done under endoanal ultrasound guidance or blindly into the IAS defects previously mapped by endoanal ultrasound.

A non-randomised study of the NASHA injection for the Food and Drug Administration in the USA in 2011 reported that 52% of the patients had over 50% reduction in incontinence episodes compared with 31% receiving sham injection. A Cochrane review in 2013 of five randomised studies concluded that long-term outcome data was not available.

Injection therapy may have a role in treating patients with mild passive incontinence.

Sphincter replacement operation

This operation involves replacing the existing sphincter with a nearby skeletal muscle, which is transposed to encircle the anal canal and acts as a neo-sphincter. The nearby muscles that have been used include gracilis, gluteus maximus, sartorius and adductor longus. The transposed muscle can be used in an electro-stimulated state or a non-stimulated state. Electro-stimulated gracilo-plasty has been the most widely used and studied operation. It is a complex and expensive operation with a success rate of up to 60% but high complication and re-operation rates of over 50%.

Other alternatives to muscle transposition are artificial bowel sphincter and magnetic anal sphincter. The artificial bowel sphincter consists of a fluid-filled silicone elastomer cuff encircling the anal canal, which is in turn connected to a pressure-regulating balloon and a pump system placed in the labial or scrotal skin. Fluid is manually pumped in and out of the cuff to close or open the anal canal for defecation. This operation is less technically demanding than gracilo-plasty, but the higher complication rate of device erosion and infection (20–45%) is a major concern. Nevertheless, it remains a useful alternative in patients with deficiency of pelvic floor muscles due to congenital anomalies or trauma.

The magnetic anal sphincter is a novel device consisting of a ring of titanium beads with internal magnetic cores. It is surgically placed around the EAS to close the anus, and during defecation the beads separate to open the anus for passage of stool. This new device is currently undergoing clinical trials and its role in faecal incontinence treatment remains undetermined.

Neuromodulation

Sacral nerve stimulation

This procedure (Figure 64.3) involves the placement of a thin electrode wire into the sacral foramen to stimulate the sacral nerve, optimally the S3 nerve roots, by an implanted nerve stimulator generator. The nerve stimulation results in contraction of the anal sphincter and pelvic floor musculature to maintain continence.

The exact mechanism of action remains unclear, but it is thought to involve neuromodulation of the sacral reflexes and parasympathetic nerves to alter rectal compliance, rectal sensitivity and anal canal resting tone. Recent brain MRI studies also implicate higher centre involvement in this neuromodulation process.

A unique and attractive feature of sacral nerve stimulation is that it is a reversible and minimally invasive procedure. There are two stages to the operation: the first is the testing phase and the second, the implantation of the permanent nerve

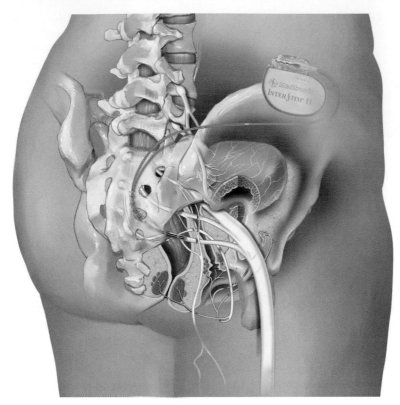

Fig. 64.3 Implantation of sacral nerve stimulation equipment consisting of a battery (IPG) and tined lead inserted into S3 foramen alongside the S3 nerve root. Source: reproduced with permission of Medtronic plc.

stimulator, is performed if the patient achieves over 50% reduction in incontinence episodes.

The first stage procedure involves the insertion of a tined lead or a temporary wire electrode into the S3 foramen to lie alongside the S3 nerve root. The electrode is then connected to an external nerve stimulator for a trial stimulation of 2 weeks. If the patient experiences a greater than 50% reduction in incontinence episodes, this is considered to be successful and the patient can proceed to the second stage. If the response is less than 50% improvement in continence, then the electrode is simply removed. The second stage involves insertion of a tined lead electrode and implantation of a permanent pulse generator (like a pacemaker) in the subcutaneous pocket in the upper buttock region. Both procedures can be performed under intravenous sedation and local anaesthetic infiltration using X-ray guidance, as day cases.

Some adverse effects of sacral nerve stimulation include infection in approximately 5% of cases and perineal pain from chronic stimulation. Longer-term effects on the nerve are unknown. Additionally, some older pulse generators may not be compatible with MRI scanners and hence patients will not be able to be investigated by MRI.

A prospective non-randomised multicentre study conducted in 14 centres across the USA, Canada and Australia reported a greater than 50% improvement in 89% of patients and complete continence in 36% at 5-year follow-up. However, a Cochrane review in 2015 of six trials assessing the effectiveness of sacral nerve stimulation concluded that the technique can improve continence in a proportion of people but longer-term efficacy data are still lacking.

Because of its reversibility, minimal invasiveness and efficacy, sacral nerve stimulation has now emerged as the treatment of choice for faecal incontinence in suitable patients. However, the high cost precludes it from wider use.

Posterior tibial nerve stimulation

This therapy involves stimulation of the posterior tibial nerve at the ankle, either percutaneously via a fine needle or transcutaneously for 30 minutes at a time for 12 treatment sessions. The rationale is that this produces retrograde stimulation of the S3 nerve roots. The results are conflicting, with some studies showing some improvement in patients with mild faecal incontinence, but long-term sustained improvement has not been confirmed in large studies.

Radiofrequency (SECCA) therapy

This therapy uses radiofrequency energy to create thermal burns in the anal canal, causing fibrosis within the internal sphincter muscle and thereby tightening the anal canal to maintain continence. The radiofrequency energy is delivered via a special endoanal probe inserted into the anal canal under sedation and local anaesthetic. There are limited long-term data on its efficacy and hence its use is limited to a few major centres.

Stoma formation

The formation of a diverting stoma, either a colostomy or ileostomy, is an effective treatment of faecal incontinence. The faecal stream is diverted from the anus to the anterior abdominal wall where a small opening is created for the colon or ileum to exit as a conduit (stoma). The faecal content is collected in a sealed plastic bag, which is disposed of in a controlled manner.

This surgical option is considered the last resort in the management of faecal incontinence and may not be acceptable to some patients who have a physical and psychological aversion to wearing a stoma bag. Furthermore, intestinal stomas are not without complications, such as leakage around the appliance, parastomal hernia, prolapse of the stoma, the odour and uncontrolled flatus. It is therefore important to counsel patients carefully and manage their expectations appropriately to ensure a satisfactory outcome.

Prevention

The old adage 'prevention is better than cure' certainly rings true in the management of faecal incontinence. Patients can reduce their risks of developing faecal incontinence by maintaining a regular bowel habit, avoiding constipation and straining at stools, avoiding injury to the rectum by foreign bodies, and practising pelvic floor exercises especially postpartum.

In obstetric practice, posterior midline episiotomy should be avoided and the posterolateral approach used, a prolonged second stage circumvented, and caesarean section considered for large babies or at-risk anal sphincters.

In general surgery, the practice of Lord's procedure has been abandoned as it involves forceful anal dilatation for anal fissure or constipation, causing internal sphincter injury and incontinence. Surgeons should be aware of the principle of sphincter identification and preservation when performing anorectal operations such as haemorrhoidectomy, sphincterotomy and fistulotomy.

Summary

Faecal incontinence is an embarrassing and debilitating symptom caused by a multitude of aetiological factors affecting the anal sphincter muscle complex, the pelvic floor musculature, pudendal nerve, rectal capacity and compliance, stool consistency, spine and central nervous system. Treatments are directed at the underlying structural or functional abnormalities and are tailored to individual needs.

Conservative therapies include dietary modification, medications, pelvic floor training and biofeedback therapy. Surgical interventions, which attempt to restore anal sphincter anatomy and function, include anal sphincter repair, post-anal repair, sphincter augmentation, artificial bowel sphincter, injection therapies, sacral nerve stimulation, posterior tibial nerve stimulation and Secca therapy. Treatment outcomes in terms of reduction in incontinence and improvement in quality of life are highly variable between techniques and less than optimal.

Sacral nerve stimulation has emerged as the least invasive and most effective treatment for faecal incontinence. However, a recent systematic review of surgical treatments for faecal incontinence concluded that high-quality evidence is still lacking to assist proper clinical decision-making and more rigorous randomised studies are required.

It can be concluded that there is currently no single cure for faecal incontinence and that this debilitating condition should be managed as a chronic disease by a combination of conservative, supportive and surgical measures through a multidisciplinary team.

Further reading

Benezech A, Bouvie M, Vitton V. Faecal incontinence: current knowledge and perspectives. *World J Gastrointest Pathophysiol* 2016;7:59–71.

Brown SR, Wadhawan H, Nelson RL. Surgery for faecal incontinence in adults. *Cochrane Database Syst Rev* 2010;(9):CD001757.

Lehur PA, Wong MTC. Incontinence. In: Phillips RK, Clark S (eds) *Colorectal Surgery*, 5th edn. Elsevier, 2014.

Norton C, Whitehead WE, Bliss DZ, Harari D, Lang J. Conservative and pharmacological management of faecal incontinence in adults. International Continence Society. Available at https://www.ics.org/Publications/ICI_4/files-book/comite-16.pdf

Paquette IM, Varma MG, Kaiser AM, Steele SR, Rafferty JF. The American Society of Colon and Rectal Surgeons' Clinical Practice Guideline for the Treatment of Fecal Incontinence. *Dis Colon Rectum* 2015;58:623–36.

MCQs

Select the single or multiple correct answers to each question. The correct answers can be found in the Answers section at the end of the book.

1 Normal faecal continence is maintained by
  a intact anal sphincters
  b normal rectal reservoir and compliance
  c functioning pudendal nerve
  d normal stool consistency
  e all the above

2 Which of the following causes of anal sphincter injury is *incorrect*?
  a childbirth injury from prolonged labour, episiotomy and use of forceps to deliver the baby
  b anorectal surgery such as haemorrhoidectomy, sphincterotomy or fistulotomy
  c chronic constipation and excessive straining at defecation
  d impalement trauma to the anus
  e type 1 diabetes mellitus

3 Which of the following statements about the pudendal nerve is *incorrect*?
  a it arises from S2–S4 nerve roots of the sacral plexus
  b it arises from L4–L5 nerve roots
  c it carries sensory nerve supply to the perineal structures
  d it carries motor nerve supply to the perineum
  e it becomes stretched during prolonged childbirth and may cause faecal incontinence in later life

4 Which of the following treatments for faecal incontinence is *incorrect*?
  a biofeedback therapy
  b sacral nerve stimulation
  c injection of anal sphincter bulking agent
  d loperamide tablet
  e subtotal colectomy

65 Rectal bleeding

Adele Burgess

University of Melbourne and Austin Health, Melbourne, Victoria, Australia

Chronic rectal bleeding

Rectal bleeding can be alarming for patients, although most causes are benign. Bleeding may be overt and noticed by the patient or occult when the blood loss can only be detected by a faecal occult blood test or its consequences noted on blood tests as iron deficiency or anaemia. Management of rectal bleeding involves exclusion of a colorectal neoplasm and finding the cause of the bleeding.

The classification and common causes of chronic rectal bleeding are given in Table 65.1.

History

A detailed history should be taken. The nature of the rectal bleeding must be determined (duration, colour and amount of blood). Macroscopic bleeding recognised by the patient usually arises from the left side of the colon or rectum. Right-sided colonic bleeding usually presents with anaemia or iron deficiency but without overt bleeding. The presence of anal pain should be inquired about. This occurs with anal fissure, strangulated haemorrhoids and some anorectal cancers. Prolapse occurs with second- and third-degree haemorrhoids and with mucosal or full-thickness rectal prolapse. Other symptoms that may be seen are mixture of blood with stool, tenesmus, alteration in bowel habit, abdominal pain or distension and weight loss.

A past and family history of colorectal neoplasm must be gained from the patient, as well as a past history of colonic diseases such as inflammatory bowel disease.

Anorectal examination

Anorectal examination is essential in any patient presenting with rectal bleeding. This should be undertaken on every patient after gaining consent and offering (or having) a chaperone. Inspection should determine the presence of anal fissure, prolapsed haemorrhoids and most anal canal cancers. During straining, look for prolapsing haemorrhoids or rectal prolapse. Digital examination is used to feel for an anal or rectal polyp or cancer. This may not be possible in the presence of an acute anal fissure because of anal sphincter spasm and pain.

Proctoscopy can be used to visualise any anal canal lesion and haemorrhoids. On rigid sigmoidoscopy the level of the rectum visualised should be recorded together with the level of any abnormality seen. The presence of blood clots or blood-stained faeces beyond the reach of the sigmoidoscope indicate a more proximal pathological process. Fibre-optic flexible sigmoidoscopy allows for an easier examination of the rectum and a variable length of the sigmoid and descending colon. In many specialist colorectal practices, this has replaced rigid sigmoidoscopy.

Special investigations

Colonoscopy is the test of choice in the majority of patients. Colonoscopy allows examination of the large bowel and the distal part of the small bowel and provides both a visual diagnosis (e.g. ulceration, polyps) and therapeutic opportunity. Small polyps can be removed, angiodysplasia can be controlled with argon plasma coagulation or cautery, and it grants the opportunity for biopsy and tattoo marking of suspected colorectal cancer lesions.

Virtual colonoscopy, which uses two- and three-dimensional imagery reconstructed from CT scans (or less commonly MRI), is also possible. This is not standard, however, because it does not allow for therapeutic manoeuvres nor visualisation of lesions smaller than 5 mm. It also does not negate the need for bowel preparation. It is usually reserved for patients in whom a colonoscopy was unable to be completed or for those unable to have sedation.

Textbook of Surgery, Fourth Edition. Edited by Julian A. Smith, Andrew H. Kaye, Christopher Christophi and Wendy A. Brown.
© 2020 John Wiley & Sons Ltd. Published 2020 by John Wiley & Sons Ltd.

Table 65.1 Classification and common causes of chronic rectal bleeding.

Classification	Common causes
Anal outlet bleeding	
Bright blood per rectum, separate from the stool and often present as a smear of bright blood on the toilet paper	Haemorrhoids, anal fissure, rectal prolapse, angiodysplasia, malignancy
Bleeding associated with defecation	
No change in bowel habits	
No past or family history of colorectal neoplasm	
Suspicious bleeding	
Dark blood or blood mixed with stool	Diverticular disease, inflammatory bowel disease, proctitis, anorectal cancer, colorectal neoplasm
Change in bowel habit or passage of mucus	
Tenesmus	
Past or family history of colorectal neoplasm	

Box 65.1 Causes of massive rectal bleeding

- Diverticular disease
- Angiodysplasia/angioma
- Ulcerated cancer
- Rare colonic causes (e.g. radiation colitis, inflammatory bowel disease, ischaemic colitis)
- Upper gastrointestinal lesions

Capsule endoscopy is an investigation to identify a bleeding source in the small bowel.

Massive rectal bleeding

The management of massive rectal bleeding involves:
- resuscitation and clinical evaluation
- investigations to locate bleeding site
- therapeutic intervention.

Resuscitation and initial assessment

Resuscitation should be immediately initiated with massive rectal bleeding while diagnostic tests are performed.

Clinical evaluation

A detailed history is important. The nature and amount of bleeding give an indication of the cause of the bleeding (Box 65.1). Massive colonic haemorrhage is dark red or plum coloured and is to be differentiated from melaena, which is black. Melaena almost invariably arises from the stomach or small bowel. A rapidly bleeding peptic ulcer may occasionally present with bright red rectal bleeding. The haemodynamic condition of the patient will also reflect the severity of bleeding. Massive bleeding indicates bleeding of more than 1500 mL

in 24 hours. In these circumstances, the patient has signs of shock on admission that demand urgent management with transfusion. Massive rectal bleeding will cease spontaneously in 80% of cases.

A prior history of a bowel disorder such as inflammatory bowel disease or haemorrhoids is ascertained. Use of anticoagulant therapy or nonsteroidal anti-inflammatory drugs may contribute to bleeding. Liver disorders with impaired coagulation are also noted. A rectal examination with rigid proctosigmoidoscopy is performed to exclude bleeding haemorrhoids or rectal tumours.

Localisation of the bleeding site and therapeutic intervention

Upper gastrointestinal endoscopy

In cases of severe rectal bleeding with shock, upper gastrointestinal endoscopy should be performed as soon as clinically feasible to exclude an upper gastrointestinal lesion, such as a bleeding peptic ulcer, oesophageal varices or aorto-enteric fistula. Alternatively, a nasogastric tube is passed to exclude blood in the stomach.

Colonoscopy

Colonoscopy has been the first-line investigation for colonic bleeding. Emergency colonoscopy is difficult with active bleeding and requires a great deal of experience. Colonoscopy is performed as soon as feasible once the patient has been resuscitated. There is debate around the use of full bowel preparation and colonic blood often works as a cathartic. Colonoscopy is the first-line choice of investigation and management in post-interventional bleeding. Once the bleeding site has been identified, treatment may include coagulation and injection with vasoconstrictors or sclerosing agents or the use of metal clips.

CT angiography

CT angiography is available in most hospitals and has the advantage of being non-invasive, readily available and requires no bowel preparation. In many centres this has now become the first line of investigation after resuscitation. A recent meta-analysis of 672 patients reported sensitivity and specificity rates of 85.2% and 92.1%, respectively.

Capsule endoscopy

This involves the patient swallowing a small videocapsule (PillCam) which will capture digitised images of the small bowel. The duration of test is limited by the battery life of the videocapsule (8 hours). This is best done in a patient who is haemodynamically stable and who has had recurrent gastrointestinal bleeding of unknown origin despite being previously investigated with upper gastrointestinal endoscopy, colonoscopy and CT angiography.

Radionuclide scan

If bleeding continues and the site of haemorrhage is not located by colonoscopy, a radionuclide scan is done using technetium-99m sulphur colloid or technetium-99m-labelled autologous red cells. One advantage of this examination is its ability to detect bleeding rates as low as 0.05–0.1 mL. The accuracy of these scans is variable, ranging from 40 to 90%.

Mesenteric angiogram

Selective angiogram of the inferior mesenteric, superior mesenteric and coeliac arteries is performed if bleeding continues and the rate is greater than 0.5 mL/min. Angiography is likely to be positive if there is active bleeding at the time of injection of contrast. If the site of bleeding is identified, haemostasis with super-selective intra-arterial embolisation can be considered.

Surgery

If bleeding continues, laparoscopy or laparotomy is performed. If the site of bleeding is not clearly localised preoperatively or intraoperatively, intraoperative endoscopy can be performed. The bowel is transilluminated during intraoperative enteroscopy in a darkened room to detect angiodysplasias or small bowel angiomas. In rare circumstances if the site of bleeding remains unclear, a subtotal abdominal colectomy is performed.

Review

If the diagnosis is unresolved despite a full investigation, the patient is observed. If bleeding recurs, a full investigation is repeated as in a new case of active bleeding. Laparotomy and intraoperative enteroscopy may be necessary if these rebleeding episodes are moderately severe.

Further reading

García-Blázquez V, Vicente-Bártulos A, Olavarria-Delgado A, Plana MN, van der Winden D, Zamora J. Accuracy of CT angiography in the diagnosis of acute gastrointestinal bleeding: systematic review and meta-analysis. *Eur Radiol* 2013;23:1181–90.

Hewitson P, Glasziou PP, Irwig L, Towler B, Watson E. Screening for colorectal cancer using the faecal occult blood test, Hemoccult. *Cochrane Database Syst Rev* 2007;(1):CD001216.

Hongsakul K, Pakdeejit S, Tanutit P. Outcome and predictive factors of successful transarterial embolization for the treatment of acute gastrointestinal hemorrhage. *Acta Radiol* 2014;55:186–94.

MCQs

Select the single correct answer to each question. The correct answers can be found in the Answers section at the end of the book.

1 Most patients presenting with massive rectal bleeding:
   a will bleed to death unless they have surgery
   b usually are found to have colon cancer
   c usually are found to have rectal cancer
   d should be appropriately resuscitated
   e should have an immediate colonoscopy

2 A patient with chronic rectal bleeding:
   a usually will be found to have a cancer
   b should always have an anorectal examination
   c will have a history of inflammatory bowel disease
   d needs virtual CT as first-line examination
   e requires immediate blood transfusion

66 Haematemesis and melaena

Wendy A. Brown

Monash University Department of Surgery, Alfred Health, Melbourne, Victoria, Australia

Introduction

Definition

Haematemesis is the vomiting of blood, either bright or altered blood (so-called 'coffee grounds' vomitus) due to the action of acid on the blood. Melaena is the passage of black tarry stools. The tarriness is characteristic and distinguishes melaena from the passage of black stools due to dietary agents, including the ingestion of iron. Haematemesis occurs from a point that is usually not distal to the duodenum but melaena may occur not only from a proximal bleeding site but rarely from a small intestinal cause.

Incidence

Haematemesis and melaena is a common and important symptom complex presenting either as an acute catastrophic illness or more electively with prolonged minor bleeding. Patients with this condition make major demands on hospital beds.

Significance

Patients with haematemesis and melaena require admission to hospital. The condition has a high mortality and demands a systematic approach to the initial resuscitation process, the diagnostic method and the therapeutic program. The overall management of this condition has been revolutionised by the introduction of new endoscopic techniques to control bleeding.

Causes of haematemesis

Swallowed blood from, for example, a bleeding site in the post-nasal space must be excluded as a cause for haematemesis.

The list of causes of haematemesis and melaena is long (Box 66.1). The common causes are:
- peptic ulcer (i.e. gastric or duodenal ulceration)
- oesophageal varices
- gastritis or duodenitis.

The site of bleeding usually lies in the oesophagus, stomach or duodenum.

Oesophagus

The most common cause of bleeding in the oesophagus is from oesophageal varices secondary to portal hypertension. Oesophageal varices are the cause of some 10–30% of major haematemesis episodes in most western countries. Less commonly, oesophagitis secondary to gastro-oesophageal reflux is associated with haemorrhage. Oesophageal cancer rarely presents with bleeding.

Stomach

Gastric ulcer is one of the most common causes of haematemesis and melaena. The ulcer may be in the

---

Box 66.1 Common causes of haematemesis and melaena

Oesophageal
Reflux oesophagitis: other associated hiatus hernia
Oesophageal varices (portal hypertension)
Oesophageal tumours
Mallory–Weiss mucosal tear

Gastric
Gastric ulcer, usually benign
Haemorrhagic gastritis
Gastric varices
Gastric cancer
Delafoy lesion

Duodenum
Duodenal ulcer
Duodenitis

Textbook of Surgery, Fourth Edition. Edited by Julian A. Smith, Andrew H. Kaye, Christopher Christophi and Wendy A. Brown.
© 2020 John Wiley & Sons Ltd. Published 2020 by John Wiley & Sons Ltd.

body or the antrum of the stomach. The pre-pyloric position is the most common. Gastric ulcer may be the site of torrential haemorrhage because of the invasion of a major vessel (e.g. the splenic artery). Gastritis is also a common cause of gastric bleeding.

The common use of non-steroidal anti-flamma-tory drugs (NSAIDs) is associated with haematemesis and melaena due to gastric ulceration in many elderly patients. Despite the use of cyclooxygenase (COX)-2 inhibitor antiarthritic agents, ulceration can still occur, particularly when these drugs are prescribed in conjunction with aspirin. A Mallory–Weiss tear is a laceration of the gastro-oesophageal junction as a result of retching, with differential intra-abdominal and thoracic pressures leading to the tear. Characteristically the haematemesis appears after initial blood-free vomit.

Gastric varices may be associated with portal hypertension and coexist with oesophageal varices. Gastric cancer is not a common cause of haematemesis and melaena but a gastric ulcer may bleed and prove to be malignant on biopsy.

Duodenum

Duodenal ulcer is traditionally the most common cause of haematemesis and melaena. The ulcer is usually on the posterior wall of the duodenum and characteristically invades the gastroduodenal artery. Haemorrhage may be profuse but is usually self-limited.

In western societies the number of patients presenting with duodenal ulcers is decreasing. However, there is an increasing number of patients presenting with gastric ulceration, particularly elderly patients on NSAIDs.

Management

Initial assessment

In most hospitals, patients with haematemesis and melaena are managed in a special unit and employ-ing a clinical pathway or algorithm to systematise management (Figure 66.1).

The circulatory state of the patient is assessed. The extent of blood loss can be estimated on the basis of the patient's clinical status. Apprehension, air hunger, cerebral changes, marked pallor, thready pulse and hypotension indicate significant blood loss (up to 50% of blood volume). Maintenance of normal peripheral circulation without cerebral

findings but with mild tachycardia and postural drop in blood pressure is consistent with 10–20% blood volume loss. This estimation of circulatory status gives an indication of the urgency of fluid replacement.

The cause of bleeding must then be diagnosed. This is often not obvious. However, the presence of a previous history of peptic ulceration or evidence of hepatic cirrhosis may indicate a likely site of blood loss.

Management of the patient

Optimal management of the patient with haematemesis and melaena involves vigorous resuscitation and early diagnosis.

Resuscitation

Intravenous therapy is started with normal saline and/or colloid (Haemaccel or 5% albumin solution). Blood is then taken for cross-matching. Depending on the clinical state of the patient, urgent cross-match can be performed and blood given immediately. Rarely, O negative blood is required for a patient *in extremis*.

Monitoring is essential to estimate the effectiveness of blood replacement. Successful resuscitation can be observed by noting improvement in the clinical state of the patient, return of blood pressure and pulse rate towards normal, and the presence of a satisfactory urine output.

Diagnosis

Early endoscopy has been shown to be a safe and effective way of making a diagnosis. Once the patient's clinical condition is stabilised, this procedure is carried out either urgently if there is concern about continuing bleeding, or on the next elective endoscopy list if there is no indication for urgent intervention.

The patient is sedated with intravenous medication and the gastroscope is passed. The oesophagus, stomach and duodenum are carefully examined. There may be some difficulty in this examination process with the presence of old blood, blood clot or fresh bleeding. Adequate suction and irrigation are required in order to define the bleeding point. Rarely the bleeding point is not identifiable. Throughout this procedure the patient requires adequate monitoring, and the airway must be controlled and oxygen administered.

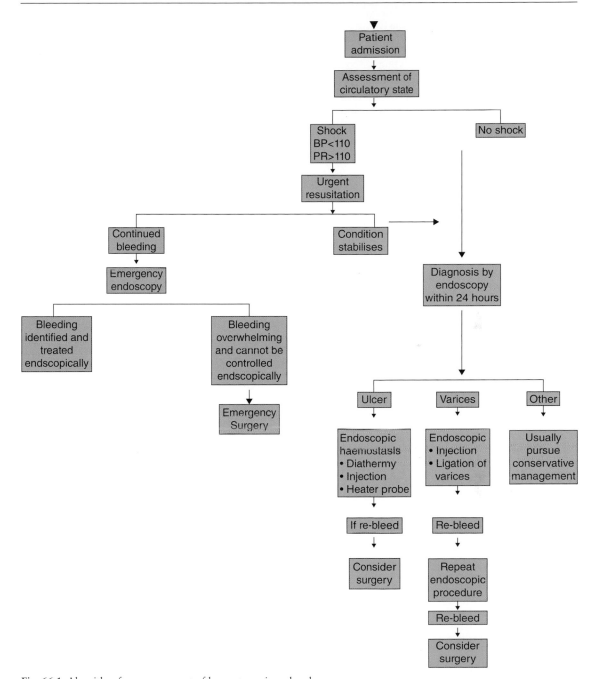

Fig. 66.1 Algorithm for management of haematemesis and melaena.

Therapy

Usually a therapeutic procedure can be carried out at the time of endoscopy. Injection of alcohol or adrenaline close to the bleeding point will usually result in cessation of bleeding. If oesophageal varices are present, these may be injected or banded.

If it is evident that a major problem exists, such as a large gastric ulcer or persistent bleeding from a large duodenal ulcer, or bleeding from oesophageal varices, then immediate consultation with the surgical team is mandatory and combined management is implemented.

There is an increasing role for radiological intervention. Angiogram and embolisation of bleeding vessels may be useful, especially if the patient is too frail for surgical intervention. Transjugular intrahepatic portosystemic shunt (TIPS) may be used to reduce portal pressures and improve bleeding from varices.

Indications for surgical intervention

The indications for surgical intervention include massive haemorrhage not responding to conservative means, patients requiring more than 6 units of blood, and elderly patients, particularly if a large ulcer is present, because they tolerate blood loss poorly.

Where a second haemorrhage occurs in hospital or there is concern about persistent ongoing bleeding, surgery is necessary.

Results of treatment

Most bleeding sites causing haematemesis and melaena stop bleeding spontaneously or with interventional endoscopy. The modern medical management of peptic ulcers, including the eradication of *Helicobacter pylori*, is so effective that surgery is to be avoided unless absolutely indicated to save life.

The results of treatment of bleeding from varices due to portal hypertension will depend on the degree of liver disease and the extent of the varices. These patients usually require an intensive care unit program of therapy. In the short term, injection or banding of varices is usually effective in stopping the bleeding. If bleeding persists, then the use of a Sengstaken–Blakemore tube or Linton balloon to apply direct pressure to the cardia will usually result in tamponade of the bleeding point and control the haemorrhage. Occasionally emergency surgery is required, with some form of direct ligation of varices or gastric disconnection in order to control bleeding. Direct ligation of varices involves opening the stomach or oesophagus and directly suturing the varices. A gastric disconnection procedure involves devascularising the stomach completely in order to interrupt the venous channels supplying the varices.

Prognosis

The prognosis from this condition will depend on the underlying cause and the clinical state of the patient. Overall, patients with haematemesis and melaena have a high mortality and morbidity rate, varying from 5 to 20% in most series. This is because most patients with haematemesis and melaena are elderly, often with cardiac and pulmonary disease. These patients tolerate surgery poorly. Thus, the balance between surgical intervention and persisting with medical management in the face of continuing haemorrhage is often very fine and the best results are obtained in dedicated units for the management of this condition.

Further reading

Fujishiro M, Iguchi M, Kakushima N *et al*. Guidelines for endoscopic management of non-variceal upper gastrointestinal bleeding. *Dig Endosc* 2016;28:363–78.

Samuel R, Bilal M, Tayyem O, Guturu P. Evaluation and management of non-variceal upper gastrointestinal bleeding. *Dis Mon* 2018;64:333–43.

Shah AR, Jala V, Arshad H, Bilal M. Evaluation and management of lower gastrointestinal bleeding. *Dis Mon* 2018;64:321–32.

Storace M, Martin JG, Shah J, Bercu Z. CTA as an adjuvant tool for acute intra-abdominal or gastrointestinal bleeding. *Tech Vasc Interv Radiol* 2017;20:248–57.

Tayyem O, Bilal M, Samuel R, Merwat SK. Evaluation and management of variceal bleeding. *Dis Mon* 2018;64:312–20.

MCQs

Select the single correct answer to each question. The correct answers can be found in the Answers section at the end of the book.

1 Which of the following statements about the passage of black tarry stools is *incorrect*?
   a is usually an indication of bleeding from the upper gastrointestinal tract
   b can be mimicked by the ingestion of iron medication
   c is commonly a symptom of a cancer of the colon
   d can be present without other symptoms
   e is often but not universally associated with haematemesis

2 Which of the following causes of haematemesis and melaena is *incorrect*?
   a oesophageal varices
   b gastric ulceration
   c epistaxis with swallowed blood
   d beetroot ingestion
   e gastritis

3 Which of the following statements about the patient who has suffered a gastrointestinal bleed is *incorrect*?
   a pale and sweaty
   b faint and has a bradycardia
   c faint and has a tachycardia
   d requires urgent resuscitation with normal saline initially
   e appears quite well with normal supine blood pressure

4 Which of the following statements about diagnosis of the cause of the bleeding episode is *incorrect*?
a is the most urgent requirement in patient management
b may be suspected from a history of NSAID intake
c can be made by early endoscopy of upper gastrointestinal tract
d can often be combined with treatment at the initial endoscopy
e surgical intervention is required for ongoing blood loss

5 Which of the following statements about haematemesis and melaena is *incorrect*?
a is a serious condition with a high mortality and morbidity rate
b now occurs in an older age group of patients
c has been eliminated with the advent of COX-2 inhibitor anti-inflammatory drugs
d when associated with oesophageal varices may require repeated interventions for control
e is best managed in a dedicated specialist treatment unit

67 Obstructive jaundice

Frederick Huynh[1] and Val Usatoff[2]

[1] Alfred Health, Melbourne, Victoria, Australia
[2] University of Melbourne and Western Health, Melbourne, Victoria, Australia

Introduction

Jaundice is a common medical presentation and can be broadly classified into:

- prehepatic
- hepatic
- posthepatic (obstructive) jaundice.

Common causes for each category are outlined in Box 67.1. This chapter addresses the assessment and management of obstructive jaundice (Figure 67.1).

History and examination

The first step to evaluating a patient with jaundice is a detailed history and physical examination. One of the key objectives is to differentiate between benign and malignant causes of obstructive jaundice.

It should be assessed whether the jaundice is associated with pain and, if present, an impression of its onset, character and pattern of radiation should be elicited. Enquiries about associated symptoms such as nausea, pale stools and dark urine should be made. Significant unintended weight loss may be associated with an underlying malignancy. Cholangitis should be highly suspected in the setting of jaundice, right upper quadrant pain and fever (Charcot's triad), and expedient investigations, treatment and decompression of the biliary tree is required.

The patient should also be assessed for risk factors associated with hepatitis, including a history of intravenous drug use, medication history and family history. The frequency and amount of alcohol intake should be evaluated. A thorough surgical history should also be obtained, as jaundice in a patient having undergone a previous cholecystectomy may represent a late presentation of a biliary injury, while prior endoscopic retrograde cholangiopancreatography (ERCP) may be due to a recurrence of the original pathology, or a stricture/stenosis secondary to the sphincterotomy. Choledocholithiasis is also less likely in a patient with an absent gallbladder.

On examination, once the bilirubin is more than double the normal level, icterus should be evident in the sclera. Skin scratch marks in response to pruritus should be noted, as should signs of chronic liver disease, such as petechiae/ecchymoses, spider naevi and gynaecomastia. The patient's general nutritional status is gauged, as cachexia may represent an advanced cancer. Abdominal examination consists of palpating for any abdominal masses and

---

Box 67.1 Causes of jaundice

Prehepatic
Increased haemolysis
Hereditary red blood cell disorders
Acquired haemolytic disorders
Autoimmune haemolytic anaemia

Hepatic/hepatocellular
Congenital abnormalities of metabolism (e.g. Gilbert's disease, Crigler–Najjar syndrome)
Medications
Viral hepatitis
Alcoholic hepatitis
Non-alcoholic steatohepatitis
Chronic liver disease/cirrhosis

Posthepatic (obstructive)
Choledocholithiasis
Primary sclerosing cholangitis
Traumatic biliary strictures
Autoimmune pancreatitis
Malignancy (cholangiocarcinoma, pancreatic carcinoma, periampullary tumours)

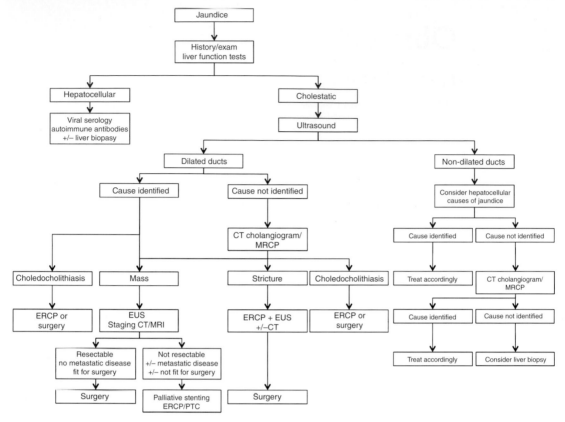

Fig. 67.1 Diagnostic and therapeutic approach to a patient with jaundice. CT, computed tomography; ERCP, endoscopic retrograde cholangiopancreatography; EUS, endoscopic ultrasound; MRCP, magnetic resonance cholangiopancreatography; MRI, magnetic resonance imaging; PTC, percutaneous transhepatic cholangiography.

evaluating the size of the liver. The presence of ascites is assessed, as is any lymphadenopathy.

Courvoisier's law states that in the presence of a palpable non-tender gallbladder accompanied by painless jaundice, the cause is unlikely to be gallstones and suggests a malignant process.

Investigations

Liver function tests

The pattern of abnormal liver function tests should be noted. Significant elevations of alanine aminotransferase (ALT) and aspartate aminotransferase (AST) are in keeping with hepatocellular injury, while derangements of alkaline phosphatase (ALP) and gamma-glutamyltranspeptidase (γ-GT), which are enzymes primarily produced by the epithelial cells of the biliary tract, are more consistent with biliary obstruction. It should be remembered that ALP levels can also be elevated in bone diseases such as Paget's disease or certain types of bony metastases, while abnormal γ-GT levels may represent excess alcohol intake. Coagulation studies

should also be performed and if there is evidence of coagulopathy secondary to hepatic impairment, this should be corrected with vitamin K.

Conjugated and unconjugated bilirubin levels may differentiate between prehepatic and hepatic causes of jaundice and also diagnose genetic abnormalities related to bilirubin metabolism (e.g. Gilbert's disease).

If liver function tests suggest a hepatocellular process, then viral hepatitis serology, autoimmune antibodies and a metabolic screen should be performed (iron studies for haemochromatosis, serum caeruloplasmin for Wilson's disease, and α_1-antitrypsin levels for α_1-antitrypsin deficiency). A liver biopsy may be required for confirmation.

Ultrasonography and computed tomography

Ultrasound is a routine and readily available initial investigation to evaluate the liver and biliary tree. Particular note should be made of the calibre of the biliary tree with any associated intrahepatic ductal dilatation, and the presence or absence of gallstones. A common bile duct diameter in excess of 5 mm is considered abnormal, although this figure rises with increasing age and in patients who have previously undergone a cholecystectomy.

Ultrasonography may also demonstrate an obstructive mass either within the head of the pancreas or along the biliary tree. If ultrasound or cholangiography demonstrates a mass, then the next step is computed tomography (CT) to further evaluate the lesion and to determine if it is potentially surgically resectable. Imaging including arterial and venous phases is needed. These scans are often performed in conjunction with ERCP/endoscopic ultrasound (EUS) to manage and determine the nature of the obstruction.

Cholangiography

Significant advances have been made in the past decade that has allowed non-invasive techniques to specifically evaluate the biliary tree. CT cholangiography relies on hepatobiliary excreted contrast agent (e.g. Biliscopin™), while magnetic resonance cholangiopancreatography (MRCP) utilises the fluid within the biliary system as a contrast agent by acquiring heavily T2-weighted images (Figure 67.2). As CT cholangiography depends on adequate hepatobiliary excretion of a contrast agent, it should generally not be used in cases where the bilirubin is above 30 mmol/L.

Intraoperative cholangiography is often performed by direct cannulation of the cystic duct at the time of cholecystectomy (Figure 67.3). If choledocholithiasis is identified during intraoperative cholangiography, this is managed by either an intraoperative bile duct exploration (transcystic or via choledochotomy) or by postoperative ERCP.

Endoscopic ultrasound and endoscopic retrograde cholangiopancreatography

EUS is an important adjunct in the investigation of obstructive jaundice. It is particularly sensitive for evaluating very small tumours and also allows sampling of any masses by fine-needle aspirate. The procedure may provide the diagnosis of autoimmune pancreatitis, a rare but important cause of obstructive jaundice that is managed with steroids rather than surgery.

ERCP is an endoscopic procedure that is both diagnostic and therapeutic, the main risks being bleeding, perforation and pancreatitis. If the cause of the obstructive jaundice is due to choledocholithiasis, the calculi can often be extracted by ERCP, usually in conjunction with a sphincterotomy of the

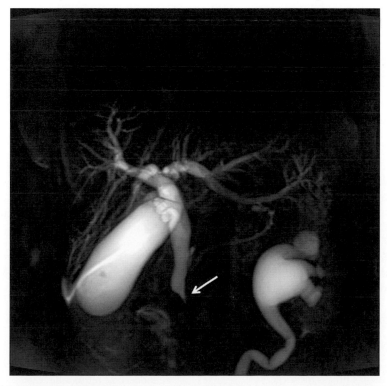

Fig. 67.2 MRCP demonstrating a dilated biliary system and gallbladder due to a common bile duct stricture (arrow) caused by adenocarcinoma at the head of pancreas.

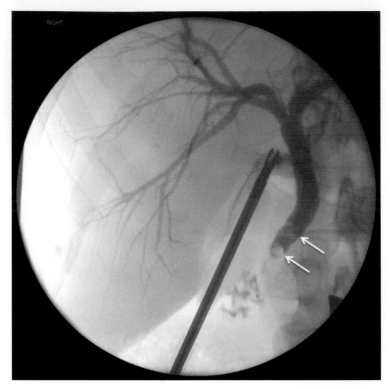

Fig. 67.3 Intraoperative cholangiogram demonstrating choledocholithiasis visualised as filling defects in the common bile duct (arrows).

ampulla of Vater. Following this, the patient is treated by a cholecystectomy, provided that the individual is fit for operation. If ERCP demonstrates a benign stricture, this is dilated or stented to improve the patient's clinical condition and then a decision should be made as to whether repeated dilatations should be performed or whether a surgical bypass/resection should be undertaken.

Malignant causes of obstructive jaundice may occur anywhere along the biliary tree, and include cholangiocarcinoma (intrahepatic, hilar or extrahepatic), pancreatic carcinoma and periampullary tumours. Distal biliary tumours are more likely to be amenable to stenting by ERCP, while more proximal tumours may require percutaneous transhepatic cholangiography (PTC). This transhepatic approach may also be required if the ampulla cannot be accessed by ERCP due to technical difficulties (previous gastrectomy, duodenal diverticulum). Stenting can be performed with plastic (temporary) stents or with metal stents, which are far more difficult to remove but have less problems with early occlusion. Once the tumour is stented, an assessment must be made about the resectability of the tumour (based on its anatomical features), the presence or absence of metastatic disease and the patient's fitness for surgery.

If the tumour is unresectable, a surgical bypass may provide better palliation, provided the patient

is expected to live beyond 6 months. This is because stents tend to occlude within 6 months, with the resultant septic episodes secondary to cholangitis having a significant impact on the patient's chemotherapy treatment and quality of life.

Further reading

Addley J, Mitchell RM. Advances in the investigation of obstructive jaundice. *Curr Gastroenterol Rep* 2012;14:511–19.

Kinney T. Evidence-based imaging of pancreatic malignancies. *Surg Clin North Am* 2010;90:235–49.

Tazuma S, Unno M, Igarashi Y *et al*. Evidence-based clinical practice guidelines for cholelithiasis 2016. *J Gastroenterol* 2017;52:276–300.

MCQs

Select the single correct answer to each question. The correct answers can be found in the Answers section at the end of the book.

1 Which of the following investigations does *not* require injection of contrast?
  a endoscopic retrograde cholangiopancreatography
  b magnetic resonance cholangiopancreatography

c computed tomography cholangiography

d percutaneous transhepatic cholangiography

e intraoperative cholangiography

2 A malignant cause for obstructive jaundice includes:

a primary sclerosing cholangitis

b autoimmune pancreatitis

c choledocholithiasis

d post-sphincterotomy stricture

e cholangiocarcinoma

3 Which of the following is *not* a component of Charcot's triad?

a palpable gallbladder

b right upper quadrant pain

c fever

d jaundice

68 The acute abdomen, peritonitis and intra-abdominal abscesses

Paul Cashin[1], Michael Levitt[2] and the late Joe J. Tjandra[3]

[1] Monash University and Monash Health, Melbourne, Victoria, Australia
[2] St. John of God Healthcare, Subiaco, Perth, Western Australia
[3] Royal Melbourne Hospital and University of Melbourne, Melbourne, Victoria, Australia

The acute abdomen

The aim of this section is to provide a broad set of guidelines for the management of patients presenting an acute abdomen. The detailed clinical, laboratory and radiological features of the numerous causative conditions are provided elsewhere in this book.

The term 'acute abdomen' should be confined to those patients with both acute abdominal pain and examination findings consistent with peritonitis. These findings often constitute a surgical emergency and should be managed as such. The term is not interchangeable with acute abdominal pain and it specifically implies the highest level of abdominal surgical emergency.

The management of patients with an acute abdomen comprises three concurrent processes – differential diagnosis, resuscitation and definitive therapy – culminating in the decision to operate or to observe (Box 68.1). These processes often compete with each other in a severely ill patient.

Diagnostic

Regardless of the severity of the presenting illness, management of patients with acute abdominal pain depends heavily on early and accurate establishment of the clinical diagnosis or, at least, a workable differential diagnosis. This clinical diagnosis requires accurate history taking, often from a number of sources, and careful examination. This is an important discipline to develop and the label 'acute abdomen' should be regarded as a flag for urgent management and not simply for review at a later time.

History and examination

Establishing a differential diagnosis or a definitive diagnosis of the acute abdomen by history and examination is achieved by two processes. The first is pattern recognition, drawn from clinical experience, and the second is probability, based on the theoretical knowledge of what is most likely to be the cause given the circumstances.

The pattern of the pain is a very important factor to explore in the history. The acuteness of onset, periodicity, site, radiation and aggravating factors are features that give hints as to cause. These need to be explored in detail. Information with regard to this may need to be sought from multiple sources (e.g. family) in the case of a severely ill patient. This accurate history taking also often brings to light precipitating factors that give clues to the likely cause.

The age, sex and past medical history of the patient give helpful indications as to the likely cause when establishing a differential diagnosis. Specific examples of clinical patterns in patients with acute abdominal pain include the following.

1 Sudden onset of pain may indicate perforation of the gut (perforated ulcer, perforated diverticulum, foreign body perforation) or a vascular event (ruptured aneurysm, vascular occlusion). The sudden change in nature of the pain (crampy to sudden exacerbation) may indicate a perforation secondary to an obstruction. In the case of right iliac fossa pain in a female, the sudden onset of pain might be more likely to indicate ovarian pathology (cyst rupture or bleed) than appendicitis.

2 Syncope or collapse associated with abdominal pain suggests acute blood loss until proven otherwise, for example a ruptured aneurysm or ruptured ectopic pregnancy.

Textbook of Surgery, Fourth Edition. Edited by Julian A. Smith, Andrew H. Kaye, Christopher Christophi and Wendy A. Brown.
© 2020 John Wiley & Sons Ltd. Published 2020 by John Wiley & Sons Ltd.

Box 68.1 Management of the acute abdomen

Diagnostic	Therapeutic
History and examination	*Resuscitation*
Assess severity	Airway and breathing
Establish a differential	control
diagnosis	Establish early intrave-
Seek information from	nous access
multiple sources	
	Symptom control
Investigations	Analgesia
Explore specific	Anti-emesis
diagnoses with directed	Nasogastric tube if
investigations	indicated
Preoperative	
investigations	*Monitoring the patient*
General investigations	Urinary catheter
	Oxygen saturation
	Invasive and non-invasive
	monitoring
	Non-surgical treatment
	Blood transfusion/
	intravenous fluids
	Intravenous antibiotics

Operate or observe

3 A combination of nausea and vomiting with abdominal pain is more suggestive of gastroenteritis. Vomiting and distension with abdominal pain is more suggestive of obstruction.

4 A colicky nature to the abdominal pain is suggestive of obstruction, and examination usually finds a relatively non-tender abdomen until either perforation or gut ischaemia intervene to give peritonitis or an acute abdomen. Patients with renal colic are usually non-tender on examination but have severe loin to groin pain.

5 A patient lying rigid in bed whereby the pain is exacerbated by movement and with associated tachycardia and often hypotension is indicative of peritonitis.

6 Pain exacerbated by movement suggests peritoneal irritation (e.g. appendicitis or a musculoskeletal cause).

Specific examples of the application of probability in the clinical setting include the following.

1 Recent onset of abdominal pain in the right side of the abdomen and anorexia in a previously well young man (acute appendicitis).

2 Left iliac fossa pain and tenderness in a 60 year old (sigmoid diverticulitis).

3 Upper abdominal pain, back pain and vomiting in a known alcoholic (acute pancreatitis).

4 Right upper quadrant pain and tenderness in a 30-year-old female (acute cholecystitis).

It is beyond the scope of this chapter to cover all the possible clinical scenarios that account for patients who present with acute abdominal pain. At the heart of their management, however, is a determination on the part of the clinician to establish an accurate clinical differential diagnosis on the basis of history and examination and to direct further investigation and/or management. Indeed, an accurate history and examination may occasionally lead to immediate surgery.

Investigations

It is not possible, at the outset, to anticipate all the investigations that might ultimately prove helpful in patient diagnosis and management. Emergency surgical management should never be delayed by investigations that may not add to the information gathered from history and examination. In the event of a confident clinical diagnosis (e.g. acute appendicitis) in a fit individual, no confirmatory or diagnostic investigations may be deemed necessary. Numerous clinical factors affect the choice of initial diagnostic investigations and some examples follow.

1 The severity of the presenting illness:
   a FAST (focused assessment using sonography for trauma) in the emergency department if an intra-abdominal catastrophe is suspected.
   b Full blood count and cross-match if haemorrhage is suspected.

2 Specific diagnostic possibilities:
   a Serum β-human chorionic gonadotropin in suspected ruptured ectopic pregnancy.
   b Serum amylase or lipase in suspected acute pancreatitis.
   c Abdominal ultrasound in cases of suspected biliary disease, obstructive uropathy, ruptured abdominal aortic aneurysm.
   d 12-lead ECG in suspected acute myocardial infarction.
   e Urine dipstick and midstream urine (MSU)/ catheter specimen of urine (CSU) should be performed, as urinary tract infections often mimic many other abdominal conditions.

3 If surgery is anticipated, prior to undergoing a general anaesthetic, certain investigations may be obtained, particularly in older patients, as a routine. This will vary from centre to centre, but such tests include urea and electrolytes, full blood count, ECG, chest X-ray as well as cross-match in appropriate cases.

4 General investigations in patients with acute abdominal pain of uncertain origin. These investigations may direct further intervention or flag a previously unrecognised degree of severity. Even before a clinical diagnosis is formulated, certain diagnostic investigations may have been instigated in anticipation of subsequent need. Many centres have routine investigation sets performed on presentation of the patient to aid efficiency. Amongst these, those most frequently of value are as follows.

a Full blood count: elevation of the white cell count is a cardinal sign of sepsis but it may also be raised by the 'stress' of pain alone; it is also mildly elevated during normal pregnancy. In general, an elevation of white cell count should never be dismissed and a very high white cell count (>30 × 10⁹/L) in the context of a patient with acute abdominal pain raises the possibility of intestinal perforation, peritonitis or ischaemia (hollow viscus perforation, mesenteric infarction, closed-loop small-bowel obstruction).

b Abdominal X-ray: a supine abdominal X-ray reveals distension of intra-abdominal gas (intestinal obstruction), thickness of intestinal wall (mesenteric ischaemia), abnormal calcification (ureteric colic, chronic pancreatitis) and outlines the psoas shadows (possibly obscured in ruptured abdominal aortic aneurysm). The erect abdominal/chest X-ray reveals fluid levels or free gas under the diaphragm (confirmation of intestinal obstruction or perforation).

c Ultrasound in experienced hands may reveal free fluid suggestive of haemorrhage or perforation.

d CT may reveal or confirm the diagnosis and is now readily available. A CT scan should not be performed in an unstable patient (where it delays definitive surgical management or endangers the patient) nor be used to replace accurate and rigorous clinical history and examination.

Therapeutic

At the same time as these diagnostic steps are being taken, concurrent therapeutic management should be undertaken. This includes the following broad groups.

Resuscitation

Unwell patients may require preliminary resuscitation before any practical diagnostic steps can be taken. Tachycardia, hypotension, pallor, sweating and cool extremities all suggest a more severe clinical presentation and the possibility of sepsis or hypovolaemia. Immediate *intravenous access* should be established and *fluid replacement* appropriate to the clinical setting commenced. Oxygen should be administered to maximise vital organ oxygenation. If conscious state is compromised, early airway management should be undertaken.

In cases of haemorrhagic shock, a *blood transfusion* should commence as soon as practicable. However, transfusion should not be allowed to delay the commencement of urgently needed surgery (e.g. ruptured abdominal aortic aneurysm) where the need to control the bleeding point outweighs the desire to restore intravascular volume by transfusion.

Symptom control

In the acute setting it is easy to overlook the need to provide basic symptom control. *Analgesia* should not be withheld pending surgical review. Analgesia requirements are usually an excellent indicator of the degree of pain being suffered by the patient; *anti-emetic therapy* usually accompanies opiate analgesics. For repeated vomiting (e.g. intestinal obstruction, acute pancreatitis) a *nasogastric tube* should be passed. This will relieve the symptoms, permit more accurate measurement of fluid loss and protect the patient from the risks of aspiration of gastric contents. Urinary retention often accompanies the acute abdomen and a urinary catheter should be inserted to also aid fluid balance monitoring.

Monitoring the patient

In the severely unwell patient, it is important to monitor the outcome of resuscitation and fluid replacement. Apart from the standard vital signs (pulse rate, blood pressure, temperature), additional information can be obtained by measuring urine output (indwelling urinary catheter) and invasive (arterial line or central venous line) or non-invasive cardiovascular monitoring. These measures are more sensitive to changes in intravascular fluid status than are the pulse rate and blood pressure.

Non-surgical therapy

Broad-spectrum *antibiotics* should be administered according to the likely clinical diagnosis. This may precede the formulation of an accurate clinical diagnosis, especially in unwell patients. Agents active against Gram-negative bacilli (aminoglycosides, third-generation cephalosporins) and anaerobic organisms (metronidazole) are generally preferred in patients presenting with acute abdominal pain.

In cases of suspected peptic ulcer complications, intravenous proton pump inhibitors (PPIs) should be administered. In the anticoagulated patient, reversal of anticoagulation may need to be considered, if possible, when bleeding is suspected or surgery is planned.

Surgery versus observation

Ultimately, an assessment needs to be made about the need for surgery. This may be clear-cut where a confident clinical diagnosis has been made (e.g. appendicitis).

In some cases, advanced age or infirmity might caution against surgery even where a confident diagnosis points to a surgical remedy (e.g. ruptured abdominal aortic aneurysm in a frail 90 year old). Significant concerns in this situation about goals of care, limitations of care and end-of-life care need to be incorporated into the clinical discussion.

Often, however, the precise diagnosis is uncertain and the need for urgent surgery is made obvious by virtue of either the clinical features of generalised peritonitis (e.g. perforated hollow viscus, mesenteric infarction, closed-loop small bowel-obstruction) or the severity of the presenting illness (e.g. associated shock). In this situation, clinical experience (pattern recognition) enables early identification of the need for prompt surgical intervention, often without further investigation.

Where the need for surgery is unclear (e.g. some cases of right iliac fossa pain or small intestinal obstruction), observation, resuscitation and non-surgical treatment of the likely diagnosis, rather than exploratory surgery, is appropriate. This involves regular clinical review conducted at a frequency appropriate to the severity of the illness; for example, review in 12 hours for a 20-year-old woman with mild right iliac fossa pain and tenderness or in 1–2 hours for a 75-year-old man with small bowel obstruction and associated abdominal tenderness. At times, such review may be augmented by further laboratory or radiological investigations. Of these, the white cell count and C-reactive protein (CRP) are most often of practical value; a rising white cell count or CRP generally indicates progression of the underlying pathological process.

Clinical example

The clinical scenario described in Box 68.2 serves as a demonstration of the dual processes – diagnostic and therapeutic – in the management of a patient with acute abdominal pain. Note especially the rapid construction of a workable differential diagnosis to permit subsequent history and examination to focus on identifying the most likely diagnosis.

Peritonitis

Peritonitis is defined as an inflammation of the peritoneum of whatever underlying cause. As previously discussed in the section on the acute abdomen, peritonitis is an essential feature of this clinical syndrome but is also a feature of other more localised diseases of the peritoneal cavity causing acute abdominal pain.

Often the peritonitis is localised to a particular area of the abdomen and this occurs due to the body's ability to contain the inflammatory process by wrapping of the omentum. This containment may eventually lead to a localised abscess (see section Intra-abdominal abscesses) or progress to generalised peritonitis and an acute abdomen. This progression may be accompanied by marked ileus, hypovolaemia, toxaemia or even septicaemia.

Cardinal signs of peritonitis are tenderness, guarding and rebound over the specific area or the whole abdomen in the case of diffuse peritonitis (see section The acute abdomen). Fever, tachycardia and dehydration are common features and movement generally exacerbates the pain.

Causes of peritonitis

Acute primary peritonitis

Acute primary peritonitis is rare and usually occurs in association with immunosuppression, such as post splenectomy, renal disease or in cirrhosis, where the proteinaceous ascitic fluid provides a good culture medium for bacteria. Sometimes it affects young girls following pelvic inflammatory disease. Commonly involved organisms include haemolytic streptococci, *Escherichia coli* and *Klebsiella* species. Acute primary peritonitis is often a diagnosis of exclusion and requires aggressive antibiotic therapy (Box 68.3).

Box 68.2 Clinical scenario

A 65-year-old man presents with the sudden onset of generalised abdominal pain and collapse. On examination, he is pale, sweaty and distressed, with pulse rate of 110 beats/min, blood pressure 90/50 mmHg and temperature 36.0°C

Diagnostic	Therapeutic

Diagnostic

1 **History and examination** (establish and explore the likely differential diagnosis)
- Ruptured abdominal aortic aneurysm
  - Pain radiating to back or groin
  - History of smoking, other vascular diseases
  - Palpate abdomen for pulsatile mass
  - Absent or reduced lower limb peripheral pulses
- Mesenteric infarction
  - History of palpitations, arrhythmia, digitalis therapy
  - Palpate pulse for atrial fibrillation
- Perforated peptic ulcer
  - History of dyspepsia, antacid therapy, NSAID ingestion
  - Board-like abdominal rigidity
- Acute pancreatitis
  - Prominent vomiting, pain referred to back
  - Alcoholic or gallstone aetiology
- Acute myocardial infarction
  - Past history of ischaemic heart disease

2 **Investigations**
- Full blood count
  - Low haemoglobin may indicate haemorrhage, high white cell count suggests infection associated with perforation or ischaemia
- Urea and electrolytes: to guide resuscitation
- Serum lactate and blood gases: measure of organ damage/ischaemia
- 12-lead ECG: changes of acute ischaemia
- Abdominal X-ray, supine and erect
  - Free intraperitoneal gas, loss of psoas shadow, calcification of abdominal aortic aneurysm, dilated loops of small intestine
- Serum amylase/lipase: >1000 U/L diagnostic of acute pancreatitis
- Cross-match: if haemorrhage is suspected and/or major surgery anticipated
- FAST scan: to confirm ruptured abdominal aortic aneurysm
- Investigations should not delay surgical management in a deteriorating patient or a patient not responding to resuscitation

Therapeutic

1 **Resuscitation**
- Adequate intravenous access (beware of over-transfusion in acute myocardial infarction)
- Oxygen mask (plus airway support if appropriate)
- Transfuse if haemoglobin <8 g/dL
- Beware the normal haemoglobin in patients with acute haemorrhage: a normal value does not rule out acute bleeding
- Consider transfusing if haemoglobin <10 g/dL and further bleeding or major surgery is planned

2 **Symptom control**
- Intravenous or intramuscular opiate analgesics
- Anti-emetic therapy
- Nasogastric tube if vomiting

3 **Monitoring the patient**
- Indwelling urinary catheter
- Oxygen saturation monitoring
- Non-invasive or invasive cardiovascular monitoring

4 **Non-surgical treatment**
- Intravenous antibiotics (suspected perforation, mesenteric ischaemia)
- High-dose PPIs

Operate or observe?

- **Ruptured abdominal aortic aneurysm**: immediate laparotomy or angiographic stenting depending on facility
- **Perforated peptic ulcer**: immediate operation (occasionally may be treated by antibiotics, PPIs and observation if abdominal signs are localised)
- **Mesenteric infarction**: immediate operation to exclude closed-loop small-bowel obstruction
- **Acute pancreatitis**: intravenous fluid replacement, analgesia, oxygen administration, nasogastric tube if vomiting, urinary catheter for fluid balance monitoring. Observe for progressive abdominal signs, features of intra-abdominal sepsis. Monitor full blood count, liver function tests, serum calcium, blood glucose level, arterial blood gases and CRP
- **Acute myocardial infarction**: monitor patient in critical care facility, specific therapy according to local protocols

Box 68.3 Common varieties of peritonitis

Acute peritonitis
  Primary (spontaneous)
  Secondary
  Acute suppurative (e.g. perforated viscus)
  Chemical-induced
Chronic (sclerosing) peritonitis
  Infections (e.g. tuberculosis, *Candida albicans*)
  Chemical-induced (e.g. surgical talc in the gloves, chlorhexidine)
  Carcinomatosis

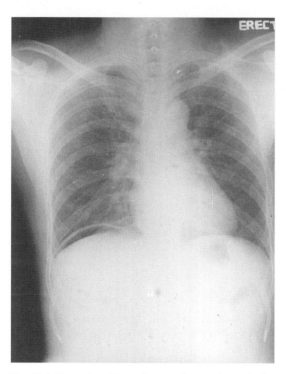

Fig. 68.1 Erect chest X-ray showing free gas beneath the right hemidiaphragm indicating likely perforation.

Secondary peritonitis

Secondary peritonitis may be suppurative, chemical or chronic sclerosing.

Acute suppurative peritonitis may occur secondary to a disease process of an intra-abdominal organ, i.e. perforation (e.g. peptic ulcer, diverticular disease, Crohn's disease, appendix or gallbladder), infection (e.g. appendix abscess, pyosalpinx) or ischaemia (volvulus, mesenteric ischaemia or strangulated hernia). Most of these cases will require urgent surgical intervention. Erect chest X-ray may show free gas beneath the diaphragm, indicating a perforated viscus and clinical findings may suggest an acute abdomen (Figure 68.1).

Chemical peritonitis may occur secondary to bile (bile leak post laparoscopic cholecystectomy) or blood (postoperative bleeding, abdominal trauma). Less commonly, urine (ureteric injury in pelvic surgery or intraperitoneal rupture of bladder) may also be the cause. Bacterial contamination and overgrowth may develop as a secondary event if the condition goes unrecognised.

Intra-abdominal abscesses

Intra-abdominal abscesses are one extreme in the spectrum of bacterial peritonitis. They are often related to the body's attempt or ability to localise infections by migration of the omentum to the site of sepsis. They require drainage in addition to antibiotic therapy. The pathogenesis requires a polymicrobial infection, often with the presence of foreign matter facilitating the development of progressive infection. The bacterial flora of the gastrointestinal tract varies from small numbers of aerobic streptococci and facultative Gram-negative bacilli in the stomach and proximal small bowel to larger numbers of these species with an increasing number of anaerobic Gram-negative bacilli (*Bacteroides* spp.) and anaerobic Gram-positive flora (streptococci and clostridia) in the distal ileum and colon. In patients who have received prolonged antibiotic therapy and in those with extended hospital stay or long-term illness, colonisation by yeasts such as *Candida* species or a variety of nosocomial pathogens may occur. Skin flora may be responsible following penetrating abdominal injuries. Pelvic abscesses in women may occur as part of pelvic inflammatory disease. Common organisms include *Neisseria gonorrhoeae* and *Chlamydia trachomatis*.

There are four functional compartments within the peritoneal cavity: pelvis, right and left paracolic gutters and the subdiaphragmatic spaces. In the recumbent patient, diffuse intraperitoneal fluid collects under the diaphragm and in the pelvis. These are the common sites for abscess formation. More localised abscesses may develop in relation to the affected viscus (e.g. abscesses in the lesser sac secondary to severe pancreatitis or a perforated peptic ulcer, or a peri-appendiceal abscess). In the paracolic gutters, local abscesses often develop in conjunction with small colonic perforations. This is usually related to diverticular disease or diverticulitis in the left colon. Solitary diverticular perforation and foreign body perforation are more common in the right colon. Perforated tumours also need to be part of any differential diagnosis in these situations. These conditions demonstrate pattern recognition in clinical assessment.

Clinical features

The clinical presentation of an intra-abdominal abscess is highly variable. In a patient with predisposing primary intra-abdominal disease or following abdominal surgery, persistent abdominal pain, focal tenderness, swinging fever, persistent paralytic ileus, elevated CRP and leucocytosis suggest an intra-abdominal purulent collection. The patient may simply fail to thrive and may have mildly abnormal liver function secondary to portal sepsis.

With a pelvic abscess, there may be urinary frequency, dysuria, diarrhoea or tenesmus due to irritation of the anatomically related organs. With a subphrenic collection, there may be shoulder tip pain, hiccups and unexplained pulmonary symptoms (pleural effusion, basal atelectasis).

Investigations

Investigations in patients with suspected intra-abdominal abscess include full blood examination, CRP, urea and electrolytes and liver function tests. Blood cultures and other appropriate cultures (urine, sputum, catheter) may also be performed.

CT scan with iodinated soluble oral contrast is useful. Spiral images are obtained from the diaphragm to the pelvis. It is particularly useful for localising small or deep intra-abdominal abscesses (Figure 68.2). Interpretation in postoperative patients can be particularly difficult, as loculated non-infected serous collections are common physiological events.

Ultrasound equipment is mobile and examinations may be readily performed in a critically ill patient in the intensive care unit. However, the quality of such studies is not as good as a CT scan

and is vastly operator dependent. Endovaginal ultrasound is particularly useful for detecting tubo-ovarian abscess complicating pelvic inflammatory disease in women

Laparoscopy is occasionally used if there is diagnostic uncertainty.

Therapy

Parenteral antibiotics

Parenteral antibiotics should be administered prior to drainage of the abscess. Initial choice of antibiotics is empirical but should provide a broad-spectrum activity against likely organisms as they pertain to the proposed source of the infection. Specific therapy is guided by the results of cultures. With adequate drainage of the abscess, it may not be necessary to treat each component of the polymicrobial flora. Commonly used antibiotics include metronidazole with a second- or third-generation cephalosporin or meropenem alone. Alternatively, combinations of amoxicillin, gentamicin and metronidazole provide additional cover against enterococci as well. In immunosuppressed patients, *Candida* species may have an important pathogenic role, and treatment with antifungals is indicated.

Percutaneous drainage

CT scan or ultrasound localises the abscess cavity and guides safe access for percutaneous drainage (Figure 68.3), avoiding adjacent viscera and blood vessels. A diagnostic needle aspiration is initially performed to confirm the presence of the abscess and to obtain pus for Gram stain and culture. A large-bore drainage catheter is then placed in the most dependent position. While percutaneous drainage is effective in a single unilocular abscess,

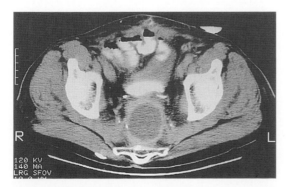

Fig. 68.2 CT scan showing a pelvic abscess.

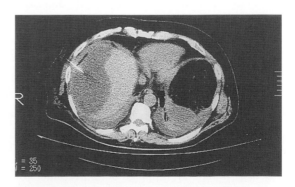

Fig. 68.3 CT scan of the abdomen showing a large subphrenic abscess that was aspirated percutaneously under CT guidance.

it is more limited in a multiloculated abscess, especially if the contents are tenacious.

Preliminary percutaneous drainage is sometimes useful in improving and reducing the sepsis, prior to definitive surgical treatment. In some cases, as for complicated diverticular disease or Crohn's disease, it may facilitate subsequent single-stage resection and primary anastomosis, rather than traditional multistage procedures with diversion. Repeat imaging with sinography or CT will often help to estimate the size of the residual cavity and any enteric communication.

Intraluminal drainage

The development of technology such as endoscopic ultrasound has seen the ability to safely drain intra-abdominal abscesses into the lumen of the gut. This is particularly useful in draining infected necrotic pancreatic abscesses, following severe pancreatitis, into the stomach. This drainage is further facilitated by the ability to insert drain tubes between the abscess and the gastric lumen or to debride necrotic material via endoscopic cyst-gastrotomy.

Surgical drainage

Surgical drainage is mainly undertaken in patients who have not improved with percutaneous drainage or in whom the collections are not appropriate for percutaneous drainage, as in multiple abscesses, severe necrotising pancreatitis or interloop abscesses with Crohn's disease. An extraperitoneal approach, if possible, is generally preferred because it limits the risk of further contamination of the peritoneal cavity. With a distally located pelvic abscess that is bulging, the drainage may be performed through the rectum or vagina. The loculae are gently broken down digitally and soft drains are placed in the most dependent position. Laparoscopic drainage of singular abscesses has also proven beneficial in many cases.

Definitive surgery

Definitive surgery is generally deferred until after preliminary drainage of the abscess. In some situations, surgery on the offending organ is performed, for example appendicectomy for appendiceal abscess, unilateral salpingo-oophorectomy for tubo-ovarian abscess, omental patch of a perforated duodenal ulcer.

Summary

Many severe intra-abdominal pathologies can present clinically in a variety of ways. The term 'acute abdomen' should be distinguished from acute abdominal pain and represent those intra-abdominal conditions at the most severe end of the clinical spectrum, requiring the most urgent treatment. Pattern recognition and application of probabilities, ascertained from rigorous clinical history taking and clinical examination, remain the mainstay in the diagnosis and subsequent management of many of these conditions.

Further reading

Almeida PRL, Leão GS, Gonçalves CDG, Picon RV, Tovo CV. Impact of microbiological changes on spontaneous bacterial peritonitis in three different periods over 17 years. *Arq Gastroenterol* 2018;55:23–27.

Colas PA, Duchalais E, Duplay Q *et al*. Failure of conservative treatment of acute diverticulitis. *World J Surg* 2017;41:1890–5.

Constantinides VA, Tekkis PP, Senapati A. Association of Coloproctology of Great Britain and Ireland. Comparison of POSSUM scoring systems and the surgical risk scale in patients undergoing surgery for complicated diverticular disease. *Dis Colon Rectum* 2006;49:1322–31.

Galbraith N, Carter JV, Netz U *et al*. Laparoscopic lavage in the management of perforated diverticulitis: a contemporary meta-analysis. *J Gastrointest Surg* 2017;21: 1491–9.

Shah TT, Herbert P, Beresford T. An atypical presentation of aortic rupture: intuition and investigation can avoid disaster. *Ann R Coll Surg Engl* 2011;93:e125–e128.

Shizuma T. Spontaneous bacterial and fungal peritonitis in patients with liver cirrhosis: a literature review. *World J Hepatol* 2018;10:254–66.

MCQs

Select the single correct answer to each question. The correct answers can be found in the Answers section at the end of the book.

1 Which of the following clinical features is often found in a patient presenting with an acute abdomen related to generalised peritonitis?
   a slow pulse rate
   b extreme restlessness and writhing around in agony
   c motionless with pain, worse with movement
   d normal bowel sounds
   e deep palpation of most abdominal organs is possible

2 Acute epigastric pain is unusual in which of the following conditions?
   a acute pancreatitis
   b acute cholecystitis
   c perforated peptic ulcer
   d acute diverticulitis
   e ruptured abdominal aortic aneurysm

3 Immediate laparotomy would not be recommended in a patient diagnosed as having which of the following conditions?
   a mesenteric infarction
   b perforated peptic ulcer with generalised peritonitis
   c acute pancreatitis
   d small bowel obstruction with peritonism
   e ruptured abdominal aortic aneurysm

4 Which of the following parameters is the most practical for monitoring progression of the underlying pathological process responsible for acute abdominal pain in a patient being initially managed non-operatively?
   a erythrocyte sedimentation rate
   b haemoglobin estimation
   c white cell count
   d white cell scan
   e serum phosphate

5 Which of the following is a common cause of post-surgical pelvic abscess?
   a cholecystectomy
   b appendicectomy
   c laparoscopic but not conventional open anterior resection
   d rectovaginal fistula
   e use of powdered surgical gloves

69 Ascites

David A.K. Watters[1,2], Sonal Nagra[1,2] and David M.A. Francis[3]

[1] Deakin University and Barwon Health, Geelong, Victoria, Australia
[2] University Hospital Geelong, Geelong, Victoria, Australia
[3] Department of Urology, Royal Children's Hospital, Melbourne, Australia and Department of Surgery, Tribhuvan University Teaching Hospital, Kathmandu, Nepal

Introduction

Ascites is an abnormal accumulation of free fluid within the peritoneal cavity. The word 'ascites' is of Greek origin (*askos*) and means bag or sac. Ascites is due to increased portal venous pressure, low plasma proteins (hypoproteinaemia), chronic peritoneal irritation, leakage of lymphatic fluid into the peritoneal cavity, or fluid overload (Box 69.1). Three-quarters of cases occur as a result of portal hypertension in the setting of liver cirrhosis, with the remainder due to infective, inflammatory and neoplastic conditions.

Ascites needs to be differentiated from other causes of abdominal distension including bowel obstruction, bleeding and huge intra-abdominal masses or cysts.

Pathophysiology of ascites

Increased portal venous pressure
(Figure 69.1)

Any cause of increased resistance to hepatic or portal venous blood flow can lead to ascites. Gross ascites occurs when increased pressure within the hepatic veins or at the post-sinusoidal level dramatically increases hydrostatic pressure within the hepatic sinusoids in the liver, and within the portal venous system. Collateral vein formation, shunting of blood to the systemic circulation and splanchnic vasodilatation (due in part to the local production of nitric oxide) develop particularly in the later stages of cirrhosis. Systemic arterial pressure is maintained by vasoconstriction and antinatriuretic factors, resulting in sodium and water retention. The increased portal pressure combined with splanchnic vasodilatation alters the capillary pressure and permeability, enabling intravascular fluid to move through pores between the vascular endothelial cells of the portal system into the extravascular space of the liver and intestine. Lymphatic flow is increased proximal to the point of vascular obstruction and, when the capacity of the lymphatic system is surpassed, the transudate moves across the surfaces of the liver, mesentery and intestine into the peritoneal cavity. Cirrhosis and schistosomal periportal fibrosis are the commonest causes of portal hypertension.

Any cause of hepatic venous outflow obstruction may cause ascites by increasing portal venous pressure (Budd–Chiari syndrome). The site of obstruction may be at the hepatic venules (haematological or liver disease), large hepatic veins, inferior vena cava or right atrium (right heart diseases).

Hypoproteinaemia

Low concentrations of plasma proteins, particularly albumin, reduce the osmotic pressure of plasma. In health, the relatively high osmotic pressure of intravascular plasma tends to draw extravascular fluid back into the intravascular space. The osmotic gradient is reduced in hypoproteinaemic states so that less fluid is removed from extravascular sites. When the capacity of the hepatic and intestinal lymphatics to remove fluid from the extravascular interstitial space is exceeded, ascites develops. This is well demonstrated in kwashiorkor where the hypoalbuminaemic state results in ascites due to the severe protein energy malnutrition.

Sodium and water retention

Reduced circulating plasma volume, as a result of loss of intravascular fluid into the peritoneal cavity and interstitial spaces (third-space fluid loss) and pooling of blood in the splanchnic vascular space

Box 69.1 Causes of ascites

Increased portal venous pressure
- Prehepatic: portal vein compression or thrombosis, schistosomiasis
- Hepatic: cirrhosis, acute hepatic necrosis, viral hepatitis
- Posthepatic: Budd–Chiari syndrome, myeloproliferative disorders, constrictive pericarditis, right heart failure, hypercoagulable states

Hypoproteinaemia
- Renal disease causing severe proteinuria: includes nephrotic syndrome
- Malnutrition and malabsorption
- Protein-losing enteropathy
- Acute or chronic liver disease
- Severe acute or chronic illness

Chronic peritoneal inflammation and infection
- Chronic infection: tuberculosis, fungal infection
- Secondary malignant infiltration (carcinomatosis peritonei)
- Post irradiation
- Serositis secondary to inflammation from chronic infection/allergic reaction

Leakage of lymphatic fluid (chylous ascites)
- Congenital
- Surgical trauma: postoperative ileus
- Primary and secondary lymphatic malignancy

Other fluids
- Pancreatic ascites
- Bilious ascites
- Urinary ascites
- Hypothyroidism: severe myxoedema

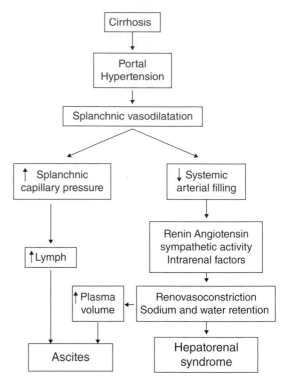

Fig. 69.1 The pathophysiology of ascites due to cirrhosis.

secondary to portal venous outflow obstruction, reduces renal blood flow and glomerular filtration. Decreased renal perfusion stimulates increased renin secretion from the juxtaglomerular apparatus in the ascending limb of the loop of Henle of the kidney. The resultant secondary aldosteronism causes retention of sodium and water. Impairment of renal excretion of water and renal vasoconstriction lead to dilutional hyponatraemia and increase the risk of hepatorenal syndrome, which comprises renal failure, portal hypertension and ascites.

Chronic peritoneal inflammation

Any chronic inflammatory process within the peritoneal cavity results in considerable increases in flow within peritoneal blood and lymphatic vessels. Peritoneal microvascular permeability increases markedly with consequent exudation of plasma proteins and fluid into extravascular spaces. When

the capacity of the lymphatics to reabsorb the fluid is exceeded, it accumulates within the peritoneal cavity. The high protein concentration of this peritoneal fluid further retards fluid reabsorption. As the inflammatory process resolves, and microvascular permeability returns to normal, less peritoneal fluid is formed and fluid is removed by absorption. The commonest cause of chronic peritoneal inflammation worldwide is abdominal tuberculosis but other peritoneal infections and foreign matter may also induce ascites.

Malignant infiltration

Metastatic deposits cause ascites by a combination of inflammation, shedding of cells, exudation, lymphatic obstruction and sometimes bleeding. Gross ascites does not usually occur until late. Gastric and ovarian cancers (Meigs syndrome) are the most notorious for causing ascites due to their ease of transperitoneal spread, but any peritoneal malignant process may be responsible.

Leakage of fluid

Leakage of fluid directly into the peritoneal cavity occurs when intra-abdominal lymphatics are transected (e.g. abdominal surgery, trauma) or obstructed (e.g. primary or secondary lymphatic malignancy, surgical ligation). Ascites forms when the rate of leakage into the peritoneal cavity exceeds the rate of absorption by peritoneal lymphatics.

Exudation of pancreatic fluid from an inflamed pancreas may occur in acute pancreatitis. If the pancreatic duct ruptures due to inflammation or surgical damage, pancreatic ascites may persist as an internally draining pancreatic fistula.

Bile leaks may be termed bilious ascites, although bile is normally very irritant to the peritoneal cavity and commonly induces more of a peritonitis/acute abdomen-type reaction.

Urine may leak into the peritoneal cavity from damage to a ureter or the bladder or from an obstructed hydronephrotic kidney.

Postoperative ascites

It is important to ensure all efforts are made to rule out bleeding, bile leak, urine leak, bowel injury and anastomotic leak prior to making a diagnosis of postoperative ascites. Most commonly, ascites presents postoperatively due to low albumin states. This is more pronounced in patients with liver impairment. Although rare, ascites has been attributed to inflammation or allergic reaction of the peritoneal surface. Postoperative patients have a negative nitrogen balance; in patients with ascites, this is further worsened with loss of protein-rich fluids in drains and through wounds.

Clinical features

Ascites should be suspected from a history of abdominal distension. Physiologically, men generally have no peritoneal fluid while women can have up to 20 mL depending on the phase of their menstrual cycle. Ascites can be detected clinically on examination of the abdomen when the volume reaches approximately 1 L. Inspection of the abdomen reveals distension, which may vary from slight fullness laterally in the flanks to gross distension predominantly in the centre of the abdomen. Sometimes a hernial sac protrudes as it becomes full of ascitic fluid, particularly at the umbilicus. Other abnormal findings on inspection may include signs of liver disease (jaundice, scratch marks because of pruritus, spider naevi, caput medusae and dilated veins on the anterior abdominal wall, hepatomegaly), para-umbilical and other abdominal hernias, pitting oedema and surgical scars.

On palpation the abdomen may feel thicker owing to the fluid asserting more than the expected degree of resistance. In cases of chronic inflammation, particularly tuberculosis, the abdomen may feel 'doughy'. Gross ascites causes tense abdominal distension that makes palpation of organomegaly challenging. Ascites is confirmed by the presence of a fluid thrill and shifting dullness on percussion.

Clinical examination should include a search for signs of heart failure such as pitting leg oedema and raised jugular venous pressure. Although rare, features of peritoneal carcinoma such as Virchow's node or a Sister Mary Joseph nodule may give a cause for the ascites. Virchow's node is the presence of left supraclavicular lymphadenopathy and results from nodular metastasis from lymphatic drainage via the thoracic duct draining into the left subclavian vein. A Sister Mary Joseph nodule is a palpable nodule at the umbilicus that arises from metastasis of a malignant cancer in the pelvis or abdomen.

Patients with a history of cancer, especially gastrointestinal cancer, are at risk for malignant ascites. Malignancy-related ascites is frequently painful, whereas cirrhotic ascites is usually painless. Patients who develop ascites in the setting of established diabetes or nephrotic syndrome may have nephrotic ascites.

Fluid thrill

Large amounts of intraperitoneal fluid, either free or encysted, may give rise to a fluid thrill. The abdomen is flicked on one side and the transmitted shock wave is palpated by the examiner's other hand, which has been placed flat on the far side of the abdomen (Figure 69.2a). An accessory hand prevents transmission of the shock wave through the subcutaneous fat of the anterior abdominal wall. A fluid thrill may also be elicited by tapping in the loin and palpating at the front (Figure 69.2b). To detect a fluid thrill in an abdomen with smaller volumes of ascitic fluid, the area of stony dullness is first determined by percussion.

Shifting dullness

Free intraperitoneal fluid gravitates to the most dependent parts of the peritoneal cavity, namely the pelvis and paracolic regions, while the gas-filled intestine tends to 'float' uppermost. Fluid-filled structures have a stony dull percussion note, while gas-filled structures are resonant or hyperresonant on percussion. Thus, when a patient with ascites lies supine, the flanks or lateral parts of the abdomen are stony dull to percussion while the periumbilical area is resonant. When the patient lies on one or other side, ascitic fluid gravitates to that side

(a)

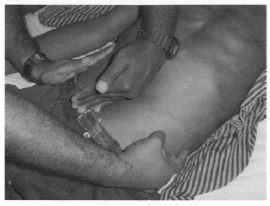

(b)

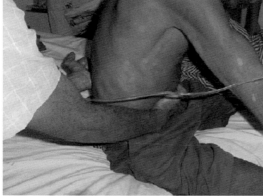

Fig. 69.2 (a, b) Clinical examination: palpating for ascites.

Ascites is a multisystem disease and the probable cause will determine which systems require investigation. The choice includes urinalysis, serum concentrations of electrolytes, urea and creatinine, total proteins and albumin, liver function tests, serology, abdominal ultrasonography (Figure 69.3a), computed tomography (CT) (Figure 69.3b), portal vein Doppler scan and echocardiography. Diagnostic aspiration of a small volume of ascitic fluid for biochemical (protein and amylase estimation), microbiological (microscopy and culture) and cytological assessment may be necessary. Laparoscopy or mini-laparotomy may be required to perform a peritoneal biopsy to diagnose abdominal tuberculosis and other inflammatory conditions. Schistosomiasis may be suspected from a history of swimming or living in endemic areas and confirmed by rectal or liver biopsy, ultrasound or serology. Plain abdominal films are not a method of diagnosing ascites but sometimes gross ascites give an appearance of ground glass.

A serum to ascites albumin gradient (SAAG) above 1.1 g/dL has 97% accuracy for diagnosis of ascites due to portal hypertension. There has been a conceptual shift from a definition that categorises ascites fluid as either transudative or exudative to one of high albumin gradient and low albumin gradient, respectively, which relate to portal hypertensive (SAAG >1.1 g/dL) and non-portal hypertensive (SAAG <1.1 g/dL) causes. (SAAG = serum albumin level – ascitic fluid albumin level in g/dL.)

Clinical outcome

Mild to moderate ascites may cause few symptoms. Large-volume ascites (more than 3–4 L) is very unpleasant for patients because it produces a constant feeling of abdominal fullness and discomfort, nausea and anorexia, limitation of movement and leg swelling. Respiratory difficulty and shortness of breath is due to elevation of the diaphragm, atelectasis and pleural effusions. Ascites may be complicated by previously unrecognised abdominal hernias and rarely by primary bacterial peritonitis. Primary or spontaneous bacterial peritonitis may be difficult to diagnose, does not always cause a lot of guarding or rigidity and patients' immune response to the infection may be impaired owing to their underlying disease, for example liver, renal or malignancy. Sometimes the peritonitis presents with general deterioration (e.g. development of hepatic encephalopathy or renal failure) rather than abdominal signs. Reduced renal blood flow and glomerular filtration, poor urine output and low urinary sodium excretion cause pre-renal

because it is then the most dependent part of the abdomen, and so the percussion note over that area becomes stony dull, while the other side becomes resonant.

Shifting dullness is elicited by percussing the abdomen and determining the point at which the percussion note changes from resonant to dull. The patient is then asked to roll about 45° to one side, and percussion is repeated after waiting for a few seconds. Shifting dullness is confirmed by a significant change in position of the area of stony dullness. It should be noted that slight changes in the percussion note may be caused by positional changes in the small intestine.

Investigation

Investigation of a patient with ascites aims to detect the cause of the fluid accumulation. This is usually evident from the history and clinical examination, including habits and previous travel or domicile. Specific investigations depend on the likely cause of the ascites (see Box 69.1).

(a)

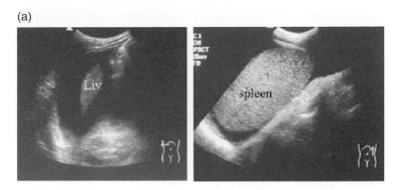

Ultrasound showing ascitic fluid (black) around liver on right
and around spleen on left.

(b)

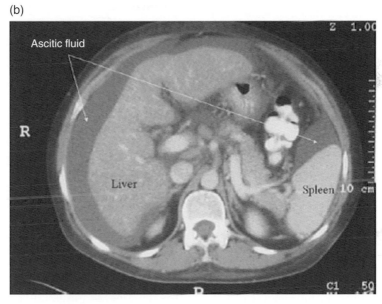

Fig. 69.3 (a) Ultrasound showing fluid (black) around the liver. (b) CT scan showing ascitic fluid, anterior abdominal distension and contrast in the loops of the bowel.

impairment with increased urea and creatinine, which may progress to acute renal failure (hepatorenal syndrome). Development of ascites in patients with chronic liver disease indicates severe liver impairment, and 1-year survival of such patients with intractable ascites is approximately 50%. Malignant ascites is most commonly due to intraperitoneal metastatic deposits of cancer originating in the ovary, stomach, breast and colon. Prognosis of these patients is poor, with a median survival of about 3 months.

Treatment

Most patients with ascites are treated non-operatively. Ascites can be classified as moderate-volume, high-volume and refractory with regard to the approach to treatment. By definition, refractory ascites does not respond to high doses of diuretics (spironolactone and frusemide). Moderate-volume ascites does not require paracentesis and large-volume ascites is controlled by a combination of medical treatment and paracentesis.

Medical management

Specific management of the cause of liver dysfunction, such as antivirals for hepatitis B and C and alcohol rehabilitation in alcohol-related cirrhosis, should be initiated. Dietary sodium is restricted to approximately one-third of the normal daily intake (i.e. to about 60–90 mEq/day). Diuretic therapy commences with an aldosterone antagonist such as spironolactone or amiloride. In recurrent or persistent ascites, this should be combined with frusemide. These two measures are successful in controlling ascites in about 60–70% of patients. In addition, a thiazide diuretic may be required. Diuretic therapy must be monitored closely to ensure that progressive renal failure and electrolyte imbalance (potassium, sodium, calcium and magnesium) do not occur. It is important to stop medications such as angiotensin-converting enzyme inhibitors, non-steroidal anti-inflammatory drugs and aminoglycosides which can worsen ascites and/or induce renal failure.

Prophylactic antibiotics are not required. Primary or spontaneous peritonitis-complicating ascites is treated with appropriate antibiotics, although sometimes a laparoscopy or laparotomy is required either for diagnosis or to wash out the peritoneal cavity. Specific causes of ascites such as tuberculosis are treated with appropriate antituberculous chemotherapy according to national guidelines. Surgical intervention is reserved for diagnosis and to treat complications such as acute bowel obstruction, bleeding or perforation due to intestinal tuberculosis.

Paracentesis

Paracentesis, or drainage of ascitic fluid, brings immediate though temporary relief to patients with symptomatic tense ascites. Paracentesis is performed under local anaesthesia and with a strict aseptic technique by inserting a cannula through the anterolateral abdominal wall, avoiding the inferior epigastric artery and the colon. It can often be performed under ultrasound or CT control. Fluid is drained into a sterile collecting system and the cannula is either removed immediately or left *in situ* for 24–48 hours. Rapid removal of large amounts of ascites may lead to serious hypovolaemia because the underlying reason for formation of ascites has not been eliminated and ascites re-forms rapidly with fluid from the extracellular space (interstitial and intravascular fluid). Volume replacement may be required during paracentesis and is undertaken cautiously with concentrated or normal serum albumin in order to avoid hypovolaemia on the one hand and fluid overload and rapid re-accumulation of ascites on the other. The complications of infection, intestinal perforation and bleeding are rare when performed with an appropriate sterile technique and a purpose-built cannula.

Relief of acute hepatic venous obstruction

When the cause of ascites is due to an acute thrombus, thrombolytic therapy or angioplasty may be performed. Where these are unsuccessful a portosystemic shunt should be considered.

Transjugular intrahepatic portosystemic shunt

Transjugular intrahepatic portosystemic shunt (TIPS) is a radiological procedure where a shunt is placed within the liver between the portal vein and hepatic vein via a transjugular route for venous access under image guidance. Accordingly, it creates a communication between the portal and systemic circulation. It may stabilise the patient while consideration is being given to liver transplantation and is judged the best management for diuretic-resistant ascites. It reduces sinusoidal and portal pressures and therefore reduces the impact of refractory ascites and the side effects of high-dose diuretics. Unfortunately, the shunts have a fairly high rate of blockage or stenosis (up to 75% after 6–12 months) and the shunt may induce hepatic encephalopathy. TIPS does not improve long-term survival as compared to repeated paracentesis.

Portosystemic shunts

If ascites is due to portal hypertension, portosystemic shunting may be performed in selected patients to reduce portal venous pressure. Shunting may be accomplished by TIPS or by making a formal anastomosis between the splenic and renal veins (lienorenal shunt) or between portal vein and inferior vena cava (portocaval shunt). These shunts do not address the problem of the underlying liver disease, but do reduce the issues with oesophageal varices. Shunt surgery may be complicated by hepatic encephalopathy and hepatorenal syndrome. The presence of ascites in patients undergoing shunt surgery for portal hypertension is a poor prognostic sign.

Peritoneovenous shunts

Symptomatic relief by draining ascitic fluid from the peritoneal cavity into the systemic venous system can be achieved by way of a peritoneovenous shunt (PVS). A PVS (Denver shunt, LeVeen shunt) consists of a silastic tube, with multiple side holes at each end and a one-way valve situated in the middle. The PVS is placed entirely subcutaneously, with one end inserted into the peritoneal cavity and the other into the superior vena cava (SVC) via a jugular or subclavian vein, so that the valve allows flow of ascites from the peritoneal cavity to the venous system. A PVS is indicated when medical therapy has failed to control ascites in patients with (i) intractable ascites in the presence of reasonably good liver function, or (ii) rapidly accumulating ascites secondary to abdominal carcinomatosis. Concern about infusing ascitic fluid laden with malignant cells into the circulation is theoretical because these patients have widely disseminated malignant disease before insertion of the PVS.

The postoperative mortality of PVS is 10–20%, reflecting the serious underlying disorder of patients requiring the procedure. However, most patients obtain useful palliation. A minor coagulopathy is common postoperatively but can be partly prevented by completely aspirating the ascites and replacing it with warmed normal saline or Hartmann's solution when inserting the PVS. Long-term complications include occlusion of the PVS (particularly with bloody or highly proteinaceous or mucoid ascites), SVC thrombosis, bacteraemia and shunt infection, which may lead to subacute bacterial endocarditis.

Surgery on patients with ascites

Surgery is liable to complications in patients with ascites. Abdominal surgery is prone to infection and there is a potential for poor wound/anastomotic healing. The patient's management is complicated by ascitic leak, wound complications, electrolyte and fluid balance difficulties and protein losses. Although not common, patients undergoing abdominal surgery may have damage to lymphatics, especially after retroperitoneal surgery, which could result in the challenging problem of lymph ascites. The underlying liver disease may cause a coagulopathy. Renal failure complicating liver disease (hepatorenal syndrome) is a major risk that can be minimised by ensuring optimal renal perfusion. Patients who have obstructive jaundice are often surgical candidates, at least for some form of bypass procedure. The presence of ascites in these patients increases the mortality, particularly from hepatorenal syndrome, and thus less invasive procedures such as biliary stenting are preferred.

Further reading

Fortune B, Cardenas A. Ascites, refractory ascites and hyponatremia in cirrhosis. *Gastroenterol Rep (Oxf)* 2017;5:104–12.

Liou IW, Kim HN. Diagnosis and management of ascites. Hepatitis C Online. University of Washington Infectious Diseases Education and Assessment. Available at http://www.hepatitisc.uw.edu/go/management-cirrhosis-related-complications/ascites-diagnosis-management/core-concept/all

Tsochatzis E, Gerbes A. Diagnosis and treatment of ascites. *J Hepatol* 2017;67:184–5.

MCQs

Select the single correct answer to each question. The correct answers can be found in the Answers section at the end of the book.

1 Which of the following statements about portal hypertension is correct?
  a there is increased portal blood volume
  b there is a decrease in portal blood pressure
  c there is increased splanchnic vasoconstriction
  d there is hypoproteinaemia due to increased renal protein losses
  e there is reduced splanchnic lymphatic flow

2 Which of the following conditions is typically associated with ascites?
  a filiariasis
  b Gilbert's disease
  c abdominal tuberculosis
  d large uterine fibroids
  e ectopic pregnancy

3 Which of the following statements about patients with ascites is correct?
  a bacterial peritonitis can be prevented by prophylactic antibiotics
  b Leveen shunts may alleviate ascites associated with portal hypertension
  c pancreatitis may develop
  d may be relieved by spironolactone
  e paracentesis gives long periods of relief, often lasting several months

4 Which of the following statements about jaundiced patients with ascites is correct?
  a there is a low risk for hepatorenal syndrome because of splanchnic vasodilatation
  b coagulation profiles are usually normal
  c systemic blood volume is increased
  d renal blood flow is increased
  e there is a poor prognosis when operating for malignant disease

5 Which of the following cancers are commonly associated with the development of ascites?
  a lymphoma
  b endometrial
  c gastrointestinal stromal tumours
  d mucus-secreting villous adenoma
  e ovarian

70 Neck swellings

Rodney T. Judson

University of Melbourne and Royal Melbourne Hospital, Melbourne, Victoria, Australia

Introduction

Swellings or lumps in the neck are a common clinical problem. Patients presenting with neck lumps are likely to be fearful that they have cancer. Neck lumps in children are common although rarely malignant, but the situation is quite different in adults. Diagnostic efforts should aim for timely exclusion of malignancy with avoidance of lengthy trials of observation or repeated futile courses of antibiotics. Diagnosis of neck lumps involves applying basic clinical methods of assessment with history and physical examination followed by selected imaging techniques and finally sampling for cytological or histological examination.

Basic knowledge

Most neck lumps can, with a little experience, be diagnosed on clinical grounds by applying knowledge of head and neck anatomy and the clinical features of the usual pathological processes affecting the structures in the head and neck (see Chapter 41). The triangles of the neck and the distribution of lymph nodes are shown in Figure 70.1. The lymph nodes can be grouped into levels and these are shown in roman numerals. Level I consists of the submandibular and submental lymph nodes. Levels II, III and IV are respectively the upper, middle and lower jugular chain nodes. Level II also contains the jugulodigastric lymph node. Level V has the lymph nodes of the posterior triangle. The following facts should be remembered.

- The jugulodigastric lymph node, draining the oral cavity and oropharynx including the tonsils, is commonly enlarged in both inflammatory and malignant conditions. In children, tonsillitis is the most common cause of swelling in this region of the neck, in young adults glandular fever or lymphomatous conditions and in adults cancers often in obscure sites such as base of tongue or tonsil.
- The lymph nodes in the posterior triangle are all distributed along the spinal accessory nerve. These nodes are most commonly involved in benign infective conditions (usually viral) in children and young adults. Metastatic involvement of posterior triangle (spinal accessory) nodes may occur with nasopharyngeal cancer and skin cancers arising on the posterior scalp, neck and shoulder region.
- Skin cancer is common in Australia and both melanoma and squamous carcinoma can metastasise to the lymph nodes in the parotid gland, those in the submandibular triangle and those in the posterior triangle.
- Approximately 80% of lateral neck lumps in adults will be due to metastatic cancer. It is important to examine the possible anatomical primary sites that may lead to metastatic disease in the neck. These include the skin of the head and neck (including the scalp), the lip, the oral cavity, the oropharynx, the post-nasal space (especially in Asian patients), the larynx and hypopharynx.
- A solitary lump, low in the neck, deep to the sternomastoid muscle in the supraclavicular fossa (level IV) is likely to be a metastasis from a primary cancer below the clavicles, i.e. lung, oesophagus, stomach or pancreas.

Clinical assessment

History

Evaluation of the patient begins with a careful history, taking into account the age of the patient and the location of the swelling as either in the lateral or anterior compartment of the neck.

The rapidity of onset of the lump provides a valuable clue as to its likely cause. A short history of

Textbook of Surgery, Fourth Edition. Edited by Julian A. Smith, Andrew H. Kaye, Christopher Christophi and Wendy A. Brown.
© 2020 John Wiley & Sons Ltd. Published 2020 by John Wiley & Sons Ltd.

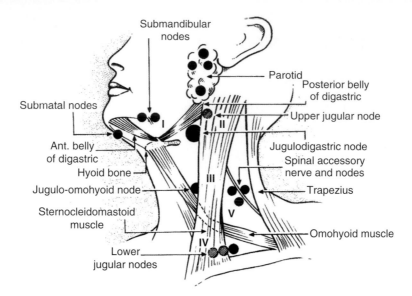

Fig. 70.1 The triangles, lymph node levels and normal lymph nodes in the neck. Diagram shows the main muscular anatomy of the neck with the sites of normal, named lymph node groups. In addition, the lymph nodes are subdivided into levels as follows: level I, submandibular and submental triangle; level II, upper jugular chain lymph nodes (including the jugulodigastric lymph node); level III, mid-jugular chain nodes (including the jugulo-omohyoid node); level IV, lower jugular chain lymph nodes (including lymph nodes overlying scalenus anterior muscle and those in the supraclavicular fossa); level V, lymph nodes of the posterior triangle, lying along the course of the spinal accessory nerve.

enlarged tender lymph nodes suggests an infective or inflammatory process, while multiple small non-tender nodes, particularly in the posterior triangle, suggests a subclinical viral infection. Long-standing swellings in children suggest a congenital problem, possibly cystic hygroma (also called lymphangioma). Painless progressive neck swellings in adults are strongly suggestive of a malignant origin.

It is also important to ascertain information about general systemic symptoms in potentially inflammatory processes and suspected lymphoma. Weight loss provides a clue to a malignant process arising below the clavicles that has metastasised to a lower cervical lymph node. Patients should also be questioned about possible past skin tumours, which may metastasise even years later to parotid, upper cervical, submental, submandibular and posterior triangle nodes.

Travel history and country of origin are important with regard to the possibility of tuberculosis. The racial group of the patient may also be important as nasopharyngeal cancer is not uncommon in Asian populations.

A smoking history is important as mucosal squamous cell carcinoma is rare in non-smokers but would be suspected as a primary site of tumour in a patient with a history of heavy tobacco and alcohol use who presents with a painless lateral neck lump.

Physical examination

The usual evaluation of lumps involves clarification of the following features: site, size, shape, consistency, deep and superficial attachments, the nature of the surface and the edge of the lump, and the presence of fluctuation, pulsation and translumination. In the neck the following issues apply.

- Which triangle of the neck is involved? Is the lump in the lateral or anterior compartment of the neck?
- Does it move with swallowing? This indicates it is deep to the pretracheal fascia and likely to be thyroid.
- Does it move with protrusion of the tongue? This applies to upper anterior neck lumps, and the physical sign refers to thyroglossal cysts.
- What is the relationship to the sternomastoid muscle? This point is important for differentiating lumps in the upper neck. Tumours in the tail of the parotid gland will lie superficial to the sternomastoid muscle and, when the muscle is contracted by turning the head to the opposite side, the lump will remain easily palpable. By contrast, an upper jugular chain (level II) lymph node, lying deep to the sternomastoid muscle, will become less obvious and more difficult to palpate when the head is turned to the opposite side.
- Where the neck lump appears to be an enlarged lymph node, either benign or malignant, the

possible sources of infection or malignancy should be searched for.

Sites of common anterior compartment swellings are shown in Figure 70.2.

Characteristic clinical features of common neck lumps

- Thyroglossal cyst: firm, tense, midline, painless swelling at or below the level of the hyoid bone, which elevates on tongue protrusion.
- Branchial cyst: smooth, often fluctuant swelling protruding at the anterior border of the sternomastoid muscle below the jaw (level II). There is usually rapid painless development of the swelling, although secondary infection and inflammation may occur.
- Plunging ranula: a soft, painless, cystic swelling in the submandibular region in continuity with a swelling in the floor of the mouth due to extravasation through the mylohyoid muscle of mucoid saliva from a disrupted sublingual gland.
- Submandibular salivary gland swelling: painful if due to obstruction of the gland or painless if due to usually benign tumour presenting as a swelling in the submandibular triangle of the neck, which is easily differentiated from a submandibular lymph node on bimanual palpation.
- Thyroid nodules: lower anterior compartment, slow-growing, painless usually smooth lumps which move upwards on swallowing.

- Metastatic lymph nodes from an upper aerodigestive tract primary squamous cell carcinoma: moderately fast growth of a painless, usually firm, often tethered upper lateral lump deep to sternomastoid occurring in middle-aged to elderly patients with a strong smoking history.
- Benign parotid tumour: long history of a very slow-growing, painless, firm, initially mobile lump behind the angle of the mandible lying superficial to the sternomastoid muscle.
- Carotid body tumour: very slow-growing, painless, deep lump in upper lateral neck with limited lateral mobility and characteristic transmitted pulsation.

Investigation

Fine-needle aspiration biopsy

Fine-needle aspiration biopsy, preferably ultrasound guided, is the single most important test in the evaluation of neck lumps, particularly in adults who may have malignancy. It is usually not necessary to carry out needle biopsy of tender lymph nodes in children; however, non-tender swellings in the central and lateral compartments of the neck in adolescents and adults should be evaluated by needle biopsy as the initial investigation. Metastatic malignancy can usually be diagnosed with a very high degree of accuracy. In general, reactive

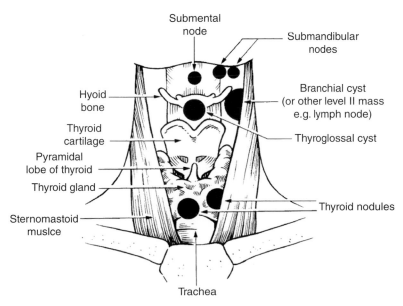

Submental node

Submandibular nodes

Hyoid bone

Branchial cyst (or other level II mass e.g. lymph node)

Thyroid cartilage

Pyramidal lobe of thyroid

Thyroglossal cyst

Thyroid gland

Sternomastoid muslce

Thyroid nodules

Trachea

Fig. 70.2 The anterior compartment of the neck showing the trachea, thyroid gland and laryngeal framework consisting of the thyroid cartilage and hyoid bone. This area is made up of the two anterior triangles of the neck, each consisting of the area bounded by the jaw superiorly, the anterior board of the sternomastoid muscle posteriorly and the midline medially. The sites of various anterior and anterolateral neck lumps are shown.

lymphadenopathy can be distinguished from lymphoma on needle biopsy; however, occasionally atypical lymphocytes are identified and it is necessary to carry out an excision biopsy of the node to clarify the diagnosis. Branchial cysts mainly occur in young adults and when they are aspirated thick creamy fluid is removed along with benign squamous cells. Under the microscope cholesterol crystals and cellular debris are visible. Branchial cysts occasionally occur in middle-aged adults, otherwise at risk of metastatic cancer, and it can sometimes be difficult to distinguish between metastatic squamous carcinoma with central necrosis and a benign branchial cyst on cytology. Excision of the lump may be necessary.

Fine-needle biopsy is also the best initial investigation of thyroid swellings. The presence of colloid, normal follicle cells and haemosiderin-laden macrophages is consistent with the presence of a colloid nodule. The presence of papillary structures raises the possibility of papillary carcinoma, while a finding of multiple follicle cells in a micro-follicular pattern with very little colloid indicates that the nodule is a solid follicular lesion. In this setting it is necessary to completely remove the lump (by thyroid lobectomy) to differentiate between follicular adenoma and follicular carcinoma.

Fine-needle aspiration biopsy is very safe and the risk of tumour implantation along the needle tract is negligible.

Ultrasound

Apart from the investigation of thyroid nodules, ultrasound is not particularly useful in the evaluation of head and neck lumps. Ultrasound can differentiate between solid and cystic masses and can indicate whether there are multiple enlarged lymph nodes or multiple nodules in the thyroid gland. While ultrasound is highly sensitive, being able to detect nodules or lymph nodes less than 1 cm in size, it is rarely diagnostic.

Computed tomography

Computed tomography (CT) is far more helpful than ultrasound in assisting with the diagnosis of neck swellings, especially when they are larger than 2 cm. CT scanning can provide an idea of the consistency of a lump along with its size and anatomical relations. Figure 70.3 shows a series of CT scans of common neck lumps, demonstrating the typical radiological appearance.

Excision biopsy

If a diagnosis cannot be confirmed on fine-needle aspiration biopsy, an excision biopsy may be necessary to confirm or exclude malignancy. Care should be taken not to spill tissue or break up a lymph node in the course of biopsy to prevent malignant cells being implanted into the surrounding tissue. The biopsy incision should be oriented in a natural skin crease in such a way that the biopsy scar can be excised in a subsequent operation. Furthermore, care must be taken not to damage related anatomical structures, for example the spinal accessory nerve in the posterior triangle and the marginal mandibular nerve in the submandibular triangle, during excision biopsy procedures.

Chest X-ray

Chest radiology is important in young adults, when lymphoma is the possibility, and in all adults. It may demonstrate mediastinal widening or primary or secondary lung neoplasms. It should be remembered that lung cancers are more common than mouth and throat cancers and that smokers, who are at risk for head and neck cancers, are also at risk of having lung cancer.

Treatment

The management algorithm for neck lumps is summarised in the decision-making flowchart shown in Figure 70.4. Following the history, physical examination and investigations, a diagnosis can usually be made. Excision of the lump may be necessary and if the lump proves to be benign, then excision biopsy is likely to be curative. Some benign lumps (e.g. reactive lymph nodes, lipomas and sebaceous cysts) may be simply observed and left untreated. Other benign lumps require removal for patient comfort, cosmesis or to avoid future problems. Branchial cysts, thyroglossal cysts, plunging ranulas, dermoid cysts, some lipomas and sebacous cysts, and benign salivary and thyroid swellings fall into this category.

Once a diagnosis of malignancy is made, definitive treatment is necessary. Lymphoma requires further staging investigations and treatment by chemotherapy, radiotherapy or both.

The treatment of metastatic cancer depends on the type of cancer and whether or not the primary site can be identified. If the primary cancer is found (skin or mucosa of the upper aerodigestive tract), it

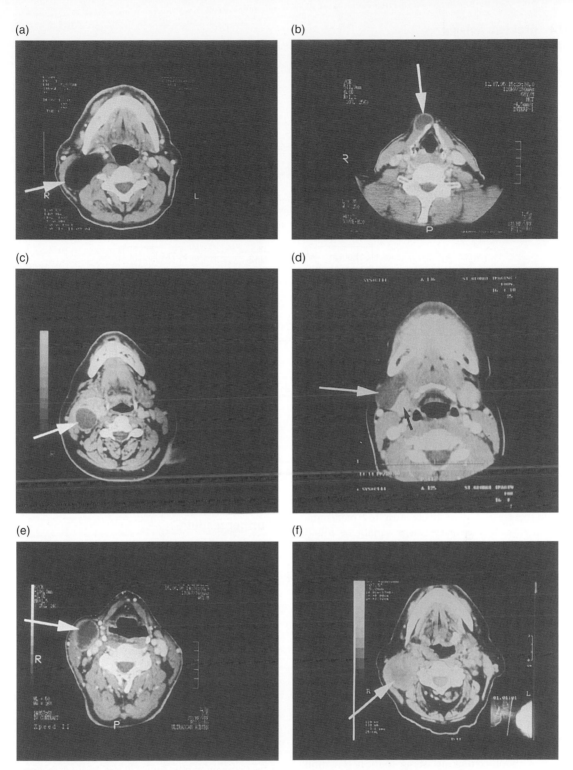

Fig. 70.3 Computed tomography scans showing common pathological processes in the neck. Each has a typical appearance. (a) Large lipoma neck deep to sternomastoid muscle and impinging on the parapharyngeal region. Note that the lesion is black, the same as the subcutaneous fat. (b) Thyroglossal cyst. Note the smooth-walled, well-circumscribed cystic mass closely attached to the anterior part of the right thyroid cartilage lamina. (c) Branchial cyst. This is a smooth-walled, well-circumscribed cyst deep to the sternomastoid muscle in the right neck in a young patient. It must be differentiated from metastatic squamous carcinoma with cystic degeneration [see (e)]. (d) Plunging ranula. This cystic swelling is more dense than subcutaneous fat but less dense than the soft tissue of the adjacent submandibular salivary gland (small black arrow). It is due to extravasation of mucoid saliva from the sublingual gland into the submandibular space and through the mylohoid muscle. (e) Metastatic squamous carcinoma of the neck with cystic degeneration. Note that this is also cystic but, unlike the branchial cyst (c), the wall of the lesion is irregular. (f) Large mass of metastatic squamous carcinoma in the right neck. This is a predominantly solid mass with little cystic degeneration.

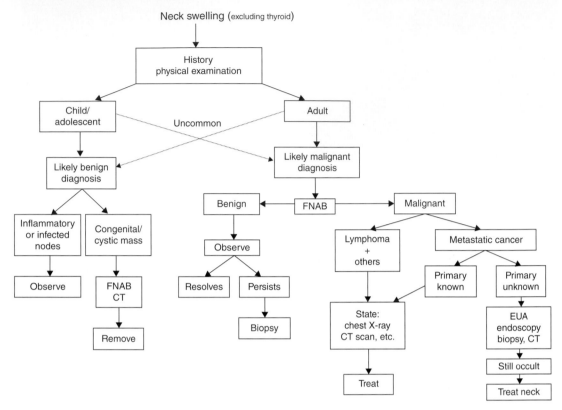

Fig. 70.4 Management algorithm for neck lumps. EUA, examination under anaesthetic; FNAB, fine-needle aspiration biopsy.

should be treated definitively with the metastatic neck disease. If a primary cancer cannot be found and the fine-needle aspiration biopsy shows metastatic squamous carcinoma, a thorough investigation of the upper aerodigestive tract should be carried out with biopsies of potential occult primary sites. These include the nasopharynx, tonsil and tongue base. When the primary site is still not identified, the metastatic disease in the neck requires treatment. This may be achieved by surgery or radiotherapy or sequential surgery followed by radiotherapy.

When metastatic adenocarcinoma is identified by fine-needle aspiration biopsy, an attempt should be made to determine whether there is a treatable primary cancer, for example in the thyroid gland or a salivary gland. Adenocarcinomas from the prostate, breast or abdomen that metastasise to the neck lymph nodes are not curable and so radical treatment to the neck may not be warranted. The operation used to treat cancer in the neck is called neck dissection. Neck dissections can vary in extent and according to which anatomical structures are preserved (see Chapter 41). Radiotherapy is given after surgery when multiple lymph nodes are involved with metastatic disease or when there is evidence of spread outside the lymph node capsule (extracapsular spread).

Further reading

Ridge JA, Glisson BS, Horwitz EM, Lango NM. Head and neck tumors. Cancer Network. Available at https://www.cancernetwork.com/articles/head-and-neck-tumors

Shah JP, Patel SG (eds) *Cancer of the Head and Neck*. Hamilton, Ontario: BC Decker, 2001, chapters 13–17.

Thompson LDR, Bishop JA (eds) *Head and Neck Pathology*, 3rd edn. Philadelphia: Elsevier, 2018.

MCQs

Select the single correct answer to each question. The correct answers can be found in the Answers section at the end of the book.

1 Which of the following neck lumps is always fluctuant?
   a carotid body tumour
   b haemangioma
   c cystic hygroma
   d branchial cyst
   e thyroid cyst

2 Which of the following is the most informative imaging technique for the assessment of a neck lump?
   a ultrasound
   b angiography
   c CT scan
   d positron emission tomography
   e radionuclide scanning

3 Which of the following statements about lymph node swellings in the neck is correct?
   a they are always characterised by their oval shape
   b multiple bilateral nodes are suspicious of lymphoma rather than a secondary carcinoma
   c are commonly associated with all skin cancers of the head and neck
   d cystic lymph node swellings are always benign
   e thyroglossal cysts do not move on swallowing

4 Which of the following is the most common cause of enlargement of the jugulodigastric lymph node in a child aged 9 years?
   a Hodgkin's disease
   b glandular fever
   c tonsillitis
   d non-Hodgkin's lymphoma
   e metastatic Wilms' tumour

5 Metastatic involvement of the posterior triangle nodes in the neck is most likely due to which of the following?
   a nasopharyngeal carcinoma
   b basal cell carcinoma of the shoulder region
   c laryngeal carcinoma
   d squamous cell carcinoma of the posterior scalp
   e carcinoma of the oesophagus

71 Acute airway problems

Stephen O'Leary

University of Melbourne and Royal Victorian Eye and Ear Hospital, Melbourne, Victoria, Australia

Introduction

Definition

Acute airway problems present as difficulty with breathing. The latter may be caused by anything that interferes with oxygenation, including respiratory or cardiovascular disease or pending airway obstruction. The surgeon's primary role is to recognise airway obstruction, determine its site within the airway, secure the airway and then treat the underlying problem.

Significance

Initial management of an acute airway problem can determine the patient's survival. A multidisciplinary team of ear, nose and throat surgeons, anaesthetists and intensivists is required to manage acute airway obstruction. The surgeon must always be prepared to provide an urgent surgical airway, such as a tracheostomy, if required.

Causes

Acute asthma and acute cardiovascular insufficiency (such as myocardial infarction) are medical causes of sudden breathing difficulty, and should always be considered. However, the emphasis of this chapter will be the identification and management of more surgically related aetiologies.

Airway obstruction, including foreign bodies

Airway obstruction can occur anywhere from the base of the tongue through to the trachea. Acute obstruction at the level of the tongue base is most often caused by *Ludwig's angina*, an infection of the floor of the soft tissue of the anterior neck. This arises from dental infection involving the molars, where the dental roots can extend beneath the mylohyoid muscle. Infection spreads into the subcutaneous tissue, pushing the tongue backwards, such that the tongue base obstructs the hypopharynx. Tumours of the base of the tongue can on occasion cause airway obstruction, but this is seldom an acute presentation. The lingual tonsils can cause acute airway obstruction in the context of acute infection or lymphoma.

Epiglottitis is the classical cause of airway obstruction in the supraglottic region. While once caused primarily by *Haemophilus influenzae* type B (HiB), since the widespread introduction of HiB vaccination *Streptococcus pneumoniae* is now the most prevalent pathogen. This too may change with the recent introduction of universal pneumococcal vaccination in children in many countries. The airway obstruction from epiglottitis is caused by swelling of the epiglottis, which narrows the glottic inlet. Critical swelling of the supraglottic airways, causing acute airway distress, may also occur during *anaphylaxis*, such as to bee stings or food allergens. It is important to recognise that these conditions can also cause acute bronchospasm and exudation of the airways, requiring management in addition to the pending airway obstruction. *Supraglottic neoplasia* may also present as an acute airway emergency. A supraglottic tumour can be relatively asympomatic, especially compared with laryngeal cancer, where the airway is narrower and vocal cord fixation is likely to cause other symptoms such as hoarseness of the voice.

Acute airway obstruction at the level of the vocal cords can arise from neoplasia, inhaled foreign bodies or following acute bilateral vocal cord palsy. The glottis is the narrowest part of the airway, which is why foreign bodies are prone to obstruct the airway at this level. Neoplasia may present as acute airway obstruction at the glottic level, but there have usually been previous indications of disease, such as bleeding, vocal hoarseness or stridor. Acute bilateral vocal cord palsy may arise from

Textbook of Surgery, Fourth Edition. Edited by Julian A. Smith, Andrew H. Kaye, Christopher Christophi and Wendy A. Brown.
© 2020 John Wiley & Sons Ltd. Published 2020 by John Wiley & Sons Ltd.

surgery to the neck, typically following total thyroidectomy. In neck surgery, the recurrent laryngeal nerve may be vulnerable. When paralysed, the vocal cords come to lie in a paramedian position, which significantly narrows the airway, causing acute obstruction. Caution must be exercised during surgery on one side of the neck, given that the contralateral vocal cord may be paralysed prior to surgery. Therefore, it is routine to assess vocal cord function prior to operations that may put the recurrent laryngeal nerve at risk, such as hemithyroidectomy or anterior surgical approaches to the cervical spine.

Acute airway obstruction at the level of the trachea is unusual, but can arise from a foreign body in the oesophagus, particularly in children. The posterior wall of the tracheal is soft tissue, with the oesophagus further posterior again. Therefore, a foreign body that is obstructed in the oesophagus can cause the anterior oesophageal wall to bulge forward, potentially causing a partial obstruction of the trachea. Foreign bodies further down the airway within a main bronchus can cause asthma-like symptoms. Consequently, a bronchial foreign body needs always to be considered in the newly diagnosed asthmatic, particularly if the clinical signs are unilateral. The right main bronchus is most likely that affected, because its vertical orientation will more likely impact a foreign body than the left.

Post-traumatic airway obstruction

The airway may be compromised after trauma due to bleeding within the respiratory tract, direct trauma to the neck, or burns. Although securing the airway is a first priority in stabilising the patient, it must be seen in the broader context of other trauma which, with airway trauma, may include injury to the cervical spine. In this situation, the need to keep the neck stable may necessitate the creation of a surgical airway.

Airway compromise may be delayed after burns, presenting 12–24 hours after the trauma. This means that high-dependency monitoring is essential for at least a day after the injury.

Post-surgical airway obstruction

The most serious risk associated with secondary bleeding following nasal surgery or a tonsillectomy is loss of control of the airway. Securing the airway in an obtunded or anaesthetised patient is made particularly difficult because in this situation blood in the pharynx obscures visualisation of the larynx. Most deaths associated with tonsillectomy are caused by loss of the airway during surgical interventions to control a post-tonsillectomy bleed. Another classical cause of airway compromise immediately after adenoidectomy or tonsillectomy is the so-called 'coroner's clot', namely a clot left in the postnasal space after the operation that is inhaled causing asphyxiation.

Bleeding into the neck following thyroidectomy carries a specific risk to the airway. This can lead to compression of the airway that can only be relieved by opening the wound and expelling the clot.

Nasal packs, placed to control nasal bleeding during epistaxis or after nasal surgery or trauma, can if displaced obstruct the airway. Airway compromise occurs when the pack is dislodged posteriorly when it may act as a foreign body. It has been said that all packs have been associated with at least one fatality, so their management is of paramount importance in postoperative care.

Assessment

The key to management of the airway is to establish the level of the obstruction within the airway. The clinical presentation will give a good indication of the site of the obstruction.

The presumptive diagnosis of an airway foreign body in a child is made on the basis of clinical suspicion. A sudden onset of airway distress, even when foreign body aspiration is not observed, is sufficient grounds to consider this diagnosis. As described, airway distress may arise after either swallowing or inspiring a foreign body. If the child is gagging, the foreign body is more likely to be in the hypopharynx. If a child cannot swallow their own saliva, then the foreign body is more likely to be in the oesophagus. Batteries are of particular concern, given that they can erode through the oesophageal or tracheal lumen within hours, so these must be removed immediately if suspected.

Additional points of history include a past history of asthma, recent exposure to an allergen or agent known to cause anaphylaxis, or a history of smoking. Progressive dysphagia, the production of blood, or dysphagia might suggest neoplasia.

Patients with airway obstruction at any location between the tongue base (e.g. Ludwig's angina) and the larynx are distressed when lying down. They present sitting upright and leaning forward to brace the shoulders in order to maintain an airway.

Stridor is a hallmark of airway obstruction, and its character can help to identify the site of lesion. Inspiratory stridor is caused by an obstruction above the level of the larynx. Biphasic stridor arises from an obstruction at the laryngeal level or in the trachea. Expiratory stridor typically arises from lower airway obstruction.

The upper airway is best assessed via nasendoscopy. This allows visualisation and identification of airway lesions to the level of the glottis, and can be done safely in most situations. Nasendoscopy is preferred over examination of the larynx with a mirror, especially in cases such as epiglottitis, when manipulation of the airway can precipitate airway obstruction.

Investigation

Imaging is seldom indicated in the initial management of acute airway distress. Lesions above the glottis can be diagnosed via nasendoscopy. Foreign bodies are managed on the basis of history alone. Unless an imaging facility is integrated into the emergency department, imaging can be dangerous and even life-threatening, because in the event of rapid progression to airway obstruction, resuscitation may not be available or optimal within the department. The better time for imaging is after the airway has been secured.

Securing the airway

Any patient with an acute airway should be given oxygen and their saturation monitored with pulse oximetry. Intravenous access is obtained, unless a foreign body is being considered in a young child when cannulation may cause distress and provoke acute airway obstruction.

In most cases, the airway will best be secured in the operating theatre, so early mobilisation of an *experienced* surgical team is necessary. Most patients will require admission to intensive care, so it is prudent to involve the intensivist in the early management.

Prior to surgery to secure the airway, it is important to keep the patient conscious if at all possible, so that the person can maintain their own airway. The management to achieve this will depend on the specific context. For example, during a post-tonsillectomy bleed there is blood in the airway and the patient may become hypovolaemic. Loss of consciousness will arise if the patient loses too much blood, so the best preoperative management (if the bleeding cannot be controlled by local measures such as cauterisation of the tonsillar bed) is to ensure that there has been adequate fluid resuscitation.

If an acute airway compromise occurs in a patient with a nasal pack, it must be assumed that the pack itself has dislodged into the pharynx and is causing the airway obstruction. An examination of the mouth may reveal a pack 'hanging down' from the post-nasal space. Urgent removal of a pack on the ward is required if it is believed to have become displaced. All packs should be taped to the face, providing a draw-cord for the rapid removal of the pack in this circumstance.

Prior to the definitive procedure to secure the airway, it is imperative that all preparations have been made meticulously. The time of greatest risk is when an anaesthetic is given, such that the patient ceases to maintain their own airway. This means that the team must have discussed all possible scenarios in advance, and have the equipment within the operating theatre before the procedure commences. This is a circumstance where team planning and communication is essential.

The approach to securing the airway will depend on the level of the obstruction. A nasopharyngeal tube will control an obstruction at the level of the tongue base. Awake fibre-optic intubation, when a nasotracheal tube is introduced through the vocal cords over an intubating bronchoscope that has been passed through the vocal cords, is an excellent technique when there is concern that the airway may be lost on induction of anaesthesia. This may be indicated for either supraglottic tumours, when there is blood in the airway, or with airway distress in a patient with a difficult (to intubate) airway.

A tracheostomy is required when there is a mass such as a tumour obstructing the glottis, in cases of bilateral vocal cord paralysis or when the neck cannot be moved as in suspected cervical fracture. Urgent tracheostomy under local anaesthesia remains the gold standard for the perilous airway that cannot be secured in another way. However, a range of new techniques can be considered as alternatives to conventional tracheostomy, such as kits for intubation via a cricothyroidotomy.

When the lesion is in the lower airway bronchoscopy will be required. Rigid bronchoscopes are designed to allow the surgeon to operate in one main bronchus and simultaneously ventilate the other. It is also possible to draw a foreign body into the rigid bronchoscope and thus remove it without the risk of causing further trauma to the airway on egress of the scope. These characteristics provide distinct advantages over flexible bronchoscopy in many circumstances.

Further reading

American College of Surgeons. *Advanced Trauma Life Support*, 10th edn. Chicago: ACS, 2018.

Kenneth M, Grundfast LF, Isolaco JL. The 10 commandments of management for acute upper airway obstruction in infants and children. *JAMA Otolaryngol Head Neck Surg* 2017;143:539–40.

MCQs

Select the single correct answer to each question. The correct answers can be found in the Answers section at the end of the book.

1 Which of the following is *not* appropriate management for a child with suspected epiglottitis?
   a provide oxygen
   b organise urgent review by ENT, anaesthetics and intensive care
   c examine the child's mouth with a tongue depressor
   d enquire about their immunisation status
   e keep the child calm, avoiding unnecessary distress

2 Which of the following types of airway support is most appropriate in the emergency setting for a patient with Ludwig's angina and acute airway distress?
   a Guedel's airway
   b nasopharyngeal airway
   c positive end-expiratory pressure
   d laryngeal mask
   e cricothyroidotomy

3 What is the safest way to maintain a patient's airway prior to definitive management (in the emergency setting) during a severe post-tonsillectomy bleed?
   a keep them conscious through adequate fluid resuscitation
   b anaesthetise and introduce a laryngeal mask
   c perform a cricothyroidotomy
   d introduce a nasopharyngeal airway
   e provide sedation

72 Dysphagia

Wendy A. Brown

Monash University Department of Surgery, Alfred Health, Melbourne, Victoria, Australia

Introduction

Definition

Dysphagia is defined as difficulty in swallowing. It is a common and important symptom. Two types are recognised.
- Oropharyngeal: involving the transfer of food from the mouth into the upper oesophagus.
- Oesophageal: involving the transport of food down the oesophagus and into the stomach.

Significance

The significance of this condition relates to its multitude of causes. Dysphagia may be caused by mild muscular spasm or incoordination due to psychological causes or, at the other end of the spectrum, may be progressive, associated with loss of weight and due to a malignant obstruction of the oesophagus. Consequently, any patient complaining of the symptom of dysphagia requires full investigation to exclude malignancy and to effectively treat the condition.

Incidence

Dysphagia is a common symptom affecting most individuals transiently at some time in life. One of the important causes of dysphagia is adenocarcinoma of the lower oesophagus. This is a tumour that is increasing in incidence throughout the western world and often occurs in middle-aged males. It is associated with long-standing gastro-oesophageal reflux and the development of Barrett's mucosa in the oesophagus (see Chapter 14).

Associated symptoms

There are a variety of other symptoms that may accompany the presence of dysphagia (Box 72.1). The presence of these symptoms helps in making a clinical diagnosis.

> **Box 72.1 Symptoms associated with dysphagia**
>
> - Chest pain due to reflux oesophagitis.
> - Odynophagia or pain on swallowing: may be associated with oesophagitis or oesophageal spasm.
> - Physical reflux of food or bile into the mouth, associated with severe gastro-oesophageal reflux.
> - Coughing and aspiration of food, indicating possible recurrent laryngeal nerve or bulbar palsy.
> - Palatal incompetence, with food being regurgitated through the nose on attempted swallowing: this is associated with bulbar palsy following cerebrovascular accident.
> - Loss of weight and anorexia often indicates a malignant obstruction.
> - Hoarseness of voice due to malignant involvement of the larynx or recurrent laryngeal nerve compression.

Causes of dysphagia

Problems within the mouth may cause difficulties in swallowing food. Simple examples include painful ulceration or abscesses, severe tonsillitis, lack of teeth, or deformity after head and neck surgery. Many of these problems can easily be excluded, and the causes of dysphagia that raise concern relate to the pharyngo-oesophageal area and the oesophagus itself (Box 72.2).

Diagnosis of the causes of dysphagia

Clinical features

The clinical history can give a major lead to the diagnosis of the cause of dysphagia. For example, difficulty in swallowing fluids rather than solids suggests a muscular incoordination problem.

Textbook of Surgery, Fourth Edition. Edited by Julian A. Smith, Andrew H. Kaye, Christopher Christophi and Wendy A. Brown.
© 2020 John Wiley & Sons Ltd. Published 2020 by John Wiley & Sons Ltd.

> ### Box 72.2 Causes of dysphagia
>
> **Pharyngo-oesophageal disorders**
> - Diminished pharyngeal propulsion: motor neurone disease; myasthenia gravis; cerebrovascular accident with dysfunction of ninth, tenth and twelfth cranial nerves.
> - Relaxation anomalies: upper oesophageal achalasia or cricopharyngeal spasm; cricopharyngeal bar.
> - Incoordination: cerebrovascular accident resulting in ninth, tenth and twelfth cranial nerve palsy; gastro-oesophageal reflux with cricopharyngeal spasm; pharyngeal diverticulum with cricopharyngeal spasm.
>
> **Oesophageal causes**
> - Motor disorders: achalasia of the oesophagus, diffuse oesophageal spasm, scleroderma.
> - Mechanical causes: luminal obstruction due to a large food bolus or bone impaction; mucosal strictures; webs (e.g. Patterson–Brown–Kelly syndrome, Schatzki ring); fibrous strictures (which result from inflammation and scarring from long-standing gastro-oesophageal reflux); ingestion of caustics (which causes fibrous scarring and predisposes to malignancy); squamous cell carcinoma; adenocarcinoma; rare tumours including lymphoma and metastatic tumours; benign tumours (rarely).
>
> **Extrinsic pressure on the oesophagus**
> - Retrosternal goitre.
> - Pharyngeal diverticulum.
> - Vascular abnormalities (right subclavian artery and right-sided aortic arteries).
> - Any mediastinal mass may cause oesophageal compression.

Progressive dysphagia for solids suggests a malignant cause. Dysphagia in the presence of retrosternal pain, associated with regurgitation of fluids, may indicate the stricture or carcinoma associated with reflux. Coughing or the aspiration of fluid into the larynx will give a guide to lesions such as cranial nerve palsies. Loss of weight is one of the most important accompanying symptoms of dysphagia and indicates malignancy. Lymph node and other masses may be palpable in the neck. However, physical signs are usually absent.

Investigations

Not all investigations need to be carried out in all cases of dysphagia, but in those cases where the diagnosis is difficult or obscure, the whole gamut of investigations may be needed (Figure 72.1).

Radiological examination

The barium swallow examination provides good views of the upper oesophagus and helps makes the diagnosis of pharyngeal pouch, webs and strictures. However, a negative barium swallow examination in the presence of persistent dysphagia demands further investigation by endoscopy.

Oesophagoscopy and gastroscopy

This is usually the first investigation for dysphagia and is done using flexible endoscopes under intravenous sedation. Care has to be taken to avoid perforation, particularly if there is suspicion of a pharyngeal pouch or if a stricture is present. The oesophagus is carefully examined for abnormalities such as inflammation and stricture. A stricture can usually be easily determined as being benign or malignant. In the absence of stricture, features such as oesophageal dilatation with food residue may suggest achalasia. Rarely, rigid oesophagoscopy is necessary if flexible endoscopy is unsuccessful.

Radiological staging

Radiological staging includes computed tomography (CT) examination and, less commonly, magnetic resonance imaging (MRI). This can help make the diagnosis in obscure cases, but its major role is helping to stage the extent of malignant disease.

Endoscopic ultrasound

Endoscopic ultrasound is a very effective way of diagnosing abnormalities within the oesophageal wall. It is not useful if there is a tight narrowing in the proximal oesophagus that prevents the passage of the instrument. It is the most precise method for detecting the depth of penetration of a cancer into or through the wall of the oesophagus.

Oesophageal transit studies

Radiolabelled (^{99m}Tc and ^{111}In) liquid, scrambled egg or porridge is given to the patient to swallow. A scintigram is performed and the level of tracer within the oesophagus is recorded at various time points until the tracer has disappeared. This allows a calculation to be made of the effectiveness of oesophageal transit.

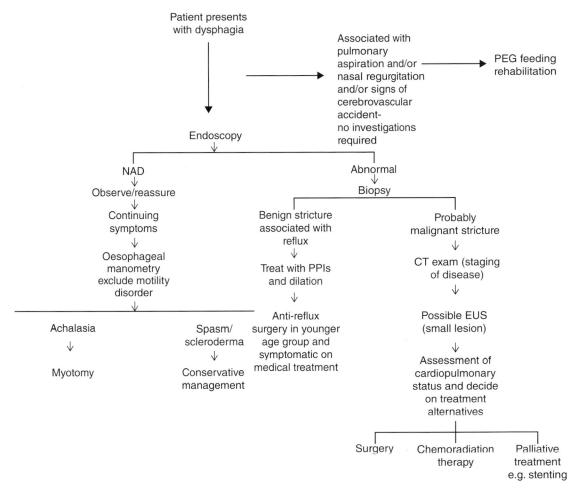

Fig. 72.1 Management of dysphagia. EUS, endoscopic ultrasound; PEG, percutaneous endoscopic gastrostomy; NAD, no abnormality detected; PPI, proton pump inhibitor.

Oesophageal motility studies

These are done via a multilumen catheter inserted into the oesophagus via the nose. Propulsive waves in the oesophagus can easily be measured and the response to a swallowing effort detected. Abnormalities can be identified in achalasia, scleroderma and oesophageal spasm.

Other investigations

Monitoring of pH over 24 hours will help document the degree of oesophageal reflux. Gastro-oesophageal reflux studies using nuclear scan techniques can be helpful in difficult cases. Reflux may be associated with fibrous stricture or oesophageal spasm, thereby causing dysphagia.

Specific causes of dysphagia

Transfer or pharyngo-oesophageal dysphagia

More correctly this is an inability to swallow and is associated with aspiration, coughing and nasal regurgitation. The common cause of this type of problem is a cerebrovascular accident. It produces major problems when attempting to rehabilitate a stroke patient with a bulbar palsy. Feeding via nasogastric tubes or gastrotomy tubes (percutaneous endoscopic gastrostomy) may be necessary to provide nourishment.

Motility disorders of the oesophagus

See Chapter 14.

Achalasia

Achalasia of the oesophagus is also known as car-diospasm and is often associated with the presence of a so-called mega-oesophagus. It occurs most commonly in the young to middle-aged (30–60 years). The incidence is 1 in 100 000 people. There are associated neural abnormalities in the ganglia but the exact cause is not known. The dysphagia is intermittent, but progressive in the longer term. It is detected by the patient as being suprasternal in position and occurs for both liquids and solids. Regurgitation is postural and aspiration pneumonitis may occur. Usually only weak oesophageal contractions occur and the condition is painless. In 10% of cases a condition known as 'vigorous achalasia' exists. This is regarded as an early stage of the disease and is associated with pain. Oesophageal manometry reveals markedly elevated lower oesophageal sphincter pressures and diminished oesophageal contractions.

Complications

In the chronic long-standing case, weight loss and chest pain occur. Pulmonary disease from aspiration of oesophageal content and the development of carcinoma within the dilated oesophagus are significant complications.

Diagnosis and treatment

Chest X-ray, barium meal and manometry examinations help to confirm the diagnosis, which may be difficult to determine. Treatment is by surgical division (myotomy) of the hyperactive lower oesophageal sphincter, usually approached laparoscopically. A thoracoscopic approach can also be used. Reflux is a complication after myotomy and an anti-reflux procedure at the time of surgery is commonly performed. An alternative treatment is by manometric dilatation using a balloon placed across the hypertensive lower oesophageal sphincter, which is then expanded causing disruption of the sphincter. The results of both methods of treatment are good in about 90% of cases.

Diffuse oesophageal spasm

This is usually a primary disorder but may be secondary and associated with:
- peptic oesophageal reflux
- ingestion of irritants
- emotion and tension
- possibly an underlying carcinoma.

Symptoms

The patient complains of dysphagia that is often worse for liquids, is intermittent and is noted in the mid-sternal region. Pain, which is retrosternal and severe, is also common, is sometimes misdiagnosed as being cardiac in origin, and is worse under emotional stress. There is rarely any weight loss. There is marked belching and other indigestion-type symptoms.

Diagnosis

The diagnosis is made on X-ray, which shows tertiary contractions in the oesophagus, and motility studies, which show simultaneous, vigorous, repetitive waves in the oesophageal body when the lower oesophageal sphincter relaxes.

Therapy

Therapy is generally simple, using simple bougienage without rupturing oesophageal muscle, and medication.

Scleroderma

This systemic connective tissue disorder is characterised by muscle atrophy, dilatation of the oesophagus and smooth muscle fibrosis. It is diagnosed by motility studies that show a non-contractile oesophagus. Oesophageal reflux is often a contributing and secondary factor causing strictures. No satisfactory therapy exists.

Chagas' disease

This is a parasitic infection, common in South America. It produces destruction of the ganglia of the oesophagus and an achalasia-type stricture.

Mechanical causes of dysphagia

The mechanical causes of dysphagia are those that are most commonly the province of the surgeon. The diagnosis depends on taking a clinical history and often requires a full investigation (see previous section) to make the diagnosis. The difficult diagnosis is often between a benign and a malignant stricture in the oesophagus (see Chapter 14). Repeated biopsies may be necessary to make this distinction. Malignant obstruction in the lower oesophagus demands either extensive surgery or combined surgery and chemoradiation if curative therapy is indicated. However, in about 30% of patients with malignancy, palliative treatment only is indicated. Intubation of the tumour or laser ablation are two effective methods of palliation.

Further reading

Gidwaney NG, Bajpai M, Chokhavatia SS. Gastrointestinal dysmotility in the elderly. *J Clin Gastroenterol* 2016; 50:819–27.

Moawad FJ, Cheng E, Schoepfer A *et al.* Eosinophilic esophagitis: current perspectives from diagnosis to management. *Ann NY Acad Sci* 2016:1380:204–17.

Philpott H, Sweis R. Hiatus hernia as a cause of dysphagia. *Curr Gastroenterol Rep* 2017;19:40.

Schlottmann F, Neto RM, Herbella FA, Patti MG. Esophageal achalasia: pathophysiology, clinical presentation and diagnostic evaluation. *Am Surg* 2018; 84: 467–72.

MCQs

Select the single correct answer to each question. The correct answers can be found in the Answers section at the end of the book.

1 Which of the following symptoms of dysphagia is *incorrect*?
   a very common and thus can be ignored in most cases
   b may be associated with reflux symptoms
   c may be associated with significant pain
   d can present acutely with total obstruction of the oesophagus
   e may be associated with diminished pharyngeal propulsion

2 Which of the following causes of dysphagia is *incorrect*?
   a classified as pharyngo-oesophageal and oesophageal
   b pharyngo-oesophageal causes are often neurological in origin, e.g. cerebrovascular accident
   c associated with altered motility of the oesophagus
   d achalasia is a disease primarily of the oesophageal musculature and is coexistent with gastro-oesophageal reflux
   e associated with an adenocarcinoma of the mucosal lining

3 Which of the following methods for identifying the causes of dysphagia is *incorrect*?
   a upper gastrointestinal endoscopy
   b barium swallow examination
   c upper abdominal ultrasound examination
   d CT examination of the chest
   e oesophageal manometry

4 With regard to patients with dysphagia, which of the following complaints is *incorrect*?
   a regurgitation of fluid and food when recumbent at night
   b difficulty with swallowing fluids more than solid food
   c difficulty with swallowing solid food more than liquids
   d may have significant weight loss
   e may have no weight loss
   f their partner may complain of snoring

5 Which of the following causes of dysphagia is *incorrect*?
   a benign strictures in the oesophagus
   b squamous carcinoma of the oesophagus
   c pharyngeal diverticulum
   d oesophageal spasm
   e uncomplicated sliding hiatus hernia

73 Leg swelling and ulcers

Alan C. Saunder[1], Steven T.F. Chan[2] and David M.A. Francis[3]

[1] Monash University and Surgery and Interventional Services Program, Monash Health , Melbourne, Victoria, Australia
[2] University of Melbourne and Western Health, Melbourne, Victoria, Australia
[3] Department of Urology, Royal Children's Hospital, Melbourne, Australia and Department of Surgery, Tribhuvan University Teaching Hospital, Kathmandu, Nepal

Introduction

Leg swelling and leg ulcers are increasingly common patient presentations, especially in our ageing populations. Most frequently, venous dysfunction, in the form of swelling, ulcers and/or varicose veins, may be immediately obvious in a coexistent way. Conversely, ulceration may occur without swelling that the patient has noticed. In either situation, it is imperative to diagnose all contributing factors and determine if the leg presentation is part of a systemic condition(s) or a local leg issue only. This chapter outlines the common causes of both leg swelling and ulceration, acknowledging that there is some clinical overlap between the two presentations and with arterial disease (see Chapter 55). This is especially the case with diabetic foot disease, presenting as Charcot foot or with foot ulcers.

It is essential that a thorough history and examination is done looking at the patient as a whole as well as the afflicted limb(s). This is a very appropriate scenario to apply the following classic surgical paradigm.
- What is it (i.e. the diagnosis)?
- What else might it be (differential diagnosis)?
- What are you going to do about it (the plan for investigations and management)?

Such an approach is an easy way to communicate with patients, families and staff what the plan is to establish a diagnosis and therefore treat the swelling and/or ulcer.

Leg swelling

Leg swelling generally occurs because of an abnormal accumulation of interstitial fluid – oedema – of the lower extremity and it may be bilateral or

---

Box 73.1 Commoner causes of leg swelling

Systemic causes
- Congestive cardiac failure
- Renal disease
- Hypoproteinaemia

Local causes
Venous conditions
- Occlusion or compression: deep vein thrombosis, abdominal or pelvic tumour, trauma, ligation, inferior vena cava plication, retroperitoneal fibrosis, ascites
- Stagnation: dependent position
- Valve incompetence: most common and need to determine superficial, deep or a combination
- Arterialisation: arteriovenous fistula

Lymphatic causes
- Primary: congenital lymphoedema, lymphoedema praecox, lymphoedema tarda
- Secondary: neoplastic obstruction, irradiation damage, surgical excision, insect bite

Inflammatory causes
- Acute infections (streptococci, staphylococci)
- Chronic infections (fungi, filariasis, mycobacteria)

---

unilateral. The commoner causes of leg swelling are summarised in Box 73.1. Lesions that result in discrete leg swellings are not discussed in this chapter. Systemic causes generally result in bilateral leg swelling and these causes should be excluded. Localised causes may result in either unilateral or bilateral swelling depending on the site of the 'localised problem'. The most common localised cause of a unilateral leg swelling is venous disease. Lymphoedema is almost always secondary to a

---

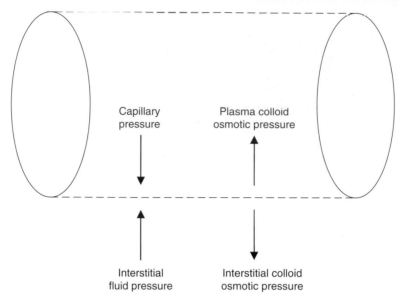

Fig. 73.1 Pressures influencing net movement of fluid in and out of capillaries. Source: Guyton AG, Hall JE. *Textbook of Medical Physiology*, 10th edn. Philadelphia: WB Saunders, 2000. Reproduced with permission of Elsevier.

disorder of lymph nodes since primary lymphoedema is a rarity (see Chapter 57).

Pathophysiology of leg swelling

There is normally a balance between the inflow and outflow of extracellular fluid as blood flows through capillaries. Figure 73.1 shows the four basic forces that determine the rate of accumulation of interstitial fluid:

- capillary pressure
- interstitial fluid pressure
- plasma colloid osmotic pressure
- interstitial fluid colloid osmotic pressure.

The capillary and interstitial fluid pressure are opposed by an oncotic gradient that is determined by the different protein concentrations of the interstitial and intravascular fluid compartments. About 90% of the fluid that leaks from the capillaries is estimated to return to the post-capillary venules, while the remaining 10% enters the lymphatic system.

Oedema can be caused by the following.

- Increased filtration pressure as a result of:
  - Arteriole dilatation
  - Venule constriction
  - Raised venous pressure
- Reduced oncotic pressure:
  - Hypoproteinaemia
  - Accumulation in interstitial space
- Increased capillary permeability
- Reduced lymphatic removal of exudate

Systemic causes of leg swelling

Congestive cardiac failure

Congestive cardiac failure (right heart failure) is a common cause of bilateral leg swelling. Venous pressure is increased due to the failing right heart, as demonstrated clinically by raised jugular and central venous pressures. Consequently, post-capillary venous pressure and intravascular hydrostatic pressure are increased. Also, fluid may be retained because of reduced glomerular filtration and secondary aldosteronism. Excessive fluid intake, which may be iatrogenic, and hypoproteinaemia also contribute to leg swelling.

Renal disease

Renal failure results in the inability to excrete water and expansion of the extracellular fluid compartment, unless fluid restriction is instituted. If renal disease is complicated by the nephrotic syndrome, hypoproteinaemia is an additional factor contributing to leg swelling.

Hypoproteinaemia

A low concentration of plasma proteins, particularly albumin, is a common cause of leg swelling in hospitalised patients. Hypoproteinaemia reduces plasma osmotic pressure and so alters the balance of opposing forces across the capillary wall in favour of fluid leaking out of capillaries into the interstitial space. Hypoproteinaemia causes a generalised oedema, but is more apparent in regions of increased hydrostatic pressure, especially gravity-dependent limbs. Hypoproteinaemia is due to increased protein loss (extensive burns, tissue catabolism, proteinuria, protein-losing enteropathy, gastrointestinal fistulas, paracentesis), decreased synthesis by the liver (acute or chronic liver disease, malnutrition, malabsorption) or fluid overload.

Local causes of leg swelling

Venous disorders

Venous hypertension or obstruction increases intravascular hydrostatic pressure and reduces movement of fluid into the venous end of capillaries, with subsequent accumulation of dilute interstitial fluid. Varicose veins secondary to saphenofemoral incompetence can be associated with lower leg oedema. Furthermore, failure of the normal calf muscle pump, due to valvular incompetence or deep vein obstruction, results in failure of the normal reduction of hydrostatic pressure within superficial veins that occurs with exercise. Incompetence of several perforating veins leads to only mild oedema because the calf pump mechanism can still lower superficial venous pressures to some extent. Gross unilateral oedema results from occlusion, such as after an occlusive iliofemoral venous thrombosis or stenosis of the femoral or iliac veins. Bilateral swelling results from occlusion or extrinsic pressure on the inferior vena cava or major pelvic veins and is uncommon. Deep vein thrombosis is discussed in Chapter 57.

Lymphatic disorders

Lymphatic obstruction reduces the clearance of fluid and protein from the interstitial space, resulting in an increased amount of interstitial fluid with a relatively high protein concentration (lymphoedema). Lymphoedema usually develops slowly. The high protein content of lymphoedema eventually leads to subcutaneous fibrosis. Movement of fluid and protein in and out of capillaries is essentially normal. Lymphatic disorders are discussed in Chapter 57.

Inflammatory disorders

As part of the inflammatory response to injury, vaso-active amines and peptides are released from damaged cells and produce vasodilatation and increased capillary permeability. Fluid and plasma proteins, in addition to cells, leak out of capillaries into the interstitial space and cause swelling. Oedema may be limited to the inflamed area but may drain by gravity to the dependent part of the limb, often causing circumferential swelling of the leg and swelling of the dorsum of the foot. Repeated acute infections (cellulitis, lymphangitis) or chronic infections (fungal infections, filariasis, tuberculosis) produce secondary lymphoedema because of lymphatic obstruction. Lymphoedema and chronic leg swelling may be complicated by infection, which increases swelling of the limb.

Assessment of the swollen leg

As with all medical problems, assessment relies on the history, examination and appropriate investigations.

History

Specific inquiry is made for symptoms suggesting disorders of the heart (chest pain, dyspnoea, paroxysmal nocturnal dyspnoea, palpitations, haemoptysis, hypertension), gastrointestinal tract (abdominal pain and distension, indigestion, vomiting, haematemesis, diarrhoea, rectal bleeding, alcohol intake, drug ingestion, jaundice) and kidneys (back pain, dysuria, haematuria, nocturia, urine volume, frothy urine, tiredness, lethargy). Recent nutritional intake must be considered, especially in hospitalised patients who may become malnourished because of long periods of anorexia, nausea, vomiting, gastrointestinal dysfunction, or fasting for investigations and treatment. Similarly, in hospitalised patients, the volume of intravenous fluid infusions must be reviewed. The duration and rapidity of onset of leg swelling must be ascertained. Family history of similar problems may be relevant. Past history of varicose veins, malignant disease, radiotherapy, surgery, previous episodes of leg swelling or infection, or deep vein thrombosis (perhaps complicating surgery or childbirth) must be identified.

Examination

A full physical examination must be performed. General points of examination include the patient's nutritional status, and abnormal pigmentation of the skin, sclera and mucous membranes. Look at the abdomen and lower limbs for the presence of suspicious skin lesions and vascular abnormalities, surgical scars, and signs suggestive of radiotherapy (skin atrophy, telangiectasia, scaly skin).

Swelling of one or both legs is confirmed by inspection and measurement at a designated point. Remember that the swollen limb may be tender to touch. Pitting oedema is determined by slow gentle pressure over the medial malleolus or the shaft of the tibia. Lymphoedema is characterised by non-pitting swelling of the leg and the foot, as well as swelling of the toes. Intradermal vesicles, weeping of the skin, dry and scaly skin and an 'elephant skin' appearance occur in long-standing cases. The legs are examined for signs of venous disease (varicose veins, venous flares, pigmentation, lipodermatosclerosis, eczema, venous ulceration). An arteriovenous fistula is characterised by a pulse, thrill and machinery bruit over dilated veins. The hip, knee and ankle joints should be examined, together with the popliteal fossa. Regional lymph node groups must be examined. Rectal and pelvic examinations may be indicated.

Signs of inflammation (erythema, heat, tenderness, swelling, reduced movement) with or without infection (pus) should be noted. Tinea pedis between the toes and on the soles of the feet leads to cracking and breakdown of the skin, and may produce the portal of entry for bacteria causing cellulitis of the legs and feet (see Chapter 9).

Investigations

These should include full blood examination, liver function tests and measurement of erythrocyte sedimentation rate and levels of serum creatinine, urea and electrolytes, glucose, plasma proteins and albumin. An ECG and chest X-ray are performed. Urinalysis for sugar, blood and protein is performed. Abdominal ultrasound scan or computed axial tomography is required to define organomegaly or tumour mass if this is suspected.

If venous disease is suspected, a Doppler study is performed to detect patency and the pattern of underlying venous incompetence. Venography is rarely required but can be used in a targeted way to demonstrate the deep veins, the extent of stenosis or obstruction, the presence of collateral circulation and some endovenous treatment options.

Lymphangiography may be attempted when venous and other diseases have been excluded. This is done using a nuclear medicine technique with technetium which provides good functional assessment of lymphatic drainage.

Treatment

The treatment of leg swelling depends on the cause. Cardiac, hepatic and renal disorders are treated

along medical lines. Protein deficiency is treated by nutritional supplementation, either orally, enterally or intravenously (see Chapter 7). Infective conditions are treated with antibiotics with or without surgical drainage. Specific treatments of venous and lymphatic diseases are discussed in Chapter 57. Non-specific measures that help in the treatment of the swollen leg include elastic support stockings, elevation and massage.

Elastic stockings

The use of elastic stockings is described in Chapter 57.

Elevation

Simple elevation of the leg relieves oedema by reducing intravascular hydrostatic pressure. The principle is to avoid having the swollen leg in a dependent position and to avoid having it still. First, patients must keep off their feet as much as possible, and elevate the affected limb above the level of the hip whenever sitting. The limb should be raised above the horizontal whenever possible and, ideally, the patient should lie on the floor with the legs vertically against a wall for 15–20 minutes several times each day. This may not be practical for many patients but should be advised and encouraged. Second, when patients are standing, they should avoid standing still and should be encouraged to exercise the calf muscles and to walk with a support stocking (usually calf length will suffice). Third, the foot of the bed should be elevated by at least 10 cm.

Massage

Massage of the limb towards the hip, using a surface skin oil, reduces subcutaneous tissue swelling and helps keep the skin and subcutaneous tissues soft and supple. This is especially so with lymphoedema.

Diuretic therapy and fluid restriction

Diuretic therapy and fluid restriction are indicated in congestive heart failure and in some renal and hepatic diseases, and may be of value in some cases of limb swelling due to local causes. However, care must be taken not to induce significant electrolyte abnormalities or dehydration.

Venous treatment options

The duplex scan may have disclosed underlying issues in a number of cases and, if suitable, the patient's venous status can be improved in many instances by ablating incompetent superficial veins, especially the great saphenous vein, using one of laser, radiofrequency, glue and less often surgery. Major deep vein thromboses, especially acute iliofemoral disease, may be suitable for endovenous treatment and subsequent stenting under the cover of anticoagulation.

Leg ulcers

Epidemiological studies have shown that leg ulcers are present in 3–4% of the population aged more than 65 years old. Management of such ulcers is often suboptimal and recurrence is common because the underlying pathophysiological mechanisms have not been correctly diagnosed and therefore treated comprehensively. Consequently, ulcers result in considerable disability and expense to the patient and the healthcare system. Improved results will follow a rigorous diagnostic approach, more specialised medical care and appropriate compression to facilitate healing, in the commonest cause, namely venous incompetence.

Aetiology and pathogenesis

Venous disease

More than 80% of lower leg ulcers will have a venous component and understanding normal venous return and hence its perturbations will allow targeted treatment to facilitate rapid healing in most cases. Musculo-venous pumps, the most important of which is the calf muscle pump, augment venous return to the heart. The pumps work best when the veins are patent, the valves competent and the pump used by regular exercise.

Venous insufficiency results from failure of the normal mechanisms returning venous blood from the lower limb, particularly incompetence of valves. Incompetence of the deep venous system may follow deep vein thrombosis (DVT) or occur spontaneously. Incompetence of the venous valves causes a reduction in the volume of blood expelled by the calf muscle pump. The calf muscle pump may also be impaired by limited ankle joint mobility caused by arthritis. With increasing obesity and a sedentary lifestyle in an ageing population, the calf muscle pump may be simply not used.

The common pathway is ambulatory venous hypertension, which leads to soft tissue damage in the leg and eventually ulceration. The overlap of leg swelling and ulceration is considerable due to venous incompetence.

Development of collateral pathways

Small venules and veins dilate in the subcutaneous venous system and may collateralise. The walls of these veins are fragile and the veins are exposed to high pressure, so they may bleed externally or rupture in the subcutaneous tissue, leading to skin pigmentation.

Impaired nutrition of the skin and subcutaneous tissue

With sustained ambulatory venous hypertension in the lower extremity, there is impaired tissue perfusion. Atrophy and fibrosis results in progressive induration of the subcutaneous tissue of the lower one-third of the leg, giving an 'inverted champagne bottle' appearance.

Ulcers

Minor injury, which may be unrecognised, can initiate leg ulceration. Healing is poor because of the impaired nutrition of the tissues and tissue breakdown follows. Ulceration can be compounded by infection, particularly streptococcal cellulitis, coincident arterial disease or diabetes.

Arterial disease

This is the predominant cause of about 20% of leg ulcer cases and a contributing factor, with venous disease, in a further 20%. As arterial insufficiency can often be corrected, it is important that arterial perfusion is checked even if the clinical appearance of an ulcer is typically venous.

Other causes

There is a miscellaneous group that comprises only 10% of patients with ulcers. Ulcers associated with hypertension (Martorell's ulcers) occur predominantly on the anterior and lateral aspects of the calf. The ulcers are distinguished from arterial ulcers by their site. Multiple ulcers may occur and may be painful. Treatment is conservative with healing often delayed.

A common injury is a fall that lifts a distally based skin flap which can leave a post-traumatic ulcer.

Diabetic foot ulcers are discussed in Chapter 55 and highlight the importance of considering peripheral neuropathy in the genesis of foot ulcers.

Several systemic diseases are associated with leg ulceration including rheumatoid arthritis, inflammatory bowel disease and vasculitis.

Finally, but most important, malignant change (so-called Marjolin's ulcer), usually squamous cell carcinoma, should be suspected in any long-standing ulcer or one with an atypical appearance or that fails to heal despite adequate management. Biopsy of the ulcer edge is then indicated.

Clinical presentation

Chronic venous insufficiency

The patient presents with ulcers, often recurrent, and the history may extend over many years. The ulcers may be painful in the early stages, relieved by elevation of the leg. The most common site is on the medial side of the lower third of the calf. On examination, the ulcer is usually irregular in outline and surrounded by eczematous and/or pigmented skin with a base of granulation tissue. Careful serial measurement, ideally using digital photography, of the size of the ulcer will help determine if healing or progressive ulceration is occurring.

Arterial disease

The ulcer may be anywhere on the lower leg, characteristically over bony prominences such as the malleoli. The pain is worse when the leg is elevated and relieved when the leg is hanging down. The ankle pulses are absent.

Investigations

General investigations

These should include a full blood examination, fasting blood glucose and serum albumin estimation.

With atypical ulcers or non-healing ulcers, markers for connective tissue disorders such as rheumatoid serology should be considered and a biopsy is mandatory.

Local investigations

Measurement of ankle blood pressure

Measurement of the ankle–brachial pressure index (ABI) should be performed to check the arterial circulation. If the ABI is abnormal, duplex ultrasound should be used to determine the site and severity of any arterial disease present. Angiography can then be performed on an intention-to-treat basis, aiming to restore arterial perfusion to normality by angioplasty or bypass surgery.

Venous duplex ultrasound

This test has supplanted venography in the assessment of chronic venous insufficiency. The veins are examined to determine the venous anatomy, patency and valvular competence. It is important to determine the pattern of venous incompetence present, as superficial incompetence can be treated very efficaciously.

Treatment

The principles of treatment have come to be applied more aggressively in recent years (Box 73.2). Such treatment should be directed to correcting the underlying cause of the ulcer, optimising healing and preventing recurrence.

Box 73.2 Management algorithm for leg ulcers

1 Define and treat cause
Measure ABI
If ABI <0.5
   Do not apply compression bandaging
   Arterial duplex scan
   Improve arterial inflow
   Angioplasty ± bypass surgery
If ABI >0.9
   Apply compression: class I–II surgical stocking or four-layered banding

2 Determine venous patency and competence
Venous duplex scan
Check deep vein patency and competence
Check saphenofemoral and short-saphenopopliteal competence

If saphenofemoral and/or short-saphenopopliteal veins incompetent, and the deep veins are patent, consider surgery to correct superficial venous incompetence
If iliac vein stenosed/occluded, consider stenting or venous bypass

3 Biopsy
Long-standing ulcers
Ulcers with atypical appearance
Ulcers that recur despite adequate initial management
Remember, a leg ulcer may be malignant *de novo*

4 Prevent recurrence
Nutritional support
Perseverance with surgical stocking support

Treatment of the underlying cause

Venous insufficiency

An immediate concern is to control oedema of the subcutaneous tissue and to minimise the sequelae. This is best done by keeping the patient ambulatory by wearing elastic stockings or using compression bandaging, although occasionally bed rest with elevation of the leg is required. Neglected or inadequate lower extremity compression is the commonest reason for failed healing or early ulcer recurrence. Elderly patients need considerable physical and emotional support to help them persevere with stockings, particularly for those with arthritis or limited mobility. It is essential that an adequate arterial supply is proven before instituting compression therapy.

Surgery has a limited place in relieving venous obstruction and restoring valvular competence. Targeted surgery, using the duplex as a 'road map', can deal with superficial venous insufficiency or perforating veins. Superficial varicose veins should be treated, unless they are forming important collateral around obstructed deep veins. Patients with only superficial incompetence and normal deep veins are an important group to identify as their tendency to ulceration can be largely controlled by a combination of endovenous or surgical procedures. Incompetent calf perforating veins, communicating between the deep and superficial venous systems, can be treated by sclerotherapy or by endoscopic surgery.

Attempts have been made to relieve venous obstruction or restore valve function by surgical means. The most successful procedure has been femoro-femoral vein bypass to relieve unilateral iliac venous obstruction. Procedures to restore valve function by applying cuffs to restore valvular competence or autotransplantion of vein segments containing competent valves into an incompetent deep vein have met with very limited success. These measures are applicable to only about 1–2% of patients with venous ulceration.

Skin grafting can hasten healing, but in almost all patients it is unnecessary. Performance of a skin graft does not remove the need for the other measures described; in particular, the need to wear supporting stockings remains an essential component of postoperative care.

The most important therapeutic measure for healing venous ulcers, supported by level 1 evidence, is external compression preferably by stockings or, alternatively, well-applied elastic bandaging. The choice of dressing is far less important, other than to cover the ulcer and protect the skin. A variety of elastic stockings are now available with application devices to make it easier for patients to put them on. These stockings are designed to provide graduated compression, greatest around the ankle, less proximally. Graduated compression should be applied with a 40 mmHg pressure gradient at the ankle level, tapering to 20 mmHg at the knee. The ankle arterial pressure should be measured before compression bandaging is applied to ensure that there will be no compromise of arterial inflow. In most cases a below-knee stocking provides adequate support.

Provide conditions to allow healing

Careful attention should be given to nutrition as elderly immobile patients with painful ulcers may neglect themselves.

Treat infection

In addition to these general measures, local skin care and antibiotic therapy for any associated cellulitis will help control infection and provide optimal local conditions for healing. It is important to distinguish between invasive infection and contamination of the wound. Prolonged courses of antibiotics should not be given because this will usually result in colonisation of the wound by strains of bacteria resistant to the antibiotics.

Provide and maintain optimum conditions for healing

The two major elements of this are to remove dead tissue and to apply appropriate dressings. Dead tissue can be removed enzymatically or surgically. Although correct application of external compression is the most important therapeutic measure, dressings are important as wounds heal best in warm moist conditions. There are now a large number of products available to provide and maintain optimum conditions for healing. The choice of dressing will depend on the depth of the wound and the amount of exudate.

Prevention of recurrence

Treatment that results in healing of an ulcer is not sufficient. The next objective is to prevent recurrence by general measures, such as lifestyle change encouraging greater mobility and weight loss, and local measures, the most important of which is perseverance with surgical stocking support.

Arterial disease

The treatment of arterial disease and diabetic foot ulcers is covered in Chapters 55 and 58.

Further reading

Fitridge RA, Thompson MM (eds) *The Mechanisms of Vascular Disease: A Reference Book for Vascular Specialists.* Adelaide: University of Adelaide Press, 2011.
Perler BA, Sidawy AN (eds) *Rutherford's Vascular Surgery and Endovascular Therapy*, 9th edn. Philadelphia: Elsevier, 2018.

MCQs

Select the single correct answer to each question. The correct answers can be found in the Answers section at the end of the book.

1 Which of the following causes of bilateral leg swelling with pitting oedema s *incorrect*?
   a reduced lymphatic removal of exudate
   b increased capillary permeability
   c decreased filtration pressure at the arteriolar end
   d reduced oncotic pressure
   e excessive fluid intake

2 A 75-year-old female underwent a right-sided total hip replacement. On postoperative day 10, she complained of discomfort and swelling over her right thigh and calf. She has been ambulating satisfactorily. Which of the following statements is true?
   a bed rest and diuretic therapy should be prescribed
   b CT scan of the lower pelvis and right hip should be done
   c Doppler study of the lower limb deep venous system should be performed
   d local complications of surgery are the most likely cause for the swelling
   e a plain X-ray of the right hip is most informative

3 Which of the following statements about acute lymphangitis of the lower limb is *incorrect*?
   a improperly managed, it may lead to lymphadenitis
   b lymphangiography is the investigation of choice in the management
   c rest and elevation of the affected limb is appropriate
   d cellulitis may be the initiating cause
   e appropriate antibiotics should include cover for streptococcal infection

4 Eight days following a low anterior resection for carcinoma of the rectum, a 65-year-old man developed unilateral gross swelling of his right lower limb. Which of the following statements is correct?
   a a diagnosis of deep venous thrombosis can confidently be made on the basis of clinical signs
   b deep venous thrombosis is unlikely as the patient had received perioperative prophylactic subcutaneous heparin
   c a past history of superficial thrombophlebitis in this patient is almost certainly related to deep venous thrombosis
   d the short saphenous vein is usually the site of origin of deep venous thrombosis
   e ilio-femoral thrombosis is likely as it commonly follows pelvic surgery

5 A 65-year-old woman has a chronic leg ulcer. Which of the following is the *least likely* cause?
   a squamous cell carcinoma
   b giant cell arteritis
   c superficial venous valvular incompetence
   d deep venous valvular incompetence
   e trauma

6 Which of the following is the most important measure for healing a chronic venous ulcer?
   a apply a dressing
   b stop smoking
   c apply compression bandaging/stockings
   d surgery to excise the ulcer
   e counselling

7 Which of the following statements about chronic leg ulcers is correct?
   a they are generally well managed
   b 80% are due to superficial venous insufficiency
   c a biopsy is best done of the ulcer edge
   d basal cell carcinoma is the commonest malignancy in the leg
   e arterial and venous ulcers are easily distinguished

8 Which of the following statements about the calf muscle pump is correct?
   a it plays no part in venous return to the heart
   b it cannot work if the valves are incompetent
   c it is the only musculo-venous pump
   d it depends on good ankle movement
   e it cannot work if arterial disease is present

74 Haematuria

Kenny Rao¹ and Shomik Sengupta²

¹ Eastern Health, Melbourne, Victoria, Australia
² Monash University, Melbourne, Victoria, Australia

Introduction

Classification

Haematuria refers to the presence of blood in the urine. It may be 'macroscopic' when it is visible to the naked eye (also known as 'gross' or 'frank') or 'microscopic' when it is only detectable on dipstick or laboratory examination of the urine. Only a small amount of blood is needed to change the colour of urine, and thus it is common to overestimate the amount of bleeding. Fresh active bleeding causes the urine to look bright red while old blood or clot results in a dark yellow or brown discoloration.

Significance

In most cases, haematuria results from benign or indeterminate causes, but it can also be the cardinal symptom of serious conditions such as urinary tract malignancy. Hence, the presence of blood in the urine should never be taken lightly and almost always warrants further investigation.

Asymptomatic microscopic haematuria in low-risk patients (age <45 years, non-smoker) does not usually require further investigation. Neither does haematuria in females that is clearly attributable to an uncomplicated urinary tract infection (UTI) and resolves with its successful treatment. It should be noted that recurrent UTIs or UTIs in males usually requires further investigation for potential predisposing causes.

Differential diagnosis

A systematic approach is necessary to assessing a patient presenting with haematuria, since various pathologies can occur anywhere along the genitourinary tract from the kidneys to the external genitalia (Table 74.1). Consideration needs to be given particularly to the serious and common causes.

Medical renal disease

A range of intrinsic diseases of the kidney can also cause haematuria but are usually managed by nephrologists (renal physicians). Typically, the presentation is with microscopic rather than visible haematuria, and can be associated with other features such as hypertension, renal impairment, proteinuria or oedema. The key distinction between renal diseases and surgical causes of haematuria is that in the former the red cells have come from within the glomeruli and on microscopy usually have a dysmorphic appearance as a result. There may also be associated red cell casts, and if these diagnoses are suspected, referral to a renal physician is required. Occasionally, low-level microscopic haematuria may be difficult to classify accurately, and both urological and nephrological evaluation maybe warranted.

Neoplasm

Tumours arising from any part of the genitourinary tract can present with haematuria, and thus represent the most serious potential cause of this symptom. Therefore, the assessment of the patient with haematuria is aimed, in large part, to the detection of any underlying neoplasm. While this is particularly important if the patient has risk factors such as smoking, metabolic syndrome, a family history or environmental exposure, such pathology can arise even in those who do not. It is crucial to note that the presence of non-malignant causes of haematuria, such as infection, does not exclude concurrent malignancy as a cause for haematuria. Therefore, a systematic protocol-based assessment is key to avoid missing serious causes of haematuria.

Textbook of Surgery, Fourth Edition. Edited by Julian A. Smith, Andrew H. Kaye, Christopher Christophi and Wendy A. Brown.
© 2020 John Wiley & Sons Ltd. Published 2020 by John Wiley & Sons Ltd.

Table 74.1 Differential diagnoses of underlying causes of haematuria.

	Kidney	Ureter	Bladder	Prostate	Urethra
Neoplasm	Renal call carcinoma Angiomyolipoma Oncocytoma Urothelial carcinoma	Urothelial carcinoma Solitary fibrous tumour	Urothelial carcinoma Adenocarcinoma Squamous carcinoma	Adenocarcinoma	Urothelial carcinoma
Inflammation	Pyelonephritis		UTI Radiation cystitis	Prostatitis	Urethritis
Congenital	Arteriovenous malformation	Arteriovenous malformation	Arteriovenous malformation		
Trauma	Renal contusion or laceration	Ureteric injury	Bladder rupture		Urethral injury
Calculi	Renal	Ureteric	Bladder		
Other	Glomerulonephritis Cyst			Benign prostatic hyperplasia	Stricture

Bladder cancer

Haematuria is the most common presentation of bladder cancer. It may be microscopic or macroscopic and is often isolated or episodic rather than continuous. It may also be associated with dysuria, recurrent UTIs, pelvic pain and voiding frequency. Bladder cancer can progress rapidly, and delays in diagnosis are known to significantly worsen outcomes and thus prompt investigation is crucial.

Renal tumours

Various renal neoplasms can cause haematuria including renal cell carcinoma, urothelial cell carcinoma, angiomyolipoma and cystic diseases. Other associated symptoms can include flank pain or a palpable mass. In current practice, however, the majority of renal malignancies are discovered incidentally on radiological imaging rather than due to symptoms.

Prostate pathology

Prostate cancer and benign prostatic hyperplasia (BPH) can each result in increased vascularity over the surface of the prostate which surrounds the urethra. These vessels are friable and may spontaneously bleed. Patients may also have concomitant lower urinary tract symptoms (LUTS) including frequency, intermittency, dribbling, hesitancy, incomplete emptying, nocturia and urgency. However, prostate cancer is most commonly diagnosed at an asymptomatic stage based on elevation of the serum marker PSA (prostate-specific antigen).

Infection and inflammation

UTI is one of the most common causes of haematuria, particularly in young adults. This can affect the bladder (cystitis) or the kidneys (pyelonephritis). The resultant inflammation and oedema can cause bleeding from the epithelium and into urine. The more typical symptoms of UTI are dysuria and LUTS, and if involving the kidney flank pain, fever and constitutional symptoms.

Various non-infective causes of cystitis can also lead to a similar presentation as UTI. Radiation therapy, often used to treat cancers of the pelvic viscera, is the commonest cause of such chronic haemorrhagic cystitis. Other causes include drug-induced (e.g. the immunosuppressant cyclophosphamide) or infiltrative (interstitial or eosinophilic) cystitis. Inflammation of the bladder mucosa causes friable neovascularisation which can bleed easily and be difficult to control. Haemorrhagic cystitis is often episodic in presentation, but when severe can be life-threatening and require urgent and major intervention.

Calculi (stones)

Urinary calculi commonly originate in the renal collecting system, where they can remain asymptomatic for lengthy periods, but presentation can be with pain or haematuria. Sometimes, stones can travel along the urinary tract, and typically present with flank pain (renal colic) caused by urinary obstruction. Renal colic is commonly associated with haematuria, often microscopic, but sometimes visible.

Bladder stones usually arise as a result of bladder outlet obstruction and urinary stasis, and thus are often identified during assessment of the associated

LUTS, but again visible or invisible haematuria can coexist.

Urethral strictures

Strictures arise as a result of scarring of the urethra, which may be secondary to prior trauma, infection or instrumentation. Strictures impair bladder emptying and commonly present with LUTS but can also cause haematuria.

Trauma

The mechanism of injury usually alerts the clinician to potential genitourinary trauma as a cause of haematuria. Blunt trauma from falls, motor vehicle accidents or sports injury are most common in Australia, but penetrating injuries from gunshots or stabbings need specific consideration.

Renal trauma occurs in a spectrum of grades, ranging from simple contusion to a completely shattered or avulsed kidney. The extent of haematuria may not provide an accurate assessment of the severity of injury since a major component of the bleeding may be confined to the retroperitoneum. Appropriate imaging by CT is the key to diagnosis and underpins further management.

Pelvic fractures can be associated with bladder and urethral injuries that can sometimes remain undiagnosed without appropriate imaging. There needs to be a high index of suspicion, with blood at the urethral meatus being a pathognomonic sign. Again, appropriate imaging by way of retrograde urethrogram and cystogram is crucial for making the diagnosis. Urological involvement is important for avoiding further exacerbation of the injury during attempted catheter placement.

Assessment

History

Haematuria may be reported by the patient on visualising their urine or be picked up incidentally on urine microscopy. The pattern of haematuria may sometimes provide clues to the source; initial or terminal bleeding is suggestive of prostatic or urethral pathology. The extent of haematuria, including the presence of clots and resulting difficulties in passing urine (sometimes resulting in so-called 'clot retention'), may have implications for management including the potential need for catheterisation to drain and wash out the bladder.

The presence of associated LUTS may provide suggestive evidence of lower urinary tract pathology, especially if they pre-date the haematuria.

However, it should be noted that the presence of blood in the bladder can itself provoke irritative LUTS, while obstructive symptoms may be caused or exacerbated by clots.

Flank pain in association with haematuria may indicate renal inflammation from pyelonephritis or obstruction from calculi or clots within the ureter. Fever, malaise and related symptoms can be indicative of sepsis from infection. Weight loss, cachexia and bony pain are symptoms that raise the concern of advanced malignancy. Renal cell carcinoma can additionally lead to a variety of paraneoplastic syndromes, including fever.

Exposure to risk factors for genitourinary malignancies should be assessed. Smoking is associated with both urothelial cancers and renal cell carcinoma. Environmental exposure to aniline dyes and aromatic amines are also risk factors for urothelial cancers and employment in the textile, dry cleaning, petrochemical, rubber and other chemical industries, trucking, painting and printing are of potential concern.

Family history may be of particular significance for some malignancies, notably prostate cancer and renal cell carcinoma, especially in the context of known cancer syndromes such as von Hippel–Lindau and Birt–Hogg–Dubé syndromes. Urolithiasis and BPH can also be associated with a familial tendency.

Past medical history, such as urolithiasis, malignancy, radiation therapy and surgery, can obviously be particularly important in directing clinical diagnosis. Comorbidities, particularly cardiovascular disease, may lead to treatment with anticoagulant and antiplatelet medications which can precipitate or worsen haematuria. It should be noted that even among patients on such medications, haematuria can be associated with underlying pathology and therefore appropriate clinical assessment and investigation is imperative.

Examination

In most cases, other than visible haematuria on a urine sample, there are few signs visible on examination. Significant blood loss or infection can present with hypovolaemic or septic shock. Chronic blood loss may occasionally manifest as signs of anaemia.

Abdominal examination can reveal masses or tenderness, which may be indicative of renal pathology (if in the flank) or lower urinary tract pathology including a full bladder or large pelvic malignancy. A digital rectal examination (DRE) in males is helpful in assessing the prostate for size and possible cancer.

The DRE (or a vaginal examination in females) can also give clues on other pelvic malignancies. Examination of the genitalia in either sex helps identify potential external sources of bleeding.

In the context of trauma, it is vital to rule out a palpable pulsatile retroperitoneal mass as this is an indication for urgent surgery for renal bleeding. Blood at the meatus is a sign of possible urethral or bladder injury, as previously discussed.

Investigations

Blood tests

- Full blood examination: searching for anaemia, infection or platelet abnormalities.
- Electrolytes, urea and creatinine: important for assessing renal function.
- Coagulation studies: assessing for bleeding diathesis.

Urine tests

- Urine dipstick: can be quick and convenient but has limitations of false positives and false negatives. Provides additional information about the presence of leucocytes/nitrates (indicative of infection), glycosuria, etc.
- Midstream urine: attention needed for appropriate collection to avoid contamination. Urine microscopy allows the detection of red cells (indicative of bleeding), while morphology is important in distinguishing nephrological causes of bleeding. White cells are indicative of infection or inflammation, microorganisms (bacteria or fungi) of colonisation or infection, casts of nephrological conditions, and crystals of risk for stone formation. Culture and sensitivity analysis provides information on possible infectious agents and thus guide appropriate antibiotic therapy.
- Urine cytology: allows assessment for malignant or atypical cells shed in the urine, typically indicative of high-grade urothelial cancer. However, relatively few cancers are actually associated with positive urine cytology, and the analysis is significantly operator-dependent and prone to both false-negative and false-positive results.

Imaging studies

- CT intravenous pyelography (CT-IVP) is the gold standard for radiological investigation of haematuria, and is usually recommended for patients considered to be at risk of serious underlying pathology. Abdominopelvic CT scans are undertaken prior to, during and after administration of intravenous contrast. This allows the detection of the full range of possible pathology (Figure 74.1): urolithiasis, renal and bladder masses and abnormalities along the collecting system (possibly indicating tumour, calculi, clots, etc.). The administration of intravenous contrast is contraindicated in patients who have an allergy to it or inadequate renal function (usually, estimated glomerular filtration rate <45 mL/min per 1.73 m^2).
- Non-contrast CT: can be used if contrast administration is contraindicated. However, the assessment of renal masses and collecting system abnormalities is very inadequate in such a scan.
- Renal tract ultrasound: provides an alternative to CT that avoids the risks of radiation and contrast exposure, of particular utility in pregnant or young females. However, ultrasound has more limited resolution than CT and can be dependant on operator skill and body habitus. Good at detecting renal masses and stones as well as the presence of hydronephrosis, but limited in assessing ureteric abnormalities. Provides fairly good anatomical detail of the lower urinary tract. Ultrasound can be used for initial imaging for patients considered to have a low risk for underlying pathology.
- Magnetic resonance imaging (MRI): provides another alternative modality for high-resolution cross-sectional imaging, although used relatively infrequently. Useful for patients who cannot have CT contrast administration due to allergy (for those with inadequate renal function, gadolinium MRI contrast also poses significant risks and is contraindicated). Sometimes utilised if findings on CT and/or ultrasound are equivocal.
- Retrograde urethrogram: undertaken by instilling contrast into the urethra. Relatively rare as an investigation for haematuria, but used if urethral stricture or injury are suspected, as discussed previously.
- Retrograde pyelogram: undertaken by instilling contrast into the collecting system at the time of cystoscopy (see next section). A specialised test that is utilised for assessment of the collecting system usually undertaken if other imaging studies have shown suspicious findings or inadequate visualisation of the collecting system. May often lead on to endoscopic examination of the collecting system if indicated (see next section).

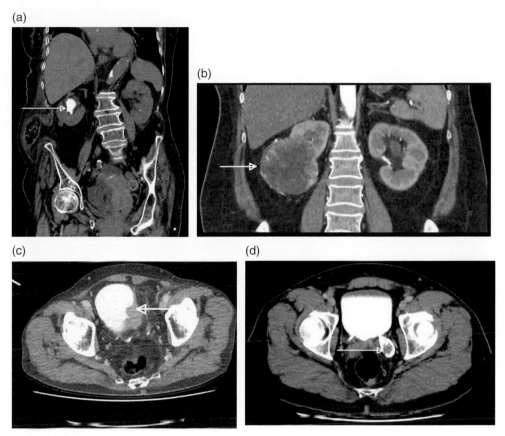

Fig. 74.1 Representative CT images: (a) calculus (arrow) within the lower pole of right kidney; (b) renal mass (arrow) consistent with renal cell carcinoma arising from right kidney; (c) filling defect within bladder lumen (arrow) suggestive of bladder tumour; (d) filling defect within left ureteric lumen (arrow) suggestive of ureteric tumour.

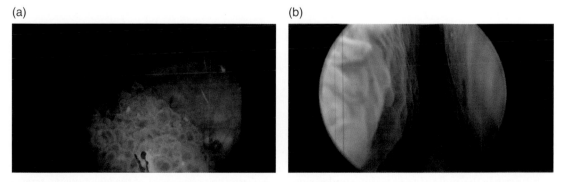

Fig. 74.2 Cystoscopic images: (a) bladder tumour; (b) enlarged prostatic lobes.

Procedural investigations

- Cystoscopy (Figure 74.2): examination of the lower urinary tract using an endoscope. This can be carried out under local anaesthetic or sedation using a flexible endoscope or under general anaesthetic using a rigid endoscope (which allows more interventions to be undertaken).

The most important role of cystoscopy in haematuria is to exclude bladder tumour, but the procedure also provides additional useful information on anatomy and pathology of the lower urinary tract. Biopsy or resection of tumours, removal of bladder calculi and performance of retrograde pyelogram (see previous section) can

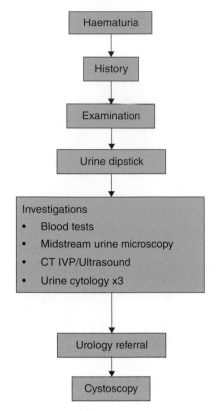

Fig. 74.3 Flowchart illustrating clinical assessment of patients with haematuria.

also be carried out at the time of cystoscopy as indicated.

- Ureteroscopy and/or pyeloscopy: endoscopic examination of the upper urinary tract. This is not a routine investigation for haematuria, but would be undertaken if a stone or upper tract tumour was found on imaging. Biopsies or laser destruction of tumours and extraction or fragmentation of calculi can be undertaken as indicated.

Conclusion

Haematuria is a common presenting symptom that can sometimes be indicative of serious underlying pathology. Every patient needs careful and systematic assessment, by way of careful history and examination and appropriate further investigation (Figure 74.3). With limited exceptions, all patients with haematuria should undergo imaging of the urinary tract and cystoscopic examination.

Further reading

Chiong E, Grossman HB. Hematuria, gross and microscopic, adult. In: Gomella LG (ed.) *The 5-Minute Urology Consult*, 2nd edn. Philadelphia: Wolters Kluwer/Lippincott Williams & Wilkins, 2010.

Ngo B, Papa N, Perera M, Bolton D, Sengupta S. Factors affecting the timeliness and adequacy of haematuria assessment in bladder cancer: a systematic review. *BJU Int* 2017;119(Suppl 5):10–18.

Sharp VJ, Barnes KT, Erickson BA. Assessment of asymptomatic microscopic hematuria in adults. *Am Fam Physician* 2013;88:747–54.

MCQs

Select the single correct answer to each question. The correct answers can be found in the Answers section at the end of the book.

1 Which of the following patients presenting with haematuria does *not* need further investigation?
   a single episode of visible haematuria in a 70-year-old male who has never smoked
   b a 55-year-old male who is admitted via emergency with clot retention
   c a 20-year-old female who has haematuria with a proven UTI that resolves after antibiotic treatment
   d a 60-year-old ex-smoker who is found to have microscopic haematuria on his urine tests during a health check

2 CT scan done for radiological assessment of the urinary tract in patients presenting with haematuria should:
   a include pre- and post-contrast scans with early and delayed phases
   b is done for patients who cannot have an ultrasound scan
   c should cover the chest abdomen and pelvis
   d all of the above

3 Cystosopic assessment of the lower urinary tract:
   a is essential to complete investigation of haematuria
   b is the best way to assess for bladder tumour
   c allows for initial treatment by resection of bladder tumours
   d all of the above

75 Postoperative complications

Peter Devitt

Department of Surgery, University of Adelaide and Royal Adelaide Hospital, Adelaide, South Australia, Australia

Introduction

The management of postoperative complications can be approached in a number of ways. Perhaps the most practical way is to consider the frequency with which various complications may occur (Box 75.1). Another strategy is to consider the problems that relate directly to the procedure and those that are more general and patient-related (Box 75.2).

This chapter will take the former approach, but obviously it is sensible that in managing any patient with a postoperative problem, the doctor considers:
- the procedure
- the general state of health of the patient before the illness/operation
- progress since the procedure.

Thus, the questions to be asked should include the following.
- What procedure was done, when was it done and why was it done?
- Is there any coexisting illness (i.e. is there a past medical history of note, such as chronic respiratory disease)?
- Is the patient on any medication?
- What has now happened to the patient to demand your attention?
- What investigations have been done (both before and after procedure)?

These will then be followed by the following questions.
- Is the cause of the problem clear-cut?
- If yes, how should I proceed with management?
- If no, what will I need to do to make a clear diagnosis?

This chapter contains a number of examples of postoperative complications. A model answer is provided for each scenario. As a learning exercise,

Textbook of Surgery, Fourth Edition. Edited by Julian A. Smith, Andrew H. Kaye, Christopher Christophi and Wendy A. Brown.
© 2020 John Wiley & Sons Ltd. Published 2020 by John Wiley & Sons Ltd.

cover each model answer and provide your own answer. Put yourself in the position of the intern.

Confusion

Example: A 67-year-old man becomes confused 2 days after a laparotomy for a perforated peptic ulcer. The operation was uneventful and 2 L of gastric contents were evacuated from the peritoneal cavity. Lavage was performed and the perforation closed. What critical piece of information would help you determine the cause of the confusion? How would you approach the problem?

Model answer: Hypoxia is the most important and common cause of confusion. If this patient has a chest infection, you may have the quick explanation for his confusion.

To approach the problem, gain all the information you can about the patient's preoperative state of health, the details of the procedure and progress since the operation. From the case notes you will hopefully glean information about the patient's past medical history, medications, examination findings and general fitness. From the past history, look for evidence of chronic respiratory disease and sustained alcohol consumption. Various investigations may have been undertaken (e.g. blood biochemistry) that may give clues as to the current problem. Any problems associated with the operation (the procedure itself or the anaesthetic) should be noted. The case records and the nursing observations since the procedure may help determine the cause of the current problem. Note any investigations that have been performed since the procedure.

Take a history from the patient, if his state of confusion allows. Examine the patient, looking particularly for evidence of hypoxia. A chest infection may explain the confusion. There may be other causes of hypoxia to consider (e.g. opiate toxicity, cardiac failure). If the patient is not obviously hypoxic, he may be septic, have a fluid and electrolyte disturbance, be suffering a drug complication or be in alcohol withdrawal.

To test some of these hypotheses, several investigations may be required. These may include arterial blood gas analysis, serum biochemistry, blood culture, an electrocardiogram (ECG) and a chest X-ray.

Before you start the investigations, some simple measures can be adopted. Ensure that the patient is given supplemental oxygen through a face mask and that intravenous fluids are being given. If sepsis is likely, you may want to start the patient on a broad-spectrum antibiotic. A pulse oximeter must be attached for monitoring and consideration should be given to further management on a high-dependency unit.

You have excluded hypoxia as a cause for the confusion and the patient does not appear to be septic. There is no apparent electrolyte disturbance and you are reasonably confident that the patient is suffering alcohol withdrawal symptoms (delerium tremens). Describe your initial plan of management.

Move the patient to a quiet well-lit room. Arrange continuous nursing care, preferably with a nurse familiar to the patient. Institute an alcohol withdrawal program. The protocol for this program will stipulate regular observations of the patient's symptoms, allocating a score to various symptom groupings and correlating the amount of sedation (if any) that needs to be given according to the score. Symptoms to be scored include nausea, anxiety, visual disturbances and agitation. The preferred sedative is oral diazepam.

Chest pain

Example: Five days after a bilateral salpingo-oophorectomy and total abdominal hysterectomy, you are asked to see a 62-year-old patient who complains of breathlessness and right-sided chest pain. What are the thoughts that go through your mind and how would you approach this problem?

Model answer: If she has had a major pulmonary embolism, the patient may have circulatory collapse and require resuscitation.

You will obviously want to know more about the current symptoms, including the type of pain, the mode of onset and severity. Her medical history will be important, particularly any pre-existing cardiorespiratory problems. Ideally, you will want to look at the case record, nursing observations and drug charts before you proceed with the history and physical examination. The conditions you will need consider include:
- pulmonary embolism
- chest infection
- pneumothorax
- pleural effusion
- cardiac problems.

Your priority will be an assessment of her cardiovascular system. Provided the patient is normotensive and not hypoxic, you can proceed with your investigations. These will include an ECG, arterial blood gas analysis, a chest X-ray and possibly a CT pulmonary angiogram (CTPA). The CTPA will allow accurate definition of the major pulmonary vasculature and can detect filling defects and obstruction. The scans are undertaken after rapid bolus administration of 100–140 mL of non-ionic contrast. This technique can be used to detect 3–4 mm clots in the second-, third- and fourth-order branches of the pulmonary vasculature.

On the assumption that the diagnosis of pulmonary embolism has been confirmed, the patient should be started on intravenous heparin.

Clinical examination of a patient with suspected deep venous thrombosis (DVT) or pulmonary embolism is relatively inaccurate and should not be relied on to determine diagnosis or treatment.

Fever

Example: A previously well 45-year-old man undergoes a laparotomy and oversewing of a perforated duodenal ulcer. Peritoneal lavage is performed to deal with the contamination from the perforation. Postoperative progress is slowed by the development of a paralytic ileus. On day 6, he is noted to have a temperature of 38.5°C, blood pressure of 110/60 mmHg, pulse rate of 100/min and a respiratory rate of 20/min. Describe how this situation should be managed.

Model answer: The measurements on the nursing chart indicate systemic inflammatory response syndrome (SIRS). In this case, the SIRS almost certainly has an infectious aetiology and, considering the timing of onset with response to the laparotomy, the site of origin of sepsis is most like to have originated at the site of the operation (rather than the chest).

First, there must be an overall assessment of the general state of health of the patient. It appears that he is about to slip into septic shock. The patient's progress since the operation must be reviewed and information sought on any pre-existing problems (e.g. diabetes) that might predispose the patient to infection. The nursing observation chart and pattern of the fever and pulse rate may give clues as to the likely cause. A spiking fever over several days could be due to an intra-abdominal abscess.

Although a chest infection may not be the cause of the fever, the chest must be examined carefully. After that, the abdomen should be inspected and the wound examined. Cannula and drain sites should also be examined for evidence of infection. Occasionally, a DVT will be accompanied by a low-grade fever, and the legs should be examined.

In this instance, the patient will require prompt resuscitation with oxygen by face mask, a bolus of intravenous fluid and empirical broad-spectrum antibiotics, Provided that there is a rapid response to this treatment, consideration can then be given to looking for the underlying cause of the problem. The patient will almost certainly have an intra-abdominal collection and this can usually be both identified and drained percutaneously under CT guidance.

Initial assessment of a patient with suspected sepsis must include an appreciation of the type of procedure undertaken and the risk of infection from that procedure. Also to be considered are the consequences should infection in that particular patient occur, for example reduced resistance to infection in an immunocompromised individual. The type of procedure and the pattern of fever will give important clues as to the site of sepsis and the causative organism. Investigations to be considered include those to:
- identify the site of infection
- diagnose the type of infection.

Oliguria

Example: A 68-year-old patient is reviewed on the ward some 6 hours after he returned from the operating suite for a sigmoid colectomy performed for perforated diverticular disease. The nursing observation charts show that he has accumulated a total of 50 mL of urine in the catheter bag since his return. The patient looks comfortable, with a blood pressure of 110/75 mmHg and pulse of 90/min. Describe an appropriate plan of management.

Model answer: While it is possible that this man's problem may be fluid retention and pump failure, it is more likely that he has received inadequate fluid replacement, either during or immediately after the operation and you are dealing with an under-filled patient.

Ideally, his urine output should be about 1 mL/kg per hour. This patient has a poor urine output and there are many reasons to consider:
- inadequate filling
- inadequate output
- renal tract obstruction.

Most cases of postoperative oliguria are due to under-filling, either during or immediately after surgery. The case notes should be studied, looking for evidence of pre-existing renal or cardiac disease. Any recent laboratory investigations (serum biochemistry) should be assessed. Details of the surgical procedure should be noted, with a calculation of how much fluid was lost during the operation and how much was given. The amount of fluid given since the time of the operation should be noted and any discharge from drains or a nasogastric tube measured. Given the scenario, this patient may have lost a considerable amount of fluid as a result of the peritonitis and may still be losing fluid into the peritoneal cavity. Not all fluid lost by a patient may be readily evident. Patients with paralytic ileus and/or peritonitis can accumulate many litres of fluid within the peritoneal cavity, so-called 'third space' losses.

Whilst less likely, a blocked catheter could be a simple explanation and a bedside bladder scan will provide rapid information; however, considering his recent surgery, this might not be a very practical manoeuvre.

It is unlikely that this patient would have been sent directly back to the ward if there had been (preoperative or perioperative) concerns about coexisting conditions that might have had a major impact on his recovery. On the assumption that the patient does not have pre-existing renal impairment or cardiac failure (the latter backed up by physical examination), in most instances it will be relatively safe to manage the problem at the bedside. The first step will be to give a bolus infusion of 500 mL of isotonic saline rapidly and observe the effect on urine output over the next few hours. Further boluses of fluid may be required and a diuretic should only be given once it can be confidently judged that the patient has had adequate fluid replacement. In more complex cases, the resources of an intensive care unit may be required to help determine the nature of the underlying problem.

Wound discharge

Example: Five days after undergoing a laparotomy and small bowel resection following an episode of adhesive obstruction, a 73-year-old patient develops a pinkish discharge from the wound. Describe how the problem should be managed.

Model answer: While there are a number of causes of wound discharge, the most urgent to consider is the possibility that this is the harbinger of disruption of the deep layers, with the consequent risk of complete wound failure.

First, the wound should be covered with a sterile dressing in the event of sudden complete disruption. The next action must be to ascertain if the patient has any risk factors for wound failure. The case records should provide information on his preoperative nutritional status. His progress since the operation should be assessed and any problems sought that might have led to an untoward increase

in intra-abdominal pressure, such as a chest infection or paralytic ileus.

During this process the patient must be kept fully informed and warned that he may need to be taken back to the operating theatre (for the wound to be resutured) if the wound has indeed disrupted. The wound must be carefully inspected. A non-inflamed wound with seepage of pink fluid is highly suggestive of acute failure of the wound. Extensive bruising around the wound might suggest discharge of a seroma, while a red angry wound would be in keeping with infection.

If there is any doubt as to the nature of the problem, the wound should be gently probed (with sterile instruments). If intestine becomes visible, there should be no further local exploration and the patient prepared for formal wound closure in the operating room.

There are a number of factors that can contribute to deep wound dehiscence (acute wound failure).
- Local: poor suturing techniques, poor tissue healing (infection, necrosis, malignancy, foreign bodies), increased intra-abdominal pressure.
- General: malnutrition, diabetes mellitus.

In most instances, acute wound failure is due to a local factor. The hallmark of deep wound dehiscence is the presence of a serosanguineous discharge some 5–7 days after the initial surgery.

Bleeding

Example: A 27-year-old man is being reviewed on the ward, having recently undergone a splenectomy for trauma. The nursing staff report fresh blood in the drain. How should this problem be approached?

Model answer: Further information is needed. The bleeding may be localised or generalised. It may be reactionary, primary or secondary. How long ago was the operation and how much blood is in the drain? A small amount of fresh blood a few hours after the operation may be of little consequence. Is the bleeding confined to the drain or is there evidence of bleeding at other sites (wound, intravenous cannula)? If the former, the problem may be haemorrhage from the operative site; if the latter, the patient may have a disorder of coagulation.

The initial assessment must include a review of the charts. In what circumstances was the operation performed? If the patient had a massive and rapid transfusion to maintain his circulatory state, then the problem may be one of a coagulation defect. What has happened since the operation? A rising pulse and falling blood pressure would suggest that the patient is still bleeding, and what is seen in the drain may only be the tip of the iceberg. In other words, there could be a considerable volume of blood collecting at the operative site, with only a little escaping into the drain. Remember that when a drain drains, positive information may be gleaned; however, an empty drain means little.

Examine the patient and look for evidence of circulatory insufficiency. The material in the drain tube and drainage bag may be fresh and not clotted, or it may be serosanguineous. A normotensive patient with old clot in the drain is probably a stable patient. It is more important to pay attention to the general state of the patient, rather than the contents of the drainage bag.

In summary, the clinical assessment of this case should include:
- the severity of the bleed
- the site of the bleed
- the cause of the bleed
- the need for further action (e.g. coagulation studies, cross-matching blood, contacting senior staff).

Shock

Example: A call is made to review a 66-year-old man on the ward who is hypotensive and confused. Twelve hours earlier he had a transurethral prostatectomy. Describe an appropriate plan of management.

Model answer: The priority will be resuscitation and to do this effectively it is important to have a clear idea of the likely cause of his collapse. The causes of shock to consider in these circumstances are:
- pump failure (cardiogenic)
- haemorrhage (hypovolaemia)
- sepsis (septicaemia)
- anaphylaxis (drug reaction).

Make a rapid assessment of the state of the patient. How profound is the hypotension and it real or a statutory call based on a nursing chart algorithm? The patient may be connected to a monitor, facilitating any changes in the ECG to be noted.

Ensure that the patient has an oxygen mask in place, running at 6 L/min, and that a pulse oximeter is attached. On the assumption that the cause of the problem is not cardiac failure, run in 500 mL of isotonic saline rapidly. While this is happening, take blood samples for assay of cardiac enzymes (creatine kinase), myocardial breakdown proteins (troponin), haematological and biochemical screens, blood cross-match and culture. Arterial blood gas analysis should be considered.

Once these things have been done, stand back and review the situation. Look at the charts. Is there a history of ischaemic heart disease or other cardiac problems? Did the patient come in with urinary retention and could he have infected urine and the present problem be septic in origin? How major was the procedure that was performed and how much fluid was used during the procedure, both intravenous administration and as irrigation? What is in the urine drainage bag? A large volume of fresh blood would suggest hypovolaemia as the cause of the collapse. Were there any complications during the procedure? How has the patient progressed since the operation? It is important to know if this has been a sudden collapse or a steady deterioration since the procedure.

In this case there is nothing of significance from the medical history, except that the patient presented in acute urinary retention after a series of urinary tract infections. The operation itself was uneventful and associated with minimal blood loss. The fluid in the bladder irrigation system is tinged with blood and there are no blood clots. The patient's vital signs were within normal limits until about 15 minutes before the call was made. The ECG monitor does not show any acute changes. Describe the further management.

The cause of the problem appears not to be hypovolaemia. It is either septicaemia or a cardiac event. A normal ECG does not exclude an acute myocardial problem and the enzyme assays and troponin levels must be studied.

It would be prudent to work on the assumption that the patient is in septic shock. In addition to the oxygen by face mask and fluid loading, antibiotics should be given. The choice of antibiotics will depend on the likely organisms. Gram-negative aerobes are an important and common cause of urinary infection, and in this case it would be logical to assume that the presumed sepsis has originated from the urinary tract. The trio of an aminoglycoside (gentamicin), metronidazole and amoxicillin remains perhaps the most effective antibiotic combination in the management of patients with Gram-negative septic shock.

Leg swelling

Example: Five days after a low anterior resection for a carcinoma of the rectum, a 75-year-old man complains of pain and swelling in his right leg. Discuss the initial assessment of the problem.

Model answer: Of prime concern is whether this patient has a DVT. Before the patient is examined, information should be sought on any medical history of venous thromboembolic disorders and any risk factors for DVT. Apart from the nature of the recent surgery, were appropriate prophylactic measures taken to minimise the risk of clot formation? The changes that may bring about DVT (Virchow's triad) focus on:

- change in flow
- change in the vessel wall
- change in the constituents of the blood.

Apart from DVT, other conditions to consider include congestive cardiac failure, dependent oedema and cellulitis. The clinical assessment for the presence of DVT is at best unreliable, but a tender swollen calf suggests that the patient may have a DVT.

In this case, the patient has an unremarkable medical history and in particular there is no history of thromboembolic problems or cardiac disease. He is not overweight and had been mobile before the operation. The patient had been classified as having a low risk for DVT and immediately before the operation had been given a dose of an unfractionated heparin preparation. A calf vein compression device had been used during the procedure. The operation itself had been uncomplicated and the patient has started to mobilise.

On examination, there is some swelling of most of the leg, with calf tenderness and some pitting oedema. From this assessment it is suspected the patient may have a DVT, based on a Wells score of 4. Describe the next step in management.

An ultrasonographic examination of the deep veins of the thigh and leg should confirm or refute the diagnosis. If the patient has a DVT, it will be important to document the extent of the clot and the degree of luminal occlusion. Extension of the clot into the femoral vein increases the risk of detachment and pulmonary embolism.

If clot is present and extends into the popliteal vein or beyond, heparin should be started and graded compression stockings applied if there is a substantial amount of leg swelling. There is no evidence that long-term use of graded compression stockings will reduce the risk of post-thrombotic syndrome. If conventional heparin is to be used, a typical regimen is a loading dose of 5000 units followed by 1000 units/hour. The patient will require monitoring with serial activated partial thromboplastin time (APTT) measurements. Alternatively, a low-molecular-weight heparin can be given. This does not require APTT estimations and can therefore be used on an outpatient basis.

Traditionally, this patient would have been anticoagulated with warfarin for 3–6 months; however, with the advent of the direct oral anticoagulants, such patients now tend to be treated with a direct factor Xa inhibitor (e.g. apixaban) or a direct thrombin inhibitor (e.g. dabigatran). The direct oral anticoagulants do not require monitoring, but care must taken in patients with any renal impairment and in those where there could be interactions with other drugs.

Further reading

Stubbs MJ. Deep vein thrombosis. *BMJ* 2018;360:k351.

MCQs

Select the single correct answer to each question. The correct answers can be found in the Answers section at the end of the book.

1 A 19-year-old man is injured in motorbike crash in which his right femur is fractured. This is treated by internal fixation and early mobilisation is encouraged. He makes satisfactory postoperative progress but on day 5 complains of sudden left-sided chest pain which makes him catch his breath. A friction rub can be heard on the left side on auscultation. Which one of the following is the most likely diagnosis?
   a fat embolism
   b pneumonia
   c pulmonary embolism
   d pneumothorax
   e cough fracture

2 A 55-year-old man with type 2 diabetes and chronic obstructive pulmonary disease undergoes a sigmoid colectomy and end-colostomy for perforated diverticular disease. His body mass index is 34. Five days after the operation a copious serosanguineous discharge is noted from the lower part of the abdominal wound. The discharge soaks through the dressing. The wound has some thickening and erythema at the margins. Which one of the following is the most likely diagnosis?
   a staphylococcal wound infection
   b streptococcal wound infection
   c small bowel fistula
   d wound dehiscence
   e liquified wound haematoma

3 You are asked to see a 65-year-old woman who feels unwell and faint. Seven days previously she underwent an elective sigmoid colectomy for carcinoma. The procedure was uncomplicated and, until now, she had been making an uneventful

recovery. On examination she has a temperature of 39.5°C, a pulse rate of 100/min and blood pressure of 90/60 mmHg. Her respiratory rate is 15 breaths/min. She has cool clammy peripheries. Her abdomen is tender in the left iliac fossa, around the wound site. Which of the following is the most reasonable explanation for her current problem?

a myocardial infarction

b pneumonia

c secondary haemorrhage

d pulmonary embolus

e septic shock

4 An otherwise fit 57-year-old man spikes a temperature of 39°C 5 days after an open appendicectomy for acute appendicitis. There is a tender, reddened and fluctuant swelling at the medial end of the wound. What is the most appropriate initial action to take?

a arrange a CT scan of the abdomen

b arrange an ultrasound scan of the wound and anterior abdominal wall

c start the patient on oral antibiotics

d open the wound to allow free drainage

e send off blood samples for a white cell count and culture

76 Massive haemoptysis

Julian A. Smith

Department of Surgery, Monash University and Department of Cardiothoracic Surgery, Monash Health, Melbourne, Victoria, Australia

Introduction

Massive haemoptysis is rare but carries with it a high mortality. Any amount of blood loss in excess of 100 mL in 24 hours may constitute massive haemoptysis. Some patients may expectorate several litres of blood per day. The risk to life is from respiratory compromise due to the tracheobronchial tree filling with blood rather than from hypovolaemia and haemodynamic deterioration. The term 'life-threatening haemoptysis' may be more appropriate.

Aetiology of massive haemoptysis

The causes of massive haemoptysis are listed in Box 76.1. The majority are benign inflammatory or infective lung disorders. Malignancy seldom presents with massive bleeding (<5%).

Box 76.1 Causes of massive haemoptysis

Infective lung conditions
  Tuberculosis
  Bronchiectasis
  Lung abscess
  Aspergillosis
  Cystic fibrosis
Pulmonary neoplasms
Pulmonary embolus
Trauma
  Pulmonary artery catheter injury
  Penetrating or blunt external
Arteriovenous malformation
Cardiac valve disease
  Mitral stenosis
  Infective endocarditis

Surgical pathology

The source of bleeding is nearly always the high-pressure bronchial circulation. These vessels are often enlarged in response to the primary pathology (e.g. bronchiectasis) or are involved in the inflammatory or necrotic process (e.g. tuberculosis). The pulmonary arterial circulation is the source of bleeding from arteriovenous malformations.

Clinical evaluation

A thorough history and examination is required bearing the possible causes in mind. Epistaxis and haematemesis must be excluded. Any anticoagulant intake should be established. A history of fever, night sweats, weight loss, previous tuberculosis or exposure to tuberculosis may suggest active tuberculosis. Recurrent pulmonary infections may point to bronchiectasis. Helpful physical signs may include finger clubbing, peripheral or cervical lymphadenopathy and localised wheeze, crepitations or consolidation. Abnormal respiratory signs may be absent if the blood is effectively expectorated.

Box 76.2 Investigations of massive haemoptysis

Haemoglobin level
Arterial blood gases
Coagulation studies
Sputum microscopy and culture
Chest X-ray
Bronchoscopy
Computed tomography
Radionuclide perfusion scanning
Angiography (CT or digital subtraction)

Investigations

The investigations for massive haemoptysis are listed in Box 76.2. A chest X-ray may be completely normal if little blood is retained within the airway. Infection or tumour may be localised but shadows of aspiration may be confusing. Serial chest X-rays may be helpful. Bronchoscopy, performed while bleeding is occurring, is the best way to localise the source (achieved in over 70% of cases). The rigid instrument provides a superior view and facilitates airway suction and bronchial toilet. Occasionally the flexible instrument may be passed through the rigid bronchoscope to visualise more peripheral lung lesions. If the patient is fit enough to tolerate computed tomography (CT) scanning, the majority of causes of massive haemoptysis will be demonstrated. CT or digital subtraction bronchial or pulmonary branch angiography and possible embolisation may have a role in high-risk surgical patients where initial bronchoscopy has been unhelpful.

Management plan

The key principles in the management of this potentially fatal condition are:
- prompt early resuscitation
- precise localisation of the bleeding source and airway protection
- definitive therapy.

The patient requires intensive care monitoring of vital signs and oxygen saturation. The patient should be positioned head down and bleeding side down (if known). Adequate amounts of blood should be available for administration via a large-bore intravenous line based on haemodynamic parameters rather than the amount of blood lost (notoriously unreliable). Broad-spectrum antibiotics should be given pending results of sputum cultures. Specific antituberculosis therapy is added in the presence of active tuberculosis.

Rigid bronchoscopy is vital for maintaining the airway, aspirating blood and secretions from the airway and for ventilation. After localising the source of bleeding, control may be obtained by ice-cold saline lavage (leading to vasospasm) or placement of an endobronchial balloon blocker and endotracheal intubation. Patients are ventilated (with positive end-expiratory pressure) and bronchoscopy is repeated 12–24 hours later to assess ongoing bleeding prior to definitive therapy.

Definitive therapy may include one or more of the following.
- Medical therapy: antibiotics, reversal of anti-coagulation.
- Rigid bronchoscopic control (local coagulation therapies).
- Surgical resection: immediate or after initial control of bleeding source.
- Angiography and arterial embolisation for arteriovenous malformations: up to 20% incidence of rebleeding, so should be followed with surgical resection.
- Radiotherapy: for non-resectable tumours or if the patient is unfit for surgery.

Massive rebleeding can occur following the initial establishment of control. Surgical resection of the lesion therefore offers the best hope of cure. All endobronchial and angiographic therapies should be considered temporary answers to this problem. Surgical resection is contraindicated in patients with severe cardiorespiratory dysfunction, uncorrectable coagulopathy, unresectable cancer and in those in whom the bleeding site is impossible to localise by any method.

Further reading

Ibrahim WH. Massive haemoptysis: the definition should be revised. *Eur Respir J* 2008;32:1131–2.

Jean-Baptiste E. Clinical assessment and management of massive hemoptysis. *Crit Care Med* 2000;28:1642–7.

Jougon J, Ballester M, Decambre F *et al.* Massive haemoptysis: What place for medical and surgical treatment. *Eur J Cardiothorac Surg* 2002;22:345–51.

Sakr L, Dutau H. Massive hemoptysis: an update on the role of bronchoscopy in diagnosis and management. *Respiration* 2010;80:38–58.

MCQs

Select the single correct answer to each question. The correct answers can be found in the Answers section at the end of the book.

1 From which of the following blood vessels does the bleeding in a patient with massive haemopytsis usually occur?
 a pulmonary artery
 b pulmonary vein
 c bronchial artery
 d bronchial vein
 e thoracic aorta

2 Which of the following lung conditions is *not* a common cause of massive haemoptysis?
  a carcinoma of the lung
  b pulmonary arteriovenous malformation
  c tuberculosis
  d lung abscess
  e aspergillosis

3 Which of the following investigations will most reliably determine the site of bleeding in a patient with massive haemoptysis?
  a chest X-ray
  b CT scan of the chest
  c radionuclide lung scan
  d bronchoscopy
  e pulmonary angiogram

4 Definitive therapy in a patient with massive haemoptysis may include which of the following?
  a broad-spectrum antiobiotics
  b surgical resection of the bleeding source
  c pulmonary arterial embolisation
  d radiotherapy
  e all of the above

77 Epistaxis

Robert J.S. Briggs

University of Melbourne and Royal Victorian Eye and Ear Hospital, Melbourne, Victoria, Australia

Introduction

Nasal bleeding or epistaxis is the most common otolaryngologic emergency and may occur in either the paediatric or adult patient. Epistaxis may be minor or more severe, requiring hospitalisation, resuscitation and surgical control. In the majority of cases the aetiology is idiopathic, although other causes such as primary neoplasms or trauma need to be identified.

Vascular anatomy

The nasal cavity and its mucosa is extremely vascular, with supply from terminal branches of both the internal and external carotid arteries and frequent anastomoses between the systems. The anterior septum is the most frequent site for bleeding, with a plexus of vessels known as Kiesselbach's area or Little's area supplied by both systems.

Epistaxis in children

Nose bleeds in children most often occur from Little's area on the septum. Bleeding is usually minor and stops spontaneously. The site of bleeding can frequently be cauterised with silver nitrate using local anaesthetic. For uncooperative or younger children, general anaesthesia is required and electrocautery may be used.

For recurrent or more severe epistaxis, it is important to exclude conditions that may cause abnormal bleeding. These include acute leukaemia, thrombocytopenia and clotting factor deficiencies. As many as 5–10% of children with recurrent epistaxis may have undiagnosed von Willibrands's disease.

Primary tumours are a rare cause of epistaxis in children that should be considered. Rhabdomyosarcoma is a malignant tumour occurring in the paediatric population which sometimes involves the nasal cavity and presents with epistaxis. Juvenile nasopharyngeal angiofibroma is a benign, highly vascular tumour that involves the posterior nasal cavity, typically affecting adolescent males and presenting with epistaxis. The diagnosis must be considered because biopsy of the tumour is contraindicated due to the potential for severe haemorrhage. The appearance on CT imaging and angiography is diagnostic.

Epistaxis in adults

The most common site for bleeding in adults is also the anterior septum, Little's area. Bleeding usually stops spontaneously and this may be facilitated by local pressure, applied by pinching the alar cartilages to occlude the nasal airway. Bleeding sites more posterior in the nasal cavity are more often associated with severe bleeding and likely to require hospitalisation, particularly in patients with hypertension.

A common predisposing factor in adults with epistaxis is the use of blood thinning agents for thromboembolic prophylaxis. Aspirin, warfarin and clopidogrel in particular are often taken alone or in combination and may complicate management of epistaxis. A high alcohol intake is also associated with a higher incidence of epistaxis.

Epistaxis may occur secondary to a variety of local or systemic factors affecting the nasal mucosa.
- Trauma, such as nose picking or nasal fracture.
- Inflammatory conditions: allergic, viral or bacterial rhino-sinusitis.
- Granulomatous diseases.

Textbook of Surgery, Fourth Edition. Edited by Julian A. Smith, Andrew H. Kaye, Christopher Christophi and Wendy A. Brown.
© 2020 John Wiley & Sons Ltd. Published 2020 by John Wiley & Sons Ltd.

- Environmental irritation.
- Iatrogenic: following nasal or sinus surgery.
- Primary neoplasms: benign or malignant.
- Drugs: topical nasal steroids or cocaine abuse.
- Osler's disease or hereditary haemorrhagic telangectasia.

Assessment of patients with epistaxis must include adequate history, examination and investigation to exclude such conditions.

Management

Initial assessment should include estimation of the amount of blood loss and whether there is a need for immediate resuscitation and blood volume replacement. Cardiac status and circulating blood volume should be assessed and intravenous access obtained if necessary. Checking and correcting any hypotension, anaemia or clotting deficiencies should be performed as required.

The key to controlling epistaxis is to establish both the site and the cause of bleeding so that the bleeding can be stopped and the cause treated.

Headlight examination with local anaesthesia

Thorough examination of the nose with adequate light and instrumentation is necessary. When bleeding is minor, or even when more severe, often the bleeding site can be identified and controlled. Chemical cautery with silver nitrate can be used, particularly for anterior septal vessels; however, bipolar or even monopolar diathermy is more effective.

If the site for bleeding cannot be seen and controlled, then packing the nasal cavity usually provides control. Most emergency departments have specialised packing devices, inflatable balloons or packing material for this purpose. Thorough topical anaesthesia is required for nasal packing, otherwise the procedure can be very painful. The pack is usually left in place for 2 days and prophylactic antibiotics administered.

Nasal endoscopy

Examination of the nasal cavity using rigid or flexible fibre-optic endoscopes is now standard when managing epistaxis. Whilst anterior sites for bleeding can be seen and controlled with a headlight, nasal endoscopes have a vital role in defining and treating posterior epistaxis.

In acute epistaxis management, active bleeding is often reduced or stopped after initial topical anaesthesia and skilled endoscopic examination

may allow identification and control of the bleeding site. During examination, unusual conditions such as tumours can be identified and dealt with after acute bleeding is controlled.

Endoscopic sphenopalatine artery ligation

If bleeding cannot be controlled after endoscopic examination and cautery and/or nasal packing, then treatment under general anaesthesia may be necessary. This provides the opportunity for better examination of the nasal cavity. In the past it was the opportunity to insert a firmer nasal pack. Currently, if direct cautery of bleeding points is not effective, then clipping or diathermy of the sphenopalatine artery is the accepted treatment for management of persistent posterior epistaxis.

Embolisation

Arterial embolisation can also be effective for control of intractable epistaxis. The procedure carries risk of significant complications and so is reserved for patients with refractory epistaxis who are unfit for surgery or in whom surgery has failed to control the bleeding.

Further reading

McGarry GW. Epistaxis. In: Gleeson M (ed.) *Scott-Brown's Otolaryngology Head and Neck Surgery*, 7th edn, Vol 2. London: Hodder-Arnold, 2008:1596–608.

Simmen DB, Jones NS. Epistaxis. In: Flint PW, Haughey BH (eds) *Cummings Otolaryngology Head and Neck Surgery*, 6th edn, Vol 1. Philadelphia: Elsevier Saunders, 2015:678–90.

MCQs

Select the single correct answer to each question. The correct answers can be found in the Answers section at the end of the book.

1 Which of the following is the most common site for bleeding in minor epistaxis?
   a posterior septum
   b inferior turbinate
   c anterior septum
   d sphenopalatine artery

2 Recurrent epistaxis in an elderly patient is *not* usually associated with which of the following?
   a hypertension
   b cardiac failure
   c aspirin
   d clopidogrel

3 Which of the following is the most likely cause for epistaxis in a child?
  a juvenile nasopharyngeal angiofibroma
  b rhabdomyosarcoma
  c nasal fracture
  d a blood vessel on Little's area

4 For a patient with intractable bleeding, which of the following is *not* a treatment option?
  a ascending pharyngeal artery ligation
  b nasal packing under general anaesthesia
  c angiography with embolisation
  d sphenopalatine artery ligation

78 Low back and leg pain

Jin W. Tee[1,2,4] and Jeffrey V. Rosenfeld[1,3]

[1] Alfred Health, Melbourne, Victoria, Australia
[2] Monash University, Melbourne, Victoria, Australia
[3] Monash Institute of Medical Engineering, Melbourne, Victoria, Australia
[4] National Trauma Research Institute, Melbourne, Victoria, Australia

Introduction

Low back and leg pain, isolated or in conjunction, are amongst the most common reasons for general practice consultations. They are mainly degenerative in cause but in some instances may be traumatic, oncological and infectious. These latter aetiologies are deemed 'red flag' conditions or neurosurgical emergencies, and awareness of red flag symptoms and signs are paramount in ensuring safe and timely medical care.

This chapter covers the management principles required to assess and treat these conditions, both in the short and long term. The most important consideration regarding the successful long-term management of low back and leg pain is that the spinal vertebrae and soft tissue structures (disc, ligaments, facet joint capsule) deteriorate with age. Acute stressors of the spine are cumulative and often in an active person, accelerate a natural tendency to symptomatic osteoarthritic degeneration. As such, treating physicians must also be aware that genetic factors, underlying structural anomalies, occupation, pain tolerance, psychological factors and social circumstances all contribute to the origin, persistence and success of the long-term management of low back and leg pain.

There are many possible pain generators in the spine, including discs, ligaments, facet (zygapophyseal) joints, nerve roots, paraspinal muscles and extraspinal structures. It is often difficult to identify the exact cause of back pain in particular, as the pain is often emanating from multiple structures at multiple segmental levels in the spine. This makes the treatment of low back pain especially problematic, particularly as much of the treatment given for back pain is not based on a strong evidence base.

Importantly, low back pain results in a large financial cost to the community, especially as it afflicts professions with repetitive lifting or very physical work such as labourers, firefighters, paramedics, nurses, police and army personnel. It is therefore an important public health issue. Prevention is therefore the most important strategy to reduce the prevalence of low back pain.

Leg pain in a dermatomal pattern is often due to nerve root compression and in most patients is benign and self-limiting. Anatomically, the leg refers to that part of the lower limb below the knee, although when discussing leg pain, it commonly refers to any part of the lower limb, i.e. the buttock, thigh, leg and foot.

There are a few terms that are regularly used when discussing leg pain: sciatica, claudication and antalgic gait being the important ones.

- *Sciatica* is a symptom not a disease. It is a syndrome characterised by pain radiating from the back into the buttock and into the lower extremity along its posterior or lateral aspect; the term is also used to describe pain in the distribution of the sciatic nerve.
- *Claudication* is a condition where the patient suffers lower limb pain on walking, possibly associated with lameness or limping. It usually resolves on rest. A neural cause is likely when the patient has a stooped posture when ambulating, and when the symptoms dissipate on sitting and not on standing. A vascular cause is likely when the symptoms dissipate on standing alone.
- An *antalgic* gait is a limping gait as a result of a painful lower limb and with avoidance of mechanical stress on the affected side.

Applied anatomy

There are seven cervical vertebrae, twelve thoracic vertebrae, five lumbar vertebrae and five sacral

---

vertebrae. The spinal cord terminates in the adult at the LI–L2 disc level, where it becomes the filum terminale. The nerve roots of the cauda equina arise from the conus medullaris and pass through the lumbar and sacral canal.

The spinal nerve roots exit through the intervertebral foramina. There are eight cervical spinal nerve roots, so for example C7 passes across the C6–C7 disc and exits the C6–C7 intervertebral foramen. A posterolateral C6–C7 disc prolapse will therefore compress the C7 nerve root. As there are eight cervical roots and with C8 passing in the C7–T1 foramen, the T1 nerve root passes out in the T1–T2 foramen.

In the lumbar spine, each nerve root passes under the pedicle of its numbered level, so for example the L5 nerve root passes inferiorly across the back of L4–L5 intervertebral disc to exit below the L5 pedicle. Therefore, a posterolateral disc prolapse at L4–L5 will compress the L5 nerve root. A posterolateral disc prolapse at L5–S1 will compress the S1 nerve root. A 'far' lateral disc prolapse may compress the lumbar root passing beneath the pedicle above, so for example a far lateral disc prolapse at L4–L5 may compress the L4 nerve root.

Pain generators

Pain arising from the bones of the spine, ligaments, muscles or intervertebral discs is often called mechanical back pain. There is a lot of crossover in segmental nerve supply in the lumbar spine between different structures. The annulus of the intervertebral disc and the facet joints are supplied with nerve fibres. Pain from the disc (discogenic pain) or facet joints is felt in the back centrally (somatic pain) but may radiate to the buttock and upper thigh (somatic referred pain). Somatic back pain may also emanate from musculoskeletal structures, bone and extraspinal or paraspinal structures. Box 78.1 lists the common differential diagnoses of low back pain.

Nerve root compression or irritation results in radicular pain, which is sharp lancinating pain radiating down the lower limb and which may pass into the foot or down the arm into the hand. It may not follow an exact dermatomal pattern. As the facet joints are innervated by the nerve roots of that level and the level above, it is often difficult to distinguish somatic referred pain from radicular pain. The overall clinical assessment and correlation with the radiological findings is important. Local anaesthetic facet joint blocks, which suppress facet joint pain, and intradiscal injections have also been used to identify the principal pain generators in patients

> **Box 78.1 Differential diagnosis of low back pain**
>
> - Pancreatic disease, e.g. pancreatitis (high lumbar region)
> - Renal disease, e.g. hydronephrosis (usually lateral loin pain)
> - Abdominal aortic aneurysm
> - Pelvic disease
> - Rectum, bladder, gynaecological disease
> - Hip disease: there is pain on moving the hip; the pain may radiate to the buttock and posterior or lateral thigh down to the knee
> - Sacroiliitis
> - Lumbosacral plexus pathology
> - Peripheral nerve pathology, e.g. schwannoma, entrapment, inflammation

with chronic back pain. Table 78.1 lists the common causes of leg pain.

Musculo-ligamentous strain

This is the commonest cause of acute back pain. Usually there is an acute event such as a twisting, bending or lifting motion. The pain is localised but may spread to the buttock and upper thigh if from the lumbar region. There is spinal stiffness, local paraspinal muscle tenderness but no abnormal neurological signs.

Intervertebral disc prolapse

This is a common problem. There is usually a background of pre-existing weakening of spinal structures due to degeneration, and coupled with occurrences of high intra-abdominal pressure and sudden flexion of the lumbar spine (repeated straining and coughing) could lead to intervertebral disc prolapse. The fibrous annulus of the disc tears, allowing the softer nucleus of the disc to herniate or prolapse. If the prolapsed nucleus separates from the disc, it becomes a sequestrated fragment and may not resolve with expectant treatment. The intervertebral disc usually prolapses in the posterolateral direction and may compress the exiting spinal nerve root, which is adjacent to it, and cause sciatica. In the acute phase, the back pain is usually a minor component. Much less common is the central disc prolapse, which compresses the spinal cord or the cauda equina nerve roots depending on the spinal level. Cauda equina syndrome is a clinical syndrome that ensues as a result a major compressive lesion within the spinal canal, in this instance an acute disc prolapse. Based on the level of compression, this

Table 78.1 Differential diagnosis of leg pain.

Clinical problem	Presentation	Region of pathology	Pathology
Neural: spinal			
Sciatica	Radiating leg pain	Nerve root compression in spinal canal or exit foramen	Disc prolapse Lateral recess stenosis Osteophyte Synovial cyst Spondylolisthesis Foraminal stenosis Tumour
Neurogenic claudication	Bilateral leg pain, pins and needles, heaviness	Multiple roots under compression in the spinal canal	Lumbar canal stenosis Facet hypertrophy Ligamentum flavum hypertrophy Diffuse disc bulge Spondylolisthesis
		Venous hypertension or ischaemia of the spinal cord	Dural arteriovenous fistula
Neural: peripheral nerve			
Meralgia paresthetica	Burning pain, numbness anterolateral thigh	Lateral cutaneous nerve of thigh	Entrapment under inguinal ligament medial to anterior superior iliac spine
Piriformis syndrome	Pain in sciatic distribution	Sciatic nerve	Entrapment by piriformis muscle
Common peroneal nerve entrapment	Weak ankle dorsiflexion and anterolateral leg pain	Common peroneal nerve	Trapped as it winds around the head of fibula
Tarsal tunnel syndrome	Burning pain in the plantar surface of foot	Posterior tibial nerve	Flexor retinaculum from medial malleolus to calcaneus
Morton's neuralgia	Pain in third web space of foot and adjacent toes	Digital nerve in foot	Compression between metatarsal heads
Vascular	Acute vascular compromise Vascular claudication Varicose vein/venous insufficiency Deep vein thrombosis		
Joint/bony	Degenerative arthritis Rheumatoid arthritis Bony pathology: fracture, infection, malignancy Soft tissue: muscle Ligament Joints: facet, sacroiliac, symphysis pubis, hip, knee, ankle, foot		
Referred	Retroperitoneal pathology Appendicitis Inguinal hernia Aortic dissection Renal colic Pelvic disease		

causes severe bilateral sciatica, lower limb weakness, paraesthesia or dysaesthesia, loss of proprioception, and bowel and bladder dysfunction. The patient may develop acute urinary retention.

Disc prolapse (Figure 78.1) is most frequent in the lower lumbar spine (L4–L5, L5–S1) and in the lower cervical spine (C5–C6, C6–C7). These are also the levels where degenerative changes are most common. Disc bulging (protrusion) occurs where there is no prolapse (or extrusion) of nucleus. This is a common finding on CT or MRI and is not necessarily the cause of back pain and sciatica. Also, thoracic disc prolapse may compress an intercostal nerve laterally and cause radiating pain in the distribution of that nerve or may cause spinal cord compression when central.

(a)

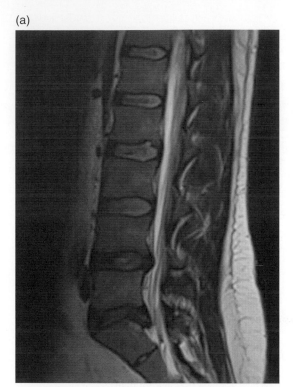

(b)

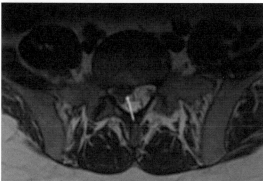

Fig. 78.1 (a) T2-weighted sagittal MRI of lumbar spine showing a smaller disc prolapse at L4/L5 and a larger disc prolapse at L5/S1. (b) T2-weighted axial MRI of lumbar spine showing a right-sided posterolateral disc prolapse (green arrow) compressing the S1 nerve root.

Infection

Osteomyelitis may be due to pyogenic infection usually by haematogenous spread, or due to tuberculosis. This will cause acute back pain (severe, unrelenting) and may cause neurological deficit due to vertebral deformity, bony instability or secondary epidural abscess. Again, acute and severe compression of the thecal sac is a neurosurgical emergency.

Primary epidural abscess may occur without osteomyelitis, particularly if bacteria are introduced into the spinal epidural space by a needle puncture or placement of an epidural catheter for analgesia. This problem has been reported following childbirth, with the mother developing severe back pain and possibly neurological deficit in the weeks following the placement of an epidural catheter for analgesia during labour. Discitis caused by a bacterial infection following surgery or systemic bacteraemia may also cause acute (and chronic) back pain.

Trauma

Trauma to the spine (Figure 78.2) may cause vertebral fractures, which may be unstable and may cause neurological injury. These injuries cause acute and often severe local pain and tenderness.

Vertebral collapse

Crushing of the anterior portion of the vertebral body in the thoracic or lumbar region is common following a hyperflexion injury to the spine. This causes wedging of the affected vertebral bodies and acute pain (severe, unrelenting). Wedging and vertebral collapse is also common in elderly patients and may be due to neoplastic infiltration (Figure 78.3), osteoporosis or, less commonly, infection.

Haematoma

An acute subdural or epidural haematoma in the thoracic spinal canal may cause acute cord compression with severe back pain and paraparesis. The cause of the bleed may be a ruptured vascular malformation or a spontaneous bleed in a patient on anticoagulants such as warfarin.

Spinal stroke

Thrombotic occlusion of the anterior spinal artery usually in a patient with diffuse atherosclerotic vascular disease causes an acute paraplegia, with severe acute back pain in the thoracic region. Myelogram or MRI does not show any compressive lesion but MRI may show cord signal hyperintensity, which indicates oedema or developing infarction.

Clinical presentation

History

A detailed history will provide a likely cause of the patient's low back and leg pain, and should help to distinguish mechanical, radicular and long tract symptoms. The age of the patient is an important factor in the analysis of cause of back pain. Back

(a) (b)

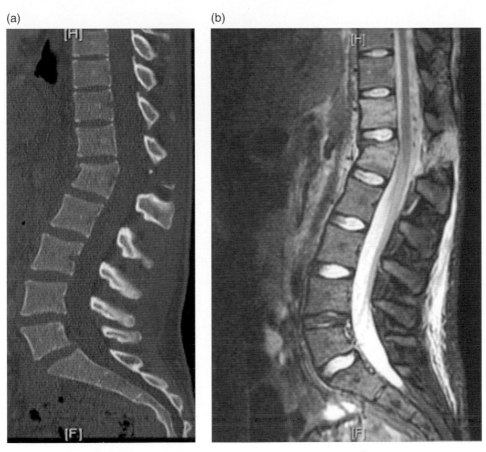

Fig. 78.2 (a) Sagittal midline CT of lumbar spine (bone windows setting) showing an L1 vertebral body compression fracture with distraction injury of the posterior elements (note the increase in superior–inferior dimensions of the T12 and L1 spinous processes and lamina). (b) T2-weighted sagittal midline MRI of lumbar spine showing the L1 fracture and distraction injury, which can be clearly seen as a hyperintensity between the T12 and L1 posterior elements.

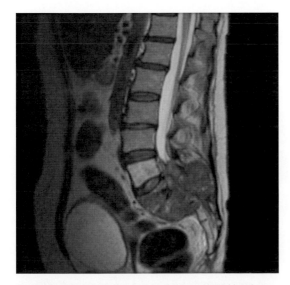

Fig. 78.3 T2-weighted sagittal midline MRI of lumbar spine showing a destructive sacral hepatocellular carcinoma metastases and pathological fracture with complete lumbar canal obliteration.

pain can be caused by disorders of organs that are not part of the musculoskeletal system (Box 78.1).

Degenerative spinal disorders

The commonest cause of sciatica is entrapment of the nerve root in the lumbar spinal canal or the exiting foramen by a disc prolapse or foraminal stenosis secondary to degeneration. The pain is usually unilateral and commonly involves one or more of the nerves from L4 to S1. Patients complain of sharp shooting pain, often originating in the buttock and radiating down the leg in the distribution of the nerve root under pressure (the sciatic nerve is not under pressure, rather a nerve root that contributes to the formation of the sciatic nerve). The pain is often associated with numbness, pins and needles and tingling, typically in a dermatomal pattern (see Figure 78.4a for dermatomal patterns). Patients can go on to develop weakness (see Figure 78.4b for myotomal patterns) in the distribution of the nerve root. Patients may occasionally develop leg pain as

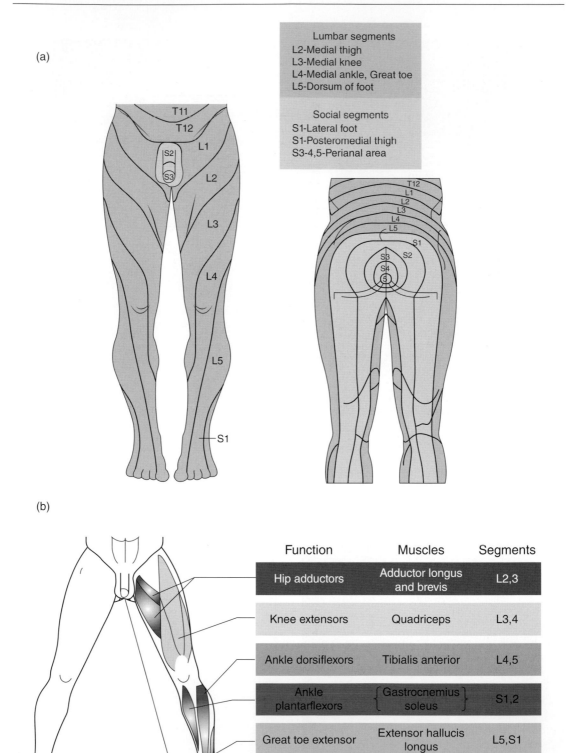

(a)

Lumbar segments
L2-Medial thigh
L3-Medial knee
L4-Medial ankle, Great toe
L5-Dorsum of foot

Social segments
S1-Lateral foot
S1-Posteromedial thigh
S3-4,5-Perianal area

(b)

Function	Muscles	Segments
Hip adductors	Adductor longus and brevis	L2,3
Knee extensors	Quadriceps	L3,4
Ankle dorsiflexors	Tibialis anterior	L4,5
Ankle plantarflexors	Gastrocnemius soleus	S1,2
Great toe extensor	Extensor hallucis longus	L5,S1
Anal sphincter	Sphincter ani externus	S2,3,4

Fig. 78.4 (a) Dermatomal pattern of sensory supply. Source: adapted from Netter FH. *The CIBA Collection of Medical Illustrations*, Vol 1. Nervous System, Part II: Neurologic and Neuromuscular Disorders, p. 183. Reproduced with permission of Elsevier. (b) Nerve root supply of muscles. Source: adapted from Netter FH. *The CIBA Collection of Medical Illustrations*, Vol 1. Nervous System, Part II: Neurologic and Neuromuscular Disorders, p. 182. Reproduced with permission of Elsevier.

a result of pressure on the L3 and rarely L2 nerve root, and this will radiate to the anterior thigh and knee.

The patient presents with an antalgic gait (where the gait is shortened on the painful side) and avoids sitting or does so with the leg straightened at the hip and flexed at the knee. This posture tends to relieve the stretch on the nerve and reduces pain levels.

Examination reveals limitation of straight leg raising, limited back movements, altered sensation, and numbness or weakness in the distribution of the nerve root. An absent reflex aids significantly in confirming the root involved.

Neurogenic claudication is characterised by bilateral leg pain, worse with walking but can be present when upright and standing still and improves with a change in posture (as compared with vascular claudication, which resolves with rest, irrespective of the posture of the patient). The pain is an ache-like discomfort, often with pins and needles, heaviness and tiredness of the legs, with variable numbness and a sense of weakness with walking. Lumbar canal stenosis is the commonest cause. Examination is often unremarkable and hyporeflexia may be the only finding. A vascular examination of skin circulation, and peripheral pulses is also required.

Thoracic or cervical myelopathy is a rare cause of leg pain. Occasionally compression or pathology in the spinal cord in the thoracic or cervical spine can result in a syringomyelia (a cavity in the spinal cord) that may result in leg pain.

Vascular

The vascular causes are described in greater detail in Chapters 55 and 57.

- *Acute arterial vascular compromise*: caused by trauma or acute arterial occlusion of a diseased artery by a thrombotic or embolic event. The patient presents with leg pain and paraesthesia with coldness, absence of pulses and pallor. Acute intervention to restore circulation is vital to preserve limb function.
- *Vascular claudication*: a well-recognised and common problem of leg pain, often calf pain. The pain is worse with walking and improves with rest. The pain is often a cramp-like pain in the muscles of the legs with a sense of tiredness and fatigue. Pain at rest is present with very severe disease. This is a result of progressive arteriosclerotic disease and the distribution of the pain reflects the site of arterial disease. Patients may benefit from bypass surgery.
- *Venous disease*: incompetence of the valves of the veins of the lower limb results in progressive

gravitational congestion of the leg. This results in a painful, achy, swollen leg that improves with rest and elevation of the leg. A major associated complication is thrombophlebitis and consequent risk of deep vein thrombosis. Surgery is indicated for major vascular incompetence.

Joint/bone pain

Joint pain as a result of acute inflammation, as seen in rheumatoid disease, connective tissue disease, gout or septic arthritis, is often acute and associated with swelling, redness and tenderness of the joint with radiation up or down the leg.

- Gout is a metabolic disorder characterised by an excess of uric acid in the blood. It usually presents in middle-aged men with rapid-onset painful swelling of a joint, usually the first metacarpophalangeal joint, which is red, hot and associated with proximal and distal pain. It must be differentiated from septic arthritis and other causes of leg pain.
- Septic arthritis is often bacterial in origin, presents with pain, swelling, redness and tenderness of a joint with radiation. Inflammatory markers are abnormal and patients require antibiotics and possibly aspiration or irrigation of the joint.
- Pain from wearing down of the cartilage of the articular surface is a progressive event and thus the pain has an insidious nature and progresses over a long period.
- An injury or inflammation of the joint capsule, tendon and muscle around a joint can also simulate joint pathology with secondary leg pain. Both muscle and joint pain can occur from metabolic and connective tissue disorder, and thus these patients may require a blood screen with measurement of erythrocyte sedimentation rate (ESR), rheumatoid factor and antinuclear factor and a rheumatology review.
- Sacroiliitis and arthritic changes in the hip, knee, ankle or arch of foot will cause local and radiating pain. Sacroiliac joint pain can radiate from the buttock into the upper thigh. Hip joint pain can radiate down to the knee.

Entrapment neuropathies

The pain is restricted to the distribution of the nerve root and thus a good history and examination can often provide the diagnosis. These syndromes (meralgia paresthetica, piriformis syndrome, tarsal tunnel syndrome, Morton's neuralgia) present primarily with pain restricted to the distribution of the nerve under pressure (Table 78.1). Medical therapies with an anticonvulsant (carbamazepine) or antidepressant (amitriptyline) can provide good control of their symptoms. The alternative is a diagnostic and therapeutic block with local anaesthesia and steroids. Should this fail, surgical decompression of the nerve should be considered.

Extraspinal pathology

Pathology of any of the structures in the abdomen, retroperitoneum and pelvis may cause local and referred pain. In most of these patients, the referred pain is likely to be non-radiculopathic, with no dermatomal pattern unless there is involvement of the lumbosacral plexus.

Emergencies

The attending physician should always be on the look out for red flag conditions presenting with acute low back and/or leg pain (Box 78.2) These conditions need urgent neurosurgical review, as they are likely to require emergency surgical decompression to treat neurological deficits, and fixation to treat instability. Nocturnal pain and pain at rest may indicate neural ischaemia from significant mechanical compression. A history of recent trauma and worsening pain on ambulation requires the exclusion of fracture. A history of weight loss and solid organ primary tumours implies metastatic spread or primary lesions unless proven otherwise. Fever, night sweats and rigors are symptoms suggestive of an infection or haematological malignancy including lymphoma.

A red flag is raised if the patient has bilateral lower limb symptoms such as numbness, weakness or pain.

Box 78.2 Key points and pitfalls

- Most back pain is benign in nature and cause, and usually resolves, even without treatment, in 3–4 weeks.
- It is important to try to differentiate radicular pain from musculoskeletal spinal pain and spinal cord compression.
- Hip pain may mimic sciatica due to compression of a spinal nerve root.
- Back pain in children should not be ignored as it often has a serious underlying cause.
- Negative plain radiographs or CT scans do not exclude the presence of serious spinal pathology.
- Make sure adequate investigation of back pain is undertaken at an early stage so that serious pathology is not missed.
- In patients with signs of spinal cord compression, do not forget to examine perineal sensation or to percuss the bladder.

Urgent MRI of the spine is mandated with any patient complaining of saddle area numbness or difficulty initiating micturition or incontinence. In these situations, a large disc prolapse or tumour causing cauda equina syndrome (compression of the cauda equina – the lumbosacral nerve roots in the lumbar spine – resulting in sacral anaesthesia plus bowel and bladder disturbance) needs exclusion. A cauda equina syndrome is a neurosurgical emergency and requires urgent neural decompressive surgery.

Examination

The examination is done in the erect, prone and supine positions. It is important to differentiate between upper and lower motor neurone lesions and to identify the level of spinal pathology.

Spine and joints

Standing

Inspection for midline skin lesions such as a pit, sinus, hairy patch, lipoma, naevus or angioma over the spine. These may indicate underlying occult spinal bifida, spinal dysraphism or tethering of the spinal cord.

Assess general posture and spinal alignment, particularly for scoliosis or kyphosis. Are both feet planted symmetrically on the ground? The cervical spine and the lumbar spine normally have a lordosis (forward curve).

Range of movement includes forward flexion, lateral flexion, rotation and extension. Examine the shoulders and upper limbs if the patient has neck pain.

Supine

Examine the movements of the hips and knees. Examine the sacroiliac joint by adduction and internal rotation of the flexed hip.

Prone

Palpate the back for tenderness, paraspinal mass, paraspinal muscle spasm. Percuss the spine for tenderness. Complete the examination of the hip joint with extension.

Motor function

Neurological examination

Even in the absence of limb pain a careful examination must be made of the limbs, as the neurological signs that may be detected will often lead you to the precise site of pathology in or around the spine.

Gait

Observe for limping, rate of movement, length of stride and need for walking aid. This will give many clues as to what is wrong and the severity.

Muscles

Muscle wasting and fasciculation imply denervation of muscles – examine all the muscle groups including the shoulder girdle and gluteal region. Muscle tone, power and reflexes including the plantars are measured to determine whether it is an upper or lower motor neurone problem, or a mixed picture (see Figure 78.4).

Sensation

If you suspect a spinal cord lesion, then full sensory testing should be performed. Test pain with pinprick (spinothalamic tracts) and light touch and proprioception (dorsal columns). Figure 78.4 shows the dermatomal distribution from T11 to S5. Do not forget to test sacral, perianal and scrotal/vulval sensation when relevant. Establish a sensory level on the trunk for a suspected case of spinal cord compression. This will help with the localisation of the pathology.

Special tests

Straight leg raising is normally to 90° with the patient in the supine position. Lift the whole lower limb passively whilst it is straight, flexing at the hip joint. This stretches sciatic nerve roots. Record the angle at which sciatica stops the movement.

Lasègue's stretch test is a test of pressure on the sciatic nerve. The ankle is dorsiflexed with the lower limb outstretched and flexed at the hip, placing extra stress on the sciatic nerve which, if already tethered by some pathology such as a disc prolapse, will cause a sharp jab of pain.

Femoral stretch test is a test of pressure on the upper lumbar nerve roots. The patient is *prone* and the lower limb is extended at the hip, placing tension on the upper lumbar roots.

Rectal examination includes prostate and pelvis, anal tone, external sphincter contraction (the patient tightens the anus with the gloved finger in the rectum), perianal and perineal sensation. Assess the abdomen for bladder fullness.

Anal reflex (S4–S5) involves contraction of the subcutaneous portion of the external sphincter in response to scratching the perianal skin.

Sacral sparing may occur within a widespread area of sensory loss caused by an intramedullary spinal cord lesion, and is due to the laminar arrangement of the fibres in the spinothalamic tract. The sacral segments are lateral in the tract. It thus means there is an incomplete spinal cord problem and may be the only sign of this.

General examination

The examination includes chest, abdomen and lymph nodes. Rectal and internal pelvic examinations are done when relevant. In a patient with back or radicular pain always consider intra abdominal and other pathologies as a cause for pain. Assess the adequacy of the arterial circulation in the lower limbs in the older patient.

Investigation

Plain X-rays

Plain X-rays are often done as an initial screen for patients with back pain but have a low sensitivity. Plain cervical X-rays are also used as a routine screen in multiple trauma patients and other regions of the spine if clinically indicated.

Dynamic (flexion–extension) views

These are plain radiographs, fluoroscopy or MRI scans used to demonstrate mechanical instability of spinal segments.

Computed tomography

Computed tomography is often ordered as the initial investigation for back pain. It shows the bony anatomy and the facet joints very clearly but is of variable and often inferior quality at showing the soft tissues, including the discs and intraspinal pathology.

Magnetic resonance imaging

MRI is now the main modality for spinal imaging and has virtually replaced CT myelography because it is non-invasive and because of the extensive information provided in different projections including the sagittal.

Myelography

The introduction of intrathecal contrast produces a myelogram that outlines the spinal roots and cord and is a dynamic study which can demonstrate a spinal block of the subarachnoid space by a mass lesion. Myelography is often followed by CT (CT myelography) which shows the contrast on the axial (horizontal) CT images. This modality is especially useful in patients with previous metal components (obscures MRI images) and especially those with MRI-incompatible cardiac pacemakers and deep brain stimulators.

SPECT-CT nuclear medicine bone scan

Single photon emission computed tomography (SPECT)-CT is a fusion between a technetium-labelled nuclear medicine bone scan and CT spine imaging. The radionuclide is detected by a gamma camera. The cameras rotate over a 360° arc around the patient, allowing for reconstruction of images in three dimensions. This allows identification of hotspots, which if correlated with clinical history and examination can lead to higher accuracy of spinal element pain generators. These areas are then injected with local anaesthetic and corticosteroids to assess response.

Discography

Discography involves injection of the intervertebral disc with contrast, which may show internal derangement of the disc and may be used as a provocative test to identify the origin of back pain. This test has rapidly gone out of favour with poor evidence for its use. Instead, injection of local anaesthetic and corticosteroid into the disc space is used occasionally to diagnose discal pain generators.

Biopsy and needle aspirate of vertebral or paraspinal disease

Biopsy and needle aspirate under CT guidance is a useful diagnostic technique that may be used when open surgery is not indicated and provides specimens for histopathology and microbiology analysis.

Blood tests

Blood tests, including blood cultures, full blood examination and inflammatory markers are performed selectively.

Treatment

Non-operative treatment

Most back pain aetiologies are benign in nature, and usually resolve in 3–4 weeks with no treatment. Degenerative disease and disc prolapse are initially managed conservatively and surgery should be considered as a last resort unless there is significant neurological deficits causing functional impairment.

Conservative treatments for acute back pain usually trialled include rest and physiotherapy, which may include massage, traction, interferential heat treatment and manipulation. Chiropractic treatment and acupuncture are alternatives, but should not be recommended when there is a spinal deformity or significant radicular symptoms. Drugs include non-steroidal anti-inflammatory drugs (NSAIDs), analgesics including opiates, nerve membrane stabilisers, muscle relaxants and steroids. Exercises such as Pilates are often not useful in treating acute back pain, but have a role once it has largely settled so as to strengthen the paraspinal and abdominal muscles, which are often weakened in patients with degenerative spinal disease and disc prolapse.

More than 80% of patients with sciatica respond to non-operative treatment. Patients also need to avoid factors that will exacerbate the pain, so should avoid heavy lifting, repetitive bending and twisting. The role of physiotherapy is to re-educate the patient in terms of posture, exercises to strengthen back, abdominal and pelvic muscles, and stretches.

The role of warm/cold therapy, massage, acupuncture or hydrotherapy in the acute stage is uncertain and unpredictable. The patient must be cautioned against manipulation as it may precipitate a larger disc prolapse and a cauda equina syndrome. In the acute setting the benefit from epidural or foraminal steroids is not predictable and more likely to succeed in patients who have a small disc bulge or a foraminal disc prolapse.

The role of non-surgical treatment for neurogenic claudication is limited in patients with significant symptoms. They may have some benefit from analgesia, NSAIDs, physiotherapy and hydrotherapy; however, in view of the mechanical compression, decompression offers the best long-term result.

Operative treatment

Surgical intervention is indicated in patients with intractable pain, in those who fail to respond to medical therapy, and in those who have a neurological deficit. Patients are usually treated conservatively for a minimum of 6 weeks unless they present with red flag conditions.

Microdiscectomy and neurolysis (freeing up the nerve root) are indicated for patients who have a disc prolapse and have failed non-operative treatment. The microdiscectomy is done with magnification of the surgeon's view, a small skin incision, minimal paraspinal muscle disruption, and minimal bony removal of lamina and adjacent ligament.

This surgery has a better than 90% success rate for control of the leg pain provided the clinical picture matches the imaging.

Patients with lumbar canal stenosis require a decompressive laminectomy, lateral recess decompression (the lateral part of the spinal canal where the nerve roots are compressed) and neurolysis. In either situation, the presence or potential of instability will require consideration of an instrumented fusion in addition to the surgical decompression.

The potential success of spinal surgery for degenerative conditions depends on many factors. Predictors of a poor outcome are smokers, patients undergoing active litigation or those who are claiming compensation within the work-cover system and having a predominant back pain symptomatology. It is crucial that all patients are given the full range of conservative management prior to surgical intervention. This will include chronic pain management if their symptoms are chronic and disabling and where the surgical indications are uncertain. They would also need to be well counselled regarding the goal of surgery, the potential complications, the lifestyle modification required to ensure longevity of their spine construct and, finally, appropriate expectations.

It is pertinent that red flag conditions are diagnosed and treated emergently. Neural decompression, restoration of neural deficits and augmentation of spinal structures conferring stability remain the mainstay of treatment of these conditions.

Acute or subacute spinal cord compression and cauda equina syndrome are serious problems that require urgent referral to a neurosurgeon. Emergency decompressive surgery may be required to preserve neurological function and reverse neurological deficit. Whether the decompression of the spinal canal is done via a posterior approach (laminectomy or costotransversectomy) or via an anterior approach (anterior cervical, thoracotomy or transabdominal) depends on the nature and site of the pathology and the experience of the surgeon. A diseased vertebral body may require excision and replacement by a prosthesis (intervertebral 'cage') and the stability of the spine may need to be restored with metallic internal fixation using rods, plates, pedicle screws and bone grafts. Following such spinal surgery the patient may require radiotherapy or chemotherapy for a neoplasm or prolonged antibiotic therapy for an infection.

An osteoporotic vertebral collapse could be treated with an injection of acrylic cement into the affected vertebral body under radiological guidance to restore the volume and strength of the bone and relieve pain. This treatment remains controversial based on a conflicting evidence base.

Further reading

Koes BW, van Tulder M, Lin C-WC, Macedo LG, McAuley J, Maher C. An updated overview of clinical guidelines for the management of non-specific low back pain in primary care. *Eur Spine J* 2010;19:2075–94.

Lewis RA, Williams NH, Sutton AJ *et al.* Comparative clinical effectiveness of management strategies for sciatica: systematic review and network meta-analyses. *Spine J* 2015;15:1461–77.

Lurie JD, Tosteson TD, Tosteson ANA *et al.* Surgical versus non-operative treatment for lumbar disc herniation: eight-year results for the Spine Patient Outcomes Research Trial (SPORT). *Spine* 2014;39:3–16.

Samanta J, Kendall J, Samanta A. 10-minute consultation: chronic low back pain. *BMJ* 2003;326(7388):535.

MCQs

Select the single correct answer to each question. The correct answers can be found in the Answers section at the end of the book.

1 An L5–S1 posterolateral disc prolapse is most likely to cause which of the following?
   a pain from the buttock radiating down the back of the thigh and to the sole of the foot
   b an L5 radiculopathy
   c weakness of foot dorsiflexion
   d weakness of extensor hallucis longus
   e an absent knee jerk

2 Which of the following statements about cauda equina syndrome is correct?
   a it is a benign clinical problem
   b requires urgent decompression
   c has no influence on bladder function
   d can only be present if the patient has severe leg pain
   e can be managed best with manipulation

3 A 30-year-old man presents with 1 week of right sciatica and has numbness on the dorsum of his right foot and weak dorsiflexion at the ankle. Which of the following is true?
   a he probably has an L4–L5 disc prolapse, with compression of the L4 nerve root
   b he needs an urgent CT myelogram
   c he can be managed initially with rest and analgesics
   d he is likely to require surgery
   e he should be encouraged to undertake spinal extension exercises

4 A 35-year-old woman presents with acute lumbar back pain, bilateral sciatica, difficulty in voiding and on examination has weakness in the ankles and feet, absent ankle reflexes and decreased sensation in the soles of both feet. Which of the following statements is *incorrect*?

a she has developed an acute cauda equina compression

b she has developed an acute spinal cord compression

c central disc prolapse at L5–S1 is a likely cause

d urgent MRI is required

e urgent surgery will be required

5 A 30-year-old diabetic presents with a severe mid and lower thoracic pain, radiation of the pain to the mid-abdomen, and on examination is tender in the thoracic spine at the level of T10, has weak lower limbs and finds it difficult to walk. Which of the following statements is *incorrect*?

a CT scan will be helpful as an initial investigation

b he should have a full blood examination and ESR

c he may have a dissecting aneursym of the aorta

d a needle biopsy is indicated initially

e MRI is indicated and urgent surgery should be considered

79 Acute scrotal pain

Anthony Dat[1] and Shomik Sengupta[2]

[1,2] Eastern Health, Melbourne, Victoria, Australia
[2] Monash University, Melbourne, Victoria, Australia

Introduction and anatomy

The scrotum is the pouch of skin that contains the testes, spermatic cords and associated structures (Figure 79.1). Embryologically, the scrotum develops by fusion of the labioscrotal swellings and the urogenital folds in the midline. The scrotum contains the dartos muscle, a smooth muscle underlying the skin which contributes to its rugosity. Deep to this are the following layers covering the testes and spermatic cord: external spermatic fascia, cremasteric muscle (over the cord) and fascia, internal spermatic fascia, tunica vaginalis and tunica albuginea. The cremaster muscle, supplied by the genital branch of the genitofemoral nerve, allows the raising and lowering of the testicle. This function allows for temperature regulation to optimise spermatogenesis (which requires a temperature slightly lower than core body temperature). The contents of the spermatic cord (vas deferens, testicular artery, pampiniform plexus, nerves and lymphatics) enter the scrotum via the inguinal canal.

Acute scrotal pain is a presenting complaint that requires a timely diagnosis. There are a number of differential diagnoses, ranging from the emergent such as testicular torsion and incarcerated inguinal hernia to epididymo-orchitis and varicocele. A presumptive diagnosis can be obtained on history and physical examination in most cases.

Differential diagnosis

Testicular torsion

Testicular torsion occurs due to twisting of the spermatic cord, a surgical emergency with an incidence of 1 in 4000 in males under than the age of 25 years. Testicular torsion leads to vascular compromise, initially causing venous occlusion with subsequent arterial ischaemia and infarction. Scrotal ultrasound, if undertaken, may demonstrate reduction of blood flow (Figure 79.2).

There are two types of torsion: intravaginal and extravaginal. Intravaginal torsion is by far the most common type (95%) with torsion of the spermatic cord within the tunica vaginalis. Extravaginal torsion occurs almost exclusively in newborns as the tunica vaginalis is not adherent to the dartos. Thus, the spermatic cord and tunica vaginalis can twist as a unit. Predisposing factors for torsion include undescended testis (cryptorchidism) and the bell clapper deformity (12% of the male population). This is a congenital abnormality where the tunica vaginalis has an abnormal fixation proximally on the spermatic cord, allowing greater mobility and hence risk of torsion.

Testicular torsion is a true surgical emergency because viability of the testis is inversely related to duration of ischaemia. Ischaemia greater than 6 hours usually results in irreversible damage and loss of the testis. Thus, the diagnosis of torsion needs to be based mainly on clinical suspicion and should lead to urgent surgical intervention to untwist the testicle and restore vascularity. This is usually undertaken by surgical exploration of the scrotum, although external detorsion can also be attempted, especially if there are unavoidable delays in organising surgery. Possible complications of testicular torsion include testicular infarction and atrophy or the development of anti-sperm antibody, both of which can lead to subfertility.

Torsion of appendages

Torsion of testicular appendages is the most common cause of acute scrotal pain in prepubertal children. The appendix testis (hydatid of Morgagni) is a remnant of the paramesonephric or Müllerian duct and is present in 92% of cases and found at the superior pole of the testis. The appendix of the epididymis is a remnant of the mesonephric or Wolffian duct and

(a)

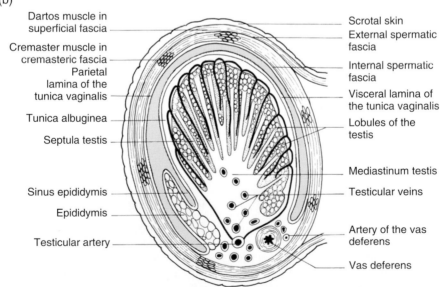

(b)

Fig. 79.1 (a) Diagrammatic view of scrotal anatomy. (b) Cross-section of testicular anatomy. Source: Ellis H, Mahadevan V. *Clinical Anatomy: Applied Anatomy for Students and Junior Doctors*, 13th edn. Oxford: Wiley Blackwell, 2013. Reproduced with permission of John Wiley & Sons.

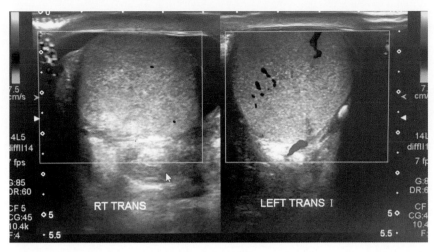

Fig. 79.2 Ultrasound images demonstrating a reduction in blood flow in the right testicle consistent with testicular torsion.

is present in about 25% of cases, usually near the head of the epididymis. The clinical presentation can be similar to testicular torsion but with a peak age of incidence between 7 and 12 years old. Torsion of appendages can sometimes present with the 'blue dot' sign, the blue infarcted appendage seen through the scrotal skin. This sign occurs in 20% of people and mainly in those with fair skin. This condition is usually self-limiting with no adverse sequelae to fertility, although scrotal exploration is often undertaken if there is any diagnostic uncertainty.

Fournier's gangrene

Fournier's gangrene is a form of necrotising fasciitis that is a surgical emergency requiring urgent debridement and broad-spectrum antibiotics. It is potentially life-threatening and most commonly arises secondarily from infections of the skin, anorectal region or urethra. Risk factors include diabetes mellitus, immunosuppression or recent urethral instrumentation. It is usually polymicrobial with a mixture of anaerobic and aerobic bacteria. Clinically, it starts as cellulitis that rapidly spreads. Extreme pain, fever and evidence of septic shock are key findings. Crepitus can be felt secondary to gas gangrene. A high clinical suspicion is necessary if there is a systemic inflammatory response syndrome or septic shock out of proportion to local findings.

Management involves intravenous fluid resuscitation, intravenous broad-spectrum antibiotics and immediate surgical debridement of all necrotic tissue. A second look for further debridement and washout should be performed 24–48 hours after the initial procedure to assess further tissue viability.

Depending on the area of involvement, temporary urinary diversion (either urethral or preferably suprapubic catheter) or diverting colostomy or rectal tube may be required. Anatomically, the infection is usually superficial to Colles' fascia of the perineum, the dartos fascia of the scrotum and Scarpa's fascia of the anterior abdomen. Orchidectomy is usually not required as the testes have their own blood supply (testicular arteries and veins) independent to that of the scrotum.

Epididymo-orchitis

Epididymo-orchitis occurs due to an ascending infection from the lower urinary tract. Most cases in younger men are due to sexually transmitted organisms such as *Neisseria gonorrhoeae* and *Chlamydia trachomatis*. Urethritis is usually present in those with a sexually transmitted infection (STI)-related cause. In older men, it is usually due to Gram-negative urinary pathogens such as *Escherichia coli*. Epididymo-orchitis can also occur secondary to a number of systemic bacterial infections such as extrapulmonary tuberculosis, syphilis, melioidosis and viral infections (e.g. mumps). On scrotal ultrasonogaphy, patients with epididymo-orchitis have increased blood flow to the epididymis or testicle (Figure 79.3). A reactive hydrocele may also be present. Antibiotics are the mainstay of treatment. Untreated epididymo-orchitis can lead to abscess formation, pyocele and infertility.

Inguinal hernia

A complicated inguinal hernia must be considered as part of the work-up of acute scrotal pain. Reducible

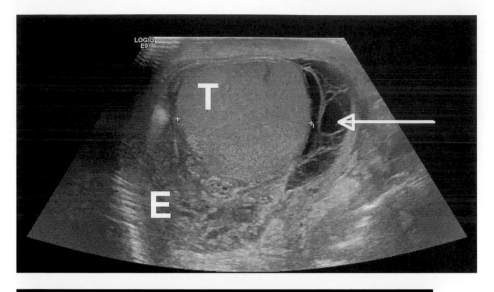

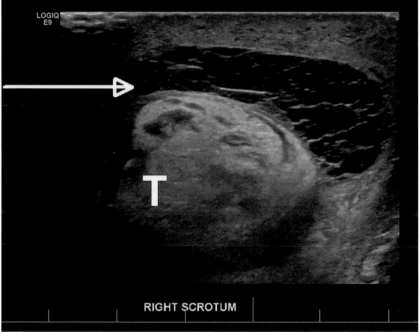

Fig. 79.3 Ultrasound images demonstrating oedema and swelling of the epididymis (E) and testis (T) and a reactive hydrocele (arrow) resulting from epididymo-orchitis.

hernias can cause discomfort, but acute pain and tenderness associated with an irreducible mass is concerning for an incarcerated inguinal hernia. Bowel contents within the hernia sac can infarct if emergency inguinal herniorrhaphy is not undertaken. A history of known hernias or previous hernia surgery may exist. Key physical examination findings to suggest an inguinal hernia as cause of a scrotal mass include the inability to get above the scrotal mass and presence of bowel sounds over the mass.

Testicular or paratesticular tumour

Characteristically, testicular or paratesticular tumours present as a painless scrotal mass, although a minority can present with pain particularly if there is acute haemorrhage or infarction within the tumour. Testicular ultrasound should be used to further characterise if there is suspicion of malignancy. Differentiation from an inflammatory mass can sometimes be difficult, in which case close temporal follow-up with repeat imaging may be needed.

Hydrocele

This is a serous fluid collection sometimes resulting from a defect in the tunica vaginalis, although most adult hydroceles are idiopathic. It should be noted that some hydroceles can occur in those with a testicular tumour. In addition, a reactive hydrocele can form secondary to infection (e.g. orchitis). Thus, clinical and radiographic examination of the underlying testicle and scrotal ultrasound is essential. Clinical presentation is usually with swelling and subacute discomfort, with acute painful presentation suggesting infection or haemorrhage. In those patients with ongoing pain and discomfort, surgery can be undertaken, whereby the hydrocele sac is excised and everted to prevent recurrence.

Epididymal cyst or sperm granuloma

These epididymal pathologies are quite common, and typically present with a palpable lump, occasionally with mild discomfort. Acute pain occurs rarely and may be indicative of infection or haemorrhage. The diagnosis is usually obvious on clinical examination, but may be confirmed by scrotal ultrasound. Surgical excision is indicated only if symptoms are bothersome.

Varicocele

Varicocele refers to the dilatation and tortuosity of the pampiniform plexus and should be seen as the testicular version of varicose veins. It can occur in up to 10% of men and is due to incompetent valves in the testicular veins. The majority of varicoceles occur on the left side. The pathophysiology is thought to be due to increased venous pressure within the left renal vein and increased risk of valvular incompetence at the junction between the left testicular vein and the left renal vein. Occasionally, it can be a presenting feature of a left renal tumour, hence the kidneys are usually assessed sonographically if a varicocele is found. An additional concern about varicoceles is that they can be associated with subfertility due to increased testicular temperature secondary to vein dilatation. Treatment in the form of a varicocelectomy or embolisation should be considered for those with demonstrably impaired sperm quality or quantity and ongoing severe pain.

Testicular trauma

The mechanism of testicular trauma can be divided into blunt, penetrating or degloving. In the Australian setting, it is predominantly blunt secondary to assaults, sporting injuries or, infrequently, motor vehicle accidents. Penetrating injuries are secondary to a projectile such as a gunshot wound. Degloving (avulsion) injuries are the least common, with scrotal skin being sheared off, for example, from clothing getting caught in machinery. In the blunt trauma setting, ultrasound can be useful for demonstrating evidence of testicular rupture. If testicular rupture is present, the goal of surgery is to debride devascularised tissue and ensure closure of the tunica albuginea. The aim is to preserve as much testicle as possible for endocrine function and spermatogenesis.

Referred pain

Referred pain from the abdomen, lower back or upper thigh can present with scrotal pain and is usually duller and not easily localised. Classic examples of this are pain from ureteric colic causing the typical 'loin to groin' pain or nerve root pain arising from intervertebral disc prolapse.

Assessment

History

The following structure can be used as a template for history taking.

History of presenting complaint

- Onset and duration of pain (testicular torsion is sudden onset and intense, epididymo-orchitis is gradual and progresses from mild to more severe). Duration is key for prognosis in those with torsion
- Prior episodes (may indicate previous intermittent torsion that resolves)
- History of trauma or symptoms of urinary tract infection (UTI) such as dysuria and frequency
- Presence of vomiting
- Concurrent fevers, chills and rigors (suggests infective cause)
- Patient fasting status, if need for theatre

Past medical/surgical/medications history

- Comorbidities and regular medications (e.g. anticoagulants/antiplatelet medication due to bleeding risk)
- History of prior testicular pathologies (e.g. tumour, varicocele)
- Previous scrotal surgery
- History of inguinal hernia

Family history

- Family history of testicular cancer

Social history

- Sexual history in those with suspected STI-induced epididymo-orchitis

Examination

Systematic examination includes the abdomen, inguinal region and finally the perineum and scrotum. Inspection should be followed by palpation.

Inspection

- Perineal or scrotal masses or wounds
- Previous scrotal and inguinal hernia surgical scars
- Presence of erythema, crepitus and swelling (marking the extent of erythema is useful in assessing response to treatment)
- Dilated varicosities for varicocele ('bag of worms'); can perform Valsalva manoeuvre to enlarge varicosities
- Lie of testicle (should be vertical)
- Check for urethral discharge

Palpation

- If scrotal mass present, characterise size, location, consistency (e.g. hard, fluctuant), transillumination with a pen torch (in case of hydrocele) and presence of concurrent tenderness
- Check inguinal ring for presence of hernia and whether reducible
- Palpate testes and epididymis for tenderness and lie (note that patients with torsion will do everything they can to prevent you from examining due to pain)
- Elicit cremasteric reflex (see following)

Testicular torsion is characterised by a high-lying testicle that is exquisitely tender and which may preclude full examination. The affected testis may also be in a horizontal orientation due to the torsion as opposed to the normal vertical lie. Testicular torsion has been associated with an absent cremasteric reflex. This reflex, mediated by the genitofemoral nerve which supplies the cremaster muscle, normally presents after the age of 2 years and is elicited by scratching the medial thigh with resultant testis elevation. It is thought that the reflex correlates with normal testicular perfusion. However, up to 10% of men with testicular torsion can

present with an intact cremasteric reflex. Thus the presence of a cremasteric reflex does not necessarily rule out a diagnosis of torsion, especially if there are other strong clinical findings of torsion present.

Investigations

In the setting of acute scrotal pain with clinical suspicion of testicular torsion, investigations should not delay emergency scrotal exploration. In those where diagnosis is uncertain and a timely ultrasound Doppler of the scrotum can be sought, it has a sensitivity of 86–100% and specificity of 75–100%. Findings consistent with torsion include testicular parenchymal heterogeneity and reduced or absent Doppler colour flow compared with the contralateral testis. Scrotal ultrasound is most useful in confirming diagnoses other than torsion, such as epididymo-orchitis.

Besides this, investigations that are useful include midstream urine for microscopy, culture and sensitivity for UTI; first-void urine sample for nucleic acid amplification testing (polymerase chain reaction, PCR) for *C. trachomatis* and *N. gonorrhoeae*; and urethral swab for Gram stain and culture for *N. gonorrhoeae* if there is suspicion of STI.

Management

When findings support or raise suspicion for testicular torsion, emergency scrotal exploration and detorsion is indicated and should not be delayed, as discussed previously. If the testicle is viable, both testes should be surgically fixed to the scrotum (orchidopexy). Orchidectomy is reserved for non-viable testicles. Time is critical in successful salvage rates. Detorsion within 6 hours results in a salvage rate of 90% and higher. This falls significantly to 20% after 12 hours and 0–10% after 24 hours.

For epididymo-orchitis, antibiotic treatment against the causative organisms is the mainstay, with selection of agents guided by local antibiotic guidelines. Sexually acquired infection should be treated with ceftriaxone 500 mg i.v. stat plus azithromycin 1 g oral stat. Subsequent maintenance treatment is doxycycline 100 mg oral 12-hourly for 2 weeks or azithromycin 1 g oral as a single dose 1 week later (if the patient is suspected to be non-adherent to doxycycline). For those with non-sexually acquired infections, trimethoprim or a quinolone (e.g. ciprofloxacin, norfloxacin) for 2 weeks is required. Symptomatic relief may be provided by scrotal support and analgesics or anti-inflammatories.

Conclusions

Acute scrotal pain has a limited range of differentials. Despite this, it has a number of important diagnoses that require timely surgical management. These include testicular torsion, Fournier's gangrene, testicular rupture and incarcerated inguinal hernia. If clinically indicated, management should not be delayed by ultrasound imaging as 'time is testis'.

Further reading

Jaison A, Mitra B, Cameron P, Sengupta S. Use of ultrasound and surgery in adults with acute scrotal pain. *ANZ J Surg* 2011;81:366–70.

Metzdorf M, Barthold JS. Torsion, testis and testicular appendages. In: Gomella LG (ed.) *The 5-Minute Urology Consult*, 2nd edn. Philadelphia: Wolters Kluwer/Lippincott Williams and Wilkins, 2010.

Srinath H. Acute scrotal pain. *Aust Fam Physician* 2013;42:790–2.

MCQs

Select the single correct answer to each question. The correct answers can be found in the Answers section at the end of the book.

1 Which of the following symptoms and signs is *not* commonly found in testicular torsion?
   a high-riding testicle
   b vomiting
   c transverse lie of testicle
   d haematuria
   e acute severe testicular pain

2 Which of the following is the most appropriate next step for a clinically suspected testicular torsion?
   a organise Doppler testicular ultrasound
   b start on intravenous antibiotics and review again in 24 hours
   c proceed to scrotal exploration and orchidopexy
   d organise computed tomography of the scrotum
   e discharge the patient and organise review in outpatient clinic in 2 weeks

3 Which of the following is *not* associated with epididymo-orchitis?
   a bell clapper deformity
   b fever
   c history of urinary tract infection
   d recent urethral instrumentation
   e sexually transmitted infection

80 Post-traumatic confusion

John Laidlaw

University of Melbourne and Royal Melbourne Hospital, Melbourne, Victoria, Australia

Introduction

The term 'confusion' is widely used but not discretely defined. In medical situations confusion typically refers to a disordered state characterised by lack of clear and orderly thought and/or behaviour. Common features include inattentiveness and altered perception of the world (disorientation in time, place and/or person, and occasionally hallucinations) with these features commonly resulting in the patient demonstrating uncooperative behaviour and agitation. Although the term 'delirium' is also often used interchangeably with the term 'acute confusional state', this adds further confusion and will not be used further in this chapter.

It must be appreciated therefore that post-traumatic confusion is a clinical finding, but not in itself a diagnosis. It is not confined to patients with brain injuries and is not uncommon following other injuries. It can occur at any age, although is more commonly identified in very young and also elderly patients. Being a clear demonstration of abnormal brain function, the need to identify and treat the pathology underlying post-traumatic confusion is of critical importance.

Aetiology and pathogenesis (Box 80.1)

Primary brain injury

Primary brain injury occurs at the time of the trauma. This includes direct neuroglial injury that can be relatively focal at the major points of impact or can occur throughout the brain following blunt head trauma, the diffuse form being referred to as diffuse axonal injury (DAI). Direct damage to the cortical vessels causing haemorrhagic contusions is also usually included in the primary brain injury group. One of the main principles of brain injury management is that not all damage to neurones is irreversible, and given an optimal cellular environment some or many of these cells can recover.

Even after relatively minor trauma, a very significant head injury can occur. Indeed, it is often not recognised that a fall from a standing position resulting in direct head impact can commonly cause a fatal brain injury. Therefore, post-traumatic confusion must always raise a high degree of suspicion for a significant head injury, with altered brain function immediately after the trauma being highly suggestive of a primary brain injury, and delayed onset suggesting secondary brain injury (e.g. hypoxia, poor cerebral perfusion, expanding intracranial haematoma).

Although a normal CT scan of the brain following trauma is somewhat reassuring, it needs to be remembered that this does not exclude a significant brain injury; indeed, DAI may have a normal early CT scan (if present, the 'pathognomonic' petechial haemorrhages seen in the subcortical regions, splenium and tectal plate are a result of small vessel shear injury, and the axonal injury is implied but not directly demonstrable on the scan).

It is also important to remember that a minor traumatic brain injury (mTBI) can sometimes fail to be identified, particularly in intoxicated patients but also in those with multiple other injuries. The terms 'concussion' and 'post-traumatic amnesia' (PTA) are often applied to mTBI patients with post-traumatic confusion and a brain CT that is normal or only has minor changes. These terms are not strictly interchangeable, and there is institutional variability in the defining criteria. Concussion is generally considered to be a predominantly transient alteration in neurological function following head trauma, with the cerebral injury being predominantly functional rather than structural. Its major features are confusion and amnesia following cerebral trauma, often following a brief period of loss of consciousness, usually associated with minimal evidence of structural

Textbook of Surgery, Fourth Edition. Edited by Julian A. Smith, Andrew H. Kaye, Christopher Christophi and Wendy A. Brown.
© 2020 John Wiley & Sons Ltd. Published 2020 by John Wiley & Sons Ltd.

Box 80.1 Causes of post-traumatic confusion

Head injury
Primary brain injury
- Diffuse axonal injury
- Cerebral contusions

Secondary brain injury
Hypoxia
- Hypoxaemia due to respiratory causes
  - Aspiration
  - Pulmonary contusions
  - Pulmonary oedema
  - Pulmonary thromboembolism
  - Pulmonary fat embolism
  - Hypoxaemia due to anaemia

Cerebral ischaemia
- Shock
- Vascular injury (particularly arterial dissection)
- Thromboembolism
  - Thromboembolic
  - Cerebral fat emboli
  - Disseminated intravascular coagulation
- Raised ICP (CPP = MAP − ICP)
  - Intracranial haematoma
    - EDH
    - Acute SDH
    - Intracerebral haematoma and enlarging contusions
    - Chronic SDH
  - Hydrocephalus
    - Obstructive
    - Communicating
  - Brain swelling
    - Vascular
      Vasodilatation
      - Post-traumatic (usually children)
      - Hypercapnia
      Venous engorgement
      - Jugular compression or obstruction
      - Sinus thrombosis or obstruction
    - Oedema
      - Vasogenic
      - Cytotoxic
      - Hyponatraemia

Infection
- Meningitis
- Epidural abscess

- Subdural empyema
- Intracerebral abscess
- Septic venous sinus thrombosis

General/metabolic
- Hypoxia
- Hypercapnia
- Acid–base problems (particularly acidosis)
  - Metabolic
    - Renal failure
    - Lactic acidosis
    - Diabetic ketoacidosis
  - Respiratory
- Electrolyte imbalance
  - Sodium
    - Hyponatraemia
    - Hypernatraemia (unusual to cause confusion)
  - Calcium
    - Hypocalcaemia
- Glucose
  - Diabetic hyperglycaemia/ketoacidosis
  - Hypoglycaemia (usually seen in treated diabetics)
- Infection
  - Septicaemia
    - Primary (iatrogenic, i.v. lines, etc.)
    - Secondary (to other infection)
  - Pulmonary
  - Urinary
  - Wound
- Nutritional
  - Vitamin B_{12} deficiency

Drug intoxication/withdrawal
- Medication
  - Sedatives and tranquillisers
  - Analgesics (particularly narcotics)
  - Steroids (although not usually indicated in trauma)
  - Anticonvulsants
  - Hypoglycaemic agents
- Non-medicinal
  - Alcohol
  - Narcotic
  - Hallucinogens
  - Cocaine
  - Solvents

CPP, cerebral perfusion pressure; MAP, mean arterial pressure; EDH, extradural haematoma; SDH, subdural haematoma.

cerebral injury on imaging, and typically has a good prognosis for spontaneous recovery. PTA has similar clinical features, but occurs also after more significant brain injuries, and does not imply minimal structural brain injury and nor does it necessarily imply a good prognosis. These terms (concussion and PTA) have been mentioned because of their widespread usage, but I would encourage clinicians in the acute clinical settings to avoid their use when possible.

Secondary brain injury

Secondary brain injury occurs after the trauma, and its prevention is the primary focus of most therapy for brain injury. The most common preventable causes are hypoxia, cerebral ischaemia secondary to hypotension or vascular injury, raised intracranial pressure (most commonly due to intracranial haematomas and brain swelling) and seizures. A host of other factors can also contribute to secondary brain injury, and these include fever, infection, hyperglycaemia, hyponatraemia and other metabolic conditions. It is also recognised that complex biochemical cascades are activated at a cellular level following trauma, and these events (e.g. free radical formation) are significant contributing factors to secondary brain injury. An important principle to recognise is the increased susceptibility of the recently injured brain to secondary insults; relatively mild hypoxia or hypotension that would be readily tolerated by a normal brain can cause significant further damage to an injured brain.

Causes of post-traumatic confusion not directly related to brain injury

Even in the absence of a brain injury, a broad range of pathologies can cause confusion in a patient following trauma. These include hypoxia and hypotension, infections, medication, non-prescribed drugs (substance effect and withdrawal), electrolyte abnormalities and metabolic problems. Confusion is commonly the first presentation and the underlying pathology not necessarily clinically obvious, necessitating a high level of suspicion and appropriate investigation.

Management of patient with post-traumatic confusion (Box 80.2)

Clinical assessment

Post-traumatic confusion is not uncommonly a sentinel for serious underlying pathology and demands rapid and detailed medical assessment. Immediate attention to 'ABC' is of course required: adequacy of the patient's airway (which must not only be patent but protected by a good cough or gag), breathing (including oxygen saturation and arterial blood gas in most cases) and circulatory sufficiency (heart rate and rhythm, peripheral perfusion and chest auscultation). The vital signs chart provides much but not all of the necessary information for this immediate assessment. The patient's conscious state needs formal assessment using the Glasgow Coma Scale (GCS; Table 80.1). Please note that 'confused' is not an adequate descriptor of conscious state, and conscious state assessment demands the GCS be documented (eye opening, best motor response, and verbal response). If previous GCS has been charted, the degree and rapidity of the change should be noted. A very rapid assessment for lateralising neurological signs should then be performed (particularly looking for pupillary inequality, gaze palsies, and obvious differences in motor function on one side).

At this point the clinician should be aware whether urgent action is required, or if a more detailed clinical assessment is appropriate. Inadequate airway, respiratory failure, or a GCS score below 9 demand urgent attention to the airway (optimally, immediate endotracheal intubation). Circulatory failure requires urgent investigation and support, with particular attention to cardiac, thromboembolic and concealed blood loss in a post-trauma patient. New lateralising neurological signs and/or a rapid fall in GCS score of 2 points or more require an urgent brain CT.

However, the vast majority of patients do not have these sentinel indicators, and in each a methodical and detailed examination should be performed. This includes a detailed general examination, with particular attention to the respiratory system and also looking for evidence of infection, and a full neurological examination (also of course looking for any evidence of meningism). The drug charts should be examined and considered, and if possible a history of alcohol and substance abuse and/or withdrawal should also be considered.

Investigation

The investigations and their urgency are dictated by the clinical assessment findings. However, the majority of cases of post-traumatic confusion require strong consideration for the following investigations.

- Arterial blood gas examination: note that normal oxygen saturation monitoring is usually not adequate alone, and measurement of Pao_2, $Paco_2$, bicarbonate, pH and base excess provide evidence not just for respiratory failure but are also rapidly available indicators suggesting other serious pathologies (e.g. pulmonary embolus, sepsis, diabetic ketoacidosis).
- Venepuncture: full blood examination (haemoglobin, red cell count, white cell count and platelet count), electrolytes, urea and creatinine, liver function, calcium and phosphate, blood glucose.

Box 80.2 Management of post-traumatic confusion

Clinical assessment
- Physical examination
  - Airway, breathing, circulation immediately, then general examination
- Neurological examination
  - Particularly note GCS, papillary inequality or other focal neurological deficit, and meningism

Investigation
- CT scan brain (urgent if GCS score falls >2 points, or focal neurological signs)
- Arterial blood gas analysis (Pao_2, $Paco_2$, bicarbonate, pH, base excess)
- Full blood examination (haemoglobin, RCC, WCC, platelets)
- Urea, creatinine and electrolytes
- Calcium/phosphate
- Septic work-up (wound swabs, blood cultures, urine analysis and culture, chest X-ray, ± CSF analysis)

General management of confused patient
- Environmental
  - Close monitoring and supervision
  - Protection
  - Quiet environment if possible
- Sedation avoided if at all possible
  - If absolutely required, best to use only short-acting parenteral (i.v.) sedatives in small doses titrated to effect, closely supervised
- Analgesia if required
  - If narcotic, only small frequent i.v. doses (e.g. morphine 1–2 mg p.r.n.) titrated carefully, with the patient closely supervised (not intramuscular or subcutaneous)

- Recognition of legal incompetency
- Relevancy to consent and refusal of treatment

Specific management of the cause of confusion
- Intracranial lesions
  - Immediate neurosurgical opinion for all
  - Usually surgical decompression if mass effect, and relatively urgent if a patient is developing lateralising signs or deteriorating GCS
  - Consider arterial dissection if lateralising neurology and normal CT/infarction
  - Perform lumbar puncture and urgent CSF analysis for meningitis (check CT normal first) if no other cause of confusion or risk factors for meningitis (compound fracture, skull base fracture, CSF leak, pneumocephalus, ICP monitor, ventricular drain, cranial surgery)
- Hypoxia and respiratory disturbance
  - Oxygen supplementation
  - Immediate intubation if:
    - Airway not patent and protected (cough and gag)
    - Respiratory failure
    - Note spinal precautions for all intubations, but do not delay for spinal investigation
- Electrolyte disturbance
  - Appropriate fluid and electrolyte therapy
- Infection
  - Appropriate antibiotic therapy instituted immediately after cultures, and modified when culture and sensitivities known
- Medications and non-medicinal drugs
  - Medications scrutinised
  - Drug and alcohol history determined

Table 80.1 Glasgow Coma Scale.

Score	Best eye opening (E)	Best verbal (V)	Best motor (M)
6			Obeys
5		Orientated	Localises pain
4	Spontaneous	Confused	Withdraws to pain
3	To speech	Inappropriate words	Abnormal flexion to pain ('decorticate')
2	To pain	Incomprehensible sounds	Extension to pain ('decerebrate')
1	None	None	None

GCS = E + V + M.
Worst score is 3, best is 15.
Use best response if differences between sides for eye opening or motor function.
GCS measures only conscious state, not neurological deficit.

- CT brain: this is urgent if there is a rapid fall in GCS score of 2 points or more, or if there are localising (lateralising) neurological signs.
- Septic work-up: blood cultures, urine microscopy and culture, chest X-ray and sputum culture, changing intravenous lines, wound swabs, and lumbar puncture if meningism and CT shows no intracranial mass lesion.

General management of the confused patient

The primary management goals are always to diagnose the causative pathology and then treat appropriately. However, there are a number of general management strategies for confused patients that warrant further discussion.

Environmental

A safe environment for a confused patient requires close supervision by experienced nursing and medical staff in order to protect the patient from harm and also to detect any further neurological deterioration in a timely manner. A busy ward environment often causes more agitation and a quiet environment is optimal, but this should not be at the expense of close supervision. Confused patients are often agitated, and this often responds to calm reassurance with minimal extraneous stimulation.

Falls are a significant risk for confused patients, and padded bed-sides and other protective strategies must be employed. A Craig bed, allowing a confused patient to be nursed at floor level with padded safety barriers, is useful for those who are medically and orthopaedically stable in the post-acute period.

On occasions physical restraint is required for patient safety, although these restraints can often frighten the patient, lead to more agitation and are not without risk. Restrained confused patients are at risk of becoming entangled, experiencing respiratory restriction, or sustaining pressure injury or other injuries arising from the restraint itself. It must be stressed that if a patient is restrained, there is a need for closer supervision not less.

Sedation

Sedation is best avoided in confused patients if at all possible and should be used only when there are serious concerns that patient agitation poses a significant risk of harm to the patient. Sedatives themselves may cause confusion, and sedation might aggravate the situation in a confused patient.

Patients with post-traumatic confusion are also commonly very sensitive to sedatives, and on occasion a relatively small incremental dose increase can cause respiratory depression and compromise airway protection. Also, in patients with raised intracranial pressure (ICP) the effect of the sedation controlling the agitation causes a reduction in the associated hyperventilation, and in doing so can trigger a cascade of escalating intracranial hypertension and cerebral herniation. Therefore, if sedation is to be used in these patients it needs to be determined that the appropriate level of vigilance and the appropriate facilities for emergency airway support are available.

A major concern with sedation is that it can mask neurological deterioration from other causes. It is therefore unwise to use sedation in confused patients who have not had dangerous intracranial (such as expanding intracranial haematoma, brain swelling, hydrocephalus, meningitis) or metabolic (particularly hypoxic) problems excluded, and even then staff should be cautioned regarding the dangers of attributing any significant deterioration in conscious state or any other neurological deterioration to the sedative. If sedation is considered necessary in the acute post-traumatic period, then a shorter-acting benzodiazepine such as clonazepam in small doses intravenously that can be titrated for immediate effect has significantly less risk than longer-acting medication (e.g. diazepam) or medication given by other routes (oral or intramuscular).

Analgesia

Analgesia is an important in management of the patient with post-traumatic confusion, particularly in those with multisystem trauma. Inadequate analgesia is unlikely to cause confusion but is likely to cause a confused patient to become agitated and uncooperative.

Patients with isolated head injuries often have headache, but it should be recognised that severe headache is the exception rather than the rule. Oral or intravenous paracetamol is commonly very efficacious for these headaches, and its regular use in the early post-traumatic period is recommended. Non-steroidal anti-inflammatory agents used in combination with paracetamol can also be very effective after the acute period, although their anti-platelet affect and gastric ulceration side effects usually preclude their consideration in the first week or so after a significant trauma.

Narcotic agents may themselves cause confusion but are at times necessary in the acute post-trauma period. It needs to be remembered that narcotic use in head injured patients has significant risks, including the sedative effect masking deteriorating conscious state from other causes, the analgesic effect hiding the headache associated with raised ICP or meningitis, and the respiratory depression (with secondary rise in ICP), vomiting (with aspiration in a poorly protected airway) and pupillary constriction. Therefore, if narcotics are used I would recomend frequent small intravenous doses that are rapid in onset and which can be titrated for immediate effect and have a predictable and short duration of action that allows for assessment of neurological deterioration. For these same reasons I would strongly argue against the use of oral, subcutaneous or intramuscular narcotics in the post-traumatic confused patient.

Orthopaedic injuries require significant analgesia, usually narcotic, at presentation. However, it must be remembered that the simple act of bracing and stabilising a fracture will provide very effective pain control. Failure to provide adequate pain relief to those with painful chest and abdominal injuries will predispose to respiratory compromise and chest infection. Clinical input from a specialist anaesthetist regarding the potential use of intercostal blocks and epidural analgesia is also valuable in these situations. In a multisystem trauma patient who has a head injury and/or is confused, my comments regarding analgesia are still very valid. Narcotics typically are required in these cases, but their associated risks are not only those mentioned in reference to the head injury, but also of obscuring the worsening pain that should alert clinicians to abdominal complications or compartment syndromes. Therefore, I reiterate the recommendation that narcotics be used only by the intravenous route in the acute period.

Legal competency

A confused patient is not legally competent and therefore cannot provide valid consent for medical procedures. Almost all legal jurisdictions have provisions to allow necessary urgent procedures to be performed in the absence of consent, and therefore any urgent treatment required for the welfare of a confused patient should not be withheld because of the absence of consent. There are provisions for another person/legal authority to be authorised to make medical decisions on the patient's behalf. However, the qualifications of that person and their relationship to the patient vary between jurisdictions and it is required that practitioners are aware of local requirements.

The inability of the confused patient to provide valid medical consent also of course implies that the patient's ability to make a valid decision to refuse treatment is also compromised. If a confused patient refuses necessary treatment or threatens to abscond or discharge themselves against medical advice, the same procedural steps should be followed as for obtaining consent in the jurisdiction. It should be stressed that refusal of treatment by a confused patient in no way absolves the clinician of the responsibility for that patient's ongoing welfare. Although at times formal declarations of legal incompetence and compulsory treatment orders are required, most situations can be resolved with quiet reassurance of the confused patient, particularly if the assistance of a trusted friend or family member can be a obtained.

Specific management of the cause of confusion

Identification of the cause and its appropriate treatment is the primary management goal in post-traumatic confusion.

Intracranial lesions

A CT scan of the brain is required for any patient with significant post-traumatic confusion, and consideration should be given to repeating that scan if there is further deterioration in the absence of another cause being identified. CT will identify the majority of readily treatable intracranial pathologies causing post-traumatic confusion, including intracranial haematomas (extradural, subdural, intracerebral and cerebral contusions), pneumocephalus and hydrocephalus. These conditions typically require surgical treatment and necessitate urgent neurosurgical consultation. Acute haematomas typically are composed of solid clot and therefore require a craniotomy (rather than a burr-hole) for evacuation. Hydrocephalus is recognised by ventricular enlargement and needs a burr-hole for cerebrospinal fluid (CSF) diversion (e.g. a ventricular drain or ventriculoperitoneal shunt). The urgency of the surgery is dictated by the patient's clinical condition, the rapidity of clinical deterioration and, for unilateral lesions, the mass effect of the lesion (particularly the amount of midline shift on an axial CT scan). Pneumocephalus, unlike the other conditions, rarely causes major mass effect and therefore does not usually require surgery for evacuation. However, it is very important to note (even if only one or two tiny intracranial air bubbles) on a post-trauma CT in that it implies a compound skull fracture, typically through the paranasal sinuses. These skull base fractures might not be obvious on a standard axial CT of the brain. Pneumocephalus (or the clinical findings of CSF rhinorrhoea/otorrhoea or CT evidence of skull base fractures) indicates that the patient is at risk of meningitis, the onset of which may be weeks, months or years after the head injury and after the resolution of all other clinical findings. There is some controversy as to whether prophylactic antibiotics are appropriate, with their use becoming less common in the absence of infection. However, pneumocephalus and/or skull base fracture indicates the need for nasopharyngeal swabs to identify potential pathogens, and also avoidance of positive pressure mask ventilation or blowing of nose (both of which can increase the risks of meningitis and also of tension pneumocephalus). Nasopharyngeal tubes are also typically avoided with skull base fractures, particularly those through the anterior fossa floor.

There are also a few important intracranial conditions that are not recognised on CT, including DAI, acute cerebral infarction and meningitis. DAI is a common association with severe head injuries and is caused by differential movement in the outer layers of the brain and the deeper layers during rotational acceleration (which commonly occurs in car accidents for example). This results in shear injuries to the axons (particularly the subcortical regions of the hemispheres, but also elsewhere including the splenium and tectal plate region). It has a poor prognosis and patients with DAI have a high mortality and survivors a relatively high risk of significant neurological disabilities. DAI itself is not recognisable on CT scan, although often there are similar shear injuries to penetrating vessels in those regions, and the secondary 'petechial haemorrhages' identifiable on CT scan are often said to be pathognomonic of DAI. There is no specific treatment of DAI other than supportive measures and prevention of secondary brain injury. Survivors with significant DAI typically have prolonged and often severe cognitive impairment, including confusion. However, my main point here is to remind the reader that the patient's clinical state is the most important prognostic factor after a head injury, and a normal CT scan does not necessarily rule out very severe primary brain injury.

Acute cerebral infarction is a diagnosis often overlooked in trauma patients, and when it does occur it is usually secondary to arterial dissection (a tear in the inner layers usually caused by a stretch-type mechanism at the time of trauma) of the carotid and/or vertebral arteries either in the neck or in the head. Although this might cause

complete arterial occlusion and immediate stroke, it is not uncommon for the intimal flap to be causing only arterial stenosis and/or platelet aggregation for some time, with later arterial occlusion or thromboembolism causing delayed stroke. It is therefore important to consider this diagnosis, particularly if there are unilateral neurological symptoms/signs and a normal brain scan, because recognition of a dissection (often using CT angiography) and timely treatment may prevent an established stroke. Acute cerebral infarction (stroke) typically does not show abnormalities on a CT scan in the first few hours, except if detailed perfusion scans are requested. After the first few hours, when the infarct is established, there is hypodensity identified in the area with, typically, swelling of this infarcted brain occurring 12–48 hours after the event. If this is a large area of the brain, the swelling itself might cause dramatic neurological deterioration and herniation and require surgical decompression for preservation of life.

Meningitis (see section Infection) is also an important and dangerous intracranial cause of post-traumatic confusion that is expected not to cause CT scan abnormalities.

A point should be made regarding MRI, which is now widely available and demonstrates some pathologies that are poorly demonstrated on CT (particularly in the case of post-traumatic confusion, early cerebral ischaemia and widespread changes often associated with DAI). However, the requirement for the patient to remain still, the long duration of the scan and the difficulty in monitoring patients in the scanner are such that it is rarely used in the assessment of post-traumatic confusion. For these reasons, CT is the primary diagnostic imaging tool in the acute post-traumatic period.

Hypoxia and respiratory disturbance

The patient's airway and breathing must be immediately assessed, and if there is cause for concern then ventilatory support and/or airway protection immediately instituted (see section Clinical assessment). If the cervical spine is unstable or its status unknown, then this should not delay endotracheal intubation, but necessitates the head and neck being held in a neutral position during the procedure.

All patients with post-traumatic confusion should be administered supplemental oxygen and, even if oxygen saturation monitoring demonstrates no abnormality, arterial blood gases should be assessed as a matter of priority (see section Investigations). Considering the increased susceptibility of an injured brain to relatively mild secondary insults, therapy should aim for Pao_2 above 100 mmHg and $Paco_2$ 35–45 mmHg, and normal pH. Hyperventilation is not recommended as although this reduces ICP it does so because of vasoconstriction, which can cause secondary cerebral ischaemia.

Electrolyte and metabolic disturbances

A full electrolyte and renal function screen should be assessed. Sodium abnormalities can cause significant confusion and are common in acute post-trauma patients. Acute hyponatraemia in particular can cause significant cerebral swelling, seizures and confusion, and should be treated with fluid restriction and/or hypertonic saline (typically the former, but this depends on hydration status and underlying cause). Iatrogenic water overload is quite a common cause of post-traumatic hyponatraemia, the syndrome of inappropriate secretion of antidiuretic hormone (which causes increased total body water) less common, and salt wasting syndrome (associated with total body water deficit) even more unusual. Differentiation is clinically difficult and specialist advice recommended. A point of caution is that rapid correction of chronic hyponatraemia has been associated with central pontine myelinosis, and therefore if the patient has had long-standing hyponatraemia (often due to medication) or if this is unknown but considered likely, then the correction should be slow (over 24–48 hours). In other cases a more rapid correction is appropriate.

Other electrolyte abnormalities, particularly hypercalcaemia, are less common causes of confusion.

Infection

Infection is a very common cause of post-traumatic confusion, and confusion is often the only early sign even in the absence of fever. Therefore, any post-traumatic patient with new-onset or worsening confusion should have a full septic work-up, including chest examination and chest X-ray, inspection of all intravenous sites and wounds (swabbing as necessary), changing of all intravenous lines, and urine microscopy and culture. Meningitis must also be seriously considered and if suggested in any way clinically or in the presence of risk factors, the patient must have an urgent lumbar puncture performed (after CT brain demonstrates it safe to do so).

Meningitis classically presents with sepsis, altered conscious state and meningism (headache, photophobia and neck stiffness), and can be rapidly fatal and cause major morbidity in survivors.

However, clinicians must also be aware that many of these classic symptoms might initially be absent, and particularly in trauma patients the onset can be heralded by post-traumatic confusion, not uncommonly with no clinical evidence of infection. A CT scan would not be expected to show any abnormality in early meningitis, but it should be performed to rule out lesions causing intracranial hypertension prior to performing a lumbar puncture. If meningitis is suspected (and it should be, particularly if there has been a history of skull base fracture/CSF rhinorrhoea/pneumocephalus, compound skull fractures or any intracranial surgery including ventricular drainage, CSF shunt or ICP monitoring), then a lumbar puncture must be performed after the negative CT brain as a matter of urgency. The CSF must be immediately analysed for cell counts, protein and glucose, and Gram stain microscopy for organisms, with a specimen being sent for culture. CSF with a high protein and low glucose concentration (<50% of blood glucose) and a raised proportion of white cells to red cells (more than 1 in 700) makes the diagnosis likely and necessitates institution of parenteral antibiotics (assuming blood and urine cultures have been collected), which should be continued until after final culture results have been assessed. As mentioned previously, meningitis secondary to a skull base fracture (dural fistula) can be very delayed, and once the meningitis has been treated elective surgical repair of the dural fistula is required to prevent recurrence.

If infection of any type is suspected clinically, then antibiotics should be commenced as soon as the culture specimens have been taken and modified if required when culture and sensitivity results are available.

Medication and non-medicinal drugs

Thorough assessment of the patient's recent medication is necessary for any confused patient, as is the history of chronic medication, alcohol or other non-prescribed drugs that have been withheld. As discussed, sedative and narcotic use in hospital and also their withdrawal can cause confusion. Alcohol withdrawal is also not uncommon and should be considered. Other medications, such as anticonvulsants, can also cause or exacerbate confusion.

One important point is that these medication/drug causes of post-traumatic confusion must be presumptive only, and the diagnosis made only after other serious causes (particularly intracranial pathology and hypoxia) have been excluded.

Further reading

Behrouz R, Godoy DA, Azarpazhooh MR, Di Napoli M. Altered mental status in the neurocritical care unit. *J Crit Care* 2015;30:1272–7.

Sharp DJ, Jenkins PO. Concussion is confusing us all. *Pract Neurol* 2015;15:172–86.

Zaal IJ, Devlin JW, Peelen LM, Slooter AJC. A systematic review of risk factors for delirium in the ICU. *Crit Care Med* 2015;43:40–7.

MCQs

Select the single correct answer to each question. The correct answers can be found in the Answers section at the end of the book.

1 Post-traumatic confusion:
   a indicates significant brain injury
   b indicates a concussional state
   c is always associated with an altered conscious state (GCS <15)
   d indicates the need to keep the patient in a quiet room with minimal disturbance
   e is rare in the absence of a direct head injury

2 In a patient with multisystem trauma demonstrating significant post-traumatic confusion, which of the following is the most immediate requirement?
   a a brain CT scan
   b formal assessment of the GCS
   c assessment of respiratory and circulatory sufficiency
   d exclusion of papilloedema
   e detailed neurological examination

3 Which of the following are typically always associated with abnormal findings on standard axial CT brain?
   a diffuse axonal injury
   b acute cerebral infarction
   c meningitis
   d cerebral contusion
   e skull-base fracture

81 Sudden-onset severe headache

Alexios A. Adamides

University of Melbourne and Royal Melbourne Hospital, Melbourne,
Victoria, Australia

Introduction

Headache is a very common symptom, the cause
often benign, the diagnosis often presumptive and
the course usually self-limiting. This is not the case
for sudden-onset severe headache where the underlying cause can be a serious life-threatening condition that must be diagnosed expeditiously and
treated appropriately (Box 81.1). Any patient presenting with a sudden-onset headache must be
assessed promptly with a detailed history and full
neurological examination, followed by targeted
investigations dictated by the clinical findings
(Box 81.2).

Subarachnoid haemorrhage

The most common cause of non-traumatic subarachnoid haemorrhage is rupture of an aneurysm
with extravasation of blood within the subarachnoid space. If the patient is conscious and able to
give a history, it is important to elicit whether the
headache was of gradual or sudden onset. The
latter occurs instantly and is of maximal intensity
at onset (thunderclap headache). Patients often
describe the headache of a subarachnoid haemorrhage as 'the worst headache of my life' or that it
resembles 'being shot in the head' or 'hit on the
back of the head with a bat'. A patient described the
moment of a subarachnoid haemorrhage as follows: 'I was in the pub having a drink when all of a
sudden I had a massive headache and I thought
someone punched me at the back of the head. I
turned around to see who it was but there was no-
one there.'

Cerebral aneurysms usually develop at branching
points of arteries from changes due to wear and
tear and therefore their prevalence and rupture
rates increase with age. Sudden-onset severe headache may be associated with collapse and loss of

---

Box 81.1 Causes of abrupt onset severe headache

- Intracranial haemorrhage: subarachnoid, subdural
  or intracerebral haemorrhage secondary to an
  underlying lesion such as a ruptured aneurysm,
  arteriovenous malformation, cavernous malforma-
  tion, arterial dissection, dural arteriovenous fistula,
  vasculitis
- Primary intracerebral haematoma
- Bacterial or viral meningitis
- Giant cell (temporal) arteritis
- Reversible cerebral vasoconstriction syndrome
- Reversible posterior leucoencephalopathy
- Pituitary apoplexy

Box 81.2 Initial management and investigations for abrupt-onset severe headache

- Initial resuscitation with attention to airway,
  breathing and circulation
- Vital observations: pulse rate, temperature, blood
  pressure, oxygen saturations
- CT brain
- Lumbar puncture if no contraindication on CT brain
  (four tubes for red cell count, oxyhaemoglobin,
  bilirubin, differential cell count, microscopy for
  Gram stain, culture and sensitivities, protein,
  glucose)
- Blood tests: full blood count, coagulation, urea and
  electrolytes, group and save, cross-match,
  erythrocyte sedimentation rate (ESR), C-reactive
  protein (CRP), pituitary hormones
- Depending on history/examination and findings
  from the above investigations, additional investigations may include CT angiography, magnetic
  resonance (MR) angiography, digital subtraction
  angiography CT/MR venogram

Textbook of Surgery, Fourth Edition. Edited by Julian A. Smith, Andrew H. Kaye, Christopher Christophi and Wendy A. Brown.
© 2020 John Wiley & Sons Ltd. Published 2020 by John Wiley & Sons Ltd.

consciousness, drowsiness, confusion, nausea and vomiting, meningism (neck stiffness, photophobia) or seizures. There may be focal neurological signs such as ipsilateral third nerve palsy with ptosis and a fixed dilated pupil from direct compression of the oculomotor nerve by the dome of an aneurysm arising from the junction of the internal carotid and posterior communicating arteries. Occasionally, an unruptured but acutely enlarging posterior communicating artery aneurysm may present with a painful third nerve palsy. Although the majority of ruptured aneurysms cause a subarachnoid haemorrhage, some aneurysms may rupture within the subdural space, causing a subdural haematoma, or within the brain parenchyma, causing an intracerebral haematoma, with or without subarachnoid blood. Associated hydrocephalus from blood within the ventricular system often accompanies subarachnoid haemorrhage.

Investigations for the diagnosis of subarachnoid haemorrhage

An urgent non-contrast CT scan of the brain will typically demonstrate blood (hyperdensity) within the subarachnoid space, including the basal cisterns and/or fissures in the majority of cases. Even a small amount of blood on a CT scan is adequate to confirm the diagnosis. Occasionally, in cases where the haemorrhage is small or if the patient presents late there may not be visible blood on CT scan (98% of patients with subarachnoid haemorrhage will have blood on a CT scan performed within the first day from the onset of symptoms, whereas 7 days after subarachnoid haemorrhage only 50% of patients will have visible blood on CT scan). In such cases, if the history is suggestive of subarachnoid haemorrhage but the CT scan is normal, a lumbar puncture is necessary before subarachnoid haemorrhage can be excluded. The initial lumbar puncture is often the one and only opportunity to establish the correct diagnosis and must be performed by an experienced practitioner, using a fine needle and adequate local anaesthesia so as not to precipitate rebleeding, which is a common and usually fatal early complication of subarachnoid haemorrhage. Ten drops of cerebrospinal fluid (CSF) are collected sequentially in four separate tubes which must be labelled according to the sequence of collection. The CSF specimen must be protected from light exposure and must be hand-delivered immediately to the pathology department for the sample to be centrifuged before red blood cell lysis occurs. The supernatant must be tested for oxyhaemoglobin and bilirubin (products of red blood cell lysis) using spectrophotometry as this is more accurate than the visual detection of xanthochromia (yellow coloration). The number of red blood cells in each tube must also be recorded and CSF must be sent to microbiology for a differential cell count, Gram stain, cultures and sensitivities, protein and glucose to exclude other pathologies such as bacterial or viral meningitis. CT angiography and/or digital subtraction angiography are only useful in identifying the source of haemorrhage but are of no use in establishing whether a haemorrhage is present or not.

Initial management of aneurysmal subarachnoid haemorrhage

Once the diagnosis of subarachnoid haemorrhage is established, it is important to secure the aneurysm as soon as practicable, either by craniotomy and clipping or by endovascular coiling so as to prevent rebleeding. Until the aneurysm is secured it is important to control systolic blood pressure to less than 140 mmHg using antihypertensives. Patients with hydrocephalus who deteriorate neurologically may require insertion of a ventriculostomy catheter to drain CSF but the sudden change in transmural pressure on drainage may precipitate rebleeding and therefore CSF diversion before the aneurysm is secured must only be performed if clinically necessary.

Non-aneurysmal causes of subarachnoid haemorrhage

Subarachnoid haemorrhage may also be secondary to arterial dissection, either spontaneous or traumatic. Occasionally, subarachnoid haemorrhage may be caused by rupture of an arteriovenous malformation (AVM), although typically an AVM presents with an intracerebral haemorrhage or a seizure. AVMs are generally thought to be congenital lesions and are therefore an important cause of abrupt-onset headache in children and young adults.

Convexity subarachnoid haemorrhage, with blood in a sulcal distribution and remote from the basal cisterns or fissures, is unlikely to be aneurysmal. Often this is due to trauma or may be secondary to vasculitis, dural venous sinus thrombosis, reversible cerebral vasoconstriction syndrome and reversible posterior leucoencephalopathy.

Reversible cerebral vasoconstriction syndrome

This is an entity that has been described relatively recently, also known as Call–Fleming syndrome. It is characterised by abrupt-onset severe headache, often recurrent, that may be associated with focal neurological deficits and angiographic evidence of multifocal segmental cerebral artery constriction that is reversible within 12 weeks. It is commoner in women, often early postpartum, and has also been associated with the use of drugs such as selective serotonin reuptake inhibitors, cocaine, ecstasy (MDMA), amphetamines and cannabis. There may be subarachnoid blood on CT scan in a sulcal distribution (but not in the basal cisterns). The vasoconstriction can lead to ischaemic complications such as transient ischaemic attack and stroke. Treatment is with avoidance of precipitants and with calcium channel blockers such as nimodipine.

Posterior reversible encephalopathy syndrome

Posterior reversible encephalopathy syndrome, also known as reversible posterior leucoencephalopathy syndrome, results in vasogenic oedema preferentially affecting the white matter of the posterior cerebral hemispheres, hence the name. Patients present with severe headache which can be of acute onset and associated symptoms include confusion, visual changes and seizures. CT or MRI of the brain may demonstrate the characteristic pattern of widespread vasogenic oedema predominantly affecting the parietal and occipital regions and there may be associated subarachnoid blood in a sulcal distribution. The syndrome has been associated with hypertensive encephalopathy, eclampsia/pre-eclampsia, autoimmune conditions and immunosuppression. Management is by treatment of the underlying cause, such as control of hypertension, delivery of the baby or withholding of immunosuppressive medication.

Other causes of intracranial haemorrhage

The commonest cause of an intracerebral haemorrhage in middle-aged/elderly patients is a spontaneous intracerebral haemorrhage, often associated with hypertension or amyloid angiopathy. Long-standing, poorly controlled hypertension may lead to micro-aneurysms of perforating arteries (Charcot–Buchard aneurysms) and a typical hypertensive haemorrhage is usually located in the basal ganglia, internal capsule, pons or cerebellum. Amyloid angiopathy is a common cause of lobar haemorrhage in elderly patients. All patients with an intracerebral haemorrhage must be resuscitated and their hypertension controlled and may require craniotomy and evacuation of the haematoma if there is significant mass effect and/or deteriorating consciousness. In all

young patients and in elderly patients in whom the haematoma is in a location atypical of a hypertensive haemorrhage (e.g. if the haematoma extends into the sylvian or interhemispheric fissures), CT angiography or digital subtraction angiography may be necessary to exclude an underlying vascular lesion.

Less common causes of intracranial haemorrhage include bleeding from a cavernous malformation, arteriovenous fistula, or hypervascular intracranial tumours such as haemangioblastoma, melanoma or renal cell metastases.

Giant cell arteritis

This is primarily seen in middle-aged/elderly Caucasian patients and is twice as common in women compared with men. It is a chronic vasculitis primarily involving the cranial branches arising from the aortic arch and if untreated may lead to blindness, stroke or arterial dissection. Headache associated with giant cell arteritis is usually of insidious onset, although occasionally it may occur abruptly. It may be generalised or located in the temporal region and there may be associated tenderness over the course of the superficial temporal arteries (hence the previous name 'temporal arteritis'). Associated features may include a variety of visual symptoms and signs, including ocular pain, amaurosis fugax (painless transient visual loss), visual field deficits and blindness (due to occlusion of branches of the ophthalmic/posterior ciliary arteries). There may be associated jaw claudication. Systemic symptoms may include fever, weight loss, fatigue, myalgia, joint pain and peripheral neuropathies. Inflammatory markers (ESR and CRP) are elevated and the diagnosis is confirmed with a temporal artery biopsy. Early treatment with corticosteroids is critical for preventing blindness.

Pituitary apoplexy

Pituitary apoplexy occurs due to sudden expansion of a mass within the sella turcica, usually from haemorrhage or infarction within a pre-existing pituitary adenoma. Patients often present with abrupt-onset severe headache with associated visual disturbance, typically bitemporal hemianopia but also ophthalmoplegias, diplopia, deteriorating visual acuity or blindness. There may be drowsiness, confusion or loss of consciousness from hydrocephalus. If the haemorrhage ruptures through the tumour capsule and the arachnoid membrane and into the chiasmatic system, there may be symptoms and signs of subarachnoid haemorrhage such as nausea and vomiting, neck stiffness and photophobia. Associated endocrinological abnormalities may result in hypotension or diabetes insipidus. CT or MRI of the brain will demonstrate haemorrhage in the sella region and CT or MR angiography are usually the minimum investigations required to exclude subarachnoid haemorrhage from a ruptured aneurysm. There may be associated compression of the optic chiasm or hydrocephalus from obstruction of the third ventricle. Management includes corticosteroid administration and urgent surgical decompression if there is sudden constriction of visual fields or deterioration of visual acuity from compression of the visual apparatus.

Meningitis

Bacterial meningitis is a potentially life-threatening infection of the meninges that must be diagnosed and treated expeditiously with antibiotics. Viral meningitis is usually self-limiting and often requires supportive therapy only. Clinical features of meningitis include headache, which can be of sudden onset, nausea/vomiting, meningism (neck stiffness, photophobia), fever, petechial rash, drowsiness, confusion and coma. There may be associated features of the original source of infection, such as upper respiratory tract symptoms, sinusitis, otitis media, mastoiditis or features of bacterial endocarditis. The diagnosis is by microbiological examination of CSF obtained by lumbar puncture. Treatment with empirical antibiotics should be administered immediately on suspicion of bacterial meningitis, even before a lumbar puncture is performed.

Further reading

Connolly ES Jr, Rabinstein, AA, Carhuapoma JR *et al.* Guidelines for the management of aneurysmal subarachnoid haemorrhage: a guideline for healthcare professionals from the American Heart Association/American Stroke Association. *Stroke* 2012;43:1711–37.

Laidlaw JD, Siu KH. Ultra-early surgery for aneurysmal subarachnoid haemorrhage: outcomes for a consecutive series of 391 patients not selected by grade or age. *J Neurosurg* 2002;97:250–8.

Tunkel, AR, Hartman J, Kaplan SL *et al.* Practice guidelines for the management of bacterial meningitis. *Clin Infect Dis* 2004;39:1267–84.

MCQs

Select the single correct answer to each question. The correct answers can be found in the Answers section at the end of the book.

1 A 49-year-old male smoker with poorly controlled hypertension presents with a 5-day history of sudden-onset severe headache and neck stiffness. On examination he is found to have expressive dysphasia and right-hand clumsiness. A CT scan of the brain does not show intracranial haemorrhage. Which of the following is correct?

a he requires urgent thrombolysis

b he requires urgent empirical antibiotics for meningitis

c the most likely diagnosis is reversible cerebral vasoconstriction syndrome

d the most likely diagnosis is posterior reversible encephalopathy syndrome

e the most likely diagnosis is delayed cerebral ischaemia after aneurysmal subarachnoid haemorrhage and a lumbar puncture is likely to show elevated oxyhaemoglobin and bilirubin on spectrophotometry

2 A 21-year-old woman presents with a 3-day history of sudden-onset headache. A CT scan of the brain shows a 2.5-cm right temporal intracerebral haemorrhage but a CT angiogram does not show any underlying lesion. While in the scanner she has a generalised tonic–clonic seizure. Which of the following is correct?

a a lumbar puncture must be performed to exclude subarachnoid haemorrhage

b a CT angiogram of the circle of Willis is adequate to exclude an underlying vascular lesion

c she requires immediate craniotomy and evacuation of the haematoma

d the clinical priority is to secure her airway and administer anticonvulsants to terminate the seizure

e the most likely cause of the haemorrhage is amyloid angiopathy

3 A 55-year-old man presents to a small country hospital with a history of headache. While in the emergency department he collapses unconscious and is found to have a fixed and dilated right pupil. A brain CT scan shows a large right temporal intracerebral haematoma and a CT angiogram shows a right middle cerebral artery aneurysm. He is air-lifted to a neurosurgical centre intubated and ventilated. Which of the following is the most appropriate management?

a urgent cerebral angiogram and coiling of the aneurysm followed by craniotomy and evacuation of the haematoma

b urgent craniotomy and clipping of the aneurysm and evacuation of the haematoma

c urgent craniotomy and evacuation of the haematoma followed by cerebral angiography and coiling of the aneurysm

d transfer to intensive care to wean sedation and assess neurology

e transfer to a palliative care ward for comfort measures

82 The red eye

Christine Chen

Monash University and Department of Ophthalmology, Monash Health, Melbourne, Victoria, Australia

Introduction

Ophthalmology is the diagnosis and management of conditions affecting the eye, orbit and visual neural pathways. To cover the entire field of ophthalmology is beyond the scope of this book, so the aim of this and the following chapter is to provide a solid foundation for recognising both common and serious conditions presenting with red eye and diplopia and for understanding the appropriate primary management prior to referral to an ophthalmologist. At the end of these chapters you should have an understanding of the relevant anatomy of the eye (see Figure 82.1), be able to take a targeted ophthalmic history based on the presenting problem and undertake a basic ophthalmic examination to identify and describe pathology. Most importantly, you should be able to identify life-threatening, eye-threatening and sight-threatening conditions and undertake emergency ophthalmic investigation and treatment where appropriate.

Basic anatomy of the eye

See Figure 82.1.

The red and/or painful eye

The red eye is one of the most common ophthalmic presentations to general practitioners and accident and emergency departments (Table 82.1). It is usually accompanied by some degree of pain or discomfort and possibly discharge. It is important to differentiate the benign self-limiting causes such as viral conjunctivitis and subconjunctival haemorrhage from sight-threatening conditions such as microbial keratitis and angle closure glaucoma.

Remember the golden rule: *Beware of the unilateral red eye.*

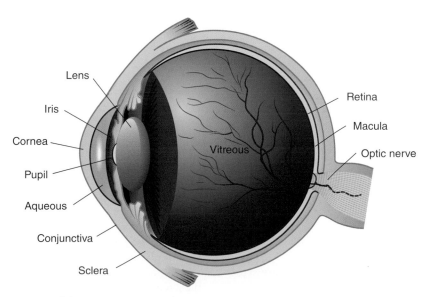

Fig. 82.1 Basic anatomy of the eye.

Textbook of Surgery, Fourth Edition. Edited by Julian A. Smith, Andrew H. Kaye, Christopher Christophi and Wendy A. Brown.
© 2020 John Wiley & Sons Ltd. Published 2020 by John Wiley & Sons Ltd.

Table 82.1 Common systemic causes of red eye.	
Causes of red eye	Associated systemic conditions
Conjunctivitis	Upper respiratory tract viral infection *Chlamydia*
Scleritis	Connective tissue disorders, e.g. rheumatoid arthritis, systemic lupus erythematosus Infectious causes: herpes zoster ophthalmicus
Uveitis	Paediatric: • TORCH infection • Juvenile arthritis Adults: • Any autoimmune condition, e.g. serum-negative arthropathies, sarcoidosis, inflammatory bowel disease • Systemic infections, e.g. tuberculosis, syphilis
Dry eye	Sjögren's syndrome Thyroid eye disease

History

Duration of symptoms

Patients with eye trauma will generally seek medical attention immediately.

Patients with viral conjunctivitis will generally present within the first 1–2 weeks after failing with over-the-counter medications such as chloramphenicol drops or ocular lubricants. Viral conjunctivitis will often start unilaterally and spread to the fellow eye. There is often a history of viral illness or contact with people with viral conjunctivitis or viral illness.

Chronic conjunctivitis is defined as conjunctivitis lasting for more than 4 weeks. The most common cause of chronic conjunctivitis is chlamydial inclusion conjunctivitis in sexually active young adults. A sexual history is therefore important.

Description of pain

- Foreign body sensation is usually associated with foreign bodies or conjunctivitis.
- Burning watery eyes and itchy eyelids are symptoms of blepharitis.
- Severe pain, not relieved by rest or simple analgesia, can indicate more sinister pathology such as keratitis.

Associated symptoms

- Vision loss: most benign causes of a red painful eye such as conjunctivitis should not affect vision.
- Discharge: watery or purulent.
- Photophobia: associated with corneal pathology such as keratitis or ocular inflammation such as uveitis.
- Headache: associated with ocular inflammation or raised intraocular pressure (IOP).

Previous ophthalmic history

- Contact lens wearers are at higher risk of infective keratitis.
- Uveitis can be recurrent and many patients will have a prior history of similar episodes.
- Recurrent corneal erosion syndrome is a condition where previous minor corneal trauma, such as a fingernail scratch, results in a healed but unstable corneal epithelium. Subsequent very minor trauma (such as rubbing or even opening of the eyes first thing in the morning) can lead to repeated, painful, corneal epithelial defects.
- Those with long sightedness and people of Asian descent are predisposed to angle closure glaucoma.

Previous medical history

Hypertension and anticoagulants predispose to subconjunctival haemorrhage.

The basic eye examination

Visual acuity

Visual acuity represents the global function of the eye and visual system and is the single most important part of the eye examination.

Distance visual acuity testing and recording

Distance visual acuity is obtained one eye at a time by occluding the fellow eye (Figure 82.2). This measures the patient's 'best corrected vision', which means that vision should be tested with the patient's habitual *distance* glasses (many patients over 50 years old may have separate distance and near/reading glasses). The eye not being tested is occluded with an occluder or the patient's palm. The test is then repeated with a pinhole over the eye being tested.

The patient should be encouraged to read the smaller letters or the next line even if they are not

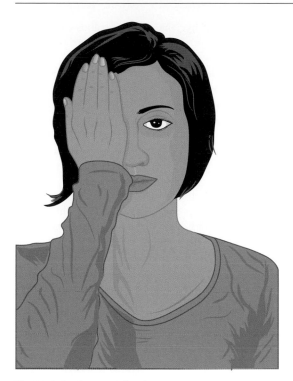

Fig. 82.2 Occlusion with palm.

confident of the letters. The distance visual acuity is recorded as a fraction, with the numerator as the distance at which the chart is positioned from the patient (in metres for Australia). Each chart is calibrated to be read at a certain distance, most commonly 6 m, and the fraction is 6/*x*. The distance can be changed

and the numerator then changes, e.g. 3/*x*, 1/*x*. The denominator (*x*) corresponds to the smallest letter line that a patient is able to read correctly. Each letter line is assigned a number (Figure 82.3). This number represents the distance at which a person without a visual deficit should be able to read those letters.

For example, vision of 6/12 is interpreted as follows. The patient was tested with a chart calibrated to be read at 6 m. He or she was only able to see the line that should be read at 12 m, i.e. the patient can see at 6 m what can be read at 12 m by a person without a visual deficit. If the patient is unable to read the top letter of the chart (60), reduce the distance to 3 m (3/60), then 2 m (2/60) and then 1 m (1/60).

If the patient is unable to read the top letter of the chart at 1 m, test their ability to count fingers at 1 m (CF), then hand movement (HM), and then the ability to perceive a very bright light source (LP). If the patient is unable to perceive a bright light source, then this is recorded as no perception of light (NPL).

An 'E' chart should be used for patients who do not recognise English alphabet characters. The patient is asked in which direction the 'arms' of the E are pointing. A picture chart can be used for children unfamiliar with alphabetical symbols.

Gross examination of the eye and adnexae

Inspect the eyelids and the surrounding tissue
- Inspect the cornea for clarity.
- Inspect the conjunctiva and sclera for redness.

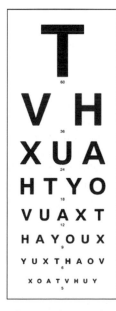
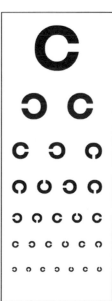
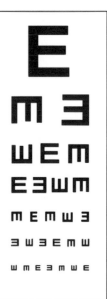

Fig. 82.3 Standard Snellen visual acuity chart, 'C' chart and 'E' chart.

Additional tests

- Tonometry to measure IOP: use a slit lamp-mounted Goldmann tonometer or a hand-held electronic tonometer such as the Tonopen™.
- Colour vision testing: with Ishihara colour plates.
- Fluorescein staining: to detect corneal epithelial defects or penetrating eye injuries. A cobalt blue illumination source, as found on direct ophthalmoscopes or slit lamps, is used to identify the fluorescein dye.
- Eversion of the upper lid: for foreign bodies.
- Examination of the eye and adnexae: a great deal of pathology can be detected on gross inspection and with a direct ophthalmoscope.

Primary management

Subconjunctival haemorrhage

Subconjunctival haemorrhage is a haemorrhage into the potential space between the conjunctiva and sclera (Table 82.2). Blood pressure should be checked. The condition is self-limiting but can take several weeks for complete resolution of the blood. Ocular lubricant may alleviate the foreign body sensation.

Blepharitis

Blepharitis or inflammation of the eyelid due to either staphylococcal infection or meibomian gland dysfunction causes symptoms disproportionate to the underlying pathology (Table 82.2). Stye and chalazion can develop as a complication of blepharitis. Treatment options include:

- lid hygiene, with scrubbing of eyelid margin with a mild, very dilute shampoo such as 'no tear' shampoo
- hot compress
- ocular lubricant.

The patient may be referred to an ophthalmologist if the symptoms are not responsive to these simple measures.

Conjunctivitis

Most mild cases of conjunctivitis are managed with simple ocular lubricant and reassurance (Table 82.2). The typical course of viral conjunctivitis is much like a viral upper respiratory infection, with worsening of symptoms without visual disturbance in the first 7–10 days and subsequent involvement of the fellow eye. The symptoms will start to improve after 7–10 days with resolution expected within 3 weeks. Viral conjunctivitis is extremely contagious and

therefore hand hygiene and meticulous cleaning of the examination room and instruments is mandatory to prevent spreading of infection.

If chlamydial conjunctivitis is suspected, azithromycin 1 g orally should be administered immediately. It is important to take conjunctival swabs for polymerase chain reaction (PCR). The patient must be reviewed to check the results and contact tracing instituted in confirmed cases.

Keratitis

Keratitis describes the inflammation of the cornea caused by either infection or inflammation (Table 82.2). Microbial keratitis is a serious and potentially sight-threatening condition. It is usually associated with decreased vision, sensitivity to light (photophobia) and pain. Examination may confirm reduced visual acuity, fluorescein staining and corneal infiltrate (Figure 82.4).

Pathogens include viruses such as herpes simplex types 1 and 2 and herpes zoster ophthalmicus; bacteria such as *Staphylococcus*, *Streptococcus* and *Pseudomonas*; and *Acanthamoeba*. These infections often occur on a background of predisposing factors which could be ocular (contact lens use or ocular trauma) or systemic (diabetes or rheumatoid arthritis).

Primary management of microbial keratitis includes prompt referral to ophthalmologists for microbiological work-up and empirical anti-infective treatment.

Episcleritis

Episcleritis is inflammation of the episclera (superficial layer of the sclera), which can be either localised or diffuse and is often idiopathic (Table 82.2). It is often self-limiting and can be treated with ocular lubricant and topical non-steroidal anti-inflammatory drugs (NSAIDs). Scleritis is a more severe condition that may be associated with systemic disease. It is classified into non-necrotising and necrotising and requires treatment with high-dose systemic anti-inflammatory agents such as NSAIDs or steroids and investigation and treatment of the underlying associated systemic conditions (see Table 82.1).

Uveitis

Uveitis describes inflammation of the uveal tract, which includes the iris, ciliary body and choroid (see Table 82.2). An anatomical classification, grading system and diagnostic criteria is published by

Table 82.2 Common differential diagnosis for a red eye.

Differential diagnosis	Discharge	Pain	Visual acuity	Pupil	Conjunctiva	Cornea	Anterior Chamber	IOP	Refer
Subconjunctival haemorrhage	No	No, FBS	Unaffected	Normal	Localised redness	Clear	Quiet	Normal	No, if visual acuity is normal
Blepharitis	Dry crusts	No, FBS	Unaffected	Normal	Diffuse redness Often bilateral	Clear. May have pinpoint staining with fluorescein	Quiet	Normal	No, if visual acuity is normal
Conjunctivitis	Yes Viral: watery Bacterial: purulent	No, FBS	Can be affected	Normal	Diffuse redness Often bilateral	Clear. May have pinpoint staining with fluorescein	Quiet	Normal	No, if visual acuity is normal
Foreign body	Yes, watery	Can be	Can be affected	Normal	Localised redness Unilateral	Foreign body or abrasion with fluorescein staining	Quiet	Normal	Yes, if unable to remove foreign body
Keratitis	Yes, watery	Yes	Affected	Normal	Diffuse redness Unilateral	Localised opacity with fluorescein staining	Possible cells	Normal	Yes
Uveitis	No	Yes	Affected	May be sluggish and constricted	Diffuse redness Unilateral	Keratic precipitates (localised deposits on endothelium) without fluorescein staining	Cells and flare	Normal or increased	Yes
Episcleritis/scleritis	No	Yes	Can be affected	Normal	Localised or diffuse redness Unilateral	Clear	Possible cells	Normal	Yes
Angle closure glaucoma	No	Yes	Affected	May be sluggish and dilated	Diffuse redness Unilateral	Diffuse cloudiness due to corneal oedema without fluorescein staining	Shallow Cells	Increased	Yes

FBS, foreign body sensation.

Source: adapted from Smith JA, Fox JG, Saunder AC, Yii MK. *Hunt & Marshall's Clinical Problems in Surgery*, 3rd edn. Chatswood, NSW: Elsevier Australia, 2016. Reproduced with permission of Elsevier.

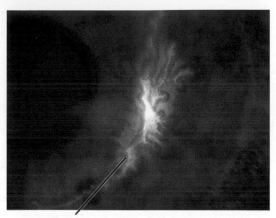

Herpes simplex virus dendrite

Fig. 82.4 Corneal dendrite caused by herpes simplex virus demonstrated by fluorescein staining. Source: Friedman NJ, Kaiser PK. *Essentials of Ophthalmology*. Philadelphia: Saunders Elsevier, 2007. Reproduced with permission of Elsevier.

the Standardization of Uveitis Nomenclature (SUN) Working Group to establish a framework for this vast and diverse condition. The patient with uveitis usually presents with a painful red eye, photophobia and reduced vision. There may be associated systemic autoimmune conditions, most commonly ankylosing spondylitis or infectious conditions such as HIV. Refer to an ophthalmologist for further assessment, investigation and management.

Acute angle closure glaucoma

Acute angle closure glaucoma is a sight-threatening emergency presenting as sudden painful loss of vision due to sudden and total closure of the iridocorneal angle (see Table 82.2). It is more common in patients with hypermetropia or long-sightedness, advancing age, of Asian race, and a positive family history. The patient usually presents with sudden onset of severe ocular pain and headache, blurred vision with halos around lights, nausea and vomiting. Examination will reveal high IOP (50–100 mmHg); mid-dilated, sluggish and irregular pupil; corneal epithelial oedema with or without stromal oedema; red eye from congested episcleral and conjunctival blood vessels; shallow anterior chamber; mild amount of aqueous flare and cells; and the optic nerve may be swollen during an attack. A definitive diagnosis depends on gonioscopy, which requires a specialised contact lens to examine the iridocorneal angle and confirm that it is closed by the iris.

Prompt referral to an ophthalmologist is required. Emergency treatment includes systemic medication such as acetazolamide and topical medication such as ocular antihypertensives including alpha-agonists, beta-blockers, prostaglandin analogues and miotics such as pilocarpine 2–4% as well as analgesia and anti-emetics. Definitive treatment consists of peripheral laser iridotomy to re-establish communication between posterior and anterior chambers. In some cases surgical treatment is required which may involve a peripheral iridectomy or cataract surgery. Prophylactic laser iridotomy for the fellow eye and screening of first-degree relatives should also be considered.

Further reading

Bagheri N, Wajda B (eds) *The Will's Eye Manual: Office and Emergency Room Diagnosis and Treatment of Eye Disease*, 7th edn. Philadelphia: Wolters Kluwer, 2017.

Bowling B. *Kanski's Clinical Ophthalmology: A Systematic Approach*, 8th edn. Elsevier, 2016.

James B, Bron A, Parulekar MV. *Lecture Notes in Ophthalmology*, 12th edn. Oxford: Wiley Blackwell, 2016.

Khaw PT, Shah P, Elkington AR. *ABC of Eyes*, 4th edn. London: BMJ Publishing Group, 2004.

MCQs

Select the single correct answer to each question. The correct answers can be found in the Answers section at the end of the book.

1 A 70-year-old man with a history of recent cold and anticoagulant use presented with a red eye and no other symptoms. On examination there is a sector of one eye that is solid red without injection of the conjunctival vessels. What is the most likely diagnosis?

 a uveitis
 b keratitis
 c subconjunctival haemorrhage
 d conjunctivitis

2 A 45-year-old Asian woman presented with a history of sudden-onset right painful red eye, blurred vision with halos around the lights, nausea and vomiting. She usually wears glasses for reading. Tonometry revealed an intraocular pressure of 55 mmHg in the right eye and 18 mmHg in the left. What is the most likely diagnosis?

 a conjunctivitis
 b scleritis
 c acute angle closure glaucoma
 d corneal foreign body

3 A 27-year-old man with a history of ankylosing
spondylitis presented with bilateral red eye,
photophobia and reduced vision. On examination,
there are cells in both anterior chambers. What is
the most likely diagnosis?
a scleritis
b conjunctivitis
c anterior uveitis
d keratitis

4 What is the definition of chronic conjunctivitis?
a conjunctivitis >1 week
b conjunctivitis >2 weeks
c conjunctivitis >3 weeks
d conjunctivitis >4 weeks

83 Double vision

Christine Chen

Monash University and Department of Ophthalmology, Monash Health, Melbourne, Victoria, Australia

Basic extraocular muscle anatomy

The extraocular muscles are divided into two groups. The first group arises from the apex of the orbit to attach to the sclera anterior to the equator of the eye. Included in this group are the rectus muscles: medial, lateral, superior and inferior. The second group consists of the oblique muscles. The superior oblique arises from the apex of the orbit and is deviated through a pulley (the trochlear ligament) in the anterior orbit so that it passes backwards and laterally above the globe to attach to the posterolateral area of the upper surface of the eye. The inferior oblique arises in the anterior orbit and passes backwards and laterally under the globe to attach to the posterolateral quadrant of the eye inferiorly.

The extraocular muscles are supplied by three cranial nerves (Table 83.1). The third cranial nerve passes forward in the lateral wall of the cavernous sinus and divides anteriorly into the superior and inferior divisions, which enter the orbit through the superior orbital fissure. The superior division supplies the levator and superior rectus, while the inferior division supplies the medial and inferior recti and the inferior oblique. The fourth cranial nerve supplies the superior oblique muscle, and the sixth cranial nerve supplies the lateral rectus. It is essential to understand the nerve pathways that supply the extraocular muscles and the pupil, a full description of which is beyond the scope of this chapter.

Extraocular muscle actions can be simply represented diagrammatically (Figure 83.1). The horizontal recti abduct (away from nose) or adduct (towards the nose). The vertical recti elevate and depress the eye in abduction. The superior oblique causes depression in adduction and the inferior oblique causes elevation in adduction. In addition, the vertical muscles have secondary actions of intorsion and extorsion.

Diplopia

Double vision (diplopia) is divided into two categories: monocular diplopia and binocular diplopia. It is important to identify the diplopia due to neurosurgical causes.

Monocular diplopia

Double vision persists in the affected eye when the unaffected eye is occluded, usually due to benign causes.

Table 83.1 Cardinal position of gaze, extraocular muscles and their cranial nerve supply.

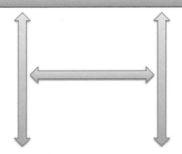

Right and up
- Right superior rectus III
- Left inferior oblique III

Right
- Right lateral rectus VI
- Left medial rectus III

Right and down
- Right inferior rectus III
- Left superior oblique IV

Left and up
- Left superior rectus III
- Right inferior oblique III

Left
- Left lateral rectus VI
- Right medial rectus III

Left and down
- Left inferior rectus III
- Right superior oblique IV

Textbook of Surgery, Fourth Edition. Edited by Julian A. Smith, Andrew H. Kaye, Christopher Christophi and Wendy A. Brown.
© 2020 John Wiley & Sons Ltd. Published 2020 by John Wiley & Sons Ltd.

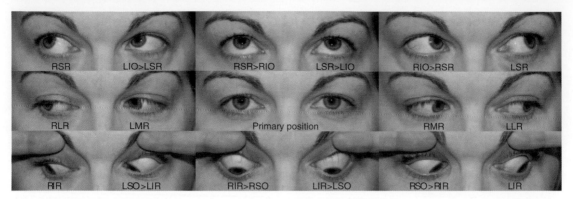

Fig. 83.1 Cardinal eye positions of gaze. The primary muscles active in each position are indicated below the associated eye. First letter indicates right (R) or left (L), and the next two letters specify the muscle. SR, superior rectus; LR, lateral rectus; IR, inferior rectus; MR, medial rectus; IO, inferior oblique; SO, superior oblique. Note the superior and inferior rectus muscles contribute to vertical eye movements in all positions of gaze. Contributions from the oblique muscles are greatest in adduction. Source: Mackay DD, Prasad S. Eye movements. In: *eLS*, July 2012. Chichester: John Wiley & Sons. DOI: 10.1002/9780470015902.a0024018. Reproduced with permission of John Wiley & Sons.

Differential diagnosis

- Refractive error: astigmatism
- Cornea: opacity or irregularity
- Lens: cataract, decentred natural or artificial intraocular lens

Binocular diplopia

Double vision is eliminated when either eye is occluded. A neurosurgical lesion must be excluded.

Differential diagnosis

Intermittent

- Myasthenia gravis
- Intermittent decompensation of an existing strabismus (squint)

Constant

- Isolated cranial nerve palsy: III, IV, VI
  - Pupil-involving third nerve palsy is highly suggestive of a compressive lesion such as cerebral aneurysm
  - Cranial nerve palsy can be a false localising sign due to cranial space-occupying lesions such as tumour or haemorrhage
- Other central nervous system (CNS) lesions: internuclear ophthalmoplegia due to multiple sclerosis
- Orbital disease: thyroid eye disease, orbital inflammation or tumour, trauma

History

- Nature of the double vision:
  - Monocular or binocular: does the double vision persist when one eye is occluded?
  - Intermittent or constant: is the double vision present all the time?
  - Horizontal or vertical: are the two images side by side or one on top of the other?
- Associated symptoms:
  - Headache: a dilated pupil with third nerve palsy and headache is a sign of cerebral aneurysm until proven otherwise
- History of trauma: orbital fracture or false localising sign due to head injury
- Previous ophthalmic history: history of squint or squint surgery
- Previous medical history: cardiovascular risk factors, Graves' disease, multiple sclerosis, myasthenia gravis

Examination

Visual acuity (see Chapter 82)

Pinhole placed in front of the affected eye will eliminate the double vision for most acquired causes of monocular diplopia.

Pupil

It is important to examine the pupil carefully for both direct and consensual responses. Pupils should be tested with the patient fixating on a distant target and a bright pen torch. Next to vision, this is perhaps the most important and easily elicited sign.

- Observe the pupil:
  - round or irregular
  - equal size in both eyes

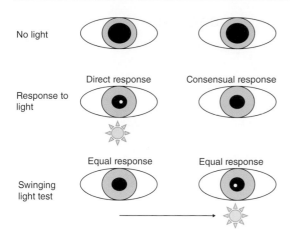

Fig. 83.2 Normal direct and consensual response.

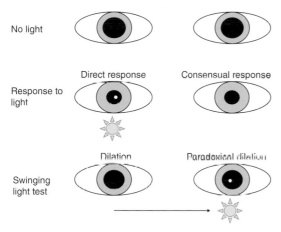

Fig. 83.3 Swinging light reflex showing relative afferent pupil defect.

- associated eyelid and or eye position/movement abnormalities
- Direct and consensual response (Figure 83.2)

Swinging light reflex (Figure 83.3)

This is to look for a difference in the afferent response of the optic nerves. It is an objective test of optic nerve function and measures the strength of one optic nerve *relative* to the other.

- If one optic nerve is damaged, on direct illumination it will transmit a lesser signal to the brainstem which will result in a lesser constriction of *both* pupils.
- When swinging the light from the unaffected to the affected side, *both* pupils will therefore dilate initially.
- When swinging the light from the affected to the unaffected side, *both* pupils will constrict because of the stronger light signal received by the brainstem.

Inspection

Observe for head posture, ptosis and eyelid swelling. To observe corneal reflections, hold the pen torch 30 cm in the midline in front of the patient and observe the corneal reflections. The corneal light reflections should be positioned symmetrically on the patient's eye. If they are not, it indicates a likely deviation.

Cover test

Determine monocular or binocular diplopia.
- In binocular diplopia, double vision is eliminated when the occluder is placed in front of either eye.
- In monocular diplopia, double vision persists when the occluder is placed in front of the unaffected eye, and is eliminated when the occluder is placed in front of the affected eye.

Eye movements

The patient is asked to follow an object in six directions, the cardinal fields of gaze. This can be best done by drawing a large imaginary 'H' in the air between the patient and yourself. If there is an obvious abnormality, the examiner should also test each eye individually, with the opposite eye occluded by the patient's palm.

If the patient is an adult, a target such as a finger or pen will suffice. If the patient is a child, a more interesting target such as a toy is required for cooperation.

In binocular diplopia, determine the following.
- Nature: horizontal, vertical or torsional diplopia. Ask the patient if the two images are side by side, one on top of the other, or rotated.
- Where: in which direction of gaze is the diplopia most pronounced?

Cranial nerve examination

Identification of any other cranial nerve involved may localise any underlying intracranial pathology.

Third nerve palsy

In third nerve palsy, one or more of the muscles that the third nerve innervates can be affected to any degree in any combination (Figure 83.4).
- Exotropia: medial rectus weakness
- Hypertropia: inferior rectus weakness
- Hypotropia: superior rectus ± inferior oblique weakness
- Ptosis: levator palpebrae superioris weakness
- Enlarged pupil: sphincter pupillae weakness

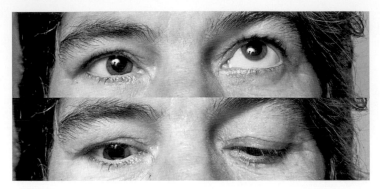

Fig. 83.4 Patient with a right third cranial nerve palsy. In the upper picture he is attempting to look up: the right eye fails to elevate. In the lower picture when he attempts to look down the upper lid elevates owing to misdirection of nerve fibres from aberrant regeneration. In this case, fibres intended for the inferior rectus are innervating the levator muscle of the upper lid.

- There may be signs of aberrant regeneration where there are changes in pupil size or eyelid position on attempted elevation, depression or adduction.

In an isolated ischaemic third nerve palsy on the affected side, the palsy should be *complete*: complete ptosis, no movement on attempted elevation, depression or adduction, with entirely normal pupil and fourth and sixth nerve function.

Fourth nerve palsy

The patient prefers their head tilted away from the hypertropic eye. On cover testing, there is a vertical and/or oblique deviation in the primary position. On motility testing there is hypertropia in primary position, which increases with ipsilateral head turn and ipsilateral head tilt. In the hypertropic eye, there is superior oblique underaction (limitation of depression in adduction) and inferior oblique overaction (upshoot in adduction). In the fixing (apparently hypotropic) eye, motility examination is entirely normal. In congenital fourth nerve palsy, there is often mild facial asymmetry.

Sixth nerve palsy

The patient exhibits horizontal diplopia that is worse for distance than near. In primary position, there is esotropia and unilateral restriction of abduction with slow abduction saccades apparent on testing movement to the side of the lesion.

Primary management

It is important to remember that binocular diplopia can be caused by life-threatening neurosurgical causes such as cerebral aneurysm.

At the end of the history and examination, one must determine whether urgent neuroimaging and neurosurgical referral is required. Magnetic resonance or computed tomography (CT) angiography should be sought, with advice from the neurosurgical team to exclude cerebral aneurysm. MRI or CT brain with contrast should be obtained if a mass-occupying lesion is suspected. CT for orbital fracture needs to specify CT orbit with fine cuts.

Presumed microvascular cranial nerve palsy does not generally require neuroimaging. Be very careful to exclude possible neurosurgical causes before making this diagnosis. The patient should be referred to a physician and ophthalmologist for follow-up.

Blood examination

Full blood examination with measurement of erythrocyte sedimentation rate (ESR) and C-reactive protein (CRP) for presence of giant cell arteritis, a bilateral blinding disease and a great masquerade. Patients presenting with binocular diplopia or reduced vision and aged over 60 years should have blood tests to exclude giant cell arteritis.

Targeted blood tests for other causes such as thyroid eye disease, myasthenia gravis and cardiovascular risk factors (e.g. fasting blood sugar and lipid profile) should be undertaken by physicians.

Ongoing management

Monocular diplopia which resolves with pinhole can be referred to community eye care providers, such as optometrists, for follow-up. Binocular diplopia not caused by neurosurgical causes should be referred to physicians and/or ophthalmologists.

Surgery for diplopia

Surgery for diplopia is performed if reversible causes have not been identified, spontaneous resolution has not occurred after at least 6 months and the condition has stabilised. The principles of surgery for double vision are:

- to strengthen weak muscles by shortening them
- to weaken overacting muscles by effectively lengthening them.

A muscle is strengthened by excising some of the tendon and then re-suturing it to its original insertion. A muscle is weakened by removing it from the globe and re-attaching it closer to its origin.

The primary intention is to at least gain single vision in the primary and depressed positions, which are the most commonly used areas of gaze, while diplopia may still remain in other position of gaze.

Further reading

Bowling B. *Kanski's Clinical Ophthalmology: A Systematic Approach*, 8th edn. Elsevier, 2016.

James B, Bron A, Parulekar MV. *Lecture Notes in Ophthalmology*, 12th edn. Oxford: Wiley Blackwell, 2016.

Pane A, Miller NR, Burdon M. *Neuro-Ophthalmology Survival Guide*, 2nd edn. Elsevier, 2018.

Snell RS, Lemp MA. *Clinical Anatomy of the Eye*, 2nd edn. Oxford: Wiley Blackwell, 2016.

MCQs

Select the single correct answer to each question. The correct answers can be found in the Answers section at the end of the book.

1 With reference to the actions of the extraocular muscles, which of the following is correct?
   a in adduction, the superior oblique elevates the eye
   b in abduction, the inferior rectus depresses the eye
   c in adduction, the inferior oblique muscle intorts the eye
   d in abduction, the inferior oblique muscle intorts the eye

2 Which of the following conditions can cause monocular diplopia?
   a refractive error
   b cataract
   c corneal irregularities
   d all of the above

3 If a patient is suspected to have a third nerve palsy, what is the most appropriate management?
   a refer patient to emergency department urgently for further assessment and investigations
   b refer patient to physician for cardiovascular risk factors work-up
   c assure patient that the double vision will resolve within 6 months
   d refer patient to ophthalmologist for squint surgery

4 A 37-year-old nurse with new-onset headache is unable to abduct the right eye and has horizontal diplopia. The diplopia resolves when she covers either eye. Which of the following is correct?
   a she may have a right sixth nerve palsy as a false localising sign
   b she has a right exotropia
   c she has thyroid eye disease
   d she has a microvascular right sixth nerve palsy

Answers to MCQs

Chapter 1
1 d
2 c
3 a

Chapter 2
1 e
2 d
3 e
4 c

Chapter 3
1 b
2 d
3 a
4 d

Chapter 4
1 d
2 c
3 c
4 e

Chapter 5
1 c
2 d
3 a
4 a

Chapter 6
1 c
2 d
3 b

Chapter 7
1 c
2 c
3 d
4 d
5 a

Chapter 8
1 c
2 e
3 a
4 d
5 b

Chapter 9
1 b
2 b
3 e
4 e
5 d

Chapter 10
1 c
2 a
3 e
4 c

Chapter 11
1 b
2 c
3 c
4 e

Chapter 12
1 b
2 e
3 e
4 b
5 d
6 c

Chapter 13
1 b
2 e
3 c

Chapter 14
1 a
2 b
3 c

Chapter 15
1 a
2 c
3 d
4 c
5 d

Chapter 16
1 b
2 d
3 c

Textbook of Surgery, Fourth Edition. Edited by Julian A. Smith, Andrew H. Kaye, Christopher Christophi and Wendy A. Brown.
© 2020 John Wiley & Sons Ltd. Published 2020 by John Wiley & Sons Ltd.

Chapter 17	Chapter 18	Chapter 19	Chapter 20
1 b	1 b	1 d	1 c
2 a	2 d	2 e	2 e
3 b	3 c	3 d	3 e
	4 a		4 e
	5 b		5 a

Chapter 21	Chapter 22	Chapter 23	Chapter 24
1 d	1 d	1 b	1 d
2 b	2 b	2 b	2 c
3 d	3 e	3 c	3 b
4 b	4 b	4 d	4 a
5 d	5 e	5 c	
6 d	6 c		

Chapter 25	Chapter 26	Chapter 27	Chapter 28
1 a	1 d	1 b	1 d
2 c	2 e	2 d	2 d
3 b	3 d	3 c	3 b
4 a	4 d	4 b	4 c

Chapter 29	Chapter 30	Chapter 31	Chapter 32
1 e	1 d	1 c	1 c
2 b	2 c	2 b	2 d
3 b	3 b	3 c	3 b
4 e	4 c	4 d	4 e

Chapter 33	Chapter 34	Chapter 35	Chapter 36
1 a	1 b	1 c	1 c
2 e	2 e	2 b	2 d
3 d	3 a	3 d	3 a
4 a	4 c	4 d	4 d

Chapter 37	Chapter 38	Chapter 39	Chapter 40
1 d	1 a	1 b	1 d
2 a	2 b	2 d	2 b
3 c	3 e	3 e	3 c
4 b	4 b	4 a	
5 e	5 d	5 c	

Chapter 41

1 b
2 b
3 e

Chapter 42

1 d
2 d
3 c

Chapter 43

1 a
2 d
3 c
4 b
5 c

Chapter 44

1 c
2 b
3 a
4 e
5 d

Chapter 45

1 c
2 d
3 e
4 b
5 e

Chapter 46

1 a
2 e
3 c
4 d
5 e

Chapter 47

1 b
2 c
3 e
4 e

Chapter 48

1 d
2 b
3 e
4 a

Chapter 49

1 c
2 d
3 a
4 e

Chapter 50

1 a
2 c
3 a
4 d
5 b

Chapter 51

1 a
2 b
3 a
4 a
5 c

Chapter 52

1 b
2 a
3 b
4 a

Chapter 53

1 c
2 d
3 a
4 c
5 d
6 d

Chapter 54

1 d
2 c
3 c
4 c

Chapter 55

1 b
2 a
3 e
4 e

Chapter 56

1 d
2 b
3 a
4 b
5 b

Chapter 57

1 d
2 a
3 e
4 d
5 e

Chapter 58

1 c
2 a
3 c
4 e

Chapter 59

1 c
2 e
3 c
4 d
5 b

Chapter 60

1 c
2 d
3 d
4 d
5 c

Chapter 61

1 a
2 b
3 e
4 e

Chapter 62

1 d
2 c
3 a
4 d

Chapter 63

1 a
2 c
3 b
4 b
5 e

Chapter 64

1 e
2 e
3 b
4 e

Chapter 65
1 d
2 b

Chapter 66
1 c
2 d
3 b
4 a
5 c

Chapter 67
1 b
2 e
3 a

Chapter 68
1 c
2 d
3 c
4 c
5 b

Chapter 69
1 a
2 c
3 d
4 e
5 e

Chapter 70
1 c
2 c
3 b
4 c
5 d

Chapter 71
1 c
2 b
3 a

Chapter 72
1 a
2 d
3 c
4 f
5 e

Chapter 73
1 c
2 c
3 b
4 e
5 b
6 c
7 c
8 d

Chapter 74
1 c
2 a
3 d

Chapter 75
1 c
2 d
3 e
4 d

Chapter 76
1 c
2 a
3 b
4 e

Chapter 77
1 c
2 b
3 d
4 a

Chapter 78
1 d
2 b
3 c
4 b
5 d

Chapter 79
1 d
2 c
3 a

Chapter 80
1 c
2 c
3 d

Chapter 81
1 e
2 d
3 b

Chapter 82
1 c
2 c
3 c
4 d

Chapter 83
1 b
2 d
3 a
4 a

Index

Page numbers in *italic* refer to figures.
Page numbers in **bold** refer to tables or boxes.

Textbook of Surgery, Fourth Edition. Edited by Julian A. Smith, Andrew H. Kaye, Christopher Christophi and Wendy A. Brown.
© 2020 John Wiley & Sons Ltd. Published 2020 by John Wiley & Sons Ltd.